PEDIATRIC EMERGENCIES

Incorporating National and International Recommendations

(IAP, NNF, GOI's DOWCD, BPNI, FOGSI, ICMR, AAP, IPA, NFI, IBFAN, WABA, ACASH, UNICEF, WHO, etc.)

Second Edition

AF662262

Edited by

Suraj Gupte

MD, FIAP

Professor and Head

Postgraduate Department of Pediatrics
Narayana Medical College and Hospitals
Nellore-524002, South India

E-mail: drsurajgupte@gmail.com, recentadvances@yahoo.co.uk
surajgupte@rediffmail.com

Honorary Director

Pediatric Education Network

Editor-in-Chief

Recent Advances in Pediatrics (International Series)
The Short Textbook of Pediatrics
Pediatric Emergencies
Neonatal Emergencies
Pediatric Gastroenterology,
Hepatology and Nutrition
Influenza: Complete Spectrum ...etc

Author

Instructive Case Studies in Pediatrics
Differential Diagnosis in Pediatrics
Pediatric Drug Directory
Influenza, Perspectives in Influenza
Speaking of Child Care etc.

E-mail: recentadvances@yahoo.co.uk
drsurajgupte@gmail.com, surajgupte@rediffmail.com

Co-editor

Asian Journal of Maternity and Child Health
(Manila, Philippines)

Section Editor

Pediatrics Today (New Delhi, India)

Editorial Adviser

Asian Journal of Pediatric Practice (New Delhi, India)

Editorial Advisory Board Member/Reviewer

Indian Journal of Pediatrics (New Delhi, India)
Synopsis: A Current Survey of World Literature in Pediatrics (Detroit, USA), Indian Journal of Pediatric Gastroenterology, Hepatology and Nutrition (Jaipur, India),
Maternal and Child Nutrition (Preston, UK),
Journal of Infectious Diseases (Turkey)

Examiner

National Board of Examinations (NBE) for DNB, New Delhi, All India Institute of Medical Sciences (AIIMS), New Delhi, Postgraduate Institute of Medical Education and Research (PGIMER), Chandigarh, Sher-i-Kashmir Institute of Medical Sciences (SKIMS) and several universities

Pediatric Faculty Selection Expert

All India Institute of Medical Sciences, New Delhi
Punjab Public Service Commission,
Jammu and Kashmir Public Service Commission,
Union Public Service Commission

PEEPEE

PUBLISHERS AND DISTRIBUTORS (P) LTD.

Pediatric Emergencies

Published by
Pawaninder P. Vij and Anupam Vij

Peepee Publishers and Distributors (P) Ltd.
Head Office: 160, Shakti Vihar, Pitam Pura, Delhi-110 034 (India)

Correspondence Address:
7/31, First Floor, Ansari Road, Daryaganj
New Delhi-110 002 (India)
Ph: 41512412, 9811156083, 23246245
e-mail: peepee160@yahoo.co.in
e-mail: peepee160@gmail.com
www.peepeepub.com

First Edition: **2006**

Second Edition: 2012

ISBN: 978-81-8445-027-9

to
my late parents
and
everybody contributing
to the care of
seriously sick children in particular
and
child health in general

CONTRIBUTORS

Robin Abrams
Consultant Pediatrician
Hospital for Sick Children
Toronto, Canada
Ch 41: Hepatic Encephalopathy

Pankaj Abrol
Associate Professor
Department of Pediatrics
Pt BD Sharma Postgraduate Institute of Medical Sciences
Rohtak, India
Ch 45: Glucose-6-Phosphate Dehydrogenase (G-6-PD) Deficiency
Ch 47: The Bleeding Child
Ch 56: Acute Glomerulonephritis

B Adhisivam
Senior Resident
Department of Pediatrics
Jawaharlal Institute of Postgraduate Medical Education and Research
Pondicherry, India
Ch 82: Naphthalene Poisoing

Shabina Ahmed
Director
Special Needs
Guwahati, India
Ch 65: Accidental Poisoning: General Management

Kamran Afzal
Lecturer
Department of Pediatrics
Jawahar Lal Nehru Medical College
Aligarh Muslim University
Aligarh, India
Ch 5: Cardiopulmonary Resuscitation (CPR)
Ch 20: Menigococcemia
Ch 21: Meningoencephalitis
Ch 62: Heat Stroke

Shazia Afzal
Resident
Department of Pediatrics
Jawahar Lal Nehru Medical College
Aligarh Muslim University
Aligarh, India
Ch 5: Cardiopulmonary Resuscitation (CRP)
Ch 20: Menigococcemia
Ch 21: Meningoencephalitis
Ch 62: Heat Stroke

Sunanda Anand
Assistant Professor
Pediatric Emergency Services
Boston Medical Center
Boston, Massachusetts, USA
Ch 4: Ethical and Legal Aspects of Pediatric Emergency Care

RA Anderson
Lecturer
Department of Pediatric Gastroenterology, Hepatology and Nutrition
Institute of Child and Adolescent Health
London, UK
Ch 39: Gastrointestinal Hemorrhage

Farooq Ansari
Consultant Pediatrician and Intensivist
Department of Emergency Pediatrics
Perth Institute of Medical Sciences
Perth, Australia
Ch 73: Mushroom Poisoning

Vineet Arora
Senior Resident
Department of Pediatrics
Dayanand Medical College and Hospital
Ludhiana, India
Ch 33: Shock

Sameer Bakhshi
Assistant Professor
Pediatric Oncology
Dr BRA Institute/Rotary Cancer Hospital
All India Institute of Medical Sciences
New Delhi 110001, India
Ch 44: Severe Anemia
Ch 46: Hemolytic Crisis

Arun Bansal
Senior Resident
Department of Pediatrics/Advanced Pediatric Center
Postgraduate Institute of Medical Education and Research
Chandigarh, India
Ch 61: Snakebite

Alpana Beri
Senior Resident
Department of Pediatrics
Dayanand Medical College and Hospital
Ludhiana, India
Ch 1: Organization and Social Aspects of Pediatric Intensive Care Unit (PICU)

B Vishnu Bhat
Professor
Department of Pediatrics
Jawaharlal Institute of Postgraduate Medical Education and Research
Pondicherry, India
Ch 77: Iron Poisoning
Ch 82: Naphthalene Poisoning

Gautam Biswas
Assistant Professor
Department of Forensic Medicine and Toxicology
Dayanand Medical College and Hospital
Ludhiana, India
Ch 71: Organophosphate and Carbamate (OPC) Poisoning
Ch 81: Phenothiazine Poisoning/Toxicity
Ch 97: Child Abuse and Neglect

Parthasarathy Biswas
Senior Resident
Department of Psychiatry
Postgraduate Institute of Medical Education and Research
Chandigarh, India
Ch 96: Psychiatric Emergencies

Tapabrata Chatterjee
Specialist Registrar (Ex)
Department of Pediatrics
Prince of Wales Hospital
Grimsby, UK
Ch 51: Diabetic Ketoacidosis

Aniece Chowdhary
Professor and Head
Department of ENT and Head and Neck Surgery
Government Medical College and Associated Hospitals
Jammu, India
Ch 87: Foreign Bodies
Ch 88: Airway Obstruction
Ch 89: Earache
Ch 90: Epistaxis
Ch 91: Caustic Ingestion
Ch 92: Faciomaxillary Trauma
Ch 93: Neck Trauma
Ch 94: Deep Neck Infections

Javed Chowdhary
Head
Department of Pediatrics
Government Medical College
Srinagar, India
Ch 52: Hyperthyroid Crisis
Ch 54: Acute Hypercalcemia
Ch 63: Electric Shock

Baljinder Singh Dhillon
Registrar
Department of Pediatrics
Dayanand Medical College and Hospital
Ludhiana, India
Ch 8: Fluid, Electrolytes and Acid-Base Balance and its Disturbances

Rajeshwar Dayal
Professor and Head,
Depatment of Pediatrics,
S N Medical College and Hospital
Agra, India
Ch 9: Multiple Organ Dysfunction Syndrome (MODS)

Akash Deep
Clinical Fellow
Pediatric Intensive Care Unit
St Mary's Hospital
London, UK
Ch 14: Increased Intracranial Pressure
Ch 15: Cerebral Edema
Ch 26: Bronchiolitis
Ch 28: Pneumothorax
Ch 60: Scorpion Sting
Ch 99: Pulse oximetry and Capnography

CM Deshmukh
Assistant Professor of Clinical Pediatrics (Ex)
Indiana University School of Medicine
Indianapolis, Indiana
Ch 38: Acute Bacillary Dysentry

Alka Dogra
Professor and Head
Department of Dermatology
Dayanand Medical College and Hospital
Ludhiana, India
Ch 95: Dermatological Emergencies

Aman Dua
Senior Resident
Department of Dermatology
Dayanand Medical College and Hospital
Ludhiana, India
Ch 95: Dermatological Emergencies

Ajay Gaur
Assistant Professor
Department of Pediatrics
G R Medical College
Gwalior, India
Ch 43: Management of Life-Threatening Complictions in Severe Malnutrition
Ch 64: Drowning

Radha Ghildiyal
Professor
Department of Pediatrics
Topiwala National Medical College and BYL Nair Charitable Hospital
Mumbai
India
Ch 26: Bronchiolitis
Ch 28: Pneumothorax

AM Graham
Clinical Professor
Center for Hemato-Oncology
Boston
Massachusette, USA
Ch 50: Oncologic Emergencies

Sheffali Gulati
Assistant Professor
Division of Pediatric Neurology
Department of Pediatrics
All India Institute of Medical Sciences
New Delhi, India
Ch 16: Acute Seizures
Ch 17: Status Epilepticus

Anupam Gupta
Registrar
Department of Pediatrics
Topiwala National Medical College and BYL Nair Charitable Hospital
Mumbai, India
Ch 60: Scorpion Sting

Gaurav Gupta
Consultant in Pediatrics
Apollo Clinics, Charak Clinics and Fortis Multispeciality Hospital
Chandigarh, India
Ch 3: Physiotherapy in Pediatric Intensive Care

Nitin Gupta
Consultant Psychiatrist
Stafordshire Healthcare NHS Trust
Margaret Stanhope Center
Burton Upon Trent
Staffordshire DE 13 ORG
UK
Ch 96: Psychiatric Emergencies

Ravinder K Gupta
Assistant Professor
Acharya Shri Chander College of Medical Sciences
Sidhra
Jammu, India
Ch 13: Dengue Hemorrhagic Fever
Ch 49: Disseminated Intravascular Coagulation (DIC)
Ch 100: Practical Procedures

Ritu Gupta
Demonstrator
Department of Physiology
Government Medical College
Jammu, India
Ch 13: Dengue Hemorrhagic Fever
Ch 49: Disseminated Intravascular Coagulation (DIC)
Ch 100: Practical Procedures

Satish Gupte
Professor and Head
Department of Microbiology
Government Medical College and Associated Hospitals
Jammu, India
Ch 37: Antibiotic-induced Diarrhea (AID)

Suraj Gupte
Director
Children's Health Center
Jammu, India.
Ch 4: Ethical and Legal Aspects of Pediatric Emergency Care
Ch 18: Infantile Tremor Syndrome
Ch 36: Diarrheal Dehydration
Ch 37: Antibiotic-induced Diarrhea (AID)
Ch 38: Acute Bacillary Dysentry
Ch 39: Gastrointestinal Hemorrhage
Ch 41: Hepatic Encephalopathy
Ch 42: Acute Severe Protein-Energy Malnutrition
Ch 50: Oncologic Emergencies
Ch 52: Hyperthyroid Crisis
Ch 53: Adrenal Crisis
Ch 54: Acute Hypercalcemia
Ch 55: Acute Hypocalcemia
Ch 61: Snakebite
Ch 63: Electric Shock
Ch 68: Kerosene oil Poisoning
Ch 69: DDT Poisoning
Ch 70: Corrosive Poisoning
Ch 72: Dhatura Poisoning
Ch 73: Mushroom Poisoning
Ch 75: Carbon Monoxide Poisoning
Ch 76: Aluminium Phosphide Poisoning
Ch 78: Lead Poisoning

Pankaj Hari
Assistant Professor
Division of Pediatrics Nephrology
Department of Pediatrics
All India Institute of Medical Sciences
New Delhi, India
Ch 58: Acute Renal Failure

Rekha Harish
Associate Professor
Department of Pediatrics
Government Medical College and Associated Hospitals
Jammu, India
Ch 27: Acute Severe Asthma

BK Jain
Professor
Department of Pediatrics
Dayanand Medical College and Hospital
Ludhiana, India
Ch 6: Oxygen Therapy

SK Jatana (Lt Col)
Associate Professor
Department of Pediatrics
Armed Forces Medical College
Pune, India
Ch 98: Sedation Analgesia

Manisha Juvekar
Senior Resident
Pediatric Intensive Care Unit
Lokmanya Tilak Municipal Medical College and General Hospital
Mumbai, India
Ch 11: Severe Malaria

Sonal Kansra
Senior Resident
Department of Pediatrics/Advanced Pediatric Center
Postgraduate Institute of Medical Education and Research
Chandigarh, India
Ch 59: Emergencies in Pediatric Rheumatology

Shailesh A Kanvinde
Pediatric Hematologist-Oncologist
Deenanath Mangeshkar Hospital
Pune, India
Ch 48: Idiopathic Throbocytopenic Purpura (ITP)

Anju Kapoor
Assistant Professor
Department of Pediatrics
PS Medical College,
Karamsad-Anand
Surat, India.
Ch 24: Coma
Ch 66: Salicylate Poisoning/Toxicity

Seema Kapoor
Assistant Professor
Department of Pediatric Medicine
Maulana Azad Medical College,
New Delhi, India
Ch 10: Anaphylaxis

RK Kaushal
Professor and Head
Department of Pediatrics
Indira Gandhi Medical College
Shimla, India
Ch 79: Mercury Poisoning

AW Koff
Professor
Department of Pediatric Endocrinology
Institute of Child and Adolescent Health
London, UK
Ch 53: Adrenal Crisis

Snehal Kulkarni
Consultant Pediatric Cardiologist
International Center for Cardiovascular and Thoracic Diseases
Chennai, India
Ch 29: Congestive Heart Failure

O Lee
Consultant
Pediatric Medicine
Singapore Medical Research Institute
Singapore
Ch 78: Lead Poisoning

Jhuma Mandal
Senior Resident
Postgraduate Institute of Medical Education and Research
Chandigarh, India
Ch 14: Increased Intracranial Pressure
Ch 15: Cerebral Edema

Mukta Mantan
Assistant Professor
Geeta Colony Children's Subspeciality Hospital
Maulana Azad Medical College
New Delhi, India
Ch 58: Acute Renal Failure

Parang N Mehta
Senior Consultant Pediatrician
Mehta Hospital
Surat, India
Ch 25: Acute Severe Pneumonia

Devendra Mishra
Assistant Officer
Geeta Colony Children's Subspeciality Hospital
Maulana Azad Medical College
New Delhi, India
Ch 23: Guillain-Barré Syndrome

Anup Mohta
Associate Professor,
Department of surgery,
University College of Medical Sciences and GTB Hospital,
Delhi, India
Ch 83: Acute Abdomen
Ch 84: Burns
Ch 85: Head Injury

Medha Mohta
Reader
Department of Anesthesiology and Critical Care
University College of Medical Sciences and
GTB Hospital
Delhi, India
Ch 84: Burns

Vaishali More
Lecturer in Pediatrics
Lokmanya Tilak Municipal Medical College and General Hospital, Sion
Mumbai 400 022, India
Ch 57: Hemolytic Uremic Syndrome

EW Nelson
Assistant Director
Institute of Toxicology
Hong Kong
Ch 73: Mushroom Poisoning

MNG Nair (Col)
Professor and Head
Department of Pediatrics
Armed Forces Medical College
Pune, India
Ch 98: Sedation Analgesia

Somashekhar Nimbalkar
Assistant Professor
Department of Pediatrics
P S Medical College
Karamsad-Anand
Surat, India
Ch 12: Tetanus

Mohinder Pal
Professor (Ex)
Department of Pediatrics
KHN Research Institute of Medical Sciences
Jammu, India
Ch 18: Infantile Tremor Syndrome
Ch 70: Corrosive Poisoning

HE Peterson
Senior Consultant
Toxicology Research Center
Bangkok, Thailand
Ch 72: Dhatura Poisoning

Puneet Pooni
Lecturer
Department of Pediatrics
Dayanand Medical College and Hospital
Ludhiana, India
Ch 6: Oxygen Therapy
Ch 7: Mechanical Ventilation
Ch 101: Drugs and Dosages in Pediatric Emergencies

VS Puri
Professor
Department of Pediatrics
Acharya Shri Chander College of Medical Sciences
Sidhra
Jammu, India
Ch 31: Paroxysmal Hypercyanotic Spells
Ch 41: Hepatic Encephalopathy
Ch 53: Adrenal Crisis

Abdul Quazi
Chief Consultant
Center for Sick Children
Kuala Lumpur
Malaysia
Ch 69: DDT Poisoning

Munni Ray
Assistant Professor
Department of Pediatrics/Advanced Pediatric Center
Postgraduate Institute of Medical Education and Research
Chandigarh, India
Ch 19: Stroke in Children
Ch 22: Bacterial Meningitis

Ghanshyam Saini
Lecturer
Department of Pediatrics
Government Medical College and Associated Hospitals
Jammu
India
Ch 36: Diarrheal Dehydration

Shiv Sajan Saini
Senior Resident
Department of Pediatrics/Advanced Pediatric Center
Postgraduate Institute of Medical Education and Research
Chandigarh, India
Ch 28: Pneumothorax

Preeti Shanbag
Professor of Pediatrics
Chief, Pediatric Intensive Care Unit and
Division of Pediatric Nephrology
Lokmanya Tilak Municipal Medical College and General Hospital
Mumbai, India
Ch 11: Severe Malaria
Ch 57: Hemolytic Uremic Syndrome

RK Sharma
Lecturer
Department of Ophthalmology
Government Medical College
Jammu, India
Ch 86: Pediatric Ocular Emergencies

Suhasini Sharma
Senior Resident
Pediatric Medicine
Maulana Azad Medical College
New Delhi, India
Ch 10: Anaphylaxis

Prajnya Shenoy
Senior Resident
Department of Pediatrics
Jawaharlal Institute of Postgraduate Medical Education and Research
Pondicherry, India
Ch 77: Iron Poisoning

Daljit Singh
Professor and Head
Department of Pediatrics
Dean Academics
Dayanand Medical College and Hospital
Ludhiana, India
Ch 1: Organization and Social Aspects of Pediatric Intensive Care Unit (PICU)
Ch 7: Mechanical Ventilation
Ch 33: Shock

Harmesh Singh
Reader
Department of Pediatrics
Dayanand Medical College and Hospital
Ludhiana, India
Ch 2: Investigations in Pediatric Intensive Care Unit (PICU)
Ch 8: Fluid, Electrolytes and Acid-Base Balance and its Disturbances

Surjit Singh
Additional Professor
Division of Pediatric Allergy and Immunology
Department of Pediatrics/Advanced Pediatric Center
Postgraduate Institute of Medical Sciences
Chandigarh, India
Ch 59: Emergencies in Pediatric Rheumatology

Utpal Kant Singh
Professor and Head
Department of Pediatrics
Nalanda Medical College
Patna, India
Ch 41: Hepatic Encephalopathy
Ch 55: Acute Hypocalcemia
Ch 68: Kerosene Oil Poisoning

Subhash Singh Slathia
B-Grade Pediatric Specialist
Directorate of Health Services
Jammu, India
Ch 40: Liver Abscess

Rita Smith
Professor
Department of General Pediatrics
Institute of Child and Adolescent Health
London, UK
Ch 4: Ethical and Legal Aspects of Pediatric Emergency Care

Praveen C Sobti
Associate Professor
Department of Pediatrics
Dayanand Medical College and Hospital
Ludhiana, India
Ch 71: Organophosphate and Carbamate (OPC) Poisoning
Ch 81: Phenothiazine Poisoning/Toxicity
Ch 95: Dermatological Emergencies
Ch 97: Child Abuse and Neglect

Ashima Taneja
Assistant Professor
Department of Obstetrics and Gynecology
Dayanand Medical College and Hospital
Ludhiana, India
Ch 97: Child Abuse and Neglect

BR Thapa
Additional Professor
Department of Pediatric Gastroenterology
Hepatology and Nutrition
Postgraduate Institute of Medical Education and Research
Chandigarh, India
Ch 35: Acute Gastroenteritis

Anu Thukral
Resident
Department of Pediatrics
All India Institute of Medical Sciences
New Delhi, India
Ch 16: Acute Seizures

Anil Vasudevan
Senior Resident
Department of Pediatrics
All India Institute of Medical Sciences
New Delhi, India
Ch 17: Status Epilepticus

Poothirikovil Venugopalan
Consultant Pediatric Cardiologist
Department of Child Health
Sultan Qaboos University Hospital
Muscat
Sultanate of Oman
Ch 30: Acute Myocarditis
Ch 32: Hypertensive Emergencies
Ch 33: Cardiac Arrhythmias

Venkataraman
Senior Resident
Department of Pediatrics/Advanced Pediatric Center
Postgraduate Institute of Medical Education and Research
Chandigarh, India
Ch 26: Bronchiolitis

Bhadresh Vyas
Assoiciate Professor
Department of Pediatrics
MP Shah Medical College and GG Hospital
Jamnagar, India
Ch 67: Paracetamol Poisoning/Toxicity
Ch 80: Barbiturate Poisoning/Toxicity

Anuj Walia
Senior Resident
Department of Pediatric Gastroenterology
Hepatology and Nutrition
Postgraduate Institute of Medical Education and Research
Chandigarh, India
Ch 35: Acute Gastroenteritis

Sanjay Wazir
Senior Registrar
Department of Pediatrics
Government Medical College and Associated Hospitals
Jammu
India
Ch 74: Opioid Poisoning

Sanjay Wazir
Senior Resident
Department of Pediatrics/Advanced Pediatric Center
Postgraduate Institute of Medical Education and Research
Chandigarh
India
Ch 99: Pulse Oximetry and Capnography

Vijaya Wali
Professor and Head
Department of Ophthalmology
Government Medical College and Assoiciated Hospitals
Jammu
India
Ch 86: Pediatric Ocular Emergencies

Preface to the Second Edition

The appearance of the second edition of the **"Pediatric Emergencies"** little over two years since it was first published in 2005 stands testimony to the warm welcome accorded to the book. In keeping with our commitment, the book has been further rendered most uptodate, state-of-the-art and informative (of course, with fresh additions and revision) and yet not exhaustive. I am confident that it shall be received with yet greater enthusiasm by the target audience.

I take this opportunity to thank the colleagues, friends, scholars and students for providing me the feedback to enhance the utility of the treatise. I do look forward to further interactions in this behalf..

Thanks are due to Mr. Pawaninder P Vij (Director), M/s Peepee Publishers and Distributors (P) Ltd. and his staff for bringing out the new edition speedily and for its excellent production qualities.

Suraj Gupte

Preface to the First Edition

For quite sometime, there has been a felt need for a textbook dealing with pediatric emergencies relevant to the Indian subcontinent and other developing countries. I recall Prof PM Udani, a pioneering pediatric academician of international eminence, wondering way back in 2001 in Jaipur during the course of the 5th International Congress of Tropical Pediatrics (ICTP) if I had done anything concrete for this challenging venture. This was a polite reminder of his earlier suggestion to me during the 8th Asian Congress of Pediatrics held in Hong Kong in 1997. This indeed set the ball rolling. Meanwhile, my experience in working on other books in the field, *Emergency Pediatrics, Criticare Pediatrics and Neonatal Emergencies* under the international series **Recent Advances in Pediatrics,** a pediatric favorite, stood me in good stead in giving concrete shape to this rather tough but quite satisfying project.

This state-of-the-art, comprehensive and yet concise first textbook of pediatric emergencies from India is the outcome of coordinated expertise, hard work and thoughtfulness of scores of distinguished contributors constituting a multidisciplinary author team drawn from India and several other countries. The chapters are written in a simple, straightforward and easy-to-understand style and to-the-point, keeping in mind the settings in the Indian subcontinent. The emphasis is on rational management with a simplified and practical approach. Nevertheless, each chapter begins with the essential background information including pathophysiology, etiopathogenesis and clinical presentation of the concerned emergency.

The reader-friendly treatise indeed is a dependable source to find complete and authoritative guidance on various pediatric emergencies. The contents, presentation and structure blend to provide a thoroughly readable, enjoyable and problem-oriented textbook of pediatric emergencies.

Taking off the ground with all important information in relation to the administrative and organizational aspects of a PICU, life-threatening situations and resuscitative aspects the treatise deals with emergencies in relation to severe tropical infections, various subspecialties such as pediatric neurology, cardiology, pulmonology and gastroenterology and superspecialities such as pediatric surgery, ENT, ophthalmology and psychiatry. Towards the end are provided chapters on emergency procedures and a compendium of pediatric emergency drug dosages. Important reference laboratory values are provided as Appendix.

The book is addressed to the pediatric residents, pediatricians dealing with pediatric emergencies in government and private hospitals/nursing homes and pediatric teachers. It shall come in handy for physicians whose practice involves childhood emergencies as well.

I wish to express my thanks to the distinguished contributors for the rich quality of its contents and for reposing confidence in my editorship.

My wife, Shamma, daughter, Novy, a prefinal MBBS student, and son, Manu, a 4th semester BE student, helped me in their own ways in working through the project successfully.

Finally, thanks are due to Mr Pawaninder P Vij of Peepee Publishers and Distributors (P) Ltd, for approaching me to undertake publication of this major project.

Suraj Gupte

Contents

VI.

CARDIOVASCULAR EMERGENCIES

VII.

EMERGENCIES RELATED TO GASTROENTEROLOGY, HEPATOLOGY AND NUTRITION

VIII.

HEMATO-ONCOLOGIC EMERGENCIES

IX.

ENDOCRINAL AND METABOLIC EMERGENCIES

X.

RENOVASCULAR EMERGENCIES

XI.

RHEUMATOLOGICAL EMERGENCIES

XII.

ENVIRONMENTAL EMERGENCIES

XIX.

PROCEDURES IN PEDIATRIC EMERGENCY COMPLEX

XX.

DRUGS IN PEDIATRIC EMERGENCIES

Section I

Organization of Pediatric Emergency Services

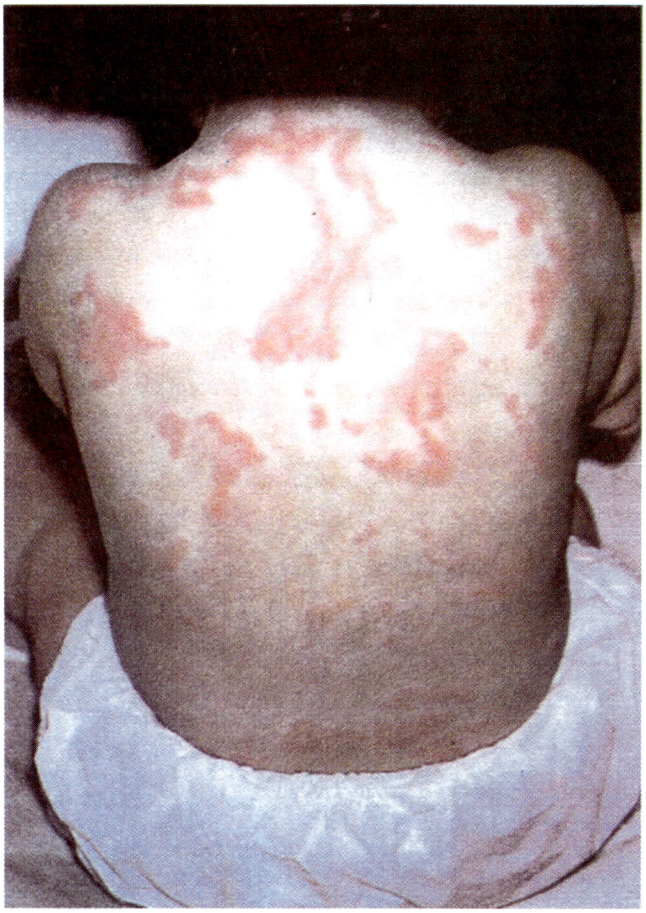

Fig. 95.1: Acute urticaria

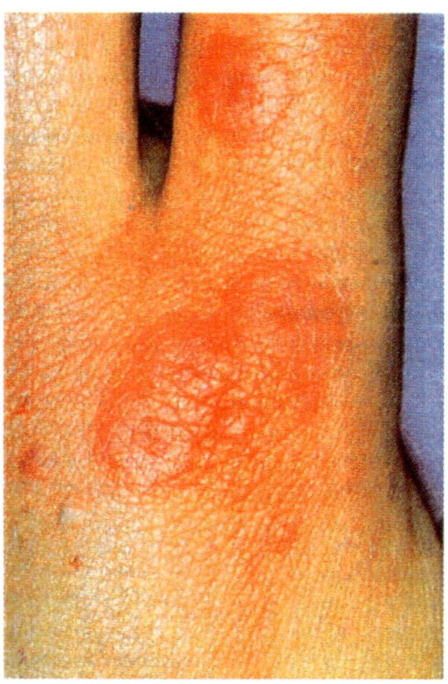

Fig. 95.2: Erythema multiforme—typical target lesions over knuckles

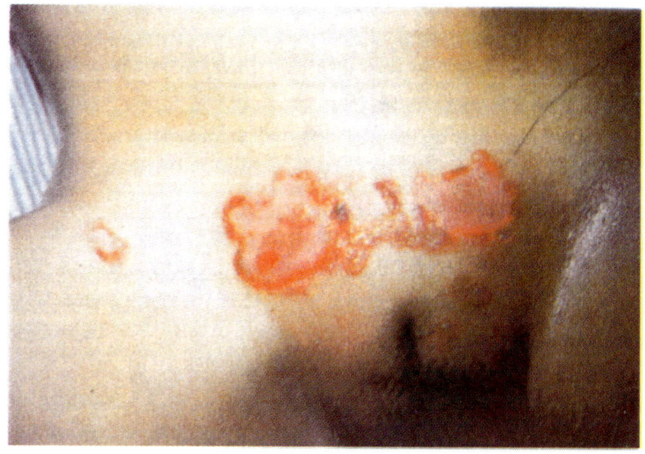

Fig. 95.3: Chronic bullous dermatoses of childhood—Cluster of jeels with new bullae forming over older lesions

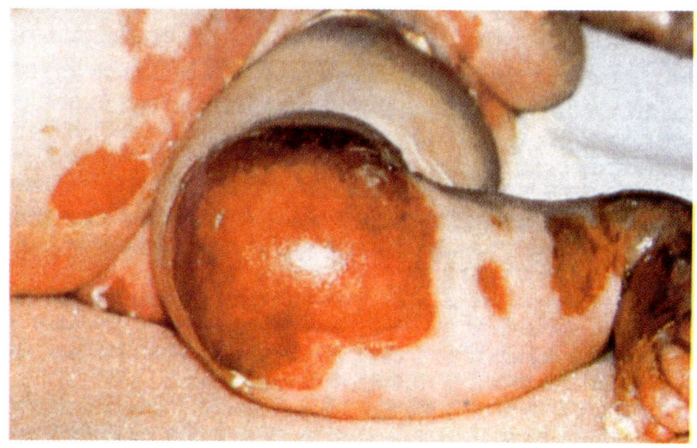

Fig. 95.4a: Extensive erosion in a neonate with Epidermolysis bullosa simplex (Dowling—Meare)

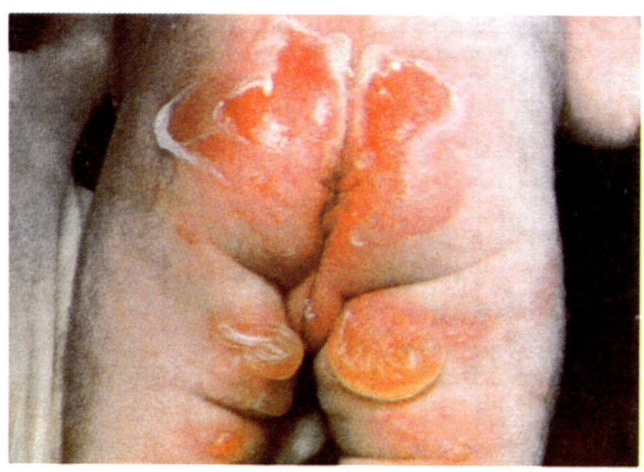

Fig. 95.4b: Junctional epidermolysis bullosa (Herlitz)

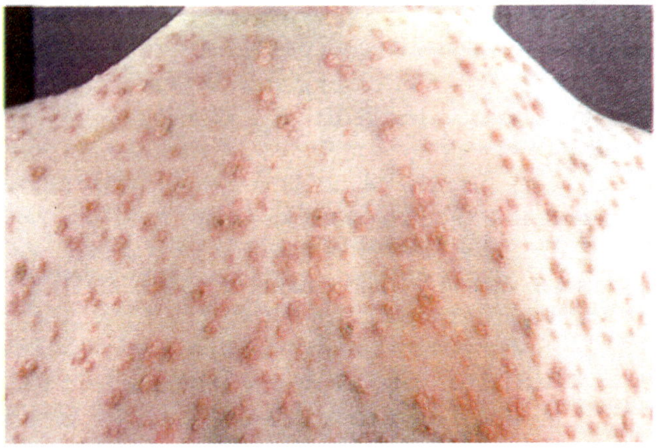

Fig. 95.5: Varicella

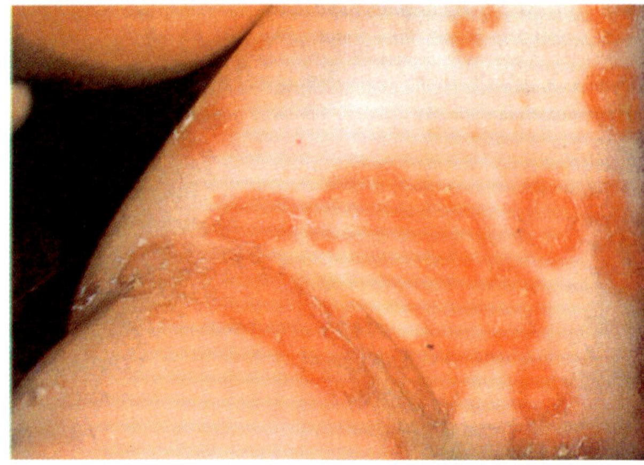

Fig. 95.6: Bullous impetigo after disruption of bullae

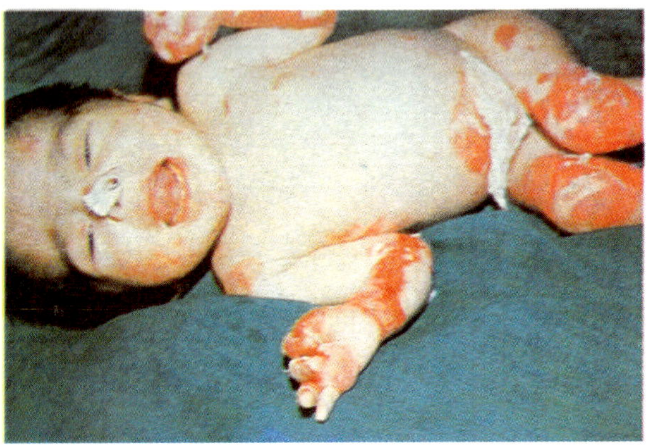

Fig. 95.7: Staphylococcal scaled skin syndrome

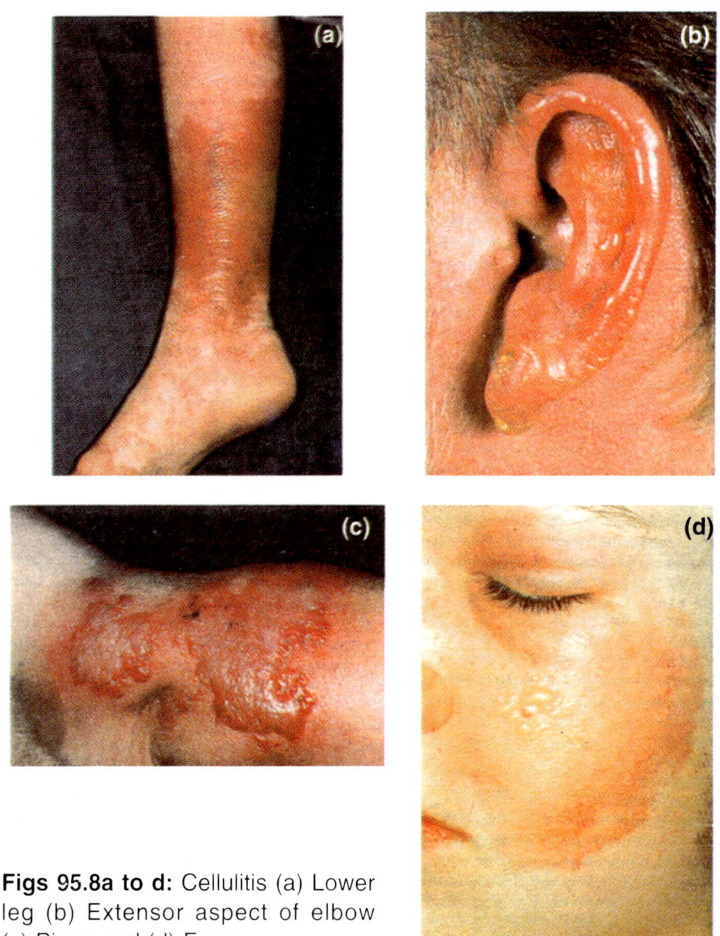

Figs 95.8a to d: Cellulitis (a) Lower leg (b) Extensor aspect of elbow (c) Pinna and (d) Face

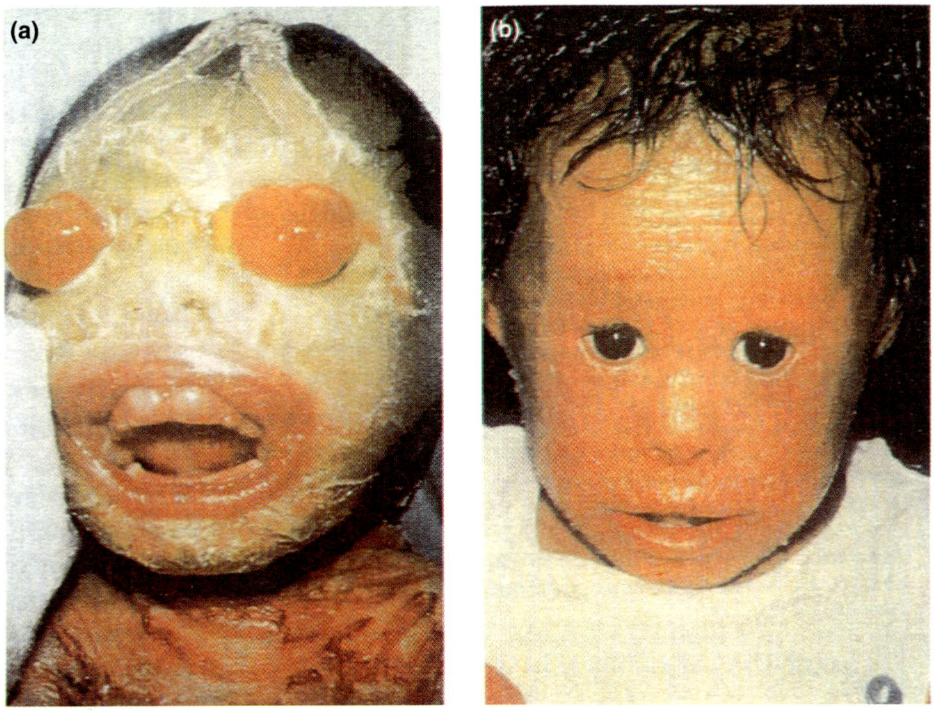

Figs 95.9a and b: (a) Harlequin ichthyosis; neonatal period (b) Same patient; aged 18 months

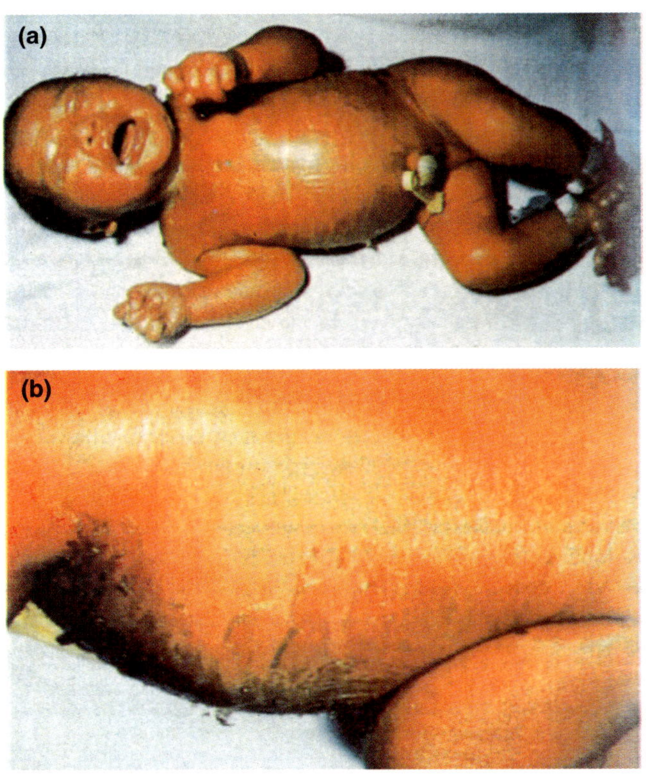

Figs 95.10a and b: (a) Collodion (lacquered) baby, aged 2 days. The membrane shed within 5 days, non-bullous ichthyosiform erythroderma was evident age 2 weeks. (b) Same patient as in (a) Peeling of collodion membrane aged 2 days.

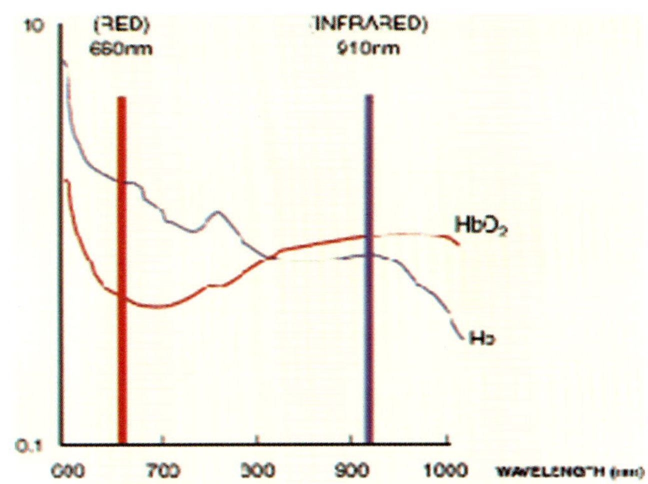

Fig. 99.1: Principle of pulse oximetry

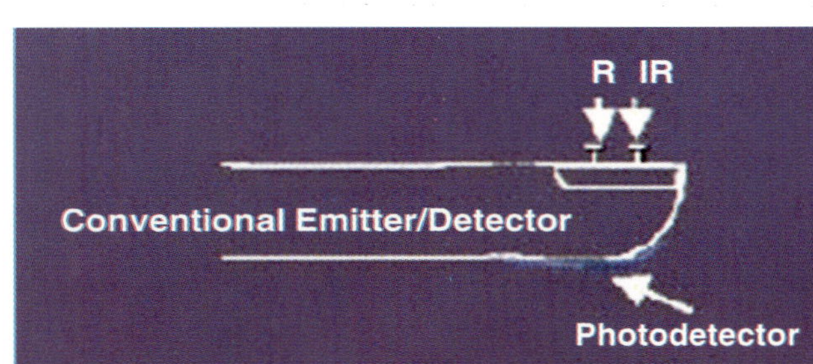

Fig. 99.2: In pulse oximetry, opposite the emitter is a photodetector

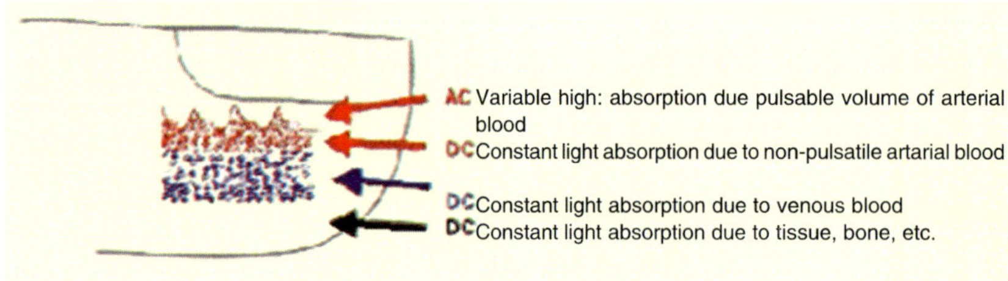

Fig. 99.3: Various light absorbers

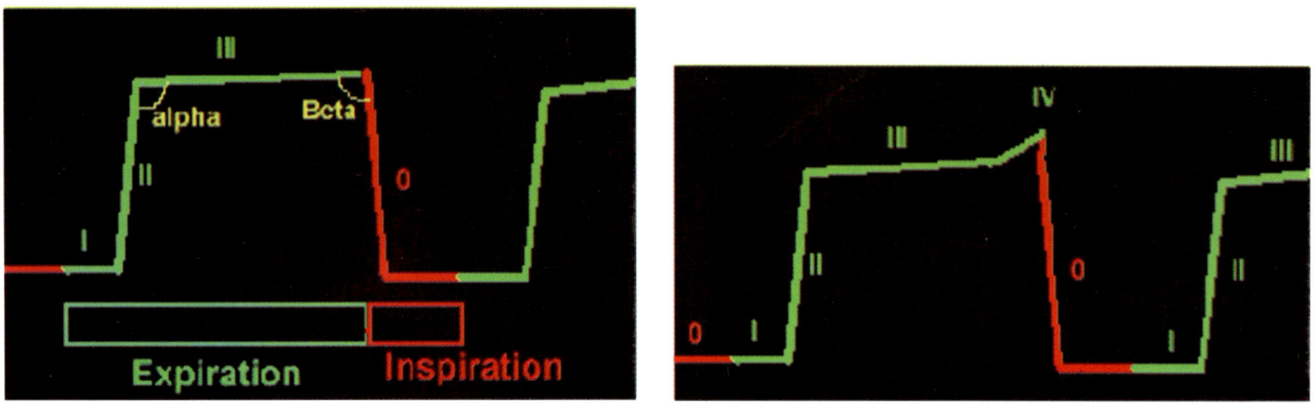

Fig. 99.4: Normal capnograph

Alpana Beri and Daljeet Singh

1 Organization and Social Aspects of Pediatric Intensive Care Unit

INTRODUCTION

Intensive care is defined as 'a service for patients with potentially recoverable disease who can benefit from more detailed observation and treatment than is generally available in the general wards and departments.' It is a low volume, high cost specialty which requires a highly trained multi-disciplinary team together with specialized tertiary expertise and diagnostic equipment.[1]

Although intensive care services for adults are well established, for children these services are still rendered in small clusters of a couple of beds within general pediatric units or within adult intensive care units. This is unfortunate because there is increasing evidence that management of sick children in discrete child centred environments and by medical and nursing staff trained in pediatrics markedly improves the outcome. Survival rates of 80-90% have been reported from advanced centres in developed countries.[2] Moreover children are not adults scaled down in size. Their relative immaturity in all respects (physiological, anatomical, functional, developmental and physiological) creates greater vulnerability to a variety of adverse influences and they should be looked after by specially trained staff familiar with the changes characteristic of each stage of development. The pattern and range of illnesses affecting children are also different. Children can become acutely ill very rapidly but have greater potential for full recovery than adults. These children have several years of normal life ahead. These facts should encourage investment of resources in intensive care of critically ill children.

Guidelines and standards for establishing PICU and standards of care have been spelled out by specifically formed expert groups from developed nations.[3-5] In the following discussion these recommendations are incorporated from the stand point of needs in our country.

PHYSICAL FACILITIES

Bed Requirement

Recommended requirement for pediatric intensive care (PIC) beds varies from 1 bed per 30,000 to 1 bed per lakh children. It is estimated that in UK 2% of all children admitted to hospital require intensive care. This compares with proportions as high as 20% in USA (patients admitted in Britain, therefore, tend to be more severely ill than those in America). As PICU is an expensive facility, it is important to use it in the most efficient and cost effective way. There are critical figures as regards the number of beds and staff. A unit smaller than 6 beds risks inefficiency and units larger than 16 beds may be difficult to manage. PICU should admit a minimum of 250 patients a year.[5-8]

Size

It is essential that minimum floor area for each bed is at least 20 sq. mt with 3-3.5 mt separating each patient. This is because, besides the bed space for individual patient, there must be sufficient area to accommodate the array of equipment, performance of procedures and provide room for family members and staff at the bed side. The total area needed for PICU is about three times the size needed for beds alone.[8]

Location

Location of the PICU should be such that there is no thorough traffic passing through the area and the transport of patient to and from the unit for diagnostic and therapeutic procedure is minimized. Keeping this in mind the PICU should preferably be situated close to the essential services and departments such as the emergency department, trauma centre, X-ray department, operating theater and laboratories.

Design and Structure

The decision to design a large open unit *vs* a unit comprising smaller rooms depends in part on the expected patient population. More critically ill patients may be better served in an open unit that affords better visibility, more flexibility in movement of patients/equipment and better use of staff but has disadvantages of increased noise, traffic and decreased privacy. The closed room design is more suitable for the population of less acutely ill patients. While it offers the advantages of privacy, there is the problem of decreased visibility, less interaction between staff resulting in a sense of isolation and less sharing of resources. A design that allows a combination of both types like closed unit designed with break-away doors, movable partitions would best meet the needs of children and staff caring for them.[9]

During designing of a PICU great care should be taken to include decorative features, paintings and color schemes so that the unit provides an environment suitable for the management of children. The unit should be double walled, sound proof, and centrally air-conditioned (temperature of 25-26°C with relative humidity of 30-60% and with at least 6 air exchanges per hr) with adequate provision of natural light. It should be provided with glazed tiles, PVC antistatic flooring, appropriate plumbing, ventilating and fire-safety features.

Facilities for Staff, Parents and Patients

Isolation facilities should be provided for infected patients and these should ideally comprise 25% of total bed complement. There should be facilities for areas for hand-washing, stocking drugs, storing equipment, performing procedures and clean/dirty supplies. There should be a intermediate care area for not so critically ill patients and continuing care of patients as they recover. PICU must have a central station which can be used for information exchange, communication, storage of notes, stationery and data management system. Facilities for staff include conference rooms for educational rounds, places for staff relief including sleep areas for physicians, eating areas and toilets.

Space to accommodate family members is essential in the design of PICU because family involvement is integral to the care of pediatric patient. Necessary areas for parents include a waiting lounge, sleep space, counseling room and areas to provide activities of daily living. Individual patient care area should have wall mounted shelves for placing electronic equipment, appropriate mechanisms for hanging of equipment for intravenous fluids and alarm system so that immediate help can be summoned when needed. There should be a minimum of 16 electrical sockets, 2 outlets each for oxygen and vacuum and 1 for compressed air (4 barr). There should also be an x-ray power socket between each pair of beds.[5,8,10] Floor plan of PICU is demonstrated in Fig. 1.1.

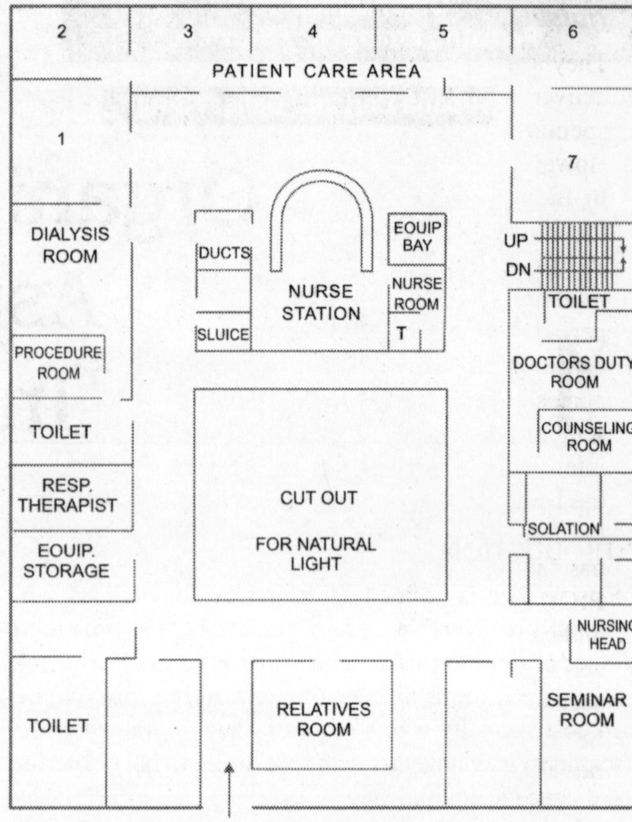

Fig. 1.1: Floor plan of a pediatric intensive care unit

Staff

Consultant Medical Staff

Each intensive care unit should be manned by 2 to 7 consultants (depending upon PICU size) one of whom will be the director of the unit. The director should be a pediatric intensivist with special training and wide experience in pediatric intensive care and has overall responsibility of the unit. He works in collaboration with the referring consultants, other medical consultants of PICU to provide complete patient care. His other tasks include organization of regular meetings for purpose of clinical audit, supervision of patient data collection, evaluation of morbidity/mortality reports, calibration and replacement of equipment, implementation of policies and organization of educational activities for unit staff. The medical consultants perform formal morning ward round, a less formal afternoon round and also provide a 24 hr consultant cover.[7]

House Staff

There should be one junior resident (preferably 3rd year postgraduate student) per four beds available throughout 24 hrs period. He should be supported round the clock by the senior resident (post-PG) with no other commitments. For purposes of training and continuity of care, the resident medical staff should be involved in all discussions concerning the clinical management of patients and should spend 3 to 6 months attached to the ICU.[10,11]

Nursing Staff

They are the most important staff in any PICU for actual delivery of critical care. It is essential to have high quality, specially trained nurses to provide 24 hrs coverage. However, at present such specialized training is not available in India. A continuing education program for nurses, therefore, must be developed within the unit.

Each patient undergoing intensive care requires a minimum of one trained nurse throughout the 24 hours period. One nurse may care for two less sick patients. Occasionally and particularly sick patients may require 2 nurses. In each shift, at least one of the nurses should be a senior staff nurse with considerable experience in pediatric intensive care. One out of the senior staff nurses is made the head nurse or clinical nurse manager. This individual (with several years of experience in pediatric intensive care) has the responsibility of providing and coordinating the PICU nursing service. The nurses should have basic understanding of commonly encountered clinical conditions and should be trained in pediatric resuscitation techniques such as respiratory care, correct usage of electronic monitoring devices, administration of life saving drugs and performance of specialized nursing procedures.

The nursing staff should be supported by nursing aides and janitors for carrying out non-nursing procedures. In India due to nursing constraints and unique socio-cultural matrix at least one of the parents should be allowed in the PICU with their critically sick child.

Other staff

Expertise and services of other specialties/sub-specialties like anesthesia, pediatric surgery, radiology, microbiology and neurosurgery are commonly required and should be constantly available. Other health care professionals needed by PICU patients and their roles are given in Table 1.1.

Table 1.1: Healthcare professionals with their role required in the PICU

Professional	Role
Physiotherapists	Prevent and treat chest problems, assist mobilization and prevent contractures in immobilised patients.
Dietitians	Advise on nutritional requirements and feeds.
Medical physics technicians	Maintain equipment including patient monitors, ventilators and blood gas analyzers.
Social workers	Provide emotional support and liaison with parents and relatives.

Equipment

An array of equipment is needed in the PICU for monitoring, provision of cardio-respiratory support, nutritional support, intravenous infusion of fluid/drugs and transport facilities (Table 1.2). Great care must be taken in selecting equipment so that it is suitable for management of critically ill children of all ages. Besides the cost, the model, reliability of the firm, the facilities provided, built-in alarm systems and maintenance services should be looked at. Enough essential accessories must also be purchased at the time of buying the equipment. The nurses and physicians must be familiar with the working and limitations of the equipment. There should be access to full time medical physics officer and ventilator/general equipment technician with a 24 hour backup. All PICU equipment should be tested for safety and proper function and retested at least quarterly with records kept.[5,11]

Table 1.2: Equipment suggested by joint commission on accreditation of health care organizations in special care units

No.	*Item*
1.	Oxygen and compressed air and the means of administration
2.	Mechanical, ventilatory assistance equipment, including airways, manual breathing bags and ventilators.
3.	Cardiac defibrillator with synchronization capability
4.	Respiratory and cardiac monitoring equipment.
5.	Thoracocentesis and closed thoracotomy sets.
6.	Tracheostomy sets
7.	Tourniquets
8.	Vascular cut down sets
9.	Infusion pumps
10.	Laryngoscopes and endotracheal tubes
11.	Tracheobroncheal and gastric suction equipments.
12.	Portable X-ray
13.	Device for weighing bed patients

FRAMEWORK OF PEDIATRIC INTENSIVE CARE IN INDIA

In India, it is desirable to adopt a two tier approach for creating PICUs. Basic PICUs should be developed at the district level and in small, medium private hospitals to tend to critically sick children with involvement of a single body system. Advanced level state of art PICUs should be established on a regional basis at tertiary care centres and major teaching hospitals. These should have facilities to manage children with life-threatening complex medical emergencies and multiorgan failure. For optimal results, it is important to have good transport facilities and timely referral of patients before they have progressed to a decompensated state.[11]

Services that Should be Available

Monitoring

An essential part of successful intensive care is the anticipation and treatment of critical problems. A PICU must, therefore, have capability to monitor on continuous basis the following:

1. *Cardiac and hemodynamic indices*
   Heart rate and rhythm
   ECG
   Blood pressure (non-invasive and invasive)
   CVP and pulmonary artery pressure
   Cardiac output
2. *Respiratory functions*
   Respiratory rate
   Oxygen saturation of hemoglobin (SaO_2)
   Blood gases
   Inspired oxygen and end-tidal CO_2 monitoring for ventilated children.
3. *Temperature:* including core temperature.
4. *Cerebral functions:* The following monitoring should be available as and when needed
   Intracranial pressure
   EEG
   Evoked potential
   Cerebral blood flow.

Therapeutic or Diagnostic Facilities

Besides the usual facilities available in pediatric wards, the following specific services should be available:

- Emergency resuscitation
- Respiratory support
- Tracheostomy
- Mechanical ventilation
- Tube-thoracotomy, thoracocentesis
- Bronchoscopy
- Cardiac support
- Defibrillation
- Temporary cardiac pacing
- Infusion pumps and pressure infusion devices
- Dialysis: peritoneal/hemodialysis
- Desirable
- Left heart support
- Intra-aortic balloon assist
- Extracorporeal membrane oxygenation.

Hyperbaric Oxygen

Support services necessary for effective functioning of PICU include 24 hrs radio-diagnosis and imaging facilities, laboratory service, centralized oxygen, compressed air and suction facility, blood bank, physiotherapy and transport system.

MANAGEMENT POLICIES

Each PICU should draw up clear management policies covering all aspects of activity. There should be written protocols for the treatment of all major conditions which are encountered in PICU. Detailed monitoring charts should be available to record vital signs, level of consciousness, input output, functional status of major body organs, progress notes etc. A prototype of the monitoring chart is illustrated in Appendix I and II. In view of limited resources and scarcity of beds admissions need to be prioritized. There should be clear policies regarding admission/discharge of patients and daily investigations to be performed (Table 1.3). In addition, there is need for policies concerning infection control (hand washing, use of slippers, limiting PICU traffic, use of asepsis during procedures, routine cultures) and health/safety at work (use of universal precautions) (Fig. 1.2).[10]

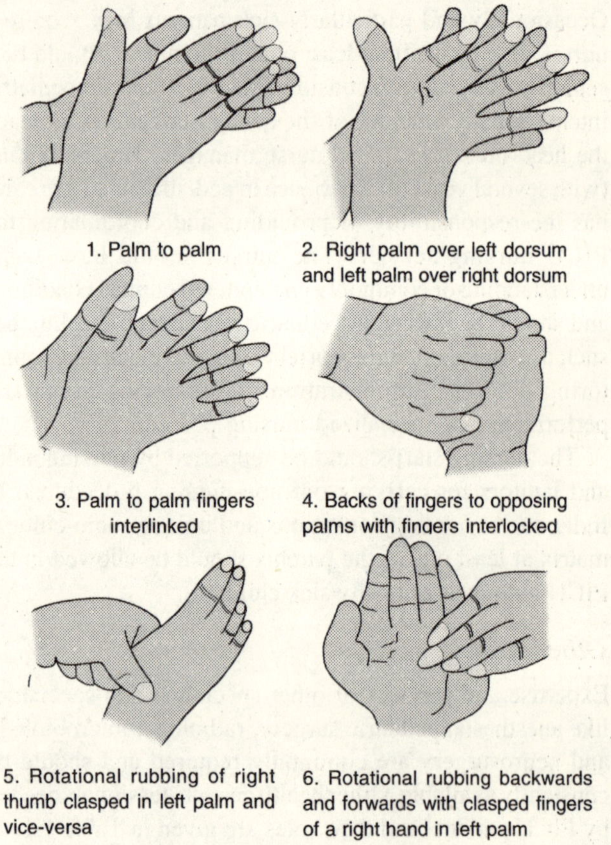

Fig. 1.2: Effective hand hygiene

Table 1.3: Indications for admissions to PICU

General: Cardiorespiratory arrest, hyperpyrexia, acute poisoning, acute hemorrhage, severe anaemia, severe dehydration and dyselectrolytemia, severe protein-energy malnutrition, diabetic ketoacidosis, near-downing, shock.

Central nervous system: Coma, intractable seizures, tetanus, acute intracranial infections, paralysis of respiratory muscles (polio/LGBS), head injury.

Cardiovascular system: Cardiac arrest, arrhythmias, pulmonary edema, intractable congestive cardiac failure, hypertensive encephalopathy.

Respiratory system: Acute respiratory distress and respiratory failure due to any cause, status asthmaticus, foreign body.

Abdomen: Upper gastrointestinal bleeding, hepatocellular failure, acute renal failure.

Data Collection and Audit

In order to assess the performance of ICU, it is necessary to collect information and undertake audit. This should include details of all admissions, collection of patient data and analysis of morbidity/mortality. Computerized data collection is desirable for ongoing evaluation and quality control. There should be regular audit meetings so that staff can be made aware of any adverse occurrence or alteration in the standard/quality of care.[10]

SOCIAL ASPECTS OF PICU

Patients, their care givers and staff are subjected to considerable physical and emotional stress in PICU (Fig. 1.3).[6,9,12]

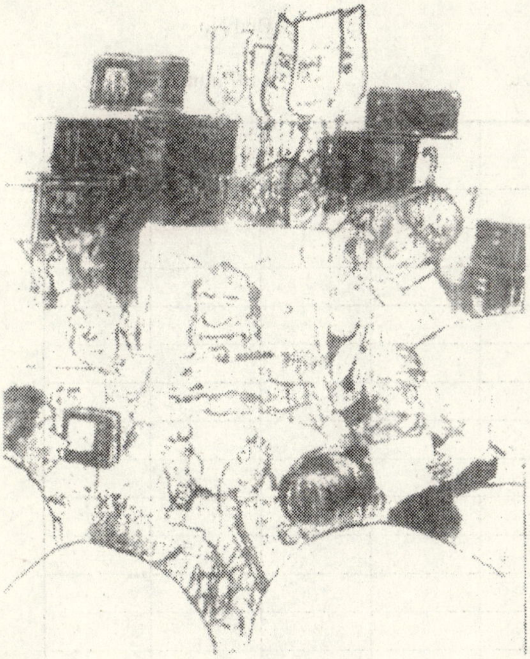

Fig. 1.3: Causes of psychological stress in ICU patients

Patients

Patients may be confused, distracted, disoriented, agitated and may have hallucinations. There may be frank delirium 'intensive care unit psychosis', acute anxiety disorders and feeling of isolation/desolation. There are numerous frightening or unpleasant stimuli such as pain, presence of endotracheal tube, sounds of ventilator and monitor alarms.

Management is aimed at prevention of these problems by emphasizing on clear difference between night and day by changing ambient light, opening windows, using large clocks with clearly visible hands and allowing patients lengthy periods of uninterrupted sleep by clustering interventions. Patients need repeated simple explanations about what is happening to them. Patients should be surrounded by familiar objects, toys and photographs. Family participation in care and conversation is encouraged. Touch and human contact by both care-givers and family are comforting and reassuring.

Family

Support of the family is crucial and requires both skill and time. Parents and relatives are often traumatized by the child's admission to PICU and require comfort, information and consideration in order to cope. The parents should be encouraged to interact verbally and physically with their child and to express their feelings/concerns. A social worker attached to PICU is in an excellent position to reassure parents and provide appropriate supportive counseling. Other steps in helping the family of the admitted child include providing orientation to the ICU, waiting area and other facilities like eating, sleeping and use of telephone. Also, referral should be made to community agencies which may help with financial and other difficulties. Help must be provided in preparing the family for the possible death of their child or only partial recovery of the child.

Staff

Close contact with critically ill patients for prolonged periods of time, staffing shortages, poorly designed work place and lack of supervision often cause the staff in PICU to experience chronic emotional stress and 'burn out'. To minimize the effects of stress on staff, it is important to provide effective leadership, positive feedback and setting defining work goals. Also there should be job autonomy, advancement potential, appropriate staffing ratios and continuing education.

Above all, it is important for proper functioning of PICU that both parents and staff keep the atmosphere positive, pleasant and as much removed from feeling of hopelessness as possible.

REFERENCES

1. Chief Nursing Officer's Taskforce report on Pediatric Intensive Care. *A Bridge to the Future Nursing Standards, Education and Workforce Planning in Pediatric Intensive Care*. London: Department of Health, U.K. 1997.
2. Singhi S. Pediatric Intensive Care: Concept and issues (editorial). Indian Pediatr 1995;32:147-157.
3. Committee on Hospital Care and Pediatric Section of the Society of Critical Care Medicine. Guidelines for Pediatric Intensive Care Units. *Pediatrics* 1983; 72:364-372.
4. Task Force on Guidelines, Society of Critical Care Medicine. Recommendation for critical care unit design. *Crit Care Med* 1988;16:796-806.
5. Task Force on Guidelines, Society of Critical Care Medicine. Recommendation for services and personnel for delivery of care in a critical care setting. *Crit Care Med* 1988;16:809.
6. National Coordinating Group. Report on Pediatric Intensive Care to the Chief Executive of NHS. *A Framework for the Future*. London: Department of Health, UK 1997.

7. Bennet D, Bion J. ABC of intensive care. Organization of intensive care. *BMJ* 1999;15:520-523.
8. Singhi S. Organization of pediatric intensive care unit In: Sachdev HPS, Puri RK, Bagga A, Choudhary P (eds) *Principles of Pediatric and Neonatal Emergency* New Delhi: Jaypee Brothers 1994;354-361.
9. Lappe D G. Pediatric intensive care nursing. In: Rogers MC (ed) *Textbook of Pediatric Intensive Care,* 3rd edn. Baltimore: Williams and Wilkins 1996; 1597-1616.
10. Anonymous. *Standards of Pediatric Intensive Care.* London: Pediatric Intensive Care Society, UK 1996.
11. Singh M. Organization of pediatric intensive care unit. In: Singh M (ed) *Medical Emergencies in Children,* 3rd edn. New Delhi: Sagar Publication 2001;1-11.
12. Adam S, Forrest S. ABC of intensive care. Other supportive care. *BMJ* 1999;15:670-683.

APPENDIX 1.1

DAYANAND MEDICAL COLLEGE AND HOSPITAL, LUDHIANA

PEDIATRIC INTENSIVE CARE UNIT

VENTILATOR MONITORING CHART

Name		Age/Sex
Dr. Incharge		C.R. No.
Unit		Bed No.
ET Size:	L.	Cuff/non cuff

Date Time								
Mode								
Tidal Volume.								
Inspiratory Time								
I:E Ratio								
Breath rate/Total								
Peak flow rate								
PIP								
PEEP/CPAP								
P-Support								
FiO_2								
MAP								
Exp Tidal Volume								
Minute Ventilation								
Temp. (Insp.)								
SPO_2								
ET Deflation								
ET Suction								
Air Entry R L								
*Sedation score								
Nasal Flaring/Acc. M								
Physiotherapy								
$pH/PaCO_2$								
PaO_2/HCO_3 (BE)								
On Sedation/M.relax								

1. Barely arousable; asleep needs shaking/shouting to arouse.
2. Asleep: eyes closed, arouse on soft voice or light touch.
3. Sleepy: eyes open but less active and responsive.
4. Awake.
5. Agitated.

APPENDIX 1.2

DAYANAND MEDICAL COLLEGE AND HOSPITAL, LUDHIANA

PEDIATRIC INTENSIVE CARE UNIT
MONITORING CHART

Name | Age/Sex
Dr. Incharge | C.R. No.
Unit | Bed No.
Wt.

Date	8	9	10	11	12	1	2	3	4	5	6	7	8
Temperature													
Heart Rate													
Respiratory Rate													
BP/CVP													
Peripheral Pulses													
SPO_2													
Colour													
CFT													
GCS/AVPU													
Pupil R L													
Posture													

INTAKE	**Regular** – Type – Amt. ordered – Level – Amt. given – Total							
	Bolus/Infusion – Type – Amt.							
	Oral/NG – Type – Amt.							
	Total							
OUTPUT	**Urine** – Amt. (ml/kg/hr)							
	Stool							
	NG/Vomit							
	Others							
	Total							

Harmesh Singh

2 Investigations in Pediatric Intensive Care Unit (PICU)

INTRODUCTION

Investigations form an essential and helpful tool of the intensive care in critically sick children. Chances of recovery and survival are much more favorable in children as compared to adults. Investigations are thus very helpful in early diagnosis and appropriate treatment in sick children.

CATEGORIES OF INVESTIGATIONS

1. *Hematological*
   - Hemoglobin
   - Complete blood counts (CBC)
   - Band cell count
   - Platelet count
   - PT, PTT
   - Micro ESR
   - Peripheral blood smear
2. *Pathological*
   - Urine routine and microscopy
   - Gastric aspirate
   - CSF cytology
   - Occult blood in stool
3. *Microbiological*
   - Blood culture
   - Urine culture
   - CSF culture
   - Serological tests
   - Viral cultures
   - Cytokines
   - Fibrin Split Products (FSP), D-Dimers
   - Other cultures– endotracheal tip, catheter tip and other secretions and body fluids
4. *Blood biochemistry*
   - ABGs
   - Blood sugar
   - Blood urea/creatinine
   - Blood lactate
   - Blood enzymes
   - CRP
   - CSF biochemistry
   - Electrolytes
   - LFT
   - Serum Ca, Mg
   - Urine ketones
5. *Radiological*
   - Skiagrams
6. *Imaging*
   - Ultrasonography
   - Echocardiography
   - CT Scan
   - MRI
7. *Others*
   - ECG
   - EEG
   - Evoked potentials
   - Oxygen saturation (Pulse oximetry)

Hematological Investigations

Hemoglobin

Hemoglobin estimation helps to know the severity of anemia and requirement of blood transfusion.

Complete Blood Counts (CBC)

The total leukocyte counts and band cell counts are helpful in the diagnosis of sepsis especially in neonates. Leukopenia (TLC <5000) has a sensitivity of up to 85% and specificity around 90%. Band cells (>20%) has sensitivity and specificity of 60-70%.[1]

Platelet Counts

Phase microscopy or electronic cell counter is used for measuring platelet counts. It can also be estimated by examination of a peripheral smear. A platelet count less than 20000/mm^3 warrants platelet transfusion. Low platelet count is seen in dengue fever, ITP, leukemia and other causes of bone marrow involvement.

Prothrombin Time (PT) and Activated Partial Thromboplastin Time (PTT)

PT and PTT measure soluble clotting proteins of the extrinsic (PT) and intrinsic (PTT) coagulation path ways. PT greater than 17 seconds and PTT greater than 45-50 seconds are considered abnormal.[2]

Micro ESR[3]

Micro ESR is estimated by taking blood sample in a preheparinized microhematocrit capillary tube of 75 mm length and 1.1 mm internal diameter and keeping it vertically for 1 hour. High micro ESR is a specific test for neonatal sepsis. Normal value is : Day of life + 3. Peak value is 15 mm.

Peripheral Blood Smear

Examination of peripheral blood smear is extremely important in critically ill children. It gives clue to different diagnostic possibilities (Table 2.1).

Table 2.1: Significance of funding in peripheral blood smear

Findings	*Possible diagnosis*
• Hemolysed RBC	Acute hemolysis, HUS
• Immature WBCs	Leukemias
• Low platelet count	Thrombocytopenia
• Malarial parasite	Malaria
• LD bodies	Kalaazar
• Basophilic stippling	Lead poisoning

Pathological Investigations

Occult Blood in Stool

Examination of stool for occult blood is helpful in the diagnosis of many disorders e.g. NEC, bleeding disorders, typhoid, dengue fever, etc. Occult blood in stools is one of the early signs of NEC in neonates.

CSF Cytology

It helps in differentiation of meningitis, encephalitis and subarachnoid hemorrhage. Elevated cell count with predominance of polymorphonuclear leukocyte indicates pyogenic meningitis. In tubercular meningitis there are more of lymphocytes in the CSF. Crenated red cells indicate subarachnoid bleed which can be differentiated from traumatic lumbar puncture by three vial test. CSF shows clearing when we proceed from vial one to vial three. CSF findings[4] in different types of meningitis are depicted in the Table 2.2.

Urine Routine and Microscopy

Routine urine examination is helpful in the diagnosis of various conditions as shown in the Table 2.3.[5]

Table 2.2: CSF findings in different types of meningites

Meningitis	*Leukocyte count (cells/mm^3)*	*Proteins (mg/dL)*	*Glucose (mg/dL)*
Acute bacterial	Hundreds-thousands Neutrophils predominate	100-500	5-40
Viral	Upto few hundred, Initially neutrophils then lymphocytes	<100	Normal
Tuberculous	25-100, rarely >500 Lymphocytes predominate	100-200 even higher	Reduced
Cryptococcal	<50, lymphocytes Predominate	20-500	Reduced
Syphilis	Average 500, lymphocytes predominate	100	Normal

Table 2.3: Routine urine examination and significance of findings[1]

Urinary findings	*Diagnosis*
Pus cells	UTI
Red cells	Acute nephritis, bleeding disorder
Proteinuria	Nephrotic syndrome, nephritis
Glucose	Diabetes mellitus
Ketones	DKA
Urinary sodium (mEq/L) :	
< 20	Pre-renal failure
> 40	Intrinsic renal failure
Urinary osmolality (mOsm/kg) :	
> 500	Pre-renal failure
< 300	Intrinsic renal failure

Microbiologic Investigations

Blood Culture

Blood culture is helpful in diagnosing or ruling out septicemia, typhoid, fungemia and nosocomial infections in sick children. Nowadays rapid method for blood culture i.e. Bectec is available which has high yield than the routine blood culture method. It helps in early initiation of appropriate antimicrobials in critically sick children. It takes about 8-12 hours as compared to 72 hours in the routine methods.

Urine Culture

ICU patients remain hospitalized for longer periods and many times they are catheterized. Hence chances of developing urinary tract infection are higher in such cases. A clean catch mid stream urine sample culture is thus required to rule out UTI.

CSF Culture

CSF culture differentiates type of microorganism and its sensitivity pattern so as to enable us to start appropriate treatment in time.

Serological Tests

Dengue Fever: MAC-ELISA test for dengue specific IgM antibodies. A positive result indicates recent infection with dengue virus.[6]

Bacterial Meningitis: Detection of bacterial antigens in CSF, blood or urine by latex agglutination or counter immuno-electrophoresis is useful in establishing the underlying causative microorganism and also in differentiating TBM from partially treated pyogenic meningitis.[7,8]

Cerebral Malaria: Tests based on detection of malarial antigens in blood by ELISA technique such as histidine rich protein 2 of p.falciparum can rapidly diagnose cerebral malaria by dipstick test.[9]

Typhoid Fever: Widal test especially the rising titres are useful in establishing diagnosis of typhoid fever and typhoid encephalopathy.

Viral Cultures: Viral isolation in blood, CSF and various body secretions may prove useful in establishing etiological cause in various viral illnesses. However, facilities for viral cultures are not available at most of the centers.

Cytokines: Interleukin 6 (IL6), tumor necrosis factor alpha (TNFa) and interleukin IB (IL-1B) have been reported as early indicators of sepsis especially in the newborn.[10,11] However a few studies have observed a high sensitivity in late onset septicemia in neonates.

FSP, D-Dimers: Elevated blood levels of fibrin split products (FSP) or D-Dimers are indicative of disseminated intravascular coagulation (DIC) which needs prompt treatment. In addition, there is evidence of acute hemolysis on peripheral smear, thrombocytopenia and prolonged PT and PTT.

Blood Biochemistry

Blood biochemistry forms a major chunk of investigations in a critically sick child. The biochemical parameters helpful in the diagnosis and monitoring of such cases are given in Table 2.4.

Radiological Investigations

Skiagram Chest

X-ray of chest may provide extremely valuable information. Both AP and lateral x-rays should be obtained. It helps in following ways:

- Position of endotracheal tube, chest tube and vascular lines
- Heart size
- Lung parenchyma, congestion and atelectesis
- Pulmonary vascular markings
- Pneumothorax and hemothorax
- Pleural effusion
- Pericardial effusion
- Diaphragmatic hernia
- HMD
- ARDS
- Fracture of ribs and bones

Table 2.4: Biochemical parameters and their significance

Biochemical parameter	*Value*	*Pathological state*	*Reference*
Blood sugar	High	Diabetes	12
	Low (< 40 mg/dL)	Hypoglycemia	
Urinary ketones	High	DKA	12
Blood urea	High	Renal failure	13
Serum creatinine	High (> 0.8 mg/dL)	Renal failure	14
Ammonia	High	Hepatic encephalopathy	15
Serum calcium	Low (< 7.0 mg/dL)	Hypocalcemia	
	High (> 11.0 mg/dL)	Hypercalcemia	
Serum magnesium	Low (< 1.2 mg/dL)	Hypomagnesemia	
Serum sodium	Low (< 130 mEq/L)	Hyponatremia	16
	High (> 150 mEq/L)	Hypernatremia	
Serum pottassium	Low (< 3.5 mEq/L)	Hypokalemia	17, 18
	High (> 5.5 mEq/L)	Hyperkalemia	
CRP	High (> 1.0 mg/dL)	Sepsis	
CSF biochemistry	High proteins (> 40 mg/dL)	Meningitis	19
	Low sugar (< 50% of blood)	Meningitis	20
	High lactate (> 35 mg/dL)	Meningitis	20
Serum proteins	Low total protein/albumin	Dengue shock syndrome	21
SGOT	High	Dengue hemorrhagic fever	22
SGPT	High	Hepatic dysfunction	23
ABGs	Low pH, PCO_2 and HCO_3	Metabolic acidosis	24
	High pH, PCO_2 and HCO_3	Metabolic alkalosis	24
	Low pH,high PCO_2 and HCO_3	Respiratory acidosis	24
	High pH,low PCO_2 and HCO_3	Respiratory alkalosis	24

Skiagram Skull

- Fracture of skull bones in unconscious child with multiple trauma

Skiagram Abdomen

- Acute abdomen
- Intestinal obstruction
- Intestinal perforation

Imaging

Ultrasound

Portable ultrasound in intensive care unit is helpful in the following situations requiring immediate attention.

- Abdominal mass
- Biliary/renal calculi
- Free fluid in the peritoneum
- Pelvic pathology especially in adolescent girls
- Pleural effusion
- Intercostal drainage under US guidance
- Intracranial hemorrhage in newborns

Echocardiography

Rapid, instantaneous, noninvasive study of dynamic cardiac functions has become increasingly possible with ultrasound technology.[25] It is now possible to study direct cardiac motion on a real time basis, to determine flows, shunts and cardiac output by using ultrasound and Doppler techniques. Noninvasive types of monitoring are particularly suitable for small children because of their small size, anatomic relationship and close distance of the heart to the chest. By echocardiography, following information can be obtained:

- Cardiac dimension
- Left ventricle and end diastolic and end systolic diameters
- Great vessel dimensions–Aorta, pulmonary artery
- Opening and closing of valvular structures
- Antegrade and retrograde flow velocity across the valve structures
- Visualization of abnormal structures e.g. thrombus [26]
- Bacterial endocarditis
- Pre-ejection and ejection times

Thus echocardiography helps to identify underlying structural abnormality as well as cardiac function in sick patients.

Other Investigations

ECG

A good 12 lead ECG is necessary in an intensive care unit. We note heart rate, PR interval, P to QRS relationship, QRS, QT duration and rhythm. In critically sick children ECG helps to differentiate various types of cardiac arrhythmias. ECG should be obtained in all cyanotic patients. Most patients with noncardiac cyanosis have normal ECG. Chronic hypoxia with corpulmonale will have right ventricular hypertrophy and right axis deviation. QT interval is prolonged in hypocalcemia. Hpothermia prolongs all intervals (R-R, P-R, QRS, Q-T).

EEG

The EEG has long been used in the evaluation and follow-up of the critically ill children. Its greatest value, lies in the assessment of the obtained, comatose or seizing patient where in it may provide diagnostic and prognostic information.[27] It may also be used to measure cerebral activity and may help to ascertain the effects of various therapeutic interventions. e.g. anticonvulsants.

The routine EEG is the most accurate means of identifying electrical discharges of seizure activity. In critically sick children it becomes necessary to identify the presence of ongoing cerebral seizure activity without clinical manifestation e.g. silent seizures, subclinical seizures or nonconvulsive status. Such epileptic disorder may represent the primary cause of encephalopathy or may accompany a variety of CNS insults. EEG is also used to define the brain death. EEG has a diagnostic as well as prognostic role in coma. Some of the EEG patterns are shown in Table 2.5.

Table 2.5: EEG patterns and their significance

EEG Pattern	*Interpretation*
• Paroxysmal seizure discharge	Status epilepticus
• PLEDS (Periodic lateralized epileptic form discharges)	Herpes encephalitis
• High voltage focal slow waves	Supratentorial lesion
• Slowing of alpha rhythm-diffuse slowing	Metabolic coma
• Triphasic paroxysmal waves	Hepatic/other metabolic coma

Burst suppression or electrocerebral silence or very low amplitude is associated with poor outcome. EEG helps in making a diagnosis of herpes encephalitis which is a treatable infection.

CT Scan and MRI

Cranial CT is an invaluable tool for assessing a comatose child with regard to potential underlying cerebral disease and need for surgical intervention. It is also particularly useful in the evaluation of cerebral edema and raised intracraneal pressure. CT also helps in grading the cerebral edema (Table 2.6).[28]

Table 2.6: CT scan grading of cerebral edema

Grade	*CT Scan features*
N	Normal
I	Loss of sulci cerebri and/or interhemispheric fissure and/or sylvian fissure and/or occlusion of body of lateral venticle.
II	Complete loss of sulci and fissures and/or chiasmatic cistern and/or quadrigeminal cistern and/or interpeduncular cistern.
III	Complete loss of sulci, fissures and all cisterns.

CT is the modality of choice for urgent neuroimaging of patients with apparently serious head injuries to reduce morbidity and mortality.

MRI is a powerful modality for brain imaging, with the ability to display the brain in exquisite details in multiple planes, distinguishes soft tissues much better than CT, detect various stages of hemoglobin degradation, assess maturity of myelination and evaluate intracranial hemorrhage. It is able to create vascular images (MRI angiography without contrast). MRI in future may be applied to critical care patients for metabolic assessment of brain functions (functional MRI and MRI spectroscopy).

Evoked Potentials

Brain stem function is assessed by the evoked potentials during coma. The absence of all wave form indicates severe neurological damage or brain death. Somatosensory evoked potentials (SEPs) are the most sensitive and reliable for evaluation of neurological outcome of coma.[29]

Applications of evoked potentials in critical care are:

- Evaluation and/or prognostication of encephalopathic child
- EPs are generally unaffected by even high levels of pharmacologic agents that may affect EEG activity.
- Some anatomic specificity is afforded by particular EPs.

Pulse Oximetry

It is one of the most important advances in the 1980s. Pulse oximetry has become a routinely used tool for monitoring the arterial oxygen saturation and in most circumstances, accurately correlates with the hemoglobin saturation as measured by co-oximetry. A miniaturized light source is applied to ear lobe, fingers, palm or arch of foot. Oxygen saturation should be maintained at more than 90%.[3]

REFERENCES

1. DaSilva O, Ohlsson A, Kenyon C. Accuracy of leukocyte indices and C-reactive protein for diagnosis of neonatal sepsis: A critical review. *Pediatr Infect Dis J* 1995;14:362-366.
2. Buchnan GR. Coagulation disorders in the neonate. *Pediatr Clin N Am* 1986;333:203.
3. Evans HE, Glass L, Mercado C. the microerythrocyte sedimentation rate in the newborn period. *J Pediatr* 1970;76:448-451.
4. Fishman RA. Cerebrospinal fluid. In: *Diseases of the Nervous System*, 2nd edn. Philadelphia: WB Saunders 1992;253-343.
5. Bagga A. Acute renal failure. In: *Medical Emergencies in Children*, 3rd edn. New Delhi: Sagar Publication 2000;372-385.
6. World Health Organization. *Dengue Hemorrhagic Fever: Diagnosis, Treatment, Prevention and Control*, 2nd edn. Geneva: WHO 1997.
7. Kumar A, Congeni B, Nankervis G. Latex agglutination test for rapid detection of bacterial antigens in body fluids. *Annals Clin Lab Sci* 1980;10:337-382.
8. Kaplan S, Fishman M. Supportive therapy for bacterial meningitis. *Pediatr Infect Dis J* 1987;6:670-677.
9. Spielman A, Perrone JB. Teklehaimanot. A et al. Malaria diagnosis by direct observation of centrifuged samples of blood. *Am J Trop Med Hyg* 1988;39:337-342.
10. Doellner H, Arntzen KJ, Haereid PE, Aag S. Austgulen R. Interleukin-6 concentrations in neonates evaluated for sepsis. *J Pediatr* 1998;132:295-299.
11. Misra PK, Kumar R, Malik GK, Mehra P, Awasthi S. Simple hematological tests for diagnosis of neonatal sepsis. *Indian Pediatr* 1989;26:156-160.
12. Becker DJ, Drash AL. Diabetic ketoacidosis. In: Dickerman JD, Lucey JF (eds) *Critically Ill Child: Diagnosis and Medical Management*. Philadelphia: WB Saunders 1985;113-128.
13. Karlowicz MG, Adelman RD. Acute renal failure in the neonate. *Clin Perinatol* 1992;1:139-158.
14. Stewart CL, Barnett R. Acute renal failure in infants, children and adults. *Crit Care Clin* 1997;13:575-590.
15. Caraceni P, Van Thiel DH. Acute liver failure. *Lancet* 1995;345:163-169.
16. Prasad SVSS, Singhi S, Chugh KS. Hyponatremia in sick children seeking emergency care. *Indian Pediatr* 1994;31:287-294.
17. Singhi S, Marudkar A. Hypokalemia in a Pediatric Intensive Care Unit. *Indian Pediatr* 1996;33:9-13.
18. Douplar SJ, Mark KP, Ralph AD. Hypokalemia. In: Allen IA, Ralph AD (eds) *Fluid Electrolyte and Acid Base* Disorders, 2nd edn. 1995;410-411.
19. Bonadio W. The cerebrospinal fluid: physiologic aspects and alterations associated with bacterial meningitis. *Pediatr Infect Dis J* 1992;11:423-432.
20. Sivakmaran M. Meningococcal meningitis revisited: normocellular CSF. *Clin Pediatrics* 1997;6:351-355.
21. Pongphanich B, Kumponpant S. Studies of dengue hemorrhagic fever, hemodynamic studies of clinical shock associated with dengue hemorrhagic fever. *J Pediatr* 1973; 83:1073-1077.
22. Pande JN, Kabra SK. Dengue hemorrhagic fever and dengue shock syndrome. *Natl Med J India* 1996;9: 256-258.
23. Acharya SK, Dasarathy S, Kumer TL et al. Fulminant hepatitis in tropical population : Clinical course, cause and early predictors of outcome. *Hepatology* 1996; 23:1448-1455.
24. Sagy M, Barzilay Z, Boichis H. The diagnosis and management of acid base imbalance. *J Pediatr Emerg Care* 1988;4:259-265.
25. Robson S, Dunlop W, Moore M, Hunter S. Combined Doppler and echocardiography measurement of cardiac output: theory and application in pregnancy. *Br J Obstet Gynaecol* 1987;93:1014-1027.
26. Horowitz M, Rossen R, Harrison D. Echocardiographic diagnosis of pericardial disease. *Am Heart J* 1979;97:420-427.
27. Bauer G. Coma and brain death. In : Niedermeyer, E, Lopes Da Sliva F (eds) *Electroencephalography: Basic Principles, Clinical Application and Related Fields*, 3rd edn. Baltimore: Williams and Wilkins 1993;445-460.
28. Tasker RC, Mathew DJ, Kendall B. Computed tomography in the assessment of raised intracraneal pressure in nontraumatic coma. *Neuropediatrics* 1990;21:91.
29. Haslam RH. Coma in childhood. In: Behrman RE, Kliegman R, Arvin A (eds) *Nelson Textbook of Pediatrics*, 15th edn. Philadelphia: WB Saunders 1996;1716-1718.
30. Scheller J, Web R. Respiratory artifact during pulse oximetry in critically ill patients. *Anaesthsiology* 1988;69:602.

Gaurav Gupta

3 Physiotherapy in Pediatric Intensive Care

INTRODUCTION

Pediatric physiotherapy is the art of supportive care facilitating early recovery in the Pediatric ICU. Young children tend to react more severely to acute respiratory infection than older people because of their narrow airways. In spite of difficulties in children, it is possible for physiotherapy to make an effective contribution in suitable cases.

ICU physiotherapy predominantly involves chest physiotherapy for critically ill children.[1-5] Active and passive limb physiotherapy may help in certain chronic conditions enhancing early physical mobilization.

The following discussion is restricted to chest physiotherapy as it forms the major chunk of the work of a physiotherapist in the Pediatric ICU.

Common conditions in which chest physiotherapy is useful include:

1. Chest infection with increased secretions.
2. Increased secretions following prolonged intubation.
3. Collapse of lung due to mucus plug or aspiration of feed.
4. Meconium aspiration.

GENERAL GUIDELINES

Before treatment, clear and honest explanations (age appropriate) are given to the child, including descriptions of what the treatment will be like and how long it will last and reassurance that it can be stopped by request at any time. Children need to be listened to, believed and given some control over what is done to them.[5]

The same physiotherapist should preferably be treating the patient throughout the stay, if possible.

The parent is encouraged to take part in child's physiotherapy as well as learn from the treatment.

ASSESSMENT FOR PHYSIOTHERAPY

Before embarking on physiotherapy, attempts should be made to assess the patient's suitability for physiotherapy.

The following points need to be assessed:

Notes, Charts and Reports provide information on the patient's age, current problem, diagnosis and all complaints apart from the daily condition. These should be thoroughly studied before planning the treatment of the patient.

Monitors in the ICU should be observed for baseline levels and for changes during treatment. This is needed to pick up any instability during the act of providing physiotherapy. In case of any marked variations from the baseline the physiotherapy regimen may be curtailed.

Auscultation may pick up wheezes and crackles though they are often easier to feel than hear. Clinical examination may help in identifying the correct positioning for effective removal of secretions.

X-ray findings may indicate atelectasis or consolidation, with the right upper lobe needing special attention due to its tendency to collapse, especially in intubated children.

TECHNIQUES OF PHYSIOTHERAPY

A trained physiotherapist would perhaps use a combination of multiple techniques like postural drainage, vibration and percussion, nasotracheal sectioning and improving lung volumes to maximize the effects of physiotherapy.[6,7]

Some techniques relevant to the pediatric patient in ICU are discussed briefly.

Postural Drainage

This involves positioning the child in such a way that drainage of chest secretions is facilitated. Side-to-side positioning, that is used for maintenance of lung volume, is usually adequate as modified postural drainage. In case of babies, postural drainage is most easily done with the baby lying on a pillow on the physiotherapist's lap (if possible). The baby feels comfortable and secure and can lie prone, supine or in half side lying position with the additional support provided by the physiotherapist's hands on his chest. Thus, all the areas of the lung can be drained with minimal disturbance. Postural drainage may not be tolerated if the child is very sick. In infants who spend much time supine, the sitting position is included to drain the apical segments.

Manual Techniques

These include the techniques of percussion and vibration of the chest wall to drain excessive or thick secretions. Percussion involves tapping gently within the confines of the lung markings while vibrations refers to gentle to-and-fro pressure being applied on the chest wall to facilitate drainage. The use of these 2 techniques is limited in children.

In babies, percussion is possible using three fingers of one hand and supporting the chest with the other. As an alternative, a small Benett (round) mask may be used for percussion. In infants vibrations with fingertips can be applied on every second or third expiration. Care should be taken to stay within the surface markings of the little lungs.

In older children the usual technique of percussion using a relaxed cupped hand can be applied. Percussion is often more soothing than vibrations. There may be a small risk of arrhythmia or compromised lung function in an unstable child during these procedures, thus adequate clinical monitoring is essential.

Methods to Clear the Secretions

Older children usually are able to spit out and blow their nose to prevent secretions from spilling into the airways at approximately four years of age. Coughing is the most spontaneous method of clearance of secretions. In infants, coughing can be stimulated by gentle inward pressure against the trachea in a circular pattern during exhalation. In an older un-cooperative child "huffing" can be encouraged, which simply refers to voluntary blowing of cotton wool, as this would enhance clearance of chest secretions.

Nasotracheal suction is usually unnecessary if the child is coughing effectively, as the cough reflex is likely to prevent aspiration in these children.

If needed, suction should be done carefully keeping in mind the level of suction pressure as it is related to mucosal damage. The following pressures are normally recommended:

- 60-90 cm H_2O for infants
- 90-100 cm H_2O for young children
- 110-150 cm H_2O for older children

Methods to Increase Lung Volume

Increasing the lung volume is important as it reduces chances of recurrent infections and improves postural drainage, thus reducing ICU stay. For this the uses of simple methods like blowing of paper balls or tissues, blowing through a straw etc., maybe effective. All these techniques utilize the deep breath that is taken before blowing out, thus helping in increasing lung volume. Use of pediatric incentive spirometers, which are enjoyable and encourage deep breathing without a subsequent deep expiration, can lead to a substantial increase in the child's respiratory reserve. Also abdominal breathing can be taught by placing a favorite toy on the abdomen and asking the child to move the toy with his breathing. This would lead to increased diaphragmatic contractility.

CONTRAINDICATIONS AND PRECAUTIONS

As with all procedures carried out in critically ill patients, certain precautions are mandated to reduce iatrogenic risk due to the procedure itself. Physiotherapy is *contraindicated* for babies who are:

- Hypothermic,
- Show cardiac instability,
- Have an undrained pneumothorax,
- Are producing fresh blood secretions.

Physiotherapy may lead to a worsening of all these problems.

The physiotherapy sessions should ideally be scheduled before feeds or at least one hour after the feeds. Both the child and the monitor should be observed before, during and after treatment so as to detect any instability or complications. Casual handling should be avoided at all costs. The physiotherapy sessions should be structured so that the child is rested before and after treatment.

A proper regimen of physiotherapy including respiratory exercises can help in reducing ICU stay, reduce mechanical ventilation time and associated morbidities, decrease infections, and also increase the patient's feeling of control over his health in an ICU setup.

REFERENCES

1. Hough A. *Physiotherapy in Respiratory Care*, 2nd edn. London: Chapman and Hall 1996;286-302.
2. Bungay C. *Cash's Textbook of General Medical and Surgical Conditions for Physiotherapists*, 1st edn. London/New Delhi: Wolfe/Jaypee 1993;355-421.
3. James I. Respiratory management in pediatrics. *Care Crit Ill* 1991;7:47-50.
4. Downs J, Parker A. Chest Physiotherapy for preterm infants. *Pediatr Nurs* 1991;3:14-17.
5. Gillespie D. Let's listen to children. *Respir Dis Pract* 1989;6:23.
6. Howard F. Endotracheal suctioning and the neonate. *Pediatr Nurs* 1994;6:14-17.
7. Shield JPH, Baum JD. Children's consent to treatment. *BMJ* 1994;308:1182-1183.

Suraj Gupte, Rita Smith and Sunanda

4

Ethical and Legal Aspects of Pediatric Emergency Care

INTRODUCTION

The term, *ethics*, originates from the Greek word *ethos* which means moral custom. In medical practice, it denotes a system of principles or standards governing medical conduct of the physician and other medicos and paramedicos. It deals with the relationship of the medical person to the patient, his family, fellow medical men and society at large.

BACKGROUND

Despite chequered history of medical ethics, its origin dates back to two monumental declarations, namely Hippocratic Oath (Box 4.1) and Declaration of Geneva (Box 4.2) which was later modified by the World Medical Association.[1]

Generally speaking, the Declaration of Geneva is followed throughout the world. In India, the Medical Council of India follows it as the *Code of Conduct*. Every doctor at the time of registration is required to submit this written declaration, duly signed, to the concerned Registrar attested by another registered medical practitioner (RMP) or the Registrar himself. A departure in following the pledges made therein is considered an unethical practice.

MEDICAL ETIQUETTES *VIS-A-VIS* ETHICS[1,2]

The term, *medical etiquettes*, denotes conventional laws and customs of courtesy that are generally followed between members of the medical profession. A doctor is expected

Box 4.1: Hippocratic Oath

An oath exacted of his students by Hippocrates, the celebrated Greek physician considered the *Father of Medicine*, because he was the first healer to record medical experiences for future references, thereby for the first time establishing the foundation for the scientific basis of medical practice;

"I swear by Apollo the physician and Aesculapius and Hygeia and Panacea and all the gods and goddesses that, according to my ability and judgment, I will keep this oath and its stipulation

To reckon him who taught me this art equally dear to me as my parents, to share my substance with him, and to relieve his necessities if required;

To look upon his off spring in the same way footing as my own brothers and to teach them this art if they shall wish to learn it, without fee or stipultion and that by precept, lecture and every other mode of instruction, I will impart a knowledge of the art to my own sons and those of my teachers and the disciples bound by a stipulation and oath according to the law of medicine, but to none other.

"I will follow that system of regimen which, according to my ability and judgment, I consider for the benefit of my patients, and sustain from whatever is deleterious and mischievous. I will give no deadly medicine to anyone if asked, nor suggest any such counsel; and in like manner I will not give to a woman a pessary to produce abortion. With purity and with holiness, I will pass my life and practice my art. I will not cut persons laboring under the stone, but will leave this to be done by men who are practitioners of this work. Into whatever houses I enter, I will go into them for the benefit of the sick and will abstain from every voluntary act of mischief and corruption; and, further, from the seduction of females and males, of freemen and slaves. Whatever, in connection with my professional practice, or not in connection with it, I see or hear, in the life of men, which ought not to be spoken of abroad, I will not divulge, as reckoning that all such should be kept secret.

"While I continue to keep this Oath unviolated, may it be granted to me to enjoy life and practice of this art, respected by all men, in all times. But should I trespass and violate this Oath, may the reverse be my lot."

Box 4.2: Declaration of Geneva

A statement adopted by the Second General Assembly of the World Medical Association in 1948

- " At the time of being admitted as Member of the Medical Profession, I solemnly pledge myself to concentrate my life to the service of humanity;
- I will give to my teachers the respect and gratitudes that is their due;
- I will practice my profession with conscience and dignity;
- The health of my patient will be my first consideration;
- I will respect the secrets which are confided in me;
- I will maintain by all means in my power the honor and the noble traditions of the medical profession;
- My colleagues will be my brothers;
- I will not permit consideration of religion, nationality, race, party politics or social standing to intervene between my duty and my patient;
- I will maintain the utmost respect for human life, from the time of conception;
- Even under threat, I will not use my medical knowledge contrary to the laws of humanity;
- I make these promises solemnly, freely and upon my honor."

to behave with his colleagues as he wishes to be behaved by them. He is not supposed to charge his professional fee from him or members of his nuclear family for the services rendered. Nevertheless, he is not legally bound to do so.

The term, *medical ethics*, refers to moral principles for the members of medical profession in their dealings with each other, their patients and the State in order to honor and maintain the noble professional traditions. In context of the first area, a doctor is not supposed to entertain a patient who is already being treated by another colleague unless okayed by the said colleague.

CONSUMER PROTECTION ACT (CPA) 1986[3-6]

According to this Act, individuals and institutions providing medical service on charging the professional fees are answerable for deficiency of service (unfair and negligent medical practices). In the case of physicians and hospitals providing medical services free of charge to all patients, CPA cannot be invoked for claiming any charges.

Despite considerable protest against the CPA by the medical fraternity (that believes that medical service has wrongly been assumed as a commodity and contract as per the spirit of the Act), CPA has come to stay.

Not that liability for doing a "wrong" is not provided in law as such. It indeed is! This Act is, therefore, a focussed means of enforcing such rights provided in the consumers of goods and services.

The general guidelines for avoiding a charge of negligence and action under the CPA are listed in Table 4.1.

Table 4.1: General guidelines to avoid a charge of negligence and action under CPA

- The healthcare professional should keep abreast of the latest advances in therapeutics.
- The diagnosis, where possible, should be confirmed by laboratory tests, including biopsy.
  Every precaution should be taken to establish early diagnosed in cases of suspected cancer.
- X-rays should be routinely advised in case of injury to bones or joints or where diagnosis is doubtful.
- Consultation with a specialist should be suggested in obscure cases.
- Immunization/prophylactic antibiotic cover should be considered a necessity where there is danger of infection.
- Sensitivity tests should be done before injection preparations likely to cause anaphylactic shock.
- The drugs to be administered by injection or otherwise should be verified.
- No procedure should be undertaken beyond one's skill.
- No experimental methods should be adopted without prior consent.
- The instruments to be used for any procedure should be properly sterilized, safe, and in proper working condition.

HOSPITAL/INSTITUTIONAL ETHICS COMMITTEE

Each hospital is supposed to have an Ethics Committee comprising unbiased, honest and knowledgeable professionals of proven standing. The Committee acts as a "watchdog" for monitoring the ethical matters with special reference to the so-called "grey areas", say lapses in treatment, declaration of death in special cases, doctor-attendant controversies in implementing consumer law, etc. The role played by such committees needs to be evaluated from time to time. In several European countries, it has been shown that often these committees, though succeeding in cutting down deficiencies in management, contribute to over treatment which too is undesirable.[1,2]

CONDUCIVE AND FRIENDLY PICU ENVIRONMENTS

Undoubtedly, PICU has got to be equipped well with technical facilities and know-how. Equally important is human warmth, compassion, optimism and friendliness. Staff should be gifted with qualities of sensitivity, compassion and genuine concern.

Though "under treatment" is undesirable, "over-treatment" too needs to be avoided. An acceptable balanced approach to treatment protocols is required. Moreover, PICU should have guidelines on admission, discharge, withdrawing/withholding life-saving system.

At least one parent/attendant should be allowed to remain with the patient. He should be taken into confidence about the progress of the patient in an understandable language on a regular and continuous basis and in a relaxed manner.

Not only that all efforts should be made by the NICU team to save the child, the parents/attendants should get a "feel" of it so that they are assured of the genuine effects being made at the PICU.

LIFE SUPPORT ISSUES

Availability of PIC Facilities

Availability of state-of-the-art PIC facilities for life threatening disorders at least in State level hospitals and, if workable, in district level hospitals is most desirable. In fact, it is a cost-effective strategy.

- The PIC staff, including doctors, should be equipped with human warmth, caring attitude, credibility and compassion.
- Overall atmosphere, despite critical nature of the subjects, should be optimistic so that the patients and the attendants feel reassured that best efforts are being put up for the welfare of the seriously sick children.
- Standard treatment protocols should be available.
- Admission as well as discharge policies should be precise.

Withholding/Withdrawing Life Support Measures

Life-support facilities should be prioritized for those critically sick in whom chances of recovery are high. It is reasonable to withhold them in those suffering from irreversible terminal conditions with no chance of recovery e.g. advanced multi-organ failure (MOF), advanced cancer, massive intracranial bleed, severe hypoxic-ischemic encephalopathy. In United States, as per the Guidelines, it is considered futile to provide such a support in persistent vegetative state (PVS).

A decision on withholding/withdrawing life-support should never be taken in haste. In fact, it should follow discussion among the experts. The family should also be taken into confidence. Not just that! It should be duly documented in the case sheet. The justification for the decision should also be recorded. The attendant's signature should be taken as a consent.

DEATH-RELATED ISSUES

Diagnosis

Generally speaking, it is fair enough to declare a critically-sick child dead when:

1. There is irreversible stoppage of circulatory and respiratory function, and
2. CPR efforts over a 30-min period have failed. This, however, cannot be the case in subjects who are maintained on life-support in the form of assisted ventilation. Here, the following criteria of brain death need to be employed:
   - Coma and apnea
   - Dilated and fixed pupils
   - Absent corneal reflex
   - No involvement of eyes or dysconjugate movements of eyes on Doll's head-eye movements maneuver
   - Lack of response to cold calorie test which consists in instilling around 20 ml of ice-cold water in each auditory canal directed towards the ear drum. Tonic deviation of both eyes towards the side being stimulated means an intact response.
   - Absent gag and cough reflex.

The following laboratory criteria for brain death are also available:

- EEG showing electrocerebral silence for at least 30 min
- Lack of brainstem evoked responses
- Radioisotopic bolus angiography
- Xenon CT
- Digital substraction angiography
- Gamma scintigraphy.

Communication with Parents/Attendants

Utmost care should be exercised in breaking the sad news of "death" to the family, especially when it is sudden and family is not prepared to face it.

- When death is very much round the corner, the family may be allowed to be at his bedside and not discouraged to communicate with the child, especially when he is conscious.
- Once the "inevitable" has in actuality happened, the family should be convinced with compassion and sympathy that "death" has occurred despite best of efforts by the doctors. There may be initial difficulties in accepting the reality by relatives. Frequently, they are likely to become hysterical and hostile with anger and shock. On the other hand, some may react with grief, guilt and depression. The support from the physician comes in handy in driving home to them the "God's will".
- If postmortem is on the card, a written permission from the family is needed. One should approach the family with the plea that autopsy is in the interest of the family as it is likely to give clues to cause of death and help in prevention of disease in siblings as also for genetic counseling.
- If a cadaveric transplant is on the card, a due permission from the parents becomes mandatory (*vide infra*).

- It is important to prepare a death certificate.
- It is desirable to arrange transportation of the dead body to family's residence.

ETHICS GOVERNING ORGAN TRANSPLANTATION

The cadaveric organ transplantation has become a fact of life in the advanced countries. A Human Organ Transplant Act 1994 exists in India too. Nevertheless, on account of the logistic difficulties, the facility has hardly taken off the ground in the Indian subcontinent.

It is important to bear in mind the ethical aspects of this area. The family should be informed, educated and convinced for organ donation if otherwise prerequisites are met with (Table 4.2). However, it shall be unethical to use pressure tactics for this even though with good intentions. The basic prerequisite is that it should be a brain death rather than death due to cardiorespiratory failure. In the latter case, there is compromise of the perfusion of the organ targeted for transplant, rendering it unsuitable for the purpose.

Table 4.2: Prerequisites for human organ transplant

• Early and reliable diagnosis of brain death.
• Absence of transmissible viral disease in the donor organ.
• Willingness on the part of the family to donate the said organ of the dead child.
• Organ is well preserved.
• Recepient is available on a short notice.

REFERENCES

1. Gupte S. Geneva Declaration, Hippocrates oath, ethics and legal issues: A pediatrician's viewpoint. *Asian J Matern Child Hlth* 2002;7:234-244.
2. Frader J, Thompson A. Ethical issues in the pediatric intensive care unit. *Pediatr Clin North Am* 1994; 41:1405-1423.
3. Parikh CK. *Parikh's Textbook of Medical Jurisprudence, Forensic Medicine and Toxicology,* 6th edn. New Delhi: CBS 1999.
4. Tiwari S, Baldwa M. Medical negligence. In: Gupte S (ed) *Recent Advances in Pediatrics,* Vol 14. New Delhi: Jaypee Brothers 2004;311-329.
5. Tiwari SK, Baldwa M. Doctors and criminal law. *Indian Pediatr* 2002;39:1119-1125.
6. Potdar RD. Consumer protection law and pediatricians. *Indian Pediatr* 1997;34:283-286.

Section II

Life-Threatening Situations and Resuscitative Aspects

Kamran Afzal and Shazia Afzal

5 Cardiopulmonary Resuscitation

INTRODUCTION

The emergency procedure, *cardiopulmonary resuscitation (CPR),* is a series of interventions aimed at restoring and supporting vital functions. The immediate goal is to reestablish substrate delivery to meet the metabolic needs of the vital organs. The overall goal is return of the child to the society without morbidity related to the underlying disease process or to the resuscitation process. Techniques of basic and advanced life support when readily available and skillfully applied contribute to the significant reduction in childhood mortality.

This chapter essentially describes the recent guidelines for CPR and Emergency Cardiovascular Care (ECC) of the American Heart Association (AHA).[1]

DEFINITIONS[2]

Cardiac arrest refers to the clinical state characterized by the absence of detectable cardiac activity, with the recognition that some children with clinical cardiac arrest may have measurable aortic pressure if an arterial line is inserted. Cardiac arrest in children is usually the result of profound hypoxemia, hypercarbia and/or ischemia.

Basic cardiopulmonary resuscitation is an attempt to restore effective circulation with external chest compressions plus expired air inflation of the lungs.

Return of spontaneous circulation (ROSC) refers to the return of any spontaneous central pulses, regardless of the duration. ROSC of 20 minutes or more is considered sustained.

Age of the victim is currently the primary characteristic which guides the decision for the application of various resuscitation techniques. For the purpose of resuscitation, *an infant* is a child under the age of 1 year. A ***child*** is aged between 1 and 8 years of age. Children above 8 years will still be subject to same resuscitation sequence as a younger child but may require adult techniques and ratios to attain effective chest compressions.

DIFFERENCES BETWEEN PEDIATRIC AND ADULT RESUSCITATION

Pediatric CPR has been based largely on the adult model of resuscitation. However, pediatric resuscitation is different from adult resuscitation for the following reasons:[3]

1. Sudden cardiopulmonary arrest in infants and children is much less common than in adults.[4]
2. Primary cardiac arrest is uncommon in children and young adults.[5] Cardiac arrest in children typically represents the terminal event of progressive shock or respiratory failure. In most circumstances, survival from documented asystolic pediatric cardiac arrest is dismal.
3. Because the cause of the arrest is mostly related to respiratory failure and because the child's myocardium is relatively resilient to hypoxemia, the rapid correction of hypoxemia may be all that is necessary to affect resuscitation.
4. Because of tremendous size variations in children, therapeutic modalities that are size-dependent require some adjustment for the individual patient. Technical demands of vascular access, airway control, and selection of pediatric equipment and drug dosages are also high. This can lead to loss of precious time when it is most critical.
5. Arrhythmia management is generally not a problem in pediatric lifesupport. As a result, antiarrhythmic medications and defibrillation are used infrequently. The most common cardiac rhythms to be recognized and managed are sinus bradycardia and asystole.
6. Often the patient has received little prehospital care leading to longer periods of hypoxia and hypoperfusion, which directly affects prognosis and morbidity. Another difficulty is that most emergency departments are unaccustomed and inept at resuscitating children.

BASIC LIFE-SUPPORT TECHNIQUES

Basic life-support (BLS) refers to the provision of CPR, with no devices or bag-mask ventilation or barrier devices until advanced life-support (ALS) can be provided. It is intended to maintain organ perfusion until definitive interventions can be instituted. There is an orderly progression through the assessment and management of the ABCs- airway, breathing and circulation in BLS (Fig. 5.1).

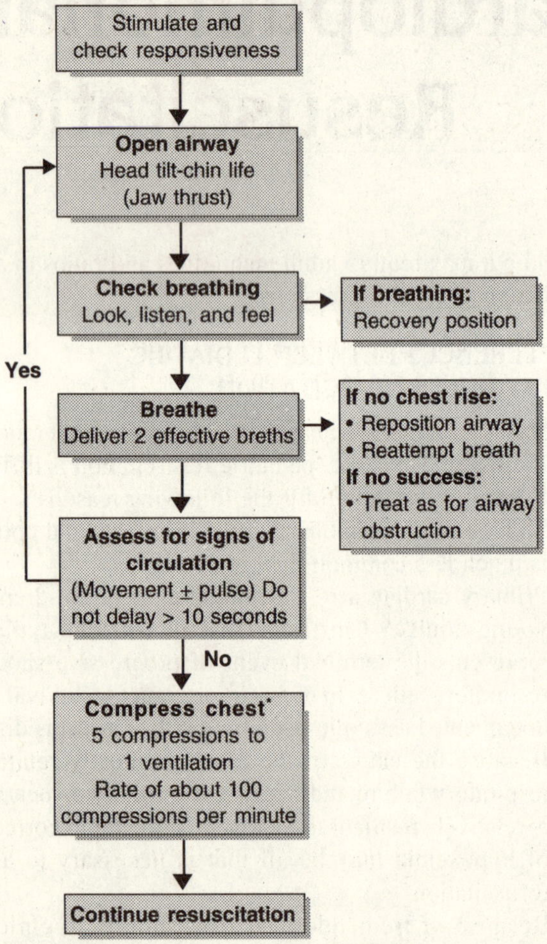

*Continue rescue breathing and CPR indicated

Fig. 5.1: Pediatric BLS algorithm[1]

Rapid Assessment

The initial steps of BLS begin when the victim is found unresponsive. The rescuer (after ensuring the safety of self and victim) should check the victim's responsiveness by gently stimulating the child and asking loudly "Are you alright?" Do not move or shake the victim with head or neck trauma (unless in imminent danger of injury), because such handling may aggravate a spinal cord injury. If trauma is suspected immobilize the child's cervical spine preventing movement of the neck and torso. If the child must be positioned for resuscitation or moved for safety reasons, rescuers should support the child's head and torso and turn as a unit (Fig. 5.2 b).

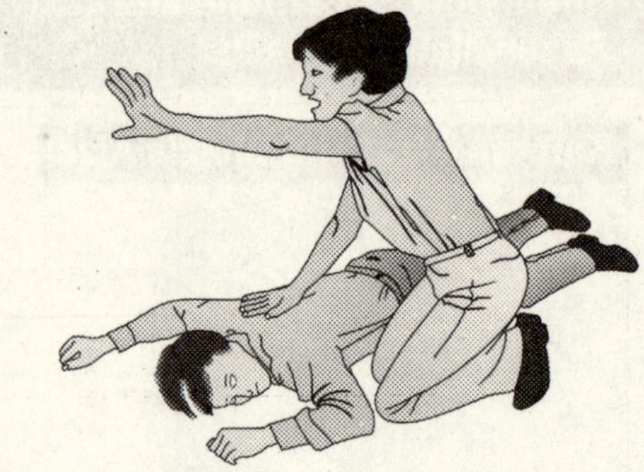

Fig. 5.2a: Cardiopulmonary resuscitation: Establishing airway and breathing. When an emergency arises, call for help

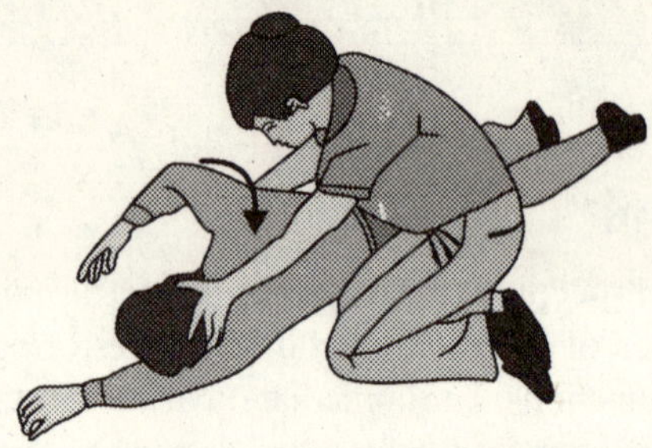

Fig. 5.2b: Cardiopulmonary resuscitation: Establishing airway and breathing. Position the victim

Airway

Evaluation: In infants, adequacy of ventilation is assessed by observing the free uniform expansion of the lower chest and upper abdomen. In contrast in older children and adolescents, one looks for uniform upper chest expansion as a sign of adequate ventilation.

Position the victim: If the child is unresponsive, turn the child as a unit into the supine (face up) position and place the child on a flat, hard surface. If trauma is suspected, the head and cervical spine should be stabilized during evaluation and management of airways by holding the head in the midline while applying gentle cephalad traction. The tongue is the most common cause of airway obstruction in the pediatric patient (Fig. 5.2c).

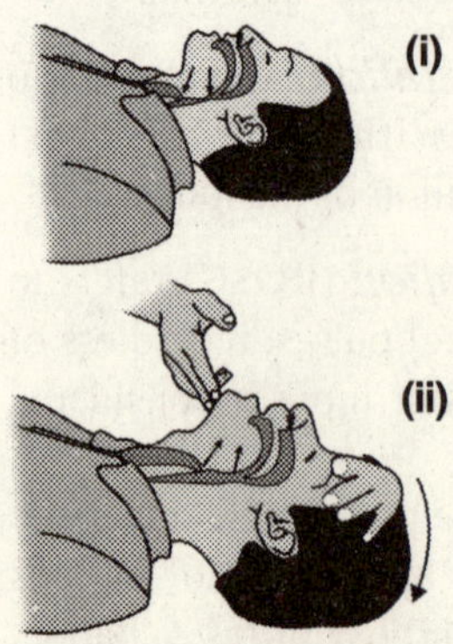

Fig. 5.2c: Cardiopulmonary resuscitation: establishing airway and breathing. Open the airway: (i) Airway obstruction produced by the tongue and the epiglottis, (ii) Relief by head-tilt/chin-lift

Management of Airway

The optimal methods of opening the airway consist of:

- *Head tilt-chin lift maneuver*: This involves:

- Tilting the head back slightly into neutral position (by gentle pressure on the child's forehead) and
- Lifting the chin forward by pushing or pulling the mandibular block of tissue forward with fingers placed near the point of chin under the bony part of lower jaw. Do not push on the soft tissues under the chin as this may block the airways (Fig 5.2c and d).

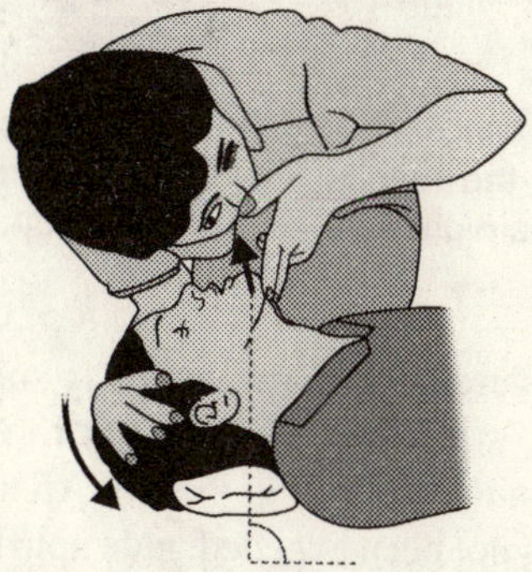

Fig. 5.2d: Cardiopulmonary resuscitation: Establishing airway and breathing—Head-tilt/chin-lift maneuver. Perpendicular line reflects proper neck extension, i.e., a line along the edge of the jaw bone should be perpendicular to the surface on which the victim is lying. One hand is used to tilt the head, extending the neck. The index finger of the other hand lifts the mandible outwards by lifting on the chin. ***Look.listen and feel*** for presence of breathing

- *Jaw-thrust maneuver* is preferred when head or neck injury is suspected. This is done by pulling the jaw forward with 2 or 3 fingers behind the angle of the jaw so that the lower central incisors are in a plane anterior to the upper central incisors (Fig. 5.2e). If a second rescuer is present, that rescuer should immobilize the spine.

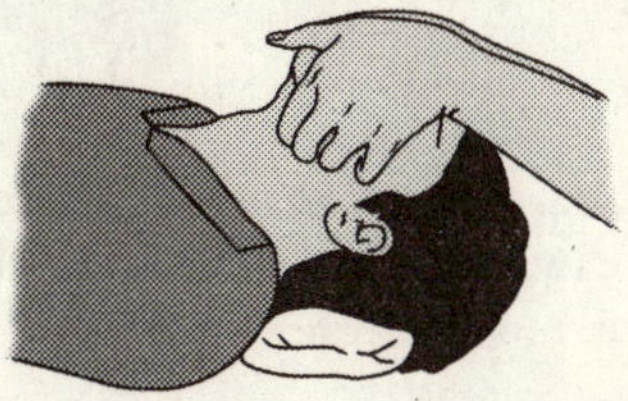

Fig. 5.2e: Cardiopulmonary resuscitation: Establishing airway and breathing. Jaw-thrust maneuver in cases with suspected spinal injury

- *Tongue-Jaw lift maneuver* is used to open airway to look for an obstructing foreign body in an unresponsive victim. In this maneuver first ensure that the patient is unresponsive. Then insert your thumb in the victim's mouth and position 2 or 3 fingers under the jaw. Grasp the tongue and lower jaw between your thumb and fingers and lift upward and outward.
- *Inspect the mouth briefly.* If secretions, vomitus or a foreign body is visible, remove it.

Breathing

Evaluation: Once a clear and stable airway has been secured look, listen and feel again for evidence of gas exchange. The physician should *look* at the chest to see whether there is chest wall or abdominal movement suggestive of breathing effort. *Listen* over the mouth and nose for the sound of exhaled breath sounds; *listen* with stethoscope over the trachea and the axilla for evidence of air movement. *Feel* for exhaled airflow from the child's mouth for no more than 10 seconds (Fig. 5.2 d). If the child is breathing adequately and there is no evidence of trauma, the child is turned to one side in a *recovery position.* For this the child is turned onto his/her side by moving the head, shoulders and torso simultaneously. The victim's leg may be bent and moved forward to provide stability. This position helps to maintain a patent airway, minimize the risk of aspiration, limit pressure on bony prominences and peripheral nerves and enables observation of the victim's respiratory effort and appearance. The recovery position is not used in head/neck trauma patients, where the supine position is preferred in case ongoing rescue breathing or CPR is needed. If there is evidence of spontaneous breathing and no evidence of gas movement through the central airways, the presumptive diagnosis is that of airway obstruction.

Management: Provide rescue breathing if no spontaneous breathing is detected even as airway patency is maintained by the above maneuvers. Take a deep breath and deliver at least 2 slow breaths (1-1½ seconds per breath) with a volume sufficient to make the child's chest rise visibly. (The current ILCOR recommendations suggest delivering between 2-5 rescue breaths initially but there is no data to support the choice of any single number of breaths).

Mouth-to-Mouth-and-Nose and Mouth-to-Mouth Breathing: In infants (<1 year old), the rescuer places his mouth over the infant's mouth and nose to create a seal and delivers the rescue breaths while maintaining good head position (Fig. 5.2 f). Inhale between rescue breaths.

The mouth-to-mouth rescue breathing where-in the rescuer pinches the victim's nose tightly with thumb and forefinger and makes a mouth-to-mouth seal before delivering the rescue breaths, is used in older children (1 to 8 years).

If the child's chest does not rise during rescue breathing, ventilation is not effective; either the airway is obstructed or greater volume or pressure is needed to provide adequate rescue breaths. Reposition the airway and reattempt ventilation. Move the child's head through a range of positions to obtain optimal airway patency (do not move if suspected head and neck trauma). If repeated attempts fail to open the airway, foreign body airway obstruction may be present.

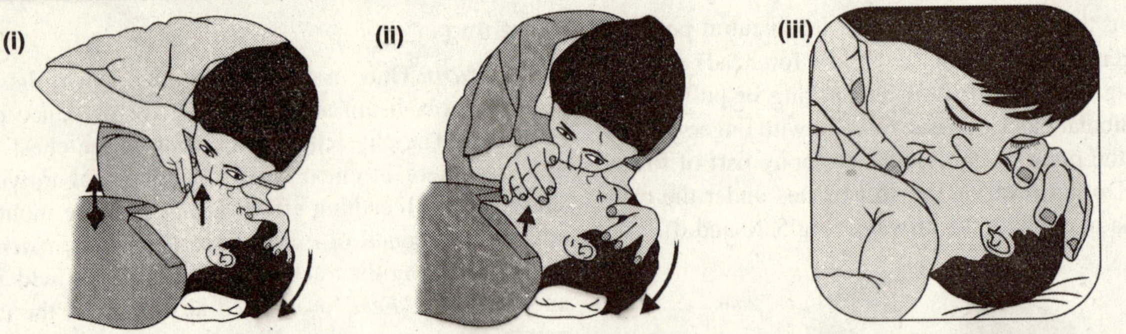

Fig. 5.2f: Cardiopulmonary resuscitation: Establishing airway and breathing—(i) Mouth-to-mouth rescue breathing in a child. Note how one hand maintains the head tilt while the rescuer looks for chest rise, (ii) Mouth-to-nose breathing in a child and (iii) Rescue breathing with an airtight seal around the mouth the nose in an infant

Generally the exposure of the rescuer to the victims is brief and infections are extremely rare after mouth-to-mouth rescue breathing.[6] Barrier devices like mask and face shields may be used if readily available but they have not been shown to reduce the risk of disease transmission.

The ideal ventilation rates are not known and are derived from normal respiratory rates for age, with some adjustments for the time needed to coordinate rescue breathing with chest compressions.

Breaths are delivered at a rate of 30 to 60/min in neonates, 15-20/min in the toddler and child, and 12-15/min in the adolescent.

. Relief of Foreign-Body Airway Obstruction (Fig. 5.3a).

Signs of foreign-body airway obstruction (FBAO) in infants and children include: sudden onset of respiratory distress associated with coughing, gagging, or stridor with no other signs of illness or infection, or if the chest does not rise in response to ventilation in an unconscious child.

Management: Three maneuvers to relieve FBAO are suggested: back blows, chest thrusts, and abdominal thrusts. For relief of FBAO in the responsive infant, back blows are delivered while the infant is supported in the prone position, straddling the rescuers forearm, with the head lower than the trunk (Fig. 5.3 b). After 5 back blows if the object has not been expelled, give upto 5 chest thrusts. This consists of chest compressions over the lower half of the sternum, 1 finger breath below the intermammary line till the foreign body is expelled or the patient becomes unresponsive. Chest thrusts in the infant are delivered while it is held supine on the rescuer's forearm, with the head lower than the body (Fig. 5.3 c).

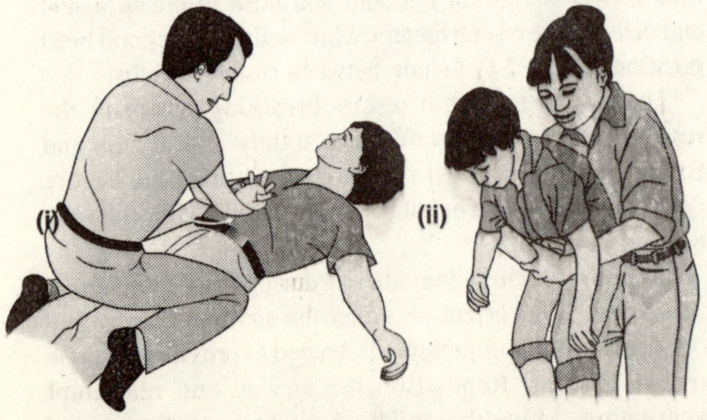

Fig. 5.3a: Foreign body airway obstruction—Subdiaphragmatic abdominal thrust (the Heimlich maneuver) :(i) Administered to a conscious or unconscious child, lying, and (ii) In a conscious child standing. A series of 5 abdominal thrusts are administered in a child older than 1 year

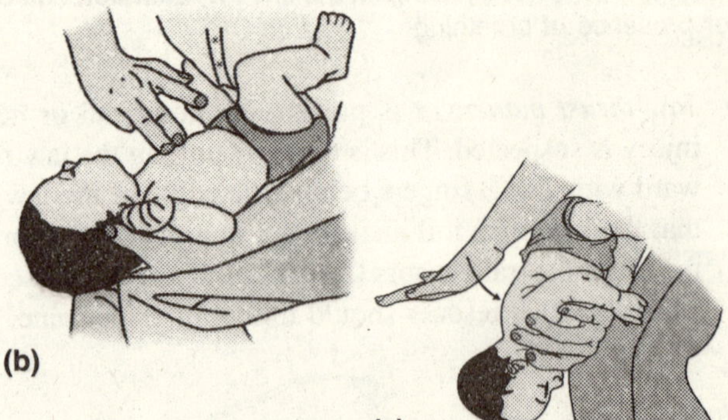

Figs 5.3b and c: Foreign body airway obstruction—(b) Chest thrust in an infant <1 year (c) Back blow: In an infant <1 year a combination of 5 back blows and 5 chest thrusts are administered

In the responsive child over 1 year with FBAO a series of 5 abdominal thrusts (Heimlich Maneuver) are used in addition to back blows and chest thrusts. Abdominal thrusts are delivered with the child in standing or sitting position if the child is conscious or in the lying down position if unconscious (Fig. 43.3 a).

In the unresponsive infant victim, the airway is opened using the tongue-jaw lift and oropharynx examined for the foreign body which is removed if visible with a finger sweep (Fig. 5.3d). Blind finger sweep should not be performed for fear of pushing the foreign body back into the airway causing further obstruction or injury to the airways. Once the foreign body is removed the airway is opened and rescue breaths delivered. If the chest does not expand, the head is repositioned and ventilation is again attempted. If unsuccessful, the sequence is repeated.

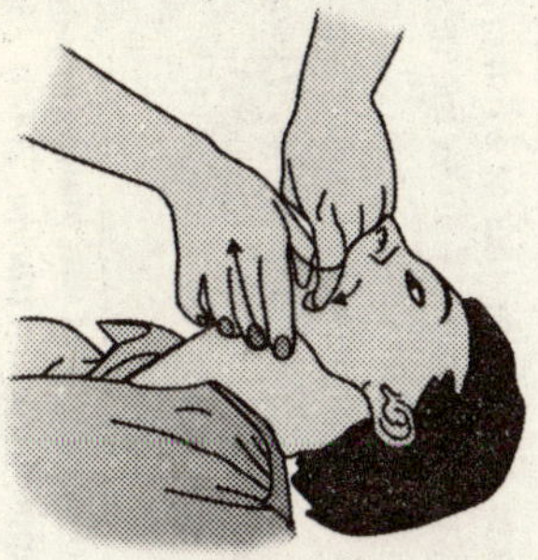

Fig. 5.3d: Foreign body airway obstruction—Finger sweep maneuver administered to an unconscious victim of foreign body airway obstruction

Circulation

Evaluation: Feel the victim's carotid (in adults and children),[7] femoral or brachial pulse with the latter site recommended in infants.[8] The short chubby neck in infants <1 year of age makes rapid location of carotid artery difficult. In addition it is easy to compress the airway while attempting to palpate the carotids pulse in the infant's neck. Hence, brachial artery is palpated in infants and the carotid pulse used for 1-8 years of age (Fig. 5.4 a).

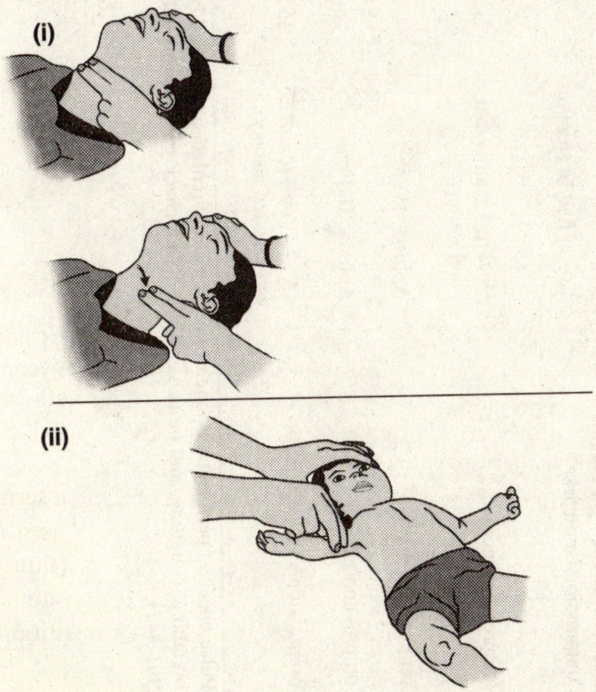

Fig. 5.4a: Cardiopulmonary resuscitation: Circulation—Locating the pulse: (i) Locating the carotid pulse in a child, (ii) Locating the brachial pulse in an infant

If the child is in cardiac arrest, begin chest compressions. For lay rescuers pulse check has poor sensitivity (90%) and specificity (60%); overall accuracy is only 65%, leaving an error rate of 35%[9]. Hence lay rescuers should not rely on the pulse check to determine the need for chest compression. Instead they should look for signs of circulation (normal breathing, coughing or movement in response to rescue breathing). Healthcare professionals should assess signs of circulation by performing both pulse-check as well as evaluate the victim for breathing coughing or movement after delivering rescue breaths. This assessment should take no more than 10 seconds. If there is no detectable pulse or other signs of circulation or if the heart rate is <60 bpm with signs of poor perfusion chest compression should be initiated. Do not delay chest compression to locate a pulse. Profound bradycardia in the presence of poor perfusion is an indication for chest compressions because cardiac output in infancy and childhood is largely dependent on heart rate, and an inadequate heart rate with poor perfusion indicates that cardiac arrest is imminent.

Management: chest compressions are serial rhythmic compressions of the chest that cause the blood to flow to the vital organs (heart, lungs, and brain) in an attempt to keep them viable until ALS can be provided. Chest compressions provide circulation as a result of changes in intrathoracic pressure and/or direct compression of the heart. Compress the lower half of sternum to a relative depth of approximately one third to one half the anterior/posterior diameter of the chest. For chest compressions to be effective the rescuer must ensure that the hands are in the proper position, allow the chest to return to its normal position after each compression and use the rate recommended for the particular age (Table 5.1, Figs. 5.4b-d). Compression should be interposed with ventilations in a ratio of 5:1. Consensus recommendations are to apply compressions for newborn at a rate of 120/min and for all other ages of children at a rate of 100/min.[1] The quality of chest compression is assessed by (1) palpation of pulses in a central artery (e.g. carotid, brachial, or femoral artery), (2) improvement of color, and (3) if possible end-tidal carbon dioxide (CO_2) and displayed arterial pressure waveform monitoring. To facilitate chest compressions, the child should be supine on a hard, flat surface. For this a resuscitation board that extends from the shoulder to the waist and across the full width of the bed may be placed beneath the patient's back. Infants with no signs of head and neck trauma may be successfully carried during resuscitation on the rescuer's forearm which supports the length of the infant's torso.

ADVANCED LIFE SUPPORT

Advanced life support is intended to achieve adequate

Table 5.1: Comparison across age groups of resuscitation interventions

CPR/Rescue breathing	*Adult and Older child*	*Child (Approx. 1-8 yrs of age)*	*Infant (Less >1 yr of age)*	*Neonate and Newly born*
Establish unresponsiveness				
Open airway (head tilt-chin lift or jaw thrust)	Head tilt-chin lift (if trauma is present, use jaw thrust)	Head tilt-chin lift (if trauma is present, use jaw thrust)	Head tilt-chin lift (if trauma is present, use jaw thrust)	Head tilt-chin lift (if trauma is present, use jaw thrust)
Check for breathing: Look, Listen, Feel) if victim breathing: place in recovery position. If victim is not breathing: give 2 effective slow breaths)				
Initial	2 effective breaths at 2 seconds/breath	2 effective breaths at 1-1½ seconds/breath	2 effective breaths at 1-1½ seconds/breath	2 effective breaths at approx. 1 second/breath
Subsequent	12 breaths/min (approx.)	12 breaths/min (approx.)	12 breaths/min (approx.)	12 breaths/min (approx.)
Foreign-body airway obstruction	Abdominal thrusts or back blows or chest thrusts	Abdominal thrusts or back blows or chest thrusts	Back blows or chest thrusts (no abdominal thrusts)	Back blows or chest thrusts (no abdominal thrusts)
Signs of circulation: Check for normal breathing, coughing or movement, pulse. If signs of circulation present: provide airway and breathing support. If signs of circulation absent, begin chest compressions interposed with breaths	Pulse check (healthcare providers)[a] Carotid	(Healthcare providers)[a] Carotid	(Healthcare providers)[a] Brachial	(Healthcare provides[a] Umbilical
Compression landmarks	Lower half of sternum	Lower half of sternum	Lower half of sternum (1 finger width below intermammary line)	Lower half of sternum (1 finger width below intermammary line)
Compression method	Heel of 1 hand, other hand on top	Heel of 1 hand	Two-thumbs-encircling hands for 2-rescuer health-care provider or 2 fingers	Two-thumbs-encircling hands for 2-rescuer health-care provider or 2 fingers
Compression depth	Approx. 1½ to 2 in	Approx. ⅓ to ½ the depth of the chest (1 to1½ in)	Approx. ⅓ to ½ the depth of the chest (½ to 1 in)	Approxi. ⅓ to ½ the depth of the chest
Compression rate	Approx. 100/min	Approx. 100/min	At least 100/min	Approx. 120 events/min (90 compressions/30 breaths)
Compression/ventilation ratio	15 : 2 (1 or 2 rescuers, unprotected airway) 5 : 1 (2 rescuers, protected airway)	15 : 2 (1 or 2 rescuers)	15 : 2 (1 or 2 rescuers)	3 : 1 (1 or 2 rescuers)

[a] Pulse check is performed as one of the 'signs of circulation' assessed by healthcare providers. Lay rescuers check for other signs of circulation (cyanosis, breathing, coughing, and movement) but do not check pulse as this delays CPR. (From: Part 9: Pediatric basic life support. *Resuscitation. 2000; 23: 46: 301-341*).

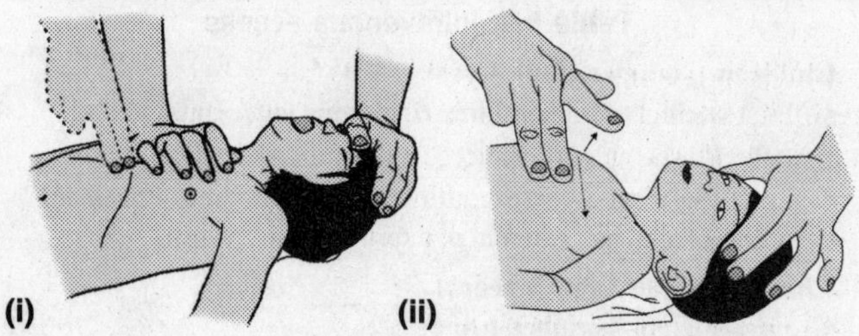

Fig. 5.4b: Cardiopulmonary resuscitation: Circulation—External chest compressions: (i) Locating the correct hand position on the lower half of the sternum in a child, and (ii) One finger width below intermammary line in an infant

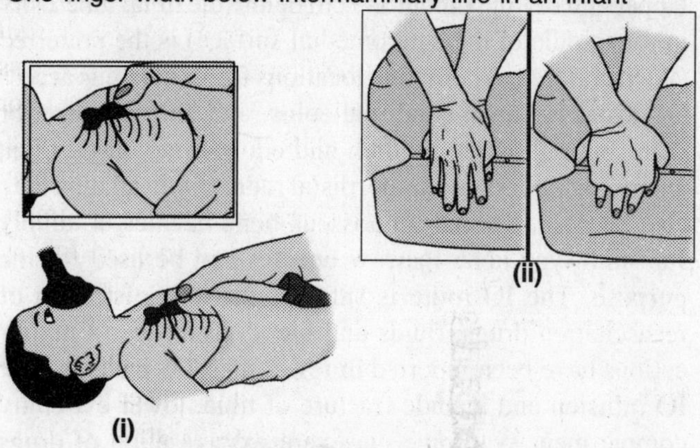

Fig. 5.4c: Cardiopulmonary resuscitation: Circulation—Hand positions for external chest compressions: (i) Hand position for chest encirclement technique for external chest compressions in neonates or infnats thumbs are side-by-side over the midsternum. In the newborn, thumbs may need to be superimposed, and (ii) Proper position of rescuer for an older child or adult: shoulders directly over victim's sternum; elbows locked. Heel of single hand is used in a child aged 1-8 years

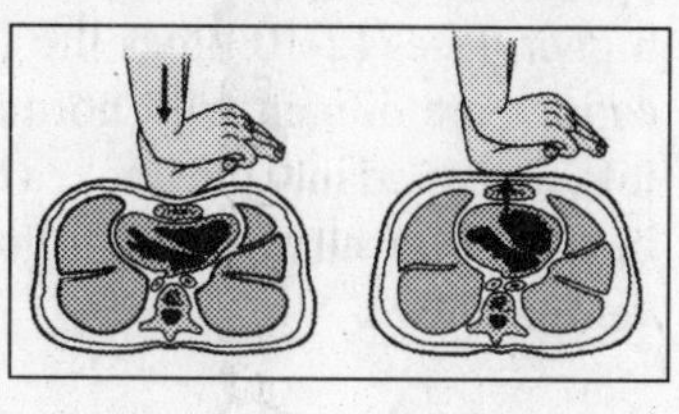

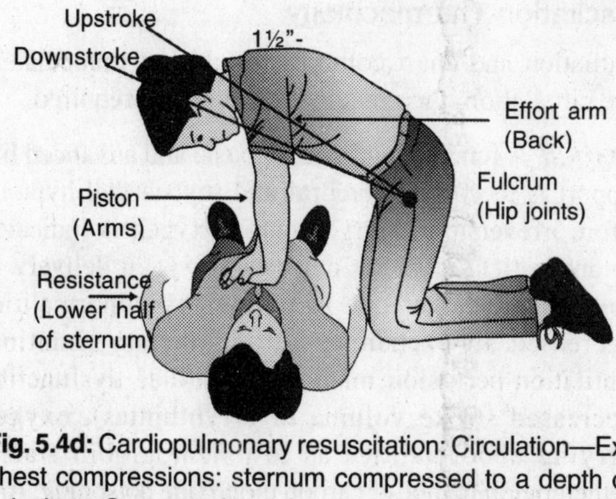

Fig. 5.4d: Cardiopulmonary resuscitation: Circulation—External chest compressions: sternum compressed to a depth of 1½-2 inches. Compression-relaxation duration must be 50 : 50 for better flow to occur

ventilation, control cardiac arrhythmias, stabilize blood pressure and cardiac output, and restore organ perfusion.

Artificial Airways

Oropharyngeal airways are used if manual manipulation of the airways fails to maintain airway patency. The airway helps to stent the mandibular block of tissue off the posterior pharyngeal wall. The proper size oropharyngeal airway can be selected by placing the airway alongside the face so that the bite block portion is parallel to the palate. The tip of the airway should just approximate the angle of the mandible.

Nasopharyngeal airways stent the tongue from the posterior pharyngeal wall and may also be used to facilitate nasopharyngeal suctioning. The length of the airway is estimated by measuring the distance from the nares to the tragus of the ear. The outside diameter of the airway should not be so large that it produces sustained blanching of the skin of the alae nasi.

Endotracheal tubes (ET) are used to (1) overcome upper airway obstruction, (2) isolate the larynx from the pharynx, (3) allow mechanical aspiration of secretions from the tracheal tree, and (4) facilitate mechanical ventilation or end-expiratory pressure. The correct tube size can be estimated using the formula based on the patient's age: Inside diameter (ID) in mm = ¼ × (16 + Age in years). Because this is only an estimate, it is prudent to have the next smaller and larger size ET tube available. Tube size may also have to be modified depending on the cause of the arrest (e.g. croup). In younger patients uncuffed tubes are used because of the normal narrowing in the trachea at the level of the cricoid cartilage which serves as a functional seal enabling satisfactory positive pressure ventilation. With patients 10 years of age and older, cuffed ET tubes should be used.

Assisted Ventilation

Mouth-to-mouth ventilation provides only 16-17% oxygen. Bag-mask ventilation provides variable amount of oxygen from room air (21% oxygen) to approximately 100% oxygen depending on the apparatus selected.

Bag-Mask ventilation: Manual resuscitator bag and mask can provide effective ventilation when used by trained personnel. There are two basic types of manual resuscitators (ventilation bags)—self-inflating and flow inflating resuscitators. Flow-inflating bags (anesthesia bags) refill only with oxygen inflow and hence supply continuous delivery of supplemental oxygen. However, they require regulation of inflow making them difficult to use. Self-inflating bags are therefore preferred and should be available in sizes appropriate for different ages. Resuscitation bags used for ventilation of full-term newborn infants, infants, and children should have a minimum volume of 450-500 mL. The rescuer should, however, use only the force and tidal volume necessary to cause the chest to rise visibly. Excessive ventilation-volume produce distension of alveoli and/or stomach, compromise cardiac output by raising the intrathoracic pressure, and increase the risk of regurgitation and aspiration.[9] Without a reservoir variable amount of oxygen and room air will enter the bag as it fills. With an oxygen reservoir, additional oxygen is provided, allowing delivery upto 95% oxygen. A minimum flow rate of 10-15 L/min is required to maintain adequate oxygen in the reservoir.

Cricoid pressure (Sellick's maneuver): gastric distention during rescue breathing may be minimized if slow rescue breaths are delivered because slow breaths will enable delivery of effective tidal volume at low inspiratory pressure. Firm but gentle pressure on the cricoid cartilage during ventilation may help compress the esophagus and decrease the amount of air delivered to the stomach.[10, 11] A nasogastric or orogastric tube may also relieve the gastric distention but this should ideally be done only after tracheal intubation to protect the airway from aspiration of gastric contents.

Vascular Access

The site of vascular access depends on the site and priorities of the patient's clinical status. The preferred site for vascular access during CPR should not interfere with resuscitative efforts.

Peripheral venous access is the vascular access method of choice in most nonemergent situations. The largest diameter vein accessible (e.g. median cubital veins at the elbow or the long saphenous vein at the ankle) and an appropriate sized catheter should be selected. Medications administered into a peripheral vein should be followed by a 5-10 mL saline flush to facilitate entry into the central circulation as blood flow in peripheral vascular beds will be poor during CPR.

Central venous cannulation is a safer and more secure route for administration of medications that may injure tissues if infiltration occurs. It also enables monitoring of central venous pressure and sampling of central venous blood for laboratory studies. Hence it is a useful option when peripheral venous cannulation cannot be achieved. The femoral vein is frequently accessed in children; external or internal jugular and subclavian (in older children) may used by skilled individuals.

Intraosseus (IO) access during pediatric CPR or treatment of severe decompensated shock, should be obtained if there is delay in achieving venous access.[12, 13] The American Heart Association recommends that if after 90 sec or three attempts to achieve venous access are unsuccessful, an intraosseus infusion should be attempted.

Table 5.2. Intravenous access

Children (younger than 5 years old)
• First attempt–peripheral line (including antecubital vein)
• After 90 seconds (if unsuccessful)–intraosseus line
• Later: saphenous vein cutdown or central line placement – (femoral, subclavian, external or internal jugular vein)
Children (older than 5 years)
• First attempt–peripheral line
• Second atempt-saphenous vein cutdown or central line placement

From: Rogers MC (ed): Textbook of Pediatric Intensive Care. 3rd edn. Baltimore: William and Wilkins; 1996.

Upper end of tibia (about 1-3 cm below the tibial tuberosity in the middle of the anteromedial surface) is the preferred site in children. Alternative locations for intraosseus access are distal femur, medial malleolus, and anterior superior iliac spine. In older children and adolescents, distal tibia, anterior superior iliac spine, distal radius or distal ulna may also be used. Special intraosseus bone needles or simply Jamshidi-type bone marrow needles can be used for the purpose. The IO route is safe for the administration of resuscitation drugs, fluids and blood products.[14] Complications have been reported in fewer than 1% patients after IO infusion and include fracture of tibia, lower extremity compartment syndrome or severe extravasation of drugs and osteomyelitis. These can be avoided by using careful technique for IO insertion.

Endotracheal route: In infants and children in whom IV or IO access is delayed, certain lipid soluble drugs may be given by the endotracheal route. These drugs include lidocaine, epinephrine, atropine, and naloxone (remembered by the mnemonic LEAN). For endotracheal administration, higher doses (2-10 times the IV dose) are used; the medications are diluted with normal saline to a volume of 3-5 mL, delivered into the trachea through a catheter positioned in the lower airway and followed with positive pressure ventilations.

Resuscitation Pharmacology

If ventilation and chest compression do not immediately restore circulation, then medications may be required.

1. *Oxygen:* A fundamental goal of basic and advanced life support is to correct cerebral and myocardial hypoxia before irreversible injury occurs. Oxygen is indicated for any patient who has decreased oxygen delivery to the tissues whether due to pulmonary abnormalities (decreased air exchange, intrapulmonary shunting, ventilation-perfusion mismatch), cardiac dysfunction (decreased stroke volume or arryhthmias), oxygen carrying abnormalities as low hemoglobin states, methemoglobinemia, or carbon monoxide poisoning. Any patient who is suspected to be hypoxemic should be

given oxygen. During resuscitation, the initial oxygen should be 100%, because the potential negative effects of high oxygen concentration are not a consideration in a life and death situation. Oxygen concentrations delivered by mouth-to-mask breathing vary from 16 to 17%. Bag-valve-mask devices deliver up to 21% oxygen. When an oxygen source is attached, bag-valve-mask devices may deliver 30 to 60% oxygen, and when a reservoir is added, 70 to 90% may be achieved. An anesthesia bag may deliver 100% oxygen.

2. *Epinephrine:* This is the drug of choice for cardiac arrest. It is an endogenous catecholamine with potent α and β-adrenergic properties. Epinephrine is indicated for bradycardia, asystole, ventricular tachycardia, ventricular fibrillation, and hypotension not related to volume depletion. For asystole, pulseless arrest or symptomatic bradycardia, the recommended initial dose of epinephrine for IV or IO administration is 0.01 mg/kg (i.e. 0.1 mL/kg of 1:10,000 solution) or tracheally in a dose of 0.1 mg/kg (0.1 mL/kg of 1:1000 solution). The higher endotracheal dose is because the endotracheal absorption of the medication is inferior to the intravenous or IO routes. The dose may be repeated every 3-5 minutes. Subsequent doses may be same as initial dose or may increase upto 10 times higher (0.1mg/kg, 1:1000, 0.1 mL/kg). Epinephrine may be a useful drug for management of shock that has not responded to volume resuscitation, especially in infants and children. The infusion is begun at the rate of 0.1 µg/kg/min and increased upto 1.0 µg/kg/min (Tables 5.3 and 5.4).

Table 5.3: Infusion medications: "Rule of 6"

Drug	*Add to 5% dextrose in water to make 100 mL*	*1mL/kg/hr delivers*
Epinephrine	0.6 mg	0.1 µg/kg/min
Dopamine or Dobutamine	60 mg	10 µLg/kg/min
Lidocaine	120 mg	20 µLg/kg/min

3. *Dopamine:* Dopamine is a precursor of epinephrine that acts on both α and β-adrenergic receptors. It has a unique "dopaminergic effect" that increases blood flow to the renal and mesenteric blood vessels. It is used for hypotension following resuscitation and shock that has not responded to fluid resuscitation. The dopaminergic effect occurs at low doses (0.5-2 µg/kg/min). It has direct β-adrenergic effects at doses above 5 µg/kg/min, while α adrenergic effect predominates as doses are raised from 10 to 20 µg/kg/min. Method for preparation of the drip is shown in Table 5.3. Dopamine is inactivated in the presence of sodium bicarbonate and may cause tissue necrosis if infiltration into the tissues occurs.

4. *Sodium bicarbonate:* With the onset of respiratory failure, the patient develops respiratory acidosis. The immediate treatment of this type of acidosis is adequate ventilation. As the patient's circulation begins to fail, there is anerobic metabolism, generation of lactic acid and resultant metabolic acidosis. Acidosis further impairs cardiac and circulatory functions and makes the catecholamines like epinephrine less effective. To correct the acidosis sodium bicarbonate may be given in a dose of 1 mEq/kg/dose by slow infusion IV or IO. Sodium bicarbonate corrects acidosis by combining with hydrogen ions to form carbon dioxide and water. This additional CO_2 must be eliminated through ventilation. Thus assurance of adequate oxygenation, ventilation and circulation is recommended before administration of sodium bicarbonate for prolonged cardiac arrest.

5. *Glucose:* It is indicated for documented hypoglycemia. A dose of 2-4 mL/kg of 25% dextrose solution (0.5-1 g/kg) is administered intravenously as infusion.

6. *Calcium:* It is indicated for documented hypocalcemia, for the treatment of hyperkalemia, hypermagnesemia, and calcium channel blocker overdose. Calcium chloride is recommended as it does not require hepatic degradation. The recommended dose is 5-7 mg/kg of elemental calcium (0.2 mL/kg IV/IO).

Rhythm Disturbances

Cardiac arrest in children is usually the end-result of progressive respiratory distress and hypoxia. In a previously well child, however, witnessed sudden collapse may result from a primary arrhythmic cardiac arrest secondary to myocarditis, congenital or acquired heart disease, severe electrolyte abnormality, drug intoxication, hypothermia, etc. Pediatric rhythm disturbances are classified into[1]:

a. *Bradyarrhythmias* (slow pulse rate): These are the most common prearrest rhythms. Clinically significant bradycardia is defined as heart rate below 60 bpm associated with poor systemic perfusion. Examples include sinus bradycardia, sinus node arrest with junctional/ventricular escape rhythms, and AV blocks. The potentially reversible causes of refractory bradycardia include the 4Hs (Hypoxemia, Hypovolemia, Hypo/Hyperkalemia, Hyperthermia) and 4Ts (Tamponade, Tension pneomothorax, Toxins/poisons/drugs, Thromboembolism). The immediate treatment of significant bradycardic rhythms is support of airway, ventilation and circulation. Therapy essentially includes epinephrine, and atropine (Table 5.4). Pacing may be done if available. Chest compressions are instituted for heart rate below 60 bpm or poor systemic perfusion.

Table 5.4: Drugs and electrical therapy used in PALS for rhythm disturbances

Drug	*Indications/Precautions*	*Dosage*
Adenosine	*Indications*: Drug of choice for treatment of symptomatic SVT *Precautions*: Very short half-life (use rapid injection technique)	IV/IO • Continuous ECG monitoring • 0.1mg/kg rapid IV push, follow with NS push • May double (0.2 mg/kg) for second dose • Maximum first dose: 0.6 mg • Maximum second dose: 12 mg
Amiodarone	*Indications:* Wide ranfe of atrial and ventricular arrythmias and shock refractory VF/VT *Precautions*: May cause bradycardia and hypotension; may prolong QT interval and increase risk for polymorphic VT; do not routinely combine with other medications that prolong QR interval (e.g. procainamide)	*For perfusing VT and SVT:* 5 mg/kg IV/IO over 20-60 minutes (repeat as needed to maximum: 15 mg/kg per day) *For refractory pulseless VT/VF*: 5 mg/kg rapid IV/IO bolus
Atropine suplfate	*Indications:* Vagally induced symptomatic bradycardia; symptomatic bradycardia refractory to oxygenation, ventilation, and epinephrine *Precautions:* Low dose may cause paradoxical bradycardia; tracheal absorption may be unreliable	IV/IO/tracheal: 0.02 mg/kg per dose; may double for second dose • Minimum dose: 0.1 mg • Maximum single dose, child: 0.5 mg (maximum total dose: 1 mg) • Maximum single dose, adolscent: 1 mg (maximum total dose: 2 mg)
Calcium chloride (10% solution = 27.2 mg/mL of elemental calcium)	*Indications*: symptomatic hypocalcemia, hyperkalemia, calcium channel blocker overdosage *Precautions:* Rapid IV push may result in bradycardia/asystole; do not mix with buffer; infiltration may cause skin to slough	IV/IO: 20 mg/kg (0.2 mL/kg of 10% solution) slow push. Repeat for documented condition
Calcium gluconate (10% solution = 9 mg/mL of elemental calcium)	——— DO ———	IV/IO: 60 to 100 mg/kg (0.6-1mL/kg of 10% solution) slow push. Repeat for documented condition
Synchronized cardio-version attempt	*Indications:* Tachyarrythmias (SVT, VT, atrial fibrillation, atrial flutter) with symptoms of cardiovascular compromise *Precautions:* Activate sync mode; provide sedation with analgesia when possible	Initial energy (shock) level: 0.5-1 J/kg Second and subsequent energy levels: 1-2 J/kg
Defibrillation attempt	*Indications:* VF/pulseless VT *Precautions:* Do not delay; use largest paddle size with good contact and no bridging	Deliver upto 3 shocks: • 2 J/kg; 2 J/kg to 4 J/kg; 4 J/kg • Subsequent energy level: 4 J/kg

Contd...

Contd...

Drug	*Indications/Precautions*	*Dosage*
Epinephrine for bradycardia	*Indications:* Sypmtomatic bradycardia refractory to oxygenation and ventilation *Precautions:*May produce profound vasoconstriction, tachyarrhythmias, hypertension; do not mix with buffer	IV/IO: 0.01 mg/kg (0.1 mL/kg of 1:10000) Tracheal: 0.1 mg/kg (0.1 mL/kg of 1:1000)
Epinephrine for asystole or pulseless cardiac arrest*	*Indications:* Pulseless arrest: asystole, pulseless electrical activity, shock refractory VF/VT *Precautions:*May produce profound vasoconstriction, tachyarrythmias, hypertension	First dose: Same as above • Subsequent doses: Repeat every 3 to 5 min during CPR • Consider a higher dose (0.1 mg/kg, 0.1 mL/kg of 1:1000)
Epinephrine infusion	*Indications:* Refractory hypotension or persistent bradycardia *Precautions:*same as above	0.1 to 1 µg/kg per minute, Titrate to desired effect
Lidocaine bolus*	*Indications:* Alternative treatment for wide complex tachycardias or VF/pulseless VT *Precautions:*High dose may cause myocardial depression and seizures; do not use if rhythm is wide-complex bradycardia (ventricular escape beats)	IV/IO/tracheal bouls: 1 mg/kg May repeat every 5 to 15 minutes
Lidocaine infusion	*Indications:* Alternative treatment for recurrent VT/VF or ventricular ectopy *Precautions:*same as above	IV/IO infusion: 20-50 µg/kg/min Administer bolus of 1 mg/kg when initiating infusion if bouls has not been given within previous 15 minutes
Magnesium sulfate	*Indications:* Torsades de pointes VT or symptomatic hypomagnesemia *Precautions:*May cause hypotension with rapid bolus	Rapid IV/IO infusion: 25-50 mg/kg (maximum 2 g) over 10-20 minutes Loading dose: 15 mg/kg IV over 30 minutes
Procainamide	*Indications:* Alternative treatment for recurrent VT/VF, SVT *Precautions:*Hypotension, bradycardia, QT prolongation Do not routinely adminster with amiodarone	
Sodium bicarbonate	*Indications:* Hyperkalemia, sodium channel blocker toxicity, and severe metabolic acidosis (documented or suspected after prolonged arrest) with adequate ventilation *Precautions:*Infuse slowly, may produce CO_2; therefore, ventilation must be adequate; do not mix with catecholmines or calcium	1 mEq/kg/dose infuse slowly and only if ventilation is adequate

In: PALS provider manual, American Heart Association, 2002; p220.

b. *Tachyarrhythmias* (fast rate): These include sinus tachycardia, supraventricular tachycardia (SVT), and ventricular tachycardia (VT). Treatment of sinus tachycardia is mainly aimed at the underlying cause; no pharmacotherapy is required. SVT is the most common tachyarrhythmia with heart rates in excess of 220 bpm producing cardiac compromise, especially in infancy. SVT with poor perfusion is treated with electrical or chemical cardioversion. SVT with adequate perfusion is treated with adenosine and/or planned synchronized cardioversion. Defibrillation is the treatment for both VT without palpable pulses as well as ventricular fibrillation (VF). For VT with signs of poor perfusion immediate synchronized cardioversion is performed. Pharmacotherapy is used for VT with pulses refractory to electrical cardioversion (see Table 5.4).

c. *Pulseless arrest (collapse rhythms):* These patients have no detectable pulses or signs of perfusion. VF, pulseless VT, asystole, and all forms of pulseless electrical activity are included under collapse rhythms.
   i. If collapse is sudden especially with known risk factors for cardiac disease, VF/pulseless VT is more likely than asystole and defibrillation should be attempted.
   ii. If arrest occurs with risk factors for hypoxia or ischemia preceding arrest, brady-asystole is more likely than VF/pulseless VT, and the emphasis should be on early support of airway and oxygenation. Asystole is a form of pulseless arrest associated with absent electrical activity in confirmed in more than one ECG lead. The etiology of asystole is usually a combination of hypoxia and ischemia, and the prognosis of intact neurologic survival is poor. Treatment is aimed at instituting immediate basic and ALS and drug therapy (epinephrine).
   iii. Pulseless electrical activity (PEA) other than VF/VT that does not produce a palpable pulse and that may degenerate rapidly into an agonal ventricular rhythm or asystole if not treated early. Treatment includes use of volume expansion, norepinehrine, dopamine or some combination of the three therapies. Identify and treat reversible causes of PEA-the 4Hs and 4Ts.

Defibrillation

Difibrillation is indicated for ventricular fibrillation and pulseless ventricular tachycardia. It is a fairly uncommon intervention in pediatric resuscitation as it is unusual for a child's heart to fibrillate. Difibrillation works by producing a mass polarization of myocardial cells with the intent that a sinus rhythm returns. The diagnosis should first be confirmed in more than one electrocardiographic leads. Acidosis and hypoxia should be treated, airway secured, ventilation with 100% oxygen provided and CPR instituted before attempting defibrillation. Vascular access should also be obtained if this does not delay defibrillation. Pediatric paddles are used for children below 10 kg while adult paddles are used for bigger children. The paddles must be prepared with electrode paste or cream, or with saline pads or electrically conductive defibrillation pads. One paddle is placed on the right side of the chest below the clavicle and the other on the left side of the chest lateral to the nipple. The initial defibrillation dose is 2 joules (J)/kg; if fibrillation persists higher dose of 4 J/kg, and if still unsuccessful 3rd dose of 4 J/kg is delivered. If these three doses are ineffective, epinephrine and lidocaine are administered and defibrillation at 4J/kg is again attempted 30-60 sec after the medications (Table 5.4).

Post Resuscitation Stabilization

Following successful resuscitation, children often require additional support to maintain stable rhythm and improve perfusion as they are hypotensive, poorly perfused, and very acidotic. Stabilization involves initiating treatment for any reversible cause of arrest and providing continuous advanced life support. The goals of postarrest stabilization

Table 5.5: Summary of postresuscitation care

Airway	: Tracheal intubation with confirmation of tracheal tube position; repeat confirmation after movement/transport. Secure tube before transport Gastric decompression
Circulation	: 100% inspired oxygen. Provide mechanical ventilation targetting normal ventilation goals (PCO_2, 35 to 40 mmHg). Monitor pulse oximetry and exhaled CO_2 (or capnography) if available.
Circulation	: Ensure adequate intravascular volume (volume titration). Optimize myocardial function and systemic perfusion (inotropes, vasopressors, vasodilators). Monitor capillary refill time, blood pressure, continuous ECG, urine output; measure arterial blood gases and lactate to assess degree of acidosis if available. Ideally maintain 2 routes of functional vascular access.
Disability	: Perform a rapid secondary survey, including a brief neurologic assessment. Avoid hyperglycemia, treat hypoglycemia (monitor glucose) If seizures are observed, administer anticonvulsant medications. Obtain laboratory studies if available: arterial blood gases, glucose, electrolytes, hemotocrit, chest radiograph.
Exposure	: Avoid and correct hyperthermia (monitor temperature) Avoid profound hypothermia (less than 33°C)

In: *PALS Provider Manual.* American Heart Association 2002.

are to preserve brain function, prevent secondary organ injury, assess and treat the cause of illness, and deliver the patient in optimum condition to a tertiary care setting. The PALS principles of rapid cardiopulmonary assessment and support of the ABCs are continued in the post-resuscitative care along with evaluation of neurologic function (**D**isability monitoring), monitor **E**xposure and **E**nvironment, and assessing and maintaining a core temperature range[1] (Table 5.5).

REFERENCES

1. Hazinski MF, Zaritsky AL, Nadkarni VM, Hickey RW, Schexnayder SM, Berg RA (ed): PALS *Provider Manual*. American Heart Association 2000.
2. Nadkarni V, Hazinski MF, Zideman D, et al. Pediatric resuscitation: An advisory statement from the Pediatric Working Group of the International Liason Committee on Resuscitation. *Circulation* 1997;95: 2185-2195.
3. Ludwig S. Resuscitation-pediatric basic and advanced life support. In: Fleisher GR, Ludwig S (eds). *Textbook of Pediatric Emergency Medicine*. 4th edn. Philadelphia; Lippincott Williams & Wilkins, 2000;3-31.
4. Young KD, Seidel JS. Pediatric cardiopulmonary resuscitation: a collective review. *Ann Emerg Med* 1999;33:195-205.
5. Hazinski MF. Is Pediatric Resuscitation Unique? Relative merits of early CPR and ventilation versus early defibrillation for young victims of prehospital cardiac arrest. *Ann Emerg Med* 1995;25:540-543.
6. Mejicano GC, Maki DG. Infections acquired during cardiopulmonary resuscitation: epidemiology and outcome. *Ann Intern Med* 1998;129:813-828.
7. Mather C, O'Kelly S. The palpation of pulses. *Anaesthesia* 1996;51:189-191.
8. Cavallaro DL, Melker RJ. Comparison of two techniques for detecting cardiac activity in infants. *Crit Care Med* 1983;11:189-190.
9. Hirschman AM, Kravath RE. Venting vs ventilating: a danger of manual resuscitation bags. *Chest* 1982; 82:369-370.
10. Petito SP, Russel WJ. The prevention of gastric inflation: a neglected benefit of cricoid pressure. *Anaesth Intensive Care* 1988;16:139-143.
11. Moynihan RJ, Brock-Utne JG, Archer JH, Feld LH, Krietzman TR. The effect of cricoid pressure on preventing gastric insufflation in infants and children. *Anaesthesiology* 1993;78:652-656.
12. Bannerjee S, Singhi SC, Singh S, Singh M. The intraosseus route is a suitable alternative to intravenous route for fluid resuscitation in severely dehydrated children. *Indian Pediatr* 1994;31:1511-1520.
13. Glaeser PW, Hellmich TR, Szewczuga D, Losek JD, Smith DS. Five-year experience in prehospital intraosseus infusions in children and adults. *Ann Emerg Med* 1993;22:1119-1124.
14. Fiser DH. Intraosseus infusion. *N Engl J Med* 1990; 322:1579-1581.

Puneet Pooni and BK Jain

6 Oxygen Therapy

INTRODUCTION

Oxygen was first isolated by Priestley in 1744 and used therapeutically by Beddoes in 1798 and was first introduced into clinical practice by Dr JS Haldane in about 1920.[1] Oxygen therapy is the administration of oxygen at concentrations greater than that in ambient air (more than 21%) with the intent of treating or preventing the symptoms, and manifestations of hypoxia.

INDICATIONS

Anoxemia not only stops the machine but also wrecks the machinery.[1] Various indications are as follows:[2, 3]

- Correction of hypoxemia, thereby decreasing the work of breathing and the myocardial workload it imposes, and promotion of adequate oxygen delivery to the tissues. Documented hypoxemia in children, and infants older than 28 days, arterial oxygen tension (PaO_2) of < 60 mmHg or arterial oxygen saturation (SaO_2) of < 90% in subject's breathing room air or with PaO_2 and/or SaO_2 below desirable range for specific clinical situation. In neonates, PaO_2 < 50 mmHg and/or SaO_2 < 88%.
- Improvement of oxygenation in patients with decreased oxygen carrying capacity e.g. anemia.
- Promotion of the reabsorption of air in body cavities e.g. small pneumothorax.
- Severe trauma.
- Short-term therapy (e.g. postanesthesia recovery).

Clinical features of hypoxemia are summarized in Table 6.1.[3]

Oxygen as a Drug

The administration of oxygen should be done with as much care and attention as the practitioner uses when administering any other drug. Oxygen, like most drugs has safe dose ranges, adverse physiologic effects, and toxic manifestations that are associated with higher doses and prolonged use. For correction of hypoxemia, enough oxygen should be administered to saturate the hemoglobin 92% or better. This will safely achieve a PaO_2 of about 60 to 70 mmHg.[4] Administering additional supplemental oxygen, once the hemoglobin is fully saturated (99% to 100%), places the patient at risk of having toxic effects of this drug.

CONTRAINDICATIONS

No specific contraindications to oxygen therapy exist when indications are judged to be present.

COMPLICATIONS[5]

Hypoventilation and Carbon Dioxide Narcosis

Oxygen-induced hypoventilation may occur because of suppression of the hypoxic respiratory drive. Normally,

Table 6.1: Signs and symptoms of hypoxemia

System	*Mild to moderate*	*Severe*
Central nervous system	Confusion, agitation	Lethargy
Cardiac	Tachycardia, ectopy, hypertension	Bradycardia, hypotension
Respiratory	Dyspnea, tachypnea, shallow respirations bradypnea or paradoxical breathing	Increasing dyspnea, tachypnea possibly
Arterial blood gases Moderate: 40-60	Mild: PaO_2 60-80 mmHg	Severe: < 40 mmHg
Skin	Cool, clammy	Cyanosis

CO_2 is the primary stimulant driving the respiratory system. However, in patients with chronic hypercapnia ($PaCO_2$ > 45 mmHg), the CNS response to an elevated CO_2 level may become blunted and hypoxemia becomes the major ventilatory stimulus. Administration of oxygen-enriched gas to these children may result in hypoventilation, hypercapnia and possibly apnea. Under these circumstances, oxygen should be administered in low concentrations (<30%) while the patient is observed for signs of respiratory depression. If oxygenation remains inadequate and respiratory depression occurs, then mechanical ventilation is necessary.

Absorption Atelectasis

It occurs when the alveoli collapse because the gas within them is absorbed into the bloodstream. Nitrogen, a relatively insoluble gas, normally maintains a residual volume within the alveolus. During the breathing of high concentrations of oxygen (>50%), nitrogen may be replaced, or washed out of the alveolus. When the alveolar oxygen is then absorbed in to the pulmonary capillary, the alveolus partially or totally collapses.

Pulmonary Oxygen Toxicity

The exposure to high oxygen can lead to pathologic parenchymal changes, which is related to the duration of exposure and oxygen tension of the inspired air, not to the PaO_2. Generally, a FiO_2 of > 0.5 is considered toxic.[6] The first signs of oxygen toxicity are due to the irritant effect of oxygen and reflect an acute tracheobronchitis. After only a few hours of breathing 100% oxygen, mucociliary function is depressed and clearance of mucus is impaired. Within 6 hours of the administration of 100% O_2, a nonproductive cough, substernal pain, and nasal stuffiness may develop. Symptoms such as malaise, nausea, anorexia and headache develop, which are reversible on discontinuation of oxygen therapy. More prolonged exposure to high oxygen tension may lead to changes in the lung that mimic acute respiratory distress syndrome (ARDS). Endothelial lining of the pulmonary circulation gets disrupted resulting in leakage of proteinaceous exudates causing lung damage. Pulmonary macrophages are also depressed, making the patient more prone to infection. This occurs because of biochemically reactive oxygen-derived free radicals. Cellular repair may result after termination of high oxygen but results in pulmonary fibrosis of varying degrees.

Retinopathy of Prematurity

In premature infants PaO_2 of > 80 mmHg should be avoided because of the possibility of retinopathy of prematurity.[7] Also increased PaO_2 can contribute to closure or constriction of the ductus arteriosus-a possible concern in infants with ductus-dependent heart lesions.

OXYGEN DELIVERY SYSTEMS

There are many ways of giving oxygen. The administration of supplemental oxygen to neonatal and pediatric patients requires the selection of an oxygen delivery system that suits the patient's size, needs, and the therapeutic goals.[8-11] Many devices are available and are classified into two general categories i.e. low-flow or reservoir and high-flow or enclosure systems (Table 6.2).

Table 6.2: Two systems of oxygen delivery

Low-flow systems	*High-flow systems*
Nasal cannula	Oxygen hood
Nasopharyngeal catheters	Oxygen tents
Simple face-mask	Venturi mask
Partial rebreathing mask,	
Nonrebreathing mask	

Low-flow systems provide an FDO_2 (fractional concentration of delivered oxygen) that varies with the patient's inspiratory flow and are classified as variable-performance oxygen delivery systems.

High-flow systems can provide a specific FDO_2 at flows that meet or exceed the patient's inspiratory flow requirement and are classified as fixed-performance oxygen delivery systems.

Enclosure systems provide a means of controlling oxygen concentration, temperature, and humidity.

Whether a system is low or high flow does not determine its capability of delivering low versus high concentration of oxygen. When choosing the appropriate technique for delivering supplemental oxygen, one must consider the device's advantages and disadvantages, the FiO_2 limits of the device, and its appropriateness for a particular patient.[11]

Low-flow Systems

Low-flow systems by definition do not provide all the gas necessary to meet the patient's total minute ventilation. These systems require that the patient draw in room air while gas enriched with oxygen be also inspired from a reservoir. With these systems, the FiO_2 delivered to the patient can only be estimated because the humidity, temperature and actual FiO_2 cannot be precisely controlled.

Nasal Cannula

Consist of two soft prongs (infant prongs 7 mm apart or pediatric prongs 12 mm apart) that arise from oxygen supply tubing. The prongs are inserted into the patient's nares, and the tubing is secured to the patient's face.[12] Oxygen flows from the cannula into the patient's nasopharynx, which acts like a reservoir. If only adult nasal prongs are available, first cut off the ends of the prongs leaving two short barrels to be inserted into the child's nostrils. It is most important to keep the child's nose clean and free of mucus. In infants flow should not be more than 1 L/min.

Advantages:

- Inexpensive
- Well tolerated, comfortable
- Patient can eat and drink

Disadvantages:

- The concentration delivered falls substantially if the child breathes through the mouth
- Nasal prongs can be easily dislodged if they are not fixed properly
- Use may be limited by the presence of excessive mucus drainage
- Contraindicated in patients with nasal obstruction
- Skin irritation may result because of the material.

Nasopharyngeal catheters are soft tubes with several distal holes. The catheter should be inserted into the patient's nose to a depth equal to the distance from the ala nasi to the tragus or be gently advanced and then withdrawn until it rests slightly above the uvula. The tube, secured to the patient's face, is connected to oxygen supply tubing. Oxygen flows from the catheter into the patient's oropharynx, which acts as an anatomic reservoir. The FiO_2 varies with the patient's inspiratory flow. Catheter sizes less than 8 Fr are less effective in oxygen delivery.[11, 13]

Advantages: Apart from advantages of nasal prongs it has additional advantages as follows:

- Lowest flow rate of oxygen is required to achieve a given concentration in the airways Blockade of nostrils do not reduce the concentration of oxygen.
- The catheter can easily be secured in place so that it is unlikely to be dislodged.
- There is no danger of hypercarbia (carbon dioxide accumulation) if the oxygen is turned off or the tubing disconnects.

Disadvantages:

- Risk of gastric distension.
- Method is in less common use because of the complexity of care.
- FiO_2 is difficult to control and measure.
- Catheter should be cleared frequently to prevent occlusion of the distal holes. The patient should be observed for evidence of catheter occlusion, and the catheter should be alternated between nares every (8-12) hour and changed daily.
- Catheter sizes less than 8 Fr are less effective in oxygen delivery.
- Lower oxygen concentrations are delivered if the catheter is placed in the nose rather than in the pharynx.
- Improper insertion can cause gagging and nasal or pharyngeal trauma.
- Excessive flow can produce pain in the frontal sinuses.
- Pneumocephalus is a rare but possible complication.
- Excessive secretions and/or mucosal inflammation can result.
- Skin irritation may result from material used to secure the cannula and/or from local allergic reaction to polyvinyl chloride.
- Occlusion of distal openings may occur.

Simple oxygen masks are plastic reservoirs designed to fit over the patient's nose and mouth and be secured around the patient's head by an elastic strap. A reservoir effect is produced by the internal capacity of the mask. Oxygen is delivered through a small-bore tube connected to the base of the mask.[11] Holes on each side of the mask provide an egress for exhaled gases and serve as room-air entrainment ports.

Simple oxygen masks are used to provide supplemental O_2 in the moderate range (0.35-0.50, depending on size and minute ventilation) for short periods of time (e.g., during procedures, for transport, in emergency situations).

Advantages

- Simple, light weight
- Can be used with humidity
- Delivery of FiO_2 unto 0.60

Disadvantages:

- Provide variable FiO_2 depending on inspiratory flow and construction of the mask's reservoir and are not recommended when precise concentrations are required.
- Are confining and may not be well tolerated.
- Interfere with feeding; may not be available in sizes appropriate for all patients.
- Require a minimum flow to avoid possible rebreathing of CO_2.
- The maximum FiO_2 attainable with a simple, non-rebreathing or partial-rebreathing mask in neonates, infants, and children has not been well documented.
- Performance is altered if the entrainment ports are blocked.
- Aspiration of vomitus may be more likely when a mask is in place.
- Irritation may result from tight application.

Partial breathing and non-rebreathing masks have a reservoir bag, with a one-way valves between the reservoir bag and the mask and over the exhalation ports of the mask, which prevents exhaled gases from entering the bag.[10,11] This design provides a higher FiO_2 than the simple masks and the nasal devices.

Advantages: Delivery of >80% oxygen is possible to severely hypoxemic patient.

Disadvantages: All disadvantages of simple facemasks as mentioned above.

High-flow Systems

Venturi Mask

An air-entrainment mask is designed to fit over the patient's nose and mouth and contains a short corrugated hose with a jet orifice that is connected to oxygen supply tubing. Oxygen under pressure is forced through a small jet orifice entering the mask. The velocity increases causing a shearing effect distal to the jet orifice, which causes room air to be entrained into the mask. The total flow provided by the mask is determined by the cross-sectional area of the entrainment ports, the diameter of the jet orifice, and the oxygen flow to the jet. The FDO_2 is determined by the dimensions of the jet and the entrainment ports. The entrainment mechanism is based on the principles described by Bernoulli.[14] A collar can be attached to the base of the corrugated hose for supplemental humidification.

Air-entrainment masks provide a flow of gas of predetermined precise oxygen concentration (24-40%) that exceeds the patient's inspiratory flow. At the 50% setting, the total flow from the device may not meet the inspiratory flow. Its advantage is of delivering predictable FiO_2 and disadvantages are the same as nonbreathing facemask.

Oxygen hoods or head box are transparent enclosures designed to surround the head of the neonate or small infant. A continuous flow of humidified oxygen is supplied to the hood. Transparent enclosures in larger sizes (so-called tent houses or huts) are available for patients who are too big for neonatal-size hoods, which need very high, flow (20-40 L/min) and not routinely used. Flows > 7 L/min[11] are required to wash out CO_2.

Advantages:

- Controlled FiO_2 in infant and small children.
- Controlled FiO_2 and/or increased heated humidity to patients who cannot tolerate other devices.
- Controlled FiO_2 when the chest, abdomen, and extremities must be accessible to caregivers.
- The oxygen concentrations necessary for oxygen challenge (hyperoxia) tests in the spontaneously breathing neonate.

Disadvantages:

- O_2 concentrations may vary within the hood or tent. O_2 concentrations should be measured as near the nose and mouth as possible. Opening any enclosure decreases the O_2 concentration.
- Devices can be confining and isolating.
- Dense fog or excessive condensation can develop, which may frighten the child and limit observation.
- Inadequate or loss of gas flow may result in hypoxia or hypercapnia.
- Temperature within enclosures should be closely monitored to reduce the potential for cold stress or apnea from overheating in neonates.
- Use of an improperly sized hood can result in irritation of the infant's skin.
- Hypercarbia (carbon dioxide accumulation) will occur if the oxygen tubing kinks or disconnects, or if the oxygen flow rate is too low (a gas flow of 2-3 l/kg/min is necessary to avoid rebreathing of carbon dioxide.

Various commonly used oxygen devices along with the flow rate and expected FiO_2 is shown in Table 6.3.[9]

Exact FiO_2 delivered varies with changes in tidal volume, respiratory rate, minute ventilation and ventilatory pattern.

Table 6.3: Inspired FiO_2 for commonly used oxygen delivery systems in infants and children

System oxygen	*Flow rate (L/min)*	*FiO_2*
Nasal cannula	0.25-6.0	0.21-0.50
Simple oxygen mask	1.0-6.0	0.21-0.50
Nonrebreathing mask	4-10	0.5. -1.0
Venturi mask	4.0-12.0	0.24-0.60
Oxygen hood	10-15	0.80-1.0

MONITORING

Patient: Clinical assessment including but not limited to cardiac, pulmonary, and neurological status and apparent work of breathing; assessment of physiologic variables using noninvasive or invasive measurement of oxygen tensions or saturation in any patient treated with oxygen should be done.[11]

Equipment: All oxygen delivery systems should be checked at least once each day. More frequent checks by calibrated analyzer are necessary in systems as these are susceptible to variation in oxygen concentration;

The change from one type of device to another is based on a change in the patient's condition or ability to use a specific device.[15] Oxygen therapy should be administered continuously unless the need has been shown to be associated only with specific situations e.g., exercise, feeding, or other stress.

HUMIDIFICATION

No subjective or objective evidence supports routine humidification of O_2 at flows < or = 4 L/min. However, it is not known whether the use of a bubble humidifier with a nasal cannula in the neonate has benefit, and the use of a bubble humidifier can verify oxygen delivery at flows < 1 L/min.[11]

INFECTION CONTROL

Low-flow systems: Under normal circumstances, low-flow oxygen systems do not present clinically important risk of infection and do not require routine replacement on the same patient. Nasopharyngeal catheters should be changed every 24 hours.[11]

High-flow systems: In the absence of definitive studies to support change-out intervals on nonintubated patients, results of institution-specific and patient-specific surveillance measures should dictate the frequency with which such equipment is replaced.[11]

Between patients, subject equipment (e.g., probes, oxygen sensors) to high-level disinfection.

All critically ill patients should receive additional inspired oxygen on a "more not less is best" philosophy.[16]

REFERENCES

1. Boothby WM. Oxygen therapy. *JAMA* 1932;99: 2026-2033.
2. Bolgiano CS, Bunting K, Shoenberger MM. Administering oxygen therapy: What you need to know. *Nursing* 1990;10: 47-51.
3. Pierce LNB. Administration of oxygen, humidification, and aerosol therapy. In: *Guide to Mechancial Ventilation·and Intensive Respiratory Care*. Philadelphia: WB Saunders 1996; 92-121.
4. Kumar H, Antony TJ, Sharma D. Oxygen therapy in pediatric practice. *Indian Pediatr* 1993;30:117-121.
5. Fisher AB. Oxygen therapy: Side effects and toxicity. *Am Rev Respir Dis* 1980;122:61-69.
6. Beers ME, Fisher AB. Oxygen toxicity. In: Carlson RW, Geheb MA (eds): *Principles and Practice of Medical Intensive Care*. Philadelphia: WB Saunders 1993;949-957.
7. Thiebault DW, Gregory GA. *Neonatal pulmonary care*, 2nd edn. Menlo Park CA: Addison-Wesley Publishing Co 1986.
8. Ryerson GG, Block AJ. Oxygen as a drug: Clinical properties, benefits, modes and hazards of administration. In: Burton GG, HodgkinJE, Ward JJ (eds): *Respiratory care: A guide to Clinical Practice* Philadelphia: JB Lippincott 1991;319-339.
9. Sivan Y, Pfenninger J, Newth CLJ. Assisted ventilatory support and oxygen treatment. In: Taussig, Landau, Lesouef, Martinez, Morgan (eds): *Pediatric Respiratory Medicine*. St Louis: Mosby 1999;311-347.
10. Martin DL, Bratton SL, Walker LK. Principles and Practice of Respiratory Support and Mechanical Ventilation. In: Roger MC (ed): *Textbook of Pediatric Intensive Care*. Baltimore: Williams and Wilkins 1996;265-330.
11. Bower LK, Barnhart SL Betit, Myers TR. Selection of an Oxygen Delivery Device for Neonatal and Pediatric Patients. AARC Clinical Practice Guideline. *Respir Care* 2002;47:707-716.
12. Rotschild A, Schapira D, Kuyek N, Solimano A. Evaluation of nasal prongs of new design for low-flow oxygen delivery to infants. *Respir Care* 1989; 34:801-804.
13. Shann F. Nasopharyngeal oxygen in children. *Lancet* 1989;1077-1078.
14. Scacci R. Air entrainment masks: Jet mixing is how they work; the Bernoulli and Venturi principles are how they don't. *Respir Care* 1979;24:928-931.
15. Singhi S. Intensive Care of pediatric patients. In: Sachdev HPS, Puri RK, Bagga A, Choudhury P (eds): *Principles of Pediatric and Neonatal Emergencies*. New Delhi Jaypee 1994:329-353.
16. Singer M, Webb A. *Oxford Handbook of Critical Care*. Oxford: Oxford University Press 1997.

Puneet Pooni and Daljit Singh

7 Mechanical Ventilation

INTRODUCTION

Respiratory support constitutes a major portion of pediatric critical care and mechanically assisted ventilation is one of the vital elements of supportive care provided to patients in ICU setting.[1] In spite of advent of a variety of newer methods like high frequency ventilation (HFV), extracorporeal membrane oxygenation (ECMO), conventional mechanical ventilation is the principal mode of respiratory support in all the age groups.

GOALS

The overall goals of mechanical ventilation, regardless of the age group remain the same, which include:[2]

1. To provide adequate alveolar ventilation, while avoiding respiratory acidosis or alkalosis.
2. Maximize ventilation to perfusion relationships, while ensuring optimal gas exchange.
3. Reduce work of breathing and enhance patient comfort, while avoiding disuse atrophy of the ventilatory muscles.
4. Accomplish the first three goals with minimal cardiovascular compromise and damage to the lung.

These goals are central to the application of ventilatory support, regardless of the specific technology employed or the particular approach used to ventilate patients.

INDICATION

The primary indication of mechanical ventilation is impending or existing respiratory failure, which is defined as an inability of the respiratory system to maintain adequate arterial oxygenation and carbon dioxide elimination. The objective clinical definition of respiratory failure means a $PaO_2 < 60$ mmHg on a $FiO_2 > 0.5$ (oxygenation), a $PaCO_2 > 50$ mmHg, with a pH of 7.25 or less (ventilation), $PaO_2/FiO_2 < 150$ or an A-a gradient >350.[3,4]

From a pathophysiologic perspective, respiratory failure can be divided into following two general categories:[5] (Fig. 7.1)

1. Hypoxic respiratory failure (failure to oxygenate). Oxygenation deals primarily with gas exchange at the alveolar level and hypoxic respiratory failure occurs due to ventilation perfusion mismatch as a result of local pulmonary changes in compliance or resistance, where because of hypoxemia respiratory drive is stimulated, and initially patient can be managed by administration of additional oxygen but may need mechanical ventilation to prevent tissue hypoxia.
2. Hypercapnic respiratory failure (failure to ventilate) Ventilation deals primarily with the movement of gases

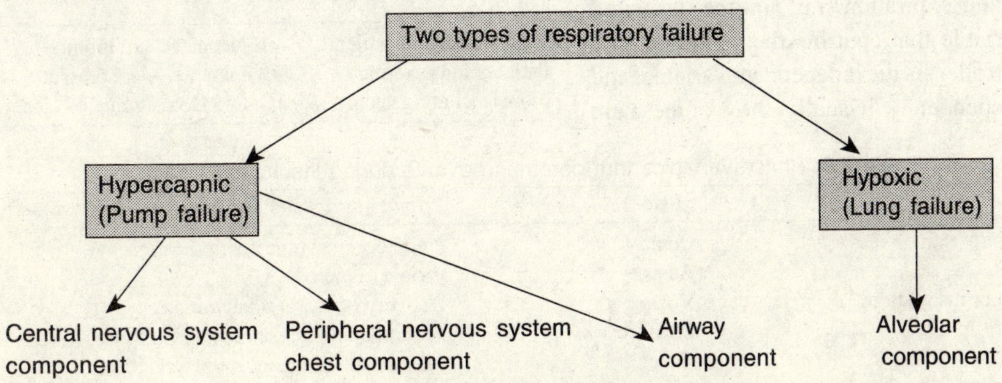

Fig. 7.1: Types of respiratory failure

in and out of the lungs. And ventilatory pump failure includes failure of any component including the muscles, cartilage, bones of chest wall and abdomen along with the neuro network that maintains control of the pump.

Clinical indicators of presence of respiratory failure include an increasing respiratory rate, decreasing tidal volume, increase in work of breathing as evidenced by clinical use of accessory muscles of ventilation, grunting and paradoxical breathing leading to exhaustion, cyanosis or desaturation <90% despite oxygen therapy. Blood gas analysis is not a must before starting mechanical ventilation.

A classification of diseases predisposing to respiratory failure is presented in Table 7.1.

Table. 7.1: Categories of intrapulmonary and extra-pulmonary disorders predisposing to respiratory failure

Category	*Examples*
CNS disorders (reduced respiratory drive)	Meningitis, encephalitis, drug overdose, cerebrovascular accident, cerebral trauma
Neuromuscular disorders	Guillain-Barre syndrome, poliomyelitis, spinal cord injury, snake bite
Musculoskeletal and pleural function disorders	Pleural effusion, pneumothorax, hemothorax, flail chest
Conductive airway disorders	Upper airway obstruction, asthma, bronchiolitis
Disorders of Gas exchanging units (alveoli and pulmonary capillaries)	Pneumonia, pulmonary edema, ARDS, aspiration, near drowning, interstitial lung disease, smoke inhalation

Such classification is required to understand the pathophysiologic process underlying the failure and suitable therapies[6]. Mechanical ventilation does not cure the condition but supports the respiratory system till the recovery of illness.

CLASSIFICATION

There are several basic modes of positive pressure ventilation (PPV), which differ by the variable used to start and end the inspiration and expiration (i.e. volume, pressure, flow, time). The variable that controls the ventilator in a specified mode (controller) is the independent variable, and the others become dependent.[7-9] Usually, three of these are set and the fourth results from the patient's compliance and resistance. Cycling is defined by what stops inspiration and starts expiration e.g. volume-cycled, pressure-cycled, time-cycled, flow-cycled. Modes are defined by what starts next inspiration e.g. controlled mode ventilation (CMV), pressure controlled ventilation (PCV), synchronized intermittent mandatory ventilation (SIMV/IMV), pressure-support ventilation (PSV) etc.[10,11] Basic ventilator types are shown in Table 7.2. Phase variables are shown in Table 7.3.

The current group of ventilators fit into one of these categories.

Pressure-cycled ventilators: These are simple machines but now rarely used in pediatric intensive care units.

Volume-cycled ventilators: Inspiratory phase terminates when the preset tidal volume has been delivered Volume ventilation in small pediatric patients is unreliable because of the variable amounts of leakage caused by the use of uncuffed tubes and relatively large compressible volume of the circuit. New pediatric circuits have been developed with small diameter, short inspiratory line, rigid tubing (compressible volume 1ml/cm H_2O compared with 4 ml/1 cm H_2O in adult tubing). Still volume loss may be significant so these ventilators are not preferred in neonates and infants.

Time-cycled: All modern ventilators are time cycled i.e inspiration stops and expiration starts when the pre-set time

Table 7.2: Basic ventilator types

Volume control	*Pressure control*
Controls	
Rate FiO2 PEEP Inspiratory time Tidal volume	Rate FiO2 PEEP Inspiratory time Peak inspiratory pressure
Relative Advantages/Disadvantages	
Known TV Risk for barotrauma risk of barotrauma	No guarantee of TV Pressure limited-decreases
Uses	
Most ventilated patients Patients in operating room (including neonates)	Neonates and infants Patients where pressure is a concern (ARDS, asthmatics sometimes)

Table 7.3: Phase variables that determine events during inspiration

Function	*Mode*	*Primary parameter (set by operator)*
Initiation of breath	Control	Predetermined time interval
	Assist	Patient triggered
Limit (end of inspiration)	Volume	Delivery of preset tidal volume
	Pressure	Attainment of preset airway pressure
	Time	Attainment of preset inspiratory time
Cycle off (start of expiration)	Volume	Preset volume achieved
	Time	Predetermined time interval passed
	Flow	Decline to preset minimal flow rate

has elapsed; in addition, these offer a volume controlled mode or a pressure controlled mode. Many present day ventilators provide both these modes.

Combined ventilators: So many newly developed ventilators can be used as either volume or time-cycled, pressure limited ventilation.

Numerous, well controlled prospective studies have demonstrated no difference in gas exchange or pulmonary mechanics when pressure or volume control were compared with total PEEP and mean airway pressure kept constant.

MODES OF VENTILATION

Once the expiratory phase has been completed, the change-over to the next inspiratory phase begins which may be initiated by the patient or by the ventilator and is the basis of classifying modes of ventilation as assisted or controlled. The goal is to select a mode that is both comfortable for the patient and allows adequate ventilation and oxygenation with minimal trauma. There are advantages and disadvantages of all the modes. There is no best mode for managing the patient in need of ventilatory support, just as there is no exact science to the application of the various modes. Experience and skill rank very high in the success of modes application.[7,9]

Pediatric critical care is unique in the sense that patients range in size from neonates to adults. Since there are a wide variety of factors to be considered, it is helpful to have sound understanding of pediatric respiratory mechanics and pediatric ventilators.[12-14]

1. Controlled Mechanical Ventilation (CMV)

With this mode the patient receives a preset number of breaths per minute, of a preset tidal volume (V_T). Patient effort will not trigger a mechanical breath. The ventilator performs all the work of breathing (WOB). These breaths may be at a preset V_T (volume controlled) or at a preset inspiratory pressure (pressure controlled, PCV).

Indications

- Patients with minimal or no respiratory effort (LGBS, spinal cord lesion).
- When negative inspiratory effort is contraindicated (flail chest).
- To provide a fail-safe method of ventilating the patient's lungs under conditions such as anesthesia or as a backup to assisted ventilation.

Advantages and Disadvantages

CMV was used widely before the advent of A/C ventilation. Because the patient cannot achieve a spontaneous breath, if he is awake and attempts to breathe, the CMV will lock him out; this leads to sensation of air hunger and significantly increased work of breathing causing patient-ventilator asynchrony. Patient who can generate spontaneous efforts must be heavily sedated or paralyzed to improve patient comfort and ventilating efficiency on this mode. Its prolonged use may result in respiratory muscle weakness and atrophy making it harder to wean the patient. Patient's peak inspiratory pressure (PIP) needs to be monitored.

2. Assist-control Ventilation (ACV)

The A/C mode is a method of ventilation in which the ventilator delivers a preset number of breaths of a preset VT. Between these machine-initiated breaths, the patient may trigger spontaneous breaths. When the ventilator senses the patient's spontaneous respiratory effort, it delivers a breath of the preset V_T, so the patient cannot vary the volume of spontaneous initiated effort. The only work the patient must perform is the negative inspiratory effort. The difference between A/C and CMV is that with A/C mode the ventilator is sensitive and responds to patient's efforts, in many ventilators these two are mentioned together.

Indications

- Normal respiratory drive, but respiratory muscles are too weak to perform WOB.
- In case where respiratory muscles are unable to perform the increased WOB, as in pulmonary abnormalities where lung compliance is decreased.
- In case of apneic patients A/C is like CMV only.

Advantages

The A/C mode allows the patient to control the rate of breathing, and still it guarantees the delivery of a minimal preset rate and volume. It allows only a minimal work of breathing and is indicated when it is desirable for the ventilator to perform the bulk of the ventilatory work. At the same settings WOB with A/C is less as compared to intermittent mandatory ventilation.

Disadvantages

These include patients tendency to hyperventilate because of anxiety, pain or neurological factors, leading to respiratory alkalosis. Hyperventilation may also lead to formation of intrinsic PEEP, because of shortened expiratory time. Variability in the patient's hemodynamic status may occur with the A/C mode because every breath is delivered under positive pressure. Patients PIP should be monitored along with exhaled tidal volume.

3. Synchronized) Intermittent Mandatory Ventilation ((S) IMV)

IMV is a mode of ventilation in which the patient receives a preset number of breaths of a preset VT. Between these mandatory breaths, the patient may initiate spontaneous breaths. The volume of spontaneous breaths is dependent on the muscular respiratory effort that the patient is able to generate. Mandatory breaths may be synchronized with a patient's spontaneous efforts (SIMV) to avoid mandatory breaths occurring during a spontaneous breath. This effect, known as "stacking" may lead to excessive tidal volumes, high airway pressure, incomplete exhalation and air trapping. Pressure support may be added to spontaneous breaths to overcome the work of breathing associated with opening the ventilator demand valve.

The main difference between the IMV and A/C mode is the volume of the patient initiated breaths. In the A/C mode the V_T is guaranteed, whereas in IMV it is variable. It was originally developed in an effort to create a mode in which the patient could interact with the ventilator, using the respiratory muscles; it would thus be useful for weaning patients from ventilatory support. The lower the IMV rate, the more spontaneous breaths the patient will initiate, therefore assuming a greater portion of the ventilatory work, so as patients efforts improve the mandatory breaths are gradually reduced.

Indications

- Normal respiratory drive but respiratory muscles unable to perform all WOB.
- In situations where it is desirable to allow patients to set their own respiratory rate and thus assist in maintaining a normal $PaCO_2$.
- Need to wean the patient from mechanical ventilation.

Advantages

- Hyperventilation is less of a problem in this mode than A/C mode because the patient can modify rate and volume of ventilation on the spontaneous breaths and therefore maintain normal $PaCO_2$ levels.
- Less respiratory muscle atrophy occurs as the patient also participates in the ventilation.
- As the mean airway pressure is also less, so less hemodynamic effects of positive pressure ventilation will occur.
- Synchronizing the mandatory breaths with the patient's readiness to breathe improves patient comfort, reduces competition between ventilator and patient, and prevents breath stacking and its potential problems, such as barotrauma and loss of V_T as a result of pressure limiting.

Disadvantages

Patients respiratory rate should be monitored, if RR increases then the V_T of the spontaneous breaths should be reassessed, which should be at least 5-8 cc/kg. If the patient is beginning to fatigue, a more shallow and rapid respiratory pattern may develop, this may lead to atelectasis, reduction in compliance, further increase in WOB and need for greater ventilatory support. If patient-ventilator dyssynchrony is a problem, especially during weaning trials, patient can be provided with some sedation, T-piece trials alternating with the use of the A/C may be another option. Also consider a mode that allows the patient more control, such as synchronized IMV with pressure support (PS) ventilation.

4. Time-cycled, Pressure-limited Ventilation

In this mode, the rate and inspiratory time (TI) (or I: E ratio) are preset. A preset PIP is determined such that excessive pressure is not produced. Preset pressure is delivered throughout inspiration, cycling being determined by time. Tidal volume (V_T) is dependent on respiratory compliance and airway resistance and high peak airway pressures can be avoided.

Indications

This is the mode of choice in neonates and infants, where tidal volume is small.[15]

Advantages

Precise control of inspiratory time and a rapid respiratory rate are possible with this mode. PIP can be limited and thus chances of barotrauma is less.

Disadvantages

Continuous monitoring of tidal volume is preferable, as with improved lung compliance the same pressure may deliver more tidal volume, so pressure has to be decreased to prevent barotrauma. Major problem associated with the use of PLV is the inability to detect airway obstruction or kinking. Unlike VCV, complete airway obstruction may not cause a rise in peak inspiratory pressure, and the high-pressure alarm may not go off.

5. Pressure-controlled, Inverse-ratio Ventilation

PC-IRV is a particular version of PCV in which all breaths are pressure limited and time cycled and the inspiration is longer than expiration. This was first applied in neonates with hyaline membrane disease (HMD), then to patients with acute respiratory distress syndrome (ARDS). Ratios of 1:1, 2:1, 3:1 are called inverse I : E ratios. IRV is most effective in conditions resulting in unstable or collapsed alveoli.[16-18] The prolonged T_I stabilizes alveoli, recruits already collapsed alveoli, and allows for more even distribution of gas resulting in improved gas exchange

Indications

The use of inverse I: E ratio with pressure–control ventilation (PCV) is restricted to specific noncompliant lung conditions in which the disease process exhibits a non-homogenous distribution and the typical patient should be considered who has progressively worsening radiographic infiltrates, increasing PIP, worsening oxygenation despite a high FiO_2 and a high level of PEEP and a high minute ventilation.

Advantages

It improves oxygenation.

The use of IRV allows for decrease in both PIP and PEEP levels. In noncompliant lungs, the short inspiratory time of a normal I: E ratio allows unstable alveoli to collapse during the relatively longer expiratory pause. The long inspiration with inverse ratio allows unstable lung units more time to fill and equilibration of volume between the alveoli as a result of collateral ventilation.

Disadvantages

This inversion increases MAP, and may cause an increase in PEEP above the set level (auto-PEEP). The patient must be sedated and paralyzed and continuously monitored. It can result in significant decrease in cardiac output.

6. Pressure Support Ventilation (PSV)

It is a mode of ventilation in which the patient's spontaneous respiratory activity is augmented by the delivery of a preset amount of inspiratory positive pressure. The VT is variable, being determined by patient effort, the amount of PS applied, and the compliance and resistance of the system.[19] PS is therefore a flow-cycled mode of ventilation, as inspiration ends on the basis of a flow criterion. The patient retains control over respiratory pattern and volume. The PS mode may be used alone or in combination with SIMV. A PS should only be used in patients who display a reliable respiratory drive, because all breaths are patient initiated. When PS is used with SIMV, only the spontaneous breaths are pressure supported, its advantage being that in the event of apnea the patient will be assured of a preselected, backup number of mandatory breaths.

Indications

- Need to wean patient from mechanical ventilation.
- Long-term mechanical ventilation. PS, by augmenting inspiratory flow, reduces the WOB associated with the artificial airway and the ventilator circuit.

Advantage

It lies in overcoming the resistance work associated with moving inspiratory flow through an artificial airway and the ventilator circuit (5-10 cm). Decreasing the WOB also increases the likelihood that the patient will better tolerate weaning. PS improves patient-ventilator synchrony and patient comfort because the patient has control over the process of ventilation.

Disadvantage

V_T is variable and therefore the alveolar ventilation. V_T would decrease if compliance decreases or resistance increases particularly in patients with bronchospasm and significant secretions.

7. Positive End Expiratory Pressure (PEEP)

PEEP is the application of a constant, positive pressure in the airways so that, at end-expiration, the pressure is never allowed to return to atmospheric pressure. PEEP is measured in centimeters of water and ranges from 5 to 20 cm H2O. The positive pressure is actually applied through out the ventilatory cycle, but is used for its physiologic effects at end-expiration. PEEP recruits atelectatic alveoli, internally splints and distends already patent alveoli, counteracts alveoli and small airway closure during expiration, and redistributes lung water, so it decreases intrapulmonary shunting, increases functional residual capacity, improves compliance, decreases the diffusion distance for oxygen and improves oxygenation. The increase in FRC by PEEP offers much more than just an increase in lung volume in pediatric patients[20]. Airway closure in young children is said to occur above the FRC level, even under normal conditions, and a slight fall in FRC can cause a significant fall in PaO_2. It can be added to every type of mechanical ventilation including spontaneous respiration where it is known as continuous positive airway pressure (CPAP).

Contraindication

PEEP of 3-5 cm is considered physiological in children; higher than this is relatively contraindicated in:

- Unilateral lung disease, as PEEP may result in alveolar over distension in the healthy lung.
- In obstructive lung disease, FRC is already increased because of air trapping, and PEEP may not increase oxygenation but may potentate barotrauma.
- Pneumothorax.
- Bronchopleural fistula.
- Intracardiac shunt,and
- Increased intracranial pressure.

In last five conditions increase in intrathoracic pressure may worsen the underlying disease.

All the major modes are shown in a graphic form in Figure 7.2.

The various modes of ventilation give the clinician the opportunity to change the therapeutic option when the patients condition changes. New knowledge continues to bring about changes in the way we perceive and use current modes. What remains the same is the clinical outcome goal: the provision of adequate oxygenation and alveolar ventilation, without compromise of pulmonary or systemic perfusion, while complications of applied therapy are prevented. Various types of pediatric ventilators available with their types and modes are shown in Table 7.4.

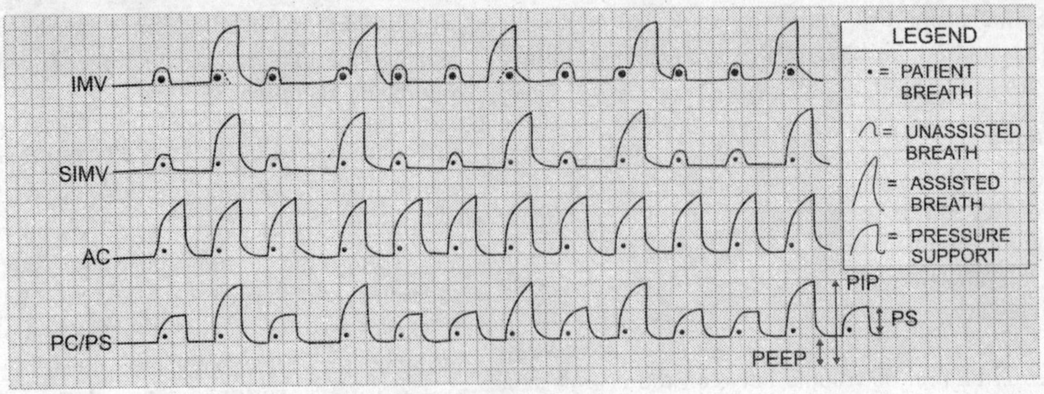

Fig. 7.2: Graphic representation of various modes

CHOOSING THE APPROPRIATE MODE

Full *Versus* Partial Ventilatory Support

There is no simple answer to the right mode of ventilation for respiratory failure of a particular cause. There are many therapeutic options. Initial ventilator support can be classified according to two general approaches: full ventilatory support (FVS) and partial ventilatory support (PVS).

In **FVS** ventilator performs all work of breathing whereas in **PVS** the patient also contributes.[14,21]

Normally FVS is the initial application of mechanical ventilation required by patients with acute respiratory failure with indications same as used for CMV.

The patient is put on **PVS** as early as possible to allow him/her to change minute ventilation and promoting use of the respiratory muscles, thereby preventing disuse atrophy. PVS can be provided by all modes described above with exception of controlled mode ventilation (CMV) and pure pressure-control (PC) ventilation, by titrating the amount of support offered.

SETTING UP THE MECHANICAL VENTILATOR[22]

Fraction of Inspired Oxygen Concentration (FiO_2)

When one is initiating mechanical ventilation for a patient in respiratory failure, it's best to start with high FiO_2 (0.7-1.0) to ensure adequate oxygenation. After the initial blood gas value is obtained, the FiO_2 may be decreased to achieve the goal of clinically acceptable PaO_2 of >60 mmHg (equivalent to oxygen saturation of 90% on pulse oximeter under normal body temperature and pH) with an $FiO_2 < 0.6$. Oxygen toxicity is minimized at FiO_2 of 0.5 or less, if higher FiO_2 is required to maintain oxygenation then addition of PEEP should be considered. Continuous monitoring of oxygenation along with titration should be done using pulse oximeter. One should wait for at least 20 minutes after a ventilator change before getting arterial blood gases.

Table 7.4: Some commonly used mechanical ventilators

Ventilators	*Types of ventilation*	*Modes*
Sechrist	Pressure	Pressure Control/ IMV/CPAP
	Volume and pressure	PC/VC/SIMV/SIMV with PS/PS
Servo 300		Numerous
VIP Bird	Volume and pressure	Numerous
Drager-babylog	Pressure	Numerous
Infant Star	Pressure	SIMV and Assist Control
LP-10	Volume and pressure	SIMV and Assist Control

Tidal Volume

Whereas V_T relative to body weight changes little; absolute V_T is significantly smaller in smaller children. The relatively large volume of ventilatory circuit (tubes, humidifiers) relative to V_T creates a large and variable compressible volume making precise tidal volume control difficult. A practical approach to determining adequate tidal volume is to evaluate desired degree of chest expansion during manual ventilation and reproduce when connected to the ventilator. Spontaneous tidal volume is 5-8 cc/kg, in mechanical ventilation conventionally 10-15 cc/kg of tidal volume is recommended to prevent progressive alveolar collapse. Smaller tidal volumes may be used when the lung is already hyper inflated as in severe bronchospasm or in disease process associated with a decrease in compliance, as in later condition larger tidal volume may result in increase in PIP, predisposing the patient to barotrauma. Exhaled tidal volume, regardless of the mode of ventilation, is the most accurate measure of the volume received by the patient.

Peak Inspiratory Pressure (PIP)

Respiratory compliance is the major determinant of the inflating pressure required. When normalized for body size comparable levels of positive inspiratory pressure are required in small children and adults. Peak pressure in volume-cycled ventilation is the end-result of factors such as delivered tidal volume and flow rate. However, in pediatric respiratory care in which volume controlled ventilation is difficult to achieve, peak pressure is not an end-result but is the factor to be controlled. The safe inspiratory pressure range cannot be defined, but upper alarm is set at 30 cm H_2O and chances of barotrauma are more if PIP remains higher that 35 cm water. In pressure controlled ventilation, PIP is increased to maintain proper oxygenation and ventilation, high PIP increases the risk of pulmonary barotrauma and may also impair pulmonary and systemic circulation. PIP is set as follows:

Normal lungs	15-19cm
Mild lung disease	20-24 cm
Moderate lung disease	25-30 cm
Severe lung disease	>30 cm

Respiratory Rate

The respiratory rate set on the ventilator should generally be as near as physiological for that age group, for example 25-30 for infants, 20-25 for children, 15-20 for adolescents. Frequent changes in the RR are often required and are based on observation of the patients work of breathing and comfort and on assessment of $PaCO_2$ and pH. Majority of the patients, initially require full ventilatory support. The respiratory rate at this time is selected on the basis of tidal volume, so that minute ventilation (RR X V_T = MV) is sufficient to maintain a normal acid-base status. As the patient begins to participate in the ventilatory work, the ventilatory RR may be decreased.

Slow rates may be useful in patients with obstructive pulmonary disease because as the rate is decreased, more time is available for exhalation and less air trapping will occur. In patients with non-compliant lungs fast rates may be useful who require ventilation with smaller tidal volumes to prevent barotraumas from increased airway pressures. In order to avoid respiratory alkalosis, it is desirable for patients to set their own RR by using a mode of ventilation that allows patient-initiated breaths (like SIMV, PS).

Flow Rate

It is the speed with which the tidal volume is delivered, which is measured in liters per minute. The flow is usually 3-4 times the minute ventilation. In volume targeted ventilation flow is kept at 1-3 L/kg/min to provide tidal volume of 10-15 ml/kg. Flow is kept higher in pressure limited ventilation 4-10 L/kg/min, to allow PIP to reach the predetermined limit early in inspiration and peak inflation pressure is held at that level until onset of expiration. The Inspiratory flow is the chief determinant of inspiratory time and thus have the I: E ratio. So the flow rate must be adjusted for each patient on the basis of the desired I : E ratio, the tidal volume, and the respiratory rate. Higher flow rates shorten inspiratory time, lengthening expiratory time (decreased I : E Ratio), which may be desirable in bronchial asthma and air trapping. However, increasing the flow rate may increase peak inspiratory pressure (PIP) and adversely affecting the distribution of gases, because flow becomes more turbulent. Slower flow rates will prolong inspiratory time, improve distribution of gases and reduce PIP as a result of more laminar flow, required in restrictive lung disease.

Inspiratory Time and Expiratory Time

An understanding of the pathophysiological processes involved is necessary before ventilating a child. The components of respiration may be divided into ventilation and oxygenation. The product of compliance and resistance is termed as time constant. This a measure of time required for an alveolar unit to reach equilibrium i.e. the time to fill up and get emptied. One time constant fills in 63% of an alveolus, two fills 87% and three 95%. Three to five time constants are required to allow complete filling or emptying of alveolar unit. If this is not allowed in expiration air trapping will occur. A normal infant has a time constant of 0.15 second. Normal inspiratory time of 0.5-1.0 seconds is kept, with an appropriate I : E ratio.

The I : E ratio is the duration of inspiration in comparison with expiration. Generally the I : E ratio is set at 1:2, that is, 33% of the respiratory cycle is spent in inspiration and 66% in the expiratory phase. This is like spontaneous respiration when lung function is normal. In cases of bronchospasm, an I : E ratio of 1:3 or 1:4 may be used to ventilate the lungs as longer expiratory times promote more complete exhalation and air trapping is reduced.

Positive End Expiratory Pressure

PEEP is generally started at a level of 3-5 cm water and increased gradually with the aim to achieve a $SpO_2 > 90\%$ with the lowest level of PEEP that allows FiO_2 to be reduced to nontoxic levels (<0.5). A very high PEEP (>15 cm water) can lead to air leaks, depressed cardiac output and barotrauma. PEEP is applied in case of most patients in pediatric critical care because of the unique characteristics of respiratory mechanics in children. Apart from PEEP, other therapies are applied to treat the underlying condition like diuresis, postural drainage, chest physiotherapy, antibiotics and body positioning.

Mean Airway Pressure (MAP)

MAP is the average airway pressure over the entire respiratory cycle and is a key determinant of oxygenation. In general, the same changes of MAP results in a similar change of PaO_2 regardless of ventilatory mode. MAP is the end-result of many variables including inspiratory pressure, PEEP, flow, inspiratory time (Fig. 7.3). It is displayed on the monitor and can be indirectly controlled by changing the parameters. Higher MAP has the negative effect of creating more positive pressure in the thorax, which may lead to hemodynamic compromise.

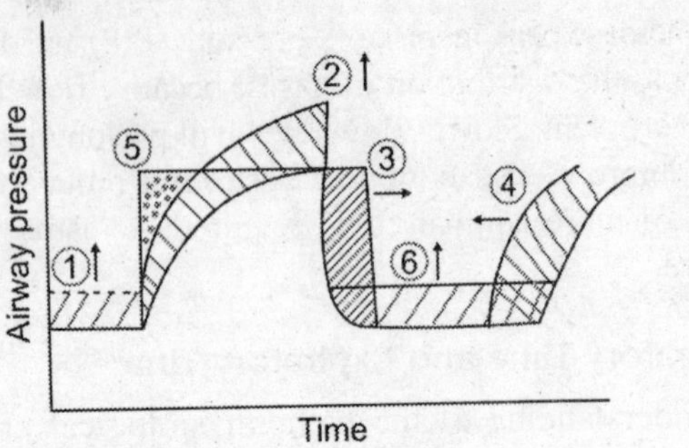

Pressure vs. time

Ways to increase MAP
1. Increase PEEP 2. Increase PIP 3. Increase Ti
4. Increase RR 5. Increase Flow

Fig. 7.3: Factors affecting the mean airway pressure (MAP)

Humidification

The absolute amount of heat and moisture loss via the respiratory tract of children is small but can potentially cause significant clinical problems, such as inadvertent hypothermia, impaired mucociliary function and drying of respiratory secretions leading to airway obstruction. Inspired gases normally are heated to body temperature and are humidified to 100% relative humidity as they pass through upper respiratory tract. Insertion of artificial airways bypasses this area. A relative humidity of 100% at 20ºC represents less than 40% relative humidity at a normal body temperature, thus a simple humidifier without heating capability is not useful in patients with artificial airways. Recommended is 80-100% humidity at 32-37ºC. Thermal injury should be avoided. Heat and moisture exchanger (HME) are not recommended in small children, particularly who are hypothermic, dehydrated and having thick secretions.

INITIATION OF MECHANICAL VENTILATION

Before starting ventilation, it is standard practice to ensure that the ventilator is clean and patient circuit sterilized. The humidifier should always be used. Ventilator parameters *viz.*, rate, volume and/or pressure and appropriate alarms are set to desired level. The patients baseline data is recorded.

After at least one minute of manually controlled ventilation with 100% oxygen by bag and mask, an orotracheal tube of appropriate diameter is inserted by direct laryngoscopy. Adequacy of ventilation is assessed by the degree of excursion of chest wall, the presence of breath sounds bilaterally and the general response of the child. Ventilation should be started in the control mode with 100% oxygen to correct hypoxia and bring blood gas values towards normal. Once the child begins to breathe spontaneously, ACV, IMV or SIMV modes may be used. The initial settings primarily depend on the nature of the lung disease as shown in Table 7.5 and subsequently changes are made depending on the blood gases (Table 7.6) and clinical assessment.[23] Alarm settings are done with FiO_2 set it 5-10% above and below the set FiO_2. Expiratory tidal volume should be set to detect any leaks. Low-pressure alarm set at 5-10 cm and high-pressure alarm at 30-40 cm water. PEEP set at lower of –3 cm of PEEP, which is kept.

Three common categories of pediatric patients requiring ventilator support are:

1. Those with little or no lung disease with a loss of respiratory drive or airway control e.g. general anesthesia, sedation, coma, neuromuscular diseases, CNS infections.
2. Those with restrictive lung (low lung volume) e.g. pneumonia, interstitial disease, aspiration pneumonia, near drowning, ARDS.

Table 7.5: Ventilatory strategy in various lung conditions

Ventilator strategy	*Normal lungs*	*Restrictive lung disease*	*Obstructive lung disease*
Cycling/limiting	Volume or pressure	Volume or pressure	Volume or pressure
Mode	Assist control or SIMV	Initially full ventilatory support	FVS for 24-72 hours
Tidal volume (VT)	12-15 ml/kg	6-10 ml/kg	8-12 ml/kg
Rate (< 1 y-25-30 bpm 1-8 y: 20-25. > 8 y: 15-20)	Age dependent	Age dependent, can increase to improve minute ventilation	Lower side, to allow longer time for expiration
PEEP	3-5 cm	5-12 cm	2-3 cm
I : E ratio	1:2	1:2 or 1:1	1:3 or more
FiO_2 adjust to keep PaO_2	80-100 mmHg	50-80 mmHg	> 60 mmHg
$PaCO_2$	Normal or lower (30-40 mmHg)	Allow to rise > 60 mmHg, if necessary	Allow to rise > 60 mmHg, if necessary
PIP	< 35 cm H_2O	< 35 cm H_2O	< 35 cm H_2O
With SIMV mode add 8-10 cm H_2O of PSV			

Table 7.6: Ventilator maneuvers to achieve desired PaO_2 and $PaCO_2$

Desired	*Parameter manipulated*					
			MAP			
Change	*FiO_2*	*Rate*	*PIP*	*PEEP*	*Ti*	*Te*
↑ PaO_2	↑	↑	↑	↑	↑	—
↓ PaO_2	↓	—	↓	↓	↓	—
↑ $PaCO_2$	—	↓	↓	—	—	↓
↓ $PaCO_2$	—	↑	↑	↓	—	↑

3. Those with obstructive lung (high lung volume) disease e.g. asthma, bronchiolitis.

Strategies to Improve Oxygenation (PaO_2)

An improvement in oxygenation can be achieved by manipulating FiO_2 and in:

Volume-cycled	*Pressure-limited*
Tidal volume	PIP
Inspiratory time	Inspiratory time
PEEP	PEEP

These components determine mean airway pressure (MAP). Final tidal volume should be adjusted at a level that gives a PIP between 25-35 cm H_2O and achieves satisfactory chest expansion and oxygen saturation. Fraction of inspired oxygen increases PaO_2 without changes in mean airway pressure. In patients with parenchyma lung disease with significant intrapulmonary shunting the major determinant of oxygenation is lung volume, which is a function of MAP.[24,25]

***FiO_2*:** It is best to keep FiO_2 below 0.5 to prevent the complications associated with high FiO_2 while keeping the PaO_2 greater than 60 mm Hg. Initially can be increased to 1.0 then gradually reduced to safe levels. Since it is desirable to keep the PaO_2 between 60-100 mmHg, an arterial blood gas analysis is obtained and the results compared to the FiO_2 being delivered. A linear relationship exists between PaO_2 and FiO_2 for any patient as long as the cardio-pulmonary status remains fairly constant. The PaO_2 and FiO_2 can be used to select the FiO_2 necessary to achieve a desired PaO_2[10]

$$\frac{\text{Known } PaO_2}{\text{Known } FiO_2} = \frac{\text{desired } PaO_2}{\text{desired } FiO_2}$$

$$\text{Desired } FiO_2 \; \frac{\text{Desired } PaO_2 \times \text{Known } FiO_2}{\text{Known } PaO_2}$$

PaO_2 targets in acute lung injury is as follows:[2]

> 80 mmHg in normal lungs,
> 70 mmHg in mild lung injury,
> 60 mmHg in moderated lung injury
> 50 mmHg in severe lung injury.

***PEEP*:** If an adequate PO_2 cannot be maintained on FiO_2 values less than or equal to 0.50, then significant shunting is present and ventilation-perfusion (V/Q) abnormalities are severe, PEEP is considered as an alternative form of therapy. High PEEP can cause decreased venous return and hypo tension which can be corrected with volume replacement and Inotropic support if need be. PEEP is increased in steps of 2 cm H_2O to maximum of 10-12 cmH_2O.

Inverse ratio ventilation: If patient still does not respond then patient needs to be put on inverse ratio ventilation with pressure control mode. I: E ratio is inverted, 1:1, 2:1, 3:1, 4:1 to improve gas distribution in the lung and increase the mean airway pressure for improvement of oxygenation. As the ventilatory pattern is altered, sedation and medical paralysis are usually necessary to maintain patient-ventilator synchrony.

Oxygenation should be continuously monitored using pulse oximeter. At a normal pH oxygen saturation correlates well with PaO_2 as shown below:

SpO_2	PO_2
100%	>150 mmHg
95-97%	80-100 mmHg
90%	60 mmHg
85%	50 mmHg
80%	45 mmHg
75%	40 mmHg
50%	25 mmHg

Hematocrit should be maintained at 40 to improve arterial oxygen content.

If PaO_2 is >100 mmHg, then the last parameter which is more traumatic should be decreased first, so I: E ratio is reversed to normal if the patient is maintaining saturation, and the mode can be changed from PC to volume cycled. Then PEEP and FiO_2 are decreased simultaneously.

STRATEGIES TO IMPROVE VENTILATION ($PaCO_2$)

Ventilation depends on two factors-respiratory rate and tidal volume.[10]

Low $PaCO_2$: When $PaCO_2$ is decreased below the patient normal value and pH reflects a respiratory alkalosis, then excessive minute ventilation is present. To decrease the ventilation in a volume-cycled ventilator, decrease the respiratory rate, then if necessary decrease the V_T but preferably not less than 10ml/kg. If the ventilator is time-cycled and pressure limited, decrease the rate first, and then the cycling pressure, if needed. In case patient is on assist ventilation then decreasing the rate will not correct respiratory alkalosis, as the patient will be able to initiate all breaths, in such a case patient should be put on SIMV mode, and may need sedation.

High $PaCO_2$: When arterial carbon dioxide partial pressure ($PaCO_2$) is increased above the patient's normal value (normal 35-45 mmHg) and the pH decreases, respiratory acidosis is present, indicating that patients minute ventilation is not adequate. When the ventilator is volume-cycled, increasing the V_T up to 15 ml/kg will decrease the $PaCO_2$. If the V_T is already at this level, then the rate can be increased. If the ventilator is pressure-limited then the cycling pressure can be increased.

Changes in RR and V_T is done as below:

Known $PaCO_2$ × known RR (or known V_T) = desired $PaCO_2$ × desired RR (desired V_T).

$$\text{Desired RR } (V_T) = \frac{\text{Known } PaCO_2 \times \text{Known RR } (V_T)}{\text{Desired } PaCO_2}$$

In case of persistent respiratory acidosis persisting after the minute ventilation has been increased can be due to the following reasons with appropriate response:

- The patency of endotracheal tube must be checked and secretions should be cleared to reduce the dead space.
- In patients with obstructive lung disease, reducing the flow or increasing the expiratory time (lower rate) may correct the situation.
- Uneven distribution of ventilation due to a pathologic problem in the lung. Sometimes repositioning the patient so the least compromised lung is in the down position will help.
- *A high I : E ratio (3:1) could be causing the problem:* Increasing the flow rate or decreasing the I : E ratio to 1:1 or 1:2 in the case of air trapping might help.
- In conditions like burns, multiple trauma, sepsis and multiple surgical procedures it is not unusual for metabolism to be high leading to increased production of CO_2. In this situation respiratory rate is already high, and further increasing the rate would increase auto-PEEP, to decrease the work of breathing pressure support (PS) should be added and higher $PaCO_2$ may be tolerated.
- In severe lung disease like ARDS permissive hypercapnia is allowed which is a deliberate limitation of ventilatory support to avoid alveolar over distension (ARDS) or auto-PEEP (asthma). As a result $PaCO_2$ rises to levels greater than normal up to 100 mmHg. It is contraindicated in cases of increased intracranial pressure, where even small increases in $PaCO_2$ increase cerebral blood flow. The primary factor limiting permissive hypercapnia is the pH produced; patients without renal or cardiovascular diseases tolerate pH of 7.20 or greater. Using alkalinizing agents to manage the acidosis induced by permissive hypercapnia is debatable.

Ventilators parameters changed to achieve desired oxygen and CO_2 levels are shown in Table 7.6.[11] All the parameters should be changed in such a way that there is overall balance of ventilatory support is optimal, it is important to develop a feel for overall balance of ventilatory support, such as shown in Table 7.7.[15]

Table 7.7: Guidelines for ventilator care

FiO_2	PEEP	PIP	RR	T_I
• 30	2-3	15-20	<30	0.3
• 40	3-4	18-25	30-35	0.4
• 60	5	25-30	35-45	0.5
• 80	6-7	25-35	40-60	0.5
• 100	7-10	30-40	40-60	0.6

MONITORING OF THE PATIENT

The initial evaluation and recording of a patient who needs assisted ventilation should include clinical and laboratory data.[26]

- Clinical data-Vital signs-RR, HR, BP, Temperature, SPO_2.
- Lab data-Chest X-ray, ECG, blood counts, biochemistry-Blood sugar, electrolytes, Urea, Creatinine, Calcium, phosphorus, magnesium, ABG, Coagulation parameters, baseline cultures.
- Intake and output chart should be monitored closely. In case of cuffed endotracheal tube, the cuff must be deflated every 4 hours for 5 minutes.
- While on ventilator, the following variables should be measured and recorded at least 2-4 hourly to assess proper functioning of ventilator and oxygen delivery or demand. FiO_2, I : E ratio, Tidal volume (both inspiratory and expiratory), minute ventilation, PIP, MAP, temperature of inspired gases, confirmation of all alarms, oxygen saturation of hemoglobin.
- Following are measured particularly when settings are changed-ABG, chest X-ray.

Regular physiotherapy and suction (maximum negative pressure limited to 50-100 mmHg) is recommended. In addition to general supportive care, intake and output should be monitored closely and twice-daily weight record kept.

Sedatives and muscle relaxants are often needed to enable effective ventilation. These medications can be used on an intermittent dosing schedule or as a continuous infusion (Table 7.8). In most patients, sedation alone is sufficient. Muscle relaxants are needed in patients requiring maximal ventilatory support and higher oxygen concentr-tions. It is important to understand that agitation frequently results from hypoxemia and correcting hypoxemia often obviates the need for further sedation.

DISCONTINUATION OF MECHANICAL VENTILATION (WEANING)

Weaning has been defined as the process whereby mechanical ventilation is *gradually* withdrawn and the patient resumes spontaneous breathing.[27,28] The ultimate goal of mechanical ventilatory support is ventilator discontinuation, and in the vast majority of cases, this is a simple process.

Table 7.8: Drugs used during mechanical ventilation

Sedatives	*Dose (mg/kg)*	*Duration*	*IV infusion*
Midazolam	0.05-0.1	2 h	Loading: 0.05 mg/kg/IV Maintenance: 0.025 mg/kg
Fentany1	2-10	30-60 min	Loading: 2-10 mg/kg/IV Maintenance: 1-5 mg/kg/h
Morphine	0.1	4 h	Loading: 0.05 mg/kg/IV Maintenance: 0.02 mg/kg/h
Lorazepam	0.05-0.1	4-6 h	
Diazepam	0.1-0.2	4-6 h	
Muscle Relaxants			
Pancuronium	0.1	50-60 min	
Vecuronium	0.1	25-35 min	0.1 mg/kg/h
Atracurium	0.5	20-30 min	0.3-0.6 mg/kg/h
Succinylcholine	1-2	5-15 min	

About 75-80% of patients who are mechanically ventilated may have the ventilator discontinued when the physiologic reason for ventilatory support is reversed. Another 15-20% of ventilated children may require the use of a specific weaning protocol applied over an 8-72 hour period before discontinuation is possible. It is the remaining 5% of mechanically ventilated patients that require a gradual weaning, sometimes requiring weeks or months before discontinuation, which is most problematic. In a small percentage of patients < 1%, they may be never be physiologically ready to wean and should be considered chronically ventilator-dependent.

There is no ideal weaning mode. Like all forms of ventilatory therapy, weaning is a learnt art rather than a science.[14,29,30] Criteria for weaning are shown in Table 7.9.

Table 7.9: Criteria for weaning from mechanical ventilation

General weaning criteria	*Specific Criteria*
Improving lung condition	$PaO_2 > 60$ with $FiO_2 < 0.4$
Stable cardiovascular system	$PaO_2/FiO_2 > 200$
Improving chest X-rays	Vital capacity > 10-15 ml/kg
Decreased secretions	Negative inspiratory
pressure of 20 cmH_2O	
Normal hemoglobin	Minute ventilation < 10l/min
Adequate Nutritional status	Tidal volume > 5 ml/kg
Normal fluid and electrolyte balance	PEEP < 5 cmH_2O
Intact airway reflexes	PIP < 20 cmH_2O
Intact ventilatory drive	RR < 10 bpm
Absence of other major organ failures	

Approaches to Weaning

In general, the major techniques of discontinuing ventilator support can be grouped into three categories:[2,9,30]

- Pressure support ventilation (PSV)
- SIMV or
- T-piece/CPAP trials, although combinations of these are also employed.

In those patients requiring a lengthy period of weaning (more than 1 or 2 days), it is important to adjust ventilatory support to ensure ventilatory muscle rest at night and a good night's sleep. Successful weaning approaches appropriately mix work and rest periods and ensure proper nutrition and sleep.

Pressure Support

Many recommend the use of gradual reduction in the level of PSV, provided the patient can maintain a target respiratory rate and VT, as the most appropriate approach to weaning. The process is begun by setting the PSV (up to 20 cmH_2O) at a level where a tidal volume and a respiratory rate consistent with the level expected on discontinuation is achieved, it is then decreases on regular basis (hours to days) until some minimum level 5-9 cm is reached, which unloads the WOB imposed by the circuit and tube, MV is then discontinued once the patient is maintaining the target gas exchange and ventilatory pattern. This approach works well with most of the patients requiring short term weaning (6-72 hours), it is problematic in patients who require weeks to wean, as it does not allow the patient to rest.

Synchronized Intermittent Mandatory Ventilation (SIMV)

This mode was introduced to facilitate weaning. Like PSV, a gradual reduction in SIMV rate to a predicted minimal level is commonly the approach used during weaning. Some patient may experience asynchrony with low SIMV. When SIMV is used during weaning of patients with longer ventilator duration, it is essential that the level of ventilatory support be increased during the night to ensure rest and sleep. Because of the WOB imposed by the ventilator and the endotracheal tube, patients should not be maintained on an SIMV rate of less than or equal to 4-10/min (dependent on age).

T-piece/CPAP Trial

The classic approach to weaning is the T-piece or CPAP trial. With this approach, increasing periods of unsupported spontaneous breathing are interspersed between periods of full ventilatory support. In long-term mechanically ventilated patients, the trial period may begin with periods as short as 5 minutes several times a day. The length of trials is then increased over time as the patient's tolerance improves, always allowing periods of complete rest between trials and at night. Patients with endotracheal tubes who can tolerate spontaneous breathing without blood gas or ventilatory pattern changes for 60 minutes should be considered weaned from ventilatory support and candidates for extubation.

Unfortunately, no single optimal approach to weaning has been defined, and there is no conclusive evidence of one method better than the other.

In pressure limited ventilation weaning is done as shown in Figure 7.4.[15]

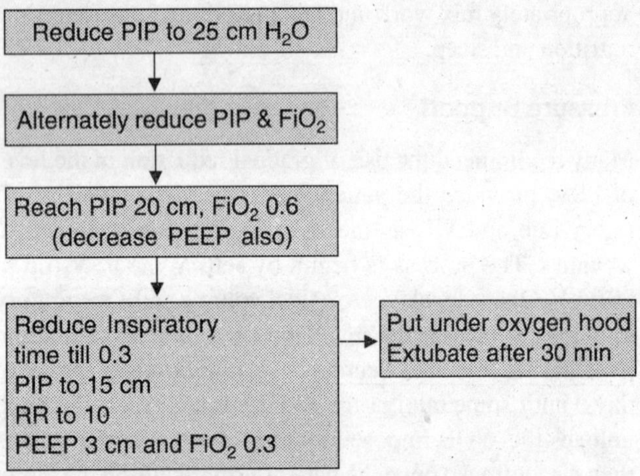

Fig. 7.4: Weaning in time-cycled, pressure-limited ventilation

At this baby can be put under oxygen hood, if ABG are normal after 20 minutes, extubate the baby. In cases of prolonged intubation, post-extubation stridor or laryngeal edema can be prevented by giving injection dexamethasone 2 mg/kg 6 hours prior to planned extubation and giving adrenaline nebulisation post-extubation.

While weaning the patient, continuous monitoring should be done and discontinue or modify the process if they appear, persist, or worsen:

1. Increasing tachypnea, associated with patient distress. A rise in the respiratory rate increases by more than 10 breaths per minute or decrease by 10 is a sign of fatigue.
2. Agitation, panic, diaphoresis, or tachycardia, unrelieved by adjustment of the mechanical ventilation system.
3. Acidemia: acute drop in pH to < 7.25 to 7.30, associated with an increasing $PaCO_2$.
4. A significant change in blood pressure (drop or rise of 20 mmHg in systolic pressure)
5. A rise in heart rate of more than 20 beats per min from the baseline.

At the present time and to our knowledge, no study has been published that has compared the optimal use of the three major techniques of discontinuing mechanical ventilation.

Table 7.10: Causes of failed weaning

- Ventilatory pump failure
  - Decreased respiratory muscle capacity
  - Decreases respiratory center output (CNS disorders)
  - Phrenic nerve injury
- Decreased muscle strength or endurance
  - Malnutrition,
  - Prolonged neuromuscular blockade,
  - Muscle fatigue,
  - Electrolyte abnormalities (hypokalemia, hypocalcemia, hypomagnesemia, hypophophatemia)
- Increased respiratory muscle load
  - Increased work of breathing Hyperinflation
  - Lower airway obstruction
  - Decreased compliance
- Increased ventilatory requirements
  - Increased CO2production (excessive carbohydrate intake)
  - Increased dead space
  - Hyper catabolic states (sepsis)

There may be many causes of failure of weaning as shown in Table 7.10.

COMPLICATIONS OF MECHANICAL VENTILATION

Although mechanical ventilation offers vital life support, its use can result in untoward or life-threatening side effects.[31,32] Many such hazards can be modified or avoided by appropriate attention to the technique of implementation.

A. **Complications of Airway Intubation**

1. *Airway Complications:* Accidental tracheal extubation or obstruction of the tracheal airway by mucus or blood can be prevented by proper airway care, adequate humidification of the inspired gas, physiotherapy of the chest and frequent suction. Prolonged intubation may lead to post-extubation subglottic bands. Vocal cord damage and palatal grooves are also long term complications of prolonged mechanical ventilation. Tube may get misplacement and dislocation. Glottic injury occurs due to repeated or prolonged intubation.
2. *Infection*: The risk of nosocomial pneumonia is increased due to the passage of pathogens via artificial airway, disruption of the coughing mechanism and mucociliary escalator causing retention of airway secretions, aspiration of pharyngeal secretions. Gram negative septicemia is the most common fatal complication in infants who require prolonged mechanical ventila-tion. The artificial airway and multiple intravascular catheters represent the route of contamination, and the hands of the professional personnel are the major vectors. Strict asepsis, daily change of the dressing and frequent changes of respiratory tubing are effective means to preventing infection. If infection develops, appropriate antibiotics should be administered, guided by culture/sensitivity patterns.

B. **Complications of PPV**

During PPV, the lungs and chest wall distend, intrathoracic pressure rises. Although considerable experimental data have been accumulated, detailed clinical information is not yet available regarding which oxygen concentrations, pressures, and ventilation patterns are safe to apply for extended periods.

1. *Barotrauma:* All forms of barotrauma have been described previously in the pediatric literature, including interstitial and subcutaneous emphysema, pneumomediastinum, pneumoperitoneum, pneumopericardium, pneumothorax, tension cysts, systemic gas embolism, and damage similar to bronchopulmonary dysplasia. It can be avoided by keeping PIP < 40 cm. By keeping small V_Ts the acceptance of any consequent elevation of $PaCO_2$
2. *Oxygen Toxicity:* High fractions of inspired O_2 (FiO_2) are potentially injurious when applied over extended periods. The combinations of O_2 concentration and duration of exposure that produce significant damage have not been firmly established in the setting of critical illness, and may well vary with disease type, severity, and individual susceptibility but preferably be kept < 0.6 s far as possible.
3. *Cardiovascular Complications:* MAP relates fundamentally to oxygen exchange, cardiovascular performance, and fluid retention. The tendency for an elevation of MAP to compromise hemodynamic performance is heightened by impaired cardiovascular reflexes and depletion of intravascular volume.

C. **Adverse Effects of Sedation and Paralysis**

Sedation and paralysis are often required to allow patient comfort and to facilitate the imposition of ventilatory patterns (*e.g.,* inverse ratio ventilation [IRV]) which would otherwise conflict with the patient's own ventilatory pattern. Sedation may result in vasodilatation that contributes to hypo tension and reduced cardiac output. Paralytic agents immobilize the patient, encouraging secretion retention, atelectasis, and muscle wasting. With breathing efforts prevented, such patients are totally dependent on the ventilation set by the clinician and provided by the machine. Inadvertent disconnection of the ventilator circuit can prove rapidly catastrophic in this setting.

D. **Other Complications**

Among the wide variety of noncardiopulmonary complications that have been described for mechanical ventilation, perhaps the most important involve mental distress and dysfunction of the renal, gastrointestinal, and central nervous systems.

1. *Renal dysfunction* during PPV is believed to be a consequence of reduced circulating blood volume. This tends to alter perfusion of the renal parenchyma, redistribute intrarenal blood flow, release antidiuretic hormone, or inhibit atrial natriuretic peptides. In any event, reduced free water clearance and generalized fluid retention are commonplace during ventilation with high pressures.
2. *Gastrointestinal consequences* of mechanical ventilation include gut distention (due to air swallowing), hypomotility, and obstipation (due to pharmacologic agents and immobility), vomiting (due to pharyngeal stimulation and motility disturbances), and mucosal ulceration and bleeding.
3. *Liver dysfunction* that occurs as a direct consequence of mechanical ventilation is rare. However, PEEP has been associated with hyperbilirubinemia and mild elevations of liver enzyme levels in the serum, possibly related to altered hepatic perfusion and impeded venous and biliary drainage.
4. *CNS*: Intracranial pressure may increase due to increase in intrathoracic pressure that elevate jugular venous and intracranial pressures, and thereby reduce cerebral perfusion pressure. Such effects assume particular importance in the setting of reduced mean arterial pressure and reduced intracranial compliance resulting from head injury or surgical intervention.

Troubleshooting

Evaluating the patient who becomes acutely hypoxic: Hypoxemia can arise as a result of mechanical complications related to the ventilator or problems related to the patient. An ICU design that allows for constant observation of the ventilated patient by nursing staff is crucial to the prevention and detection of mechanical mishaps. Following algorithm should be followed.[33,34]

High Pressure Alarms: An audible and visual alarm will be activated on most ventilators if the pressure exceeds a limit usually set at 5 to 10 cmH_2O above the PIP reading. It may be due to increased resistance (secretions, block or bronchospasm) or decreased compliance (worsening lung condition or development of pneumonia), patient may be coughing or biting the tube, water from condensation may have accumulated.

Low pressure alarm: When PIP has fallen below the desired limit of 5-10 cmH_2O below ventilating pressures, due to leak due to disconnection or improved lung condition

Newer modes of ventilation: Mandatory minutes ventilation and minimal mandatory ventilation ensure delivery of a preset minute volume either by spontaneous breathing or assisted ventilation regardless of the respiratory drive. High frequency ventila-tion provides very high respiratory rates of 5-25 Hz (300-1500 breaths per minutes) with very small tidal volumes. High frequency ventilation is primarily used as a rescue therapy for neonates failing on conventional ventilation. Liquid ventilation by instilling a perfluoro

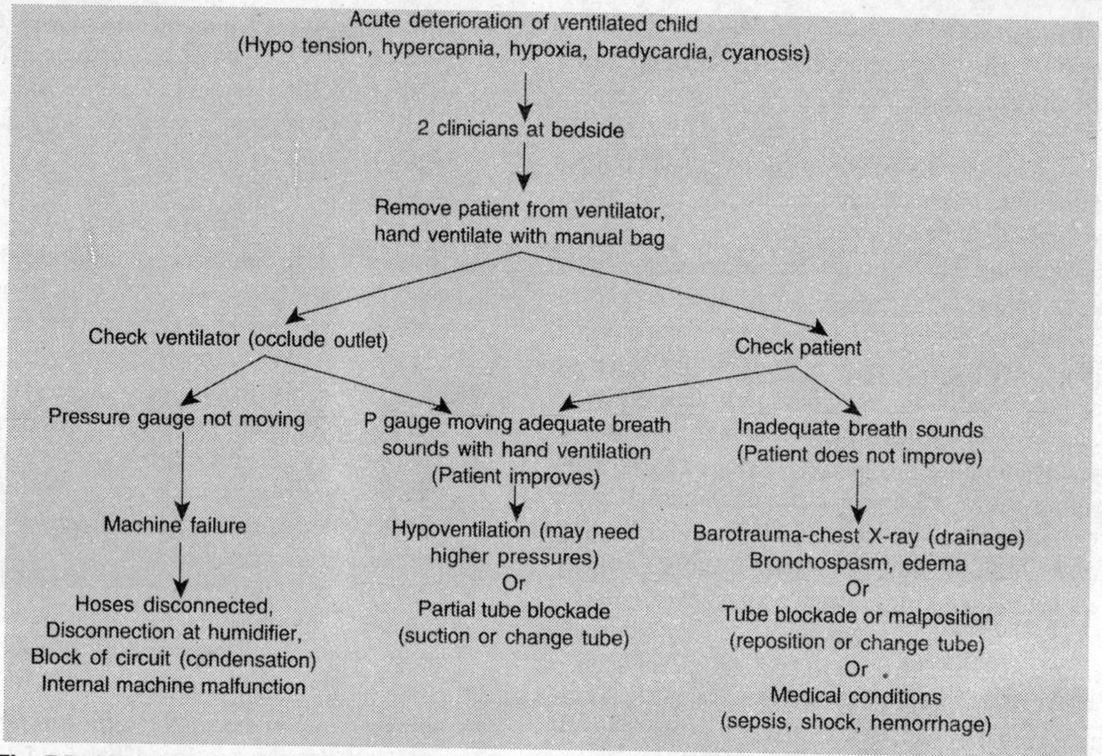

Fig. 7.5: Algorithm demonstrating approach to the ventilated infant with sudden, acute deterioration

chemical in which both oxygen and carbon dioxide are highly soluble is an experimental method for achieving pulmonary gas exchange. Elimination of the gas liquid interface reduces surface tension resulting in increased pulmonary compliance and homogenous gas exchange.

The outcome of mechanical ventilation bears a direct relationship to the etiology of the primary physiologic impairment, available facilities and professional competence of the physicians and nursing staff. The survival rate of patients presenting with primary respiratory failure is high in experienced hands using standard equipment[11]. In contrast, respiratory failure secondary to either circulatory or neurologic failure shows lower survival. Among survivors, nearly 1% develop chronic respiratory failure, which is defined as requiring mechanical ventilation for more than one month. Proper understanding of the physiologic concepts in mechanical ventilation with continuous monitoring of the patients decreases the mortality

REFERENCES

1. Salyer JW. Outcome of pediatric mechanical ventilation. *Resp Care Clin N Am* 1996;471-485.
2. Kaemarek R, Custer JR, Fugate JH. Mechanicla ventilation. In: Todres F (ed): *Critical Care of Infants and Children.* Battimore: Lippincott, Williams and Wilkins 1996:155-178.
3. Stoller JK. Determining the need for mechanical ventilation. In:Pierson DJ, Kaemarek RM (eds): *Foundations of Respiratory Care.* New York: Churchill Livingstone 1992:212-218.
4. Bone RC. Acute respiratory failure: Definition and overview. In: Bone RC (ed): *Pulmonary and Critical Care Medicine.* St Louis: Mosby-Year Book 1993;1-7.
5. Aldrick TK, Prezant DJ. Indications for mechanical ventilation. In:Tobin MJ (ed): *Principles and Practice of Mechanical Ventilation.* New York: McGraw-Hill 1994;155-189.
6. Pierce LNB. Mechanical Ventilation:Indications, basic principles of ventilator performance of the respiratory cycle and initiation. In: *Guide to Mechancial Ventilation and Intensive Respiratory Care.* Philadelphia: WB Saunders 1996;147-174.
7. Pierce LNB.Modes of mechanical ventilation. In: *Guide to Mechancial Ventilation and Intensive Respiratory Care.* Philadelphia WB Saunders 1996;175-205.
8. American Assocation for Respiratory Care. Consensus Statement on the Essentials of Mechanical Ventilators. *Respir Care* 1992;37:1000-1008.
9. Chatburn RL. Classification of mechancal ventilators. *Respir Care* 1992;37:009-1025.
10. Pilbeam SP. *Mechanical Ventilation-Physiological and Clinical Applications.* St Louis: Mosby Year Book 1992.
11. Tripathi VN, Misra S. Mechanical ventilation in pediatric practice. *Indian Pediat* 2001;38:147-156.
12. Branson RD, Chatburn RL. Technical description and classification of modes of ventilator operation. *Respir Care* 1992;37:1026-1044.
13. Kacmarek RM. Methods of providing mechanical ventilatory support. In: Pierson DJ, Kacmarek RM (eds): *Foundations of Respiratory Care.* New York: Churchill Livingstone 1992;953-971.
14. Martin DL, Bratton SL, Walker LK. Principles and practice of respiratpory support and mechancial ventilation. In: Roger MC

(ed): *Textbook of Pediatric Intensive Care.* Baltimore: Wiliams and Wilkins 1996;265-330.

15. Spitzer AR, Fox WW. Positive-Pressure ventilation:Oressure-limited and time-cycled ventilators. In: Goldsmith JP, Karotkin EH, Siede BL (eds): *Assisted Ventilation of the Neonate* 3rd edn. Philadelphia: WB Saunders 1996;167-186.
16. Brathwaite CEM, Borg U. Ventilator support: Use of pressure modes in critically ill patients. *Crit Care Report* 1990;1:300-307.
17. Lessard MRE et al. Effects of pressure-controlled with different I : E ratios versus volume-controlled ventilation on respiratpry mechanics, gas exchange and hemodynamics in patients with adult respiratory distress. *Anesthesiology* 1994;80:983-991.
18. Gurevitch MJ, Van Dyke J, Young ES, et al. Improved oxygenation and lower peak airway pressure in severe adult respiratory distress syndrome. Treatment with inverse ratio ventilation. *Chest* 1986;89:211.
19. Brochard L. Pressure support ventilation. In MJ Tobin (ed): *Principles and Practice of Mechanical Ventilation.* New York: McGraw Hill 1994;239-257.
20. Tyler DC. Positive end-expiratory pressure: A review. *Crit Care Med* 1985;13:851-854.
21. McWilliams BC. Mechanical ventilation in pediatric patients. *Clin Chest Med* 1987;8:573-581.
22. Kanter RK, Blatt SD, Zimmerman JJ. Initial mechanical ventilator settings for pediatric patients, *Am J Emerg Med* 1987;5:113.
23. Derish MT, Frankel LR. Mechanical Ventilation. In:Behrman RE, Kleigman RM, Jenson HB (eds): *Nelson Textbook of Pediatrics* 16th edn. Philadelphia: WB Saunders 2000;268-271.
24. Dettenmeier PA, Johnson TM. The art and science of mechanical ventilator adjustments. *Crit Care Nurs Clin North Am* 1991;3:575-583.
25. Singer M, Webb A. *Oxford Handbook of Critical Care*. Oxford: Oxford University Press 1997.
26. Singhi S. Intensive care of pediatric patients. In: Sachdev HPS, Puri RK, Bagga A, Choudhury P *Principles of Pediatric and Neonatal Emergencies*. New Delhi: Jaypee 1994;329-353.
27. Boegne E. Modes of ventilatory support and weaning parameters in children. *Crit Care Nurs* 1990;378-186.
28. Price E. Robinson EA. *Trends in Ventilaory Support*, 2nd edn. London: Smith and Smith 2002.
29. Pierce LNB. Weaning from mechanical ventilation. In: *Guide to Mechancial Ventilation and Intensive Respiratory Care.* Philadelphia: WB Saunders 1996; 288-311.
30. S. Krishnan. Weaning from mechanical ventilation. In: Singhi S (ed): *Current Concepts in Pediatric Intensive Care.* Chandigarh: Postgraduate Institute ofMedical Education and Research. 1999;31-35.
31. Pierce LNB.Complication of mechanical ventilation. In: *Guide to Mechancial Ventilation and Intensive Respiratory Care.* Philadelphia : WB Saunders 1996: 206-242.
32. Parker JC, Hernandez LA, Peevy KJ. Mechanism of ventilator induced injury. *Crit Care Med* 1993;21: 131-144.
33. Campbell RS. Managing the patient-ventilator system: System checks and circuit changes. *Respir Care* 1994;39:227-236.
34. Gottsschalk SK, King B, Schuth CR. Basic concepts in positive pressure ventilation of the newborn. *Perinatol Neonatol* 1980;4:15.

Harmesh Singh and Baljinder Singh Dhillon

8 Fluid, Electrolytes and Acid-Base Balance and its Disturbances

INTRODUCTION

The infants and young children have high total body water, basal metabolic rate and daily turnover of water. Understandably, therefore, an uninterrupted supply of water, electrolytes and an energy source is extremely important. Inadequate intake or excessive loss may result in dehydration and electrolyte imbalance. Left untreated this can lead to an altered level of consciousness, vascular collapse, renal failure and death. Young infants with diarrhea are particularly vulnerable to dehydration and electrolyte imbalance. In various disease states the balance of water and electrolytes is a must.

DISTRIBUTION OF BODY FLUIDS

Water constitutes almost 60% of body weight of adult and as high as 70-80% of normal and premature neonate respectively. Total body water (TBW) is comprised of two major compartments: extra cellular fluid (ECF) and intracellular fluid (ICF). At birth TBW, ECF and ICF comprise approximately 79%, 45% and 34% of body weight, respectively. By puberty, TBW, ECF and ICF reach their adult values of approximately 60%, 20% and 40% of body weight, respectively.[1] The ICF is two thirds of the TBW and represents all the cellular fluid contents of the body. The ECF comprises one third of the TBW {plasma (intravascular) and interstitial fluid} constitute 4% and 16% of body weight, respectively. Lymph is interstitial fluid and comprises approximately 2% of body weight. The ECF compartment, also includes the transcellular compartment (cerebrospinal, pleural, pericardial, peritoneal, intraocular, synovial fluids, and gastrointestinal tract secretions).[2]

The distribution of the TBW into the ECF and ICF compartments is determined by the number of osmotically active particles (solute) in each compartment. In the ECF, sodium is the principal cation while chloride and bicarbonate are the major anions. More than 90% of the total solute of the ECF is formed by these ions. Their concentrations in the plasma and interstitial fluid are quite similar because these compartments are separated only by the vascular endothelium permeable to low molecular weight ions. Proteins are present predominantly in the plasma (intravascular space).[2] In the ICF, potassium is the predominant cation, and magnesium is present in high concentrations as well. The major intracellular anions are phosphate, sulfate, and protein.[3]

Sodium accounts for the majority of the plasma osmolality, which regulates the size of the ECF. During hyperosmolar states, water moves out of the ICF into the ECF to restore normal osmolality. Conversely, a decrease in plasma osmolality results in water movement out of the ECF into the ICF. Solutes which exert an osmotic force across cell membranes and initiate water movement in and out of cells are referred to as effective osmoles. In ECF and plasma, sodium, glucose, and urea (as measured by blood urea nitrogen [BUN]) are the major effective osmoles. Sodium and glucose, in the absence of insulin, are also called impermeable solutes because they are relatively confined to the ECF. In contrast, urea is a permeable solute and is distributed evenly between the ICF and ECF. Osmolality reflects the concentration of both permeable and impermeable solutes. Therefore, plasma osmolality can be estimated by the following formula:

$$P_{osm} = 2 \text{ (sodium [mmol/L])} + \text{glucose (mg/dL)}/18 + \text{BUN (mg/dL)}/2.8$$

The normal plasma osmolality ranges from 280 to 295 mOsm/kg H_2O.

WATER AND ELECTROLYTE REQUIREMENTS

Infants and Children

Maintenance requirements of water and electrolytes are directly related to a child's metabolic rate which depends on the child's age, body weight, type of activity, temperature, and presence of illness.[3] Water and electrolytes lost through the skin and the respiratory tract are called insensible or evaporative losses. Insensible losses account for one-fourth to one-third of the maintenance requirements, while urinary losses account for the remaining two thirds.[5]

According to Holliday and Segar[3] the rate of caloric expenditure of infants and children could be determined from body weight as given in Table 8.1. Assuming normal renal function and under ordinary homeostatic conditions, an allowance of 50 mL/100 cal/day of water will replace insensible losses, and 66.7 mL/100 cal/day will replace the average urinary losses so that the total water requirement is 116.7 mL/100 cal/day. As the water of oxidation will supply approximately 16.7 mL/100 cal/day, the remaining 100 mL/100 cal/day must be supplied to replace renal and extra renal water losses.

Table 8.1: Maintenance requirement of water and electrolytes

Body weight	*Caloric expenditure*
Upto 10 kg	100 kcal/kg/24 hour
10-20 kg	10000 kcal + 50 kcal/kg/24 hour for weight > 10 kg
> 20 kg	1500 kcal + 20 kcal/kg/24 hour for weight > 20 kg
Water	100 ml/100 kcal/24 hour
Sodium	3-mmol/100 kcal/24 hour
Potassium	2-mmol/100-kcal/24 hour

Newborns[4]

Neonates are born with an excess of TBW, primarily ECF, which needs to be removed. Term neonate bodies are 75% water (40% ECF, 35% ICF), and term neonates usually lose 5-10% of their weight in the first week. Preterm neonates have more water (at 23 weeks' gestation, 90% water composed of 60% ECF and 30% ICF), and they may lose 5-15% of their weight in the first week.

Insensible water loss (IWL) is water loss that is not readily measured, and IWL is water lost via evaporation through the skin (two-thirds) or respiratory tract (one-third). IWL depends on gestational age; the earlier the gestational age of the preterm infant, the greater the IWL. The magnitude of IWL also depends on the postnatal age. Since skin thickens with age, the IWL decreases as neonates age. All other measurable sources of fluid and electrolyte losses need to be considered as well. Sources include stool (e.g., diarrhea and ostomy), nasogastric (NG) or orogastric (OG) drainage, and cerebrospinal fluid (CSF), including ventricular drainage.

Total fluid equals maintenance requirements (IWL plus urine plus stool water) plus growth requirements. In the first few days, IWL is the largest component of lost fluids. Later, as the renal solute load increases, the amount of water the kidneys need to excrete this load increases (80-120 cal/kg/d equals 15-20 mOsm/kg/d, which means that 60-80 mL/kg/d is needed to excrete wastes). Stool requirement usually is 5-10 mL/kg/d. As infants add tissue, they also need to add water to maintain normal ECF and ICF volumes. Since weight gain is 70% water, an infant growing 30-40 g/d requires 20-25 mL/kg/d of water. As the skin matures postnatally, the IWL decreases. Elevated body and environmental temperatures increase IWL. Radiant warmers increase IWL by 50%, phototherapy increases IWL by 50%, and the use of a plastic heat shield reduces IWL by 10-30%. Environmental humidification decreases IWL from the skin and respiratory mucosa by up to 30%. Skin breakdown and skin defects (e.g. omphalocele) increase IWL proportionally to the area affected.[5,6]

For the first 12-24 hours, sodium, potassium, and chloride usually are not required. Later in the first week, needs are 1-2 mEq/kg/d for potassium and 2-4 mEq/kg/d for sodium and chloride. During the active growth period after the first week, needs for potassium increase to 2-3 mEq/kg/d, and for sodium and chloride to 3-5 mEq/kg/d. Some of the smallest preterm infants have sodium requirements as high as 6-8 mEq/kg/d because of the decreased capacity of the kidneys to retain sodium.

DEHYDRATION[7]

The negative fluid balance causing dehydration results from decreased intake, increased output (renal, gastrointestinal, or insensible losses), or fluid shift (ascites, effusions, and capillary leak states such as burns and sepsis). The decrease in total body water causes reductions in both the intracellular and extracellular fluid volumes. Clinical manifestations of dehydration are most closely related to intravascular volume depletion. As dehydration progresses, hypovolemic shock ultimately ensues, resulting in end organ failure and death.

Dehydration is categorized according to serum sodium concentration as follows:

- Isonatremic (130-150 mEq/L)
- Hyponatremic (<130 mEq/L)
- Hypernatremic (>150 mEq/L)

Isonatremic dehydration is the most common (80%). It occurs when the lost fluid is similar in sodium concentration to the blood. Sodium and water losses are of the same relative magnitude in both the intravascular and extravascular fluid compartments.

Hyponatremic (hypotonic) dehydration constitutes 5-10% and occurs when the lost fluid contains more sodium than the blood (loss of hypertonic fluid). Relatively more sodium than water is lost. Because the serum sodium is low, intravascular water shifts to the extravascular space, exaggerating intravascular volume depletion for a given amount of total body water loss.

Hypernatremic (hypertonic) dehydration (5-10%) occurs when the lost fluid contains less sodium than the blood (loss of hypotonic fluid). Relatively less sodium than water is lost. Because the serum sodium is high, extravascular water shifts to the intravascular space, minimizing intravascular volume depletion for a given amount of total body water loss.

During hypernatremic dehydration, water is osmotically pulled from cells into the extracellular space. To compensate, cells can generate osmotically active particles (idiogenic osmoles) that pull water back into the cell and maintain cellular fluid volume. During rapid rehydration of hypernatremia, the increased osmotic activity of these cells can result in a large influx of water, causing cellular swelling and rupture, with cerebral edema being the most devastating consequence. Patients presenting in shock from severe dehydration should be treated as a medical emergency. The goal of initial therapy is to rapidly expand the intravascular volume by intravenous administration of isotonic fluids such as normal saline or Ringer's lactate. Once intravascular volume is restored, therapy should be directed at further correction of water and electrolytes deficits and replacement of ongoing losses.[6]

Management[7]

Dehydration leads to a loss of effective circulating blood volume and it constitutes a medical emergency. The initial aim of treatment is to expand the effective circulating blood volume and to restore nutrient delivery and gas exchange at cellular level.

Estimation of Deficit

Findings on history, physical examination and laboratory studies often provide information required to quantify degree of volume depletion. History should include questions about Intake of fluids:

- Urine output, including the frequency of voiding.
- Stool output, frequency of stools, stool consistency, presence of blood or mucus in stools.
- Emesis, including frequency and volume and whether bilious or nonbilious, hematemesis.
- Underlying illnesses, especially cystic fibrosis, diabetes mellitus, hyperthyroidism, renal disease, fever, appetite patterns, weight loss, travel, recent antibiotic use.

A complete physical examination is essential to determine the underlying cause of the patient's dehydration and to define the severity of dehydration. The clinical assessment of severity of dehydration determines the approach to management. Table outlines the physical findings in various grades of dehydration.[8,9,10]

Parenteral Rehydration [12-16]

pH is recommended if the patient is in shock, too sick to drink or unconscious. The first phase of treatment is to expand the vascular volume rapidly, with the goals of preventing shock when a circulatory deficit is severe and improving renal function. Intravenous normal saline or Ringer lactate (10 to 20 mL/kg) should be given over 1 hour. This infusion should be subtracted from the proposed total volume for the day. The benefit of normal saline or Ringer lactate is a transient expansion of the intravascular space, but this benefit dissipates as the crystalloid solution equilibrates with the remainder of the extravascular interstitial fluid. Compared with normal saline, Ringer lactate has a more physiologic Na^+ to Cl^- ratio (1.17:1); has a slightly lower Na concentration (130 mEq/L); and contains calcium, potassium, and lactate.[11]

The aim of treatment is to correct the deficit, provide maintenance, and replace ongoing abnormal losses, if any. In severe depletion, it is appropriate to give one half of the calculated deficit over the first 8 hours and the second half over the next 16 hours; maintenance needs are provided at a steady rate. During this phase, 5% glucose should be used as the stock solution; NaCl is added according to the estimated need. Children who have isonatremic dehydration require 8 to 10 mEq of Na^+ per kg of body weight for repletion of deficit and 3 mEq/kg per day for maintenance. This Na^+ is given in a volume consisting of the calculated maintenance for water and the estimated water deficit (Table 8.3).

Once urine flow is verified, KCl is added at a concentration of 20 mmol/L to prevent the clinical effects of K^+ depletion. Intravenous K^+ administration should not be greater than 4 mEq/kg per day to avoid exceeding the capacity for cellular uptake of K^+, thereby inducing hyperkalemia. In most infants who have diarrheal dehydration, diarrhea subsides rapidly with therapy, presumably from "bowel rest." However, for patients who have continued heavy diarrhea, stool volumes should be measured to maintain an appropriate intake relative to output; such losses should be replaced volume for volume. Normal saline or two-thirds normal saline with 20 mmol/L of KCl may be used safely to replace most fluid losses from gastric or intestinal drainage.

Oral Rehydration[17,18]

The oral rehydration solution should be administered in small volumes very frequently to minimize gastric distention and reflex vomiting.

HYPONATREMIC DEHYDRATION [19-21]

Hyponatremia is defined as a serum sodium concentration of less than 130 mEq/L. This is the most common electrolyte abnormality encountered in clinical practice. While assessing a child with hyponatremia it is necessary to determine whether it is true or fictitious. It is equally important to ascertain the volume status of the patient (i.e., hypovolemia, hypervolemia,or euvolemia). This enables to distinguish between hyponatremia caused by sodium loss or that by water excess.

Table 8.2: Assessment of degree of dehydration

Symptom/Sign	*Mild Dehydration*	*Moderate Dehydration*	*Severe Dehydration*
Level of consciousness	Alert	Lethargic	Obtunded
Capillary refill	2 Seconds	2-4 Seconds	Greater than 4 seconds, cool limbs
Mucous membranes	Normal	Dry	Parched, cracked
Tears	Normal	Decreased	Absent
Heart rate	Slight increase	Increased	Very increased
Respiratory rate	Normal	Increased	Increased and hyperpnea
Blood pressure	Normal	Normal, but orthostasis	Decreased
Pulse	Normal	Thready	Faint or impalpable
Skin turgor	Normal	Slow	Tenting
Fontanel	Normal	Depressed	Sunken
Eyes	Normal	Sunken	Very sunken
Urine output	Decreased	Oliguria	Oliguria/anuria

Table 8.3: Amount of fluid deficit in different degrees of dehydration

Severity	*Infants (weight <10 kg)*	*Children (weight >10 kg)*
Mild dehydration	5% or 50 mL/kg	3% or 30 mL/kg
Moderate dehydration	10% or 100 mL/kg	6% or 60 mL/kg
Severe dehydration	15% or 150 mL/kg	9% or 90 mL/kg

Causes

i. Euvolemic hyponatremia
- Fictitious hyponatremia
- Pseudohyponatremia
- Syndrome of inappropriate ADH
- Adrenal insufficiency
- Hypothyroidism
- Excess free water intake: inappropriate free water administration, inappropriately mixing formula, iatrogenic administration of hypotonic fluids

ii. Hypovolemic hyponatremia
- GI: vomiting and diarrhea
- Skin: sweat and burns
- CSF: ventriculostomy, CSF drains
- Third space: pancreatitis, peritonitis, burns and bowel obstruction
- Renal: diuretics, recovery phase of acute renal failure, postobstructive, salt-losing nephropathy inadequate salt intake: low-sodium diet

iii. Hypovolemic hyponatremia

Edema forming states:

Nephrotic syndrome

Congestive heart failure

Cirrhosis

Acute or chronic renal failure

Symptoms and signs of hyponatremia are related to the absolute level and rate of fall of serum sodium from baseline. Symptoms do not correlate with specific sodium levels. However, symptoms may appear when the serum sodium concentration is less than 125 mEq/L. Understanding the pathophysiology and treatment options is important because the morbidity and mortality of untreated hyponatremia are significant. Central nervous system (CNS) symptoms include apathy, nausea and vomiting, headache, seizures, or coma; the musculoskeletal symptoms include cramps and weakness. Thus, infants who have hyponatremic dehydration may appear quite ill, because fluid loss in combination with hyponatremia leading to circulatory insufficiency causes a disproportionate reduction in ECF volume. As serum osmolality falls, water moves into cells, causing musculoskeletal dysfunction and putting the brain at risk for swelling. The brain adapts to hyponatremia by pushing interstitial fluid into the cerebrospinal fluid and by extruding cellular solutes, primarily K^+ and amino acids. The relevance of this point is to stress that rehydration puts the brain at risk for dehydration, or even injury, if the correction of fluid and electrolyte losses is much more rapid than the rate at which the brain can recover solute. In severe hyponatremia, it is advisable to effect a correction in plasma Na^+ concentration of no more than 10 to 12 mEq/L per day to avoid undue fluid shifts.[22]

Management

Regardless of the mechanism of hyponatremia, the therapy and rapidity of correction of hyponatremia depend on the etiology and severity of clinical manifestations. Patients who present with severe neurologic symptoms (e.g. seizures or coma) should be aggressively treated with hypertonic saline to rapidly raise their serum sodium concentration to 125 mmol/L. The sodium deficit may be estimated by the following formula:

TBW (L) = body weight (kg) × 0.6 (L/kg) Sodium deficit

(mmol) sodium = TBW x [desired sodium- measured (mmol/L)]

where the desired sodium is 125 mmol/L.

In patients with neurologic symptoms such as seizures, the amount of sodium required to raise the serum sodium to 125 to 130 mmol/L should be calculated using the above formula and administered over 10 to 15 minutes in the form of 3% hypertonic saline. If hypertonic saline is not readily available, sodium bicarbonate (1 mEq sodium/mL) can be used for the initial sodium replacement. The remainder is corrected over a 48-hour period. Asymptomatic patients are corrected by merely replacing the deficit plus maintenance and ongoing losses, correcting no faster than 25 mmol/L in the first 48 hours. Rapid correction of hyponatremia can be associated with central pontine myelinolysis, a demyelinating disorder mainly restricted to the central pons[16]. It is most commonly seen following rapid correction of chronic hyponatremia. Symptomatic patients have findings of quadriplegia, pseudobulbar signs, and swallowing dysfunction. Diagnosis can be confirmed by magnetic resonance imaging of the brain.

Fluid restriction is the mainstay of therapy for SIADH. This may be accomplished by limiting fluid intake to 50% to 75% of maintenance. However, in the presence of signs of severe water intoxication, more aggressive therapy is indicated. Infusion of 3% hypertonic saline (513 mmol/L) with or without administration of a potent diuretic (i.e. furosemide at 1 to 2 mg/kg) may be used to induce ECF volume loss. Six milliliters of 3% saline per kilogram body weight will raise serum sodium level approximately 5 mmol/L.

Patients with hypovolemic hyponatremia require sodium and volume replacement with sodium-containing solutions. Primary disturbances such as adrenal insufficiency, diabetic ketoacidosis, renal or cerebral salt wasting syndromes, and diuretic and mannitol use should be identified and appropriately treated. Hyponatremia associated with increased volume status usually requires both water and sodium restriction. Correction of underlying cardiac, hepatic and renal dysfunction must also be addressed.

HYPERNATREMIC DEHYDRATION[23-29]

Hypernatremia occurs in the following ways:

- Pure water depletion (e.g., diabetes insipidus)
- Sodium excess (e.g., salt poisoning)
- Water depletion exceeding sodium depletion (e.g., diarrhea)

The increased extracellular sodium raises the plasma tonicity which in turn results in removal of fluid from within the cells, resulting in cell desiccation. Extracellular volume remains normal at the expense of intracellular dehydration, which is responsible for the clinical manifestations of hypernatremia.

Causes

i. Euvolemic hypernatremia
   - Sodium bicarbonate administration
   - Formula errors
   - Use of high-sodium dialysate
   - Use of hypertonic saline

ii. Hypovolemic hypernatremia
   - Net loss of water in excess of sodium
   - GI: vomiting and diarrhea
   - Skin: sweat and burns
   - Lungs: hyperventilation
   - Renal: osmotic diuresis (mannitol, diabetes mellitus), postobstructive diuresis, diuretics, intrinsic renal disease and diabetes insipidus

iii. Hypervolemic hypernatremia
   - Sodium bicarbonate administration
   - Formula errors
   - Use of high-sodium dialysate
   - Use of hypertonic saline
   - Mineralocorticoid excess

Infants, because of certain physiologic characteristics, are predisposed to dehydration. They have larger surface area in relation to height or weight than adults and have relatively large evaporative water losses. Infants are unable to concentrate urine beyond 700 mOsm/L in the early months of life.

Clinical signs and symptoms of hypernatremia with associated hypertonicity are directly related to cerebral cell dehydration resulting from water movement from the ICF to the ECF. Neurologic manifestations include varying degrees of depressed sensorium, ranging from lethargy to coma. The majority of patients exhibit marked irritability, a high-pitched cry and seizure activity. Muscle tone may be normal or increased and may be accompanied by hyperreflexia or twitching. Examination of the cerebrospinal fluid may show an elevated protein without pleocytosis. Some patients may also have hyperglycemia, hyperkalemia, hypocalcemia and/or metabolic acidosis. With extreme hypertonicity and resultant water movement from brain cells into ECF, the entire brain can shrink away from the cranium and produce rupture of cerebral vessels. Consequently, focal intra cerebral and subdural hemorrhages and venous thrombosis may occur.

Since the central nervous system is particularly vulnerable to hypertonicity, the brain cells adapt within hours by increasing intra cellular osmolality with resultant movement of water back into the brain cells.

Glucose, myoinositol, taurine, and other amino acids may be the solutes (idiogenic osmoles) responsible for normalizing brain water content. If hypertonicity develops rapidly, idiogenic osmoles may not be generated fast enough to prevent brain cell shrinkage. Therefore, the severity of clinical manifestations of hypernatremia and associated hypertonicity is relative to its degree and rate of development.

Treatment

Whenever possible, therapy should be directed at the underlying disease process (e.g., administration of vasopressin analogues in DI). In the presence of shock or severe ECF volume contraction, restoration of the intravascular volume takes precedence over normalization of plasma osmolality. In this setting, isotonic solutions are the recommended fluid replacement to restore circulating blood volume.

The speed of correction of hypernatremia depends on the rate of its development and the accompanying clinical presentation. Correction of hypernatremia should be accomplished slowly, except in the setting of acute massive salt poisoning. Rapid lowering o serum sodium may result in water movement from the ECF into the brain cells, resulting in cerebral edema and possible herniation. When serum sodium acutely exceeds 175 mmol/L (as in salt poisoning), dialysis may be performed to rapidly lower serum sodium. Once serum sodium concentration is at 170 mmol/L, further reduction should be carried out over 48 hours, with the aim of lowering serum sodium no greater than 1 mmol/L/hour.

Assuming no ongoing losses, the amount of water required in the therapeutic management of hypovolemic hypernatremia may be estimated using the following series of formulas:

$$\text{TBW (L)} = \text{body weight (kg)} \times 0.6\ \text{(L/kg)}$$

$$\text{Water required (L)} = \frac{\text{Actual sodium–desired sodium (mmol/L)}}{\text{Desired sodium (mmol/L)} \times \text{TBW}}$$

The desired sodium is assumed to be 140 mmol/L. Serum sodium should be monitored closely to ensure that the rate of drop is not excessive.

POTASSIUM

Potassium is the primary or intracellular cation and plays a key role in intracellular volume regulation. Total body potassium is approximately 53-55 mEq/kg of body weight, as determined by evaluating gamma emissions of radionuclide-tagged potassium. Almost 100% of body potassium is contained in the intracellular fluid space, most in skeletal muscle. A balance between intake and excretion maintains plasma potassium levels within a narrow range (3.5-4.5 mEq/L). Less than 10% of potassium is excreted through sweat and stools, while more than 90% is excreted by the kidneys.

Hypokalemia[30,31]

Hypokalemia is generally defined as a serum potassium level less than 3.5 mmol/L. Clinically, the etiology of hypokalemia can be divided into two broad categories:

1. Reduction of total body potassium and
2. Re-distribution into the intracellular space.

Total body potassium may be reduced secondary to inadequate dietary intake or increased potassium losses. In general, abnormal losses of potassium play a more significant etiologic role in hypokalemia than decreased intake.

Etiology

- Hypokalemia may be due to a total body deficit of potassium, which may occur chronically with the following: Prolonged diuretic use, Inadequate potassium intake, Laxative use, Diarrhea, Hyperhidrosis, Hypomagnesemia
- Acute causes of potassium depletion include: Diabetic ketoacidosis, Severe gastrointestinal losses from vomiting and diarrhea, Dialysis and diuretic therapy
- Hypokalemia may also be due to excessive potassium shifts from the extracellular to the intracellular space, as seen in: Alkalosis, Insulin use, Catecholamine use, Sympathomimetic use, Hypothermia
- Other recognizable causes of hypokalemia include the following:
  - Renal tubular disorders
  - Type I or classic distal tubular acidosis
  - Periodic hypokalemic paralysis
  - Hyperaldosteronism
- Other states of mineralocorticoid excess that may cause hypokalemia include the following:
  - Cystic fibrosis with hyperaldosteronism from severe chloride and volume depletion, Cushing syndrome, Exogenous steroid administration
- Other conditions that may cause hypokalemia include acute myelogenous, monomyeloblastic, or lymphoblastic leukemia
- Drugs that may cause hypokalemia include the following:
  - Theophylline, Verapamil (with overdose), High-dose penicillin, Ampicillin, Carbenicillin, Drugs associated with magnesium depletion, such as aminoglycosides, amphotericin B, and cisplatin

In general, signs and symptoms of hypokalemia are not exhibited unless the serum potassium level drops below 3 mmol/L. Clinical manifestations are result of aberrations in membrane potential affecting the function of excitable tissues such as nerve and muscle. Neuromuscular findings may include weakness, fatigue, tetany and cramps. Muscle weakness resulting in respiratory insufficiency does not usually occur unit the plasma potassium is less than 2.5

mmol/L. Hypokalemia also affects gastrointestinal function by reducing motility, with symptoms ranging from constipation to ileus.

Its effect on the heart may include arrhythmias and abnormal electrocardiographic finding. The electrocardiographic changes that are produced with hypokalemia are primarily related to delayed ventricular repolarization. These findings include flattening of the T wave, ST segment depression, prominence of U waves, and prolongation of the QT interval. With more several hypokalemia, the P wave becomes more prominent, the PR interval becomes prolonged and the QRS complex widens.

Treatment

Potassium replacement is the mainstay of treatment for hypokalemia. Whenever possible, the oral route rather than the intravenous route should be used. The risk of inducing hyperkalemia must always be kept in mind when correcting hypokalemia; thus, it is generally prudent to replace deficits slowly. The oral dose of potassium is 2 to 4 mmol/kg/day in two to four divided doses. If the intravenous route must be used, potassium chloride may be given through a peripheral vein in concentrations not to exceed 40 mmol/L. The risk of precipitating cardiac arrhythmias should always be kept in mind when administering potassium via a central venous line. The recommended rate of infusion ranges from 0.25 to 0.5 mmol/kg/h (maximum 10 to 20 mmol/h). Continuous electrocardiographic monitoring and frequent determinations of serum potassum levels are essential to avoid the risk of iatrogenic hyperkalemia.

Hyperkalemia[31,32]

Hyperkalemia is a life-threatening emergency. Patient's electrocardiograms (ECGs) should be continuously monitored and therapy should be initiated while ascertaining the etiology of the elevated serum potassium concentration. The first step in determining the cause of hyperkalemia is to rule out laboratory error. The most common cause of pseudohyperkalemia is hemolysis, resulting from the release of potassium from red blood cells. Hemolysis commonly results from heel stick and finger stick specimens. Other causes of spurious hyperkalemia are thrombocytosis (release of potassium from the platelets during clotting), leukocytosis (intracellular release when there is delay in separating the serum or plasma from the cellular elements) and as ischemic blood draw (potassium release from muscles after prolonged application of the tourniquet).

Once a true potassium level is established, the next step is to determine whether hyperkalemia results from redistribution, excessive potassium load, or inadequate excretion. In clinical practice, the majority of cases of hyperkalemia secondary to potassium retention are due to compromised renal function, or inability of the kidney to handle a substantial potassium load. The causes of hyperkalemia are as under:

Causes

- *Pseudohyperkalemia:*
  Release of potassium from cell lysis: Leucocytosis, Thrombocytosis, Hemolysis (improper collection)
  Redistribution: changes in pH, Hypertonicity, drugs e.g.diogoxin toxicity, beta blockers, succinylcholine, chemotherapeutic agents, nifedipine etc.
- *True hyperkalemia:*
  Decreased renal excretion—Renal insufficiency or failure, drugs that block potassium excretion, hypoaldosteronism, congenital renal defects, sickle cell disease, addisons disease, diabetes mellitus, SLE, renal allograft
- *High potassium intake:*
  Toxic ingestion of potassium preparations, intravenous potassium administration, rapid infusion of old blood
  Inhibition of tubular secretion
  Drugs–spironolacton, triamterene,amiloride

As with hypokalemia, the most serious clinical manifestation of hyperkalemia results from aberrations in membrane polarization of cardiac tissue. Peaking or tenting of the T wave is the earliest ECG abnormality. As hyperkalemia progresses, there is flattening of the P wave, prolongation of the PR interval, widening of the QRS complex, development of a sine wave, and ultimately, ventricular fibrillation or cardiac arrest. Acidosis, hyponatremia, and hypocalcemia potentiate the dangerous effects of hyperkalemia and must be corrected.

Treatment

The first step in the treatment of hyperkalemia is to stop the administration of potassium-containing fluids and potassium-sparing diuretics. Therapeutic strategies are directed to counteract the cardiac toxicity, promote the intracellular movement of potassium, and remove excessive potassium from the body. Intravenous calcium chloride 10 to 25 mg/kg or calcium gluconate 50 to 100 mg/kg will antagonize the hyperkalemic effects on cardiac conduction but have no effect on the serum potassium concentration. Continuous cardiac monitoring is imperative during the treatment of hyperkalemia. Alkalinization (raising the pH) with sodium bicarbonate promotes movement of potassium into the cells in exchange for H^+ ion. Dosing of sodium bicarbonate starts with 1 to 2 mmol/kg intravenously over 10 minutes. Alternatively, alkalinization can be induced by increasing the minute ventilation and lowering the partial pressure of arterial carbon idoxide (PCO_2). The latter is simple and quickly accomplished in patients who are receiving mechanical ventilation. Like bicarbonate, insulin also favors the cellular uptake of potassium. To prevent hypoglycemia, insulin (0.1 U/kg) is combined with glucose (0.5 g/kg). Sodium potassium exchange resins (Kayexalate) eliminate excess of potassium in the gut in exchange for sodium ions. Kayexalate (1 to 2 g/kg) may be given orally or as a retention enema. It should be kept in mind that Kayexalate also binds magnesium and calcium and, therefore, symptoms related to the deficiency of these ions must be addressed. Additionally Kayexalate exchanges sodium for potassium and therefore hypernatremia and hypervolemia may develop. b-Adrenergic agonists such as epinephrine and isoproterenol also promote the intracellular movement of potassium, and their use has been suggested as a temporizing strategy for the treatment of hyperkalemia. In patients with intact renal function, loop diuretics with mannitol may increase potassium losses in the urine. Finally, in the setting of severe acute renal failure and worsening hyperkalemia, hemodialysis must be considered. Peritoneal dialysis is not as effective in quickly removing potassium

ACID-BASE HOMEOSTASIS[33]

Maintenance of a normal pH is essential for intracellular health. The critical care physician's challenge is to preserve this relatively narrow normal range of hydrogen ion concentration ([H^+] when the body is stressed by increased requirements of metabolism or alterations of natural adaptation. pH is the negative logarithm of the [H^+]; it is considered normal in the 7.35 to 7.45 range (corresponding to a [H^+] of 35 to 45 mEq/L). Although changes in the pH reflect a relatively linear change in the [H^+] between 7.20 and 7.50, it is of particular importance to remember the logarithmic relationship outside this range. Large changes of [H^+] outside this relatively narrow range of pH are reflected in comparatively small changes in the pH.

ACID-BASE DISTURBANCES[35]

Acid-base abnormalities are the result of primary changes in either P_aCO_2 or bicarbonate concentration. In general, increase or decrease in P_aCO_2 result in acid-base disturbances that are referred to as respiratory acidosis or respiratory alkalosis, respectively. Likewise, increase or decrease in bicarbonate concentration result in metabolic alkalosis or metabolic acidosis, respectively. In each of the four primary acid-base abnormalities, the initiating process not only changes the acid-base balance, but also triggers compensatory physiologic mechanisms to restore the HCO_3^-/P_aCO_2 ratio and eventually return the pH to normal.

Respiratory Acidosis[36]

Primary respiratory acidosis is the consequence of alveolar hypoventilation or excessive carbon dioxide production resulting in an inadequate ratio of carbon dioxide excretion relative to carbon dioxide production. The etiologies of respiratory acidosis are given in Table 8.4. Signs and symptoms of respiratory acidosis and symptoms of respiratory acidosis depend on the duration and severity of the acidosis, the degree of compensation, and the patient's level of consciousness. Initially, compensation is by the nonbicarbonate intracellular buffers. The secondary rise in serum HCO^-_3 occurs by that increased excretion of H^+ in the urine as titratable acid and as ammonium. This begins at 6 to 12 hours and probably takes several days to reach its maximum compensation capacity. During this time the serum HCO^-_3 rarely rises above 32 mEq/L. In the setting of acute respiratory acidosis, a mixed respiratory acidosis-metabolic alkalosis disorder with higher HCO^-_3 values should be suspected although values of up to 45 mEq/L are seen in chronic respiratory acidosis. It is also of interest that even in chronic respiratory acidosis the serum pH can usually be corrected for Pco_2 values up to 70 mmHg. Higher values of Pco_2 values up to 70 mmHg. Higher values of Pco_2 in this state are usually associated with serum pH values below 7.35.

Table 8.4: Causes of respiratory acidosis

Ventilatory failure is the primary cause of CO_2 retention.
CNS depression may be due to trauma, infections, tumor, cerebrovascular accidents, and drug overdose.
Neuromuscular disorders include poliomyelitis and Guillain-Barré syndrome.
Thoracic disorders include hydrothorax, pneumothorax and flail chest.
Lung disorders include upper or lower airway obstruction, asthma, emphysema or chronic bronchitis (chronic obstructive airway disease), pulmonary edema and bronchopulmonary dysplasia.

Treatment

Respiratory acidosis is a disorder for which the therapy is relatively simple. Regardless of the cause, the therapy is ventilatory support of some kind. Institution of mechanical ventilation is the mainstay of treatment of hypercapnia. In certain cases, however, tromethamine (THAM) may be helpful. Dose may be calculated as:

mL of 0.3 M solution = lean body weight (kg) × the base deficit (mEq/L) × 1.1 Infusion rate not to exceed 3-16 mL/kg/h; titrate according to serum pH

Respiratory Alkalosis[37,38]

Primary respiratory alkalosis is the consequence of alveolar hyperventilation which results in carbon dioxide excretion exceeding carbon dioxide production. In the beginning intracellular buffers compensate it and after a longer period of 12 to 24 hours, renal compensation corrects serum pH by excretion of HCO^-_3 along with sodium and potassium excretion by the kidney occurs. After 24 hours of renal compensation for respiratory alkalosis, potassium balance is restored.

Table 8.5: Causes of respiratory alkalosis

- **Hypoxia and hypoxemia:** Any condition associated with a fall in the PaO_2 below 65 mm Hg or with decreased oxygen delivery to the tissues increases minute ventilation:Altitude/ low fraction of inspired oxygen (FiO_2), Anemia, Hypotension, Lung disease
- **Pulmonary disorders:** Embolism, Airway obstruction/ inflammation, Pneumonia: A classic presentation of *Pneumocystis* pneumonia is hypoxemia with respiratory alkalosis, interstitial lung disease.
- **Mechanical ventilation:** Respiratory alkalosis could result from a too high ventilatory rate or tidal volume or from the patient triggering excessive additional breaths.
- **Extrapulmonary disorders:** In a child with normal lung function with an overriding ventilatory stimulus: Anxiety, stress, Neurologic disease (e.g., stroke, infection, trauma, tumor), Hormones/drugs (e.g., catecholamines, progesterone, methylxanthines, salicylates/doxapram, nicotine), Pregnancy, Hyperthermia, Liver failure, especially with hepatic encephalopathy, Sepsis, Recovery from metabolic acidosis

Treatment

Therapy should be directed at correction of the underlying problem.

Metabolic Acidosis[39,40]

Metabolic Acidosis results from the addition of acid or the removal of alkali from body fluids, and it compensatory response is in form of increased alveolar ventilation (respiratory alkalosis) and a fall in PCO_2. This adaptation, hyperpnea (defined as deep, pauseless respirations), does not lead to complete normalization of pH, but it occurs rapidly, beginning within minutes. The clinical manifestations of acidosis include depressed myocardial contractility, arrhythmias, arteriolar dilatation, hypotension, and even pulmonary edema.

Diagnosis

The diagnostic approach to metabolic acidosis is remarkably simplified when examined in terms of the anion gap. The anion gap is derived from the following formula: AG (mmol/ L) = sodium – [Cl^- + HCO_3^-].

The normal range is 8 to 16 mmol/L (mean 12). Acidosis associated with an increased anion gap result from overproduction of endogenous acids (lactate and keto-anions), decreased excretion of fixed acids (renal failure), or toxic ingestions (salicylates, methanol, ethylene glycol). Normal anion gap acidosis can result from the net loss of base through the gut and kidney or from infusion of acidifying agents.

Treatment

The main goals of therapy should be directed at correction of the underlying process, and maintenance of tissue perfusion and renal function by restoring adequate intravascular volume. In the presence of severe metabolic acidosis (pH < 7.1), alkali therapy may be reasonable. Sodium bicarbonate is the agent of choice in acute acidosis requiring intervention. No matter what the cause, bicarbonate should be given when plasma HCO^-_3 is < 5 mmol/L. Bicarbonate should be added to a hypotonic solution and given as a continuous infusion over 1 hour. The amount to infuse may be calculated by using the following formula:

$$\text{Dose (mEq)} = \text{Body Wt (Kg)} \rightarrow (15\text{-Observed } HCO_3^-) \times 0.5$$

In diarrhea, the severity of the acidosis varies according to the etiology. With severe watery diarrhea, the stool HCO_3^- concentration may reach 40 mEq/L, resulting in moderate-to-severe metabolic acidosis. In addition to volume replacement, which is the principal arm of therapy, it may be necessary to add HCO_3^- to the intravenous fluid. Before giving HCO_3^-, the serum K^+ concentration must be determined. If it is normal or low, treatment with HCO_3^- may induce or worsen hypokalemia and lead to neuromuscular complications.

Children who have type 1 RTA need 5 to 15 mEq/kg per day of supplemental alkali. Oral sodium citrate is more palatable than bicarbonate salt. The maintenance dose is highly variable and is titrated to normalize the patient's plasma HCO_3^- concentration. A fixed HCO_3^- loss persists, even when the serum HCO_3^- concentration is low, so these infants are at risk for severe acidosis when they cannot maintain oral alkali supplementation. After age 6 years, affected children exhibit a reduction in urinary HCO_3^- loss, allowing a reduction in the dose of alkali. Prior to appropriate treatment, renal K^+ and Ca^+ losses may occur. Children who have type 2 RTA may require up to 20 mEq/kg of supplemental alkali as well as oral potassium supplements. Children who have type 4 RTA require administration of NaCl and possibly mineralocorticoid replacement. Hyperkalemia responds to restriction of oral intake of K^+; low doses (1 to 2 mEq/kg per day) of HCO_3^- may be required for correction of acidosis.

In DKA, therapy with fluids and insulin allows for the ketoacids to be metabolized and for acid to be excreted by the kidneys, thus regenerating HCO_3^-. Therefore, administration of bicarbonate is not required for most patients who have DKA. Moreover, the potential complications of bicarbonate therapy include rebound hypokalemia, "overshoot" metabolic alkalosis, hypernatremia, and paradoxic CNS acidosis. However, many recommend administering bicarbonate if the pH is below 7.0.

In severe lactic acidosis, the mainstay of treatment is correction of the underlying process. However, administration of bicarbonate offsets the negative inotropic and arrhythmogenic effects of academia.

However, the amount of sodium bicarbonate needed to achieve a pH greater than 7.1 is difficult to predict. Furthermore, sodium bicarbonate infusions may be fraught with theoretical adverse effects such as hyperosmolality, paradoxical intracellular and cerebrospinal fluid acidosis, and alkalemia resulting in increased affinity of hemoglobin for oxygen and consequent tissue hypoxia.

Metabolic Alkalosis[41-45]

The etiology of metabolic alkalosis may be classified based on the urinary chloride concentration and the response to chloride administration. The chloride-responsive group is usually associated with ECF volume contraction whereas the chloride-resistant group is associated with ECF volume excess. The symptomatology of metabolic alkalosis may be the consequence of its effect on the neuromuscular system (confusion and muscle weakness), on cardiac conduction (refractory supraventricular and ventricular arrhythmias), and on oxygen delivery (tissue hypoxia secondary to shift of the oxygen-hemoglobin dissociation curve to the left).

Treatment

Therapy is centered on identifying and treating the underlying pathology. In mild-to-moderate alkalosis, provision of Cl^- will allow the kidney to excrete the excess base. In severe alkalosis, hydrochloric acid administration may be necessary. Alternative choices for therapy are ammonium chloride or arginine monohydrochloride, although these are contraindicated in hepatic and renal disease, respectively. In obstructive vomiting or nasogastric aspiration, providing an adequate supply of chloride salt, 1 to 2 mEq/kg per day, may offset the loss of acid. Such patients often have a deficit of potassium, which should be corrected. In hyperaldosteronism, an antagonist such as spironolactone will correct the hypertension and the hypokalemia and restore a normal acid-base status. Amiloride may be equally effective. Hypokalemia and alkalosis are observed in Bartter syndrome, which is characterized by hyperreninemic hyperaldosteronism and hypersecretion of renal prostaglandins. These may respond to indomethacin, but additional KCl may be needed. In Cushing syndrome, therapy is directed at the underlying process.

REFERENCES

1. Rosaleah VB, Joseph E Segeleon, Steven E Haun. Fluid and Electrolyte issues. In: Tobias JD (ed) *Pediatric Critical Care: The Essentials*. New Delhi: Orient Longman 2000;287-309.
2. McKeown JW. Disorders of total body sodium. In Kokko JP, Tannen RL (eds) *Fluids and Electrolytes*. Philadelphia: WB Saunders 1986;63-117.
3. Holliday MA, Segar WE. The maintenance need for water in parenteral fluid therapy. *Pediatrics* 1957; 19:823-832.
4. Simmons CF Jr. Fluid and electrolyte management. In: Cloherty JP, Stark AR (eds) *Manual of Neonatal Care*. 4th ed. New York: Lippincott Raven 1997;87-100.
5. Denne SC, Clark SE, Poindexter BB. Nutrition and metabolism in the high-risk neonate. In: Fanaroff AA, Martin RJ (eds) *Neonatal-Perinatal Medicine: Diseases of the Fetus and Infant*. 6th edn. St Louis: Mosby 1997;562-621.
6. Hellerstein S. Fluids and electrolytes: Physiology. *Pediatrics in Review*. 1993;14:70-79.
7. Humes DH. Disorders of water metabolism. In: Kokko JP, Tannen RL (eds) *Fluids and Electrolytes*. Philadelphia: WB Saunders 1986;118-149.
8. Gorelick MH, Shaw, KN, Murphy, KO. Validity and reliability of clinical signs in the diagnosis of dehydration in children. *Pediatrics* 1997;99:E6.
9. MackenzieA, BarnesG, Shann F. Clinical signs of dehydration in children. *Lancet* 1989;2:605-607.
10. Duggan C, Refat M, Hashem M. How valid are clinical signs of dehydration in infants? *J Pediatr Gastroenterol Nutr* 1996;22: 56-61.
11. Brown RG. Disorders of water and sodium balance. *Postgrad Med* 1993;93:227-8,231-4:239-240 passim.
12. Segar WE. Parenteral fluid therapy. *Curr Prob Pediatr* 1972;3:3-40.
13. Holliday M. The evolution of therapy for dehydration: should deficit therapy still be taught? *Pediatrics* 1996; 98:171-177.
14. Kallen RJ, Lonergan JM. Fluid resuscitation of acute hypovolemic hypoperfusion states in pediatrics. *Pediatr Clin North Am* 1990;287-294.
15. Reid SR, Bonadio WA. Outpatient rapid intravenous rehydration to correct dehydration and resolve vomiting in children with acute gastroenteritis. *Ann Emerg Med* 1996;28:318-323.
16. Watkins SL. The basics of fluid and electrolyte therapy. *Pediatr Ann* 1995;1:16-22.
17. Casteels HB, Fiedorek SC. Oral rehydration therapy. *Pediatr Clin North Am* 1990;37:295-311.
18. Goepp JG, Katz SA. Oral rehydration therapy. *Am Fam Physician* 1993;4:843-851.
19. Avner ED. Clinical disorders of water metabolism: hyponatremia and hypernatremia. *Pediatr Ann* 1995;24:23-30.
20. Berry PL, Belsha CW. Hyponatremia. *Pediatr Clin North Am* 1990;37:351-363.
21. Gruskin AB, Sarnaik A. Hyponatremia: Pathophysiology and treatment, a pediatric perspective. *Pediatr Nephrol* 1992;6: 280-286.
22. Zarinetchi F, Berl T. Evaluation and management of severe hyponatremia. *Adv Intern Med* 1996;41:251-283.
23. Avner ED. Clinical disorders of water metabolism: Hyponatremia and hypernatremia. *Pediatr Ann* 1995; 24:23-30.
24. Brown RG. Disorders of water and sodium balance. *Postgrad Med* 1993;93:227-228.
25. Conley SB. Hypernatremia. *Pediatr Clin North Am* 1990;37: 365-372.
26. Finberg L. Hypernatremic (hypertonic) dehydration in infants. *N Engl J Med* 1973;26:196-198.
27. Palevsky PM. Hypernatremia. Semin Nephrol 1998; 18(1): 20-30.
28. Paneth N. Hypernatremic dehydration of infancy: An epidemiologic review. *Am J Dis Child* 1980;134:785-792.
29. Gruskin AB, Baluarte HJ, Prebis JW, *et al*. Serum sodium abnormalities in children. *Pediatr Clin North Am* 1982;29: 907-932.

30. Tannen RL. Potassium disorders. In: Kokko JP, Tannen RL. *Fluids and Electrolytes.* Philadephia: WB Saunders 1986; 150-228.
31. Khilnani P. Electrolyte abnormalities in critically ill children. *Crit Care Med* 1992;20:241-250.
32. Moreno M, Murphy C, Goldsmith C. Increase in serum potassium resulting from the administration of hypertonic mannitol and other solutions. *J Lab Clin Med* 1967;76:291-298.
33. Kravath RE. Pathophysiology of hydrogen ion disturbance. In Finberg L, Fleischman AR (eds) *Water and Electrolytes in Pediatrics.* Philadelphia: WB Saunders 1982;90-107.
34. Al-Awqati Q. The cellular renal response to respiratory acid-base disorders. *Kidney Int* 1985;28:845–855.
35. Adrogué HJ, Madias NE. Management of life-threatening acid-base disorders. *N Engl J Med* 1998;338:26-34.
36. Goldstein B, Shannon DC, Todres ID. Supercarbia in children: Clinical course and outcome. *Crit Care Med* 1990;18:166-168.
37. Shapiro BA, Peruzzi WT: Clinical approach to interpretation. In: *Clinical Application of Blood Gases*, 5th edn. St Louis: Mosby-Yearbook 1994: 69-83.
38. Krapf R, Beeler I, Hertner D, Hulter HN. Chronic respiratory alkalosis: The effect of sustained hyperventilation on renal regulation of acid-base equilibrium. *N Engl J Med* 1991;324: 1394-1401.
39. DuBose TD Jr. Hyperkalemic hyperchloremic metabolic acidosis: Pathophysiologic insights. *Kidney Int* 1997;51:591-602.
40. Madias NE, Bossert WH, Adrogué HJ. Ventilatory response to chronic metabolic acidosis and alkalosis in the dog. *J Appl Physiol* 1984;56:1640-1646.
41. Finberg L, Kravath RE, Hellerstein S. Metabolic alkalosis. In: *Water and Electrolytes in Pediatrics: Physiology, Pathophysiology, and Treatment.* Philadelphia: WB Saunders 1993;97-98.
42. Kokko JP, Tannen RL. Metabolic alkalosis. In: *Fluids and Electrolytes.* Philadelphia: WB Saunders 1990; 356-376.
43. Maxwell MH, Kleeman CR. Metabolic alkalosis. In: *Clinical Disorders of Fluid and Electrolyte Metabolism.* New York: McGraw-Hill 1994;213-220.
44. Shapiro BA, Harrison RA, Cane RD. Clinical Application of Blood Gases. St. Louis: Mosby 1989.
45. Sabatini S, Kurtzman NA. Metabolic alkalosis: Biochemical mechanisms, Pathophysiology, and treatment. In: Suki WN, Massry SG (eds) *Therapy of Renal Diseases and Related Disorders.* Boston: Kluwer Academic Publishers 1997; 189-210.

Rajeshwar Dayal

9 Multiple Organ Dysfunction Syndrome (MODS)

INTRODUCTION

The past three decades have witnessed the emergence of a new syndrome termed "multiple organ dysfunction syndrome" which today represents one of the most common causes of death in pediatric intensive care units.

The reasons for increased incidence during the past three decades are better critical care in early phase of severe illness and increase in high risk patient population being cared for in PICU. So, this syndrome is a product of progress in critical care and life-saving technology.

MODS was first noticed by Tilney in 1973. The terms MOF and MSOF were coined by Fiseman and Foy, respectively.[1]

DEFINITION

To overcome the haphazard definitions and for better understanding of clinical course of MODS, American College of Chest Physicians (ACCP)/Society of Critical Care Medicine (SCCM) outlined the definitions of MODS and concerned terminology in 1992.[2]

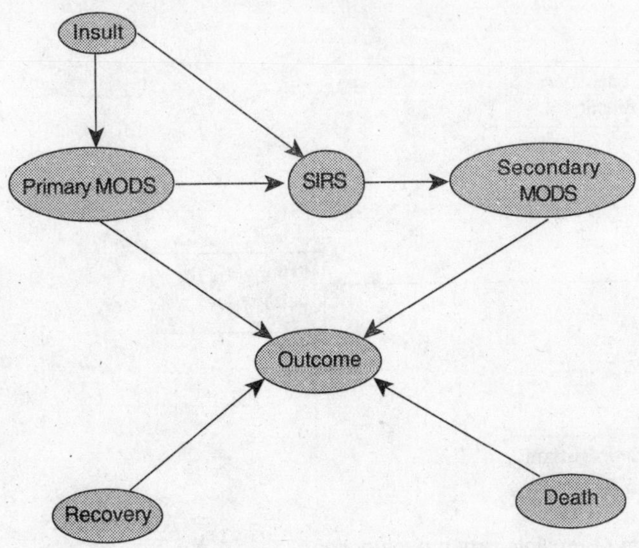

Fig. 9.1: Primary and secondary MODS

Accordingly, MODS has been defined as "altered organ function in a acutely ill patient so that homeostasis cannot be maintained without intervention."

CLASSIFICATION

Primary MODS

It is the direct result of a well-defined insult in which organ dysfunction occurs early and can be attributable to the insult itself.

Secondary MODS

It is a consequence of host response that is characterized by a generalized activation of inflammatory reaction in organs remote from initial insult.

Any major injury or insult results in the development of primary MODS or it may lead to development of SIRS which leads to secondary MODS. The outcome may be recovery or death, depending on the prognosis.

PATHOPHYSIOLOGY

MODS at its most basic level is a cellular disease mediated by proteins and lipid molecules.

Organ injury in MODS is not directly due to exogenous factors such as bacteria or toxins but is largely a consequence of the host's own endogenously produced mediator leading to damage to distant organs in addition to directly injured one.

Basic pathophysiology of this syndrome remains to be fully elucidated. Multiple hypothesis have been proposed to explain the development of MODS.

Macrophage Hypothesis

According to this hypothesis, excessive or prolonged activation or stimulation of macrophages ultimately results in excessive production, surface expression and liberation of cytokines and other products which through a cascade effect involving additional humoral and cellular effector systems (like Nitric oxide, bradykinin etc.) exert local and systemic deleterious effects. IL-1, IL-6, TNFa, IF-g are main cytokines involved. Among these, TNF-a appears to be the most important messenger which initiates and orchestrates the septic response.

Microcirculatory Hypothesis

According to it, organ injury is related to ischemia or vascular endothelial injury. Shock leads to vascular congestion and sludging resulting in formation of microthrombi, interstitial oedema and increased capillary permeability. Although prolonged ischemia causes cell death, but main injury occurs after reperfusion due to production of O_2 free radicals, the main source being xanthine oxidase and leucocytes. Endothelial- leucocyte interaction is a common pathway for tissue injury in response to various initiating factors. There occurs a phenotypic change in endothelium towards the more proinflammatory state as shown by pronounced and persistent increase in plasma VCAM-1 (vascular cell adhesion molecule-1) and ICAM-1 (Intercellular adhesion molecule-1).[3]

Gut Hypothesis

It states that intestinally derived bacteria or endotoxins serve as triggers to initiate, perpetuate and exacerbate septic state and development of MODS. In critically ill patients:

a. gut barrier is disrupted due to ischemia and hypoxia,
b. normal gut flora is replaced by gram-negative bacteria due to antibiotic usage and
c. patient is immunocompromised leading to spread of endotoxins to portal circulation. Also impaired hepatic RES activity potentiates systemic effects of gut barrier failure by allowing gut bacteria to reach systemic circulation where they cause generalised inflammatory response.

All the three hypothesis i.e. macrophage, microcirculatory and gut hypothesis function in an integrated way to cause MODS. This is shown clearly in Figure 9.2.

Apoptosis Hypothesis

According to this hypothesis, increased apoptosis rate at parenchymal and microvasculature level is involved in organ dysfunction in MODS4.

Two Hit Phenomenon

According to it, initial insult primes the host so that on a second or subsequent insult, the host response is greatly amplified.[1] Examples include

a. shock leading to ischemia-reperfusion injury.
b. hypoxia → priming of macrophages and neutrophils → tissue injury and amplified response during any subsequent injury like infection and endotoxemia.

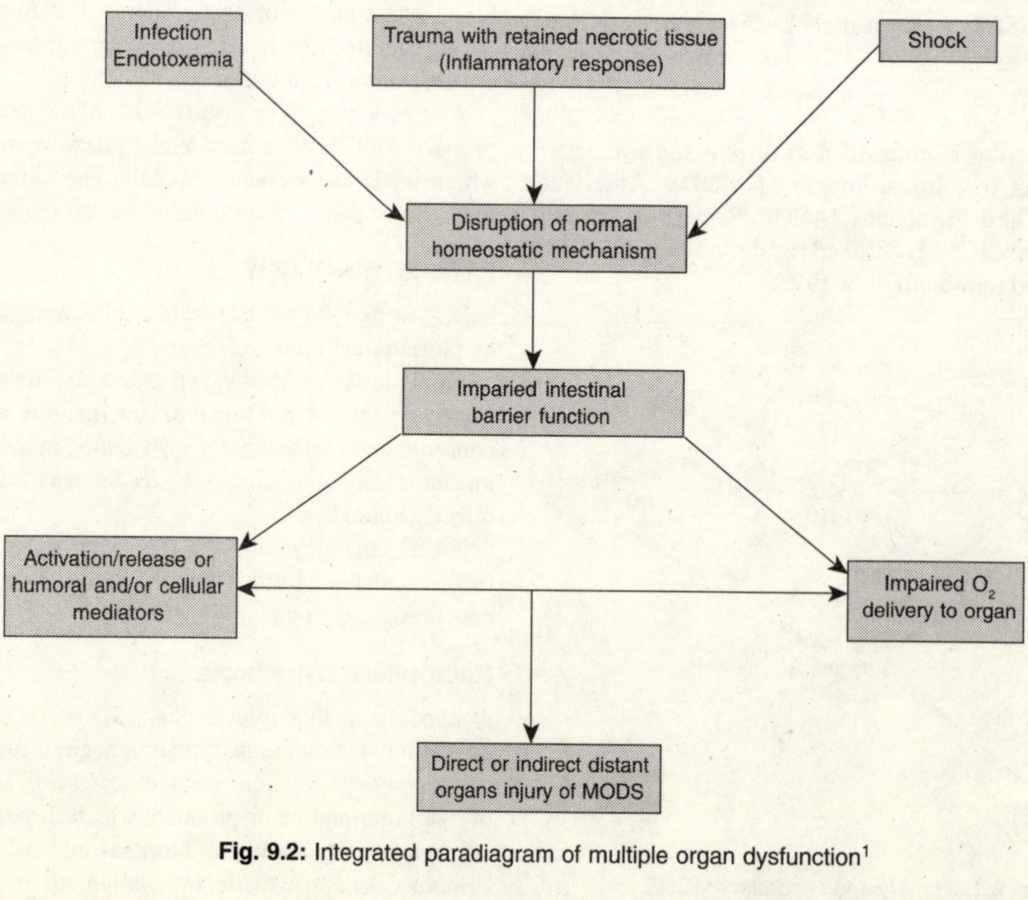

Fig. 9.2: Integrated paradiagram of multiple organ dysfunction[1]

Table 9.1: Risk factors for MODS [6,7]

Infections
Peritonitis and intraabdominal infections
Pneumonia
Necrotising soft tissue infections
Endocarditis
Meningitis
Candidiasis
Plasmodium species
Extensive miliary tuberculosis
Disseminated hematogenous tuberculosis in immunocompromised patient
Fulminant salmonella infection
Fulminant amebic infection
Viral agents
Inflammation
Pancreatitis
Injury
Burns
Multiple trauma
Ischemia
Ruptured aneurysm
Hypovolumic shock
Aortic occlusion
Haemorrhage
Mesenteric vascular occlusion
Immune reactions
Autoimmune disease
Transplant rejection
Graft versus host disease
Administration of interleukin-2
Iatrogenic factors
Delayed or missed injury
Blood transfusion
Total parentral nutrition
Intoxication
Drug reactions
Salicylate intoxication
Arsenic intoxication
Acetaminophen overdosage
Idiopathic
TTP (Thrombotic thrombocytopenic purpura)
Pheochromocytoma

Regardless of the cause, MODS follows a predictable course beginning with lung and followed by hepatic, intestinal, renal, hematological and cardiac failure in that order. Onset of CNS alteration can occur either early or late. This classical sequential order of organ failure may be modified, however by presence of pre-existing disease or by nature of precipitating clinical event. Clinical manifestations of various organ system involvement is as follows:

In lungs, ARDS (acute respiratory distress syndrome) develops. There occurs tachypnea, chest wall retraction, grunting and frothy serosanguinous fluid from nose, mouth and ET tube with increasing severity.

Severe liver dysfunction and hepatic encephalopathy is uncommon in previously healthy children with acute illness leading to MODS but common in immunocompromised children with indolent sepsis.

In intestine, occult or frank GIT haemorrhage, intolerance to enteral feeding, abdominal distension, ileus, diarrhoea, GI ulcerations and over growth of Gram –ve bacilli and Candida commonly occurs.

In renal system involvement, oliguria and fluid over load can occur. Most survivors have complete recovery.

In hematological system, widespread petechiae, purpura, ecchymosis and haemmorhagic diathesis, DIC and bone marrow failure can occur.

In central nervous system, disorientation, agitation, confusion, lethargy or obtundation occurs. The child may also show inconsolable irritability, lack of interaction with parents or inability to be aroused. However significant encephalopathy is unusual. Peripheral neuropathy and muscle weakness has also been seen.

In CVS, poor myocardial contractility, decreased cardiac output, tachycardia, tachypnea, poor capillary refill, abnormal hemoregulation, cool and vasoconstricted peripheries and hypotension occurs.

The outlined criteria in Table 9.2 serve as good diagnostic and prognostic markers.

MANAGEMENT

The aim should be to prevent MODS. Prompt administration of antibiotics for bacterial infection should be ensured after taking suitable samples for culture and sensitivity. Immediate definitive management of all treatable injuries to limit inflammatory response should be done. Early reparative surgery to remove necrotic tissue should be done. Early drainage of abscesses should be performed. Antimalarials for plasmodium falciparum infection should be administered.[10]

Continuous monitoring is the most essential part of management of MODS. Pulse oximetry, continuous electrocardiography, continuous BP, temperature, urine output, CVP and oxygen saturation, pulmonary artery pressure and oxygen saturation , cardiac output and glucose and calcium should be monitored. According to the organ involved in MODS, the relevant investigations and monitoring should be done.[11]

Hypovolemia should be treated quickly. Vascular access should be rapidly attained. Interosseous access should be established if venous access cannot be established rapidly. In newborns, umbilical arterial or venous catheter is prefered. If this is not possible, peripheral arterial or peripherally positioned central catheter is to be placed. Central venous catheter should be placed for vasoactive infusions. Type of fluid used depends on cause of hypovolemia, amount of fluid required, availability and cost. For patients with diarrhoea and vomiting NS or RL 20 ml/kg may be used

Table 9.2: Criteria for specific organ system dysfunction[9]

Organ systems	*Criteria*	*MODS index*
Cardiovascular system	Systolic BP < 40 mm Hg (< 12 mth) Systolic BP < 50 mm Hg (> 12 mth) HR < 50 or > 220 beats/mt (< 12 mth) Cardiac arrest Serum pH < 7.2 with normal $PaCO_2$ Continuous vasoactive infusion to maintain BP	1
Respiratory system	RR > 90/mt (< 12 mth) RR > 90/mt (> 12 mth) $PaCO_2$ > 65 mm Hg PaO_2 < 40 mm Hg PaO_2/FiO_2 < 200 Mechanical ventilation (> 24 hours post operative) Tracheal intubation for airway obstruction	1
Neurological system	Glasgow Coma Scale < 8 Fixed, dilated pupils	1
Hematological system	Hb < 50 g/lt WBC < 3 × 109/lt Platelets < 20 × 109/lt Disseminated intravascular coagulapathy (DIC) (PT > 2.0 or PTT > 60s presence of fibrin split products)	1
Renal system	Serum urea nitrogen > 36 mmol/lt Serum creatinine > 177 mmol/lt Dialysis	1
GI system	Blood transfusion > 20 ml/kg 24 Haemorrhage Hr attributable to GI	1
Hepatic system	Total bilirubin > 60 mmol/It LDH > 2 × normal Hepatic encephalopathy > Grade 2	1

MODS index : Sum of points/7 and is expressed as percentage.

while observing for development of rales, gallop rhythm, hepatomegaly and increased work of breathing. The average requirement can be up to and over 40-60 ml/kg in the 1st hour. In newborns, fluid bolus of 10 ml/kg should be infused and up to 60 ml/kg may be infused in 1st hour. In septic shock, initially use isotonic crystalloids followed by isooncotic colloids like 5% albumin. Packed RBCs transfusion should be given in children with Hb < 10 gm%. Adequacy of fluid replacement in Ist hr. correlates to prognosis in septic shock. The goal should be to attain normal perfusion and BP.

In case of myocardial insufficiency, if after giving adequate fluid hemodynamic status is not restored, inotropic support is given by dopamine or dobutamine or both. Dose is adjusted according to clinical response.

In neonates, septic shock should be suspected in presence of maternal history of chorioamnionitis or prolonged rupture of membranes. Cardiogenic shock caused by closure of PDA should also be considered in newborns with hepatomegaly, cyanosis, cardiac murmur, differential upper and lower extremity BP and peripheral pulses. In refractory cases epinephrine infusion should be used for cold shock and norepinephrine for warm shock.

Adrenal insufficiency should be suspected in catecholamine resistant hypotensive shock in children with history of CNS abnormality or chronic steroid use or with purpura fulminans. Hydrocortisone should be used in a dose of 1-2 mg/kg for stress coverage to 50mg/kg for shock followed by same dose as 24-hr infusion. After achievement of normal BP, reduce after load to improve tissue perfusion. Nitroprusside or nitroglycerine are the first line vasodilators used. Continuous arterial B.P. monitoring should be done. Milrinone can also be used as an inodilator. Cardiac index of 3.3-6.0 Lt/min/m2 should be maintained. Children with catecholamine refractory shock must be suspected to have unrecognized morbidities like pericardial effusion, pneumothorax, hypoadrenalism, hypothyroidism, ongoing blood loss, and others.

Newborns suspected of having cardiogenic shock should be started on PGE1 until complex congenital heart disease is ruled out by echocardiographic analysis. Newborn septic shock is accompanied by persistent pulmonary hypertension which can cause right ventricular failure.

PPHN is treated by hyperoxygenation initially with 100% oxygen, and then metabolic alkalinization (up to pH 7.50) with $NaHCO_3$ or trimethamine is instituted. Mild hyper-

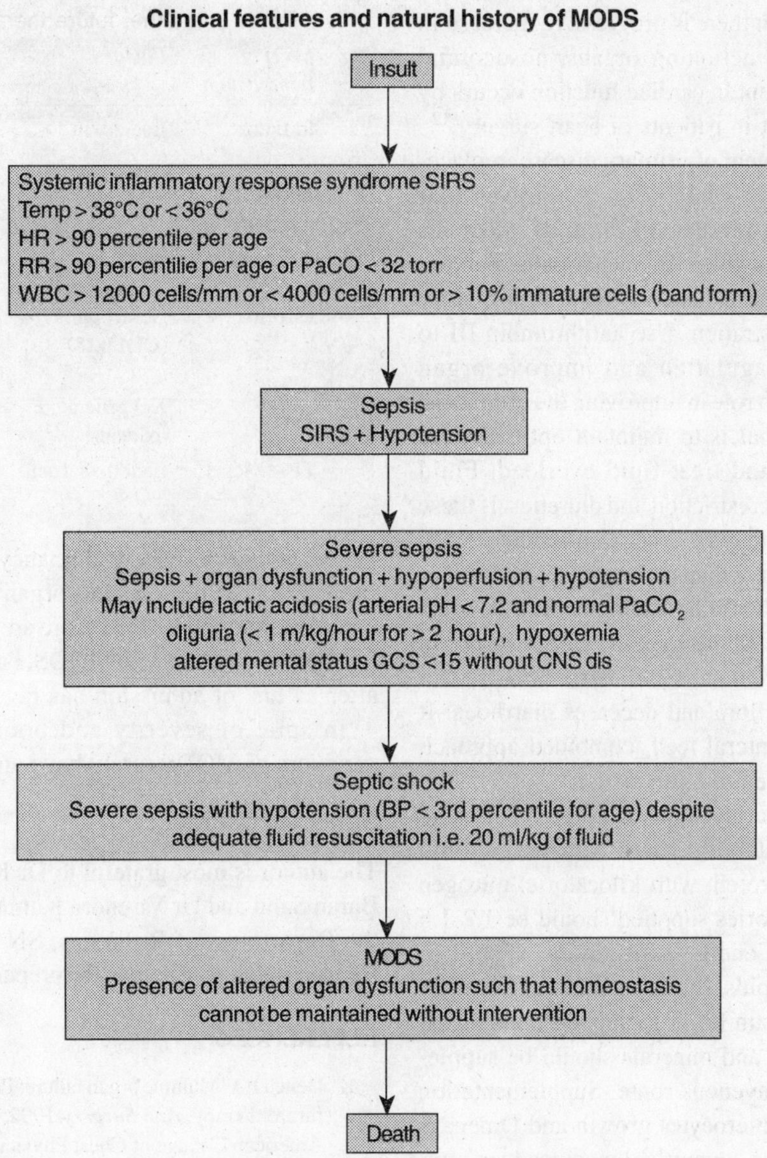

Fig. 9.3: Natural history of MODS[8,9]

ventilation can also be instituted until 100% oxygen saturation and <5% difference in preductal and postductal saturations are obtained. Therapeutic narcosis with fentanyl and paralysis with neuromuscular blocker should be considered to reduce pulmonary blood pressures in ventilated patients without response to the PPHN therapy outlined above. Inhaled nitric oxide should be considered when available.

O_2 delivery should be optimal in MODS patients. Oxygen delivery at 600 ml/mt/m^2 and O_2 consumption at 170 ml/mt/m^2 should be maintained. SaO_2 should be maintained at > 95%. Patients with respiratory distress and SPO_2 < 95% despite supplemental O_2 and clinical impression of respiratory fatigue are intubated electively and mechanically ventilated. In acute conditions, O_2 should be administered in as high concentration as possible and risk of O_2 toxicity should be neglected

PEEP allows decrease in FiO_2 and minimizes toxicity associated with prolonged use of O_2. Gradual increase in PEEP upto 8 to 10 cmH_2O is reasonable if each stepwise increase in PEEP is associated with increase in PaO_2. In conventional mechanical ventilation, protective ventilation strategy should be used with PEEP just above critical opening pressure, low tidal volume and permissive hypercapnia. High frequency ventilation improves gas exchange in some patients with ARDS not responding to conventional mechanical ventilation. HFJV (High frequency jet ventilation) and HFO (High frequency oscillation) are two main techniques for high frequency ventilation.

ECMO (Extracorporeal membrane oxygenation). Some patients who fail to respond to mechanical ventilation have improved oxygenation with ECMO. It should be started before irreversible lung injury occurs. ECMO withdrawal should be considered when there is progressive increase in number of abnormally functioning organs, nosocomial infection or no improvement in cardiac function occurs by 250 hrs of ECMO support in patients of heart surgery.[12]

DIC is treated by treatment of primary disease, replacement of clotting factors and inhibition of intravascular coagulation. Fresh frozen plasma (FFP) at 20 ml/kg for replacing clotting factors is given. If coagulopathy persists double volume exchange transfusion is done followed by FFP and platelets administration. Use antithrombin III to inhibit intravascular coagulation and improve organ perfusion.[14] Heparin has no role in improving the prognosis.

In renal failure, the goal is to maintain optimal fluid volume and to prevent and treat fluid overload. Fluid overload is treated by fluid restriction and diuretics. If these are not effective, dialysis may be used. Continuous hemodiafiltration is more effective than peritoneal dialysis.[15]

Early enteral feeding should be attempted as it bolsters antibacterial host defences, blunts hypermetabolic response to trauma, maintains mucosal mass and barrier and prevent disruption of normal gut flora and deceases diarrhoea. It patients cannot tolerate enteral feed, combined approach of enteral and parenteral feeding can be used.

In MODS, there is hyperglycemic, hypermetabolic and immunocompromised catabolic state. Nutrition should provide 1.5 to 2.5 g/kg protein with kilocalorie: nitrogen equal to 150-300:1.[16] Calories supplied should be 1.2-1.5 times the predicted basal energy expenditure. 2530% of calories are provided by lipids. Burns patient requires extra calories. Diet should contain fibres to support commensal flora of gut. All vitamins and minerals should be supplemented by enteral or intravenous route. Supplementation of glutamine to support enterocytes growth and Omega-3 and Omega-6 fatty acids to support colonocytes is recommended. Bile salts to neutralise gut bacterial toxins and arginine to support immune system should also be used.

Newer Therapeutic Strategies

Various newer therapeutic strategies are under trial for treatment of MODS. Some of these are mentioned in Table 9.3.

Other unproven strategies include-cyclo-oxygenase blockade, calcium channel antagonists, immunomodulators-IFN g, GM-CSF, PAF.

PROGNOSIS

It is related more to the number of organs involved than to any other variable, including underlying process initiating MODS. Length of time patient has had MODS also correlates directly with mortality rate. The clinical disease causing MODS also has strong influence on outcome.

Table 9.3: Other future therapeutic strategies

No.	Level of Intervention	Factor	Strategy
1.	Initiator	Endotoxin	Antibody mediated neutralisation
2.	Mediator	TNF a	Antibody mediated neutralisation
		IL-1	Target cell receptor blockade
3.	Effector	Neutrophils (CD11/18)	Antiadherence monoclonal antibodies, antioxidants
		XO generated oxidants	Antioxidants, inhibitors. inactivators of XO
4.	Tissue level	Endothelial cell	Anti ELAM-1 or anti ICAM-1 antibodies

Patient with underlying malignancy, malnutrition, immunosuppression or pre-existing organ dysfunction have poor outcome. Age and PRISM score are independent risk factors for death in children with MODS. Fall of procalcitonin levels after 24 hrs. of admission has favourable prognosis.[17]

In spite of severity and poor outcome of MODS, survivors of MODS rarely have any long-term sequelae.

Acknowledgements

The author is most grateful to Dr Kamal Singal, Dr. Timir Baran Sahu and Dr Virendra Kumar, all junior residents of the Department of Pediatrics, SN Medical College, Agra for their invaluable help in the preparation of this manuscript.

REFERENCES

1. Deitch EA. Multiple organ failure: Pathophysiology and potential future therapy. *Ann Surgery* 1992;216: 117-134.
2. American College of Chest Physicians/Society of Critical Care Medicine Consensus Conference. Definitions for Sepsis and Organ failure and guidelines for use of innovative therapies in sepsis. *Crit Care Med* 1992;20:864-875.
3. Whalen MJ,Doughty LA, Carlos TM, Wisnlewski SR. Intercellular adhesion molecule-1 and vascular cell adhesion molecule-1 are increased in the plasma of children with sepsis-induced multiple organ failure. *Crit Care Med* 2000;28:2600-2607.
4. Elizabeth DE, Moynihan JA, Ackerman MH. Does programmed cell death (apoptosis) play a role in development of multiple organ dysfunction in critically ill patients? A review and a theoretical framework. *Crit Care Med* 2000;28:537-549.
5. Metinz PGH, Fischer M, Bartens C, Stelzer H. Impact of acute renal failure on antioxidant status in multiple organ failure. *Acta Anaesthesiol Scand* 2000;44:236-240.
6. Fischer JE, Nussbaum MS, Chance WT, Luchette F. Mutiple organ failure syndrome. In: Schwartz's *Principles of Surgery,* 7th edn. New Delhi: Mc Graw Hill 1999;1074-1076.
7. Modebe O, Jain S. Multisystem failure in Plasmodium vivax malaria: Report of a case. *Ann Trop Med Para* 1999;93:409-412.

8. Powell KR. Sepsis and shock. In: Berman RE, Kliegman RM, Jenson HB (eds): *Nelson Textbook of Pediatrics*, 16th edn. Singapore: Harcourt Asia 2000; 747-751.
9. Goh A, Chan P, Lum L. Sepsis, severe sepsis and septic shock in pediatric multiple organ dysfuction syndrome. *J Pediatr Child Health* 1999;35:488-492.
10. Border. Multiple systems organ failure. *Ann Surgery* 1992;216: 111-116.
11. Carcillo JA, Fields AI. Clinical practice parameters for hemodynamic support in pediatric and neonatal patients in septic shock. *Crit Care Med* 2002;30: 1365-1378.
12. Montgomery VL, Strotman JM, Ross MP. Impact of multiple organ system dysfunction and nosocomial infections on survival of children treated with extracorporeal membrane oxygenation after heart surgery. *Crit Care Med* 2000;28:526-532.
13. Parker MM. Blood pressure support in patients with multiple organ failure: Is more better? *Crit Care Med* 2000;28:1223-24.
14. Dschietzig T, Alexiou K, Laule M et al. Stimulation of pulmonary big endothelin-1 and endothelin-1 by antithrombin III: A rationale for combined application of antithrombin III and endothelin antagonists in sepsis- related acute respiratory distress syndrome? *Crit Care Med* 2000;28:2445-2449.
15. Lowrie LH. Renal replacement therapies in pediatric multiorgan dysfunction syndrome. *Pediatr Nephrol* 2000;4:6-12.
16. Ronald ES, Wilson A. *Resuscitation through Rehabilitation in Trauma*. London: Smith and Smith 2002.
17. Hatherill M, Tibby SM, Turner C, Ratnavel N, Murdoch IA. Procalcitonin and cytokine levels: Relationship to organ failure and mortality in pediatric septic shock. *Crit Care Med* 2000;28:2591-2594.

Seema Kapoor and Suhasini Sharma

10 Anaphylaxis

INTRODUCTION

Anaphylaxis is a severe clinico-immunological reaction which has a potential to be fatal. In clinical practice and literature, the term 'anaphylaxis' has been used variably to connote the acute constellation of symptoms after exposure to an allergen, or to indicate the immunopathogenic mechanism consisting of an 'immediate' IgE-mediated hypersensitivity response.[1] In many cases of severe life-threatening reactions, however, antigen-specific IgE-antibody cannot be demonstrated. These reactions involve direct activation of mast cells which is independent of the IgE antibodies or complement cascade. Because these reactions are identical clinically, they are often termed 'anaphylactoid'. Example of this category is reaction to radiology contrast material and vancomycin.

The American Academy of Allergy, Asthma and Immunology defines anaphylaxis as "a collection of symptoms affecting multiple systems in the body." The most dangerous symptoms include breathing difficulties and a drop in blood pressure or shock, which are potentially fatal.[2] Thus, anaphylaxis is a *syndrome* with a multiplicity of inciting etiological agents and a variety of pathogenic mechanisms.

ETIOLOGY AND PREDISPOSING FACTORS

The materials capable of eliciting the systemic anaphylactic agents are given in Table 10.1.

Table 10.1: Causative agents implicated in anaphylaxis[3,4]

IgE mediated reactions

1. Protein drugs-insulin, ACTH, vasopressin
2. Non-protein drugs (haptens)–antibiotics; penicillin, sulfonamides, cephalosporins
3. Vaccines-pertussis, Typhoid
4. Foods-Eggs, fish, nuts, chocolate, fruits
5. Venoms-bee, wasp, snake
6. Foreign protein agents-tetanus antitoxin, gamma globulin, venom antitoxin
7. Enzymes-Trypsin, chymotrypsin, penicillinase
8. Allergen extracts-pollen, mould, animal dander
9. Chemicals-ethylene oxide gas, formaldehyde
10. Parasite-hydatid cyst rupture
11. Latex-Surgical gloves, catheter tip

Non-IgE mediated reactions

1. Opiates
2. Antibiotics
3. Plasma expanders
4. Muscle relaxants
5. Chemotherapeutic agents
6. Barbiturates
7. Radiocontrast media

Food induced anaphylaxis accounts for one-third to one-half of anaphylaxis cases treated in the emergency departments of North America, Europe and Australia;[1] it seems to be uncommon in Asian countries.[5] The food stuffs commonly implicated are peanuts, tree nuts, shellfish, milk, eggs, and the bisulfite additives to many foods. These food allergies can be fixed or cyclic. Many persons can lose their reactivity to a food allergen if the food is identified and eliminated from the diet for approximately 2 years and such sensitivity is known as cyclic food allergy. Allergic reactions to antibiotics occur frequently. Estimates of anaphylaxis caused by penicillin predict that 1 per 10,000 administrations will result in anaphylaxis.[6] In the hospital setting, anaphylaxis to latex has become one of the major causes of anaphylaxis perioperatively (Table 10.2).[7]

Age, race, sex, occupation, geographic location, and season of the year are not truly risk factors but they contribute to the eliciting agent. The risk for anaphylaxis increases with the length and frequency of exposure to a specific antigen. Repeated interrupted courses make one more susceptible. Administration of drugs by parenteral route is associated with an increased likelihood of developing a reaction as compared to the oral route. Atopy does not appear to be a risk factor for developing anaphylaxis by

Table 10.2: Hospital objects potentially containing G latex

Blood pressure cuffs
Stethoscopes
Gloves
Surgical caps
Catheters
Oral and nasal airways
Tourniquets
Intravenous tubing
Syringes
Electrode pads
Band aids
Rubber tops of multidose vials
Dental mouth guards
Surgical drains
Anesthesia facemasks
Endotracheal tubes
Household Objects Potentially Containing Latex
Automobile tires
Carpeting
Swimming goggles
Shoes
Dish washing gloves
Hot water bottles
Earphones
Pantyhose
Rubber balls
Balloons
Chewing gum
Cosmetics
Baby bottle nipples
Pacifiers
Rubber bands
Erasers
Adhesive tape
Stamps
Condoms
Elastic in clothes (especially in waistbands)

certain triggers e.g., bee stings and medications but is for others like food, latex and radiocontrast media.[4] Reactions to foods occur in patients who are highly allergic and the presence of asthma appears to be a risk factor for more severe outcomes.[8] Many forms of exercise, with or without the ingestion of certain foods, can cause an anaphylactic reaction. Vigorous anaerobic activity is more likely to precipitate an event than less strenuous activities. Fortunately, the number of episodes tends to stabilize or decrease over time. Treatment consists of exercise modification and avoidance of any food precipitants that can be identified as cofactors.

CLINICAL FEATURES

The syndrome of anaphylaxis can include any or all of the symptoms listed in Table 10.3.

Table 10.3: Clinical features of anaphylaxis[1]

Oral:
Pruritus of lips, tongue and palate and edema of lips and tongue; metallic taste in the mouth
Cutaneous:
Flushing, pruritus, urticaria, angioedema, morbilliform rash and pilor erecti
Gastrointestinal:
Nausea, abdominal pain, vomiting (large amounts of 'stringy mucus'), and diarrhea
Respiratory:
Laryngeal: pruritus and tightness in throat, dysphagia, dysphonia and hoarseness, dry 'staccato' cough
Lungs: dyspnoea, chest tightness, wheezing
Nose: pruritus, congestion, rhinorrhea, and sneezing
Cardiovascular:
Feeling of faintness, syncope, chest pain, dysrhythmia, hypotension
Other:
Periorbital pruritus, conjunctival erythema, aura of "doom"

Typically the reaction begins to develop within minutes of exposure and usually reaches its maximum within 15 to 30 minutes. However, in some cases symptoms may not become severe until hours later. Lower respiratory tract symptoms, such as wheezing and shortness of breath, are almost exclusively seen in patients with underlying asthma.[4] The development of cardiovascular symptoms and airway obstruction is of greatest clinical significance. Hypotension and vascular collapse may be primary events or secondary complications of asphyxia or cardiac dysrhythmias.[3]

The onset of symptoms, however, is a good indicator of the severity of the reaction. Generally, sooner the onset of symptoms, the more severe is the reaction. Anaphylaxis may be divided temporally into isolated immediate, biphasic, and protracted reactions. Isolated immediate reactions usually resolve within hours of their onset. Biphasic reactions are characterized by an initial onset of symptoms, partial or complete resolution of these symptoms, and a subsequent late response that mimics the initial response but occurs hours later. Protracted reactions consist of symptoms that are refractory to all forms of therapy for hours or days. The biphasic pattern is estimated to occur in 5% to 20% of anaphylactic reactions, with a similar rate reported for protracted cases. The biphasic or protracted patterns of anaphylaxis are more likely to occur after oral administration of antigen or when symptoms begin 30 minutes or more after exposure to the stimulus.[9,10]

PATHOPHYSIOLOGY

Most cases of anaphylaxis are IgE mediated. Following previous exposure to an antigen, IgE antibodies are released into the circulation by plasma cells derived from B-lymphocytes, under the influence of helper T-cells. These antibodies bind to glycoprotein receptors on tissue mast cells or blood-borne basophils, thereby sensitizing them.

Subsequent re-exposure to the antigen cross-links the Fab portions of two surface-bound IgE molecules, activating the cell and triggering the release of chemical mediators. Mast cell and basophil activation results in the release of preformed and generated mediators (Table 10.4).

Table 10.4: Preformed mast cell mediators

1. Vasoactive mediator-Histamine
2. Chemotactic mediators- Neutrophil chemotactic factor, Eosinophil chemotactic factor
3. Enzymes-Tryptase, Chymase, Beta-glucuronidase, Beta-hexosaminidase, Arylsulphatase-A
4. Proteoglycans-Heparin, Chondroitin sulphate
Mediators generated as a result of mast cell activation
1. Arachidonic acid metabolites: cyclooxygenase pathway-Prostaglandin D_2, Thromboxane A_2, Lipoxygenase pathway-Leukotreines LTB_4, LTC_4, LTD_4, LTE_4
2. Platelet-activating factor (PAF)
3. Cytokines-Interleukins, Tumor necrosis factor
4. Adenosine

The action of these mediators may be divided into 3 categories. First, histamine, PAF, tryptase and bradykinin are inflammatory activators that induce vasodilation and edema. Secondly, histamine, prostaglandin D_2, LTC_4 and LTD_4 are agents that cause bronchial smooth muscle contraction, increased mucous production and mucosal edema. Thirdly, neutrophil chemotactic factor, eosinophil chemotactic factor and LTB_4 are chemotactic agents which recruit other inflammatory cells (neutrophils, eosinophils, lymphocytes, monocytes, mast cells and basophils). These newly recruited cells in turn release secondary mediators of anaphylaxis such as histamine releasing factor, major basic protein and lysosomal enzymes causing more inflammation and tissue destruction. A further wave of mast cell degranulation is induced, leading to a vicious cycle of ongoing inflammation associated with increased vascular permeability.

However, some of the secondary mediators released, in particular by eosinophils, inhibit anaphylaxis. For instance, histaminase breaks down histamine, arylsulphatase B inactivates leukotrienes, and phospholipase D destroys PAF. Thus the anaphylactic process may be self-limiting in less severe reactions.[3]

Anaphylactoid reactions are non-IgE mediated and are caused by mediator release that is triggered independently of reaginic antibodies. These reactions do not require prior exposure and patients may not react on every occasion. Anaphylactoid reactions may be due to direct release of mediators from mast cells by medications and physical factors (e.g. morphine, exercise); disturbances of leukotriene metabolism (e.g. aspirin, NSAIDs); immune aggregates and complement activation (blood products); probable complement activation (e.g. radiocontrast dyes).[11]

DIAGNOSIS

The history and physical examination remain the mainstay of diagnosis. Elucidating a temporal relationship between onset of symptoms and possible antigen exposure should be the focus of the history in a suspected episode of anaphylaxis. Serum analysis of tryptase levels is valuable in confirming an anaphylactic reaction, although treatment of a suspected reaction should not be postponed while waiting for assay results. Tryptase is a preformed mediator released by mast cells on antigen exposure and has a half-life of several hours. Histamine, on the other hand, has a half-life of minutes and can be measured by immunoassay only if blood is drawn very early in an acute event. Optimally, a mast cell tryptase assay should be taken within the first hour of an attack and then repeated at 2, 12, and 24 hours

DIFFERENTIAL DIAGNOSIS

A diagnosis of anaphylaxis is usually readily apparent because of its abrupt onset, temporal association to the causative agent, and dramatic physiological features. In practical terms, it is not necessary to differentiate between anaphylactic and anaphylactoid reactions at the time of patient presentation as both respond to the same treatment, however anaphylactic shock must be differentiated from other causes of circulatory collapse. The differential diagnoses of anaphylaxis is presented in Table 10.5.

Table 10.5: Differential diagnosis of anaphylaxis[12]

Acute Respiratory Decompensation
Severe asthma, foreign body aspiration, pulmonary embolism
Loss of Consciousness
Vasovagal reaction, seizure disorder, myocardial infarction, arrhythmias
Disorders Resembling Anaphylaxis
Systemic mastocytosis, carcinoid syndrome, hereditary angioedema
Non-organic disease
Hyperventilation syndrome, panic attacks, vocal cord dysfunction

Vasovagal collapse is the condition that most frequently needs to be differentiated from anaphylaxis. It is usually preceded by an anxiety-provoking or a painful situation and leads to an abrupt syncopal episode. Associated features include pallor, diaphoresis and complaints of nausea before collapse. Distinguishing features include lack of pruritus and respiratory difficulties, maintenance of blood pressure, bradycardia and resolution of symptoms with recumbency.

Hyperventilation syndrome occurs frequently in adolescents at times of stress, especially during athletic events, and can be associated with breathlessness and collapse. Again differentiation can be made by noting that blood pressure and pulse are maintained and that numbness of the lips and extremities, tetany and chest pain can be associated findings.

Hereditary angioedema should be considered when laryngeal edema and abdominal pain are part of the presenting symptoms, especially if the symptoms are slowly progressive, there is a lack of urticaria and hypotension and a positive family history can be elicited.[4,13]

TREATMENT

Anaphylaxis is a medical emergency which requires immediate treatment. Establishing a patent airway and providing adequate oxygenation and ventilation are the first priorities. Effective ventilation may be compromised by the development of laryngeal edema, necessitating endotracheal intubation. Supplemental oxygen should be provided to ensure a PaO_2 of at least 60 mmHg. The mainstay of treatment for anaphylactic shock is oxygen, adrenaline and fluids.[3]

Adrenaline

Adrenaline should be given to all patients with significant hypotension, airway swelling or bronchospasm. The actions of adrenaline reverse all features of anaphylaxis. α-adrenegic stimulation increases peripheral vascular resistance and coronary artery perfusion raising the blood pressure, reverses peripheral vasodilation and decreases angioedema and urticaria. β_1 adrenergic stimulation has positive inotropic and chronotropic effects on cardiac muscle, and β_2 adrenergic stimulation leads to bronchodilation. b-adrenergic receptors also increase the production of intracellular cyclic AMP which inhibits further mast cell mediator release.[14] The dose is 0.01 ml/kg, upto a maximum 0.3 ml of a 1:1000 dilution. Recent research has established the intramuscular route to be superior to the subcutaneous route.[15,16] Adrenaline can be reinjected every 5-15 minutes until there is a resolution of the anaphylaxis or signs of hyperadrenalism (including palpitations, tremor, uncomfortable apprehension and anxiety occur. Intravenous adrenaline (1:10,000 dilution) should be administered only in severe hypotensive shock because of its potential for tachyarrhythmias.

Although some reports suggest that inhalation of racemic epinephrine may be an effective alternative form of therapy for anaphylaxis,[17] a recent controlled trial failed to confirm the efficacy of this therapeutic approach in children.[18] If wheezing is prominent, then an aerosolied β-adrenergic agent (e.g. salbutamol) is recommended intermittently or continuously, depending on the patient's symptoms.

Once therapy is initiated, a continuous infusion of adrenaline can be started if no improvement is seen with bolus doses. Infusion rates of 0.1 mg/kg/min are advised, increasing in increments of 0.1 mg/kg/min. Patients on β-blockers or on chronic treatment with β-agonists, who may have down-regulation of their β-receptors, may not respond as well to treatment with adrenaline and may need higher doses to achieve the same physiological effects. Attention to acid-base and electrolyte status is important because abnormalities could prevent successful treatment by decreasing the action of sympathomimetics and interfering with cardiac function.

In the patient who has been receiving β-blockers and who is not responding well to sympathomimetics, glucagon administration may be of benefit. Glucagon increases myocardial contractility and heart rate without interacting with β-receptors, presumably because of its ability to stimulate adenyl cyclase directly, leading to increases in intracellular cAMP.[14]

Fluid Therapy

Placement of a large-bore intravenous line for medication administration and restoration of the hypovolemia produced by vasodilation and increased permeability is another major objective of successful therapy of anaphylactic shock. Crystalloid solutions such as normal saline or Ringer's lactate may be given rapidly at 10-20 ml/kg. Alternatively, colloids including albumin, dextran 70, and gelatin preparations may be given, also at 10-20 ml/kg. Large volumes of fluid are required. Measurement of central venous pressure and packed cell volume helps in guiding treatment. Although both solutions have been used successfully, the 3-6 fold extra requirement with crystalloids, their dilution of the colloid oncotic pressure, and the longer lasting capillary leakage which prolongs resuscitation are factors favoring the use of colloids in anaphylactic shock.[1,4,14]

Antihistaminics

Antihistaminics cannot have a central role in the management of anaphylaxis, as the concentration of histamine in the vicinity of a mast cell after degranulation is so great, that by the time anaphylaxis is diagnosed, it is too late for a competitive blocker to be of value. Their role is subsidiary to that of oxygen, adrenaline and fluids. Current recommendations are to administer H_1 and H_2 antihistaminics agents in combination, because H_1 and H_2 blockade is more effective than H_1 blockade alone in preventing the symptomatology of anaphylaxis in experimental models.[19] The pediatric doses are diphenhydramine 1 mg/kg and cimetidine 5 mg/kg or ranitidine 1-2 mg/kg.

Steroids

The role of steroids in the management of acute anaphylaxis is limited to the prevention or shortening of protracted reactions, particularly those associated with bronchospasm. This is despite their many theoretical benefits, which include an increase in tissue responsiveness to β-adrenergic agonists, inhibition of mediator release, down regulating cell activation, prevention of neutrophil and platelet aggregation, and decreasing IgE receptor expression. Even if given intravenously, steroids may take upto four to six hours to be maximally effective. The recommendation is intravenous hydrocortisone 5 mg/kg followed by 2.5 mg/kg 6 hrly; or methylprednisolone 2 mg/kg loading followed by 1 mg/kg/dose 6 hrly; or prednisolone 1 to 2 mg/kg/day orally divided 6 hourly.[3,14]

Observation

Despite adequate response to therapy initially, some patients may go on to develop late-phase responses. Therefore, patients must be kept under close observation for at least 8 to 12 hours to facilitate prompt treatment of any subsequent reaction, should it develop.

Table 10.5: Emergency management of anaphylaxis

Rapid clinical assessment
1. Airway management
2. Supplemental oxygen
3. Adrenaline: 0.01 ml/kg intramuscularly
4. Intravenous access and fluid expansion
5. H1 antagonist: Diphenhydramine i.v, i.m, or oral
6. H2 antagonist: Ranitidine i.v. or oral
7. Corticosteroids: Hydrocortisone or methylprednisolone i.v., or oral prednisolone
8. Nebulized salbutamol
9. Post reaction treatment: H1 antagonist- Cetirizine, Fexofenadine, Loratidine for 3 days
Steroid-oral prednisolone 1 mg/kg/day for 3 days

PREVENTION

The first step in the prevention of anaphylaxis is identification of the causative agent, if possible. Confirmation of the cause requires referral to an allergist for a skin prick test and when deemed necessary, *in-vitro* assessment for the presence of specific IgE antibodies. Referral for skin prick testing is particularly important when no causative agent can be clearly identified by history or for bee or wasp stings, because confirmation of IgE mediated reactivity is necessary to offer potentially curative immunotherapy.[20,21] In the case of drug or food allergy, not only must the offending substance be avoided, but the potential for cross-reactivity (e.g., cephalosporins in the case of penicillin allergy) must also be recognized.[6]

SUMMARY

Anaphylaxis is a syndrome with clinical manifestations that can range in severity from localized urticaria to death. Precipitating factors are numerous, as are the potential immunological, biological, and physiological mechanisms responsible for the initiation, propagation and target organ preference for the clinical response. Successful recognition and treatment of anaphylaxis represent one of the most challenging and gratifying elements of patient care because the time interval between life and death in many patients may only be a matter of minutes.

REFERENCES

1. Sampson HA. Anaphylaxis and Emergency treatment. *Pediatrics* 2003;111:1601-1608.
2. AAAAI Board of Director. Anaphylaxis in schools and other child-care settings. *J Allergy Clin Immunol*. 1998;102:173-176.
3. Broun AFT. Anaphylactic Shock: mechanisms and treatment. *J Accid Emerg Med* 1995;12:89-100.
4. Ritter M, Lemanske RF. Anaphylaxis. In : Fuhrman BP, Zimmerman J (eds): *Pediatric Critical Care*, 2nd edn. St Louis: Mosby 1998;1129-1140.
5. Hill OJ, Hosking CS, Heine AG. Clinical spectrum of food allergy in children in Australia and South-East Asia: identification and targets for treatment. *Ann Med* 1999;31:272-281.
6. Saxon A, Beall GN, Rohe AS et al. Immediate hypersensitivity reactions to beta-lactam antibiotics. *Ann Int Med* 1987;107: 204-215.
7. Slater JE. Latex allergy. *J Allergy Clin Immunol* 1994;2:139.
8. Sampson HA, Mendelson L, Rosen JP. Fatal and neat fatal anaphylactic reactions to food in children and adolescents. *N Engl J Med* 1992;327-380-384.
9. Stark BJ, Sullivan TJ. Biphasic and protracted anaphylaxis. *J Allergy Clin Immunol* 1986;78:75.
10. Douglas DM, Sukenick E, Andrade WP, et al. Biphasic systemic anaphylaxis: an inpatient and outpatient study. *J Allergy Clin Immunol* 1994;93: 977-985.
11. Smapson HA, Leung DYM. Anaphylaxis. In Berhman RE, Liegman KM, Jenson HB (eds): *Nelson Textbook of Pediatrics*, 17th edn. Philadelphia: WB Saunders 2004;781-783
12. Ellis AK, Day JH. Anaphylaxis: diagnosis and treatment. *Allergy Asthma* 2000;13:22-35.
13. Ellis AK, Day JH. Diagnosis and management of anaphylaxis. *CMAJ* 2003;104:307-312.
14. Brown AFT. Therapeutic controversies in the Management of acute anaphylaxis. *J Accid Emerg Med* 1998;15:89-95.
15. Simons FE, Roberts JR, Ger X, Simons KJ. Epinephrine absorption in children with a history of anaphylaxis. *J Allergy Clin Immunol*. 1998;101:33-37.
16. Simons FER, Gu X, Simons KJ. Epinephrine absorption in adults: Intramuscular versus subcutaneous injection. *J Allery Clin Immunol* 2001;108:871-873.
17. Heilboun H, Hjemdahl P, Daleskog M, Adamsson U. Comparision of subcutaneous injection and high dose inhalation of epinephime: implications for self-treatment to prevent anaphylasis. *J Allergy Clin Immunol* 1986;78:1174-1179.
18. Gu X, Simous KJ, Johuston L, Gillesoie C, Simous EF. Can epinephrine inhalations be substituted for epinephrine injections in children at risk for systemic anaphylaxis? *Pediatrics* 2000;106: 1040-1044.
19. Lieberman P. The use of antihistaminics in the prevention and treatment of anaphylaxis and anaphylactoid reactions. *J Allergy Clin Immunol* 1990;86:684-686.
20. Reisman RE. Venom Insect Stings. *N Engl J Med* 1994;331: 523-527.
21. Sturm G, Kranks B, Rudolf C, O Aberer W. Rush hymenoptera venom immunotherapy: A safe and practical protocol for high risk patients. *J Allergy Clin Immunol* 2002;110:928-933.

Section III

Acute Severe Tropical Infections

Preeti Shanbag and Manisha Juvekar

11 Severe Malaria

INTRODUCTION

Malaria remains a devastating global health problem. Worldwide, an estimated 300 to 500 million people contract malaria each year, resulting in 1.5 to 2.7 million deaths annually.[1,2] *P falciparum* is a major cause of death in tropical areas.[2] The other three species cause acute febrile illnesses, that although unpleasant, rarely cause severe morbidity. Rarely, *P vivax* or *P ovale* produces serious complications, debilating relapses, and even death.[3] The virulence of *P falciparum* is attributed to its propensity to produce heavy parasite burdens and its ability to cytoadhere to the vascular endothelium, which leads to sequestration of parasitized red blood cells in the microvasculature of vital organs, whereas the other malarias seldom parasitize more than 2% of the erythrocytes and do not sequester. *P falciparum* and *P vivax* account for most clinical cases worldwide. *P falciparum* predominates in sub-Saharan Africa; *P vivax* predominates in Latin America. There are also many areas of mixed species transmission.[4]

Severe and complicated malaria is a serious systemic disease characterized by multiorgan failure, much in the same way as bacterial septicemia. Severe malaria reflects one end of a spectrum of disease severity in malaria and has a treated mortality rate of 15 to 30%, even with intensive care management. The overall mortality rate of acute, uncomplicated falciparum malaria is 200 times lower, approximately 0.1%.[5]

PATHOPHYSIOLOGY

The pathophysiology of severe malaria results from destruction of erythrocytes, the liberation of parasites and erythrocyte material into the circulation and the host reaction to these events.

Cytokines

An increasing body of evidence from both murine models and human studies indicates that cytokines, along with T cells, natural killer (NK) cells, and macrophages, contribute either to the resolution of malaria infection or to a persistent increase in concentrations of malaria parasitemia, which leads to complicated malaria such as cerebral malaria.[6,7] *P falciparum* is considered an intracellular pathogen, since it can be seen within hepatocytes during the exoerythrocytic stage and invades red blood cells during the intraerythrocytic stage of disease. As with other intracellular pathogens—including *Listeria monocytogenes, Salmonella typhimurium,* and *Toxo plasma gondii*—the rapid production of proinflammatory and phagocyte-activating cytokines by natural killer (NK) cells is a key factor of early host resistance against intracellular infection.[8, 9]

Resolution of *P falciparum* malaria may be dependent on a very early and effective activation of macrophages, stimulated by various malarial antigens to produce and secrete proinflammatory cytokines like interleukins (IL) 12 and 18, tumor necrosis factor (TNF) α, and interferon γ. Transforming growth factor (TGF) β sems to be an important cytokine for maintaining the balance between protection and progression towards severe malaria. Omer et al[10] reported that TGF β has proinflammatory activity at low concentrations, whereas high concentrations of TGF β are associated with anti-inflammatory activity as seen in severe *P falciparum* malaria.

Thus, it seems that an early proinflammatory cytokine response, including IL12, IL18, and TGF β (at low concentrations) mediates protective immunity, whereas a persistent and late anti-inflammatory cytokine response, including TNF α and TGF β (at high concentrations) contributes to severe and complicated *P falciparum* malaria.

Sequestration[11]

The process whereby erythrocytes containing mature forms of *P falciparum* adhere to microvascular endothelium ('cytoadherence') and, thus, disappear from circulation is known as sequestration. Sequestration is thought to be central to the pathophysiology of falciparum malaria. Cytoadherence begins at the middle of the parasites' 48-hrs asexual life cycle. Mature malarial parasites are rarely seen on blood smears in falciparum malaria, and if seen indicate serious infection. Sequestration occurs predominantly in the venules of vital organs. It is not distributed uniformly throughout the body, being greatest in the brain, particularly the white matter, prominent in the heart, liver, kidneys, intestines and adipose tissue, and least in the skin. Cytoadherence and the related phenomenon of 'rosetting' (i.e. adherence of erythrocytes containing parasites to uninfected erythrocytes) lead to microcirculatory obstruction in falciparum malaria. The consequences of microcirculatory obstruction are reduced oxygen and substrate supply, leading to anaerobic glycolysis and lactic acidosis.

Immunological Processes[11]

Immune mechanisms have not been proven to have a role in the pathogenesis of malaria. Malarial infections induce both cellular and humoral immune responses and there is evidence of complement activation in acute malaria. In severe malaria there is evidence of a broader immune suppression, with defects in monocyte and neutrophil chemotaxis, reduced monocytic phagocytic function and a tendency to bacterial superinfection. In the nephrotic syndrome associated with chronic *P malariae* infections, malarial antigen and immune complexes can be eluted from the kidney

Permeability [11]

There is evidence of a mild generalized increase in systemic vascular permeability in severe malaria. It is now clear from imaging studies that the majority of adults and children with cerebral malaria have no evidence of cerebral edema. Studies of computerized tomography or magnetic resonance imaging have generally shown slight brain swelling in cerebral malaria (compatible with an increased intracerebral blood volume) but no evidence of cerebral edema. Thus, raised intracranial pressure probably arises from an increase in cerebral blood volume, independent of permeability.

The major complications of severe malaria include cerebral malaria, pulmonary edema, acute renal failure, severe anemia, and/or bleeding. Acidosis and hypoglycemia are the most common metabolic complications. Any of these complications can develop rapidly and progress to death within hours or days.[12] In many patients, several of these complications exist together or evolve in rapid succession within a few hours. In clinical practice, patients must be assessed for any of these signs or symptoms that suggest an increased risk for developing complications and must be treated immediately.[13-15] In tropical countries with a high transmission of malaria (hyperendemic areas), severe malaria is predominantly a disease of young children (1 month to 5 years of age).[15]

In 1990, the World Health Organization (WHO) established criteria for severe malaria in order to assist future clinical and epidemiological studies.[16] In 2000, the WHO revised these criteria to include other clinical manifestations and laboratory values that predict a poor prognosis based on clinical experience in semi-immune patients. These are summarized in Table 11.1.

Patients with severe malaria should be treated in an ICU. Should clinical deterioration occur, it usually develops 3 to 7 days after fever onset, although there have been rare reports of nonimmune patients dying within 24 hours of developing symptoms. Severe malaria may develop even after initial treatment response and complete clearance of parasitemia due to delayed cytokine release.

Neurologic Complications

Cerebral malaria is the most common clinical presentation and cause of death in adults with severe malaria. The onset may be dramatic with a generalized convulsion, or gradual with initial drowsiness and confusion, followed by coma lasting from several hours to several days. The strict definition of cerebral malaria requires the presence of *P falciparum* parasitemia and the patient to be unrousable with a Glasgow Coma Scale score of 9 or less, and other causes (e.g. hypoglycemia, bacterial meningitis and viral encephalitis) ruled out.[16] From a practical standpoint, any alteration in mental status should be treated as cerebral malaria. A lumbar puncture should be performed to rule out bacterial meningitis. To distinguish cerebral malaria from transient postictal coma, unconsciousness should persist for at least 30 min after a convulsion. The deeper the coma, the worse is the prognosis. The Blantyre Coma Scale should be used in infants and small children (Table 11.2.).[16]

In an unconscious patient, a drop in score from 2 to 0 may be the only clinical clue to the development of a complication e.g. hypoglycemia on examination of the nervous system.

On examination, neurologic abnormalities resemble those of a diffuse symmetric encephalopathy, similar to a metabolic encephalopathy. Nuchal rigidity and focal neurologic signs may occur but are rare. In patients with profound coma, corneal reflexes and 'dolls eye' movements may be absent and there may be abnormalities of conjugate gaze. The pupils are usually mid-size and non reactive and the fundus is unremarkable. Papilloedema is rare but retinal hemorrhages may be seen in 15.1% of cases more if indirect opthalmoscopy is used. The hemorrhages are often flame-shaped, and may have a pale center resembling Roth spots. Corneal reflex may be lost with deep coma in children (a poor prognostic sign). There may be forced jaw closure with repetitive spontaneous teeth grinding (bruxism).[11] The jaw jerk is sometimes brisk and there is often a pout reflex.

Table 11.1: Indicators of severe malaria and poor prognosis

Manifestation	*Features*
Initial World Health Organization criteria 1990 [16]	
Cerebral malaria	Unrousable coma not attributable to any other cause, with a Glasgow Coma Scale score = 9. Coma should persist for at least 30 min after a generalized convulsion
Severe anemia	Hematocrit <15% or hemoglobin < 50 g/l in the presence of parasite count >10 000/µl
Renal failure	Urine output <400 ml/24 hours in adults (<12 ml/kg/24 hours in children) and a serum creatinine>265 µmol/l (> 3.0 mg/dl) despite adequate volume repletion
Pulmonary edema and acute respiratory distress syndrome	The acute lung injury score is calculated on the basis of radiographic densities, severity of hypoxemia, and positive end-expiratory pressure
Hypoglycemia	Whole blood glucose concentration <2.2 mmol/l (<40 mg/dl)
Circulatory collapse (algid malaria)	Systolic blood pressure <70 mmHg in patients > 5 years of age (< 50 mmHg in children aged 1-5 years), with cold clammy skin or a core-skin temperature difference >10°C
Abnormal bleeding and/or disseminated intravascular coagulation	Spontaneous bleeding from gums, nose, gastrointestinal tract, or laboratory evidence of disseminated intravascular coagulation
Repeated generalized convulsions	≥ 3 convulsions observed within 24 hours
Acidemia/acidosis	Arterial pH < 7.25 or acidosis (plasma bicarbonate < 15 mmol/l)
Macroscopic hemoglobinuria	Hemolysis not secondary to glucose-6-phosphate dehydrogenase deficiency
Added World Health Organization criteria 2000 [12]	
Impaired consciousness	Rousable mental condition
Prostration or weakness	
Hyperparasitemia	> 5% parasitized erythrocytes or > 250 000 parasites/µl (in nonimmune individuals)
Hyperpyrexia	Core body temperature > 40°C
Hyperbilirubinemia	Total bilirubin > 43 µmol/l (> 2.5 mg/dl)

Table 11.2: Blantyre coma scale [16]

	Score
a. Best motor response	
• Localizes painful stimulus	2
• Withdraws limb from pain	1
• Non-Specific or absent response	0
b. Verbal response	
• Appropriate cry	2
• Moan or inappropriate cry	1
• None	0
c. Eye movements	
• Directed (e.g., follows mother's face)	1
• Not directed	0

Other frontal release signs are very unusual, cranial nerve abnormalities are rare. Abnormalities of posture are often seen.[16, 17]

The abdominal reflexes are invariably absent, the cremasteric reflexes often preserved and the plantar responses are extensor in approximately half the patients. Patients may exhibit phasic increases in tone with extensor posturing of the decorticate, or more usually, decerebrate type. The back may arch in opisthotonos (which may misleadingly suggest a diagnosis of tetanus and meningitis) with sustained usual upward and lateral ocular deviation.

The duration of coma varies considerably but is overall shorter (average of 1 day) in children. Monoplegia, hemiplegia, tremors and signs of cerebellar involvement may be present.[18] Convulsions are usually generalized, with nonspecific abnormalities on electroencephalographic examination. Computed tomography or magnetic resonance imaging often shows evidence of mild cerebral swelling; marked edema or focal lesions are unusual. Delirium, agitation, and even transient paranoid psychosis may develop as the patient recovers consciousness.

Several hypotheses have been proposed to explain the pathophysiology of cerebral malaria, but none is completely satisfactory. The excellent neurologic recovery argues against ischemia alone being the culprit. Raised intracranial pressure, at least in nonimmune adults, appears not to play an important role in the pathogenesis of cerebral malaria. The mortality of cerebral malaria ranges from 10 to 50% with treatment. Most survivors (>97% adults and >90% children) have no neurologic abnormalities on hospital discharge.[19]

Post-Malaria Neurological Syndromes

In approximately 10% of children there is a persistent neurological deficit following cerebral malaria.[17] In children this is associated with profound and protracted coma, anemia, hypoglycemia and prolonged convulsions. In approximately 60% of cases there is a hemiparesis and variable hemisensory deficit sometimes hemianopia, ataxia 43%, hemiplegia 42%, speech disorders 28% behavioral disorders 24%, epilepsy 24%, blindness 8%, and diffuse cortical damage 6%. Tremor and occasionally cranial nerve palsies may occur.[11]

Hematologic abnormalities [11]

The pathogenesis of anemia is multifactorial. There is obligatory destruction of red cells containing parasites at merogony. There is also accelerated destruction of non-parasitied red cells that parallels disease severity. The rapid hemolysis of unparasitized red cells is a major contributor to the decline in hematocrit. The hemolytic anemia is compounded by bone marrow dysfunction; dyserythropoeisis persists for days or weeks following acute malaria and reticulocyte counts are usually low in the acute phase of disease. Immune-mediated hemolysis has also been suggested as a mechanism of anemia. Red cell survival is shortened. Severe anemia is more common in children in highly endemic areas due to repeated or chronic Plasmodium infections.

Thrombocytopenia is common, but usually not associated with bleeding. Disseminated intravascular coagulation is reported in fewer than 10% of patients with severe malaria.

There is an accelerated coagulation cascade activity with accelerated fibrinogen turnover, consumption of antithrombin III and increased concentrations of fibrin degradation products.

Renal Complications

Acute renal failure is usually oliguric or anuric, rarely nonoliguric, and may require temporary dialysis.[20] In severe cases, acute tubular necrosis may develop secondary to renal microvascular obstruction consequent to sequestration in the kidney.[21] The term 'blackwater fever' refers to passage of dark red, brown, or black urine secondary to massive intravascular hemolysis and resulting hemoglobinuria. This occurs even in patients with normal G-6-PD levels and has been associated with use of quinine, though the mechanism is poorly understood. Significant glomerulonephritis is very rare.

Pulmonary Complications

Acute lung injury usually occurs a few days into the disease course. It may develop rapidly, even after initial response to antimalarial treatment and clearance of parasitemia. The first indications of impending pulmonary edema include tachypnea and dyspnea, followed by hypoxemia and respiratory failure requiring intubation. Pulmonary edema is usually noncardiogenic and may progress to acute respiratory distress syndrome (ARDS) with an increased pulmonary capillary permeability.[22] Acute lung injury is defined as the acute onset of bilateral pulmonary infiltrates with an arterial oxygen tension/fractional inspired oxygen ratio of 300 mmHg or less, a pulmonary artery wedge pressure of 18 mmHg or less, and no evidence of left atrial hypertension. ARDS is defined as acute lung injury and an arterial oxygen tension/fractional inspired oxygen ratio of 200 or less.[23] Volume overload and hypoalbuminemia may aggravate pulmonary capillary leakage. Chest radiograph abnormalities range from confluent nodules to basilar and/or diffuse bilateral pulmonary infiltrates. Noncardiogenic pulmonary edema rarely occurs with *P vivax* and *P ovale* malaria.

Hypoglycemia[24,25]

Hypoglycemia is a common feature in patients with severe malaria. It may be overlooked because all clinical features of hypoglycemia (anxiety, dyspnea, tachycardia, sweating, coma, abnormal posturing and generalized convulsions) are also typical of severe malaria itself.

It is associated with hyperlactatemia and shares the same pathophysiological etiology.

- Increased peripheral requirement of glucose secondary to anaerobic glycolysis.
- Increased metabolic demands of the febrile illness.
- The obligatory demands of the parasites which use glucose as their major fuel.
- Failure of hepatic gluconeogenesis and glycogenolysis
- Hepatic glycogen is exhausted rapidly, stores in fasting adults last approximately 2 days, but in children only for 12 hours.
- In patients treated with quinine, this is compounded by quinine-stimulated pancreatic b-cell insulin secretion.

Quinine-induced hyperinsulinaemia causes hypoglycemia which tends to occur after the first 24 hours of treatment whereas malaria-related hypoglycemia (with appropriate suppression of insulin secretion) is often present when the patient with severe malaria is first admitted. Hypoglycemia contributes to nervous system dysfunction and in cerebral malaria is associated with residual neurological deficit in survivors.

Circulatory Collapse (Algid Malaria)[11]

Most patients with shock exhibit a low peripheral vascular resistance and elevated cardiac output. Cardiac pump function appears remarkably well preserved despite intense sequestration of parasitized erythrocytes in the microvasculature of the myocardium. Postural hypotension may be secondary to autonomic dysfunction. Circulatory collapse may occur suddenly without any warning if there is associated severe dehydration, Gram-negative septicemia and massive gastrointestinal bleed.

Liver Dysfunction[11]

Jaundice is common with severe malaria and there is other evidence of hepatic dysfunction with reduced metabolic clearance of the antimalarial drugs and a failure of gluconeogenesis which contributes to lactic acidosis and hypoglycemia. There is sequestration in the hepatic microvasculature and in very severe infections liver blood flow is reduced. Jaundice in malaria appears to have hemolytic, hepatic and cholestatic components. Cholestatic jaundice may persist well into the recovery period.

Fluid, Electrolyte and Acid-base Disturbances[11]

Total body water and extracellular volume are normal. Plasma renin activity, aldosterone and antidiuretic hormone concentrations are elevated, reflecting an appropriate activation of homeostatic mechanisms to maintain adequate circulating volume in presence of general vasodilatation and a falling hematocrit. Hyponatremia is common and is thought to be as a result of intravascular volume expansion occurring as a compensatory response to vasodilatation caused by malarial endotoxins. Serum potassium concentrations are usually normal.

Arterial, capillary, venous and CSF concentrations of lactate rise in direct proportion to disease severity. Indeed the venous lactate concentration 4 hours after admission to hospital is the best prognostic indicator in severe malaria. Lactic acidosis is an important cause of death. Triglyceride and free fatty acid levels are also elevated in acute malaria, and plasma concentrations of ketone bodies are raised in patients who have been unable to eat.

Bacterial Infection

Patients with severe malaria are vulnerable to bacterial infections, particularly of the lungs and the urinary tract (following catheterisation), spontaneous gram-negative septicaemia may occur but is rare. However salmonella septicaemias are an important complication of otherwise uncomplicated falciparum malaria in African children.[26]

LABORATORY FINDINGS

Thrombocytopenia is the most common laboratory abnormality (60% of cases), followed by hyperbilirubinemia (40%), anemia (30%) and elevated hepatic aminotransferase levels (25%).[27] The leukocyte count is usually normal or low, but neutrophilia with a marked increase in band forms (left shift) is present in the majority of cases. The erythrocyte sedimentation rate and C-reactive protein, are almost invariably elevated.

There may be mild hyponatraemia, serum bicarbonate is often reduced and the anion gap widens in proportion to the acidosis. Hypoglycaemia may occur in absence of quinine usage. Low and falling serum albumin is an important index of hepatic dysfunction.

Lactate levels in arterial or venous blood or CSF are elevated in proportion to the disease severity.

The CSF is usually normal in cerebral malaria but moderately raised concentrations of protein are common (sometimes upto 200 mg/dl). There may be up to 10 cells/ml, and on occasions upto 50 cells are seen (all lymphocytes). The CSF lactate concentration is raised in proportion to disease severity and glucose is often slightly low relative to blood.

When the urine is dark red or black and the urine analysis dipstick test is positive for hemoglobin, the absence of microscopic hematuria suggests either hemoglobinuria or myoglobinuria.

Conventional Microscopy

Light microscopy of thick and thin stained blood smears remains the standard method for diagnosing malaria.[28] Thick smears are 20 to 40 times more sensitive than thin smears for screening of Plasmodium parasites, with a detection limit of 10 to 50 trophozoites/ml. Thin smears allow one to identify malaria species (including the diagnosis of mixed infections), quantify parasitemia, and assess for the presence of schizonts, gametocytes, and malarial pigment in neutrophils and monocytes. The diagnostic accuracy relies on the quality of the blood smear and experience of laboratory personnel. Before reporting a negative result, at least 200 oil immersion visual fields should be examined on both thick and thin smears, which has a sensitivity of 90%. The level of parasitemia may be expressed either as a percentage of parasitized erythrocytes or as the number of parasites per microliter of blood. In nonfalciparum malaria, parasitemia rarely exceeds 2%, whereas it can be considerably higher (>50%) in falciparum malaria. In nonimmune individuals, hyperparasitemia (>5% parasitemia or >250 000 parasites/ml) is generally associated with severe disease.[29]

In falciparum malaria, parasitized erythrocytes may be sequestered in tissue capillaries resulting in a falsely low parasite count in the peripheral blood ('visible' parasitemia).[11] In such instances, the developmental stages of the parasite seen on blood smear may help to assess disease severity better than parasite count alone. The presence of more mature parasite forms (>20% of parasites as late trophozoites and schizonts) and of more than 5% of neutrophils containing malarial pigment indicates more advanced disease and a worse prognosis.[30] One negative blood smear makes the diagnosis of malaria very unlikely (especially the severe form). However, smears should be repeated every 6 to 12 hours for 48 hours if malaria is still suspected.

Alternative Diagnostic Methods

Although examination of the thick and thin blood smear is the 'gold standard' for diagnosing malaria, important advances have been made in diagnostic testing, including fluorescence microscopy of parasite nuclei stained with acridine orange, rapid dipstick immunoassay, and polymerase chain reaction assays. Sensitivity and specificity of some of these methods approach or even exceed those of the thin and thick smear.[31]

Rapid dipstick immunoassays detect species-specific circulating parasite antigens targeting either the histidine-rich protein-2 of *P falciparum* or a parasite-specific lactate dehydrogenase.

Although the dipstick tests may enhance diagnostic speed, microscopic examination remains mandatory in patients with suspected malaria, because occasionally these dipstick tests are negative in patients with high parasitemia, and their sensitivity below 100 parasites/ml is low.[32]

Tests based on polymerase chain reaction for species-specific Plasmodium genome are more sensitive and specific than are other tests, detecting as few as 10 parasites/ml blood.[33]

Antibody detection has no value in the diagnosis of acute malaria. It is mainly used for epidemiologic studies.

TREATMENT

Severe malaria is a medical emergency and calls for expert medical and emergency care. The key to successful outcome for malaria in children is prompt diagnosis with species identification and early treatment.

Principles of management are as follows[12]

- Early suspicion of diagnosis, rapid clinical assessment and transfer to the highest level of care available or referral.
- Early antimalarial chemotherapy using optimal doses of an appropriate agent administered by the parenteral route.
- Prevention, or early detection and treatment, of complications (e.g., convulsions, hypoglycaemia, hyperpyrexia).
- Correction of fluid, electrolyte and acid-base balance.
- Avoidance of harmful ancillary treatments (e.g., corticosteroids).

Initial Management of A Patient With Severe Malaria[12]

1. Clear and maintain the airway.
2. Position semi-prone or on side.
3. Weigh the patient, calculate dosage.
4. Take blood for diagnostic smear, monitoring of blood sugar ('stix' method), hematocrit and other laboratory tests.
5. Start antimalarial chemotherapy.
6. Make rapid clinical assessment.
7. Exclude or treat hypoglycaemia.
8. Assess state of hydration.
9. Measure and monitor urine output. If necessary insert urethral catheter. Measure urine specific gravity.
10. Plan first 8 hours of intravenous fluids – including diluent for antimalarial drug, glucose therapy and blood transfusion.
11. Consider inserting central venous pressure catheter to monitor fluid replacement.
12. If rectal temperature exceeds 39°C, remove patient's clothes, use tepid sponge, fan, cooling blanket and consider antipyretic.
13. Lumbar puncture to exclude meningitis or cover with appropriate antibiotic. Consider other infections.
14. Consider need for anticonvulsant and additional drugs (antimicrobials, vitamin K etc.).

Nonimmune patients with *P falciparum* malaria should be treated as a medical emergency and be considered for hospital admission, regardless of disease severity at presentation. All patients with severe malaria (Table 11.1) and those who are unable to tolerate drugs orally should initially receive parenteral treatment immediately (Table 11.3) and be admitted to the ICU.[34] In these patients, gastrointestinal intolerance and erratic intestinal absorption make the oral route of administration unreliable. To prevent medication errors it is important to check whether the recommended dose relates to a base or salt. Patients with severe malaria should always receive a full treatment dose, including those with breakthrough malaria and those who received some prior antimalarial medication.

Monitoring Treatment Response

When reliable blood smear results are not immediately available and malaria is suspected on clinical grounds, empiric treatment for falciparum malaria should be administered without delay. Treatment response should be assessed by parasite count daily until clearance of all trophozoites is achieved. Parasitemia may rise during the first 12 to 24 hours, because available drugs do not inhibit schizont rupture and release of merozoites. Rising parasitemia beyond 36 to 48 hours after the start of antimalarial treatment indicates treatment failure, usually because of high-level drug resistance.[35] Because nonimmune hosts may exhibit a high pre-treatment total parasite burden, it may take up to 6 days to achieve complete elimination of *P falciparum* trophozoites from the blood, even with fast-acting antimalarial agents (e.g. quinine, artemisinin derivatives). A rising gametocyte count does not indicate treatment failure. Persons with partial immunity can tolerate low parasitemia (<10000 parasites/ml) without clinical symptoms.[29] Therefore, in a proportion of semi-immune individuals parasitemia may not be responsible for current signs and symptoms. In 5 to 10% of patients with falciparum malaria, treatment failure will occur, with recurrence of symptoms usually within 1 month of treatment. Hence, a repeated blood smear examination at 7 and 28 days after completion of therapy is recommended.[36]

Table 11.3: Recommended regimens for initial parenteral treatment of severe falciparum malaria

Drug	*Loading dose*[1]	*Maintenance dose*	*Comments*
Regimen 1			
Quinine dihydrochloride salt reconstituted in 5% glucose or normal saline	7 mg salt/kg iv over 30 min followed immediately by maintenance dose or 20 mg salt/kg over 4 hr, followed 8 hours later by maintenance dose hours[2]	10 mg salt/kg diluted in 10 ml/kg isotonic fluid iv over 4 hours repeated every 8 hours	If hemodialysis is performed, then quinine is administered after dialysis. Monitor blood glucose because of risk for developing hyperinsulinemic hypoglycemia
PLUS (either concurrently or immediately thereafter) Doxycycline[3]	Not required	2 mg/kg (max.100 mg) po or iv every 12 hours for 7 days	Should not be given to pregnant or breastfeeding women or children < 8 years old
		OR	
Clindamycin	10 mg/kg iv	5 mg/kg every 8 hours till blood is clear of a sexual parasites	Should be given when patient is unable to take doxycycline No loading dose if patient has received quinine or mefloquine in the past 24 hours.
Regimen 2			
Artesunate	2.4 mg/kg iv bolus	1.2 mg/kg iv daily[4]	Artesunic acid 60 mg is dissolved in 0.6 ml 5% sodium bicarbonate, diluted to 3–5 ml 5% glucose, and given immediately by iv bolus injection
Regimen 3			
Artemether	3.2 mg/kg im	1.6 mg/kg im daily[4]	

[1]Loading dose should not be administered to patients who received quinine, halofantrine, or mefloquine within the preceding 12 hours. [2]Intravenous quinine should be given for at least 24 hours but oral antimalarial treatment should be substituted as soon as the patient is stable and can take oral therapy to complete the treatment course. If intravenous treatment is continued past 48 hours, then the maintenance dose should be reduced by 30–50%. In renal failure and in dialysis patients, the maintenance dose of quinine should be reduced by 30–50%. [3]Clindamycin 5 mg/kg (usually 300 mg) po or iv every 8 hours can be administered if the patient is unable to take doxycycline. [4]Parenteral artesunate or artemether should be given for at least 3 days but oral antimalarial treatment should be substituted as soon as the patient is stable and can take oral therapy to complete the treatment course. im = intramuscularly; iv = intravenously; po, orally.

Quinine

Intravenous quinine is currently the most widely used agent in the treatment of severe falciparum malaria, usually formulated as a dihydrochloride salt. Quinine may cause cinchonism (bitter taste, dysphoria, tremor, tinnitus, reversible high-tone hearing loss, headache, nausea, vomiting, and abdominal pain) or pruritus, which should not lead to dose reduction. The drug has a narrow therapeutic window. Severe toxicities include cardiac arrhythmias, hypotension, blindness, deafness, and hyperinsulinemic hypoglycemia.[12, 37]

An initial loading dose of quinine should be administered as soon as possible, followed by the maintenance dose. Both drugs should be given by a rate-controlled intravenous infusion (infusion pump), and never by a bolus injection, which may cause fatal hypotension or cardiac arrhythmia. Without a loading dose, it takes more than 24 hours to achieve therapeutic drug concentration. This delay may allow sequestration of trophozoites causing major organ dysfunction. The loading dose should not be administered to patients who received quinine, quinidine, halofantrine, or mefloquine within the preceding 12 hours. If intravenous treatment is continued past 48 hours, the maintenance dose should be reduced by 30 to 50%. In renal failure (clearance <10 ml/min) and in dialysis patients a normal loading dose should be administered, but the maintenance dose should be reduced by 30 to 50%. If hemodialysis is performed, quinine should be administered after dialysis. Electrocardiographic monitoring is mandatory with quinine infusion if the patient has acute renal failure or if mefloquine or halofantrine have been administered in the previous 2 weeks. If the QRS complex lengthens by more than 25% beyond baseline or the QTc interval increases to more than 500 ms, the infusion should be slowed or discontinued. Monitoring of plasma quinine concentrations does not predict cardiotoxicity; electrocardiography may be a more accurate approach for monitoring cardiotoxicity.[38] Apart from lengthening of the QTc interval, common electrocardiographic abnormalities include suparventricular and ventricular ectopic beats, sinus bradycardia (<50 beats/min), and ventricular tachycardia.[39]

Artemisinin Derivatives

Although artemisinin derivatives clear parasites from blood about 20% faster than quinine dihydrochloride, improved survival was observed only in regions of South-East Asia with recognized quinine resistance.[40] Furthermore, recovery from coma may be delayed and the incidence of seizures is higher than with quinine dihydrochloride.[12,41,42] At present, artemisinin derivatives are recommended for treatment of quinine-resistant *P falciparum* infections. There are four artemisinin formulations: dihydroartemisinin, artesunate (a water-soluble compound for intramuscular injection), arteether, and artemether (an oil-soluble compound for intravenous injection). Artesunate and artemether are metabolized to the biologically active metabolite dihydroartemisinin. Artemisinin derivatives are well tolerated. Side effects include nausea, vomiting, pruritus, and fever; bleeding and cardiac arrhythmias rarely occur. Despite reports of brainstem neurotoxicity with high doses in animal studies, this side effect has not been observed in humans to date. Artemisinin and its derivatives may be administered by the rectal route. Suppository formulations of artemisinin developed originally in China have proved highly effective in clinical tests. Artesunate rectocaps are also available.

Parenteral chloroquine is currently not recommended for the treatment of severe malaria in India.

Oral Treatment

When patients with severe falciparum malaria show significant clinical improvement (after at least 24 hours of parenteral therapy) and can tolerate tablets, they should be switched to oral medication (Table 11.4).

The choice of oral antimalarials is guided by the susceptibility pattern of the plasmodia. Higher blood levels are reached when oral antimalarials are given with or after food intake.

Basic Supportive Care

The intravascular volume should be maintained at the lowest level sufficient for adequate systemic perfusion. In hypotension early use of inotropic support is indicated rather than overhydration. Negative fluid balance is critical to avoid exacerbating acute lung injury, but is balanced against the risk for precipitating acute renal failure.[42] The patient may need to be intubated because of impaired consciousness or because of acute lung injury. Mechanical ventilation with lower tidal volume improves the clinical outcome.[44] A higher positive end-expiratory pressure may be needed to maintain optimal arterial oxygenation. In respiratory acidosis, the plateau pressure should be in excess of 25 cm H_2O and the ventilator rate should be increased.

Comatose patients should be placed in a semirecumbent position to reduce the risk for aspiration. Serum sodium concentration, arterial carbon dioxide tension, blood glucose, and arterial lactate concentration should be monitored frequently.

Seizures should be treated promptly with anticonvulsants, but their prophylactic use is still in dispute.[12] Diazepam, initial dose of 0.3 mg/kg (rate not to exceed 2 mg/min) is used. Intrarectal administration is an alternative, at a dose of 0.5 mg/kg. Treatment may be repeated cautiously after 15 min if initial treatment fails. If diazepam or paraldehyde cannot control seizures, phenytoin or phenobarbitone should be used. The efficacy of hypertonic mannitol in treatment of cerebral edema is not proven.

Intravenous glucose is preferred for rapid correction of hypoglycemia in markedly symptomatic or comatose patients. It should be administered as D25W in a dose of 2–4 ml/kg/dose (0.5–1 /kg of sugar) intravenously slowly D50W (1 to 2 ml/kg/dose) may be used for children over three years of age. Maintenance of adequate glucose homeostasis and fluid balance is achieved with 10% glucose in 0.2 NS at a rate to deliver about 7 mg/kg/minute.

Early institution of renal replacement therapy may avoid the development of ARDS.[45] Acidosis is usually multifactorial in origin, with causes including tissue hypoxia, liver dysfunction, and impaired renal handling of bicarbonate.[46] Blood transfusion should be considered if the hematocrit falls below 20%, but volume overload should be avoided.

Antimicrobial Therapy

Bacterial infections often complicate the course of patients with severe malaria. Common infections include aspiration pneumonia and sepsis. Parasite factors stimulate the

Table 11.4: Recommended oral treatment for severe falciparum malaria after initial parenteral therapy for at least 24 hours when clinical improvement is evident and the patient can tolerate oral medication

Drug	*Dose*	*Comments*
Artemether /lumefantrin	80 mg arthemeter/480 mg lumefantrin once daily for 3 days	Well tolerated, faster parasite clearance, but longer fever resolution time
Quinine (sulfate salt)	10 mg salt/kg (600–650 mg) every 8 hours to complete7 days of treatment (total duration)	Side effects include cinchonism and pruritus

production and release of cytokines such as tumor necrosis factor (TNFa) and interleukin-1 by macrophages, resulting in fever, chills, and hyperkinetic hemodynamic changes. The clinical and laboratory characteristics of severe malaria are similar to those of sepsis. Therefore, a bacterial infection in a patient with malaria may not be recognized initially. Repeated microbiologic sampling of appropriate body fluids such as blood, sputum, cerebrospinal fluid, and urine may help to diagnose and treat a possible infection early.

Exchange Blood Transfusion and Red Cell Exchange (Erythrocytapheresis)

Death in patients with malaria is related to the level of parasitemia, with significant mortality when parasitemia exceeds 5% despite appropriate parenteral antimalarial therapy.

Exchange transfusion may rapidly reduce parasitemia, decrease the risk for intravascular hemolysis, improve blood flow, decrease cytokines, and improve oxygen-carrying capacity. Although there are no sufficiently powered, randomized, controlled studies, exchange blood transfusion has been suggested in patients with severe malaria, especially for those with hyperparasitemia (> 5%).[12] Some authors recommend exchange transfusion only in countries with well equipped and staffed ICUs and safe blood supplies.[47] Published data about the effectiveness of this method is controversial. A meta-analysis involving eight studies,[48] in which groups of patients with severe malaria who received adjunct exchange transfusion were compared with patients who received antimalarial chemotherapy alone, found no difference in survival rates between groups. However, patients who received transfusions had higher parasitemia and were much more ill according to WHO criteria for severe malaria.

Cytokines such as TNFa and interleukin-1 probably contribute to the pathogenesis of severe malaria, and some authors have suggested that plasma exchange, plasmapheresis, and hemodialysis are effective alternatives to exchange transfusion.[49]

Unproven Treatments

Therapy with monoclonal antibodies against TNFa shortens the duration of fever, but has no impact on mortality in patients with severe and complicated malaria, and may increase morbidity due to neurologic sequelae.[50] Although corticosteroids were used in the past to treat patients with cerebral malaria, a controlled trial has shown that they are harmful. Those who received dexamethasone had a longer duration of coma and worse outcome than did patients who received antimalarial chemotherapy alone.[51] Results of studies of antipyretics, pentoxifylline, hyperimmune serum, and iron chelators (deferoxamine) have shown no effect on outcome.[26]

SUMMARY

Malaria represents a medical emergency because it may rapidly progress to complications and death without prompt and appropriate treatment. Severe malaria is almost exclusively caused by *Plasmodium falciparum.*

The case fatality rate remains high despite progress in intensive care and antimalarial treatment. Clinical deterioration usually appears 3 to 7 days after onset of fever. Complications involve the nervous, respiratory, renal, and/or hematopoietic systems. Metabolic acidosis and hypoglycemia are common systemic complications.

Intravenous quinine is the most widely used drug in the initial treatment of severe falciparum malaria, whereas artemisinin derivatives are currently recommended for quinine-resistant cases. As soon as the patient is clinically stable and able to swallow, oral treatment should be given. The intravascular volume should be maintained at the lowest level sufficient for adequate systemic perfusion to prevent development of acute respiratory distress syndrome. Renal replacement therapy should be initiated early. Exchange blood transfusion has been suggested for the treatment of patients with severe malaria and high parasitemia.

For early diagnosis, it is important to consider malaria in every febrile patient, especially in endemic areas.

REFERENCES

1. Muentener P, Schlagenhauf P, Steffen R. Imported malaria (1985 to 1995). Trends and perspectives. *Bull World Health Organ* 1999;77:560-566.
2. Sachs J, Malaney P. The economic and social burden of malaria. *Nature* 2002;415:680-685.
3. Svenson JE, MacLean JD, Gyorkos TW, Keystone J. Imported malaria. Clinical presentation and examination of symptomatic travelers. *Arch Intern Med* 1995;155:861-868.
4. Kain KC, Keystone JS. Malaria in travelers. Epidemiology, disease and prevention. *Infect Dis Clin North Am* 1998;12: 267-84.
5. Kain KC, Harrington MA, Tennyson S, Keystone JS. Imported malaria: Prospective analysis of problems in diagnosis and management. *Clin Infect Dis* 1998; 27:142-149.
6. Taylor-Robinson AW. Regulation of immunity to malaria: Valuable lessons learnt from murine models. *Parasitol Today* 1995; 11:334-342.
7. Winkler S, Willheim M, Baier K et al. Reciprocal regulation of Th1- and Th2-cytokine-producing T cells during clearance of parasitemia in Plasmodium falciparum malaria. *Infect Immun* 1998;66:6040-6044.
8. Hunter CA. How are NK cell responses regulated during infection? *Exp Parasitol* 1996;84:444-448.
9. Bancroft GJ. The role of natural killer cells in innate resistance to infection. *Curr Opin Immunol* 1993;5: 503-510.
10. Omer F, Kurtzhals J, Riley E. Maintaining the immunologic balance in parasitic infections: role for TGF-beta. *Parasitol Today* 2000;16:18-23.
11. White NJ. Malaria. In Cook GC, Zumla AI, Weir J (eds) *Manson's Tropical Diseases.* Philadelphia : WB Saunders 2003;1205-1295.

12. World Health Organization. Severe falciparum malaria. *Trans R Soc Trop Med Hyg* 2000;94(Suppl 1):S1-S90.
13. Bruneel F, Hocqueloux L, Albert C et al. The clinical spectrum of severe imported falciparum malaria in the ICU: Report of 188 cases in adults. *Am J Respir Crit Care Med* 2003;167: 684-689.
14. Blumberg L, Lee RP, Lipman J, Beards S. Predictors of mortality in severe malaria: A two year experience in a non-endemic area. *Anaesth Intensive Care* 1996; 24:217-223.
15. Schwartz E, SadetzkiS, Murad H, Raveh D. Age as a risk factor for severe falciparum malaria in non-immune patients. *Clin Infect Dis* 2001;33:1774-1777.
16. World Health Organization. Severe and complicated malaria. *Trans R Soc Trop Med* 1990;84(Suppl 2):S1-S65.
17. Molyneaux ME, Taylor TE, Wirima JJ, Borgstein A. Clinical features and prognostic indicators in pediatric cerebral malaria. A study of 131 comatose Malawian children. *Q J Med* 1989;71:441-459.
18. Shendurnikar N, Gandam DS. Cerebellar ataxia in malaria. *Indian J Pediatr* 1985;52:261-267.
19. Brewster DR, Kwiatkowski D, White NJ. Neurological sequelae of cerebral malaria in children. *Lancet* 1990;336:1039-1043.
20. Prakash J, Gupta A, Kumar O, Rout SB, Malhotra V, Srivastava PK. Acute renal failure in falciparum malaria: Increasing prevalence in some areas of India, a need for awareness. *Nephrol Dial Transplant* 1996; 11:2414-2416.
21. Mehta KS, Halankar AR, Makwana PD, Torane PP, Satija PS, Shah VB. Severe acute renal failure in malaria. *J Postgrad Med* 2001;47:24-26.
22. Gachot B, Wolff M, Nissack G, Veber B, Vachon F. Acute lung injury complicating imported Plasmodium falciparum malaria. *Chest* 1995;108:746-749.
23. Bernard GR, Artigas A, Brigham KL et al. Report of the American-European consensus conference on ARDS: definitions, mechanisms, relevant outcomes and clinical trial coordination. The Consensus Committee. *Intensive Care Med* 1994;20: 225-232.
24. Taylor TE, Molyneux ME, Wirima JJ, Fletcher KA, Morris K. Blood glucose levels in Malawian children before and after administration of intravenous quinine for severe falciparum malaria. *N Engl J Med* 1998; 319:1040-1047.
25. White NJ, Warrell DA, Chanthavanich P et al. Severe hypoglycemia and hyperinsulinemia in falciparum malaria. *N Engl J Med* 1983;309: 61-66.
26. Warrell DA. Management of severe malaria. *Parasitologia* 1999; 41:287-294.
27. D'Acremont V, Landry P, Mueller I, Pecoud A, Genton B. Clinical and laboratory predictors of imported malaria in an outpatient setting: an aid to clinical decision making in returning travelers with fever. *Am J Trop Med Hyg* 2002;66:481-486.
28. Moody AH, Chiodini PL. Methods for detection of blood parasites. *Clin Lab Hematol* 2000;22:189-201.
29. Torres JR. Malaria and babesiosis. In Baddour LM, Gorbach SL (eds): *Therapy of Infectious Diseases.* Philadelphia: WB Saunders 2003;597-613.
30. Nguyen PH, Day N, Pram TD, Ferguson DJ, White NJ. Intraleucocytic malaria pigment and prognosis in severe malaria. *Trans R Soc Med Hyg* 1995;89:200-204.
31. Lee SH, Kara UA, Koay E, Lee MA. New strategies for diagnosis and screening of malaria. *Int J Hematol* 2002;76(Suppl 1): 291-293.
32. Moody A. Rapid diagnostic tests for malarial parasites. *Clin Microbiol Rev* 2002;15:66-78.
33. Hanscheid T, Grobusch MP. How useful is PCR in the diagnosis of malaria? *Trends Parasitol* 2002;18: 395-398.
34. Murphy GS, Oldfield III EC. Falciparum malaria. *Infect Dis Clin North Am* 1996;10:747-775.
35. Watt G, Shanks GD, Phintuyothin P. Prognostic significance of rises in parasitemia during treatment of falciparum. *Trans R Soc Trop Med Hyg* 1992;86: 359-360.
36. Canadian recommendations for the prevention and treatment of malaria among international travelers. Committee to Advise on Tropical Medicine and Travel (CATMAT). Laboratory for Disease Control. *Can Commun Dis Rep* 2000;26(Suppl 2): 1-42.
37. Bonington A, Davidson RN, Winstanley PA, Pasvol G. Fatal quinine cardiotoxicity in the treatment of falciparum malaria. *Trans R Soc Trop Med Hyg* 1996; 90:305-307.
38. Sukontason K, Karbwang J, Rimchala W, et al. Plasma quinine concentrations in falciparum malaria with acute renal failure. *Trop Med Int Health* 1996; 1:236-242.
39. Bethell DB, Phuong PT, Phuong CX, et al. Electrocardioscopic monitoring in severe falciparum malaria. *Trans R Soc Trop Med Hyg* 1996;90:266-269.
40. Pittler MH, Ernst E. Artemether for severe malaria: a meta-analysis of randomized clinical trials. *Clin Infect Dis* 1999;28: 597-601.
41. Tran TH, DayNP, Nguyen HP, et al. A controlled trial of artemether or quinine in Vietnamese adults with severe falciparum malaria. *N Engl J Med* 1996; 335:76-83.
42. Murphy S, English M, Waruiru C, et al. An open randomized trial of artemether versus quinine in the treatment of cerebral malaria in African children. *Trans R Soc Trop Med Hyg* 1996; 90:298-301.
43. Blum PG, Stephens D. Severe falciparum malaria in five soldiers from East Timor: A case series and literature review. *Anesth Intensive Care* 2001;29: 426-434.
44. The Acute Respiratory Distress Syndrome Network. Ventilation with lower tidal volumes as compared with traditional volumed for acute lung injury and the acute respiratory distress syndrome. *N Engl J Med* 2000;342:1301-1308.
45. Wilairatana P, Westerlund EK, Aursudkij B, et al. Treatment of acute renal failure by hemodialysis. *Am J Trop Med Hyg* 1999; 60:233-237.
46. Day NP, Phu NH, Mai NT, et al. The pathophysiologic and prognostic significance of acidosis in severe adult malaria. *Crit Care Med* 2000;28:1833-1840.
47. Panosian CB. Exchange blood transfusion in severe falciparum malaria: the debate goes on. *Clin Infect Dis* 1998;26:853-854.
48. Riddle MS, Jackson JL, Sanders JW, Blazes DL. Exchange transfusion as an adjunct therapy in severe Plasmodium falciparum malaria: a meta-analysis. *Clin Infect Dis* 2002;34: 1192-1198.
49. White NJ. What is the future of exchange transfusion in severe malaria? *J Infect* 1999;39:185-186.
50. Kwiatkowski D, Molyneux ME, Stephens S, et al. Anti-TNF therapy inhibits fever in cerebral malaria. *Q J Med* 1993;86: 91-98.
51. Warrell DA, Looareesuwan S, Warrell MJ, et al. Dexamethasone proves deleterious in cerebral malaria. A double-blind trial in 100 comatose patients. *N Engl J Med* 1982;306:313-319.

Somashekhar Nimbalkar

12 Tetanus

INTRODUCTION

Tetanus is an important cause of death worldwide and is associated with a high case mortality. Modern intensive care management can prevent death from acute respiratory failure but cardiovascular complications as a result of autonomic instability and other causes of death remain problematic. Satisfactory management of tetanus requires intensive care facilities that are not easily available. Tetanus has been aptly described as a third world disease which requires first world technology to treat.

There are between 800,000 and 1 million deaths due to tetanus each year, of which about 400,000 are due to neonatal tetanus. Eighty per cent of these deaths occur in Africa and South East Asia and it remains endemic in 90 countries worldwide. The clinical course of tetanus is often unpredictable and patients should be closely monitored throughout their illness.[1]

ETIOLOGY

Clostridium tetani is the causative organism of tetanus. The clostridia genus is a diverse group of anaerobic spore forming gram positive bacilli. They are widely distributed in the environment, and are found in the intestinal flora of domestic animals, horses, chickens, and humans. Endospores are produced which are wider than the bacillus, giving rise to the characteristic drumstick shape.[1] *Clostridium tetani* is an anaerobic motile gram positive rod that forms an oval colorless terminal spore resembling a tennis racket or drumstick. Germination and toxin production takes place in wounds with a low oxidation-reduction potential such as those with devitalized tissue, foreign body or active infection. Tetanospasmin is the toxin primarily responsible for the clinical manifestation of tetanus.[2] Carried into wounds along with soil, spores may not germinate immediately because of unfavorable tissue conditions. They may activate well after the wound has healed, which accounts for the cases of tetanus that have no identifiable source. When conditions such as gross contamination or tissue injury favor anaerobic proliferation, the spores germinate into mature bacilli, which then form the toxins tetanolysin and tetanospasmin. Tetanolysin has an uncertain role in clinical tetanus; it may contribute to an anaerobic environment by damaging viable tissue.[3] Older organisms lose their flagella after the development of a spore. The spores are extremely stable, and although boiling for 15 minutes kills most, some will survive unless autoclaved at 120°C, 1.5 bar, for 15 minutes, which ensures sterility. Tiny amounts of the toxin are thought to be present in a typical infection. Rethy and Rethy estimated the human lethal dose to be approximately 500 pg/kg e.g. 25 ng/70 kg adult.[1]

TETANUS TOXIN AND PATHOGENESIS

The toxin gene is encoded on a 75 kb plasmid and synthesized as a single polypeptide with a molecular weight of 150,000. The polypeptide undergoes post-translational cleavage into two disulfide-linked fragments, the light (L) and heavy (H) chains. The carboxyl terminal portion of the H chain, termed HC, mediates attachment to gangliosides (GD1b and GT1b) on peripheral nerves, and subsequently the toxin is internalized. It is then moved from the peripheral to the central nervous system by retrograde axonal transport and trans-synaptic spread. The entire toxin molecule is internalized into presynaptic cells in a process requiring the HN fragment and the L chain is released from the endosome. The L chain is a zinc metalloprotease, which cleaves synaptobrevin. A single base pair mutation in the light chain abolishes this proteolytic activity. Synaptobrevin is an integral membrane component of synaptic vesicles and is essential for the fusion of synaptic vesicles with the presynaptic membrane. Cleavage by tetanus toxin L chain prevents release of their contents, the inhibitory neurotransmitter ã-aminobutyric acid (GABA), into the synaptic cleft. The α motor neurons are therefore under no inhibitory control and undergo sustained excitatory discharge causing the characteristic motor spasms of tetanus. The toxin exerts its effects on the spinal cord, the brain stem, peripheral nerves, at neuromuscular junctions, and directly on muscles. To what extent cortical and subcortical structures are involved remains unknown.[1]

Unlike the diagnosis of most infections, the diagnosis of tetanus is based almost entirely on clinical observations. The action of the toxin, tetanospasmin, helps explain the clinical manifestations. The toxin reaches the central nervous system by intraaxonal transport, moving at a rate of 75 to 250 mm per day. In the central nervous system, the toxin produces presynaptic blockade of the synapses of inhibitory Renshaw cells and 1a fibers of alpha motor neurons that handle the transmission of-aminobutyric acid and glycine, but not of the synapses of Renshaw cells that handle acetylcholine transmission.[3]

This results in a the lack of inhibition at brain stem and spinal cord level resulting initially in increasing resting muscle tone or rigidity and later reflexes spread widely and inappropriately resulting in spasms. The toxin binding appears to be irreversible, recovery depending on the sprouting of new axonal terminals, probably explaining the long duration of the disease which cannot be reduced by treatment.[5] Instability of the autonomic nervous system also occurs. This is because it also affects preganglionic sympathetic neurons in the lateral gray matter of the spinal cord.[2] Tetanospasmin also causes loss of inhibitory control of catecholamine secretion by the adrenal medulla at the spinal level, resulting in a hypersympathetic state.[6] The toxin binding appears to be irreversible; recovery depends on the sprouting of new axonal terminals. Once the toxin is synthesized it moves from the contaminated site to the spinal cord- a process that takes 2 to 14 days. With facial injuries the interval is short. Once the toxin reaches the spinal cord, localized or cephalic tetanus may occur initially, followed by generalized tetanus. The patient is usually afebrile, unless there is concurrent local infection. With severe tetanus, all muscles contract, with the stronger overpowering the weaker.[4]

Tetanolysin is the other toxin produced by *C. tetani*. This toxin damages cell membranes and tissues, thereby providing an environment suitable for further growth and proliferation of the organism.[6]

Cardiovascular complications are postulated to result from the effects of tetanus exotoxin with:

- Brain stem damage resulting in fatal cardiac and respiratory failure.
- Myocardial depression or toxic myocarditis, believed to be due to excessively high levels of circulating catecholamines, or
- Widespread disinhibition of autonomic nervous system in the CNS which may lead to sympathetic nervous hyperactivity and/or parasympathetic overactivity.

In 1968, Kerr et al described the syndrome of sympathetic nervous hyperactivity " sustained but labile hypertension and tachycardia, irregularities of cardiac rhythm, peripheral vascular constriction, profuse sweating, pyrexia, increased carbon dioxide output, increased catecholamine excretion, and in some cases, the late development of hypotension." These signs and symptoms if they occur, usually develop towards the end of the first week. They may occur spontaneously or in response to minor stimuli, as in the case with tetanic spasms, and cannot be alleviated through pain control and sedation. Most such patients' manifest elevated plasma catecholamine levels. Prolonged sympathetic activity may end with profound and preterminal bradycardia and sinus arrest, salivation and increased bronchial secretions. Direct damage to the vagal nucleus has been implicated as well as local damage to the sinus node, and to reflex excessive vagal tone.[7]

CLINICAL FEATURES AND MANAGEMENT

Tetanus occurs in four major clinical forms:

- Neonatal tetanus
- Local tetanus
- Cephalic tetanus and
- Generalized tetanus.

Neonatal Tetanus

Neonatal tetanus is generalized tetanus that occurs in the newborn around the first week of life. Symptoms begin with nonspecific irritability and poor feeding and rapidly progresses to generalized spasms. The portal of entry is the freshly cut umbilical cord. The risk of contracting neonatal tetanus is directly related to the cleanliness of delivery conditions and to maternal immunizations because passive transfer of maternal immunoglobulins is protective. Mortality is very high, 50 to 100%, due to the high load of toxin per body weight in neonates. Seizures, meningitis and sepsis are differential diagnosis.[3,6,8] Its details are beyond the scope of this book and are provided in *Textbook of Neonatal Emergencies (Book 2).*

Local Tetanus

Local tetanus presents as persistent muscle rigidity close to the site of the injury. The rigidity may linger for weeks to months and often resolves without sequelae. A caveat of what appears to be localized tetanus may instead be the first symptom of generalized tetanus. The incidence is 13% and the fatality rate is about 1%.[3,8]

Cephalic Tetanus

Cephalic tetanus is a type of local tetanus characterized by cranial nerve palsies. It has a higher mortality than localized tetanus. It commonly involves the facial nerve and is associated with ear infections or head wounds after trauma. It has an incidence of 6%. Cephalic tetanus uniquely results in nerve palsies as well as muscle spasms. The seventh cranial nerve is most often involved, followed by the 6th, 3rd, 4th and 12th in decreasing order of frequency. Cephalic tetanus also presents with trismus, but in 42% of cases cranial nerve deficits precede the onset of tetanus. In such cases cephalic is easily misdiagnosed. With its predilection for the 7th cranial nerve, it commonly mimics Bell's Palsy. Head trauma and otitis media are commonly cited etiologies. About two thirds of the patients progress to generalized tetanus and the overall mortality is 15-30%.[3]

Thus both local and cephalic tetanus have the potential to be generalized.

Generalized Tetanus

Generalized tetanus is the most common form of the disease, and presents with pain, headache, stiffness, rigidity, opisthotonus, and spasms, which can lead to laryngeal obstruction.[1] The hematogenous spread of toxin from the initial site to other myoneural junctions results in the generalized form of tetanus. Trismus is an early presenting sign followed by risus sardonicus and opisthotonus. Autonomic dysfunction such as fever, extreme blood pressure fluctuations, arrhythmia's, and excessive salivation often occur during the second week of illness.[6]

Tetanus typically follows deep penetrating wounds where anaerobic bacterial growth is facilitated. The most common portals of infection are wounds on the lower limbs, postpartum or postabortion infections of the uterus, non-sterile intramuscular injections, and compound fractures. However, even minor trauma can lead to disease and in up to 30% of patients no portal of entry is apparent. Tetanus has been reported after a myriad of injuries, including intravenous and intramuscular injections, acupuncture, earpiercing, and even from toothpicks. It can follow from chronic infections such as otitis media, and has been reported via a decubitus ulcer. Tetanus acquired after intramuscular injection with quinine is associated with a higher mortality than other modes of acquisition. The disease when following intramuscular quinine injections has a significantly higher mortality than tetanus due to other causes.[1] The usual formulation available for intramuscular injection is acidic (pH 2) and may cause local vasoconstriction and necrosis which lowers the redox potential at the injection site providing a favourable milieu for rapid sporulation and growth of the organism.[5]

Early on the patient may report a "sore throat" with dysphagia. Contraction of the facial muscles produces the grimacing, the so-called "risus sardonicus". With severe tetanus there is opisthotonus, flexion of the arms, extension of the legs, periods of apnea due to spasm of the intercostal muscles and diaphragm, and rigidity of the abdominal wall. Late in the disease autonomic dysfunction develops, with hypertension and tachycardia alternating with hypotension and bradycardia.[4] The incubation period (the time from inoculation to the first symptom) can be as short as 24 hours or as long as many months after inoculation with *C tetani*. This interval is a reflection of the distance the toxin must travel within the nervous system, and may be related to the quantity of toxin released.[1] The period of onset is the time between the first symptom and the start of spasms. These periods are important prognostically, the shorter the incubation period or period of onset the more severe the disease. Trismus (lockjaw)—the inability to open the mouth fully owing to rigidity of the masseters—is often the commonest presenting symptom.[1] Other presenting symptoms could be backache and abdominal pain but trismus soon follows.[5] With severe tetanus all muscles contract with the stronger overpowering the weaker. Rigidity progresses in a descending manner, with dysphagia, risus sardonicus and neck stiffness, the short cranial nerves being affected first. With severe tetanus there is opisthotonus, flexion of the arms, extension of the legs, rigidity of the abdominal wall, followed by rigidity of the trunk and limbs.[5] These may be induced by minor stimuli such as noise, touch, or by simple medical and nursing procedures such as intravenous and intramuscular injections, suction, or catheterization. The spasms are excruciatingly painful and may be uncontrollable leading to respiratory arrest and death. Spasms are most prominent in the first 2 weeks, autonomic disturbance usually starts some days after spasms and reaches a peak during the second week of the disease. Rigidity may last beyond the duration of both spasms and autonomic disturbance. Severe rigidity and muscle spasm necessitates paralysis for prolonged periods in severe tetanus.[1]

As an aid in clinical diagnosis, Apte and Karnard[9] described a bedside spatula test for tetanus. A spatula is carefully inserted into the pharynx. If the patient gags and tries to expel the spatula, the test is negative for tetanus; if the patient bites the spatula because of reflex muscle spasm, the test is positive for tetanus. They reported 94% sensitivity and 100% specificity. The authors found the test most useful in the early phase of tetanus, before the onset of generalized spasms, when the diagnosis may not be obvious. The test may have limitations in areas where tetanus is less common. It should be used in caution in patients who may not be able to protect their airway.[3, 5] Spasms with intervening rigidity (being greater in the trunk than the limbs) occur both spontaneously and on stimulation and varies in severity. Arching the trunk-(opisthotonos) is a feature during the established disease. Periods of apnea may occur due to spasm of the intercostal muscles and the diaphragm.[5]

Autonomic dysfunction occurs in the more severe cases and sets in a few days after the onset of spasms due to the slower intraaxonal transport to the lateral horn cells. It consists of a basal sympathetic activity characterised by a resting tachycardia and depression of bowel motility and bladder dysfunction. Episodes of severe sympathetic overactivity (SOA) which includes fluctuating tachycardia, labile hypertension, sweating and pyrexia takes place both with and without stimulation. Profuse salivation and bronchial secretions due to increased parasympathetic activity also occur. All these signs do not necessarily occur concurrently and its severity varies from patient to patient. Episodes of bradycardia and hypotension some times lead to cardiac arrest. These signs have been explained on the basis of increased parasympathetic activity, but many attribute it to sudden withdrawal of sympathetic activity as the bradycardia does not always respond to atropine. Cardiac arrest in tetanus has also been attributed to myocardial damage caused by high catecholamine levels and toxic damage to the brainstem.[5]

Prior to the early 1950s the main cause of death in tetanus was respiratory failure secondary to spasms, obstruction by secretions, exhaustion and pulmonary aspiration. The development of modern intensive care techniques, muscle relaxation and artificial ventilation led to a dramatic decrease in these deaths only to reveal severe cardiovascular complications with high mortality due to autonomic dysfunction. Autonomic dysfunction is seen as increased basal sympathetic activity and episodes of sympathetic overactivity (SOA) or "crises" involving both alpha and beta receptors, evidenced by high circulating levels of norepinephrine and loss of inhibition of the adrenal medulla. During the crises, there is an outpouring of catecholamines in amounts comparable with pheochromocytoma. Other postulated contributory causes are the direct inhibition by tetanus toxin of the release of endogenous opiates and the increased release of thyroid hormone.[5]

DIAGNOSIS

The diagnosis of tetanus must be made on clinical grounds alone. There are no laboratory tests that can diagnose or rule out tetanus. A protective serum antibody level, commonly accepted as 0.01 U/ml (in vivo) or 0.15 U/ml (in vitro), makes the diagnosis of tetanus very unlikely, but not impossible. There are case reports of tetanus in immunocompromized individuals with protective antibody levels.[3]

DIFFERENTIAL DIAGNOSIS

The differential diagnosis includes tetany, strychnine poisoning, rabies, generalized convulsive seizures, black widow spider bite, meningitis, subarachnoid hemorrhage, sepsis, progressive fluctuating muscular rigidity (stiff-man syndrome), peritonitis, drug withdrawal, conversion syndrome and orofacial infection. In neonates the differential diagnosis would also include hypocalcemia, hypoglycemia, meningitis and meningoencephalitis, and seizures.[1,6] The differential diagnosis also includes acute local infections (dental or masseter) with trismus, acute temperomandibular disease in the early stages, meningitis and dystonic reactions following neuroleptic drugs (which typically involve lateral turning of the head often with protrusion of the tongue-symptoms which are rarely seen in tetanus.[5]

SCORING SYSTEMS

Several scoring systems are used to guide severity and prognosis of patients with tetanus. The scoring systems developed by Phillips, Dakar, Ablett and Patel and Joag are most commonly used.[2] Some groups have attempted to devise scoring systems to assess prognosis; the Dakar score and the Phillips score (Tables 12.1 and 12.2) are two examples. Both these scoring systems are relatively straight forward schemes, which take into account the incubation period and the period of onset as well as neurological and cardiac manifestations. The Phillips score also factors in the state of immune protection. The diagnosis is a clinical one, relatively easy to make in areas where tetanus is seen often, but often delayed in the developed world where cases are seen infrequently.[1] Ablett devised a useful method of grading the severity of tetanus for the purposes of management and study (Table 12.3). The more clinical grading system developed by Patel and Joag[10] (Table 12.4) is also useful.

Table 12.1: Prognostic scoring systems in tetanus: Dakar score

Prognostic factor	*Dakar score*	
	Score 1	*Score 2*
Incubation Period	< 7 days	> = 7 days or unknown
Period of Onset	< 2 days	> = 2 days
Entry Site	Umbilicus, burn, uterine, open fracture, surgical wound, intramuscular injection	All others and unknown
Spasms	Present	Absent
Fever	> 38.4 C	< 38.4°C
Tachycardia	Adult > 120 beats/min Neonate > 150 beats/min	Adult < 120 beats/min Neonate < 150 beats/min
Total Score		

Table 12.2: Prognostic systems in tetanus: Phillips score

Factor	*Score*
Incubation time:	
< 48 hours	5
2-5 days	4
5-10 days	3
10-14 days	2
> 14 days	1
Site of Infection	
Internal and Umbilical	5
Head, Neck and body wall	4
Peripheral proximal	3
Peripheral distal	2
Unknown	1
State of Protection	
None	10
Possibly some or maternal immunisation in neonates	8
Protected > 10 years ago	4
Protected < 10 years ago	2
Complete protection	0
Complicating factors	
Injury or life threatening illness	10
Severe injury or illness not immediately life threatening	8
Injury or non life threatening illness	4
Minor injury or illness	2
ASA Grade 1	0
Total Score	

Table 12.3: Ablett classification of severity of tetanus

Grade	*Clinical Features*
I	*Mild:* Mild to Moderate trismus; general spasticity; no respiratory embarrassment; no spasms; little or no dysphagia
II	*Moderate:* Moderate trismus; well-marked rigidity; mild to moderate but short spasms; moderate respiratory embarrassment with an increased respiratory rate greater than 30; mild dysphagia
III	*Severe:* Severe trismus; generalized spasticity; reflex prolonged spasms; increased respiratory rate greater than 40; apnoeic spells; severe dysphagia; tachycardia greater than 120
IV	*Very Severe:* Grade III and violent autonomic disturbances involving cardiovascular system. Severe hypertension and tachycardia alternating with relative hypotension and bradycardia, either of which may be persistent

TREATMENT

Treatment of tetanus consists of:

1. Eradication of the organism
2. Neutralization of the toxin

Table 12.4: Modified Patel and Joag criteria for grading tetanus

Sign(s)/Symptoms(s)	*Points*
Rigidity	
Neck	1
Abdomen	1
Limb	1
Trismus	1
Spasms	
Less than 1/hour	2
More than 1/hour	4
Continuous/Laryngeal	6
Vital Parameters	
Temperature > 38°C	2
Pulse > 120/min	2
Respiratory rate > 40/min	2

Grade–Mild: < 3; Moderate: 4-10; Severe: >10

3. Symptomatic treatment of the effects of the toxin; namely control of
   a. Muscle spasms
   b. Autonomic dysfunction
4. Supportive measures
5. Active immunization.

Eradication of the Organisms

In patients with a deep wound thorough debridement and toilet are critical to reduce the anaerobic conditions that bacteria thrive in. The wound must be cleaned with wide excision of devitalised tissue under anaesthesia.[1] Metronidazole is preferred as the antibiotic of choice by some because of its effective penetration of devitalised tissue, wounds and abscesses and its activity against anaerobes. It also has a better safety profile and negligible central nervous system irritability.[1-3,6] By the time symptoms develop the frequent absence of the wound or damaged tissue makes treatment based solely on adequate wound care futile and urgent attention must be given to other measures particularly to neutralisation of toxin.[5]

Penicillin remains the standard therapy for tetanus in most parts of the world, although antibiotics for *Clostridium tetani* probably play a relatively minor part in the specific treatment of the disease. The dose is 100000–200000 IU/kg/day intramuscularly or intravenously for 7 to 10 days in four doses per day. The structure of penicillin, distant to the β-lactam ring is similar to ã-aminobutyric acid (GABA) the principal inhibitory neurotransmitter in the CNS. Penicillin therefore acts as a competitive antagonist to GABA. Penicillin does not readily cross the blood-brain barrier, but in high cumulative doses it can cause CNS hyperexcitability. In tetanus this side effect of penicillin could synergize with the action of the toxin in blocking transmitter release at GABA neurons. Metronidazole is a safe alternative, and hence may now be considered as the first line therapy. After rectal administration metronidazole is rapidly bioavailable and causes fewer spasms than repeated intravenous or intramuscular injections. Ahmadsyah and Salim[11] were the first to compare penicillin and metronidazole, and showed a reduction in mortality in the metronidazole group (7% compared with 24%). In a much larger study Yen et al[12] recruited over 1000 patients and showed that there was no significant difference in mortality between the penicillin and metronidazole group. However, the 533 patients randomized to metronidazole required fewer muscle relaxants and sedatives compared with 572 patients randomized to penicillin. This may be explained by the action of penicillin at GABAergic synapses and may therefore apply to the third generation cephalosporins. The structure of these drugs is similar to that of penicillin and ceftazidime has been shown to induce absence seizures with spike and wave discharges. If metronidazole is available and applicable this should be considered as the drug of choice in the treatment of tetanus. The dose is 10 mg/kg rectally every 6 hours, or 11 mg/kg orally every 6 hours or intravenously for 7–10 days or upto 14 days. Erythromycin, tetracycline, vancomycin, clindamycin, doxycycline, and chloramphenicol would be alternatives to penicillin and metronidazole if these were unavailable or unusable in individual patients. There is little or no indication for the use of other antibiotics in the management of tetanus.[1-3, 6]

NEUTRALISATION OF TOXIN

Neutralization of toxin should be undertaken as early as possible since the toxin becomes inaccessible to antitoxin after it enters the central nervous system; as once the toxin is bound and internalized it would clearly have no effect. Human tetanus immune globulin (HTIG) i.m. should be injected in a dose of 500 units as the traditional much larger doses of 3000-5000 units are of questionable benefit. 500 units intramuscularly is considered the preferred dose and adult and pediatric doses being the same as the burden of tetanospasmin within the patient determines the amount of HTIG needed, not the patients weight. The weight based dosage for HTIG is 4 units/kg in children. In the absence of HTIG anti tetanus horse serum (ATS) after sensitivity tests will suffice in a dose of 5000 units i.m. and 5000 infiltrated around the wound. HTIG or ATS should be injected within 24 hours of diagnosis.[3,5,6] Passive immunisation with HTIG will shorten the disease course and reduce mortality. The human antiserum is isolated from a pool of plasma derived from healthy human tetanus immune donors, and has a half life of 24.5 to 31.5 days. Maximum concentration is reached in 24 to 48 hours and lasts for 10 to 15 days. The equine (or bovine) form has a higher incidence of anaphylactic reactions and a half life of only 2 days, but is much cheaper to produce. Human antiserum should be administered, if available. Yet in most parts of the world equine antitoxin is the standard. In established cases patients should receive 500–1000 IU/kg equine antitoxin intravenously or intramuscularly.

Anaphylactic reactions occur in 20% of cases; in 1% they are severe enough to warrant adrenaline, antihistamines, steroids, and intravenous fluids. Local infiltration around the wound is of no proven value. Passive immunization with human or equine tetanus immunoglobulin shortens the course and may reduce the severity of tetanus. Anti-tetanus toxin was first used in 1893, and there was a dramatic fall in the incidence of disease among soldiers in the first world after its introduction. Although the antiserum will have an effect only on circulating and unbound toxin (demonstrated in serum samples of only 10% of cases at presentation and in 4% of CSF samples, it should be administered to all patients with tetanus. Whether it should also be infiltrated locally at the portal of entry is unclear. For prophylaxis 1500–3000 IU equine or 250–500 IU human anti-tetanus immunoglobulin should be given. It is not easy to assess the optimal dose of antiserum to give for prophylaxis. Extrapolation from animal work would suggest that 50,000 IU would afford greater protection; however, at such doses the incidence of side effects is higher. The side effects can be either acute anaphylactic reactions or delayed serum sickness. The incidence of immediate reactions can be reduced by simultaneous (or 15 minutes before use) injection with an antihistamine (promethazine). The use of the Besredka rapid desensitization method does not necessarily prevent anaphylactic reactions.

The use of human tetanus immunoglobulin is very rarely associated with anaphylactic reactions, creates a longer duration of protective immunity, and lower doses can be used (500–1000 IU). It is the passive immunization of choice. Complete human immunoglobulin now can be engineered in vitro and designed for specific antigens. This raises the possibility of producing human antibodies specific for the tetanus toxin, free from the risks of infection, easy to store, and potentially available at a affordable cost. Owing to its smaller size it is possible that the antigen binding domain of the immunoglobulin, the Fab fragment, may gain better access to the toxin, and so enhance neutralization. Fab fragments can be produced from donors, but the engineered approach to antibody production would facilitate this.[1] It is important that the toxoid and tetanus immunoglobulins are administered at two different sites when used concomitantly, to prevent the risk of interaction.[2] Immunologic response may diminish with the simultaneous administration of HTIG with live virus vaccines (e.g., measles, mumps, rubella and oral polio). To avoid this interaction, delay live virus vaccination for 3 months after tetanus immunoglobulin is given.[6]

Attempts have been made to inactivate the toxin that is bound to nervous tissue by administering the anti toxin intrathecally thereby reducing the mortality from 70 to 18%. In a comparison HTIG was given to 97 patients, in an intrathecal dose of 250 i.u. to 49 patients and an intramuscular dose of 1000 i.u. to the remaining 48. There were only 3 deterioration's (including one death) with the intrathecal administration and 15 deterioration's (including 10 deaths) with the intramuscular administration. However a meta-analysis on intrathecal therapy in neonatal tetanus failed to provide convincing evidence that intrathecal therapy with either the equine serum or HTIG is of major benefit in neonatal tetanus although clinically important treatment effects in some subtypes cannot be excluded indicating a need for more definite studies.[1, 5]

Control of Spasms

Spasms may lead to compromised ventilation, exhaustion, and often aspiration of gastric contents, all of which are life threatening. Heavy sedation was the mainstay of treatment but lost its importance with the introduction of muscle relaxants and continued to be used only as an adjunct to provide patient comfort and tolerance to therapy.

Muscle relaxants then became the mainstay of treatment of spasms in tetanus.[5] Traditionally the long acting agent Pancuronium has been used for muscular paralysis.

Pancuronium is an inhibitor of catecholamine reuptake and as such could worsen autonomic instability in severely affected patients. There have been isolated reports of worsening hypertension and tachycardia associated with its use in tetanus.[1] The initial dose is 0.08 to 0.1 mg/kg. The maintenance dose is approximately 20% of the initial dose. The infusion dose commonly used is 0.4 to 0.6 microgram/kg/min. The dose requirement is typically titrated through clinical judgement, although neuromuscular monitoring techniques such as train of four response is recommended. Depending on the clinical response and stabilization of the basic disease, this drug should be used for the shortest possible period. The doses should be spaced out after two weeks and stopped after 3 weeks. Tachycardia, hypertension and increased cardiac output are related to vagal blockade and norepinephrine release. Prolonged use of this drug is associated with delayed recovery from paralysis and persistent need of ventilation.[2] Alternatives include the older agents d-tubocurarine and alcuronium which have been reported to reduce hemodynamic instability, but may also be a cause of hypotension through histamine release. Vecuronium has been proposed as it is "cardiovascularly clean" but is relatively short acting.[1] An initial dose of 0.08 to 0.1 mg/kg is given followed by a maintenance of an infusion in a dose of 0.8 to 2 microgram/kg/min. Vecuronium is devoid of vagolytic or histamine-releasing actions though the long term toxicity of pancuronium is shared. Metabolites are 50 to 70 % as effective as the parent drug and have a tendency to accumulate, causing prolonged paralysis. Because of renal elimination, the drug must be used with caution in renal failure.[2] Longer acting agents are preferable as they lend themselves to administration by intermittent bolus rather than requiring infusion of the newer agents pipercuronium and rocuronium are long acting and "clean" but are expensive compared with older drugs. Atracurium is an intermediate acting neuromuscular blocking agent that is associated with histamine release at higher doses. It possesses the unique metabolic trait of being inactivated by ester hydrolysis and Hoffman elimination; therefore renal and hepatic dysfunction does not affect the duration of blockade. The initial dose is 0.5 mg/kg. For infusion, a dose of 4 to 12 microgram/kg/min is used.[2] Individual drugs have not been compared in randomized trials.[1,8] Vecuronium is considered the drug of choice due to the absence of cardiovascular effects but proves to be very expensive in the long term. Atracurium has been used as an infusion with no serious accumulation of metabolites. Pancuronium is better avoided in patients with severe sympathetic activity, but these effects are not very prominent in the dosages used, and are still popular in many institutions due to the cost factor. The disadvantage of muscle relaxants is the need for long term artificial ventilation (2- 4 weeks) which carries with it complications of pulmonary infection, barotrauma, difficulty in weaning and deep venous thrombosis.[5]

Dantrolene has been used in place of muscle relaxants for the control of spasms in tetanus without the need for artificial ventilation. It produces skeletal muscle relaxation by a direct action on excitation contraction coupling, presumably by decreasing the amount of calcium released from the sarcoplasmic reticulum. Avoidance of the need for artificial ventilation is a tremendous advantage, but dantrolene does not suppress autonomic dysfunction and has to be supplemented with heavy sedation in the more severe cases. Dantrolene is an expensive drug, which, in the long term is a major disadvantage.[5] The directly acting muscle relaxant dantrolene has been reported in one case in which spasms were difficult to control. Paralysis was unnecessary after administration of dantrolene, spasms reduced, and patient condition improved.[1, 8]

The need for heavy sedation is, however, rapidly regaining ground on the basis that muscle relaxants alone with minimal sedation are associated with severe autonomic dysfunction. A variety of drugs are used for this purpose, namely barbiturates, diazepam, chlorpromazine morphine and recently even isoflurane and propofol. In the absence of glycinergic agonists, gamaaminobutyric acid agonists have been used for the control of spasms. Diazepam as a GABA agonist has gained a traditional place in the control of spasms in tetanus. As an adjunct to muscle relaxants it was used in doses of 10–30 mg/6–8 hourly. It has also been used as the sole agent for the control of spasms. The use of doses as high as 3400 mg/day have been reported. Metabolic acidosis may occur with these large doses probably due to the effects of the solubilizing vehicle propylene glycol. The sedative agent propofol may also have useful muscle relaxant properties. Sedation with propofol allowed control of spasms and rigidity without additional relaxant. Examination of EMG and neuromuscular function during propofol boluses showed an 80% reduction in EMG activity without alteration of neuromuscular function. However, drug concentrations were closer to anaesthetic than sedative doses and mechanical ventilation would be required.[1, 5, 8] Ventilatory support is not always necessary but the airway needs to be secured and the prolonged after effects of these large doses are a major disadvantage. Midazolam has also been used for the same effect with less prolonged duration of after effects, but its cost is a limiting factor. Diazepam has been often used in combination with other sedatives such as chlorpromazine and morphine to control spasms in severe tetanus without the need for muscle relaxants or ventilation, but control of basal rigidity is poor and mouth care and limb physiotherapy require intermittent muscle relaxation. When given in large doses, diazepam prolongs the stay in the ICU due to the presence of active metabolites with long half lives. However in the more severe forms muscle relaxants become a necessary adjunct.[5]

Control of Autonomic Dysfunction

Autonomic disturbance with sustained labile hypertension, tachycardia, vasoconstriction, and sweating is common in severe cases. Profound bradycardia and hypotension may occur and may be recurrent or preterminal events. Involvement of the sympathetic nervous system was recognized in 1968. Basal catecholamine concentrations rise but noradrenaline (norepinephrine) rises more markedly than adrenaline (epinephrine). Noradrenaline concentrations may rise 10-fold, spontaneously or in response to stimulation, leading to a "sympathetic storm". These rises are similar to those found in pheochromocytoma. Sympathetic neuronal overactivity is generally more prominent than adrenal medullary overactivity and hypertension is accompanied by a rise in systemic vascular resistance without large changes in cardiac index. Histological changes in the hearts of patients dying from tetanus are strikingly similar to those of patients with pheochromocytoma and the likely cause in both is persistently raised concentrations of catecholamines. Sedation, which is useful for controlling spasms and rigidity, is also the first step in reducing autonomic instability.[1] A regimen is required that will stabilize the cardiovascular system whilst preserving compensatory mechanisms and avoiding sudden collapse and death. A variety of drugs have been used with varying success and none of them entirely fulfils the above criteria.

Two different approaches have been used in the management of sympathetic over activity-peripheral adrenergic blockade and suppression of the release of catecholamines with sedation, both of which have been used as an adjunct to relaxants and artificial ventilation.

Chlorpromazine is a traditional sedative but was especially useful due to its alpha blocking action. It has been used in conjunction with diazepam in doses of 50-100 mg 8 hourly, but unacceptable hypotension sometimes occurred.[1,5] Phenothiazines, particularly chlorpromazine, are useful sedatives with α-adrenergic and anticholinergic effects.[1]

Propranolol, with or without concomitant alpha blockers, was the first drug used and was reported as effective; but in the late 1970s several workers reported fatal cardiovascular failure and irreversible cardiac arrest in patients treated with propranolol. Concern over unopposed alpha stimulation led to the addition of specific alpha blockers and then to the use of labetalol which (combined alpha and beta block) was used successfully, only to be implicated in irreversible cardiac arrest. The short acting beta blocker esmolol has been useful in suppressing crises but this does not solve the problem as the catecholamine levels remain high. The use of adrenergic blockade without the preservation of some response to changes in sympathetic activity can therefore be effective, but unpredictably dangerous. The combined alpha and beta blockade effectively denervates the cardiovascular system rendering the pressure support difficult during hypotensive episodes. The release of catecholamines is unaffected and these high levels can cause myocardial damage, which could be implicated in the irreversible cardiac arrest.[5] Mortality was not markedly reduced by these treatments and concerns about â blockade and sudden death have been raised. Sudden falls in catecholamine concentrations after "sympathetic storms", catecholamine induced cardiac damage, negative inotropism, β-blocker induced vasoconstriction, and unopposed parasympathetic activity are all plausible mechanisms. Epidural or spinal bupivacaine have also been reported to improve hemodynamic instability. Unfortunately, most reports are either case reports or small series and there are few adequate trials that have compared treatments or examined important outcome data. Intrathecal Baclofen (a GABAB agonist) has been reported in some small series with varying success. Doses have ranged from 500 to 2000 mg/day and have been given as boluses or infusion. Larger doses and boluses are associated with more side effects. In all reports a significant number of patients developed coma and respiratory depression necessitating ventilation. In some cases adverse effects were reversible with the GABAA antagonist flumazenil, but this is not reliable. The technique is invasive, costly, and facilities for ventilation must be available immediately. Tetanus patients are at risk of sepsis and may require anticoagulation which makes repeated or continuous spinal techniques a significant risk.[1] In one series Baclofen a GABA agonist was given by intermittent intrathecal injections to avoid artificial ventilation, but ventilatory depression occurred in 5 out of the 10 cases possibly due to overdosage (as baclofen is 600 more times potent by the intrathecal route). This overdosage could be avoided with continuous intrathecal infusion placed in L3-L4 space. The drug has been used for an average period of 7 to 14 days. Practical considerations are the risk of infection with external infusions devices (less costly) and the high cost of the implantable infusion device.[2, 5] There have been reports of successful management of autonomic disturbance with intravenous atropine. Doses of up to 100 mg/h were used in four patients. The basis being that tetanus is a disease of acetylcholine excess and used these high doses to achieve muscarinic and nicotinic blockade providing autonomic blockade, neuromuscular blockade, and central sedation. Blockade of the parasympathetic nervous system was reported to markedly reduce secretions and sweating. Oral or parenteral clonidine has been used with variable success. In one report of 27 patients treated over 12 years, the group randomized to receive clonidine had a significantly lower mortality.1

With the recognition of sympathetic over activity and the danger of using adrenergic blocking agents, heavy sedation has been re-introduced in an attempt to block the exaggerated response to stimuli, and thus control the endogenous autonomic dysfunction by suppressing catecholamine release. This has been recognized as a more logical method of suppressing autonomic dysfunction. Varying degrees of success have been claimed for a variety of drugs such as barbiturates, chlorpromazine, benzodiazepines, and volatile anesthetics.[5] Benzodiazepines augment GABA agonism by inhibiting an endogenous inhibitor at the GABA A receptor. Adequate sedation is essential in tetanus but is a double edged sword. Benzodiazepines are the most commonly used sedative agents. Diazepam has a wide margin of safety, has a rapid onset of action, can be given orally, rectally, or intravenously, and is a sedative, an anticonvulsant, and a muscle relaxant. It is also cheap and available in most parts of the world. However, it has a long cumulative half life (72 hours) and has active metabolites, in particular oxazepam and demethyldiazepam. Invariably, in the doses required to achieve adequate control of spasms (often up to 3–8 mg/kg/day) respiratory depression, coma, and medullary depression are common. Establishing the correct therapeutic window is extremely difficult, particularly in patients requiring prolonged support.[1, 5] The drug can be given daily divided iv or an infusion. Doses as high as 120 mg/kg/day can be administered. For mild spasms, a dose of 5 to 10 mg orally every 4 to 6 hours may be effective. Individual dose titration is mandatory. The drug is continued during the acute phase of the disease, when spasms and rigidity are severe. Typically spasms are more prevalent in the first 1 to 2 weeks of the illness. The drug is then gradually tapered off. However, low doses of the drug may be continued for a longer duration if autonomic dysfunction ensues.[2] Midazolam is an alternative, but it is usually not available or not affordable. Phenobarbital has been widely used since the 1960s. Morphine is particularly effective as sedation and cardiovascular stability may be achieved without compromising cardiac performance. Important actions in reducing cardiovascular instability include replacing depleted endogenous opioids and histamine release.[5] Morphine is used with an average dose of 0.1 mg/kg every 4 to 6 hours. The dose is tailored according to the presence of hypotension, hypertension or bradycardia. It is given for a duration of 7 to 10 days.[2] With all these drugs enormous doses may be required.[1] The use of morphine for the control of autonomic dysfunction is considered effective and is probably due to replacement of the deficiency in endogenous opioids found in tetanus. The only disadvantage is the depression of bowel motility which limits the use of enteral feeding. However heavy sedation does not reliably control the sympathetic over activity in all cases especially that which occurs in response to stimulation. Other drugs such as magnesium sulfate and clonidine have been used as an adjunct to heavy sedation.[5]

The use of intravenous magnesium sulfate infusions as the sole agent for the control of spasms in patients with severe tetanus has been tried in some places.[5] It has been used both in ventilated patients to reduce autonomic disturbance and in non-ventilated patients to control spasms. Magnesium is a presynaptic neuromuscular blocker, blocks catecholamine release from nerves and adrenal medulla; reduces receptor responsiveness to released catecholamines, and is an anticonvulsant and a vasodilator. It antagonizes calcium in the myocardium and at the neuromuscular junction and inhibits parathyroid hormone release so lowering serum calcium. In overdose it causes paralysis and probably sedation or anesthesia, although this is controversial.[1, 2] It is administered in an infusion pump following a loading dose. The dose is increased until spasms are relieved or patellar reflex is elicited. Evidence of hypocalcemia is extracted using clinical markers (e.g., chvostek's sign and trousseau's sign) and by measuring total serum, magnesium and calcium concentrations.[2] Magnesium sulfate is able to control spasms and minimize rigidity without the need for artificial ventilation. Since it is used as the sole agent (without muscle relaxants and heavy sedation) it is possible to titrate the dose against clinical signs (control of spasms and rigidity, with preservation of the patellar reflex) which makes it much easier than titrating the dose against serum magnesium levels. With this method of titration magnesium concentrations are found to be maintained within the therapeutic range. The striking features of magnesium therapy is that it can be titrated to control spasms without compromising ventilation as hypoventilation occurs at higher concentrations than that required to control spasms. The absence of sedation and immobility avoids the danger of deep vein thrombosis and helps considerably in overall management. Magnesium has the special advantage of combining control of spasms by neuromuscular blockade without the need for artificial ventilation and cardiovascular instability by suppressing catecholamine release. Whether this form of therapy will control autonomic dysfunction in more severe forms of tetanus remains to be seen.[5] In a paper by James and Manson,[13] patients with very severe tetanus were studied and magnesium was found to be inadequate alone as a sedative relaxant but an effective adjunct in controlling autonomic disturbance. Serum concentrations were difficult to predict and regular monitoring of serum magnesium and calcium concentrations were required. Muscular weakness was readily apparent and ventilation was required in all cases. Attagyle and Rodrigo[14] studied patients at an earlier stage of the illness yet all cases were probably severe. They used similar doses of magnesium to try to avoid sedatives and positive pressure ventilation and reported successful control of spasms and control of rigidity. Magnesium concentrations were predictable and readily kept within the therapeutic range by using the clinical signs of the presence of a patella tendon reflex. In both studies the absence of hypotension and bradycardia was by contrast with results with â blockade. Both groups agreed that tidal volume and cough may be impaired and secretions increased: tracheostomy is mandatory and ventilatory support must be readily available. More work is necessary to define the role of magnesium both with regard to the physiological effect it exerts on neuromuscular function in the presence of tetanus and secondly to establish what role if any it has in the routine management of severe tetanus.[1]

The difficulty in finding a drug which controls autonomic dysfunction in all cases of tetanus could be due to the variation in plasma concentrations achieved, individual variation in response or the varying degrees of severity of the disease. As yet no single drug which controls spasms and autonomic dysfunction in all patients has been found and the search continues. A regime which controls spasms without the need for artificial ventilation is a much sought after treatment modality in tetanus.[5]

Supportive Measures

Patients suspected of having tetanus should initially be managed in the ICU. To minimize the risk of precipitating reflex tetanic spasms, the patient should be monitored in a dark, quiet area and unnecessary patient manipulation and procedures should be avoided.[2] The intensive care management of tetanus requires not only the provision of ventilatory support but also the support of all organs systems which are dysfunctional as a result of the disease and its therapy. This includes respiratory complications (from aspiration of oral and gastrointestinal contents), cardiovascular dysfunction, depression of gastro intestinal motility, and the recognized effects of immobility namely thromboembolism, fluid retention due to inappropriate secretion of anti diuretic hormone, and nosocomial infections from prolonged invasive instrumentation.[5]

Airway

Early tracheostomy helps to isolate the trachea and facilitate ventilation without undue stimulation of the upper airway. The endotracheal tube inserted as an emergency is best converted to tracheostomy as soon as possible for the incidence of complications with long term endotracheal intubation are high and clearance of secretions is easier with tracheostomy. Careful management of the cuff allowing a small leak must be ensured at all times.[2, 5] Percutaneous tracheostomy is now a routine technique on many intensive care units. It is particularly suitable for patients with tetanus. Patient transfer to and from an operating theatre (entailing unnecessary stimulation) is avoided. Other potential advantages over traditional open surgical techniques include reduced blood loss, reduced operative morbidity and reduced long term sequelae. The single step forceps dilatational method is rapid and can be used for emergency airway management and the serial dilation technique is useful for intubated patients requiring tracheostomy.[1]

Care of the Lung

Regular physiotherapy (lung and limbs) and tracheal suction are mandatory, as lung complications are a common cause of morbidity and mortality. Secretions and salivation are special problems and are evidence of increased parasympathetic activity. Nebulisation with ipratropium can help to reduce bronchial secretions considerably.[5] Regular nontraumatic suction (premedication may be needed to prevent spasms) under strict aseptic technique, tracheostomy site cleaning, a propped up position to 15° to 30°, and chest physiotherapy are essential to prevent aspiration, atelectasis and pneumonia.[2]

ENTERAL FEEDING

Should be commenced as soon as possible through the nasogastric tube since nutrition is particularly important during long-term ventilation. Weight loss is universal in tetanus. Contributory factors include inability to swallow, autonomic induced alterations in gastrointestinal function, increased metabolic rate from pyrexia and muscular activity and prolonged critical illness. Enteral nutrition is associated with a lower incidence of complications and is cheaper than parenteral nutrition. Percutaneous gastrostomy may avoid the complications associated with nasogastric tube feeding[8] i.e. avoiding the stimulation and reflux associated with a nasogastric tube. In those patients unable to tolerate enteral feeding cytoprotection is best achieved with sucralfate or ranitidine.[5]

Ventilation

Respiratory failure is the commonest direct cause of death from tetanus when artificial ventilation may not be available. Where it is available attempts should be made to anticipate and detect patients at risk from hypoxia and airways obstruction, aspiration hypoventilation, pneumonia, and respiratory arrest. Early airways protection and ventilatory support is often needed. The effects of different modes of assisted ventilation in tetanus have not been evaluated. The modes used will often be limited by the complexity of the ventilators available in the intensive care unit. In the early stages of the disease when rigidity and spasm are prominent muscular paralysis and controlled mandatory ventilation are necessary. Poor compliance and oxygenation due to muscular rigidity or pulmonary complications may be overcome by a combination of pressure controlled ventilation and positive end expiratory pressure (PEEP). In the later stages of the disease modes of ventilation that allow spontaneous ventilation (synchronized intermittent mandatory, continuous positive airway pressure and biphasic positive airway pressure ventilation) are generally preferred. These may optimize the respiratory pattern, reduce sedation requirements, minimize muscle wastage, and reduce the likelihood of acquired critical illness neuropathy or myopathy. However, there is little evidence base in tetanus for these advanced modes of support.[1]

The staff must take special precautions to prevent nosocomial infections and prophylactic administration of thrombolytic therapy is important to avoid deep vein thrombosis. Meticulous hygiene and basic care of central and peripheral venous access sites and urinary catheters must be emphasized. Heparin or other anticoagulants may be administered to prevent thrombosis and embolic events. Once spasms are controlled, physiotherapy should be encouraged to minimize the risk of contractures. Intercurrent infections should be recognized at the outset and diligently managed.[2]

COMPLICATIONS

Secondary infections are a frequent complication, most commonly associated with the lower respiratory tract, urinary catheterization, and wound sepsis. Attempts must be made to prevent secondary infection and much is achieved by attention to detail in basic care. Maintaining adequate spacing between beds and general standards of cleanliness such as regular hand washing by staff and visitors are simple effective measures.

Tracheostomy site cleaning, strict sterile technique during tracheal suction, and basic care of peripheral or central venous access sites and the urinary catheter are all fundamental to good treatment.

Respiratory complications from aspiration and hypoventilation are common and may be reduced by early tracheostomy, avoiding nasogastric tubes where possible, and nursing patients in a 15°-30° sitting up position. Gram negative organisms, particularly Klebsiella and Pseudomonas are common, and staphylococcal infections are also often encountered. Meticulous mouth care, chest physiotherapy, and regular tracheal suction are essential to prevent atelectasis, lobar collapse, and pneumonia particularly as salivation and bronchial secretions are greatly increased in severe tetanus.

Adequate sedation is mandatory before such interventions in patients at risk of uncontrolled spasms or autonomic disturbance and the balance between physiotherapy and sedation may be difficult to achieve.

Tracheal stenosis can be a problem in children.

Measures to avoid serious thromboembolic complications include compression stockings, subcutaneous heparin, and limb physiotherapy. There is very little information on follow up of patients after tetanus, particularly for cognitive function. In one of the few studies to examine this question, Anlar et al found enuresis, mental retardation, and growth delay to be frequent sequaelae after neonatal tetanus.

A list of complications is listed in Table 12.5.[8]

PROGNOSIS

Mortality figures depend on the availability and quality of intensive care, and the age of the patient. Before ICU's were established, 80% of historical controls died from early acute respiratory failure. After introduction of ICU care reduction of mortality occurred from 44 to 15%. Of these 40% of the deaths were due to sudden cardiac death and 15% were the result of respiratory complications. In Africa mortality from neonatal tetanus was reported as 82% in 1960.[8] A mortality of 10% is often quoted as reasonable in developed countries but is in fact higher in most centers. In the US a mortality rate of 11% was recorded from 1995 to 1997. In Malaysia a mortality rate of 18% has been reported. In PGIMER, Chandigarh a mortality rate of 18% is reported. Mortality typically was seen in grade 3 tetanus with autonomic instability and in patients with nosocomial infections. The course of tetanus extends more than 4 to 6 weeks, requiring ventilatory support for almost 3 weeks during that period. Increased tone and minor spasms may persist for months, nut recovery is usually complete.[2]

ACTIVE IMMUNIZATION

In addition to passive immunization, active vaccination needs to be administered to all patients, so called active-passive immunization. This adds to the short-term immunity (passive), and to long term humoral and cellular immunity (active). As the first is declining the second appears and thus avoids a window of non-protection. From experimental work in animals it is clear that the toxoid starts acting a few hours after injection and before a humoral response is detectable. Presumably the toxoid saturates the ganglioside receptors and prevents wild type toxin binding. The toxoid and the human (or equine) anti-tetanus immunoglobulin should be administered at different sites on the body to prevent interaction at the injection site. If both are to be administered together no more than 1000 IU human or 5000 IU equine anti-tetanus immunoglobulin should be administered, higher doses can neutralize the immunogenicity of the toxoid. Tetanus toxoid for vaccination is produced by formaldehyde treatment of the toxin and its immunogenicity is improved by adsorption with aluminium hydroxide. Alum adsorbed tetanus toxoid is very effective at preventing tetanus with a failure rate of 4/100 million immunocompetent people. Serum antitoxin concentrations above 0.01 U/ml are considered protective, although there have been patients reported with protective serum antibody concentrations. A protective antibody concentration is attained after the second dose, but a third dose ensures longer lasting immunity. To maintain adequate concentrations of protection additional booster doses should be administered every 10 years. Reactions to the tetanus toxoid are estimated to be 1 in 50,000 injections, although most are not severe; local tenderness, edema, flu-like illness, and low grade fever are the most often encountered. Severe reactions such as Guillian-Barré syndrome and acute relapsing polyneuropathy are rare. Neonatal tetanus can be prevented by immunization of women during pregnancy. Two or three doses of adsorbed toxin should be given with the last dose at least 1 month before delivery. Immunity is passively transferred to the fetus and protective antibodies will persist long enough to protect the baby. Research on tetanus vaccines has concentrated on a single dose vaccine, using technology such as micro encapsulation. This would be of most use in countries where a three dose regime results in management difficulties. Strategies involving expression of the immunodominant HC domain in attenuated strains of *Salmonella* followed by oral immunization have been successful in animals, and may form the basis of future multivalent oral vaccines.[1] Refer to Table 12.6 for brief guide to prophylaxis.

REFERENCES

1. JJ Farrar, LM Yen, T Cook, et al. Tetanus. *J Neurol Neurosurg Psychiatry* 2000;69:292-301.
2. Prabhakar S, Grover VK. Tetanus. *Curr Treat Options Infect Dis* 2002;4:473-484.
3. Hsu SS, Groleau G. Tetanus in the emergency department: A current review. *J Emerg Med* 2001;20:357-365.
4. Sanford JP. Tetanus: Forgotten but not gone. *N Engl J Med* 1995;332:812-813.
5. Attygalle D, Nalini, Prasanna Tetanus: Other Aspects of Tetanus. Egroup of Tetanus updated April 2000 Available from: ttp://www.geocities.com/tetanus_ tetanus/general.html accessed in February 2004.
6. Abrahamian FM. Management of Tetanus: A Review. *Curr Treat Options Infect Dis* 2001;3:209-216.
7. Abdelmoneim T, DeNicola LK, Hasan MY. Tetanus: Complications and Management in a Pediatric Intensive Care Unit. in The Rare Case Registry of Peds CCM: The Pediatric Critical Care Web Site, September 16, 1997. Available from: http://PedsCCM.wustl.edu/RARE/Tetanus.html accessed in February 2004.
8. Cook TM, Protheroe RT, Handel JM. Tetanus: A review of the literature. *Br J Anaesth* 2001;87:477-487.
9. Apte NM, Karnad DR. Short report: the spatula test. A simple bedside test to diagnose tetanus. *Am J Trop Med Hyg* 1995; 53:386-387.
10. Patel JC, Joag GG. Grading of tetanus to evaluate prognosis. *Indian J Med Sci* 1959;13:834-840.
11. Ahmadsyah I, Salim A. Treatment of tetanus: an open study to compare the efficacy of procaine penicillin and metronidazole. *BMJ* 1985;291:648–650.
12. Yen LM, Dao LM, Day NPJ, et al. Management of tetanus: A comparison of penicillin and metronidazole. *Symposium of Antimicrobial Resistance in Southern Vietnam* 1997.
13. James MFM, Manson EDM. The use of magnesium infusions in the management of very severe tetanus. *Intensive Care Medicine* 1985;11:5–12.
14. Attygalle D, Rodrigo N. Magnesium sulphate for control of spasms in severe tetanus. *Anaesthesia* 1997;52:956–962.

Ravinder K Gupta and Ritu Gupta

13 Dengue Hemorrhagic Fever

INTRODUCTION

Dengue is the most important of the arboviral infections of humans. Dengue hemorrhagic fever (DHF)/dengue shock syndrorne (DSS) is a severe, often fatal, febrile disease caused by dengue viruses, limited to children in some South-East Asian countries, including India.[1-4]

DHF is believed to be a hypersensitive response to a repeat attack with dengue fever virus. It is characterized by capillary permeability, abnormalities of hemostasis and in severe cases, a protein losing shock syndrome.

Dengue fever has become a major international public health concern.[5-8] Annually, there are 50-100 million cases of dengue fever and 0.25-0.50 million cases of DHF in the world. DHF was reported for the first time from Philippines in 1957 and subsequently it was reported in India, Nepal and Myanmar.

ETIOPATHOGENESIS

The causative virus has 4 antigenic types 1,2,3 and 4 belonging to Flavivirdae family. The dengue virus gets transmitted by mosquitoes of Stegomyia family. Aedes aegypti (dominant in India) and Aedes albopictus are the principal vectors. A. aegypti, a day time biting mosquito, is highly urbanized and breeds in water stored for drinking or bathing and in rainwater collected in any container. Since A. aegypti has a limited range, spread of an epidemic occurs mainly through viremic human beings and follows the main lines of transportation. Where dengue is endemic adults become immune and children and susceptible foreigners may be only persons to acquire overt disease. DHF occurs where multiple type of dengue virus are simultaneously or sequentially transmitted. DHF can occur during primary dengue infection, most frequently in infants whose mothers are immune to dengue.

The pathogenesis of DHF is incompletely understood. What is well-known is that it is usually associated with second infection with dengue types 1-4. Non-neutralizing antibodies promote cellular infection and enhance severity of the disease. There is rapid activation of complement system in the acute stage of secondary dengue infection. Soluble tumor necrosis factor receptor, infection, interferon-g, and interlukin 2 are elevated during shock. C1q, C3, C4, C5-C8 and C3 proactivators are depressed and C3 catabolic rates are elevated. The endothelia cell may get interacted with these factors and produce increase vascular permeability through the nitric oxide final pathway. The blood clotting and fibrinolytic system get activated, and levels of factor XII (Hageman factor) are depressed. A mild degree of DIC, liver damage, and thrombocytopenia may operate to cause bleeding in DHF. Fluid, electrolytes, small proteins and in some instances red cells leak into extravascular spaces due to capillary damage. This internal redistribution of fluid together with deficits caused by fasting, thirsting and vomiting results in hemoconcentration, hypovolemia, increased cardiac work, tissue hypoxia metabolic acidosis and hyponatremia.

Death may be due to gastrointestinal or intracranial hemorrhage.

CLINICAL MANIFESTATIONS

Incubation period is 1-7 days with a variation of 3 to 15 days. The differentiation between dengue fever and DHF is difficult early in the course of illness. Fever, maliase, vomiting, headache, anorexia and cough is followed after 2-5 days by rapid clinical deterioration and collapse. The child usually has cold clammy extremities, a warm trunk flushed face, diaphoresis, restlessness, irritability and mid-epigastric pain. Petechiae on the forehead and extremities, spontaneous ecchymoses, easy bruising and bleeding at venipuncture sites are common. There is rapid and labored respiration. The pulse becomes weak, rapid, thready and the heart sounds faint. There is tender hepatomegaly.

In the epidemic of DHF/DSS seen during fall and autumn of 1993 at Jammu, winter capital of the State of Jammu and Kashmir, gastrointestinal hemorrhages dominated the scene.[7,8] Generally speaking, hemetemesis is the most common bleeding manifestation reported in Indian children. After a 24 to 36 hour period of crisis, convalescence is fairly rapid in the subjects who recover. Bradycardia and venticular extrasystoles are common during convalescence.

DIAGNOSIS

The diagnosis of DHF is derived from high index of suspicion. The world Health Organization (WHO) criteria for DHF are fever, minor or major hemorrhagic manifestations, thrombocytopenia (≤ 1 lac/mm^3) and objective evidence of increased capillary permeability (Hematocrit increased by 20%), pleural effusion (by chest radiograph) or hypoalbuminemia. WHO grading of DHF is given in Table 13.1.

Table 13.1: WHO grading of DHF[3]

Grade 1	Fever, nonspecific constitutional symptoms, positive Hess (tourniquet) test.
Grade 2	Features of Grade 1 + spontaneous bleeding into the skin and/or from other sites.
Grade 3	Circulatory failure manifested by rapid weak pulse, hypotension or low pulse pressure, cold clammy skin, restlessness.
Grade 4	Profound shock manifested by unrecordable BP and pulse.

Serology and virus isolation, though ideal are time consuming. IgM anti-body estimation, mosquito inoculation and indirect immuno-fluorescent test also give early results. Viral RNA can be detected in blood or tissues by specific complementary DNA probes or amplified first by the polymerase chain reaction.

LABORATORY FINDINGS

The tourniquet test is positive only infrequently.

Metabolic acidosis, hemoconcentration (≥ 20% increase in hematocrit) thrombocytopenia, prolonged bleeding time, and moderately decreased prothrombin level are common. Fibrinogen levels may be subnormal and fibrin split products elevated.

Consumption of complement, hyponatremia, hypochloremia, hypo-albuminemia, elevation of serum transaminases are also seen. Roentgenograms of the chest may reveal pleural effusion.

The rapid IgM-IgG capture ELISA test, has become the standard for serological diagnosis of dengue fever.

DIFFERENTIAL DIAGNOSIS

Meningococcemia, typhoid fever, scrub typhus, leptospirosis, yellow fever, many rickettsial diseases and other severe illnesses (including severe malaria) caused by a variety of agents may produce a clinical picture similar to DHF.[3,5-8]

Table 13.2: Criteria for diagnosis of DHF/DSS[3,7]

Clinical
- Acute onset of high fever
- Hemorrhagic manifestations
- Hepatomegaly
- Shock

Laboratory
- Threombocytopenia with platelet count < 100,000/mm^3
- Hemoconcentration with hematocrit > 20% more than normal

Note: Two clinical parameters plus one laboratory parameter are enough for labelling the case as DHF/DSS provisionally.

TREATMENT

Management of DHF/DSS is, by and large, symptomatic and supportive.[7-11]

Evaluation of vital signs and hemoconcentration, dehydration and electrolyte imbalance are immediate steps in management and pave the way for appropriate therapeutic intervention.

- High fever should be controlled using tepid sponging and/or paracetamol. Since stronger NSAIDs (aspirin in particular) are likely to predispose to mucosal bleeding, these should be avoided.
- Oxygen is indicated in most cases.
- Rapid intravenous replacement of fluids and electrolytes are important. Ringer lactate infusion is the IV fluid of choice.
- Transfusion of fresh blood or platelets suspended in plasma may be useful in subjects who remain unresponsive. It is good to remember that lack of improvement may well be due to bleeding, both occult and overt.
- Plasma, plasma colloid preparations or platelet infusion are to be considered in case of overt uncontrolled bleeding despite the above-mentioned measures. This mode of therapy is particularly useful in cases complicated by DIC.[11]

Steroids (including high dose methylprednisolone) do not shorten the duration of disease[10] and are best avoided.[8]

Prevention

Attack on the vector mosquito population and personal protective measures are needed.

Attenuated dengue type 1, 2, and 4 vaccines are being developed in Thailand. Dengue vaccination may sensitize a recipient, resulting in DHF after a subsequent dengue infection.

Prognosis

Mortality is around 40 to 50%. Energetic and intensive care should bring down mortality to as low as 2% (Table 13.3).

In survivors, there remains risk of residual brain damage caused by prolonged shock or occasionally by intracranial hemorrhage.

Table 13.3: Factors contributing to reduction in mortality

• Early recognition of illness, particularly shock
• Careful monitoring
• Appropriate fluid therapy

REFERENCES

1. Rasul CH, Ahasan HAMN, Rasid AKMM, Khan MRH. Epidemiological factors of dengue hemorrhagic fever in Bangladesh. *Indian Pediatr* 2002;39:369-372.
2. Narayanan M, Aravind MA, Thilothammal N, *et al.*, Dengue fever epidemic in Chennai–A study of clinical profile and outcome. *Indian Pediatr* 2002;39:1027-1033.
3. World Health Organisation. *Dengue Hemorrhagic Fever: Diagnosis, Treatment, Prevention and Control.* 2nd edn. Geneva: World Health Organization 1997.
4. Aggarwal A, Chandra J, Aneja S, Patwari AK, Dutta AK. An epidemic of dengue hemorrhagic fever and dengue shock syndrome in children in Delhi. *Indian Pediatr* 1998;35:727-732.
5. Pushpa V, Venkatadesi Kalu M, Mohan S, Cherian T, John TJ, Ponnuraj EM. An epidemic of dengue hemorrhagic fever/dengue shock syndrome in tropical India. *Ann Trop Pediatr* 1998;18:289-293.
6. Dutta AK, Aggarwal A. Dengue Fever. In: Gupte S (ed) *Recent Adv Ped (Special Vol 1: Tropical Pediatrics).* New Delhi: Jaypee Brothers, 1998.
7. Gupte S. Pediatric viral infections. In: Gupte S (ed) *The Short Text book of Pediatrics*. 9th edn. New Delhi. Jaypee Brothers 2001:174-176.
8. Gupte S. DHF/DSS: Recounting observations from 1993 experience. *Bull Trop Med Hyg* 2002; 14:67-69.
9. Halstead SB: Dengue fever/Dengue Hemorrhagic fever. In Behrman RE, Kliegmann RM, Jenson HB (eds*) Nelson Text book of Pediatrics 16th edn*. Philadelphia: WB Saunders 2000:1005-1007.
10. Tassniyon S, Vaanawathan S, Chirawatkal V, Rojansuphot S. Failure of high dose methylprednisolone in established dengue shock syndrome. A placebo-controlled double-blind study. *Pediatrics* 1993;92:111-115.
11. Kabra SK, Jain Y, Madhulika, Tripathi P, Singhal T, Broor S, et al. Role of platelet transfusion in dengue hemorrhagic fever. *Indian Pediatr* 1998;35: 452-454.

Section IV

Neurological Emergencies

Neurological Emergencies

Akash Deep and Jhuma Mandal

14 Increased Intracranial Pressure

INTRODUCTION

The management of children who have known or presumed increased intracranial pressure (ICP) requires recognizing that two mechanisms of injury uniquely coexist in this situation. The primary injury is the inciting event, which leads to intracranial hypertension in the first place. Potential primary injuries include head injury with an acute mass lesion or hematoma, anoxic-ischemic injury as occurs in near-drowning, brain tumors, and other inciting events that lead to increased ICP, This injury may or may not lend itself to specific therapy directed at the lesion itself, such as removal of the brain tumor or hematoma, The focus of this discussion, however, is directed towards preventing a secondary injury from the intracranial hypertension itself. This secondary injury is caused by the inability of the cerebral vasculature to deliver oxygen and glucose to the neurons because of poor cerebral perfusion pressure (CPP). When the degree of decrease in CPP is only moderate and its duration brief, reversible neuronal dysfunction occurs. When the decrease in CPP is severe or prolonged, irreversible neuronal death occurs and, if extensive enough, leads to irreversible brain injury or death.

Elevated ICP may lead to brain damage or death by two principal mechanisms:

1. Global hypoxic-ischemic injury, as a consequence of reduced cerebral perfusion pressure (CPP) and cerebral blood flow.
2. Mechanical distortion and compression of brain tissue as a result of intracranial mass effect and ICP compartmentalization. All ICP therapies have as a goal, reduction of intracranial volume.

GENERAL CONCEPTS

Intracranial pressure (ICP) is normally thought of as the pressure within the intracranial vault that results from the interaction of the brain, the cerebral blood volume (CBV), and the cerebrospinal fluid (CSF). These components may undergo alterations in their individual volumes but the total volume of the intracranial contents must remain fixed. Thus, alteration in the volume of one compartment must be compensated for by opposite changes in another compartment in order for the ICP to remain the same. This concept is known as the modified Monro-Kellie doctrine.

Effect of O_2 and CO_2

The effect of arterial blood gases on CBF is important in the management of patients with elevated intracranial hypertension and therefore will be covered in detail. Although oxygen and carbon dioxide are really metabolic components, it is advantageous to discuss their proposed mechanisms separately as they are easy to manipulate in the Pediatric Intensive Care Unit (PICU) setting. Changes in oxygen pressure have been shown to produce significant effects on vascular smooth muscle. Hypoxia has been shown to greatly increase CBF by vasodilatation. Rises in oxygen content have also been shown to produce vasoconstriction but to a lesser degree. It is unclear if oxygen's effect on vascular smooth muscle is by a direct mechanism or by production of various metabolic substrates. No matter the mechanism, it is clear that maintenance of an adequate PaO_2 is essential in the management of intracranial hypertension.

$PaCO_2$ has also been shown to have a significant effect on CBF with hypercapnia increasing flow upto 350% of normal and hypocapnia producing smaller reductions in flow.[1] Again, these changes appear to be accomplished via an indirect method; alterations in tissue pH producing changes in arteriolar diameter. Carbon dioxide has been shown to readily cross the blood-brain barrier and lower CSF pH via its reaction with carbonic anhydrase. The changes in pH occur rapidly as does the resultant change in vessel diameter. These mechanisms are preserved even when normal autoregulation has been lost. Therefore changes in $PaCO_2$ are often used by the clinician to alter ICP. It is important to realize that the response to sustained hyperventilation appears to be lost after 24 hours because of accumulation of lactic acid and alterations in the bicarbonate buffer system.

Initially, hyperventilation was thought to be beneficial to the injured brain by restoring brain pH, restoring cerebral autoregulation, and increasing cerebral perfusion by reductions in ICP. Hyperventilation has since been shown to produce cerebral ischemia, hypoxia and local inverse steal phenomenon.[2-4] Several recent studies have shown prolonged hyperventilation to have an adverse effect on outcome in head-injury patients.[5] The liberal use of hyperventilation in children with increased ICP must be approached with caution because of the concerns mentioned in this section. One should maintain $PaCO_2$ between 30-35 mm Hg in head-injured patients.

Cerebral Perfusion Pressure

Fundamentally important to understanding and management of ICP is the role of CPP.

Autoregulation of the cerebral arterioles normally maintains CBF constant across a wide range of CPP (50 to 100 mmHg).[6] However, this process becomes dysfunctional in certain pathologic conditions such as trauma and stroke. When autoregulation is impaired, CBF tends to approximate a straight-line relationship with CPP, and therefore CBF may become insufficient even with minor reductions in CPP. CPP should be continuously maintained > 70 mmHg in patients with raised ICP, as reduction below that level may lead to secondary hypoxic-ischemic injury.[12] CPP must only be measured with the arterial pressure transducer at the level of the external auditory meatus, to accurately reflect the pressure on entry to the brain. The CPP should not be allowed to go higher than 120 mmHg, because above that level hyperperfusion and aggravation of brain edema may occur.[8]

Clinical Features

In the awake patient:

Irritability, headache, variable drowsiness, neck retraction, opisthotonic posturing, tense fontanelle by palpation (in those in whom the fontanelle is open) and sixth nerve palsy may all be presenting features, either alone or in combination.

In the already obtunded or comatose patient:

Consider raised intracranial pressure especially in a child with head injury, suspected meningitis/encephalitis or suspected non accidental head injury (child abuse). The following features strongly suggest the possibility of raised intracranial pressure:

- Abnormal posturing: decortication or decerebration, affecting one or more limbs (do not mistake such posturing for seizures)
- Pupillary dilatation, especially if unilateral and the pupils are non-reactive (requires emergency treatment)
- Hypertension/bradycardia
- Abnormalities of respiration: periodic respiration, hyperventilation, irregular respiration (requires emergency treatment)
- Sixth nerve palsy
- Papilloedema/retinal hemorrhages.[9]

Indication for Intracranial Pressure Monitoring

Invasive monitoring of ICP is generally indicated in patients who meet all three of the following criteria:

1. The patient is suspected to be at risk for elevated ICP.
2. The patient is comatose (Glasgow Coma Scale score of 8).
3. The prognosis is such that aggressive ICU treatment is indicated.

Head injury is the most frequent indication for ICP monitoring. However, ICP monitoring may also be useful in other conditions such as encephalitis.[10] Reye's syndrome,[11] hepatic encephalopathy,[12] intracerebral hemorrhage, sagittal sinus thrombosis,[13] and various causes of hydrocephalus.[14] Suspicion of increased ICP is usually based on clinical signs and the results of neuroimaging studies, which may show an intracranial mass lesion with midline shift, severe hydrocephalus, or cerebral edema with effacement of the basal cisterns.

Therapy of Raised Intracranial Pressure

Emergency Treatment

Appropriate early intervention to stabilize intracranial pressure may prevent the disastrous consequences of raised intracranial pressure and allow for transportation, if necessary, for definitive diagnosis and treatment.

Goals of emergency therapy are two-fold

- To maintain adequate cerebral perfusion pressure
- To prevent herniation of the brain

Measures taken to control intracranial pressure include:

- Ensure a patent airway to avoid hypercarbia and hypoxia. Airway obstruction and inadequate respiratory drive, both leading to hypercarbia and hypoxia, can aggravate/lead to increased intracranial pressure.
- Monitor blood gases and check the electrolytes.
- Assist ventilation if necessary to maintain effective oxygenation and normocarbia. The $PaCO_2$ can be maintained at approximately 30 mmHg. More intense hyperventilation to achieve lower levels can be done for short periods if the situation warrants it, ideally only after discussion with a pediatric intensivist. Maintain adequate cerebral perfusion pressure. A mean blood pressure of at least 50 mmHg is usually required.
- Raise headend of bed to 30 degrees.

- Control seizures as they may further raise the intracranial pressure and cause brain shifts in those with non-compliance. Phenytoin may be preferred to a benzodiazepine or phenobarbitone to minimize sedative effects and the risk of apnea.
- Normalize temperature.
- Use only isotonic IV solutions (normal saline or Ringer's lactate).
- Mannitol 0.25-0.50 gm/kg over 15-30 minutes may be a valuable temporary adjunct for reducing raised intracranial pressure.
- Dexamethasone 1.5 mg/kg with a maximum of 8 mg; empirical dosage, is particularly effective if tumor is a cause. The role of dexamethasone in other situations of acute encephalopathy remains uncertain. Thiopental can reduce the intracranial pressure especially in those with head injury. In children, acute head injury may be complicated by markedly increased cerebral blood flow). Treatment should only be done if ventilation is assisted/controlled, adequate oxygenation assured, arterial carbon dioxide ($PaCO_2$) kept at low normal, normal blood pressure maintained and there is the ability to monitor blood gases and blood pressure. Typically, such treatment should be done under the supervision of a pediatric intensivist.

In addition:

- In children who have shunt and in whom raised intracranial pressure is suspected, every attempt should be made to contact a neurosurgeon immediately. In critical situations, pump the shunt mechanism repeatedly. Tapping the shunt should be attempted if expertise allows and if precleared with the neurosurgeon. The use of Mannitol requires discussion with a neurosurgeon. All the other measures outlined above should be put into place.
- Lumbar puncture should not be performed unless discussed with a pediatric intensivist, if raised intracranial pressure is suspected. If bacterial meningitis is strongly suspected, initiate antibiotic therapy and transfer.
- Avoid rapid hydration especially in a child with hypernatremia; in those with meningitis, inappropriate ADH secretion may be present and fluids should be restricted.

Physiological Basis for Medical Control of ICP

General Measures

Temperature Control

The increased metabolic demand that results from fever can increase in CBF, CBV and ICP. Increased CBV and pressure may lead to worsening of cerebral edema, reduced CBF and deterioration of the brain's oxygen supply and demand ratio. Therefore, it is imperative that hyperthermia be aggressively treated when increased ICP is present.

Temperature control may be accomplished with cooling mattresses and the administration of rectal acetaminophen. Shivering, which can increase ICP by increasing intrathoracic pressure, can be prevented by muscle paralysis. Overcooling to the point of hypothermia is to be avoided; rather. The goal is normothennia. Rectal, esophageal, or pulmonary arterial (via a Swan-Ganz catheter) temperature probes should be used to provide continuous temperature monitoring.

Head Position

Keeping the headend of the patient's bed flat or raising the head to a 30 degree angle may have different theoretical effect on optimizing CPP. Specifically, remembering that CPP = MAP-ICP, the mean arterial pressure to the brain is highest in the supine position, while the ICP is lowest when the head is elevated. The question is: Which position has the predominant effect on influencing CPP. To address this issue, Feldman et al.[15] studied 22 head injured patients and concluded that keeping the head of the bed elevated to 30 degrees provided the optimal benefit for ICP control. In an earlier study, Durward et al.[16] concluded that moderate head elevation to 15 to 30° optimized cerebral perfusion pressure. At head elevation levels above 30^0 the arterial pressure measured at head level failed to maintain cerebral perfusion which was significantly reduced.[17]

Another important issue concerning head position is preventing inadvertent neck constriction secondary to cervical collars or endotracheal tube tape. These maneuvers maximize jugular venous outflow and improve ICP control. Once the cervical spine has been cleared radiographically (usually by fluoroscopic flexion-extension views), the patient may be log rolled side to side at one to two hour intervals to prevent pressure sores on the body or back of the head.

Seizure Control and Prophylaxis

During seizure activity, the brain's metabolic rate, blood flow and oxygen consumption increase significantly,[18] thus diminishing its capacity for maintaining a normal ICP. The brain is injured and has loss of autoregulatory activity, seizures can result in dangerous ICP elevations and need to be treated aggressively. Ongoing seizures may be treated with lorazepam 0.1 to 0.2 mg/kg IV repeated twice every five minutes or until the seizures cease. At the same time, the patient should be loaded with either phenytoin 20 mg/kg IV and repeated in 30 minutes in the dose of 10 mg/kg (if the patient is over 2 years of age) or phenobarbital 20 mg/kg IV and also repeated in 30 minutes (if the patient is under 2 years of age).

Prophylactic administration of antiepileptic drugs is an important part of preventing unwanted ICP elevations. However, this is a complex topic, and no study has been able to define clear-cut risk groups for which prophylactic anticonvulsant therapy is indicated. High risk groups seem to include patients with parenchymal abnormalities such as contusions, lacerations, or surgical evacuation sites, acute subdural hematoma and posttraumatic epilepsy. If a patient is being treated for increased ICP and still has sustained unexplained ICP elevations, subclinical seizures must be considered as a cause and EEG evaluation is warranted.

Fluid Management

Traditional views of head injury management have advocated restricting fluid and sodium administration in hopes of preventing cerebral edema in area of injured brain and subsequently, increased ICP.[19] However in a recent study, Schoemaker et al[20] indicated that patients kept normovolemic during the period of increased ICP fare just as well as those kept deliberately hypovolemic. In the first study of its kind they retrospectively reviewed the fluid and sodium intake of 57 adults with severe head injury. They found that maintenance of normovolemia does not predispose head injured patients to uncontrolled ICP. This is in contrast to the old concept of "drying out" a head injury patient by restricting fluids and giving large amounts of osmotic diuretics. Current practice based on this new concept has so far met with encouraging results in several centers.

The type of intravenous maintenance and replacement fluid to use is subject to debate, although we prefer using an isotonic fluid such as Ringer's lactate or 0.9% saline with 20 mEq/L of KCl. Relatively hypotonic fluids such as 0.45% saline are often used in pediatric patients, but one must be vigilant that hyponatremia does not occur. D_5W is never indicated except in the circumstance of fluid replacement for significant hypernatremia as a result of neurogenic diabetes insipidus.

Sedation

Patient sedation is a key factor in ICP control, and is often overlooked. In patients with reduced intracranial compliance, struggling against restraints and/or ventilators can increase ICP by elevating intrathoracic and jugular venous pressures. Hypertension and tachycardia as part of a sympathetic anxiety response also may contribute to raising ICP. In addition, anxiety and fear have been shown to increase cerebral metabolic rate and blood flow in normal subjects.[21] Before other measures are instituted, agitated patients with raised ICP should be sedated until they are motionless and quiet. Since parenteral sedatives can cause both apnea and hypotension, patients receiving them must be intubated and have arterial pressure monitors. Propofol is an ideal sedative for patients with neurological disease because of its short half-life. This permits quick and frequent clinical assessments. Furthermore, this agent has anti-epileptic properties and acts as a free-radical scavenger. Paralytic neuromuscular blocking agents must be avoided in patients with neurological disease because it can obscure the proper assessment of nervous system function and are rarely needed.

Dosages are approximate and should be titrated to the patient's level of agitation and ICP. Combinations of agents may be more effective than the use of a single agent.

Blood Pressure Management

If both MAP and ICP remain elevated after sedation, lowering the systemic blood pressure may lead to a reduction of ICP. This especially is true in states of disordered autoregulation. If CPP is > 120 mm Hg and ICP is > 20 mmHg, a shortacting antihypertensive agent should be administered until CPP reaches approximately 100 mm Hg. Extreme caution must be exercised not to allow CPP to go below 70 mm Hg because of the risks of cerebral hypoxia, reflex cerebral vasodilatation, and plateau wave formation. This threshold may be even higher in chronically hypertensive patients. Labetolol and nifedipine are the favored agents to use in patients with increased ICP. Nitroprusside should be avoided if possible because it has been shown to induce cerebral vasodilation and may further raise ICP.

In the case where CPP < 70 mm Hg and ICP > 20 mm Hg, the appropriate strategy is to increase MAP using a short acting vasopressor such as dopamine. By increasing MAP (and therefore CPP), hypoxic drive for cerebral vasodilation is removed, vasoconstriction can occur and thus both CBV and ICP become reduced. This is more likely to occur when cyclic ICP waves (A and B) are present, since their presence indicates exhaustion of intracranial reserve.

CSF Removal

External Ventricular Drains

An external ventricular drain (EW) has therapeutic potential by allowing CSF removal once the ICP has reached a dangerous level. Removing CSF in this fashion is a physiological way to reduce ICP and avoid unwanted side effects from medications. Obviously, the ventricle needs to be large enough to cannulate, but in experienced hands, this problem is usually surmounted. The benefits of EVD insertion for control seem to far outweigh the potential risks (such as intracranial hematomas or infection), although no controlled study has addressed this issue.

Lumbar Drains

Once medical therapy for ICP control has been exhausted and barbiturate coma therapy is being considered, further CSF removal via a lumbar drain may produce dramatic and long-lasting changes in ICP. This has been documented by Baldwin and Rekate.[22]

Osmotic Agents and Diuretic Therapy

Mannitol

Mannitol is an osmotic diuretic: It is excreted by the kidneys and its mechanism of action is to increase the osmotic gradient across the distal tubule, thereby drawing free water with it. Since it does not cross the blood brain barrier on first pass, it has as its main effect, the rapid dehydration of brain tissue. This effect causes prompt reduction in brain volume caused by either cytotoxic or vasogenic edema, and thereby lowers ICP.[23] The second way mannitol may reduce ICP is through a prolonged dehydrating effect on the brain, caused by secondary hyperosmolality. A third mechanism of action of mannitol may be related to its ability to reduce blood viscosity, which may transiently increase CBF, resulting in reflex vasoconstriction and a decrease in CBV.

The initial dose of 20% mannitol solution should be 1.0 g/kg, followed by dose of 0.25 to 0.5 g/kg as needed. Repeated doses should be given as needed for ICP > 20 mm Hg, not on a standing basis. The effect of a single bolus of mannitol on ICP begins within 10 minutes, peaks between 20 and 60 minutes, and has a duration of 4 to 6 hours. A single dose can occasionally be effective for up to 24 hours, but may be required as frequently as hourly. With repeated doses it is possible that mannitol may accumulate in the brain and lead to rebound ICP elevation,[24] but this is not common. There may be important systemic complications of aggressive mannitol use. These include congestive heart failure from initial volume expansion, later volume contraction from diuresis, hyperkalemia, and acute tubular necrosis related to hyperosmolarity. Patients who receive repeated mannitol dosing require frequent measurements of serum electrolytes, serum osmolality, and careful recording of volume input and output. Urinary volume loss should be repleted with 0.9% saline. Prolonged use of mannitol is reported to lower its effectiveness,[25] particularly when osmolality surpasses 320 mOsm/kg, however, there are exceptions and therapy should be individualized.

The loop diuretic furosemide is also helpful when managing increased ICP. Two proposed mechanisms of action are responsible for furosemide's effect on ICP. They include:

1. Interference with CSF formation and sodium, and water movement across the blood-brain barrier and
2. Preferential excretion of water over solute in the distal renal tubule.[26] It has been documented that furosemide and mannitol work better together than either one used alone, It has also been shown that giving mannitol 15 minutes before furosemide has the largest effect on ICP control.[27]

Although the carbonic anhydrase inhibitor acetazolamide is often discussed in ICP management, it is most often used as a temporizing measure for control of CSF production in hydrocephalic patients. It is almost never used in the ICU setting except for premature infants with post-hemorrhagic hydrocephalus from an intraventricular/germinal matrix hemorrhage.

Hyperventilation

Hyperventilation sufficient to lower pCO_2 to levels of 30 mmHg can lower ICP within minutes. Alkalosis causes cerebral vasoconstriction through a direct effect on the vascular endothelium. The response is rapid and the vasoconstriction leads to decreased CBV and thereby decreased ICP.[28] The peak effect of hyperventilation is achieved within 30 minutes. Over the next 1 to 3 hours, the effect diminishes as compensatory acid-base buffering mechanisms correct the CSF alkalosis.[29] Once ICP is stabilized, hyperventilation should be tapered slowly over 6 to 12 hours, because abrupt cessation can lead to vasodilation and rebound increase in ICP. Profound hyperventilation must be avoided because of its potential to cause cerebral ischemia through excess vasoconstriction.[30] Prolonged hyperventilation may occasionally be necessary in cases where increased ICP is due to severe cerebral hyperemia.

High Dose Pentobarbital

Barbiturates induce a decrease in CBF and brain metabolism[31] and in high doses can lower CBV and ICP. Clinical trials have shown that pentobarbital infusion, using a loading dose of 5 to 20 mg/kg, followed by a 1-to 4 mg/kg/hr maintenance dose, can produce a lowering of uncontrolled ICP that had been refractory to other measures. In a carefully controlled randomized trial reported by Eisenberg et al,[32] 73 patients whose ICP could not be controlled by sequential treatment with intracranial mass removal, CSF removal, head elevation, hyperventilation, and mannitol infusion were randomized to either receive high dose pentobarbital infusion or continued standard treatment. Although the literature supports the notion that high dose pentobarbital can lower ICP in patients who have failed to respond to the previously outlined therapies, careful attention must be paid to maintaining CPP > 70 mm Hg throughout the infusion, as barbiturates can markedly lower MAP. Those patients whose outcome worsened suffered a $SjvO_2$ < 45% during pentobarbital infusion, despite the fact that CPP and MAP were maintained. This suggests an overactive vasoconstriction response to pentobarbital infusion in some patients with raised ICP, which could limit the utility of high dose pentobarbital therapy. In patients treated with pentobarbital for ICP control, vasopressor support to maintain CPP > 70 is mandatory, and $SjvO_2$ monitoring is advisable.

Steroid Therapy

Steroids with their anti-inflammatory and cell membrane stabilization effects have long been used in the management of increased ICP. Their effect is most commonly seen in the reduction of vasogenic edema surrounding tumors, abscesses or hematomas. In this setting steroids are useful, and in some instances, life saving. However, as with barbiturate therapy, there is no evidence that steroids, even in high doses, improve ICP control or outcome in severe head injuries.

Steroids also have significant side effects, including gastrointestinal bleeding, glucose intolerance, and increased risk of infection. It is unclear to what degree steroids increase the risk of GI hemorrhage over and above the risk associated with head injury alone.

Hypothermia

Induced hypothermia has been shown to decrease cerebral metabolism, and may thereby reduce CBF, CBV, and thus ICP.

Cooling can be achieved by cooling blankets applied to the body, and in some cases ice-water gastric lavage. It has been demonstrated that whole body cooling is more effective than isolated head cooling at lowering brain temperature.

REFERENCES

1. Darby JM, Yonas H, Marion DW, Latchaw RE. Local "inverse steal" induced by hyperventilation in head injury. *Neurosurgery* 1988;23:84-88.
2. Kennealy JA, McLennann. JE Loudon RG, McLaurin RL. Hyperventilation induced cerebral hypoxia. *Am Rev Respir Dis* 1980;122:407-12.
3. Michenfelder JD, Sundt TM. The effect of $PaCO_2$ on the metabolism of ischaemic brain in squirrel monkeys. *Anesthesiology* 1973;38:445-453.
4. Strandgaard S, Paulson OB. Cerebral autoregulation. *Stroke* 1984;15:413-416.
5. Jennet WB, Harper AM, Meller JD, et al. Relationship between cerebral blood flow and cerebral perfusion pressure. *Br J Surg* 1970;57:390-397.
6. Shinnoj E, Strangaard S. Pathogenesis of hypertensive encephalopathy. *Lancet* 1973;1:461-462.
7. Rosner MJ, Becker DP. Origin and evolution of plateau waves: experimental observations and a theoretical model. *J Neurosurg* 1984;60:312-324.
8. Barnett GH. Ropper A. Romeo J. Intracranial pressure and outcome in adult encephalitis. *J Neurosurg* 1988;65:585-588.
9. Kindt GW, Woldman J, Kohl, S, et al. Intracranial pressure in Reye's syndrome: monitoring and control. *JAMA* 1975;231:822-828.
10. Nora LM, Bleck, TP. Increased intracranial pressure complicating hepatic failure. *J Crit Illness* 1989;4:87-96.
11. Ropper AH, Randall BK. Intracranial pressure monitoring in comatose patients with cerebral hemorrhage. *Arch Neurol* 1984;41:725-728.
12. Hanley DF, Feldman E, Borel CO, et al. Treatment of sagittal sinus thrombosis associated with cerebral hemorrhage and intracranial hypertension. *Stroke* 1988;19:903-909.
13. Feldman Z. Kanter MJ. Rohertson CS. et al. Effect of head elevation on intracranial pressure. Cerebral perfusion pressure and cerebral blood flow in head-injured patients. *J Neurosurg* 1992;76:207-211.
14. Durward QJ, Amacher AL, Del MR, Sibbald WJ. Cerebral and cardiovascular responses to changes in head elevation in patients with intracranial hypertension. *J Neurosurg* 1983;59:938.
15. Palafox, BA. Johnson MN. McEwen DK, Gazzaniga AB. ICP changes following application of the MAST Suit. *J Trauma* 1981;21:55.
16. Lassen NA. Control of the cerebral circulation in health and disease. *Circ Res* 1947;34:749-760.
17. McLaurin HL, King LR, Elam EB. Metabolic response to craniocerebral trauma. *Surg Gynecol Obstet* 1960;110:282-286.
18. Schmoker JD, Shackford SR, Wald SL, Pietropaoli JA. An analysis of the relationship between fluid and sodium administration and intracranial pressure after head injury. *J Trauma* 1992;33;476-481.
19. Lassen NA, Christensen MS. Physiology of cerebral blood flow. *Br J Anaesth* 1976;48:719-734.
20. Murphy PG, Myers DS, Davies MJ, et al. The anti-oxidant potential of propofol (2,6-diisopropylphenol). *Br J Anaesth* 1992;68:613-618.
21. Baldwin HZ. Rekate HL. Preliminary experience with controlled external lumbar drainage in diffuse pediatric head injury. *Pediatr Neurosurg* 1991; 17(3):115-120.
22. Muizelaar JP, Wei EP, Kontos HA, et al. Mannitol causes compensatory cerebral vasoconstriction in response to blood viscosity changes. *J Neurosurg* 1983;59:822-828.
23. Kaufmann AM, Cardoso ER. Aggravation of vasogenic cerebral edema by multiple dose mannitol. *J Neurosurg* 1993;44:584-589.
24. Pollay M Fullenwider C, Roberts PA, Stevens FA. Effect of mannitol and furosemide on blood-brain osmotic gradient and intracranial pressure. *J Neurosurg* 1983;59:945.
25. Roberts PA, Pollay M, Engles C, Pendleton B, Reynolds E, Stevens FA. Effect on intracranial pressure of furosemide combined with varying doses and administration rates of mannitol. *J Neurosurg* 1987;66:440-446.
26. Lassen NA. Control of cerebral circulation in health and disease. *Circ Hes* 1974;34:749-760.
27. Muizelaar JP, Marmarou A, Ward JD, et al. Adverse effects of prolonged hyperventilation in patients with severe head injury: a randomized clinical trial. *J Neurosurg* 1991;75:731-739.
28. Ropper AH. Treatment of intracranial hypertension. In: Ropper AH (ed) *Neurological and Neurosurgical Intensive Care*, 3rd edn. New York: Raven Press. 1993;29-52.
29. Ishii S. Brain swelling: studies of structural, physiologic, and biochemical alterations, in Caveness WF, Walker AE (eds) *Head Injury*. Philadelphia: JB Lippincott, 1966;276-283.
30. Cruz, J. Adverse effects of pentobarbital on cerebral venous oxygenation of comatose patients with acute traumatic brain swelling: relationship to outcome. *J Neurosurg* 1996;85:758-761.
31. Cushing H. Peptic ulcers and the interbrain. *Surg Gynecol Obstet* 1932;55:1.
32. Mellergard P. Changes in human intracerebral temperature in response to different methods of brain cooling. *Neurosurgery* 1992;31:671-677.

Jhuma Mandal and Akash Deep

15 Cerebral Edema

INTRODUCTION

The term, *cerebral edema,* denotes an abnormal accumulation of fluid in the cerebral tissue which may be located primarily in extracellular space or within the cells of the brain.

PATHOPHYSIOLOGY

The intact blood brain barrier (BBB) is composed of endothelial cells of the microvasculature which posses some unique features. These are:

1. Formation of tight intercellular junctions under the influence of some factor (or factors) released by astrocytes;
2. Few pinocytotic vesicles within the endothelial cytoplasm;
3. Greater numbers of mitochondria per unit cell volume than what occur in other endothelial cell.

Its biochemical characteristics, its size, its ionization at the physiological pH, its lipid solubility and the extent of its binding to plasma proteins are all important. This is a cascade of events involving loss of integrity of the BBB, setting up of a vascular hydrostatic gradient, increased tissue pressure, decreased cerebral blood flow with resulting tissue acidosis. Chemical changes include glutamate serotonin, components of kallikrein- kininogen, fatty acids.

The following mechanisms may operate in opening the blood brain barrier;

1. Separation of the inter endothelial tight junctions;
2. Endothelial vesicular transport and the formation of transendothelial channels,and
3. Biochemical and structural alteration of the endothelial plasmalemma resulting in increased permeability of that membrane.[2]

BBB has both cerebral (cholinergic and aminergic) and peripheral (sympathetic and parasympathetic) innervation.

TYPES OF CEREBRAL EDEMA AND PATHOGENESIS

1. Vasogenic edema
2. Cytotoxic edema
3. Osmotic edema
4. Hydrostatic edema/interstitial edema

Vasogenic Edema

The type of cerebral edema encountered most frequently in clinical practice is vasogenic edema in which an incompetent blood brain barrier (BBB) allows the extravasation of plasma like fluid into the extra cellular space. This is the type of edema that occurs in the vicinity of brain tumors, intracerebral haematomas, cerebral abscess and contusions.

In vasogenic edema the fluid in the extra cellular space has a high content of plasma protein; the fluid spreads by bulk flow rather than by diffusion, the rate of spread being proportional to the capillary hydrostatic pressure.

The edema fluid has a predilection for white matter and tends to extend from gray matter along adjacent tracts in the white matter.[2] This type of edema is seen in response to trauma, tumors, focal inflammation and late stages of cerebral ischemia.

Cytotoxic Edema

It results from a disturbance in cell membrane permeability and produces an accumulation of fluid within cells. An early response of brain tissue to injury is swelling of astrocytes. This form of edema is seen in ischaemic–hypoxic brain damage, although there may also be an element of vasogenic edema at the margins of an infarct. In essence, however this form of edema is intracellular and is therefore much more prominent in gray than in white matter.[2] Cytotoxic edema is seen in various intoxications (dinitrophenol, triethylene, hexachlorophene, isoniazid) Reye's syndrome, severe hypothermia and ischemia.[1]

Osmotic Edema

Normally CSF and ECF osmolality in the brain is slightly greater than that of plasma. When plasma is diluted by SIADH, water intoxication, hemodialysis, there is a passage of water down abnormal gradient creating cerebral edema. In case of an osmotic insult cerebral cells modify their active osmotic molecular contents in order to limit volume variation. In the event of plasma hypotonicity cerebral cells expel active osmotic molecules to reduce the osmotic gradient and water movement thereby reducing cerebral edema. The opposite reaction is observed in the case of hypertonic insult. It explains, for example, why patients with chronic and severe hyponatremia could be asymptomatic. Severe osmotic oedema is observed mainly in water intoxication, acute hyponatremia or too rapid reduction of hyperosmolarity. Hyponatremia, even modest, could modify cerebral blood volume and impair osmoregulation. In the presence of cerebral lesion, osmoregulation operates only in areas of preserved BBB. The pathological zones are therefore exposed to osmotic oedema (even in cases of moderate hyponatremia) with deterioration of both clinical status and intracranial pressure. Hyponatremia constitutes an authentic secondary cerebral insult of systemic origin.

Hydrostatic Edema

Even if vascular endothelium remains intact, a sudden increase of intravascular pressure or of transmural pressure can overcome cerebrovascular resistance, producing high pressure flooding of the capillary bed. This can occur when arterial pressure suddenly becomes high during craniotomy, or when an intracranial mass lesion that has been causing severe intracranial hypertension is abruptly decompressed. The congestive brain swelling that occurs immediately is followed after some minutes by extravasations of protein poor fluid into and through the extra cellular space of the brain. A particularly severe example of this form of oedema may be seen in patients with a very high ICP in whom a bony decompression is carried out, leading to rapid external herniation of the brain.

In patients with acute obstructive hydrocephalus there is an increase in the water content of the periventricular tissues. In such cases it appears that fluid under high pressure is forced through damaged ependyma into the per ventricular white matter. Fishman termed this process interstitial edema.[2]

PATHOLOGY

The edematous brain is softer than normal and often appears to overfill the cranial vault. In generalized edema, the gyri are flattened, the intervening sulci are narrowed and the ventricular cavities are compressed. As the brain expands, herniation may occur.

Herniations result from an increase in the volume of one area of the brain either from swelling of that area or from displacement of that area by a growing mass. Distortion of the brain results in the local area being forced beyond the normal retaining barriers created by the dense fibrous tracts with in the cranium or the bony edges of the calvarium. The displaced brain tissue impinges on vessels, leading to impairment of venous return, additional swelling, and ischemic injury. The following vicious cycle develops, which, if untreated, can be fatal:

Cerebral edema → Vascular occlusion
Cellular injury ← Brain ischemia

Five types of herniation are summarized in Table 15.1.

Table 15.1: Signs in different types of herniation

Herniation type	*Signs*
Sub falcial	None
Transtentorial lateral	Ipsilateral pupillary dilation Contralateral or occasionally ipsilateral hemiparesis
Transtentorial central	Agitation or somnolence, central neurogenic hyperventilation, B/L pupillary dilatation late
Upward from posterior fossa mass	Disordered level of consciousness and abnormal extraocular movement
Tonsillar	Cheyne stokes or gasping respirations, bradycardia hypertension

Time Relationships in the Development of Cerebral Edema

When an insult to the brain has taken place the clinical features of cerebral edema may develop over a period of hours or days. Thus immediately after a head injury within 24 to 72 hours profound stupor or even coma may develop due to cerebral edema. Diffuse edema, such as may occur in association with hypoxia or hypernatremia, can render a patient comatose within a few hours. The time course over which cerebral edema reaches a peak depends on a number of factors:

1. The nature of the edema-producing process.
2. The rate at which the pathologic process develops. Very rapidly developing edema will not permit effective accommodative mechanisms to act, whereas slowly progressive edema initially is obscured by the accommodative shifts in intracranial fluid compartments.
3. The volume of brain tissue involved in edema formation (very focal cerebral edema may not be clinically apparent, massive cerebral edema of the entire brain, such as occurs after hypoxia, would produce symptoms rapidly).
4. Measures taken to offset the development of cerebral edema.

It is important to recognize that there is an interval between a temporally discrete cerebral insult and the development of maximal cerebral edema. Prophylactic measures are most effective during this critical period.

CLINICAL ASPECTS

Clinical manifestations may range from irritability, headache, and confusion to nausea, vomiting, lethargy, stupor or coma in severe and wide spread edema.

Localizing neurological symptoms and signs such as hemiparesis or aphasia may be present when cerebral edema is confined primarily to one hemisphere or a portion thereof. Seizures usually do not occur as a result of cerebral edema perse, although the hypoxic event or electrolyte imbalance responsible for the cerebral edema may result in seizure activity.

Head retraction can be seen as a result of increased ICP, particularly if the posterior fossa is involved. Fundoscopic examination may not reveal papilledema when cerebral edema has developed only hours before, is very focal and small in extent or has occurred so gradually as to permit the cranial sutures to separate. In contrast to the percussion sound of the enlarged head due to hydrocephalus the patient with cerebral edema will have a normal percussion sound.

When ICP is markedly elevated compensatory elevation of systolic blood pressure may be seen together with widening of pulse pressure (cushing effect). Respirations may be slowed but rapid or irregular respirations are noted instead. But this sign is only inconsistently observed in only 1/5 to 1/3 of patients with documented cerebral edema.

DIAGNOSTIC EVALUATION

1. *CT scan* is the most useful non invasive technique in the assessment of lesions of brain including cerebral edema. The CT scan may demonstrate perifocal edema around a tumor or abscess. Imaging abnormality may be equally important diagnostically in the presence of clinical cerebral edema. Infants and small children often require sedation or anesthesia during the scanning procedure to avoid movement of the head.
2. *Cranial X-ray* in unilateral cerebral edema shows lateral displacement with dislocation of the pineal gland. In bilateral brain edema the pineal gland is displaced in caudal and occipital direction.
3. *Lumbar puncture* should not be performed unless it is essential to establish or rule out associated conditions such as meningitis or encephalitis. If the procedure has been performed in the case of diagnostic evaluation, the CSF pressure will be found to be elevated.
4. *Electroencephalography* often is normal or reveals slight low voltage. In severe cases a non-specific decrease in frequency and high voltage slow waves can be seen.
5. *A technetium 99m brain scan* is unremarkable in cerebral edema except in the presence of a focal edema-generating lesion such as a brain abscess or tumor.

PROPHYLACTIC VS CORRECTIVE THERAPY

Therapy may be considered prophylactic in 2 situations.

1. Preoperatively where the operative procedure is known to be associated with hazards of cerebral edema.
2. When a patient has been exposed to an edema producing insult such as hypoxia or head injury but symptoms of cerebral edema have not yet developed i.e., when the patient is within the therapeutic interval.

Therapy is considered corrective when edema from any cause has already developed and must be reduced to prevent herniation or permanent brain injury from increased pressure.

Prophylactic Treatment

A successful prophylaxis of brain edema can be expected only from rapid and immediate elimination of the most relevant causal factors and their insidious effects on the central nervous system.

Prophylaxis of cerebral edema is based upon:

1. Assurance of sufficient oxygen supply to the brain by providing for optimal respiration and eliminating respiratory disorders.
2. Control of heart and circulatory functions.
3. Control of water and electrolyte metabolism.
4. Prevention of metabolic and enzymatic disturbances of the energy–dependent water–and ion transport functions of the CNS. Prevention of cerebral edema still must be regarded as the best therapy.[9]

Management of Cerebral Edema Must

1. Include an effort to eliminate the etiological agent, so as to prevent further edema from developing, and
2. Treat cerebral edema per se. Specific measures for removing the cause of cerebral edema include correction of hypernatremia, treatment of meningitis, surgical removal of a brain tumor, drainage of an abscess, and evacuation of a hematoma. Lead encephalopathy should be treated with agents capable of binding lead and of facilitating its excretion. Water intoxication requires water restriction or other measures to restore fluid and electrolyte balance, and conditions producing hypoxia should be corrected as quickly as possible. Measures for the treatment of cerebral edema are listed in Table 15.2.

Physiological Methods

Fluid Restriction

It is important to prevent fluid overloading both in prophylactic and corrective management of cerebral edema although fluid restriction is probably more effective in prevention than in the treatment of existing cerebral edema. Patients with deranged thirst mechanisms, high fever, and impaired renal function, individuals on intravenous fluid replacement, and unconscious patients pose far more

Table 15.2: Treatment of cerebral edema

Physiological	
	Fluid restriction
	Blood pressure control
	Hypothermia
	Hyperventilation
	Hyperbaric oxygen
Pharmacological	
	Steroids
	Osmotically active agents
	Diuretics
Surgical	
	Craniectomy
	CSF diversion

difficult problems. Dehydration in infants and children with cerebral edema must be corrected gradually. Indeed, excessively rapid rehydration may precipitate seizures as well as increase cerebral edema. However patients with cerebral edema with hypovolemic or septic shock must be managed aggressively with fluids preferably with CVP monitoring as hemodynamic compromised can read to vital organ dysfunction including brain and heart. Therefore, shock resuscitation must gain preference to management of cerebral edema.

Fluid administration should follow a formula include the following:

1. Maintenance fluid intake, including an increment for patients with fever.
2. Selection of the proper fluid for replacement therapy. Lactate Ringer's solution or 5% dextrose in half-normal (0.45%) saline are preferable to hypotonic solutions of rapidly metabolized glucose in water. The latter actually adds to volume of extra cellular fluid and thus aggravates cerebral edema. "Normal" (0.9%) saline provides an excess of sodium ion to the tissues and is, therefore, not desirable for fluid replacement in patients with cerebral edema.[1] Fluid restriction when indicated, as in water intoxication, should be carried out with great care in infants and small children. The aim should be to avoid fluid over loading, since this may well aggravate cerebral edema when a predisposing cause for its development exists.[2] However, in the case of fever and diarrhea, excessive dehydration can lead to hypernatremia which itself is a cause of cerebral edema.

However in a recent study, it has been shown that patients kept normovolemic during their period of increased ICP management fare just as well as those kept deliberately hypovolemic. D_5W is never indicated except in the circumstance of fluid replacement for significant hypernatremia as a result of neurogenic diabetes insipidus.[3]

Blood Pressure Control

Unnecessary elevation of blood pressure should be avoided. Such evaluation can be caused by excessive volume replacement of any type, including over transfusion, as well as by drugs capable of elevating blood pressure, carbon dioxide retention during anesthesia, pain, and over distention of the urinary bladder. It is important, however, not to mistake the compensatory elevation of blood pressure that occurs with increased intracranial pressure for any of the above. Deliberate lowering of elevated blood pressure, when this elevation is an auto regulatory response to increased intracranial pressure, reduces cerebral perfusion and aggravates cerebral edema.

Hypothermia

Hypothermia acts to reduce brain bulk and is useful adjunct in the management of severe and extensive cerebral edema[15,16] Hypothermia reduces the metabolic needs of the brain and this is desirable when cerebral perfusion is being threatened by increased intracranial pressure. Hypothermia also reduces systemic blood pressure, and the protective volume-reducing effect could be secondary to lowering of blood pressure, which would, inturn, reduce edema formation. Maintenance of normal body temperature and prevention of fever with its increased metabolic demands and increased cerebral blood flow will be of great help. Thus, hypothermia is a useful adjunct in the management of cerebral edema associated with encephalitis or meningitis, insults or head trauma. Body temperature should not be reduced below 32°C, as lower temperatures increase the chance that cardiac irregularities will develop and aggravate such problems as acidosis associated with hypothermia. Shivering can offset some of the beneficial effects of hypothermia and is best treated with chlorpromazine.

Hyperventilation

Hyperventilation reduces intracranial pressure by constricting cerebral vessels, decreasing cerebral blood flow, and thus concomitantly decreasing the volume of blood within the cranial cavity. Reduction of the arterial PCO_2 from a normal value of 40 mm Hg to 20 mm Hg will result in a 40 to 50% decrease in cerebral blood flow.[6] One of the obvious disadvantages resulting from diminished cerebral blood flow that accompanies hyperventilation is the danger of hypoxia, and great care must be taken to ensure adequate oxygenation during hyperventilation. If arterial PCO_2 becomes elevated, cerebral blood vessels will dilate and intracranial volume will increase. This situation is to be avoided. Therein lies the importance of assuring an adequate airway and the occasional necessity of performing a tracheostomy on a patient whose life is threatened by increasing intracranial pressure.

Pharmacological Methods

Steroids

Glucocorticosteroids are the most important pharmacological adjunct to the treatment of cerebral and spinal cord edema available at this time. They have been particularly useful in the management of the various types of vasogenic edema, both in the prophylactic and corrective phases of therapy.

The response of cerebral edema to steroid administration seems to be most dramatic when there has been little disruption of neural tissue i.e., perifocal edema surrounding tumor or abscess.[7] Such edema is most prominent in the cerebral white matter. Steroids are also used widely in the treatment of cerebral edema following anoxic insults. Minimizing the time interval between the insult and the beginning of steroid therapy is very important.

Preoperative prophylactic steroid therapy is most effective in protecting neural tissue from edema associated with surgical removal of tumors, vascular malformations, or other lesions from brain or spinal cord. Steroids are also recommended in the treatment lead encephalopathy.[8]

The exact mechanism by which steroids produce their beneficial effect in cerebral edema is still under investigation.[7] Increased leakage of the protein through the "blood-brain barrier", reflected in elevated cerebrospinal fluid protein levels, seems to be reversed by steroids.[8] From the aspect of intracranial mass dynamics, steroids reduce the volume of the tissue compartment by reducing edema fluid.

Steroid therapy is most effective when administered prophylactically prior to a surgical procedure associated with reactive edema formation. In such situations therapy should be initiated 24 to 48 hours preoperatively at full therapeutic doses. Dexamethasone has been the preferred steroid preparation in the management of cerebral edema, although other steroids have been used. When administered to reduce existing cerebral edema (peritumor, periabscess) or to minimize edema formation after a focal insult trauma), an initial loading dose of dexamethasone (1.0 to 2.0 mg young children, up to 4.0 mg in older children, and up to 8.0 mg in adolescents) should be given intravenously or intramuscularly as soon as possible, followed by a maintenance dose of 0.25 to 0.50 mg/kg/day in four divided doses given at six-hour intervals. Maintenance doses may be given intravenously, intramuscularly, or orally, depending upon the availability of an infusion site and the patient's general condition. Because of the potential hazards of gastrointestinal hemorrhage and ulceration, antacids should be given by mouth, usually in liquid form, during the course of steroid therapy. Appropriate antibiotics also should be administered to the patient treated for cerebral edema associated with bacterial infection meningitis, brain abscess). Long-term steroid administration may, of course, produce the changes seen with Cushing's syndrome. Other complications of steroid therapy include electrolyte imbalance, fluid retention and activation of infections.

When the cause of edema can be surgically corrected (excision of tumor of abscess), steroid therapy should be maintained until the patient is well on the road to recovery. Similarly, steroid therapy should be continued in patients with meningitis and water intoxication until clinical signs of cerebral edema have largely subsided. When steroids are decreased or discontinued prematurely, reinstitution of medication at the previous dose often does not result in return to the previous clinical status. Some fluid extravasates during the interval and is not readily reabsorbed. The rule that edema tends to reach its maximum about three days after operation or trauma serves as a useful guide to therapy. After this period of time, edema begins to recede. Complete resolution of swelling after a period of cerebral edema may take several weeks.

Steroid medication must be tapered gradually over a seven to ten-day period once it is appropriate to discontinue the medication. Tapering of steroids over the usual period of time in such patients may be followed by signs of increased intracranial pressure, necessitating an increase in dosage and, subsequently, a much more gradual decrease. Antacid medication may be stopped concurrently with the termination of the steroids.

Osmotically Active Agents

Unlike glucocorticosteroids, osmotically active agents do not act specifically against cerebral edema but produce cellular dehydration of normal as well as of abnormal CNS tissue. They are, however, potent in reducing intracranial pressure. The mechanism by which these agents act is to produce a shift of fluid, probably from glial cells and the intercellular compartment, to the vascular system and CSF. Thirty percent urea (in 10% invert sugar) and 20% mannitol, the most commonly used agents, produce a dramatic decrease in CSF pressure (30 to 60% and greater) within one half to one hour of administration, depending on the rate at which the drugs are given. Urea and mannitol are, therefore generally used only when the process causing cerebral edema can be eliminated within a short time, i.e., surgically, as for instance just before evacuation of a hematoma or abscess or the removal of a brain tumor. In critical situations, osmotic agents may be given together with the initial dose of corticosteroids immediately before the infant or child is taken to the operating room. Osmotic diuretics also may be helpful initially in the treatment of patients with water intoxication and lead encephalopathy.

IV 20% mannitol is given at 1g per kg over 30 to 60 minutes. Rarely, a second dose of mannitol or urea may be administered within a period of a few hours. In general, when the intracranial pressure is so high as to require repeated acute administrations of osmotic diuretics, few individuals will be helped unless the potential for significant surgical decompression of the brain can be quickly realized. Repeated mannitol therapy has recently been employed in patients with extensive post-traumatic cerebral edema, with monitored intracranial pressure measurements serving as a guideline. Careful monitoring of serum electrolytes, of osmolarity, and fluid balance is necessary as part of such regimen. Hypernatremia associated with long-term hyper-osmolar therapy has been treated successfully with furosemide.[11]

Mannitol is generally considered to produce less of an "overshoot" because it essentially remains confined to the extracellular space.[12] Mannitol also would be the preferred agent in patients with renal disease. For long-term osmotic dehydration of the brain, oral glycerol (1 g/kg every six hours) has been suggested. Glycerol is said to produce little water or electrolyte loss and would be expected to produce less of an "overshoot" of CSF pressure than the other osmotic diuretics.[11] Recently however, secondary elevation of CSF pressure has been reported following the long-term administration of glycerol.[12] Unconscious patients and anesthetized patients require an indwelling catheter during osmotic dehydration therapy.

Diuretics

The various classes of diuretics have so far found little practical use in the management of cerebral edema. Exceptions should, however, be noted. Acetazolamide (Diamox) is carbonic anhydrase inhibitor and reduces formation of CSF.[26] The mechanism of this particular action is still not precisely known. Acetazolamide has not been used on a large scale in the treatment of perifocal or other cerebral edema. As noted previously, furosemide (Lasix) has recently been used as an adjunct to long-term mannitol therapy in patients with post-traumatic cerebral edema. Bergland et al[32] recently reported on the use of furosemide both for the treatment of cerebral edema and in the course of neurosurgical procedures.

Surgical Adjuncts to the Treatment of Cerebral Edema

It has been emphasized that removal of the edema-generating focus is the most effective way to reverse edema, although in some situations this may not be possible. In addition, certain nonspecific surgical procedures directed specifically at the relief of compression caused by cerebral edema deserve mention.

In the years before steroids and osmotic diuretics became available, subtemporal decompression was employed to permit the swollen brain to decompress itself externally. The decompression afforded by these small craniectomies underlying the temporalis muscle is, however, relatively ineffective. Today, with improved adjuncts for extensive surgical procedures, even in the pediatric age group, large craniectomis are performed occasionally for such conditions as severe post-traumatic cerebral edema[27,28] and lead encephalopathy.[15,16] Such surgical measures are indicated only when medical forms of therapy are inadequate to manage the increase in intracranial pressure.

CSF drainage, either as a closed system external drainage into a bottle or in the form of internalized shunt from the ventricles to the vascular system or peritoneal cavity, may occasionally find use in the treatment of extensive cerebral edema that does not respond adequately to medical therapy. Because of the risk of infection, external ventricular drain-age cannot be maintained for more than a few days and, if continued ventricular drainage is indicated, the shunt should be internalized at that time. CSF shunting occasionally finds use in the treatment of pseudotumor cerebri.[23]

REFERENCES

1. Harrigan MR. Cerebral salt wasting syndrome. *Neurosurgery* 1998;38:152-160.
2. Boulard G, Marguinaud E, Sesay M. Osmotic cerebral edema: The role of plasma osmolarity and blood brain barrier. *Ann Fr Anesth Reanim* 2003;22:215-219.
3. Plum F, Posner JB. *The Diagnosis of Stupor and Coma*, 2nd edn. Philadelphia: FA Davis 1972.
4. Teele DW, Dash EB, Klein JO. Meningitis after lumbar puncture in children with bacteremia. *N Engl J Med* 1982;306:609-610.
5. Snyder CH: Practical scheme for fluid and electrolytes therapy in children. *JAMA* 1955;158:1004.
6. Stern WE. Problems in fluid replacement and cerebral edema in the management of surgical lesions of the central nervous system. *Am J Surg* 1960;100:303.
7. Hooshmand H, Dove J, Houff S, Suter C. Effect of diuretics and steroids on CSF pressure. *Arch Neurol* 1989;21:499.
8. Schmoker JD, Shackford SR, Wald SL, Pietropaoli JA. An analysis of relationship between fluid and sodium administration and intracranial pressure after head injury. *J Trauma* 1992;33:476-481.
9. Rosomoff HL. Effect of hypothermia and hypertonic urea on distribution of intracranial contents. *J Neurosurg* 1961;18:753.
10. Rosomoff HL. Pathophysiology of the central nervous system during hypothermia. *Acta Neurochir* 1964;13(Suppl):172.
11. Maxwell RE, Long DM, French LA. The clinical effects of a synthetic gluco-corticoid used for brain edema in the practice of neurosurgery. In, Reulen HJ, Schurmann K (eds) *Steroids and Brain Edema*. New York: Springer Verlag 1972:219.
12. Goodyear E, Wilson AW. Trends in management of cerebral edema. *Bull Child Neurol* 2001;10:66.
13. Goodyear E. Steroids and brain edema: Issues.*Bull Child Neurol* 2003;12:342.

14. Siegel BA, Studer RK, Potchen EJ. Steroid therapy of brain edema. *Arch Neurol* 1872;27:209.
15. Shenkin HA, Coluboff B, Haft H. The use of Mannitol for the reduction of intracranial pressure in intracranial surgery. *J Neurosurg* 1962;19;997.
16. Tourtellotte WW, Reinglass JL, Newkirk TA. Cerebral dehydration action of glycerol. *Clin Pharmacol Ther* 1972;13:159.
17. Guisado R, Tourtellotte WW, Arieff AI, et al. Rebound phenomenon complicating cerebral dehydration with glycerol: A case report. *J Neurosurg* 1975;42:226.
18. Withrow CD, Woodbury DM. Some aspects of the pharmacology of adrenal steroids and the central nervous system. In: Reulen HJ, Schurmann K (eds) *Steroids and Brain Edema*. New York: Springer Verlag 1972:41.
19. Bergland RM, Page RB, Howland WS. Furosemide: A nonosmotic diuretic for neurosurgical use. *Annual Meeting of the American Association of Neurological Surgeons*, Miami Beach, Florida 1975.
20. Ransohoff J, Benjamin MV, Gage EL, Epstein F. Hemicraniectomy in the management of acute subdural hematoma. *J Neurosurg* 1971;34:70.
21. Kjellberg RN, Priet A. Bifrontal decompressive craniotomy for massive cerebral edema. *J Neurosurg* 1971;34:488.
22. McLaurin RL, Nichols JB. Extensive cranial decompression in the treatment of severe lead encephalopathy. *Pediatrics* 1957;20:653.
23. Vander Ark CD, Kempe LG, Smith DR. Pseudotumor cerebri treated with lumbar-peritoneal shunt. *JAMA* 1971;217:1832.

Neurological Emergencies

Sheffali Gulati and Anu Thukral

16 Acute Seizures

INTRODUCTION

Epilepsy was described by Hippocrates and its history spans that of medicine itself. **Seizure** is defined as a paroxysmal involuntary disturbance of brain function that may manifest as an impairment or loss of consciousness, abnormal motor activity, behavioral abnormality, sensory disturbances or autonomic dysfunction. Seizures affect 4-7% of children.

Seizures which occur during the course of an acute illness are termed as **provoked seizures**. Febrile seizures are the most important cause of provoked seizures and affect 3-5% of all children. **Epilepsy** is defined as two or more unprovoked seizures. It has been estimated that about 1% of children will have at least one afebrile seizure by age 14 years and 0.4 to 0.8% will have epilepsy by age 11 years.[1] The prevalence of epilepsy is 4-9/1000 population in the developed countries. The prevalence may be higher in developing countries like ours due to high incidence of neurocysticercosis, CNS (central nervous system) infections, birth asphyxia and consanguinity related metabolic diseases.

BACKGROUND

Seizure Versus Non-Seizure

Each paroxysmal event is not seizure. Misidentification of these events can lead to potential harmful treatment. Epidemiological studies suggest that between 10-13% of seizure suspects turn out to have other disorders.[2,3] About 15-30% of referrals to tertiary referral centers turn out to have non-epileptic disorders.[4] An exception is from a Kerala study where only a small number of intractable epileptics had been misdiagnosed.[5] **The first step in approaching a child with seizure disorder is to determine whether the event in the patient is truly a seizure or not.** Disorders mimicking seizures are detailed in Table 16.1.

Table 16.1: Disorders mimicking seizures [2]

Neonates
- Jitteriness
- Apnea
- Benign neonatal sleep myoclonus
- Stiff baby/hyperekplexia

Infants
- Breath holding spells-cyanotic/pallid
- Shuddering attacks
- Paroxysmal torticollis
- Extrapyramidal drug reactions, dystonia
- Benign myoclonus of early infancy

Childhood and adolescence
- Syncopal attacks
- Night terrors
- Cardiac arrhythmias
- Pseudoseizures
- Complicated migraine
- Hyperventilation attacks
- Tics
- Sleep disorders

A sequenced account of the event, precipitating factors, reproducibility, the gain expected out of the event are helpful in establishing the diagnosis. The timing of the events, injury, specific distribution and pattern of abnormal movements, post event deficits and loss of consciousness point toward a true seizure. Observation of the child during an episode, electroencephalography (EEG) and sometimes a video EEG may be helpful.

Breath holding spell is the most common misdiagnosed identity. They are self-limited and subjects generally outgrow them by school age. They may be cyanotic (wherein the child cries, stops breathing in expiration and becomes cyanosed) or pallid attacks (where child gasps, becomes apneic and pale). Iron therapy is effective in the treatment of breath holding spells and should be given irrespective of the degree of anemia since it aids in the neurotransmitter function and catecholamine metabolism.

Shuddering attacks (characterized by normal consciousness, stiffening, adduction of knees and flexion of head), syncopal attacks, night terrors, migraine, tics, hyperventilation attacks, hysterical seizures, benign paroxysmal vertigo, hypoglycemia drug "blackouts" tetany, pseudoseizures, narcolepsy, transient cerebral vascular insufficiency, paroxysmal dyskinesia are other important differentials-which must be considered in the respective settings and age groups.[6]

Provoked Vs Unprovoked Seizures

Provoked or acute symptomatic seizures or situation related seizures are seizures occurring in close temporal association with an acute systemic, metabolic, or toxic insult or in association with an acute CNS insult.[7] Common causes include febrile seizures, metabolic events including hypoglycemia, dyselectrolytemias-hypocalcemia, hypomagnesemia, hyponatremia and hypernatremia, CNS infections like meningitis, encephalitis, drug intoxication, hypoxia, cerebrovascular accident and head trauma.

Unprovoked seizures may belong to two possible categories: Symptomatic seizures or epilepsies (of presumed remote cause) and seizures or epilepsy of unknown causes. Identification of the cause may depend on the degree of investigation, which also depends on availability of ancillary tests.[7] Unprovoked seizures may occur in relation to a well-demonstrated antecedent condition, substantially increasing the risk of epileptic seizures. Two major subgroups may be categorized: Remote symptomatic unprovoked seizures owing to conditions resulting in a static encephalopathy due to an insult to CNS such as infection, cerebral trauma, or cerebrovascular disease. Symptomatic unprovoked seizures may arise due to progressive CNS disorders. Cases of unprovoked seizures for which no clear antecedent etiology can be detected can be further classified into idiopathic epilepsies or cryptogenic epilepsies.[7] In idiopathic epilepsies, there is no underlying cause other than a possible hereditary predisposition. Cryptogenic epilepsies are presumed to be symptomatic, but the etiology is not known.[8]

CLASSIFICATION

Classification of seizure disorders has evolved considerably over several decades. Use of such terms as "grand mal" or "petit mal" epilepsy has largely been supplanted by more detailed classifications based on specific clinical manifestations, mode of onset (i.e. focal or generalized) and discrete clinical syndromes.

According to ILAE (International League Against Epilepsy) International Classification of Epileptic Seizures (ICES) divides seizures into **generalized, partial and unclassifiable.** The further subdivisions of these types are shown in Table 16.2.[9] The advantages of this classification are that the patients can be classified early and relatively easily. Further choice of antiepileptic drug is often dictated by seizure type.

Table 16.2: ILAE classification of epileptic seizures (1981)[9]

I. Partial seizures
- *Simple partial seizures*
  1. With motor signs
  2. With somatosensory or special sensory hallucinations
  3. With autonomic symptoms and signs
  4. With psychic symptoms
- *Complex partial seizures*
  1. Simple partial onset followed by impairment of consciousness
  2. With impaired consciousness from onset
- *Partial seizures evolving to secondarily generalized seizures*
  1. Simple partial seizures evolving to generalized seizures
  2. Complex partial seizures evolving to generalized seizures
  3. Simple partial seizures evolving to complex partial evolving to generalized seizures

II. Generalized seizures
- Absence
- Atypical absence
- Myoclonic
- Clonic
- Tonic clonic
- Atonic

III. Unclassifiable

It was observed that many types of epilepsy may express themselves as a single seizure type or one epileptic disorder may present as various types of seizures. Therefore, a classification system that goes beyond seizure type may be useful. These considerations paved the way for the ILAE Classification of Epilepsies and Epileptic Syndromes (ICE) which was proposed in 1985 and finally approved by the ILAE in 1989. This is detailed in Table 16.3.[8] This classification was meant to supplement and not replace the existing ICES classification. **Epileptic syndrome** is defined as an epileptic disorder characterized by a cluster of signs and symptoms occurring together. These features include type(s) of seizure(s), etiology, anatomy, precipitating factors, age of onset, chronicity, severity, possible diurnal/circadian variation, response to drugs and prognosis. Therefore, if a 'syndromic' diagnosis can be made it provides far more information about the patient's epileptic disorder like juvenile myoclonic epilepsy, West syndrome (infantile spasms) and Lennox Gastaut syndrome.

Recently a didactic diagram was proposed by Tich et al (Fig. 16.1) that could be used as a teaching tool to provide an overview of the epilepsies.[10]

ETIOLOGY

Recurrent seizures are thought to result from a genetic predisposition, underlying neuropathologic changes and chemico-physiologic alterations in the nerve cell and its connections. Attributed causes for epilepsy in children and adolescents are detailed in Table 16.4.

Table 16.3: ILAE classification of epilepsies and epileptic syndromes (1989)[8]

1. Localization related epilepsies and syndromes
   - 1.1. Idiopathic (with age related onset)
     - benign childhood epilepsy with centrotemporal spikes
     - childhood epilepsy with occipital paroxysms
     - primary reading epilepsy
   - 1.2. Symptomatic
     - Chronic progressive epilepsia partialis continua
     - Syndromes characterized by seizures with specific modes of precipitation
     - Temporal/frontal/parietal/occipital lobe epilepsies
   - 1.3. Cryptogenic
2. Generalized epilepsies and syndromes
   - 2.1. Idiopathic (with age related onset–listed in order of age)
     - benign neonatal familial convulsions
     - benign neonatal convulsions
     - benign myoclonic epilepsy of infancy
     - childhood absence epilepsy
     - juvenile absence epilepsy
     - juvenile myoclonic epilepsy
     - epilepsy with grand mal seizures on awakening
     - epilepsies with seizures precipitated by specific modes of activation
     - other generalized idiopathic epilepsies not defined above
   - 2.2. Cryptogenic or symptomatic (in order of age)
     - West syndrome (infantile spasms)
     - Lennox Gastaut syndrome
     - epilepsy with myoclonic astatic seizures
     - epilepsy with myoclonic absences
   - 2.3. Symptomatic
   - 2.3.1 Non specific etiology
     - early myoclonic encephalopathy
     - early infantile epileptic encephalopathy with suppression burst
     - other symptomatic generalized epilepsies as defined above
   - 2.3.2. Specific syndromes–diseases in which seizures are a predominant or presenting feature
3. Epilepsies and syndromes undetermined whether focal or generalized
   - 3.1. With both generalized and focal seizures
   - neonatal seizures
   - severe myoclonic epilepsy of infancy
   - epilepsy with continuous spike waves during slow wave sleep
   - acquired epileptic aphasia
   - other undetermined epilepsies not defined above
   - 3.2. Without unequivocal generalized or focal features
4. Special syndromes
   - 4.1. Situation related seizures
   - febrile convulsions
   - isolated seizures or isolated status epileptics
   - seizures accompanying an acute toxic metabolic event

Table 16.4: Attributed causes for epilepsy in children and adolescents

• **Congenital**	
	CNS malformations
	Cerebral palsy
	Mental retardation, developmental delay
	Phacomatoses
• **CNS infections**	
• **Toxic/metabolic**	
• **CNS neoplasms**	
• **Perinatal**	
	Birth trauma
	Asphyxia/hypoxia
	Other perinatal
• **Traumatic**	

The etiologies, which underlie the development of epilepsy in childhood, vary in an age-dependent fashion. Seizures in neonates, infants, and toddlers most frequently result from perinatal brain injury, congenital CNS malformations, and metabolic derangements.[11] CNS infection, genetic epilepsies, and neurodegenerative disorders are more likely to present with seizures beginning in later childhood.

CLINICAL PROFILE

Childhood seizures represent paroxysmal clinical events characterized by abnormal, excessive discharges originating from populations of cortical neurons and resulting in some clinically evident alteration of function or behavior. Therefore, the clinical manifestations of childhood seizures need not include recognizable motor activity such as tonic-clonic movement; possible clinical manifestations may include staring, drop attacks, behavioral changes, or even autonomic disturbance.

Generalized seizures include absence, tonic-clonic, myoclonic and atonic seizures.

Absence Seizures

Typical absence seizures can be subtle or distinct, and they always recur during the course of several hours or days. Absence seizures typically begin in young school-aged children. They consist of brief (3-30 seconds) staring spells, accompanied by a cessation of activity. Sometimes eye fluttering, mild lip movements, or twitches occur. There is no postictal state after a typical absence seizure.

Hyperventilation may precipitate absence seizures and is an important, simple and quick diagnostic test. To perform an adequate hyperventilation test, the patient is asked to breathe in and out deeply for up to 3 minutes. Some younger patients need an aid, such as a piece of paper to blow with each breath. The patient is observed carefully during hyperventilation for any lapses in rhythmic breathing or

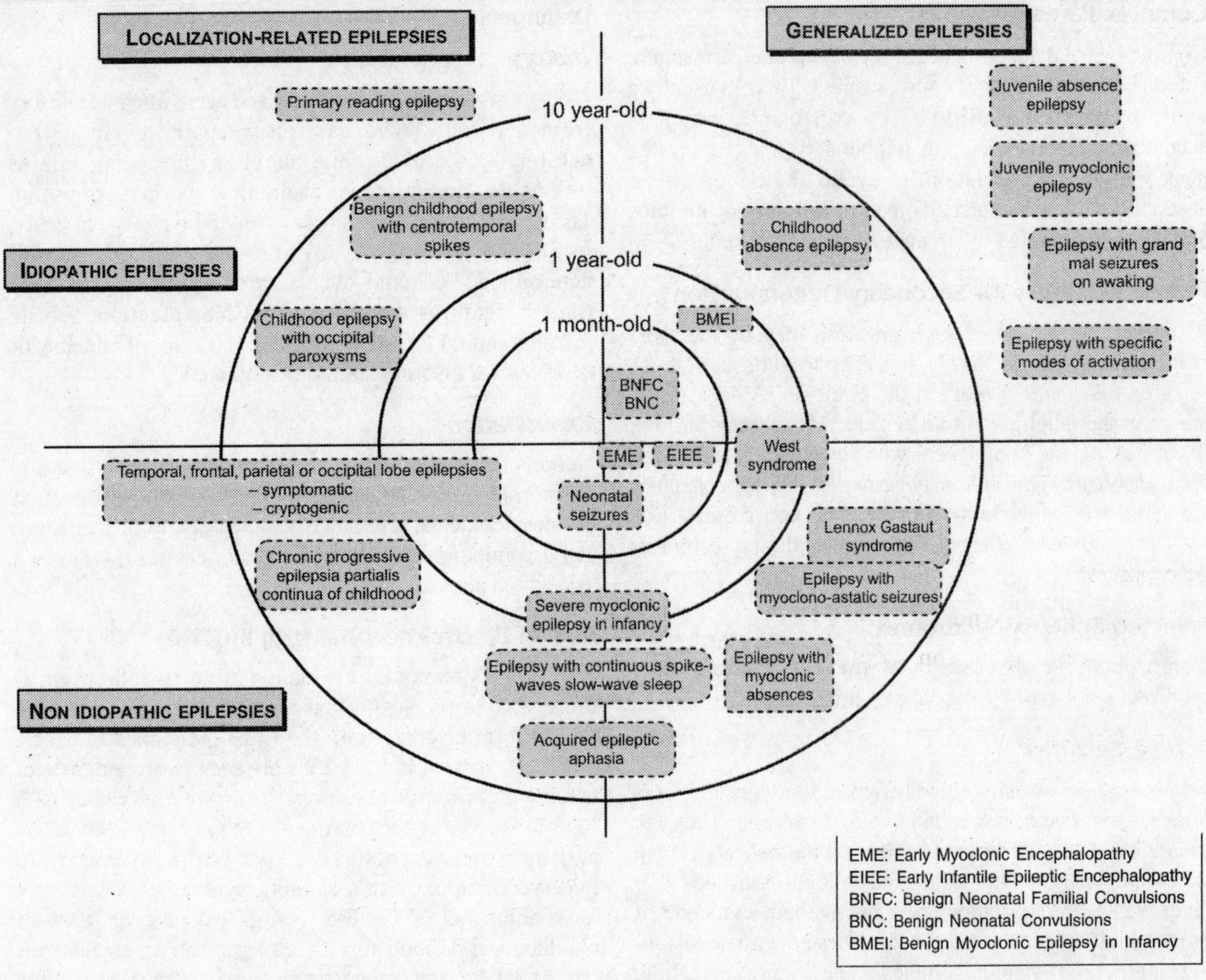

Fig. 16.1: Schematic diagram of the international classification of epilepsies and epileptic syndromes[10]

staring. At the completion of hyperventilation, the patient is asked to count to 30—this is most revealing as the stream of speech and content is interrupted by an absence seizure.

Tonic-Clonic Seizures

Tonic refers to continuous stiffening of the extremities. Clonic refers to the rhythmic alternating contraction and relaxation of the muscles. A tonic-clonic seizure is one that starts with continuous tonic stiffening and is then followed by a clonic phase of rhythmic jerks. Most tonic-clonic seizures are accompanied by loss of bladder control and are followed by a postictal state characterized by confusion, fatigue, headaches, muscle aches, and no memory of the seizure event. Note that partial seizures may have such rapid secondary generalization that they may be clinically indistinguishable from true primary generalized tonic-clonic seizures.

Myoclonic seizures are brief body jerks, often occurring in irregular flurries.

Atonic (akinetic) seizures are drop attacks. They are so brief that consciousness has been regained by the time the child strikes the floor.

Partial Seizures

Partial seizures are classified into three types; simple partial, complex partial, and partial seizures with secondary generalization. Simple and complex partial seizures may be quite subtle with little noticeable change in appearance, or they may be readily apparent to any observer. Do not neglect to take a careful history from teachers, school nurses, and even the young child, who may be able to draw a picture or enact the event.

Simple Partial Seizures

Simple partial seizures begin focally in one hemisphere and do not impair the level of consciousness. They may consist of virtually any task of which the brain is capable, such as jerking of just one extremity or abnormal sensation of one part of the body.

Complex Partial Seizures

Complex partial seizures begin focally in one hemisphere and do impair the level of consciousness. There is usually a well-defined aura followed by confusion, which is accompanied by lip smacking, fumbling, twisting or turning, neck motion, eye deviation, or eyelid fluttering. Unlike absence seizures, these spells tend to last several minutes and are accompanied by an aura and postictal state.

Partial Seizures with Secondary Generalization

Although the secondary generalization may be the most striking feature to the family, it is the partial onset of these seizures that matters most to the clinician. A Jacksonian march is the label given to a seizure that spreads through the cortex of one hemisphere with resultant spread of the clinical seizure. The child may be aware of this focal march along one side of the body, and then lose consciousness as the seizure spreads to the other hemisphere during secondary generalization.

Selected Epilepsy Syndromes

Comprehensive discussion of the specific epilepsy syndromes is beyond the scope of this chapter.

Febrile Seizures

Febrile seizures usually occur between 3 months and 5 yrs of age; most occur at 6 months to 3 yrs of age. They are usually brief and self-limited.[12] They are defined as an event in neurologically healthy infants and children associated with fever > 38°C rectal temperature but without evidence of intracranial infection as a defined cause and with no history of prior afebrile seizures. Simple febrile seizures constitute up to 85% of febrile seizures. They are generalized seizures, lasting less than 15 minutes, not recurring within 24 hours, and with no postictal neurological abnormalities. Complex febrile seizures are focal, prolonged or recurrent within 24 hours or associated with postictal neurological abnormalities including todd paresis. They constitute around 15% of febrile seizures.

The average **recurrence rate after a first febrile seizure** is 30-40% but this is dependent on complex interplay between genetic and environmental factors. Of these, 75% of recurrences would occur within 1 year of first episode. Best predictor of recurrence is early age at seizure onset and positive family history of febrile seizures.[13] Other risk factors include a low temperature at seizure onset and a shorter duration of temperature before febrile seizure. The overall **risk of subsequent epilepsy** after febrile seizures is 2-2.5%. The risk factors are: complex febrile seizures (each complex feature of febrile seizures is an independent predictor of later afebrile seizures), pre-existing neurologic or developmental abnormality and a family history of epilepsy.

Diagnosis

History

A diagnosis of epilepsy is clinical and needs a detailed history from a witness who has observed the event. Often questioning the older child about any preceding aura as well as the circumstances at the time maybe very useful. The seizure semiology, single or mixed type, age at onset, frequency and history of status epilepticus should determined. Perinatal events, previous history of head trauma, features suggestive of CNS infection, febrile seizures should be enquired. Family history of epilepsy or neurological disorder should be obtained.

Examination

Neurocutaneous markers, abnormal skull shape/size and dysmorphic facies should be looked for. CNS examination and developmental assessment should be performed in detail. Hyperventilation to provoke absence seizures if suspected as detailed above.

Role of Electroencephalography (EEG)

EEG is really part of the evaluation of any episodic event as there is a fairly strong association between interictal epileptiform discharges on the EEG and clinical seizures. However, normal initial EEGs are seen in around 50% of those with infrequent seizures.[14] The yield increases with repeated records (90% by the 4th EEG), sleep deprivation and activation procedures like photic stimulation/ hyperventilation. Certain epileptic syndromes consistently have abnormal EEGs like benign rolandic epilepsy of childhood, childhood absence epilepsy and west syndrome. On the other hand epilepsies in older children from deep regions like the mesial temporal or the basal frontal areas may not show abnormalities at all. On the other hand 2.2-3.5% of normal individuals have interictal discharges and on follow up there is only 5% risk of seizure.[14] The other major problem in India is that though EEG services are widely available and used, the technical quality and interpretation reliability is often questionable especially in childhood. Indications include.[6,15]

i. Differentiate seizure from non-epileptic paroxysmal events
ii. Classification of seizures-partial/generalized/partial with secondary generalization
iii. Assist to categorize patients into specific epilepsy syndromes
iv. Monitoring response to treatment
v. Localization and lateralisation of epileptic focus as a part of presurgical work up in intractable epilepsy
vi. Aiding the decision making process for discontinuation of treatment, once seizure remission is achieved
vii. Monitoring of status epilepticus, establishing the diagnosis of non convulsive status

viii. *Investigation of acute and chronic encephalopathies*: Diagnostic clues (Subacute sclerosing panencephalitis), prognostication.

Role of Neuroimaging

In a tropical country like India, imaging forms a part of diagnostic work up in outpatient; reason being the high incidence of inflammatory granulomas. Computed tomography (CT) scan adequately picks up inflammatory lesions and is superior to Magnetic resonance imaging (MRI) in picking up calcifications.[16] MRI utility is in subtle lesions like cortical dysplasia and hippocampal sclerosis. MRI can detect live cysts of neurocysticerci, especially subarachnoid and intraventricular cysts better than CT.

ILAE recommendations for neuroimaging of patients with epilepsy:[17,18]

Aims and Rationale

- To identify underlying pathologies that merit specific treatment.
- To aid the formulation of syndromic and etiological diagnoses and to give accurate prognosis.

MRI is clearly the structural imaging modality of choice for investigating patients with epilepsy and is superior to radiographic CT in terms of both sensitivity and specificity for identification of small lesions and abnormalities of the cerebral cortex. Imaging should include T_1- and T_2-weighted sequences to cover the whole brain.

In the **acute situation** of seizures developing in the context of a neurological insult such as head injury, intracranial hemorrhage, or encephalitis, radiographic CT scan is an appropriate initial investigation if MRI is not readily available or cannot be performed.

In the **nonacute situation**, **ideal practice** is to obtain structural neuroimaging with MRI in all patients with epilepsy, **except in patients** with a definite electroclinical diagnosis of idiopathic generalized epilepsy (benign myoclonic epilepsy of infancy, childhood absence epilepsy, juvenile absence epilepsy, juvenile myoclonic epilepsy), or benign epilepsy of childhood with centrotemporal spikes. MRI is **particularly indicated** in situations which are detailed in Table 16.5. **Appropriate minimum standards** vary between different countries and societies. Radiographic CT scanning is an alternative procedure if MRI is not available or cannot be performed for technical reasons. The Commission on Tropical Diseases of the International League Against Epilepsy considers the label "idiopathic" unacceptable in the tropics till a CT has been done due to wide prevalence of inflammatory lesions.[18] **Essential indications** for the performance of MRI scans are enumerated in Table 16.5.

Functional Neuroimaging

The main utility of Functional magnetic resonance imaging, Magnetic resonance spectroscopy, Single photon emission computed tomography and Positron emission tomography is in intractable epilepsy and not in acute situation of a seizure.[16]

APPROACH TO MANAGEMENT

Recurrence Rates in Children

After a **first unprovoked seizure** prospective studies have shown a recurrence of a second seizure in 37-54% by 2 years and 72% of those with a second seizure will have a third. [19] About 29% will have more than 10 seizures. In a prospective study of 407 children with first unprovoked seizure, the cumulative risk of a second seizure was 29%, 37%, 43%, and 46% at 1, 2, 5, and 10 years, respectively. The cumulative risk of a third seizure was 57%, 63%, and 71% at 1, 2, and 5 years, respectively, after the second seizure. After a third seizure, the cumulative risk of another seizure was 69%, 72%, and 81% at 1, 2, and 5 years, respectively.[20] The median time to recurrence was 5.7 months, with 53% of recurrences occurring within 6 months, 69% within 1 year, and 88% within 2 years.

On multivariable analysis, **risk factors** for seizure recurrence included a remote symptomatic etiology, an abnormal EEG, a seizure occurring while asleep, a history of prior febrile seizures, and Todd's paresis. In cryptogenic cases, the risk factors were an abnormal EEG and an initial seizure during sleep. In remote symptomatic cases, risk factors were a history of prior febrile seizures and age of onset younger than 3 years. Risk factors for late recurrences (after 2 years) were similar to the risk factors for early recurrence.[21]

Camfield et al reported that in children treated with carbamazepine for 1 year after a first afebrile seizure, the

Table 16. 5: ILAE recommendations for neuroimaging of patients with epilepsy[17]

MRI is particularly indicated in:

- Onset of seizures at any age with evidence of a partial onset on history or EEG.
- Onset of unclassified or apparently generalized seizures in the first year of life or in adulthood.
- Evidence of a focal fixed deficit on neurological or neuropsychological examination.
- Difficulty in obtaining control of seizures with first-line antiepileptic drug treatment.
- Loss of control of seizures with antiepileptic drugs or a change in the seizure pattern that may imply a progressive underlying lesion.

Essential indications for MRI:

- Partial or secondarily generalized seizures, and apparently generalized seizures, that do not remit with antiepileptic drug treatment.
- Development of the progressive neurological or neuropsychological deficits.

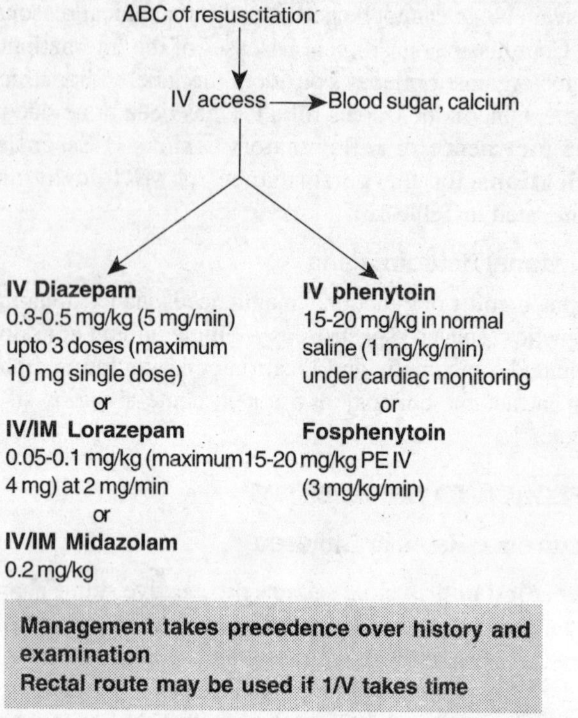

Fig. 16.2: Management of an acute seizure episode

subsequent clinical course and remission rates were not improved in comparison with a no-treatment strategy.[22] This is made amply clear in developing countries where the 'treatment gap' (% of patients not treated with any anti-epileptic drug (AED) is large. Many of these untreated patients remit spontaneously over time.

Immediate Management

The management of an acute episode of seizure is detailed in Figure 16.2. The rest of protocol in case seizure is not controlled is detailed in the chapter on Status epilepticus.

Management Issues after An First Episode of Seizure

They are detailed in Table 16.6. Idiopathic generalized, all symptomatic epilepsies and those presenting with status epilepticus or seizure clusters are more likely to be treated. Older age of onset may also bias towards treatment, as teenagers often want to drive and be independently mobile. In one study 90% of patients were on treatment by the end of the first year of seizure onset and benign partial epilepsies remained the only group where 50% of children remained untreated.[23]

Table 16.6: Management issues–First seizure

- *Provoked seizure:* Acute symptomatic treatment only. In cases of acute CNS infection, head trauma maintenance AED therapy may be given during acute stage of illness
- *Generalized tonic clonic:* Withhold antiepileptic drugs (AED) unless mentally retarded, neurological deficit, inflammatory granuloma, first episode is status epilepticus, early medical help is inaccessible
- *Partial:* Evaluate and treat
- *Absence:* Treat
- *Myoclonus:* Evaluate and treat

Antiepileptic Drugs Available[6,24-27]

Conventional Antiepileptic Drugs

Phenytoin: (Dose 5-8 mg/kg/day). It acts by altering Na^+, K^+, and Ca^{2+} conductance, membrane potentials and concentrations of amino acids, norepinephrine, acetylcholine and GABA. Its half-life varies from 12-36 hrs. It is useful in tonic and clonic convulsions, control symptomatic convulsions. It also prevents spread of partial seizures into generalized ones. It is used IV in status epilepticus and to treat digoxin-induced arrhythmias due to its membrane-stabilizing effects. **Fosphenytoin sodium** injection is a new prodrug intended for parenteral administration. It is safer and better tolerated than phenytoin and can be infused 3 times faster than intravenous phenytoin. Side effects include ataxia, tremors, nystagmus, gastrointestinal upset, gingival hypertrophy, hirsutism, dermatitis, blood dyscrasias, liver damage, lymphadenopathy, interferes with calcium metabolism, encephalopathy, folate deficiency, hypersensitivity reactions, teratogenecity-hare lip, and cleft palate.

Phenobarbitone and related drugs: (Dose 3-8 mg/kg/day). It enhances GABA receptor-mediated current by prolonging openings of chloride channels, block excitatory response induced by glutamate. It has complete but slow oral absorption, inducer of liver enzymes, t½ being 70-100 hr. Indications include tonic-clonic convulsions, continuous prophylaxis of febrile seizures. Side effects include sedation, ataxia, diplopia, drowsiness, hyperactivity, depression, decreased concentration, hypersensitivity

Carbamazepine: (Dose 10-30 mg/kg/day). It inhibits high frequency repetitive firing by blocking sodium channels at therapeutic concentration, thereby limiting the focus and the spread of discharges. It has slow oral absorption; half-life with single dosing is 25-50 hr; multiple dosing about 7-12 hr. Used in partial seizures, temporal lobe seizures whether or not these seizures undergo generalization, grand mal seizures, manic-depressive disorders, and trigeminal neuralgia. Side effects include diplopia, nystagmus, antidiuretic effect, hypersensitivity reactions, gastrointestinal disturbances, ataxia, hepatitis, skin rash, bone marrow depression, sedation, urinary retention.

Sodium valproate: (Dose 10-60 mg/kg/day). It appears to increase potassium conductance and hyperpolarize the membrane, hence decrease seizure discharge from focus and inhibit the spread. It is well absorbed orally, half-life is 8-15 hrs. Indications are absence seizures, myoclonic seizures, generalized tonic-clonic seizures. Side effects include idiosyncratic reaction, alopecia, weight gain, sedation, gastrointestinal disturbances, hepatotoxicity, leucopenia, thrombocytopenia, headache, hyperammonemia. spina bifida in neonates born to mothers consuming the same during pregnancy. An IV form of valproate is available. It is well tolerated and its bioavailability is similar to that of the oral preparation. The T_{max} after IV VPA is at the end of 1-hour infusion, and thus the drug should be administered every 6 hours.

Ethosuccimide: (Dose 15-40 mg/kg/day). Its indicated in absence seizures, myoclonic seizures. Side effects include ataxia, anorexia, drowsiness, sleep disturbances, rashes and blood dyscrasias.

Clonazepam: (Dose 0.01-0.2 mg/kg/day). It has higher affinity for the GABA-A receptor site than diazepam and binds to GABA-A receptors that do not bind with other benzodiazepines. It is indicated in myoclonic seizures and subcortical myoclonus. It also is effective in generalized convulsions and, to a lesser extent, in partial epilepsies. Side effects include sedation, ataxia, hyperactivity, restlessness, irritability, depression, cardiovascular or respiratory depression and hypersalivation.

Newer Antiepileptic drugs

Vigabatrin: (Dose-50-80 mg/kg/day, can increase upto 120-150 mg/kg/day [28]). Its indications include infantile spasms in west syndrome and partial seizures. It is less effective against primarily generalized tonic-clonic seizures and also may worsen myoclonic seizures or generalized absence seizures. Side effects include demyelination and intramyelinic vacoulation in the nervous system, hyperkinesias, and agitation..

Clobazam: (Dose 0.1-1 mg/kg/day). Indications include-complex partial seizures, atypical absence seizures, myoclonic seizures, generalized tonic clonic seizures, Lennox gastaut syndrome, used both as an add on and monotherapy. Side effects include sedation and behavior disturbance

Lamotrigine: (Dose 2-10 mg/kg/day; 0.5-5 mg/kg/day with Valproate; 5-15 mg/kg/day with enzyme inducing antiepileptic drugs). Indications include-Atonic seizures, atypical absence seizures, myoclonic seizures, generalized tonic clonic seizures, Lennox gastaut syndrome. Side effects include sedation, somnolence, severe drug rash may occur.

Oxcarbazepine: (Dose-10-45 mg/kg/day). It is approved for monotherapy or adjunctive therapy in partial, secondary generalized seizures and generalized tonic clonic seizures. It was developed in an attempt to hold on to the benefits of carbamazepine while avoiding its auto-induction and drug interaction properties. Side effects include ataxia, lethargy, dizziness, somnolence, headache, rash, hyponatremia, weight gain, gastrointestinal disturbances, and alopecia.

Primidone: (Dose-<8 years: 10-25 mg/kg/day; > 8 years: 125-1500 mg/day). This drug is metabolized to phenobarbitone and phenylmethylmalonamide. It can be used for partial onset and secondarily generalized seizures. The major adverse effects are intense sedation, dizziness, and nausea.

Gabapentin: (Dose-30-60 mg/kg/). It can be used as an add on and monotherapy in partial seizures and secondarily generalized tonic-clonic seizures. Side effects include rash, neutropenia, somnolence, dizziness, ataxia, nystagmus, headache, tremor, diplopia, rhinitis, and nausea or vomiting .It can cause behavior problems.

Zonisamide: (Dose- starts with 2-4 mg/kg/day; can go upto 8 mg/kg/day). It is mostly useful in partial seizures but also can be used in generalized seizures including atypical absence, myoclonic epilepsy, and Lennox gastaut syndrome and Landau Kleffner syndrome. Adverse reactions include dizziness, anorexia, headache, ataxia, confusion, speech abnormalities, mental slowing, irritability, tremor, weight gain, anhydrosis and renal calculi.

Felbamate: (Dose 15-45 mg/kg/day). Sidelined due to side effects of aplastic anemia and serious hepatitis. Its use is restricted to patients with severe partial epilepsy or Lennox-Gastaut syndrome who do not respond to other medications.

Topiramate: (Dose 6-11 mg/kg/day).It is used for partial onset and secondarily generalized tonic-clonic seizures, primary generalized tonic-clonic seizures, and Lennox Gastaut syndrome. The common adverse effects in children are somnolence, anorexia, fatigue, and nervousness. It also has a propensity to cause renal calculi.

Tiagabine: (Dose-4-8 mg/day upto 32 mg/day; 0.4-1 mg/kg) It can be used as second-line add-on therapy in patients with partial or secondarily generalized seizures refractory to treatment. Adverse effects include dizziness, asthenia, nervousness, tremor, depressed mood, and emotional lability.

Levetiracetam: (Dose: 500 mg twice a day upto 3000 mg/day; 40-60 mg/kg) It may be used in patients with refractory partial epilepsy and perhaps juvenile myoclonic epilepsy and generalized epilepsies. The most significant adverse effects are somnolence, asthenia, dizziness, headache and a flu-like syndrome.

Choice of Antiepileptic Drugs

It depends upon the seizure type, age and gender of the patient, epileptic syndrome diagnosis if possible, premorbid conditions, cost of therapy and safety profile. A recent study comparing valproate, carbamazepine, phenobarbital and phenytoin in newly diagnosed uncomplicated epilepsy in 161 children showed a 1 year remission rate of around 70% with no significant difference in efficacy among the four antiepileptic drugs.[29] Side effects were least with valproate and carbamazepine and these therefore remain the drugs of first choice in developed countries. In our setup in view of lower cost, ease of administration and fewer side effects phenytoin is the drug of choice. Western consensus data suggest valproate followed by lamotrigine as the most appropriate treatment for idiopathic and symptomatic generalized epilepsies.[30] The rational choice of conventional antiepileptic drugs in various seizure types in our setting is detailed in Table 16.7. Newer drugs are rarely used as first line drugs though controlled studies have demonstrated efficacy with clobazam, lamotrigine, oxcarbazepine and gabapentin. Rarely etiology would decide treatment like in the case of vigabatrin (VGB) in infantile spasms due to tuberous sclerosis. The indications of newer antiepileptic drugs are summarized in Table 16.8.

Table 16.7: Rational choice of AED (modified)[6]

Seizure type	*Conventional drugs*
Generalized tonic clinic	Phenytoin° carbamazepine° sodium valproate
Partial	Simple: Carbamazepine, phenytoin Complex: Carbamazepine, phenytoin, sodium valproate
Absence	Sodium valproate, ethosuccimide
Myoclonus	Sodium valproate, benzodiazepines
Atonic sodium valproate	
Infantile spasms	ACTH, sodium valproate, benzodiazepines
Mixed	Sodium valproate

Age, sex and presence of other disorders may also influence the choice of antiepileptic drugs. For instance, phenytoin induces significant coarsening of facies, hirsutism and gingival hyperplasia making it undesirable in adolescent girls. Benzodiazepines often worsen behaviour in mentally challenged/autistic individuals and may worsen drooling in children with cerebral palsy.

Rational AED Therapy

According to a recent consensus survey initial use of a single drug as monotherapy at a lowest possible dosage is best.[30] Seizure control is used as a yardstick to increase the dosage till side effects occur or control is achieved. It is best to avoid increasing doses according to weight ('mg/kg') after seizure control is achieved. If the first drug fails as happens in about 30-40% a second monotherapy trial is given and the first drug is gradually withdrawn. If this fails appropriate combinations are used as rational polytherapy. This would involve using drugs with different mechanisms of action and without significant interactions or additive adverse effects. Some combinations may be synergistic like valproate and lamotrigine.

Dispersible tablets and controlled release formulations allowing twice daily dosing are preferable for ensuring good compliance. Syrups and suspensions should be shaken prior to use. Once the formulation has been selected it may be best not to switch to other brands as this often leads to loss of control.

A recent randomized controlled trial in 180 patients concluded that routine therapeutic drug monitoring during monotherapy made no difference in seizure free outcome with most commonly used drugs.[31] Phenytoin however is an exception. In polytherapy regimens when drugs with interactions are used it might be of importance.

Parental Counseling

One of the most frightening occurrences for parents is to witness their child having a seizure. Explain the nature of disease and alleviate fears of supernatural involvement. Explain precipitants like fever, sleep deprivation, fasting, and photosensitivity. In vast majority of cases (80%) epilepsy would improve with drug therapy. Regular drug therapy is the corner stone of management. They should be explained the domiciliary management of seizures and importance of follow-up.

Domiciliary Management of Seizures[6]

Place the patient in head down, semi prone position. Clear the mouth of secretions, do not put anything between patients

Table 16.8: Newer antiepileptics and indications (Modified) [27]

	Partial/Sec generalized	*Primary generalized*	*Myoclonic spasm*	*Absence*	*Infantile*
Vigabatrin	+	+/–	–	+/–	+
Lamotrigine	+	+	+	+	+
Gabapentin	+	+/–	–	–	–
Felbamate	+	+	+	+	+
Clobazam	+/–	+	+	+	–
Topiramate	+	+	+	+	+
Oxcarbazepine	+	+/–	–	–	–
Tiagabine	+	–	–	–	–
Zonisamide	+	+/–	+	+	+
Levetiracetam	+	+	+	–	–

Efficacious = +, Mixed results = +/–, No proven efficacy = –

teeth. Stand by the patient and terminate the seizure by giving per rectal (PR) diazepam. Diazepam is rapidly absorbed from the rectal mucosa. Blood levels peak within 15 minutes. There is no respiratory depression. Preparations which can be used include injection Diazepam 5 mg/ml, Diazepam syrup 2 mg/5 ml in a dose of 0.5-1 mg/kg (max. 10 mg). Insert a size 8 feeding tube after lubricating with xylocaine/paraffin, per rectum upto 4 cm. Inject the required dose of injection/syrup through the feeding tube and then flush it with tap water. The dose may be repeated once after 5 minutes if one dose has not been able to abort the seizure. **Other drug options** include buccal midazolam 0.3 mg/kg [10 mg] (introduced between the gums and cheek) or intranasal midazolam (0.2 mg/kg) which is socially more acceptable. Sodium valproate [20 mg/kg] may be given as a enema (syrup 200 mg/5 ml) diluted in tap water. Rectal administration of lorazepam is safe at a dose of 0.1-0.4 mg/kg. Sublingual lorazepam at dose of 0.05-0.1 mg/kg may be used. The tablet is placed under the patient's tongue. Take to the nearest medical facility if the seizure does not respond to home treatment: 10 minutes for the first seizure, or 2 minutes longer than the usual length of seizure, or when a second seizure occurs without the child regaining consciousness.

Life-style

Patients should be informed to maintain normal lifestyle. School teachers should be informed about the nature of disease and should be specifically told not to be biased against these children. If possible, facility of acute management of seizures should be available at school. Some caution is advocated in possibly dangerous activities such as cycling, swimming and activities near fire particularly in the first year of remission. The extent of these special precautions will depend on the type and frequency of the seizure. Children who are subject to daily seizures should not be permitted to engage in activities in which they might be injured. These children should have side rails on beds with the hard surfaces padded if there is danger that they could hurt themselves. Children who have infrequent seizures or who are relatively free of seizures will have few restrictions on their activities.

Discontinuing AED

Most epileptics remit, all drugs have some side effects and there is a risk of teratogenicity in young women. Thus the need for discontinuation of AED. Around 70% of epilepsies with onset in childhood will remit over the long term.[19] In a 30-year follow-up of 245 epileptic children, 64% were seizure-free for more than 5 years and 47% were off AEDs.[32] The most important factors influencing remission were etiology, epilepsy syndrome, early response to therapy and seizure frequency. The chance of remission was 85-90% in idiopathic syndromes, 60% in cryptogenic syndromes and only about 25-30% in remote symptomatic syndromes.

The Connecticut study reported that by 2 years after diagnosis 53% have a 'good' outcome while 8% have a 'bad' outcome. Half of the remaining 'indeterminate' group goes on to have a 'good' outcome 2 years later (4 years from diagnosis) while 8% of them become 'bad'. Hence it appears that by two years if you have had no seizures then it is likely that you will do well even without AEDs and it may be time for a trial of AED discontinuation. In the not so good groups one could wait an additional 2 years to decide.[33] Only 1-year treatment may be enough in idiopathic syndromes like benign rolandic epilepsy. Acute symptomatic epilepsy due to inflammatory granulomas may allow earlier tapering.

Relapse after Discontinuing AED

Berg et al.in a meta-analysis reported that there was a 25% risk of relapse at 1 year and a 29% risk at 2 years. [34] This was irrespective of the fact that a 2 or 4-year seizure free criteria had been used prior to discontinuation. The factors associated with risk of relapse include etiology, age of onset and EEG findings at the time of AED withdrawal. The risk is less than 15% in patients with an idiopathic or cryptogenic syndrome, with a normal EEG and an age of onset < 12 years. Remote symptomatic syndromes have a worse risk; however approximately 50% will remain free on AED withdrawal suggesting that this should be attempted even in this higher risk group. Adolescent age of onset of epilepsy is consistently associated with a high recurrence risk following AED withdrawal. An abnormal EEG was associated with a relative risk of relapse of 1.45 [34] The majority of relapses occur early with half within 6 months and 60-80% within 12 months. In case of relapse the prognosis for control remains favorable after re-initiation of AEDs.

Tapering AED

The AEDs can be withdrawn within 6 weeks. Tennison et al reported that the risk of seizure recurrence during drug tapering and after discontinuation of antiepileptic drug therapy in children with epilepsy was not different whether the medications are tapered over a 6 week or 9 month period.[35]

Prognosis

The long-term mortality is increased in epileptics. This increase in mortality is more evident with children having their epilepsy within the first year of life. Mortality was much more in the remote symptomatic cases while it was not different from the general population in the idiopathic group.[32] There also seems to be an adverse long-term impact of chronic epilepsy on education, employment, marriage and fertility.

Management of a Child with Febrile Seizures

Evaluation

History aims to rule out possible CNS infections, determine cause of fever, describe seizures semiology, ascertain family risk factors, determine neurodevelopment of the child. Clinical examination includes observation of postictal phase, to look for CNS infections like meningitis and to look for signs of raised intracranial pressure.

During the Seizure: Any child with a febrile seizure needs to be managed as for any other acute seizure as mentioned already. Rectal diazepam (0.5 mg/kg) has also been found to be safe and effective. Nasal/buccal midazolam has also been used in acute seizure control.

Investigations: They are oriented towards finding the cause of fever and to rule out meningitis. Serum electrolytes, blood glucose, calcium, magnesium and blood counts are not routinely needed.

Lumbar Puncture (LP): LP is indicated whenever a doubt of meningitis exists. After the first seizure with fever in **infants younger than 12 months**, performance of a LP should be strongly considered, because the clinical signs and symptoms associated with meningitis may be minimal or absent in this age group. In a **child between 12 and 18 months of age**, a LP should be considered, because clinical signs and symptoms of meningitis may be subtle. In a **child older than 18 months**, although a lumbar puncture is not routinely warranted, it is recommended in the presence of meningeal signs and symptoms (i.e., neck stiffness and Kernig and Brudzinski signs), which are usually present with meningitis, or for any child whose history or examination suggest the presence of intracranial infection. In infants and children who have had febrile seizures and have **received prior antibiotic treatment**, clinicians should be aware that treatment can mask the signs and symptoms of meningitis. As such, a lumbar puncture should be strongly considered.[36]

EEG and neuroimaging need not be performed in the routine evaluation of a neurologically healthy child with a first simple febrile seizure.

Long Term Management

The primary goal of long-term management of febrile seizure is to prevent recurrences. Treatment options include : (a) Intermittent prophylaxis; (b) Prolonged daily prophylaxis.

Antipyretics are not effective in preventing recurrent febrile seizures, but are useful in making the child more comfortable. Tepid water sponging is advised if temperature remains high, despite drug therapy.

Intermittent Diazepam Prophylaxis

Diazepam administered intermittently either rectally or orally at the onset of fever has been shown to be effective in preventing recurrence of febrile seizures. By either route, generally a dose of 0.3 to 0.5 mg/kg (max 10 mg) is used and repeated every 8-12 hours if temperature is 38°C or more. Intermittent clobazam (1 mg/kg/day) given orally has also been found to be useful in preventing febrile seizure recurrences. In a randomized controlled study in 150 children with 559 febrile episodes done by the senior author, oral clobazam was found to be superior to oral diazepam in preventing febrile seizure recurrence.[37] Buccal or intranasal midazolam may be used. This therapy does not decrease the incidence of later epilepsy in children with febrile seizures. Duration of prophylaxis is 2 years seizure free period or 5 years of age whichever is earlier.

Continuous Prophylaxis

Indications for continuous prophylaxis include recurrent complex seizures with failed intermittent prophylaxis, abnormal neurodevelopment and positive family history of epilepsy. Phenobarbital is effective in preventing the recurrence of simple febrile seizures. Long-term phenobarbital treatment appears to influence cognition and behavior, a large price for prevention of benign condition. Sodium valproate is as effective as phenobarbitone in preventing recurrent, simple febrile seizures. Draw backs to therapy with valproate include side effects like hepatotoxicity, thrombocytopenia, weight loss and gain, gastrointestinal disturbances and pancreatitis. Sodium valproate is preferred to phenobarbitone. Neither of them is effective in reducing the risk of epilepsy in children with febrile seizure.

Patient Education

Domiciliary care should be explained. A doctor should be consulted if the seizure lasts for more than 15 minutes or if the post ictal drowsiness persists for more than 30 minutes.

On the basis of the risks and benefits of the effective therapies, neither continuous nor intermittent antiepileptic therapy is recommended by the American Academy of Pediatrics for children with one or more simple febrile seizures.[38] In those situations in which parental anxiety associated with febrile seizures is severe, intermittent oral diazepam at the onset of febrile illness may be effective in preventing recurrence. But in developing countries like ours it is preferable to give intermittent prophylaxis with oral clobazam or diazepam. The former has been reported to be better. Evidence is not convincing, however, that any therapy will alleviate the possibility of future epilepsy.

REFERENCES

1. Hauser WA, Hesdorffer DC. *Epilepsy: Frequency, Causes, and Consequences*. New York: Demos Publications 1990.
2. Paolicchi JM. The spectrum of nonepileptic events in children. *Epilepsia* 2002;43(Suppl 3):60-64.
3. Mani KS, Rangan G. The yelandur model for rural epilepsy control in India. In: Singhal BS, Nag D (ed) *Epilepsy in India*. Gurgaon: Delta Press, 2000;16-32.
4. Srinivas HV. Diagnosis of epilepsy. In Singhal BS, Nag D (ed) *Epilepsy in India*. Delta Press 2000;190-204.
5. Radhakrishnan K, Nayak SD, Kumar SP, Sarma PS. Profile of antiepileptic pharmacotherapy in a tertiary referral center in South India: a pharmacoepidemiologic and pharmacoeconomic study. *Epilepsia* 1999; 40:179-185.
6. Kalra V Ed. Assisted by Gulati S. Seizure disorders and epilepsy. In: Kalra V, Gulati S (eds) *Practical Pediatric Neurology*, 1st edn, New Delhi: Arya Publishers 2002;49-77.
7. Commission on Epidemiology and Prognosis, International League Against Epilepsy. Guidelines for epidemiologic studies on epilepsy. *Epilepsia* 1993;34:592-596.
8. Commission on Classification and Terminology of the International League Against Epilepsy. Proposal for revised classification of epilepsies and epileptic syndromes. *Epilepsia* 1989;30:389-399.
9. From the Commission on Classification and Terminology of the International League Against Epilepsy. Proposal for revised clinical and electroencephalographic classification of epileptic seizures. *Epilepsia* 1981;22:489-501.
10. Tich SNT, Pereon Y. Letter to the editor. *Epilepsia* 1999; 40: 531-532.
11. Hirtz DG. Generalized tonic-clonic and febrile seizures. *Pediat Clin of N Am* 1989;36:365-382.
12. Consensus Development Conference on Febrile Seizures, National Institutes of Health. Proceedings. *Epilepsia* 1981;22: 377-81.
13. Berg AT, Shinnar S, Hauser WA, Leventhal JM. Predictors of recurrent febrile seizures: A meta-analytical review. *J Pediatr* 1990;116:329-337.
14. Thaddeus SW, Jayakar P. Interictal EEG. In J Engel, Jr, TA Pedley. *Epilepsy. A Comprehensive Textbook*. New York: Lippincott-Raven press 1998:831-848.
15. Prasad A, Daoust Roy J. EEG-Rational use and newer innovations in pediatric epilepsy. *Indian J Pediatr* 2003;70:S20-S30.
16. Gulati S, Gaikwad SB, Kalra V. Rational use of Anatomic and functional neuroimaging in epilepsy. *Indian J Pediatr* 2003;70:S55-S63.
17. Neuroimaging Commission of ILAE. Recommendations for neuroimaging of persons with epilepsy. *Epilepsia* 1997;38: 1255-1256.
18. Commission on tropical diseases of the International League Against Epilepsy. Relationship between epilepsy and tropical diseases. *Epilepsia* 1994;35:89-93.
19. Shinnar S, Pellock JM. Update on epidemiology and prognosis of pediatric epilepsy. *J. Child Neurol* 2002;17(Suppl 1): S4-S17.
20. Shinnar S, Berg AT, O'Dell C, Newstein D, Moshe SL, Hauser WA. Predictors of multiple seizures in a cohort of children prospectively followed from the time of their first unprovoked seizure. *Ann Neurol* 2000;48:140-147.
21. Shinnar S, Berg AT, Moshe SL, et al. The risk of seizure recurrence after a first unprovoked afebrile seizure in childhood: An extended follow-up. *Pediatrics* 1996;98:216-225.
22. Camfield P, Camfield C, Smith S, Dooley J, Smith E. Long-term outcome is unchanged after a first seizure: A 15 year follow–up from a randomized trial in childhood. *Epilepsia* 2002;43: 662-663.
23. Berg AT, Levy SR, Testa FM, Shinnar S. Treatment of newly diagnosed pediatric epilepsy: A community–based study. *Arch Pediatr Adolesc Med* 1999;153: 1267-1271.
24. Bazil CW, Pedley TA. Advances in the medical treatment of epilepsy. *Annu Rev Med* 1998;49:135-162.
25. Perucca E. The new generation of antiepileptic drugs: advantages and disadvantages. *British Journal of Clinical Pharmacology* 1996;42:531-543.
26. Bialer M, Johannessen SI, Kupferberg HJ, Levy RH, Loiseau P. Perucca E. Conference Report: Progress report on new antiepileptic drugs: a summary of the fourth Eilat Conference (EILAT IV). *Epilepsy Research* 1999;341.
27. Singhi PD. Newer antiepileptic drugs and non-drug therapies. *Indian J Pediatr* 2003;70:S39-S44.
28. Haines ST, Casto DT. Treatment of infantile spasms. *Annals Pharmacother* 1994;28:779-90.
29. de Silva M, MacArdle B, McGowan M, et al. Randomised comparative monotherapy trial of phenobarbitone, phenytoin, carbamazepine or sodium valproate for newly diagnosed epilepsy. *Lancet* 1996;347:709-713.
30. Karceski S, Morrell M, Carpenter D. The expert consensus guideline series. Treatment of epilepsy. *Epilepsy & Behaviour* 2001;2:A1-A50.
31. Jannuzzi G, Cian P, Fattore C, Gatti G, Bartoli A, Monaco F, Perucca E. A multicenter randomized controlled trial on the clinical impact of therapeutic drug monitoring in patients with newly diagnosed epilepsy. The Italian TDM Study Group in Epilepsy. *Epilepsia* 2000;41:222-30.
32. Sillanpaa M, Jalava M, Kaleva O, Shinnar S. Long-term prognosis of seizures with onset in childhood. *N Engl J Med* 1998;338: 1916-1918.
33. Berg AT, Shinnar S, Levy SR, Testa FM, Smith-Rapaport S, Beckerman B, Ebrahim N. Defining early seizure outcomes in pediatric epilepsy: The good, the bad and the indeterminate. *Epilepsy Res* 2001;43:75-84.
34. Berg AT, Shinnar S. Relapse following discontinuation of antiepileptic drugs: A meta-analysis. *Neurology* 1994;44:601-608.
35. Tennison M, Greenwood R, Lewis D, Thorn M. Rate of taper of antiepileptic drugs and the risk of seizure recurrence in children. *N Engl J Med* 1994;330:1407-1410.
36. American Academy of Pediatrics Practice Parameter: The neurodiagnostic evaluation of the child with a first simple febrile seizure. American Academy of Pediatrics Provisional Committee on Quality improvement, Sub committee on Febrile Seizures. *Pediatrics* 1996;97:769-775.
37. Gulati S, Saini D, Pandey RM, Kalra V. A randomized controlled trial to compare efficacy of Oral clobazam with Oral diazepam for prophylaxis of febrile seizures. *National Conference, Indian Academy of Pediatrics*, Chennai 2004.
38. Baumamm RJ, Dufner PK. Treatment of children with simple febrile seizures. The AAP practice parameter. *Pediatr Neurol* 2000:23:11-17.

Sheffali Gulati and Anil Vasudevan

17 Status Epilepticus

INTRODUCTION

Status epilepticus (SE) is a common pediatric medical and neurological emergency. It may be life-threatening to the patient and a challenge to the treating physician. Status epilepticus is estimated as affecting approximately 1:150,000 cases per year in United States.[1] It is more frequent in children, following acute neuroinfections, dysmetabolic states, hypoxia, brain damage and antiepileptic drug (AED) withdrawal. It is estimated that 1.3 to 16% of all patients with epilepsy will develop SE at some point in their lives.[2]

If this life threatening condition is not managed promptly, it may result in significant morbidity and mortality. Although there has been lot of advances in the management, the pathophysiology of status epilepticus continues to be incompletely understood.

DEFINITION

In 1981, the International League Against Epilepsy defined status epilepticus as a single seizure or recurrent seizures lasting for more than 30 minutes during which time consciousness is not regained.[3] Lately, it is becoming increasingly recognized that seizure duration of more than 10 minutes can lead to brain damage and duration of seizure activity in definition of status epilepticus is being reduced. The longer the SE is present, more difficult is the control and more is the risk of permanent neurological damage. Immediate intervention is important whenever the patient has SE. Few authors recommend an operational definition of status epilepticus: either continuous seizures lasting at least 5 minutes or two or more discrete seizures between which there is incomplete recovery of consciousness.[4] Status epilepticus equivalents include:[4]

- Five minutes of continuous convulsive seizure.
- Three discrete convulsions within one hour.
- Thirty minutes of continuous seizure or lack of recovery between discrete seizure for focal, complex partial seizure, absences and other non-convulsive seizure.

CLASSIFICATION[3]

Status epilepticus is broadly classified as:

- Convulsive (includes tonic-clonic, tonic, clonic and myoclonic)
- Non-convulsive (includes absence status)
- Partial status epilepticus (includes elementary, somatomotor, dysphasia)
- Complex partial (includes fugue states, psychomotor)
- Unilateral status (hemiclonic, hemiconvulsion-hemiplegia).

Of these, generalized tonic-clonic seizures are the most common. Status epilepticus usually implies generalized convulsive status epilepticus. It has the highest potential for complications and even death.

ETIOLOGY

The causes of status epilepticus in various series are detailed in Table 17.1.[6-8] The causes can be effectively grouped into three broad categories: prolonged febrile seizures, idiopathic status epilepticus (seizure develops in absence of an underlying CNS lesion or insult) and symptomatic status epilepticus (seizure occurs as a result of underlying CNS insult or metabolic abnormality). Symptomatic can be acute or remote (chronic process).

Status epilepticus occurs most frequently in children aged 5 years or younger (85%).[9] Although individuals with a history of epilepsy constitute a group that is particularly at risk of developing status epilpeticus, approximately 50% of cases occur in the absence of previous epilepsy.[10] Among children with a first unprovoked seizures, 9% had status epilepticus.[11,12]

The causes of SE are age dependent. Febrile SE is most common in children less than 5 years of age.[13] Chronic CNS injury and idiopathic SE frequently cause SE in older children.[14] Severe hypoxic encephalopathy and inborn errors of metabolism may present with SE in newborns. Infants

Table 17.1: Causes of status epilepticus (modified)[6,8]

Acute Neurological (26%-49%)
• CNS* infections (meningitis, encephalitis, cerebral malaria)/sepsis syndrome
• Electrolyte disorders (hyponatremia, hypocalcemia, hypomagnesemia)
• Toxins/metabolic causes (Reye's syndrome, IEM, lead, uraemia)
• Trauma (including surgery)
• Acute anoxic insults
• Cerebrovascular accidents
Chronic Neurological Disorders (11%-21%)
• Neonatal nonprogressive insult
• Space occupying lesions (tumors, abscess, neurocysticercosis, bleed)
• CNS malformations
• Progressive encephalopathy
Cryptogenic or Idiopathic (46%-58%)
• Febrile
• Afebrile
*Central nervous system

with pre-existing neurologic abnormalities (lissencephaly or schizencephaly) may have recurrent episodes of SE.

The important risk factors for SE are: history of epilepsy, low antiepileptic drug (AED) level, younger age, genetic predisposition and acquired brain insult.[15]

The important precipitating factors include febrile illness, inadequate or irregular AED therapy, sudden discontinuation of AED, sleep deprivation, fatigue, emotional upset, metabolic, drugs (theophylline, amphetamines, isoniazid, organophosphorous compounds), hyperventilation, intermittent photic stimulation, AED (AED overdose, carbamazepine in non-convulsive SE). The search for a precipitating factor is of fundamental importance, as it will dictate appropriate therapy.

In a study at AIIMS, New Delhi on 30 children with SE by the author, sixteen patients (53.3%) presented with SE as first presentation without prior history of seizure activity. Among these 16 patients, 11 patients (68.7%) were less than 60 months age. Predisposing factors for SE included fever in 16, upper respiratory tract infection in 7, gastroenteritis in 2, hypoxia in 2, uremia in 2 and premature withdrawal of AED in 1 case.[16]

PATHOPHYSIOLOGY

Status epilepticus results from inability to normally abort an isolated seizure due to ineffective inhibition or due to abnormally persistent, excessive excitation. Excessive activation of excitatory amino acid receptors or excessive release of glutamate can cause prolonged seizures.[17] Drugs and compounds that antagonize the effects of G-amniobutyric acid (GABA), the main inhibitory neurotransmitter of the brain, may cause status epilepticus.[18] The most vulnerable areas include the limbic system, cerebellum, middle cortical area and the thalamus.

At cellular level, ischemic cellular changes due to increase in metabolic demand, depletion of glucose stores and oxygen supply are the earliest histologic finding, followed by neuronophagia, microglial proliferation cell loss and astrocyte proliferation.

Prolonged seizure activity (lasting more than 1 hour) results in hypotension, hyperkalemia, hypoglycemia, lactic acidosis, myoglobinuria, acute tubular necrosis and death. Experimental evidence suggests that neuronal injury increases and seizure activity may be refractory to treatment if it lasts for more than 60 minutes.

CLINICAL FEATURES

The child may present to the emergency with frank seizures. With time, the clinical manifestations become subtle and the child may have only small amplitude twitching movements of face and limbs or nystagmoid jerking of eyes. The child may have tachycardia, arterial hypertension and features of raised intracranial pressure (ICP). The differential diagnosis of convulsive status epilepticus includes rigors due to sepsis, myoclonic epilepsy, dystonias and pseudostatus epilepticus. In the latter condition, consciousness is often retained during convulsions.[19]

In nonconvulsive status epilepticus, clinical features include altered sensorium that may fluctuate, agitation, abnormal eye movements (including ocular deviation and nystagmus), aphasia and abnormal limb posturing. Diagnosis, therefore, requires a high degree of suspicion and can only be confirmed definitively by electroencephalography (EEG).[19] In a recent study, 8% of patients in coma were diagnosed as non-convulsive status epilepticus.[20]

LABORATORY EVALUATION AND IMAGING

Blood is obtained for complete blood count (CBC), determination of electrolytes, blood glucose, calcium and magnesium levels, creatinine, liver function tests (LFT), arterial lactate, creatine kinase and anticonvulsant levels. If indicated, blood and urine may be obtained for metabolic studies and toxicology. Hypoxia and acidosis should be ruled out by doing an arterial blood gas (ABG).

Cerebrospinal fluid (CSF) examination is mandatory if meningitis or encephalitis is considered. It may be performed (if crucial for diagnosis) after exclusion of raised ICP. Note that approximately 20% of patients have CSF pleocytosis with a white blood cell count of up to 80×10^6/L following SE, so called benign postictal pleocytosis. Such patients should be treated for suspected meningitis until the diagnosis is excluded by culture or other means.[3]

Fundus examination is done for papilledema (a sign of raised ICP). Computerized tomography (CT) or magnetic resonance imaging (MRI) scan be considered on an emergent basis if seizures are refractory to treatment, progressive neurological findings are present on serial examination, partial seizures, worsening focal findings on the EEG, suspicion of increased ICP, after head trauma and in cases in whom surgery is being considered. The yield of CT or MRI scan in a child with normal neurologic examination and EEG is less than 5%.[5]

Continuous EEG monitoring is required in cases of refractory status epilepticus, nonconvulsive status and pyridoxine dependency. Tests and procedures required for evaluation of SE are summarized in Table 17.2.[21]

Table 17.2: Tests and procedures for evaluation of status epilepticus(modified)[21]

To be done in all	*To be considered on clinical evaluation*
Pulse oximetry	Lumbar puncture
Cardiac monitoring	Antiepileptic drug levels
Blood glucose	Toxicology screen
Electrolytes	LFT/RFT*
Calcium	Ammonia level, arterial lactate, urine for metabolic screen
Magnesium	Creatine kinase
CBC	Blood culture
ABG	EEG
	CT/MRI

*Renal function tests

APPROACH TO MANAGEMENT

The goals of treatment include:

- Ensuring adequate brain oxygenation and cardiorespiratory function.
- Termination of seizures clinically and electrically as rapidly as possible.
- Prevention of seizure recurrences.
- Identification of precipitating factors.
- Correction of metabolic imbalance.
- Prevention of systemic complications.
- Management of underlying cause of status epilepticus and its complications.

It has been shown in experimental status in animals that the risk of permanent brain damage is directly related to the duration of the status epilepticus.[3] The algorithm for the initial management is detailed in Figure 17.1.

Prompt and appropriate pharmacological therapy can reduce mortality and morbidity. It requires a clear plan, which includes initiating ABCs of life support, prompt administration of effective drugs in adequate doses and identifying and treating the underlying cause.

Initial treatment begins with the standard measures applicable to any acute medical emergency, supporting respiration, maintaining blood pressure and gaining an IV access.

An oral airway should be inserted and airway secured. Excessive oral secretions are removed by gentle suction. Oxygen should be provided by nasal cannula or mask. Endotracheal intubation should be considered if there are signs of respiratory failure. It also prevents the pulmonary aspiration of gastric contents. Nasogastric tube is placed in position and two IV catheters are immediately inserted to allow fluid therapy and pharma–cotherapy.

If detected to be hypoglycemic or a blood glucose determination is unavailable, a rapid infusion of 5 ml/kg of 10% dextrose or 2 ml/kg of 25% dextrose is administered.

Cerebrovascular resistance falls and cerebral autoregulation is severely impaired during SE, making cerebral perfusion directly dependent on systemic blood pressure. Systolic blood pressure should be maintained at normal or high normal levels during prolonged seizures, using vasopressors if needed.[3]

All patients with SE have some degree of cerebral edema and raised ICP. Raised intracranial pressure was earlier

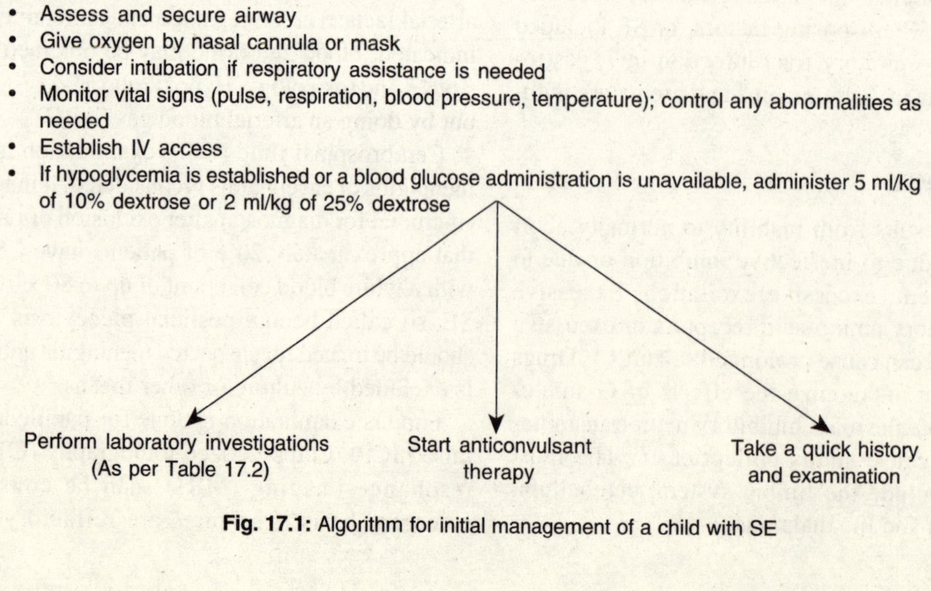

Fig. 17.1: Algorithm for initial management of a child with SE

managed by fluid restriction in an effort to avoid increasing brain water. It was later discovered that hypovolemia can rapidly lead to decreased cerebral perfusion pressure and thus global hypoxic ischemic injury. Also there is no evidence that fluid restriction reduces cerebral edema. Thus, hypovolemia must be assiduously avoided. Hypotonic intravenous fluids should be avoided because they can precipitate a fluid shift into the brain compartment and exacerbate cerebral edema. A 5% dextrose solution with half normal saline, normal saline, or Ringer's lactate is preferred. The patient should be monitored closely for the syndrome of inappropriate secretion of antidiuretic hormone (SIADH), with measurements of serum and urine osmolality. Fluid intake should be kept at maintenance levels but lowered if the syndrome of inappropriate secretion of antidiuretic hormone begins to appear. Bicarbonate should only be given if it is low enough to be of immediate concern. It can be given to half correct an acidosis when the pH is less than 7.2.

Urinary catheterization and temperature monitoring should also be instituted. Hyperthermia should be treated promptly with passive cooling. Blood is obtained for necessary investigations as described earlier. If seizures are refractory to the frontline anticonvulsants, continuous EEG monitoring is preferable.

A quick physical examination including neurological assessment should be done concurrently to detect the following: evidence of trauma, detect raised ICP (papilledema, bulging anterior fontanel or focal neurological signs), manifestation of sepsis or meningitis, retinal hemorrhages that may indicate a subdural hematoma, irregular respiration signifying brainstem dysfunction, pupillary size abnormalities suggesting toxin or drug ingestion. Further investigations can be planned after a detailed history and systemic examination.

Pharmacologic Therapy

Over half of the patients with SE will respond to therapy with a single antiepileptic drug. It is difficult to predict at presentation who will respond to the initial drug treatment. But status associated with an acute or progressive neurological disorder is more likely to be refractory. Conversely, when a patient has refractory status, the search for an acute or progressive cause should be intense. Experimental data indicate that failing to treat SE early increases the likelihood that the patient may not respond to one or even two medications.[3]

Drugs should always be administered IV. In case of difficult access, per rectal diazepam, lorazepam, valproate or paraldehyde may be used. Midazolam can be given intranasally and bucally. Sublingual lorazepam may be used. Care should be given with regard to how the anticonvulsant is administered. There is no ideal drug and a compromise between effective therapy and its inevitable side effects often has to be accepted. A recent 5-year randomized multicentric trial compared 4 options for the initial intravenous therapy. Lorazepam 0.1 mg/kg was effective as initial therapy in 65% of patients, phenobarbital 15 mg/kg in 58%, diazepam 0.15 mg/kg followed by phenytoin 18 mg/kg in 56% and phenytoin 18 mg/kg in 44%. Only the difference in efficacy between lorazepam and phenytoin was statistically significant.[22] This trial did not include a lorazepam plus phenytoin treatment combination which is a favored regimen.[23] Major drugs used are summarized in Table 17.3.

Benzodiazepines (Diazepam, lorazepam, midazolam): These drugs act as agonists at $GABA_A$ receptors and potentiate inhibition of neuronal firing. They are potent and fast acting drugs which are used as the initial therapy. Benzodiazepines, however, should be administered to patients with active seizures. If seizures have already stopped, longer-acting agents such as phenytoin or phenobarbitone are preferred.[3]

Lorazepam is, increasingly being preferred as the drug of choice for initial therapy. The dose is 0.05-0.1 mg/kg IV. Mean time for seizure cessation is 3 minutes. Duration of antiseizure effect is 12-24 hours. Its has recurrence rates probably similar to phenobarbitone or phenytoin when used

Table 17.3 : Doses, infusion rates and side effects of various drugs used in SE

Drugs	*Dose*	*Rate of administration*	*Time to stop status (min)*	*Maximum single dose*	*Duration of action*	*Side effects*
Diazepam	0.1-0.3 mg/kg IV	5 mg/min	1-3	10 mg	15-30 min	Respiratory depression, sedation, hypotension
Lorazepam	0.05-0.1 mg/kg IV	2 mg/min	6-10	4 mg	12-24 hour	Respiratory depression, sedation, hypotension
Phenytoin (fosphenytoin)	20 mg/kg IV (20 mg/kg PE IV)	1 mg/kg/min max. 50 mg/min (3 mg/kg/min) max. 150 mg/min	10-30 min	1500 mg/day (1500 mg PE/day)	24 hour	Cardiovascular collapse, hypotension, cardiac arrhythmia (less risk for hypotension, phlebitis)
Phenobarbital	20 mg/kg IV	2 mg/kg/min	20-30 min max. 100 mg/min	1000 mg/day	> 48 hours	Respiratory depression, hypotension especially if used after benzodiazepines

as initial therapy.[22] If seizures are controlled with lorazepam, it becomes less imperative to use additional long-acting drugs immediately, such as phenytoin or phenobarbitone.

Diazepam is a short-acting drug but as effective as lorazepam. Its short duration of action is because of rapid redistribution to body fat stores. It must, therefore, be followed within 20 minutes of administration by a long-acting drug such as phenytoin. It should be given directly into the vein (not the tubing). The dose is 0.1-0.3 mg/kg at rate not greater than 2 mg/min for a maximum of 3 doses.

Midazolam may also be used as the initial drug. The dose is 0.2 mg/kg and it is short acting. It can be administered by the intravenous, intranasal, buccal, rectal or intramuscular routes. Whether midazolam can be a suitable first-line agent in the treatment of SE is unclear. Its potent antiepileptic effect, relative safety record, and ease of administration by various routes clearly makes midazolam a potentially important and useful drug in the treatment of SE inside and outside of the hospital. Its optimal dosing, safety and clinical usefulness in various settings needs further evaluation.

Adverse effects of intravenous benzodiazepines include respiratory depression, hypotension and impaired consciousness. Repeated doses have a cumulative effect.

Phenytoin and Fosphenytoin

Phenytoin (or fosphenytoin) remains the drug of choice for second-line therapy in status epilepticus that does not respond to lorazepam. It is used for maintaining antiseizure effect after the initial therapy with benzodiazepine like diazepam. The loading dose is 20 mg/kg. As much as 30 mg/kg may be required (given in 5 mg/kg increments) to stop seizures in some patients. It is diluted in saline (dextrose is avoided) and given at rate of 1 mg/kg/min. Concurrent administration of other drugs should be avoided as there is a risk of precipitation. Therapeutic serum concentration is attained within 10 minutes. It is highly lipid soluble and reaches peak brain levels within 15 minutes after intravenous administration. Adverse effects include cardiovascular collapse with rapid IV infusion, hypotension and cardiac arrhythmias. The maintenance dose is 5-8 mg/kg/day in one or two divided doses.

Fosphenytoin is a prodrug of phenytoin. It is water soluble and causes less infusion site reactions (phlebitis and soft tissue damage). It also has less risk for hypotension The dose is in phenytoin equivalents (PE). It can be given at rate of 3 mg/kg/min. This drug is not available in India as yet.

Phenobarbital

It is used when phenytoin fails to control seizures. In a small randomized study, phenobarbital was as effective as the combination of diazepam and phenytoin.[24] It is given as a loading dose of 15-20 mg/kg over 10-30 min. The maintenance dose is 3-5 mg/kg/day in one-two divided doses. It may depress respiration and level of consciousness especially if benzodiazepines have also been given.

Valproic Acid

Intravenous valproic acid has been recently introduced in the market. In a study, it was found to be effective in controlling status epilepticus.[25] The dose is 25 mg/kg (3 mg/kg/hr). Per rectal valproate can be given at a dose of 20 mg/kg.

Paraldehyde

It is relatively safe for administration in children. The loading dose is 150-200 mg/kg IV slowly over 15-20 min. Maintenance dose is 20 mg/kg/hr in 5% concentration in a glass bottle. A 5% solution is prepared by adding 1.75 ml of paraldehyde to D5W to a total volume of 35 ml. The per rectal dose of paraldehyde is 0.3-0.5 ml/kg (max 5 ml) diluted 1:1 in vegetable oil. This dose can be repeated at 20 minute intervals if seizures persist.[3] Glass syringes should be used while administering the drug as it is not compatible with plastics.

Tiagabine

Other drugs include Tiagabine but no trials in children have been reported.[26]

General Anesthesia

It can be used as adjunct to the management of status epilepticus if conventional drug therapy fails to control seizures and when barbiturate coma is not on the card. Continuous EEG monitoring is desirable to direct effective and rational therapy.

Treatment of Refractory Status Epilepticus

The classical definition of refractory status epilepticus includes seizure that has not responded to sequential treatment of lorazepam, phenytoin and phenobarbitone or seizure continuing > 60-90 minutes in spite of adequate treatment. Intravenous infusions of midazolam, propofol or barbiturates are considered. The management options are detailed in Table 17.4. Midazolam infusions have been shown to be successful in terminating refractory status epilepticus in children with an average time to seizure control of 47 minutes and a mean infusion rate of 2.3 μg/kg/min (range 1-18 μg/kg/min).[27] When midazolam is not available diazepam infusion can also be used at doses of 0.02-0.04 mg/kg/min.[28] Intravenous valproic acid has also been used in refractory SE in a loading dose of 20-40 mg/kg diluted 1 : 1 in normal saline or 5% dextrose water administered over 1 to 5 minutes (repeated after 10-15 minutes, if necessary) followed by an infusion of 5 mg/kg/hr.[29]

Table 17.4 : Management of refractory status epilepticus[23]

- Intubate and ventilate the patient
- Place EEG monitor
- CVP lines may be inserted
- Administer either

  Midazolam 0.2 mg/kg IV stat followed by continuous infusion at dose of 0.75 to 18 μg/kg/minute or

  Propofol at dose of 1 to 2 mg/kg stat followed by 2 to 10 mg/kg/hr The infusion is maintained for 12-24 hours or

  Pentobarbital at 5-15 mg/kg as initial IV bolus and continue at 0.5-5 mg/kg/hours or

  Thiopental infusion loading at 2-8 mg/kg in increments of 2 mg/kg followed by infusion of 1-10 mg/kg
- Continue maintenance doses of phenytoin and phenobarbitone.
- Use vasopressors (dopamine) to treat hypotension

Thiopental is a rapidly acting intravenous barbiturate used in refractory SE. Peak brain levels are reached after 30 seconds but the drug rapidly redistributes to the lipid-dense tissues and the infusions are, therefore, difficult to manage. Pentobarbital, itself an anticonvulsant, is one of the major metabolites of thiopental. Thiopental causes hypotension, often necessitating lowering of the infusion rate and/or vasopressor administration. Propofol has gained popularity as an alternative. It has barbiturate-like and benzodiazepine-like effects at the $GABA_A$ receptor and has a potent anticonvulsant action at clinical doses. Its infusion may cause hypotension but this can be minimized by adequate intravascular filling and the use of modest doses of vasopressor drugs. Other drugs used in refractory SE include paraldehyde, lidocaine, clonazepam and chlormethiazole. Anaesthetic agents used include thiopental, pentobarbitone sodium, isoflurane, etomidate and propofol.

Figure 17.2 provides a simplified algorithm for pharmacotherapy of status epilepticus.

Treatment of Non-Tonic-Clonic Forms of SE

Other forms of SE have received much less attention because of their relatively rapid response to treatment and lack of proven increased morbidity and mortality with SE of long duration.

- *Typical absence SE:* IV benzodiazepine or IV valproate
- Complex partial status and atypical absence status: Oral benzodiazepine or IV valproate
- *Partial SE:* First choice: phenytoin, carbamazepine, phenobarbitone; Others: corticosteroids, gammaglobulin, surgery.
- SE in myoclonic syndromes: ACTH, valproate, ethsuximide, acetazolamide, nitrazepam, corticosteroids.

Drug Toxicities in SE

Knowledge of the potential drug toxicities occurring during the treatment of SE is essential, not least because they are almost always iatrogenic. An important distinction to make is between an AED-related toxicity and that produced by a drug which has also induced seizures. Treatment in the latter case will be helped by the withdrawal of the implicated agent(s). These include:

- *Antimicrobials:* Isoniazid, penicillins, nalidixic acid, metronidazole
- *Anesthetics, narcotics, analgesics*: Halothane, enflurane, cocaine, fentanyl, meperidine, ketamine
- Psychopharmaceuticals: Antihistaminics, antidepressants, antipsychotics, tricyclic antidepressants.

Out of Hospital Management

Status epilepticus frequently occurs outside the hospital. Rectal, intranasal, buccal and sublingual routes of drug administration may be used. Midazolam can be given intranasally (0.2 mg/kg) and bucally (0.3 mg/kg). Rectal administration of diazepam or lorazepam is safe. The doses are 0.5-1mg/kg (max. 10 mg) and 0.1-0.4 mg/kg respectively.[31] Sublingual lorazepam at dose of 0.05-0.1 mg/kg may be used. The tablet is placed under the patient's tongue.

COMPLICATIONS AND THEIR MANAGEMENT

Complications of status epilepticus include hypotension, shock and cardiac arrhythmia. Prolonged seizures may result in hypoxia, acidosis and acute tubular necrosis. Hypoglycemia may accompany uncontrolled seizures. The child may have pooling of secretions in oropharynx and emesis which can result in aspiration pneumonia. They may have respiratory failure, pulmonary hypertension and edema. Violent muscle contraction of seizures may cause head trauma, tongue bite, rhabdomyolysis, myoglobinuria and hyperkalemia. They may develop cerebral hypoxia, cerebral edema, cerebral hemorrhage and cerebral venous thrombosis. Multiple organ dysfunction syndrome (MODS) and disseminated intravascular coagulopathy may occur.

Management is symptomatic and supportive and includes ventilatory support, control of hyperthermia, optimal fluid management, use of vasopressors, treatment of arrhythmias, and management of raised intracranial pressure. Forced diuresis and urinary alkalinization should be considered in the presence of myoglobinuria, in an attempt to prevent acute tubular necrosis and renal failure. Occasionally, seizures may continue unabated, despite seemingly adequate AED therapy, until specific cerebral edema therapy is given (mannitol 0.25 g/kg stat dose). In patients in whom SE is a symptom of underlying brain insult, regular mannitol or even neurosurgery may be necessary.

0-5 min	inj. Lorazepam (0.1 mg/kg IV@2mg/min)# **or** inj Diazepam (0.3 mg/kg IV @ 5 mg/min) max. 3 doses+
↓	seizure persisting after lorazepam or even if controlled with diazepam **A (RSE)*** **B,C**
5-25 min	Phenytoin (20 mg/kg IV@ 1 mg/kg/min) OR Fosphenytoin (20 mg/kg PE IV @ 3 mg/kg/min**
↓	seizure continuing
25-35 min	Phenytoin or Fosphenytoin (additional 5-10 mg/kg) Upto a total of 30 mg/kg
↓	seizure persists **B(RSE)**
35-55 min	Phenobarbital (20 mg/kg IV)
↓	seizure uncontrolled
55-60 min	Phenobarbital (additional 5-10 mg/kg)
↓	seizure continuing **C (RSE)**
> 60 min	Midazolam infusion OR Propofol infusion OR Barbiturate coma.

Lorazepam is the preferred first line drug
+ Midazolam may be used
*Refractory status epilepticus(midazolam, propofol, barbiturate coma)
** IV valproate is emerging as a new alternative.
C The classic protocol by Epilepsy Foundation of America's Working Group on SE[3]
B Lowenstein and Alldredge suggested skipping the phenobarbitone arm in patients developing SE in intensive care units, severe metabolic compromise or seizure duration > 60-90 minutes.[23]
A In a recent Veteran Affairs status Epilepticus Cooperative Group study this was further modified, directly proceeding to RSE management if seizure duration was more than 60 minutes as little was gained by adding phenytoin or phenobarbitone.[30]

Fig 17.2: Algorithm for pharmacotherapy of status epilepticus

PROGNOSIS

The consequences of convulsive SE are related to etiology, duration, associated systemic abnormalities, age of the patient, and the type of treatment. All are important, but seizure etiology and duration are key determinants.[3] The mortality and morbidity among patients with prolonged febrile seizures and idiopathic status epilepticus are low. Status epilepticus owing to other causes has a much higher mortality rate. In a study at AIIMS, New Delhi, seizure duration > 45 minutes ($p > 0.001$) and presence of septic shock ($p < 0.001$) were associated with significantly more mortality in children with SE.[16] The overall mortality rate of status epilepticus is approximately 5%. Long-term sequelae include epilepsy in 20-40%, encephalopathy in 6-15% and focal neurological deficits in 9-11%. Aicardi and Chevrie[6] found that permanent neurologic sequelae occurred in 20% and mental retardation in 33%. Refractory seizures may occur in 26% of children with SE.[32]

LONG-TERM ANTIEPILEPTIC DRUG USE

The use of anticonvulsant therapy after status epilepticus is controversial. Long-term therapy is maintained in children with progressive neurological disorder, structural brain lesions or patients with known epilepsy.[3,33] Chronic AED therapy is not indicated in patients with SE solely due to transient metabolic disturbances or in febrile SE. However, the parents should be taught intermittent febrile seizure prophylaxis in the latter case scenario. Between these two extremes, whether treatment is necessary is debatable. When SE is the child's first seizure and no cause is found, the decision to initiate long-term AED therapy should be individualized. Risk factors indicating a higher risk may influence the decision. In our setting, it is preferable to start AED after first episode of SE due to inaccessible medical help in many situations.

CONCLUSION

The mortality and morbidity associated with generalized convulsive status epilepticus have decreased with organized approach and prompt management. Acute CNS injury still contributes significantly to the mortality rate. The use of intramuscular, rectal, intranasal or buccal routes may circumvent vascular access problems in children. Prevention of status is equally important. Promotion of domiciliary management will contribute towards decreasing the burden of status epilepticus in the community.

REFERENCES

1. DeLorenzo RJ, Pellock JM, Towne AR, Boggs JG. Epidemiology of status epilepticus. *J Clin Neurophysiol* 1995;12:316-325.
2. Hanhan UA, Fiallos MR, Orlowski JP. Status epilepticus. *Pediatr Clin North Am* 2001;48:683-694.
3. Working Group on Status Epilepticus. Treatment of convulsive status epilepticus. Recommendations of the Epilepsy Foundation of America's Working Group on Status Epilepticus. *JAMA* 1993;270:854-859.
4. Heidi LR, Frank WD. Seizures. *Neurol Clin North Am* 1998;16:257-284.
5. Gastaut H. Classification of status epilepticus. In: Delgado AV, Porter RJ, Wasterlain CG (eds) *Status Epilepticus: Mechanisms of Brain Damage and Treatment*. New York: Raven Press 1982;15-36.
6. Aicardi J, Chevrie JJ. Convulsive Status epilepticus in infants and children: A Study of 239 cases. *Epilepsia* 1970;11:187-197.
7. Phillips SA, Shanahan RJ. Etiology and mortality of status epilepticus in children. A recent update. *Arch Neurol* 1989;46:74-76.
8. Shinnar S, Maytal J, Krasnoff L, Moshe SL. Recurrent status in children. *Ann Neurol* 1992;31:598-604.
9. Moe PG, Seay AR. Neurologic and Muscular Disorders. In: Hay WW (ed) *Current Pediatric Diagnosis and Treatment*, 16th edn. New York: Lange Medical Books, 2003;717-792.
10. Hesdorffer DC, Logroscino G, Cascino G, Annegers JF, Hauser WA. Incidence of status epilepticus in Rochester, Minnesota 1965-1984. *Neurology* 1998; 50:735-741.
11. Shinnar S, Berg AT, Moshe SL, et al. The risk of seizure recurrence following a first uprovoked seizure in childhood: a prospective study. *Pediatrics* 1990; 85:1076-1085.
12. Shinnar S, Berg AT, Moshe SL, et al. The risk of seizure recurrence following a first unprovoked seizure in childhood: An extended follow-up. *Pediatrics* 1996;98:216-225.
13. Maytal J, Shinnar S. Febrile status eplepticus, *Pediatrics* 1990;86:611-616.
14. Shinnar S, Pellock JM, Moshe SL, et al. In whom does status epilepticus occur: Age related differences in children. *Epilepsia* 1997;38:907-913.
15. Fountain NV. Status epilepticus: Risk factors and complications. *Epilepsia* 2000;41(Suppl 2):23-30.
16. Gulati S, Kalra V, Sridhar MR. Status epilepticus in Indian children in a tertiary care centre: Clinical profile and immediate outcome. *Indian J Pediatr* (under publication).
17. Kothman E. The biochemical basis and pathophysiology of status epilepticus. *Neurology* 1990;40(Suppl 2):13-23.
18. Kapur J, Macdonald RL. Rapid seizure-induced reduction of benzodiazepine and Zn^{2+} sensitivity of hippocampal dentate granule cell GABA receptors. *J Neurosci* 1997;17:7532-7540.
19. Chapman MG, Smith M, Hirsch NP. Status Epilepticus. *Anaesthesia* 2001;56:648-659.
20. Towne AR, Waterhouse EJ, Boggs JG, Garnett LK, Smith JR, De Lorenzo RJ. Prevalence of nonconvulsive status epilepticus in comatose patients. *Neurology* 2000;54:340-345.
21. Tunik MG, Young GM. Status Epilepticus in Children: The Acute Management. *Pediatr Clin North Am* 1992;39:1007-1030.
22. Treiman DM, Meyers PD, Walton NY, et al. A comparison of four treatments for generalized convulsive status epilepticus. Veterans Affairs Status Epilepticus Cooperative Study Group. *N Engl J Med* 1998;339:792-798.
23. Lowenstein DH, Alldredge BK. Status epilepticus. *N Engl J Med* 1998;338:970-976.
24. Shaner DM, McCurdy SA, Herring MO, Gabor AJ. Treatment of Status epilepticus: A prospective comparison of diazepam and phenytoin versus phenobarbital and optional phenytoin. *Neurology* 1988;38:202-207.
25. Yu KT, Mills S, Thompson N, Cunanan C. Safety and efficacy of intravenous valproate in pediatric status epilepticus and acute repetitive seizures. *Epilepsia* 2003;44:724-726
26. Kalviainen R. Long term safety of Tiagabine. *Epilepsia* 2001; 42(Suppl 3):46-48.
27. Rivera R, Segnini M, Baltodano A, et al. Midazolam in the treatment of status epiletucus in children. *Crit Care Med* 1993;21:991-994.
28. Singhi S, Murthy A, Singhi P, Jayashree M. Continuous midazolam versus diazepam infusion for refractory convulsive status epilepticus. *J Child Neurol* 2002;17:106-110.
29. Uberall MA, Trollmann R, Wunsiedler U, et al. Intravenous valproate in pediatric epilepsy patients with refractory status epilepticus. *Neurology* 2000; 54:2188-2189.
30. Treiman DM. Treatment of status epilepticus if First drug fails: Veterans Affairs Status Epilepticus Cooperative Study Group. *Epilepsia* 1999;40:243.
31. Haafiz Allah, Kissoon N. Status epilepticus: current concepts. *Pediatr Emerg Care* 1999;15:119-129.
32. Maytal J, Shinnar S, Moshe SL, et al. Low morbidity and mortality of status epilepticus in children. *Pediatrics* 1989; 83:323-331.
33. Berg AJ, Shinnar S. The risk of recurrence following a first unprovoked seizure in childhood: A quantitative review. *Neurology* 1991;41:965-972.

Suraj Gupte and Mohinder Pal

18 Infantile Tremor Syndrome (ITS)

INTRODUCTION

The movement disorder, *infantile tremor syndrome (ITS)*, is characterized by coarse tremors, anemia, and regression of motor and mental milestones in subjects around one year of age.[1] Though once believed to be restricted to a few pockets in India, this clinical entity is beginning to receive attention globally following its discussion at international neurological and nutrition meets. Those not familiar with this entity often confuse it with status epilepticus. Hence, its incorporation in this textbook dealing with pediatric emergencies.

HISTORICAL BACKGROUND

Dikshit[2] is credited for first reporting of ITS in 1957 from Hyderabad. Since most of his cases were malnourished and anemic and tremors were superimposed on the clinical manifestations, he gave this condition the new designation, "nutritional dystrophy and anemia". Subsequently, Pohowalla and associates[3] from Indore claimed to have seen similar cases in 1953. This group provided a more precise and clear description of the disorder and named it "infantile meningoencephalitic syndrome".

In the subsequent decades, the condition has been widely reported from across the country as also from other countries.

EPIDEMIOLOGY

Geographical Distribution

ITS is primarily reported from India though there are reports of its occurrence (or occurrence of identical cases) in rest of the developing world (Afghanistan, Pakistan, Nepal, Sri Lanka, Somalia, Nigeria, Southern Turkey, Bangladesh, Myanamar), America and Italy. In India, cases have been reported from the length and breadth of the country. Nevertheless, Jammu and Kashmir (Jammu to be more precise), Delhi, Punjab, Chandigarh, Himachal Pradesh (Shimla to be more precise), Uttar Pradesh, Madhya Pradesh, Tamil Nadu, Andhra Pradesh, etc. are the areas from where a large chunk of cases are reported.[2-31]

Sementics employed for ITS by different workers are given in Table 18.1.

Table 18.1: Sementics employed for infantile tremor syndrome in the literature

Author(s)	*Sementic(s) Employed for ITS*
Dikshit[2]	Nutritional dystrophy and anemia
Pohwalla *et al*[3]	Infantile meningoencephalitic syndrome
Jadhav *et al*[4]	Vitamin B_{12} deficiency in Indian infants
Kaul *et al*[5]	Syndrome of tremor in infants
Schdeva *et al*[6]	Syndrome of tremor, mental regression and anemia in infants
Deshpande and Ingle[13]	Tremor syndrome
Agarwal *et al*[32]	Nutritional tremor syndrome
Srikantia and Reddy[7]	Megaloblastic anemia of infancy
Sharda and Bhandari[25]	Infantile neuro-motor-pallor-pigmentation syndrome
	Indian childhood tremor syndrome.

Incidence

Until 1970s, ITS accounted for 1 to 2 percent of the pediatric admissions in some hospitals that had started recognizing this condition.[1] In 1971-74, it formed 1.9 percent of the admissions to the pediatric inpatient department of the Snowdon Hospital.[18] During 1975-77, it accounted for 1.1% of our pediatric admissions at the Goverment Children Hospital, Jammu.[22,24] Subsequently, the incidence showed considerable decline. In a pilot study conducted in mid 1990s, we found its incidence to be 0.2 percent in hospitalized infants and children.

In late 1990s and early 2000s, we have noticed a remarkable hike in the number of cases of ITS admitted with us. One time in mid-summer of 2000, we had as many as 15 cases in our wards. The sudden spurt in cases couldn't be convincingly accounted for by a reasonable explanation.

Age

Six months to 18 months age group, with a peak at 9 to 15 months, is the classical span for occurrence of ITS. As high as 80% cases are seen in this age profile. A few cases may be upto 24 months. Though it is unusual to see cases outside this age range, we vividly recall a 3-year-old and another 5-year-old with characteristic features of ITS.

Sex

Slight predominance of males is obvious in a large majority of the studies. But, not much need be read in this observation since male children get the priority when it comes to seeking medical advice and care.

Nutritional Background

A kinship of prolonged breastfeeding (usually without introduction of semisolids and solids) as such or with top feeds and a concomitant malnutrition is nearly a rule in most of the infants with ITS even though they appear plump and chubby. The latter observation seemingly had led many earlier workers to miss the *camoflauged* malnutrition in these infants.

Socioeconomic Status

A vast majority of cases come from poor families, hailing from rural or periurban slum stock.

Birth Order

Most of the subjects are second, third or fourth born.

Seasonal Variation

Most of the ITS cases are encountered during the period February to June. During winter and rainy seasons, the incidence is minimal.

ETIOLOGY

Notwithstanding four decades of experience since its first recognition in 1957 in Hyderabad, a final word concerning the etiology of ITS remains to be said. It continues to be a theory-based disorder, the speculations ranging from nutritional deficiency to viral encephalitis and degenerative process. Yet, the massive weight of evidence strongly supports the "nutritional theory" (*vide infra*).

Nutritional Theory

Quite a few earlier documentations obliquely suggested that ITS appeared to be the result of megaloblastic anemia which responded to administration of vitamin B_{12} satisfactorily. This theory received support from the following observations:

- In the experience of protagonists of this theory, megaloblastic anemia was always present in ITS
- Vitamin B_{12} levels were found to be always reduced in ITS by them
- The administration of vitamin B_{12} to these cases caused regression of major manifestations of ITS
- The syndrome resembled cases of megaloblastic anemia with neurologic manifestations observed in Italy and America.

In the subsequent years, experience has indicated that only a proportion of infants with ITS have megaloblastic anemia. In fact, in some studies, there has not been even a single infant with ITS showing megaloblastic anemia. Our experience which is now duly supported by many other workers has convincingly established that there are certainly ITS cases who demonstrate purely iron-deficiency anemia. Furthermore, even those suffering from megaloblastic anemia may well need folic acid alone or in conjunction with vitamin B_{12} for an adequate response. Yet, ITS infants without megaloblastic anemia may not need (in fact, usually they do not) vitamin B_{12} and folic acid in therapeutic doses and still show cure with correction of iron-deficiency anemia and improvement in the overall nutritional status.

Magnesium deficiency has been pointed out as a possible etiologic factor in ITS. Some workers have found significantly reduced magnesium in CSF of infants suffering from ITS. Low levels of serum magnesium too have been reported.[32] Such neurologic manifestations as tremors and rigidity of ITS could well be related to magnesium deficiency. This deficiency, however, fails to explain occurrence of hair changes, skin pigmentation, mental dullness, etc. which are important features of ITS.

Some workers have hypothesized that such micronutrients as selenium, copper and cadmium may well be deficient in ITS subjects and, thus, have an etiologic role. However, such a deficiency state has not so far been convincingly demonstrated in ITS.

Zinc deficiency as an important etiologic factor in ITS is now catching up attention of the contemporary workers. Zinc reduction in body tissues and fluids has been found by us and others. Table 18.2 shows hair zinc levels in ITS in relation to controls kwashiorkor and marasmus found by us in a recent investigation.[33,34] The levels in ITS were significantly lower than in normal controls (Table 18.2).[33,34] In view of the fact that zinc deficiency is known to cause such manifestations as growth retardation, mental dullness, tremors, skin changes, irritability, susceptibility to infections and emotional disturbances,[35] the role of zinc deficiency in causation of ITS seems to be quite probable. Our clinical observations have demonstrated gratifying response to zinc supplements along with overall nutritional rehabilitation in ITS, resulting in reduced morbidity and mortality in the last around 15 years or so.[28-31] We strongly suggest further well-controlled clinical trials in different centers in order to

Table 18.2: Hair zinc levels in ITS, kwashiorkor, marasmus, and normal controls as per study conducted in Government Medical College, Jammu, Jammu and Kashmir, India

Category of subjects	*No of subjects*	*Hair zinc level (mcg/g)*	*Significant(p) value*	*Comments*
Normal controls	50	162.53 ± 7.32		
ITS	85	125.32 ± 22.53	< 0.001	Highly significant
ITS with kwashiorkor	32	123.02 ± 17.16	< 0.001	Highly significant
Kwashiorkor	43	147.44 ± 9.45	< 0.01	Just significant
Prekwashiorkor	34	142.73 ± 10.42	< 0.01	Just significant
Marasmus	30	163.11 ± 10.56	> 0.005	Insignificant

Adopted from Gupte S, Sangra KR, Pal M, Gupta SK: Infantile tremor syndrome: Perspectives and projections. In: Gupte S (ed) *Recent Advances in Pediatrics (Special Vol 9: Neurology)*. New Delhi: Jaypee Brothers 2001

establish a cause and effect relationship between zinc deficiency and ITS.

Our recent work[36-38] shows that only infants with severe ITS reveal electroencephalographic (EEG) alterations in the form of high voltage sharp waves and spikes that are consistent with seizure activity. These EEG changes fail to revert soon after full cessation of the tremors. How long these take to disappear is yet to be studied by us through an extension of this particular study. Right now, we are of the opinion that this sort of EEG pattern is also quite indicative of nutritional factor(s) as its cause in ITS.

This raises a vital question: Why do some ITS infants show EEG changes while others do not?

In order to answer this question, it is important to understand that to produce electrophysiologic disturbances in the cortical neurons to the tune of being recorded as EEG changes, there has got to be some threshold level of stimulus or insult for these neurons. In case this threshold level is attained, the EEG records changes from the scalp surface as we observed in some of our cases of ITS (the severe ones, of course). Once the stimulus or insult restricts itself to the subthreshold level only, the EEG may not record changes as was the case with majority of our cases of ITS (pretremor state, mild to moderate severity cases). In other words, or perhaps, indirectly, one can speculate that greater the brain insult, severe the tremors during active tremor phase and, thereby, more the EEG abnormalities that are recorded. The recovery from this insult may be very gradual and even incomplete. Hence, persistence of EEG changes even after the tremors are fully controlled.

Viral Theory

According to this hypothesis, ITS may well be a sort of viral encephalitis. Acute onset of tremors, their occurrence after intravenous drip or blood transfusion in certain instances, seasonal variation and common accompaniment of respiratory infection are often cited in support of this hypothesis. However, no, viral agent has so far been isolated from these subjects. The skin changes, hair changes and anemia too are difficult to ascribe to a viral agent. Moreover, absence of any consistent CSF change and course of the disease do not favor this hypothesis.

Degenerative Theory

The presence of cortical atrophy in brain biopsies and pneumoencephalographic studies and patchy fibrosis of muscle tissue and demyelination and swelling of the myelin sheath of nerves have suggested that ITS may well be a degenerative disorder. This view has not been substantiated.

Metabolic Theory

On the basis of the work carried out in Nagpur, it was postulated that a transient defect in tyrosine metabolism may be responsible for the hair changes in ITS and through involvement of the *substantia nigra* cause tremors and parkinsonian appearance with expressionless facies. This theory too has not received much support.

CLINICAL MANIFESTATIONS

Classically speaking, a typical case of ITS is an infant who is apparently plump in spite of presence of malnutrition. The striking plump look often camoflauges the infant's signs of malnutrition. In fact, this factor contributed to erroneous observation by some workers[25] in the past that these infants are usually adequately nourished. Quite a proportion of the patients have clinically demonstrable edema over the pretibial region. In addition, they are characteristically listless, apathetic, and disinterested in the surroundings.

Scalp hair is characteristically sparse and light-colored (hypochromotrichia) as in kwashiorkor or prekwashiorkor.

Brownish dark pigmentation (reticular pigmentation) of skin is present, more so over the dorsal aspects of hands (especially over terminal phalanges close to the nailbeds), feet, knees, ankles, buttocks, axillae, lower abdomen and medial aspect of thighs. Table 18.3 gives the frequency of pigmentation observed by us and some other investigators.

Though some of the subjects have delayed developmental milestones, perhaps from early months, in a vast majority there is a regression of motor and mental milestones in the

Table 18.3: Frequency of pigmentary changes in ITS in different studies

Investigator(s)	*Distribution*	*Incidence (%)*
Gupte[28]	Dorsum of hands	100.0
	Dorsum of feet	75.5
	Thighs	60.3
	Generalized	12.5
Ramkumar and Pandove[21]	Dorsum of hands	53.6
	Dorsum of feet	50.5
	Thighs	56.8
	Generalized	7.3
Agarwal *et al*[32]	Dorsum of hands	93.0
	Dorsum of feet	90.0
	Thighs	56.0
	Generalized	10.0

recent past. The infant has a dull expressionless (masklike) face with open mouth, drooling of saliva and listlessness. He fails to recognize mother and shows poor response to bright color objects.

The onset of tremors is usually preceded or accompanied by an acute stress in the form of an acute lower respiratory tract infection (LRTI), gastroenteritis, pertussis or measles (Table 18.4).

Table 18.4: Relative frequency of dominant precipitating/ aggravating factors in ITS in author's experience

Factor	*Frequency*
URTI	20%
LRTI	50%
AGE	20%
Infectious illnesses (measles, pertussis, chickenpox)	10%

Table 18.5: Relative incidence of concomittant infections/nutritional deficiencies

Tuberculosis	20%
Intestinal parasitosis	30%
Skin infections	25%
PEM	100%
Anemia	100%
Vitamin def	75%

Tremors, as a rule, have an acute onset. Initially, these are intermittent but become continuous in a few days. These are more prominent in distal parts of the limbs, head, face and tongue. Even trunk may be involved. A tremulous cry resembling the bleating of a lamb is quite characteristic. There is a tendency for the tremors to diminish or disappear during sleep. Tremors may be generalized or may involve one or more limbs, tongue, head, face in various combinations. The frequency of tremors varies between 60 and 140/minute. The site of origin of tremors appears to be cortical neurons.

Anemia is usually moderate. It may be of any morphologic type: microcytic-hypochromic, normocytic-normochromic, macrocytic/magaloblastic or dimorphic.

Hypotonia with flabbiness of the muscles, especially involving thighs, is common. In a small proportion of cases, there may be hypertonia. In some, muscle tone remains unaffected.

In addition to the associated protein-energy malnutrition, incidence of variable *nutritional deficiencies* is high. In quite a significant proportion of cases, presence of pitting edema in pretibial *reagion* justifies the concomitant diagnosis of kwashiorkor. Interestingly, literature from other centers hardly makes mention about the concurrent occurrence of ITS and kwashiorkor (not even prekwashiorkor). This situation must not be confused with the so-called "Kahn's syndrome" which is characterized by coarse tremors, parkinsonian rigidity, bradykinesia and myoclonus. The most remarkable thing about this transient state is that it occurs 6 to several days after initiating nutritional rehabilitation in infants and children with advanced protein-energy malnutrition. The ITS, on the other hand, is a phenomenon that occurs before - rather much before- nutrition correction is instituted.

Incomplete forms of ITS, including the so-called "pretremor state" (all the cardinal features of the syndrome minus tremors), are too encountered. In our experience, left untreated, these infants are quite likely to develop tremors and, thereby, the full-blown ITS. We have made this observation time and again.[28-31]

According to contemporary thinking, it is advisable to identify ITS as a syndromal state comprising three phases, namely "pretremor", "tremor" and "posttremor" (Table18.6).[1,27]

Table 18.6: Three phases of infantile tremor syndrome (ITS)

Pretremor (Prodromal) phase
Regression of motor and mental milestones as such or on top of "delay" right from the very early weeks or months of life, anemia, pigmentation, hair changes, plumpiness despite existence of malnutrition, expressionless facies with open mouth and drooling.
Tremor (Classical) phase
Appearance of parkinsonism-like coarse rhythmic tremors on top of the clinical features of pretremor phase. To begin, tremors are seen only on crying or feeding and involve fingers, face and tongue and are intermittent. Subsequently, these often become continuous and generalized.
Post-tremor (Recovery) phase
Regression of tremors and other features of the syndrome. Mental dullness continues for several months and, in a large proportion of cases, for quite a few years.

Diagnosis

By and large, ITS is a clinical entity. A high index of suspicion and familiarity with the clinical profile of ITS constitute the cornerstone of its diagnosis. Invariably, the clinical picture is so striking that a clinician who has seen such a case earlier is able to recognize infants with ITS. No laboratory finding is, in any way, specific for this condition.

Investigations should, therefore, be limited to those directed at:

- Finding the extent and morphology of anemia through hemoglobin, peripheral blood film and bone marrow
- Finding the nutritional status
- Detecting coexisting infection/infestation through X-ray of the chest and multiple stool microscopy.

Occasionally, a lumbar puncture may become necessary to rule out a CNS infection. Else, there is absolutely no need to carry out LP as a routine in ITS (Table 18.7).

Table 18.7: Investigations required in ITS

Usually recommended
- Hemoglobin
- Peripheral film/total and differential counts
- Serum proteins
- Bone marrow
- Chest X-ray
- Tuberculin (Mantoux) test/BCG diagnostic test
- Stool examination for ova and cysts

Occasionally recommended, especially when in doubt
- EEG
- CSF
- CT scan

Electroencephalogram (EEG) may reveal changes in ITS with gross tremors. These are similar to those seen in seizure disorder and are in the form of high voltage sharp waves and spikes with a slow background activity of delta range.

Management

Anemia

The cornerstone of effective management of ITS is adequate treatment of accompanying anemia and nutritional deficiency states together with good nursing care. Zinc in therapeutic doses is very much in order. However, the earlier practice of giving high doses of vitamin B_{12} to every infant with ITS by some workers needs to be discouraged. The morphologic type of anemia should dictate the choice of hematinic(s) that are to be employed.

Some cases with severe anemia may need a blood transfusion.

Other Nutritional Deficiencies

It is usual to find direct or indirect evidence of associated nutritional deficiencies (say protein-energy, vitamin A and D, vitamin C and B-complex) which should be promptly treated for adequate response.

Tremors

Unless the tremors are mild, it is desirable to administer oral phenobarbital (3 to 5 mg/kg/day). The drug reduces the intensity of tremors and may even control these in due course. Furthermore, it protects the infant from endless exhaustion and provides much needed psychologic relief to the anxious parents. With its use, the period required for control of tremors too is likely to be reduced.

In case of poor response of tremors to phenobarbital (a situation which is quite infrequent in our experience, provided that we do not get impatient), alternative agents like chloropromazine, propranolol, carbamazepine, valproic acid, etc. (Table 18.8) may be employed.[1,30,39]

Table 18.8 : Drugs used in controlling tremors in ITS

Drug	*Dose*
Phenobarbital	3-5 mg/kg/day (O) in divided doses
Chlorpromazine	2-3 mg/kg/day (O) in divided doses
Carbamazepine	10-20 mg/kg/day (O) in divided doses
Valproate	20-30 mg/kg/day (O) in divided doses
Propranolol	0.5–1.0 mg/kg/day (O) in divided doses

Their use should, however , be considered as “second line” tremor-control therapy.

Associated Infections/Infestations

Over and above these measures, the infant must receive adequate treatment for associated infections, including URTI and LRTI, intestinal parasitosis, tuberculosis, etc. One of the vital factors contributing to poor control of tremors is inadequacy of treatment of coexisting infection(s). A noteworthy observation made by us and several other workers[27] is that response of ITS-associated pneumonia to conventional antibiotic therapy is often unsatisfactory, warranting institution of more energetic chemotherapy and other measures. These are the instances where the course of tremors may well be unduly prolonged, causing temptation to the attending physician to put the child on a stronger alternative agent for controlling the tremors.

Whereas onset of tremors is usually abrupt, their cessation is a slow process. To begin with, there is a gradual reduction in their amplitude and severity. Then, these become intermittent and finally stop. At times, these may persist in one extremity or more for a longer period than the rest of the body. Eventually, all cases become tremor-free in due course.

PROGNOSIS AND COURSE

The earlier impression that ITS is by and large a self-limiting condition does not appear to be entirely true in the light of recent experience. Though some of the cases with mild disease may show recovery with cessation of tremors without any medical intervention in 1 to 4 weeks time, severe illness usually needs correction of nutritional anemia and associated deficiencies together with phenobarbital and control of precipitating and or superimposed infection(s). The cessation of tremors is, as a rule, slow. Pigmentary changes in skin and scalp hair take longer time to clear—usually around 3 months or so. Respiratory infections are not only common but take longer time to respond to adequate treatment.

Mental dullness and sluggishness last much longer. By now, we have a follow-up of several adequately treated cases spread over several years, including *asome* who are in their 20s. Most of them continue to be relatively dull and physically retarded in relation to their peers from the same stock.

Electroencephalographic changes, encountered in advanced ITS, perhaps, take longer time to regress than the tremors. We are currently endeavoring to evaluate this aspect of ITS.[40]

No doubt, ITS *per se* is not a fatal disease. Nevertheless, fatalities as a result of a precipitating or superimposed illness such as bronchopneumonia, gastroenteritis, pertussis, measles, etc. are not infrequent.

With better understanding of its different aspects and improved care, the mortality rate has fallen over the years. This is borne out by our wide experience in relation to this movement disorder as summarized in Table 18.9.[41]

Table 18.9: Mortality in ITS observed in Government Medical College, Jammu

Representative period	*No. of Cases*	*No. of Deaths*	*Mortality (%)*
1975-78	75	11	14.6
1985-88	69	7	10.1
1995-98	60	3	5.0
1998-2001	66	3	4.2
2001-2002	74	3	4.0

REFERENCES

1. Gupte S. Miscellaneous and unclassified issues. In: Gupte S (ed) *The Short Textbook of Pediatrics* 10th (Silver Jubilee) edn. New Delhi: Jaypee Brothers 2004;713-730.
2. Dikshit AK. Nutritional dystrophy and anemia. *Indian J Child Halth* 1957;6:132-136.
3. Pohowalla JN, Koul KK, Bhandari NR, *et al.* Infantile meningoencephalitic syndrome. *Indian J Pediatr* 1960;27:49-57.
4. Jadhav M, Webb JKB, Vaishnava S. Vitamin B_{12} deficiency in Indian infants: A clinical syndrome. *Lancet* 1962;2:903-906.
5. Kaul KK, Prasan N, Choudhary RM. Some clinical observations and impressions on a syndrome of tremors in infants from India. *J Pediatr* 1963;63:1158-1166.
6. Sachdev KK, Manchanda SS, Lal H. The syndrome of tremors, mental regression and anemia in infants and young children: A study of 102 cases. *Indian Pediatr* 1965;2:239-251.
7. Srikantia SG, Reddy V. Megaloblastic anemia of infancy and vitamin B_{12}. *Br J Hematol* 1976;13:949-953.
8. Bajpai PC, Misra PK, Tandon PN. Serum vitamin B_{12} in infantile tremor syndrome. *Indian J Med Res* 1968;56:1398-1405.
9. Bajpai PC, Misra PK, Tandon PN. Further observations on infantile tremor syndrome. *Indian J Pediatr* 1968;5:297-302.
10. Bajpai PC, Misra PK, Tandon PN, *et al.* Infantile tremor syndrome. *Indian Pediatr* 1969;6:249-253.
11. Garg BK, Srivastava JR. Infantile tremor syndrome. *Indian J Pediatr* 1969;36:213-228.
12. Mathur GP, Dayal RS, Prasad R, *et al.* Tremors, mental and physical retardation, light-colored hair and anemia in malnourished children. *Indian Pediatr* 1969;6:483-487.
13. Deshpandey TV, Ingle VN. Tremor syndrome in children. *Indian Pediatr* 1969;6:550-555.
14. Misra PK, Tandon PN, Bajpai PC. Infantile tremor syndrome. *Indian Pediatr* 1971;8:62-64.
15. Mahajan CM, Walia BNS, Dutta BN. Infantile tremor syndrome: Some aspects of serum biochemistry and liver histology. *Indian Pediatr* 1971;8:831-833.
16. Chhaparwal BC, Singh SD, Mehta S, *et al.* Magnesium levels in serum and in CSF in meningoencephalitic syndrome (tremor syndrome). *Indian J Pediatr* 1971;38:331-33.
17. Kaul KK. Syndrome of tremors in Indian infants. *J Indian Med Ass* 1972;59:473-477.
18. Gupte S, Pada V, Mullick DN. Infantile tremor syndrome in Chandigarh and Simla. *Indian Pract* 1973;26:45-49.
19. Agarwal SP, Katiyar GP. Infantile tremor syndrome. *Pediatr Clin India* 1972;7:203.
20. Sharma U, Saxena S. Infantile tremor syndrome. *Indian Med Gazette* 1974;14:140.
21. Ramkumar L, Pandove SP. Infantile tremor syndrome. *Indian J Pediatr* 1975;42:215-225.
22. Manchanda SS, Gupte S. Infantile tremor syndrome. In: Gupte S (Ed): *Newer Horizons in Tropical Pediatrics,* 1st edn. New Delhi: Jaypee Brothers, 1977;297-301-307.
23. Gupta BD, Maheshwari RK, Miglani N. Infantile tremor syndrome. *Indian J Pediatr* 1978;45:221-228.
24. Gupte S, Pal M: Infantile tremor syndrome: Observations on north Indian children. *Indian Pract* 1979; 32:369-375.
25. Sharda B, Bhandari B. Infantile tremor syndrome. *Indian Pediatr* 1987;24:415-421.
26. Gupte S. Infantile tremor syndrome. *Indian Pediatr* 1987;24:1159.
27. Sharda B. Infantile tremor syndrome. In: Gupte S (ed): *Recent Advances in Pediatrics,*Vol 3. New Delhi: Jaypee Brothers, 1993;155-164.
28. Gupte S. Infantile tremor syndrome: A growing Asian problem. *5th Intern Congr Child Neurol* Tokyo, 1990.
29. Gupte S. Perspectives in infantile tremor syndrome. *30th Nat Conf, Indian Acad Pediatr* Calcutta, 1992.
30. Gupte S. Infantile tremor syndrome: Newer insights. *Conjoint Meeting, Child Neurology Society/Intern Child Neurol Ass* San Francisco, 1994.

31. Gupte S, Pal M. Infantile tremor syndrome-1995. *9th World Congress of Pediatrics* London, 1995.
32. Agarwal R, Gupta BD, Agarwal DK, *et al.* A clinical study of nutritional tremor syndrome. *SDMJ* 1989; 13:185-190.
33. Gupte S, Bhave R, Mary J. Hair zinc in infantile tremor syndrome. *Asian Med News* 1995;9:7.
34. Gupte S, Bhave R, Mary J, *et al.* Hair zinc in kwashiorkor, infantile tremor syndrome and other forms of malnutrition. *Asian Med News* 1997;11:15.
35. Gupte S. Zinc deficiency. *Am J Clin Nutr* 1976;29: 235.
36. Sangra KR, Gupte S, Pal M, Gupta SK. EEG changes in infantile tremor syndrome. *5th Intern Congs Trop Pediatr* Jaipur, 1999.
37. Gupte S, Pal M. Pediatric movement disorders (with special reference to ITS) in north India (Guest lecture). *6th Asian-Oceanian Congress of Neurology,* Singapore, 1999. Abstract No AOCN-V/39.
38. Gupte S. Infantile tremor syndrome (ITS). In: Gupte S (ed): *Recent Advances in Pediatrics (Special Vol. 6: Gastroenterology, Hepatology and Nutrition.* New Delhi: Jaypee Brothers 2000:509-517.
39. Kalra V, Marwaha RK. Propranolol in infantile tremor syndrome. *Indian J Pediatr* 1981;49:341-343.
40. Gupte S, Sangra KR, Pal M, Gupta SK. Infantile tremor syndrome: Perspectives and projections. In: Gupte S (ed) *Recent Advances in Pediatrics (Special Vol 9 : Neurology)* New Delhi: Jaypee Brothers 2001.
41. Gupte S. Guest lecture: Movement disorders with special reference to ITS. *6th International Symposium on Child Neurology*, Sydney 2003.

Neurological Emergencies

Munni Ray

19 Stroke in Children

INTRODUCTION

Pediatric stroke is probably more common than once suspected, although fewer children are affected by stroke than adults.[1,2] It has been reported in all racial and ethnic groups. Studies show that the overall average annual stroke incidence rate for children through 14 years of age is 2.52 to 3.5/100,000 per year.[3,4] It occurs more frequently in the younger child (less than two years of age), becomes less common with advancing age and shows no sex bias.[5] The incidence of stroke is presumed to have risen as a result of increased survival in disorders that might predispose to stroke and were lethal in the past, such as cardiovascular anomalies and malignancies. The causes of stroke have also changed over time. In the past, infections like Haemophilus influenza meningitis were a common cause of stroke in children. Today, congenital heart disease, sickle cell anemia, coagulation disorders, extracranial carotid dissection, and varicella infections are common causes. However, in more than a third of cases, no causes are found.[6-8]

The advent of improved neuroimaging and metabolic techniques has resulted in a better understanding of the etiology and pathophysiology of childhood stroke and has increased the possibility of therapeutic intervention in acute cases. Approximately 44 to 61% of the cases are of ischemic origin whereas the rest are hemorrhagic in nature.[4,6,9]

More than half of the survivors of stroke develop some neurologic or cognitive problem, one third have a recurrence and 5-10% of affected children die. Stroke mortality in children < 1year of age has remained the same over the last 40 years.[10]

DEFINITION

Childhood stroke is defined as a cerebrovascular event that occurs between 30 days and 18 years of age causing a focal neurological deficit lasting more than 24 hours. A similar episode lasting for a shorter period of time is considered to be a transient ischemic attack. The term "reversible ischemic neurological deficit" has been coined to cover those episodes where deficit lasts more than 24 hours but the patient eventually recovers fully.[11]

TYPES OF STROKE AND CLINICAL PRESENTATIONS

Pathophysiologically, stroke can be classified into three main groups: embolism, thrombosis and hemorrhage. In children, ischemic type is more common than hemorrhagic type. Though it is difficult to distinguish between thrombotic and embolic phenomenon, stroke is largely due to cardiovascular lesions. At times it may be the first symptom to appear. Cerebral embolism classically presents with sudden loss of function, maximal at its onset and may be followed by reperfusion of the infracted cerebral tissue leading to incomplete improvement or by a secondary intracerebral hemorrhage. This is usually associated with cardiac disease. Cerebral thrombosis is more commonly arterial than venous. It takes a longer time to develop than embolism and often shows a stuttering course. Venous thrombosis is rare and it presents with features of raised intracranial pressure with or without focal neurodeficits. Hemorrhagic infarction may be either intracerebral or subarachnoid, and as in adults has a catastrophic presentation in older children with severe headache, vomiting and progressive loss of function. In younger children and infants however large lesions may even produce minimal neurological abnormalities.

The signs and symptoms appear to be vague in children. Hence, it is often difficult to pinpoint the etiology. Irrespective of the type of stroke, the older child generally present with an acute onset hemiplegia which may be accompanied by other signs such as visual field defects, dysphasia and a movement disorder whereas an younger child presents with seizures and coma which are followed by hemiplegia. The differential diagnosis of acute focal neurologic deficit in childhood is diverse. The differential diagnosis in a child presenting with an acute hemiparesis includes tumour, traumatic extradural or subdural hematoma, central nervous system infection (focal encephalitis, abscess), and demyelinating conditions like acute disseminated encephalomyelitis, as well as Todd's paresis and migraine. A deterioration of consciousness in a child with stroke is common in case of cerebral hemorrhage, large middle cerebral territory infarct or posterior fossa strokes.

Whenever assessment of a child with stroke is made, the primary aim should be to confirm the diagnosis and its type and most importantly to identify the underlying cause. The relevant features in history and the specific points in examination are shown in Table 19.2 and Table 19.3. After examination a clue to the site of thrombosis should be obtained. The anterior circulation is the most commonly affected and the occlusion of the middle cerebral artery territory causes hemiplegia and upper limb predominance, hemianopia and dysphasia in contrast to the anterior cerebral artery occlusion, in which the lower limb is particularly affected. Occlusion of the posterior circulation generally presents as vertigo, ataxia, nystagmus and lower cranial nerve palsies as well as hemiparesis and hemianopia.

ETIOLOGY

Stroke in young people is an unexpected event. It's causes are more heterogeneous than in the older population. Moreover, its diagnosis must exclude a large number of other diseases.[12] Causes of ischemic stroke in children and adults are distinct.[13]

Stroke in children is commonly associated with a combination of multiple risk factors, both genetic and acquired. In one-third of them, stroke is idiopathic in nature.[1,14-16] Awareness of etiologic factors is essential because recurrence is significant and disabilities are frequent, endangering quality of life.[1]

The pediatric causes of stroke are shown in Table 19.1. Risk factors for cerebrovascular accidents in children include congenital heart malformations, vasculopathies, infectious diseases and collagen tissue diseases, as well as some rate inherited metabolic disorders.[4,5,11] Reported prothrombotic abnormalities include cardiolipin antibody, lupus anticoagulant, deficiencies of protein C, protein S, antithrombin, and plasminogen. New hypercoagulable states are being identified as risk factors for ischemic stroke in childhood: the presence of abnormal activated protein C resistance (or Factor V Leiden G 1691A), Factor II G 2021A variant, and thermolabile variant of methylenetetrahydrofolate reductase (MTHFR C677T), raised concentrations of lipoprotein (a).[17-19]

Cardiac disease is a common cause of stroke in children accounting for up to 50% of cases in a series. Several cardiac disorders, which are associated with stroke in children, are cyanotic congenital heart disease like Fallot's tetralogy and transposition of the major arteries, intracardiac defects, cardiac procedures and acquired heart disease. Most children are known to have cardiac disease at presentation whereas there are some who have subtle lesions that are diagnosed only after the stroke.

Hematological and metabolic disorders constitute the next most common group of causes. Seventeen percent of children with sickle cell disease can have stroke and younger ones are at a higher risk. Ischemic stroke in these young children is due to a combination of intimal thickening in the large cerebral vessels, perfusion failure and intravascular sickling leading to occlusion and infarction. In older children with sickle cell disease there is risk of developing intracerebral and subarachnoid hemorrhage and occasionally they have unrelated aneurysm or vascular malformation. Five coagulation abnormalities are associated with thrombosis in children including deficiencies in protein C, protein S, and antithrombin III and the fVL and prothrombin 20210A mutations. Antiphospholipid antibodies were associated with childhood stroke in 75% of children with cerebral ischemia.[20] Metabolic disorders which commonly lead to thromboembolic stroke are homocystinuria and mitochondrial disorders like MELAS (mitochondrial encephalomyopathy, lactic acidosis and stroke like episodes) and Leigh's disease. Fabry's disease, X linked sphingolipidosis, branched chain amino acid disorders; sulphite oxidase deficiency and carbohydrate deficient glycoprotein syndrome are rare metabolic disorders, which may also present with stroke.

Acute and chronic infections appear to be an important trigger in children and young adults; tonsillitis has long been considered a possible association and dental infection may also play a role. *Mycoplasma pneumoniae, Borrelia burgdorferi, Chlamydia pneumoniae, Helicobacter pylori* and hemolysing streptococcus are specific pathogens but a wide variety of bacteria, viruses and fungi have been implicated. Among the infectious agents, tuberculosis should be remembered as an important cause in countries where the disease is endemic. Children with postvaricella angiopathy have characteristic findings of intracranial arterial stenosis within the distal internal carotid and proximal cerebral arteries with associated subcortical infarctions.[21] Multisystem inflammatory disorders like polyarteritis nodosa, systemic lupus erythematous, Behcet's disease and Takayasu arteritis may also present with stroke in children.

Vasculopathies, which lead onto stroke, occur due to dissection of vessels and Moyamoya disease. Dissection of carotid arteries may arise due to trivial blunt or penetrating trauma to the head or neck. Vertebral artery dissection may be associated with atlantoaxial dislocations and cervical

Table 19.1: Predisposing causes for pediatric ischemic stroke

Embolism	
Cardiogenic embolism from congenital heart disease e.g. ventricular septal defect, atrial septal defect, patent ductus arteriosus, coarctation of aorta, tetralogy of Fallot Septic embolism, eg. From bacterial endocarditis Complication of arterial dissection	
Thrombosis	
Vascular dysplasia	Moyamoya disease
Struge Weber syndrome	
Vascular trauma	Neck injury / intraoral trauma Arterial dissection
Vasculitis	Related to head and neck infections, eg. tonsillitis, meningitis Related to systemic infections,e.g. Postvaricella, AIDS, coxsackie A9 virus Autoimmune disorders e.g. SLE, Polyarteritis nodosa. Takayasu arteritis Isolated angitis of the central nervous system
Vasospasm	Associated with drug abuse, e.g. Cocaine abuse
Hematological	Polycythemia, e.g. From cyanotic heart disease, from dehydration
	Sickle cell disease Thrombocytosis Presence of antiphospholipid antibodies e.g. Lupus anticoagulant, anticardiolipin antibodies Abnormal anticoagulation e.g. Protein C deficiency, protein S deficiency, antithrombin III deficiency, factor V Leiden mutation, plasminogen deficiency Hypercoaguable state, e.g. Lymphoreticular cancers, disseminated intravascular coagulation
Metabolic disorders	Homocystinuria
	Mitochondrial encephalopathy, lacticacidosis and stroke like episodes Carbohydrate- deficient glycoprotein disorder Organic academia Hyperlipidemia
Hemorrhagic	
Vasculopathy	Fibromuscular dysplasia Arteriovenous malformations Aneurysms
Coagulopathies	Congenital factor deficiencies e.g. Factor VIII, IX Acquired: hepatic disease, malabsorption causing vitamin K deficiency
Thrombocytopenia	Idiopathic thrombocytopenic purpura

Table 19.2: Points in history which are important in children with stroke

- Trauma to head or neck
- Drug ingestion
- Developmental status
- Mental retardation
- Regression
- Seizures
- Family history
- Hematology
- Metabolism
- Premature vascular disease

Table 19.3: Examination of children with stroke

Skin	Birthmarks Abnormal pigmentation Nodules Rashes Signs of trauma
Cardiovascular system	Murmurs Abnormal heart sounds Blood pressure Head and neck bruits
Fundii	Retinal pigmentation Hemorrhages Papilledema

injury. Moyamoya means something hazy like a puff of smoke drifting in the air and simply describes the angiographic appearance of the telangiectatic collateral vessels at the base of the brain.[22] It occurs either unilaterally or bilaterally and is a form of occlusive arterial disease. Most cases of Moyamoya disease are idiopathic in nature whereas others are related to neurofibromatosis, tuberous sclerosis, sickle cell disease, Down's syndrome, Williams syndrome, connective tissue disorders and cranial irradiation.

Sinovenous thrombosis can also cause stroke in children particularly in those less than one year of age. This generally involves the superior sagittal sinus with or without the lateral sinus. The risk factors leading onto this condition are head and neck infections, dehydration, perinatal complications and coagulation disorders. Many of these cases have a multifactorial etiology.[23]

Hemorrhagic stroke is less common than ischemic stroke in children and the identified risk factors include vascular malformations, malignancy and trauma. It can also result from primary coagulation disorders including hemophilia A, hemophilia B and deficiencies of factors I, V, VII, X, XI and XIII. The severity of factor deficiency rather than the factor *per se* is responsible for the likelihood of bleeding. Acquired coagulation defects may result due to liver failure, malabsorption, disseminated intravascular coagulation, leukemia, and hemolytic uremic syndrome and warfarin therapy. Abnormalities of platelet numbers or function may also predispose to stroke; thrombocytopenia is usually associated with intracranial hemorrhage and thrombocythemia with cerebral thrombois.[5]

Arteriovenous malformations are the most common cause of hemorrhagic stroke in children and result due to failure in the formation of the capillary bed between primitive arteries and veins in the brain during the first trimester of fetal life. Aneurysms and cavernous malformations may also lead to hemorrhagic stroke in children. Fibromuscular dysplasia of medium and small sized arteries although rare in children is an important cause of spontaneous intracranial hemorrhage.

INVESTIGATIONS

The investigations in a child with stroke should aim to identify the underlying risk factors. They should be minimally invasive, high yield tests with rapidly available results.

Table 19.4 gives an outline of appropriate investigations for the diagnosis of stroke in children.

TREATMENT OF ACUTE STROKE

Important differences in stroke in newborns and children compared with adults, as well as a paucity of clinical trials, create challenges in the diagnosis and the management of pediatric arterial ischemic stroke.[24] The treatment of stroke in children has been primarily directed toward stabilizing systemic factors and management of the underlying causes. The initial management of the patient should focus on stabilizing the patient along with treatment of seizures and correction of metabolic problems. The management of stroke thereafter depends upon the underlying etiology. Treatment recommendations are based on small case series or have been adapted from adult stroke studies. There are no evidence-based data on efficacy in children. The main focus of management of stroke in adults is to minimize the effect of the initial stroke by using either thrombolysis or neuroprotection. Given that no clinical trials have been completed in pediatric stroke to date, treatment is by and large empiric.

In adults, stroke in the acute stage within the first 3-6 hours of onset can be managed by tissue plasminogen activation (t-PA).[25] Use of this in children is controversial. Although children with a stroke often present to a doctor within three hours, because of the rarity of stroke, the low sensitivity of CT for diagnosing acute infarction, and the wide differential in this age group, the diagnosis is rarely made with any degree of certainty at this stage. In addition, mortality is lower and most children presenting with stroke can probably expect to lead independent lives as adults. Therefore, it is difficult to see a major role for t-PA in this age group at the present time. Nevertheless, this therapy may occasionally be justified in children known to be at risk and who suffer a stroke in hospital.[5]

Volume of infarction and outcome appear to be related to the body temperature during the first few days after the stroke in adults.[26] Initial neuroprotective strategies aim to reduce the size of the infarct. Thus, apart from preventing fever, there is no neuroprotective strategy available at the present time that could be recommended for use in children.[27]

It is vital to differentiate between hemorrhagic and ischemic stroke. In case of hemorrhagic stroke neurosurgical intervention may be required for evacuation of a hematoma or excision of an AVM or both. Where the AVM is accessible to catheterization, embolization may be required.

In children with cardiac disorders underlying embolic stroke, therapy includes use of anticoagulation, use of antiplatelet agents and surgical correction of cardiac anomaly. In children with Moya moya disease, several drugs like aspirin, anticoagulants, steroids and calcium channel blockers have been tried to optimize the existing collateral circulation.

Surgical modalities like encephalomyosynangiosis and encephaloarteriosynangiosis are the two most commonly performed procedures for creating new anastomosis in this condition. Management of fibromuscular dysplasia is still

Table 19.4: Investigations for etiology of stroke[11]

Neuroimaging of brain and vessels
- Magnetic resonance imaging (MRI) and MR angiography (MRA) to:
  - Exclude hemorrhage
  - Define extent and territory of infarct
  - Define vascular anatomy of circle of Willis and neck vessels
  - T1 weighted spin echo with fat saturation sequence to exclude dissection
- Computed tomography (CT) scan to exclude hemorrhage in MR not available acutely
- Conventional angiography in hemorrhage without caoagulopathy or MRA normal

For patients with hemorrhage
- Basic coagulation studies and platelets
- Conventional angiography if no bleeding diathesis

For those with no infarct
- Electroencephalogram (unihemispheric slowing in hemiplegic migraine)

For those with an infarct in a vascular distribution and /or cerebrovascular disease
- Precordial echocardiography
  - Consider transesophageal if normal
  - Consider transcranial Doppler ultrasound with bubble contrast

Blood tests
- Full blood count, differential white cell count, and ESR
- Iron, folate, red cell folate, and hemoglobin electrophoresis if appropriate ethnic group
- Protein S*(total and free) and Protein C*
- Antithrombin III* heparin cofactor II* plasminogen, von Willibrand factor antigen,
- Factor VIII* factor XII* and lupus anticoagulant
- Anticardiolipin antibodies*
- Factor V Leiden and activated protein C resistance
- Prothrombin 20210 gene
- Total homocysteine*
- Fasting cholesterol and triglycerides and Lp (a) lipoprotein
- Infection screen, including mycoplasma, chlamydia, helicobacter and borrelia titres
- Aspartate aminotransferase

Serum and cerebrospinal fluid to look for intrathecal production of antibodies to varicella zoster Sleep study

For those with infarction in the territory supplied by the vertebrobasilar system (in addition)
- X-ray cervical spine in flexion and extension

For those with infarction not in a typical vascular distribution
- Cerebrospinal fluid lactate
- Plasma ammonia and aminoacids
- Urine organic acids

* If performed acutely, must be repeated after 3 months

controversial. Surgical techniques like balloon dilatation; endarterectomy and bypass procedures have been used along with antiplatelet antiaggregates and anticoagulants. Corticosteroids with or without other immunosuppresives are used to manage strokes due to inflammatory vasculitidis. In metabolic disorders, antiplatelet drugs may be beneficial. Coenzyme q10, idebenome and dichlorobenzene may be used to treat mitochondrial diseases.

Treatment of children with coagulopathies presenting with thrombosis includes prompt anticoagulant treatment and subsequent long-term prophylaxis. Anticoagulation with heparins (e.g. low-molecular-weight heparin or warfarin) may be indicated in children with cardioembolic stroke, arterial dissection, or persistent hypercoagulable states.[28] The use of anticoagulant therapy appears to be increasing in pediatric acute ischemic stroke. Low-dose aspirin appears to be relatively safe.

Children with sickle cell disease should be treated with exchange transfusion acutely. Prophylaxis should be done by keeping the hemoglobin S below 30% by using repeated blood transfusions, which reduce the recurrence rate for stroke to less than 10%.

Irrespective of underlying etiology and specific treatment, all children should have early intensive rehabilitation to optimize recovery. Genetic counseling including prenatal diagnosis may be required depending on the cause of the stroke.[5]

CONCLUSION

Pediatric stroke has received special attention in the recent literature. It is now recognized as an important cause of mortality and morbidity in pediatric population. Varied and poorly specific symptomatology as well as overlapping risk factors makes the diagnosis of stroke in childhood challenging. Therapy remains controversial. The use of anticoagulation and thrombolysis in the management of acute stroke in children has not been systematically studied. Use of heparin in ischemic stroke is very promising. Thrombolytic therapy is under trial. For older children antithrombotic agents are given to reduce the 20 to 30% risk of recurrence. Mortality after stroke in children ranges from 20% to 30% depending on the location and the underlying cause. Residual neurological dysfunction is present in more than 50% of survivors.

Box 19.1: Key Learning Points

- Children presenting with an acute onset focal neurological deficit with altered sensorium should be referred urgently for immediate management.
- Cerebrovascular disease presenting as stroke in children can be diagnosed by appropriate neuroimaging (magnetic resonance or conventional angiography).
- Strokes in children can be due to multifactorial etiology and diagnosis of underlying risk factors is required for both acute management as well as prevention of recurrence.

REFERENCES

1. Riela A, Rooach E. Etiology of stroke in children. *J Child Neurol* 1993;8:201-220.
2. Cheng WW, Ko CH, Chan AKH. Pediatric stroke: Case series. *Hong Kong Med J* 2002;8:216-220.
3. deVeber G, Roach ES, Riela AR, Wiznitzer M. Stroke in children: recognition, treatment and future directions. *Semin Pediatr Neurol* 2000;7:309-317.
4. Schoenberg BS, Mellinger JF, Schoenberg DG. Cerbrovascular disease in infants and children: a study of incidence clinical features and survival. *Neurology* 1978;28:763-768.
5. Nicolades P, Appleton RE. Stroke in children. *Dev Med Child Neurol* 1996;38:173-180.
6. Eeg-Olofsson O, Ringheim Y. Stroke in children. Clinical characteristics and prognosis. *Acta Paediatr Scand* 1983;72: 391-395.
7. Williams LS, Garg BP, Cohen M, Fleck JD, Biller J. Subtypes of ischemic stroke in children and young adults. *Neurology* 1997;49:1541-1545.
8. Al Sulaiman A, Bademosi O, Ismail H, Magboll G. Stroke in Saudi children. *J Child Neurol* 1999;14:295-298.
9. Giroud M, Lemesle M, Gouyton JB, Nivelon JL, Milan C, Dumas R. Cerebrovascular disease in children under 16 years of age in the city of Dijon, France: A study of incidence and clinical features from 1985 to 1993. *J Clin Epidemiol* 1995;48: 1343-1348.
10. Lynch JK, Hirtz DG, DeVeber G, Nelson KB. Report of the National Institute of Neurological Disorders and Stroke Workshop on perinatal and childhood stroke. *Pediatrics* 2002;109:116-123.
11. Kirkham FJ. Stroke in childhood. *Arch Dis Child* 1999;81: 85-89.
12. Uggetti C. Stroke in young people: imaging. *Neurol Sci* 2003; 24:S15-S16.
13. Wraige E, Hajat C, Jan W, Pohl KR, Wolfe CD, Ganesan V. Ischaemic stroke subtypes in children and adults. *Dev Med Child Neurol* 2003;45:229-232.
14. Andrews P, Ryan M, Kandt R. Genetic causes of pediatric stroke. In Alberts M (ed) *Genetics of Cerbrovascular Disease*. New York: Futura Publishing Company, 1999;261-311.
15. Riikonen R, Santavuori P. Hereditary and acquired risk factors for childhood stroke. *Neuropediatrics* 1994;25:227-233.
16. Barreirinho S, Ferro A, Santos M, Costa E, Pinto- Basto J, Sousa A, et al. Inherited and acquired risk factors and their combined effects in pediatric stroke. *Pediatr Neurol* 2003;28: 134-138.
17. Ganesan V, Kelsey H, Cookson J, Osborn A, Kirham FJ. Activated protein C resistance in childhood stroke. *Lancet* 1996;347:260.
18. Zenz W, Bodo Z, Plotho J, et al. Factor V Leiden and prothrombin gene G 20210A variant in children with stroke. *Thromb Haemost* 1998;80:763-766.
19. Heller C, Becker S, Scharrer I, Kreuz W. Prothrombotic risk factors in childhood stroke and venous thrombosis. *Eur J Pediatr* 1999;158:S117-S121.
20. Angelini L, Ravelli A, Caporali R, Rumi V, Nardocci N, Martini A. High prevalence of antiphospholipid antibodies in children with idiopathic cerebral ischemia. *Pediatrics* 1994;94:500-533.
21. Askalan R, Laughlin S, Mayank S, et al. Chickenpox and stroke in childhood: A study of frequency and causation. *Stroke* 2001;32:1257-1262.
22. Suzuki J, Takaku A. Cerbrovascular 'moyamoya" disease. *Arch Neurol* 1969;20:288-289.
23. deVeber G, Andrew M. Cerebral sinovenous thrombosis in children. *N Engl J Med* 2001;345:417-423.
24. deVeber G. Arterial ischemic strokes in infants and children: an overview of current approaches. *Semin Thromb Hemost* 2003;29:567-573.
25. The National Institute of Nerurological disorders and Stroke rt-PA Stroke Study Group. Tissue plasminogen activatior for acute ishemic stroke. *N Engl J Med* 1995;333:1581-1587.
26. Reith J, Jorgensen HS, Pedersen PM, et al. Body temperature in acute stroke severity, infarct size, mortality and outcome. *Lancet* 1996;347:422-425.
27. Ginsberg MD, Busto R. Combating hyperthermia in acute stroke: A significant clinical concern (review). *Stroke* 1998;29: 529-534.
28. Nowak-Gottl U, Gunther G, Kurnik K, Strater R, Kirkham F. Arterial ischemic stroke in neonates, infants, and children: An overview of underlying conditions, imaging methods, and treatment modalities. *Semin Thromb Hemost.* 2003;29:405-414.

Kamran Afzal and Shazia Afzal

20 Meningococcemia

INTRODUCTION

Meningococcal infection remains an important health problem in children, with significant mortality and morbidity despite major advances in understanding the pathogenesis, developments in pediatric intensive care and universal availability of effective antibiotics. The disease usually occurs sporadically but it may be endemic or epidemic. Acquisition of the organism can result in asymptomatic pharyngeal colonization or invasive disease. Dissemination of meningococci into the blood stream defines meningococcemia and is a medical emergency, with potentially rapid progression, making early recognition of the disease essential. While an effective vaccine is now available to prevent serogroup C diseases, there is at present no effective vaccine against serogroup B infection. Prompt recognition and aggressive early treatment are, therefore, the only effective measures.

ETIOLOGICAL AGENT

The causative organism of meningococcemia, *Neisseria meningitidis* or meningococcus, belongs to the family neisseriaceae. It is a gram-negative, aerobic, capsulated diplococcus, forming 1-2 mm non-pigmented, non-hemolytic transparent colonies on blood or chocolate agar. They are oxidase and catalase positive and produce acid from a few carbohydrates (glucose and maltose but not sucrose or lactose). The organism produces a polysaccharide capsule, which is the basis of the serogroup typing system. Meningococci can be segregated into at least 13 serogroups: A, B, C, D, X, Y, Z, E, W-135, H, I, K and L. Serotypes A, B, C, W-135 and Y account for more than 90% of the cases of meningococcal disease.[1] Serogroup A strains are associated with epidemics in sub-Saharan Africa and other developing countries. Serogroup B, C, and Y cause most cases of sporadic and epidemic meningococcal disease in industrialized countries.[2]

As maternal antibody levels wane disease attack rate increases and peaks from 3 to 9 months of age. Second peak occurs among teenagers. In temperate climate peak incidence coincides with the winter peak of viral illnesses. In sub-Saharan meningitis belt it is common in the middle to end of the dry season. The carriage of *Neisseria meningitidis* in the nasopharynx in otherwise healthy humans is more common than invasive disease. Healthy adults carrying virulent strains of *N meningitidis* are the main reservoir of infection. Transmission occurs among humans by respiratory secretions. There are several predisposing factors for the infection (Table 20.1).[1,3]

CLINICAL PROFILE

The two most common forms of meningococcal disease are meningitis and meningococcemia. Clinically meningococcal meningitis is indistinguishable from other forms of bacterial meningitis. In meningococcemia, bacteria and its products are found primarily within the systemic circulation. Severe meningococcemia or meningococcal sepsis is a fulminant form of Gram negative sepsis typified by rapidly spreading purpuric rash (purpura fulminans), hemodynamic instability and rapid progression to shock, coma, disseminated intravascular coagulation (DIC), and often death.

The clinical course of severe meningococcemia is rapidly progressive, with the time from onset of fever to death often as short as 12 hours. The initial symptoms are nonspecific and consist of fever, vomiting, headache, abdominal pain, lethargy and myalgia. Meningismus may or may not be present. Seizures occur in 20% of the cases.[4] The characteristic petechial rash may be subtle to start with and usually begins when the patient's mental status is normal. If the disease is recognized and treated early, patients may recover without progression of the disease. Alternatively patients may progress rapidly to hemodynamic collapse, disseminated intravascular coagulation (DIC),

Table 20.1: Factors predisposing for meningococcal infections[1,3]

1. Lack of bactericidal and/or opsonizing antibodies
2. Lack of properdin or late complement components (C5 to C9).
   (Inheritance of properdin deficiency is X-linked, and leads to more severe disease involving mostly teens or young adults. complement deficiency is inherited as autosomal recessive, occurs in older age group, and is associated with recurrent although less severe meningococcal infection).
3. Polymorphism of the Fcγ-receptor II and Fcγ-receptor III on phagocytic cells
   (Associated with reduced binding of antibody-coated bacteria → severe meningococcal disease)
4. Low levels of mannan-binding lectin, a calcium-dependent opsonizing, acute phase protein
   (Associated with one-third of all meningococcal cases in England and Ireland)
5. Preceding Influenza A infection predisposes to invasive meningococcal disease.
   (Mycoplasma and rubella infections have also been associated with outbreaks)
6. Overcrowding/residence with a carrier or case of meningococcal disease.
7. Active or passive exposure to tobacco smoke.

multisystem organ dysfunction and coma followed by either full recovery, recovery with sequelae or death. Some patients are admitted in fulminant shock with ischemic extremities. These patients either die or survive with significant neurologic, orthopedic and/or emotional sequelae.[5] Waterhouse-Friderichsen syndrome (acute hemorrhagic destruction of both adrenal glands resulting adrenal crisis) is an example of DIC-induced microthrombosis, hemorrhage, and tissue injury. Although overt adrenal failure is infrequent, partial adrenal insufficiency may be seen.

Wolfe and Birbara have described four clinical presentations:[6]

1. *Bacteremia without sepsis*: These patients are admitted for an upper respiratory illness or viral exanthema, recover without antibiotic treatment but results of blood culture are reported as positive for *N. meningitidis*.
2. *Meningococcemia without meningitis*: In these cases patient is septic and the signs of leukocytosis, skin rashes, generalized malaise, weakness, headache, and hypotension develop on admission or shortly thereafter.
3. *Meningitis with or without meningococcemia*: In these patients headache, fever, and meningeal signs are present with a cloudy spinal fluid. The state of sensorium may vary from fully alert to completely depressed. The deep tendon and superficial reflexes are present.
4. *The meningoencephalitic presentation*: These patients are profoundly obtunded with meningeal signs and septic spinal fluid. The deep tendon and superficial reflexes are altered (either absent or rarely hyperactive).

Variations of these manifestations can occur and the patient can progress from one to the other, during the course of disease. Most children presenting with meningococcal infection have features of meningitis alone, 7-10% have features of septicemia alone and 40% present with a mixed picture of septicemia with meningitis.[5-8]

The signs of meningococcal disease can vary widely. Petechial lesions are a common harbinger of this infection, but they can be easily missed if examination is done cursorily or if the examination of mucous surfaces such as the palpebral conjunctiva is omitted. Petechiae or purpura were seen in upto 80% cases with meningococcal infection in one prospective study; the remainder of cases had either a maculopapular rash (13%) or no rash (7%).[9] The petechial rash are discrete 1-2 mm in diameter, seen most frequently on the trunk and lower portions of the body especially over pressure areas; they may also occur on face, arms and mucous membranes. The petechial lesions often coalesce to form larger ecchymotic lesions or hemorrhagic bullae. The petechiae correlate with degree of thrombocytopenia and early in the course of treatment, the progression of petechiae is important to follow both as an index of the effectiveness of therapy and of whether additional therapies are needed.

Sometimes a non-pruritic maculopapular rash that lasts for less than 2 days is also noted and may be confused with viral exanthems.[10] Both patients with maculopapular rash and those without rash can develop severe disease.[9]

Uncommon manifestations are endocarditis, purulent pericarditis, pneumonia, septic arthritis, endophthalmitis, mesenteric lymphadenitis, and osteomyelitis.[11] Chronic meningococcemia that lasts for 6-8 weeks occurs rarely, and is characterized by intermittent symptoms of fever, arthralgia, headache and rash similar to gonococcal infection in a non-toxic appearing child. Untreated cases may develop meningitis.

INVESTIGATIONS

Confirmation of clinical meningococcal disease is essential for management of patients, contacts, and outbreaks.

Definitive Diagnosis

It requires recovery of the organism from blood (positive in 50% cases of disseminated meningococcemia), CSF, and sometimes the synovial fluid. Blood culture are positive in 40-50% cases of meningococcal septicemia, but < 10% if antibiotics have been given.[12] Bacteria (diplococci) may also be observed in Gram stain of buffy coat layer in patients with fulminate septicemia. Sometimes culture or Gram stain of petechial or papular lesion may be positive especially in cases of meningococcemia.[13] Positive nasopharyngeal cultures are not diagnostic of disseminated disease as it may be a normal commensal at this site.

CSF

In meningococcemia, CSF is similar to that in acute bacterial meningitis–marked pleocytosis with elevated proteins, decreased level of glucose and sometimes intra- and extracellular Gram negative diplococci detected on direct microscopy. CSF culture can be positive in patients of meningococcemia even without clinical evidence of meningitis. On the other hand prior treatment may render it sterile within 2 hours of parenteral antibiotics.[14] Lumbar puncture should, however, be avoided in patients with raised intracranial pressure (ICP), cardiorespiratory insufficiency, or coagulopathy.[15]

Latex Particle Agglutination Test

It can detect meningococcal capsular polysaccharide in CSF, serum, joint fluid or urine and is important in establishing diagnosis in culture negative partially treated cases. Current latex agglutination tests however, do not detect group B meningococcus infection, a common cause of endemic disease in some countries.

Serology

Serology may be helpful if a rising *titer* is later demonstrated in the convalescent phase.

Polymerase Chain Reaction

Meningococcal DNA detection in blood and CSF is a rapid method for diagnosing meningococcal disease and may be the only positive test in upto a fifth of clinically diagnosed cases.[16] Meningococcal PCR of CSF obtained at delayed lumbar puncture has a sensitivity of 81%.[17] Thus, it may be used to supplement blood and CSF culture and rapid antigen detection test.

Supportive Laboratory Tests

- Elevated C-reactive protein and sedimentation rate
- Haemogram and platelet count: leukocytosis/leucopenia, thrombocytopenia
- Urine examination: proteinuria, hematuria
- Coagulation studies: PT, APTT are prolonged in patients with DIC.

APPROACH TO MANAGEMENT (Fig. 20.1 and Table 20.2)[18,19]

Disease Recognition

The key to improvement in disease outcome is early recognition of disease and aggressive therapy. The most common features are a non-blanching rash, meningitis, and/ or septicemia.[3] Symptoms of meningitis include headache, fever, vomiting, photophobia, lethargy and neck-stiffness. Septicemia is characterized by fever, rash, vomiting, headache, myalgia, abdominal pain, tachycardia, cool peripheries and hypotension. Differentiation of early stages of meningococcal disease from more benign conditions as viral infections is difficult. Absence of irritability, lethargy, or decreased peripheral perfusion makes the diagnosis of meningococcal disease unlikely.[20] However this may still risk missing some early cases, and hence every child with fever and petechiae should have meningococcal disease entertained as a possible diagnosis unless proved otherwise.[19] Other cause of gram negative sepsis or rashes such as bacterial endocarditis, autoimmune vasculitis and viral infections especially by Echoviruses and Coxsackie virus should be considered in the differential diagnosis.

Prehospital Management

Parenteral penicillin (Table 20.3) should be administered to all patients on the first suspicion of meningococcemia (provided they are not allergic to the drug), especially patients residing far from health care facilities or those with rapidly evolving symptoms leading to compromised circulation and extensive hemorrhagic skin lesions. They should be stabilized and then referred to a centre with facilities for pediatric intensive care. Studies in patients with meningococcemia have shown that patients receiving antibiotics prior to transfer to a tertiary care centre have a better prognosis than those transferred without receiving antibiotics[16,21]. Strang and Pugh noted 24% deaths in the 33 patients admitted without prior treatment as against no deaths in the 13 cases with history of parenteral penicillin administered before referral to the hospital. Cartwright and colleagues also observed a substantial reduction in mortality (from 12 to 5%; relative risk 0.5, 95% confidence interval 0.2 to 1.5) in children with fever and rash who had been given parenteral antibiotics before referral. Treatment with antibiotics, however, made isolation of meningococci from blood and CSF less likely but did not affect nasopharyngeal carriage.

Initial Assessment and Management in Hospital

Maintenance of Airway and Breathing

Ensure a patent airway and adequate breathing at first assessment. Early rapid sequence elective endotracheal intubation and mechanical ventilation may be required to protect the airway, reduce the risk of pulmonary edema, facilitate adequate oxygenation, and reduce the work of breathing and oxygen consumption. Indications for elective intubation to protect the airway are decreased consciousness (Glasgow coma score < 8), signs of raised intracranial

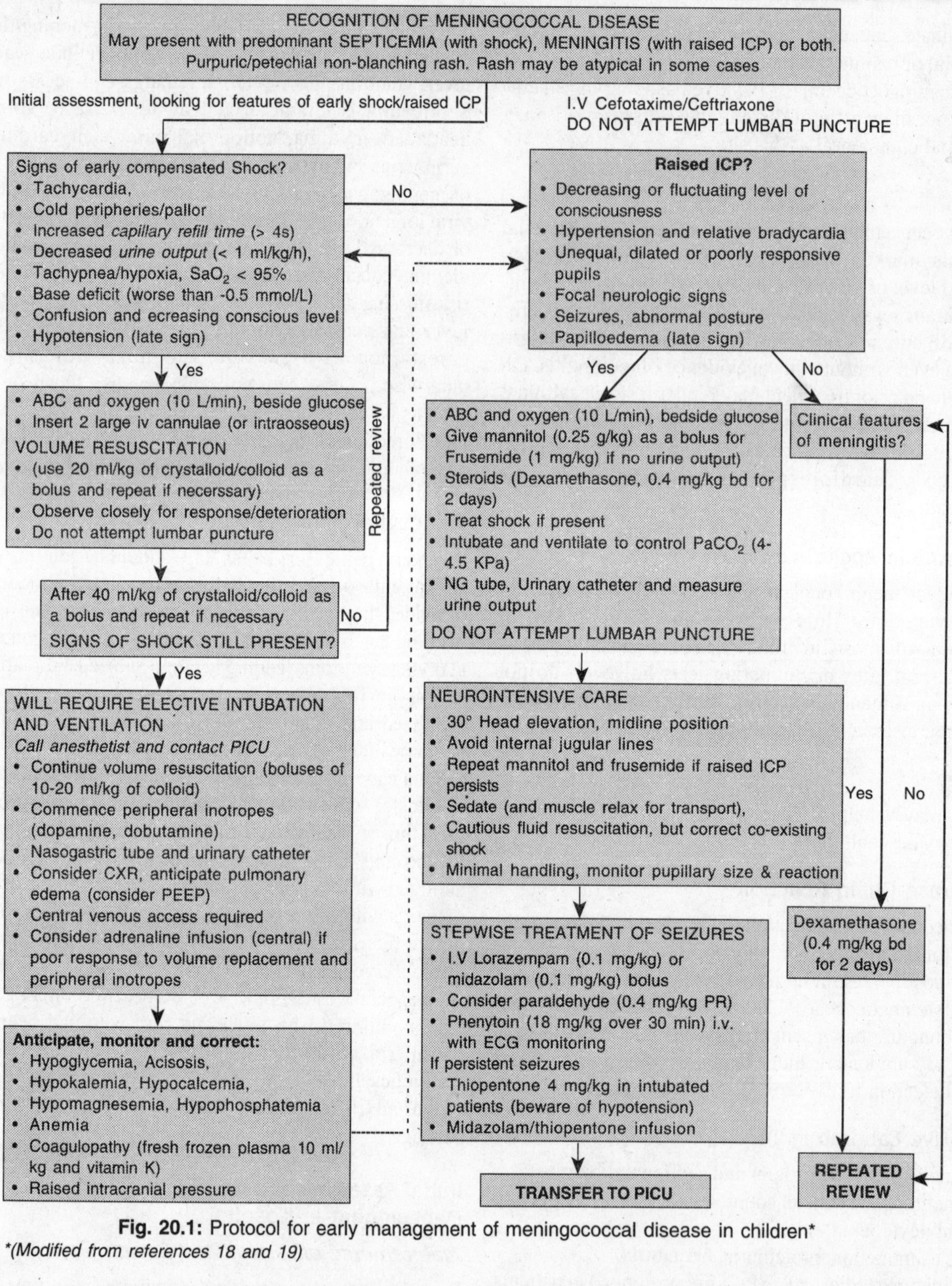

Fig. 20.1: Protocol for early management of meningococcal disease in children*

(Modified from references 18 and 19)

pressure, hypoxia and/or respiratory failure, pulmonary edema, and hypotension (decompensated shock requiring more than 40 ml/kg of volume resuscitation).

Recognition and Management of Shock

Pathogenesis of shock in meningococcemia Shock in meningococcemia is septic shock and results from loss of circulating blood volume due to increased vascular permeability, maldistribution of intravascular volume due to changes in vasomotor tone, impaired myocardial function,[21] and impaired cellular metabolism.[18] The pathogenesis of myocardial dysfunction in septic shock is multifactorial.[22] Metabolic derangements (hypoxia, acidosis, hypokalemia, hypocalcemia, hypophosphatemia,

Table 20.2: Information to complement algorithm in Figure 20.1*

Estimate of child's weight (1-10 years)

Weight (kg) = 2 x (age in years + 4)

Systolic blood pressure = **80 + (age in years x2)**

NB. Low BP is a preterminal sign in children

Conscious level		Normal values	
Alert			
Responds to voice	Age	Respiratory rate	Heart rate
Responds to pain	<1	30-40	110-160
Unresponsive	1-2	25-35	100-150
	2-5	25-30	95-140
	5-12	20-25	80-120
	≥12	15-20	60-100

Observe HR, RR, BP, Perfusion, Conscious level
Cardiac monitor and pulse oximetry. Take blood for glucose, FBC, Clotting, U&E, Ca^{2+}, Mg^{2+}, PO_4, Blood cultures, Blood gas (bicarb, base deficit), Cross-match
Colloid bolus (20 ml/kg)
4.5% Human Albumin Solution (or Fresh frozen plasma or Haemaccel) i.v. or intraosseus
Inotropes
Dopamine or Dobutamine at 10-20 mcg/kg/min. Make up 3 × weight (kg) mg in 50 ml 5% dextrose and run at 10 ml/hr = 10 mcg/kg/min; (these dilute solutions can be used via a peripheral vein)
Start adrenaline via a central line only at 0.1 mcg/kg/min. Make up 300 mcg/kg in 50 ml of normal saline at 1 ml/hour = 0.1 mcg/kg/min
Intubation (call anaesthetist)
Atropine 20 mcg/kg (max. 600 mcg) AND Thiopentone 3-5 mg/kg AND Suxamethonium 2 mg/kg (caution, high potassium)
ETT size = age/4 + 4, ETT length (oral) = age/2 + 12, Then: morphine (100 mcg/kg) and midazolam (100 mcg/kg) every 30 mins
Hypoglycemia (Glucose < 3 mmol/l)
5 ml/kg 10% dextrose bolus i.v. and then dextrose infusion at 80% of maintenance requirements over 24 hours
Correction of metabolic acidosis pH < 7.2
1 mmol/kg $NaHCO_3$ i.v. = 1 ml/kg 8.4% $NaHCO_3$ over 20 mins or 2 ml/kg 4.2% $NaHCO_3$ in neonates
If K^+ < 3.5 mmol/l
Give 0.25 mmol/kg over 30 mins with ECG monitoring; Caution if anuric
If total calcium < 2 mmol/l or ionized Ca^{2+} < 1.0
Give 0.1 ml/kg 10% $CaCl_2$ (0.7 mmol/ml) over 30 mins i.v. (max 10 ml) or 0.3 ml/kg 10% Calcium gluconate (0.22 mmol/ml) over 30 mins (max 20 ml)
If Mg^{2+} < 0.75 mmol/l
Give 0.2 ml/kg of 50% $MgSO_4$ over 30 mins i.v. (max 10 ml)
Prophylaxis for household contacts
Give Rifampicin (bd for 2 days): <1 yr: 5 mg/kg; 1-12 yrs: 10 mg/kg; >12 yrs: 600 mg
OR Ceftriaxone (single i.m dose): <12 yrs: 125 mg; >12 yrs: 250 mg
OR Ciprofloxacin as single 500 mg dose (adults only)
Diagnosis
Blood culture, throat swab, whole blood (EDTA specimen) for PCR, rapid antigen test, Aspirations/scrapings from skin showing hemorrhagic rash
Serology
For suspected cases with no isolate or where PCR does not identify serogroup, clotted blood is obtained and serum separated; (acute within 72 hrs and convalescent 10-28 days after presenting symptoms)

*(Modified from references 18 and 19)

hypomagnesemia, hypoglycemia, and disturbed fatty acid metabolism) may also have an important role. In addition, bacterial mediators, host inflammatory response (TNF-α, nitric oxide, IL-1β), and an ill-defined circulating myocardial depressant factor have been proposed as contributing to myocardial depression.[22,23,24]

Recognition of shock The shock is recognized by the development of increased heart rate and respiratory rate for age, unexplained metabolic acidosis, reduced urine output (< 1 ml/kg/h), hypoxia and often an alteration of mental status, resulting from reduced end-organ perfusion. Prolonged capillary refill time and cool skin and peripheries

Table 20.3: Doses of prehospital antibiotic to be administered in suspected cases of meningococcal infection[3]

Age	*Dose*
< 2 years	300 mg (0.5 × 10^6 IU) benzylpenicillin intramuscularly
2-7 years	600 mg (1× 10^6 IU) benzylpenicillin intramuscularly
> 7 years	1.2 g (2 × 10^6 IU) benzylpenicillin intravenously or intramuscularly

may be present. Hypotension is a late manifestation since children can compensate for upto 25-40% reduction in blood volume without developing hypotension.[25]

Treatment of shock: Treatment of shock requires stabilization of the airway and breathing, obtaining intravenous access, and replacement of circulating volume. Isotonic saline 10-20 ml/kg is given as rapid bolus (over 5 minutes). If signs of shock persist, further fluid boluses upto 60 ml/kg may be safely administered in the first hour to optimize circulating blood volume, without increased risk of cerebral or pulmonary edema.[26] However, as myocardial depression generally accompanies severe volume depletion, inotropes such as dopamine and dobutamine should be initiated in patients with persistent shock requiring more than 40 ml/kg of fluid. Improvement is objectively assessed by noting changes in heart rate, urine output, metabolic acidosis and skin perfusion. Although there is controversy about the use of human albumin solution for volume replacement treatment,[27,28] 4.5% human albumin solution remains a useful resuscitation fluid in meningococcal patients with profound capillary leak.[19]

Recognition and management of raised intracranial pressure: While patients with meningococcal septicemia present mostly in shock, those with meningococcal meningitis may develop raised ICP. Evidence of raised ICP include fluctuating or altered sensorium, normal or high blood pressure with slow or normal heart rate, unequal, dilated, or poorly reacting pupils, focal neurological signs, or abnormal posturing, seizures and papilledema. In the absence of shock, cautious diuretic therapy using mannitol and furosemide may reduce cerebral edema and improve cerebral blood flow. Anticonvulsants are used to control any seizures.

Antibiotics: Cefotaxime (200 mg/kg divided q 6-8 hr; max. 12 g/day) or ceftriaxone (100 mg/kg divided q 12-24 hr; max. 4 g/day) intravenously for 7 days is preferred as initial treatment in patients with clinical diagnosis of meningococcal disease. Aqueous Penicillin G (250,000-300,000 U/kg/24 hr, I.V. divided q 6 hourly) is an acceptable alternative but the exact status of penicillin resistance of *N. minigitidis* in India is not known, and the possibility remains until microbiologic confirmation has been received. Moreover, since purpura fulminans may rarely be caused by *Streptococcus pyogenes, Staphylococcus aureus* and Gram negative organisms, treatment may preferably be started with the 2nd generation cephalosporins till culture results are available. Those treated with cephalosporin require no further treatment. Those given only penicillin also require rifampicin to eliminate nasopharyngeal carriage (see below). Chloramphenicol may be used for penicillin allergic patients (75-100 mg/kg/d, I.V. divided q 6-8 h).

Steroids: The use of corticosteroids in meningococcal septic shock is controversial. In most fatal cases of meningococcal infection, plasma cortisol levels are normal or high. However, serial measurements and adrenal stimulation tests suggest relative deficiency. Even so, corticosteroids are not recommended routinely for meningococcemia unless a deficiency is documented.[3] The benefit of steroids in meningococcal disease has not been established. However, dexamethasone in a dose of 0.4 mg/kg twice daily for two days (or 0.15 mg/kg four times a day for four days) is given with the first dose of antibiotics in patients with meningococcal meningitis, to reduce incidence of neuronal damage.

Transfer to intensive care unit: After initial stabilization, some children require intensive care and need to be transferred to a Pediatric intensive care unit. These include children who require intubation and ventilation after administration of 40 ml/kg of fluid within an hour, or who require ongoing treatment of raised ICP. However, because of potential instability of these patients, transport should only be carried out by specialized and experienced personnel.

Ongoing Management of Complications

a. *Metabolic:* Aggressive correction of metabolic derangements like hypoglycemia, hyperglycemia, acidosis, hypokalemia, hypomagnesemia, and hypocalcemia are needed to maintain optimal organ function.
b. *Coagulation and hematology:* Anemia, thrombocytopenia, and coagulopathy are common requiring transfusion of packed cells, platelets, and fresh frozen plasma.
c. *Renal:* Acute renal failure occurs due to renal hypoperfusion, usually secondary to shock. If renal functions do not recover after adequate fluid resuscitation or in the presence of severe pulmonary edema or massive fluid requirements, renal replacement therapy in the form of peritoneal or hemodialysis/hemofiltration may be required.
d. *Gastrointestinal:* Enteral feeding (nasogastric/nasojejunal) should be tried wherever possible. Gut ischemia and gastrointestinal bleeding prevent enteral feeding; in that case parenteral nutrition may be considered.
e. *Surgical Care:* Arterial occlusion caused by intravascular clotting in the extremities may require amputation. Hypoperfused areas of skin are vulnerable to pressure damage. Compartment syndrome may threaten blood supply of underlying muscles. Fasciotomy and amputation should only be considered after extensive multidisciplinary discussion involving the orthopedic and plastic surgeons to salvage as much of the limb as possible.

Newer Treatment Options

Adjunctive treatments that may modulate the disease outcome are being developed and evaluated although none is routinely used in clinical practice. The most promising of these are endotoxin agents (e.g. bactericidal permeability increasing protein (BPI)),[29] agents which inhibit both the activation of coagulation and inflammation (e.g. activated protein C),[30, 31] and methods to improve cytokines and other inflammatory mediators (e.g. high volume hemofiltration).

PROGNOSIS

Under optimal conditions mortality should not exceed 8-10%.[10] The prognosis of patients with meningococcal meningitis is substantially better than fulminant menogococcemia (case fatality rate 3-10% *vs* 20-40% respectively).[1] Poor prognostic factors include shock, purpura fulminans, seizures, leukopenia, DIC, acidosis, increased serum levels of endotoxins and TNF-α, petechiae, hyperpyrexia and absence of meningitis.[11]

Numerous disease specific scores have been developed for meningococcal disease.[32] The most commonly used prognostic score is the Glasgow meningococcal septicemia prognostic score (Table 20.4) devised by Sinclair et al.[33] Originally 100% mortality was suggested in cases with GMSPS >8 although later studies noted survival even with higher scores.[5]

Table 20.4: Glasgow meningococcal septicemia prognostic score[33]

Parameter	*Points*
Blood pressure < 75 mmHg systolic, age < 4 year	3
Blood pressure < 85 mmHg systolic, age = 4 year	
Skin/rectal temperature difference > 3°C	3
Modified coma scale score < 8, or deterioration of 3 or more points in 1 hour	3
Deterioration in hour before scoring	2
Absence of meningismus	2
Extending purpura or widespread ecchymoses	1
Base deficit > 8	1
Maximum score	**15**

FOLLOW-UP AND LONG-TERM COMPLICATIONS

About 5% cases have neurologic sequelae, most common being sensorineural deafness.[34] Hence, all patients should have a hearing test at the time of discharge. Another 2-5% may suffer limb or digital ischemia leading to amputation, or extensive necrosis requiring grafting. These children require long-term multidisciplinary rehabilitation.

Secondary Prophylaxis

Household contacts of an index case have a 100 to 1000 times increased relative risk for developing meningococcal infection. The index case remains infectious, requiring droplet isolation for 24 hours after initiation of intravenous cefotaxime or ceftriaxone treatment. All close contacts exposed within 7 days before the onset of illness should have eradication treatment with rifampicin (Table 20.2). Recently ciprofloxacin 500 mg or ofloxacin 400 mg, as a single dose has been used in persons 18 years of age and above. Alternatively ceftriaxone single intramuscular injection in a dose of 125 mg for children below 12 years and 250 mg for older children, adults, as well as pregnant women is equally effective.

Vaccination

Quadrivalent capsular polysaccharide vaccine (A, C, Y, W-135) is available but its efficacy is unreliable in children below 2 years of age. The dose is 0.5 ml given subcutaneously and repeated every 3 years. There is no currently available effective vaccine for the prevention of group B disease. Limited efficacy has been shown with meningococcal outer membrane vaccines in children 4 years and older.[35] Polysaccharide conjugate vaccines are more immunogenic in children and are being evaluated. Indications for vaccination include:[11]

- Anatomic or functional asplenia or complement deficiencies beyond 2 year of age,
- Traveler to countries with increased incidence of meningococcal disease,
- Sustained local outbreaks of meningococcal disease caused by one of the vaccine serogroups.

REFERENCES

1. Munford RS. Meningococcal infections. In: Braunwald E, Fauci AS, Kasper DL, Hauser SL, Longo DL, Jameson JL (eds) *Harrison's Principles of Internal Medicine*, 15th edn. London: McGraw-Hill 2001;927-931.
2. Booy R, Kroll JS. Bacterial meningitis and meningococcal infection. *Curr Opin Pediatr* 1998;10:13-18.
3. Brandtzaeg P. Meningococcal infections. In: Warell DA, Cox TM, Firth JD, Benz Jr EJ (eds) *Oxford Textbook of Medicine*, 4th edn. New York: Oxford University Press 2003;478-485.
4. Steven M, Wood M. The clinical spectrum of meningococcal disease. In: Cartwright K (ed) *Meningococcal disease*. Chichester: John Wiley and Son, 1995;177-205.
5. Kirsch EA, Barton RP, Kitchen L, Giroir RP. Pathophysiology, treatment and outcome of meningococcemia: A review and recent experience. *Pediatr Infect Dis J* 1996;15:967-978.
6. Wolfe RE, Birbara CA. Meningococcal infections at an army training center. *Am J Med* 1968;44:243-255.
7. Edwards MS, Baker CJ. Complications and sequelae of meningococcal infections in children. *J Pediatr* 1981;99:540-545.
8. Nadel S, Levin M, Habibi P. Treatment of meningococcal disease in childhood. In: Cartwright K (ed) *Meningococcal Disease*. Chichester: John Wiley and Sons, 1995;207-243.
9. Marzouk O, Thompson APJ, Sills JA, Hart CA, Harris F. Features and outcome in meningococcal disease presenting with maculopapular rash. *Arch Dis Child* 1991;66:485-487.

10. Apicella MA. Neisseria meningitidis. In: Mandell GK, Bennett JE, Dolin R (eds) *Mandell, Douglas and Bennett's Principle and Practice of Infectious Diseases,* 4th edn. New York: Churchill Livingstone 1995;1896-909.
11. Woods CR. Neisseria meningitidis (meningococcus). In: Behrman RE, Kliegman RM, Jenson HB (eds) *Nelson Textbook of Pediatrics*, 17th edn. Philadelphia: Saunders; 2004;896-899.
12. Cartwright K, Reilly S, White D, et al. Early treatment with parenteral penicillin in meningococcal disease. *Br Med J* 1992;305:143-147.
13. van Deuren M, van Dijke BJ, Koopman RJJ, et al. Rapid diagnosis of acute meningococcal infections by needle aspiration or biopsy of skin lesions. *Br Med J* 1993;306:1229-1232.
14. Kanegaye JT, Soliemanzadeh P, Bradley JS. Lumbar puncture in pediatric bacterial meningitis: defining the time interval for recovery of cerebrospinal fluid pathogens after parenteral antibiotic pretreatment. *Pediatrics* 2001;108:1169-1174.
15. Berkowitz ID, Berkowitz FE, Newton C, Willoughby R, Ackerman AD. Meningitis, Infectious encephalopathy and other central nervous system infections. In: Rogers MC (ed) *Textbook of pediatric Intensive Care.* Baltimore: William and Wilkins 1996;1039-1090.
16. Cartwright K, Reilly S, White D, Stuart J. Early treatment with parenteral penicillin in meningococcal disease. *Br Med J* 1992;305:143-147.
17. Borrow R, Claus H, Guiver M, et al. Non-culture diagnosis and serogroup determination of meningococcal B and C infection by a sialyltransferase (siaD) PCR ELISA. *Epidemiol Infect* 1997; 118:117-117.
18. Pollard AJ, Britto J, Nadel S, DeMunter C, Habibi P, Levin M. Emergency management of meningococcal disease. *Arch Dis Child* 1999;80:290-296
19. Welsch SB, Nadel S. Treatment of meningococcal infection. *Arch Dis Child* 2003;88:608-614.
20. Brogan PA, Raffles A. The management of fever and petechiae: making sense of rash decisions. *Arch Dis Child* 2000;83: 506-507.
21. Strang JR, Pugh EJ. Meningococcal infections: reducing the case fatality rate by giving penicillin before admission to hospital. *Br Med J* 1992;305:141-143.
22. Parillo JE. Pathogenetic mechanisms of septic shock. *N Engl J Med* 1993;328:1471-147.
23. Mercier JC, Beaufils F, Hartmann JF, Azema D. Hemodyanamic patterns of meningococcal shock in children. *Crit Care Med* 1988;16:27-33.
24. Pathan N, Faust SN, Levin M. Pathophysiology of meningococcal meningitis and septicemia. *Arch Dis Child* 2003;88: 601-607.
25. Tobin JR, Wetzel RC. Shock and multi-organ failure. In: Rogers MC, ed. *Textbook of Pediatric Intensive Care.* Baltimore: William and Wilkins 1996;555-605.
26. Carcillo JA, Fields AI, Task force committee members. Clinical practice parameters for hemodynamic of pediatric and neonatal patients in septic shock. *Crit Care Med* 2002;30:1365-1378.
27. Cochrane injuries group albumin reviewers. Human albumin administration in critically ill patients: systematic review of randomized controlled trials. *Br Med J* 1998;317:235-240.
28. Nadel S, De Munter C, Britto J Levin H, Habibi P. Albumin: saint or sinner. *Arch Dis Child* 1998;79: 384-385.
29. Levin M, Quint Pa, Goldstein B, et al. Recombinant bactericidal/permeability-increasing protein (rBPI21) as adjunctive treatment for children with severe meningococcal sepsis: a randomized trial. rBPI21 Meningococcal Sepsis Group. *Lancet* 2000;356: 961-967.
30. Bernard GR, Vincent JL, Laterre PF, et al. Efficacy and safety of recombinant human activated protein C for severe sepsis. *N Eng J Med* 2001;344:699-709.
31. Siegel JP. Assessing the use of activated protein C in the treatment of severe sepsis. *N Eng J Med* 2002;374: 1030-1034.
32. Thorburn K, Baines P, Thompson A, Hart CA. Mortality in severe meningococcal disease. *Arch Dis Child* 2001;85:382-385.
33. Sinclair JF, Skeoch CH, Hallworth D. Prognosis of meningococcal septicemia. *Lancet* 1987;2:38.
34. Fellick JM, Sills JA, Marzouk O, et al. Neurodevelopmental outcome in meningococcal disease: a case-control study. *Arch Dis Child* 2001;85:6-11.
35. Pollard AJ, Moxon ER. The meningococcus tamed? *Arch Dis Child* 2002;87:13-17.

Kamran Afzal and Shazia Afzal

21 Meningoencephalitis

INTRODUCTION

Viral infections of the developing and mature nervous system contribute substantially to neurologic morbidity. Aseptic meningitis is a misnomer frequently used to refer to a benign, self-limiting, viral infection that causes inflammation of the leptomeninges, resulting predominantly in signs of meningeal irritation- neck stiffness, photophobia, vomiting and irritability. Encephalitis results from infection of brain parenchyma with changes of mental state and deterioration of consciousness occurring early in the evolution of the syndrome, to be followed by seizures and focal signs in a substantial proportion of cases.[1] Some viruses produce true encephalitis e.g. rabies virus. Most cases of viral encephalitis, however, have concomitant meningeal inflammation; hence the compound term meningo-encephalitis is often used.

Although infections with certain neuropathic viruses, such as mumps, measles, and rubella viruses have become less frequent because of vaccination in the western world, these and other viral species remain potential threats to the well being of children throughout most regions of the world. Nevertheless, encephalitis is an unusual consequence of common viral infections, occurring in only a minority of patients with systemic viral infections.

ETIOLOGY

Approximately 100 different viruses from 13 different families have been associated directly or indirectly with disorders of the central or peripheral nervous system.[2] The important ones are listed in Table 21.1 Several viruses are responsible for both aseptic meningitis and encephalitis (Table 21.2). Non-polio enteroviruses account for more than 80% of all cases of aseptic viral meningoencephalitis.[3] Arboviruses like Japanese encephalitis virus and Equine encephalitis viruses are transmitted by arthropods (most commonly by mosquitoes and ticks), which spread the disease to humans and other animals as horses, cattle, birds, etc. Several members of herpes family of viruses are also implicated in the causation of viral encephalitis. These include HSV-1 which produces encephalitis with focal signs in children and adults, HSV-2 meningoencephalitis in neonates who contract it from their mothers during delivery and Varicella-zoster virus which produces acute encephalitis or cerebellar ataxia. Mumps meningoencephalitis is mild but deafness can occur due to 8th nerve damage. Cytomegalovirus (CMV) usually affects immunocompromised patients. Other organisms include rubella, measles, rabies and Epstein-Barr virus (EBV) and Human immunodeficiency virus (HIV).

Table 21.1: Viruses associated with human neurologic disease

DNA viruses	
Family	*Examples*
Herpesviridae	Herpes simplex virus, cytomegalovirus, varicella zoster virus, Epstein-Barr virus, Human herpesviruses 6 and 7
Adenoviridae	Adenovirus 7
RNA viruses	
Family	*Examples*
Picornaviridae§	Poliovirus types 1-3, coxsackie A and B viruses, Echoviruses, enteroviruses 70 & 71
Togaviridae	Eastern and Western equine encephalitis viruses*, rubella virus
Flaviviridae*	Japanese and St. Louis encephalitis viruses, West Nile fever virus
Bunyaviridae*	California encephalitis virus
Reoviridae*	Colorado tick fever virus
Paramyxoviridae	Mumps and measles viruses
Orthomyxoviridae	Influenza A and B viruses
Rhabdoviridae	Rabies virus
Arenaviridae	Lymphocytic choriomeningitic virus
Retroviridae	Human immunodeficiency virus, HTLV-1

* Arboviruses; § Enteroviruses

EPIDEMIOLOGY

Worldwide statistics suggests that encephalitis develops in several thousand persons annually and many thousands

Table 21.2: Viruses associated with meningitis and encephalitis

Encephalitis	*Meningitis*
Herpes simplex virus type 1 and 2	Non-polio enteroviruses
Eastern and Western equine encephalitis viruses	Herpes simplex viruses 1 and 2
St. Louis encephalitis virus	Mumps virus
Japanese encephalitis virus	Adenoviruses
LaCrosse encephalitis virus	Polioviruses
Rabies virus	Lymphocytic choriomeningitis virus
Human immunodeficiency virus	Epstein-Barr virus
Tick-borne encephalitis viruses	Human immunodeficiency virus
Varicella zoster virus	St. Louis encephalitis virus
Enterovirus 71	Tick-borne encephalitis viruses
Colorado tick fever virus	

more experience aseptic meningitis. The incidence of encephalitis ranges between 3-8 cases per 100,000 patients, with highest rates among children at a rate more than 16 per 100,000 patients.[4-6]

Arboviruses are the leading cause of encephalitis in the USA. Japanese B encephalitis (JE) and rabies constitute the majority of cases of encephalitis outside North America[7] including India.[8] Japanese encephalitis is a leading cause of viral encephalitis in Asia that has been controlled effectively through national vaccination programs in several countries like Japan, Korea, China and Thailand.[9,10] It is endemo-epidemic in some regions in India.[11,12] In the last decade, there has been a major upsurge of JE in Assam, Andhra Pradesh, Bihar, Goa, Karnataka, Manipur, Maharashtra, Madhya Pradesh, Tamil Nadu, Uttar Pradesh, Pondichery and West Bengal.[13] JE is the only virus so far implicated in epidemics of encephalitis in India with high mortality (20-50%) and neurologic sequelae in as many as 50% of the survivors; other viruses cause sporadic cases.[14-17] Many epidemics have occurred in India since 1955.[9,11] Rabies is endemic in India and affects an estimated 3 per 100,000 persons, annually.[8]

CLINICAL MANIFESTATIONS

The spectrum and severity of neurologic signs and symptoms depend on several factors, including neurovirulence (capacity to cause disease within the nervous system) and neurotropism (propensity to infect specific cell groups of the nervous system) of the viral pathogen, as well as the nature of the host immune responses. There is often a prodrome of several days of non-specific illness reflecting systemic viremia with fever, vomiting, diarrhea, headache, malaise, fatigue and myalgia in the older child and irritability, and lethargy in infants.

Aseptic meningitis is the most frequent CNS disorder due to viral infections characterized by intense headache, irritability photophobia and signs of meningeal irritation including neck stiffness, Kernig's sign (involuntary spasm of hamstring muscles provoked by knee extension in a supine patient) or Brudzinski's sign (flexion of knees provoked by passive flexion of the neck). In young infant classic signs of meningeal irritation are often absent or minimal. Systemic features like skin rash, lymphadenopathy, hepatosplenomegaly, or parotid gland enlargement, occasionally provide useful etiologic clues. Non-polio enteroviruses often produce erythematous skin rash or oral lesions. Cutaneous herpetic lesions are usually absent in patients developing HSV encephalitis. Hepatosplenomegaly is common in disorders due to EBV, CMV and possibly HIV. Parotid enlargement and orchitis may be associated with mumps virus infection.

Most of the clinical features of encephalitis are common to all varieties of viruses. In addition to headache, vomiting and systemic complaints common to aseptic meningitis, there may be variable progression to stupor, coma, seizures, bizarre movements, and neurodeficits. Exanthems may precede or accompany neurological involvement in cases of coxsackie, echovirus, measles, rubella and VZV infections. Seizures are seen in 15-60% of infants and children and may be generalized or partial.[18] Partial seizures and focal neurologic deficits are more commonly, but not exclusively, associated with HSV encephalitis. Hyperreflexia, ataxia, cognitive disturbances, dysphasias, hemiparesis and in severe cases signs of raised intracranial pressure [ICP] including pupillary, respiratory, and postural abnormalities may be seen.

Outcome varies considerably depending on the virulence of the pathogen, immune competence of the host, and the availability of supportive and specific antiviral therapy.

Diagnosis: is generally based on clinical presentation and supported by CSF findings. Epidemiologic factors provide important clues in identifying the etiologic agent particularly: (a) age of the patient (e.g. JE is common in <15 years of age), (b) season of the year (arboviruses and enteroviruses are common during summer and early spring; mumps during winter and spring), (c) geographic location (JE is more common in rice growing areas) and travel history, and (d) possible exposure to animal bites (rabies), rodents and ticks. Various infectious and non-infectious disorders that produce neurological signs and symptoms should be considered in the differential diagnosis (Table 21.3), and excluded by relevant investigations.

INVESTIGATIONS

CSF examination should be performed in all cases of viral meningoencephalitis unless contraindicated by the presence

Table 21.3: Differential diagnosis in viral encephalitis and meningitis

Infectious	*Bacterial*	Partially treated bacterial meningitis, CNS abscess, parameningeal infections Mycoplasma, Chlamydia spp., Spirochetes, Rickettsia, Brucella, Toxin mediated
	Fungal	Candida, Histoplasma, Candida, Blastomyces, Aspergillus, Coccidiodes
	Protozoa and parasites	Echinococcus, Plasmodium spp., Toxoplasmosis, Acanthamoeba spp., Naegleria
Post infectious	*Viral post infectious*	Measles, VZV, Influenza, parainfluenza, RSV
Non-infectious	*Fluid and electrolyte imbalance*	Hyponatremia, hypernatremia, acidosis, alkalosis, water intoxication
	Poisonings and toxins	Heavy metals (lead, mercury, arsenic), insecticides, Reye's syndrome, Drug ingestion
	Vascular insult or trauma	Cerebrovascular accident or subarachnoid hemorrhage
	Tumor	Brain tumors, CNS lymphomas, Secondaries in the brain
	Metabolic	Uremic encephalopathy, hepatic encephalopathy, diabetic ketoacidosis, hypoglycemic coma, inborn errors of metabolism

Table 21.4: Cerebrospinal fluid profiles in CNS infections[18]

	Organism			
Parameter	*Virus*	*Bacterium*	*Mycobacterium*	*Fungus*
Cell number*	N to ↑	↑ to ↑↑↑	↑ to ↑↑	N to ↑↑
Predominant cell type	Lymphocyte	Polymorphonuclear	Lymphocyte	Mixed
Protein content ‡	N to ↑	↑ to ↑↑↑	N to ↑↑	N to ↑↑
Glucose content§	N to ↓	↓ to ↓↓↓	N to ↓	N to ↓

* Cell number: N, <5 cells/mm^3; ↑, 10 to 100/mm^3; ↑↑, 100 to 1000/mm^3; ↑↑↑, >1000/mm^3
‡ Protein content: N, <50 mg/dl; ↑, 50 to 100 mg/dl; ↑↑, 100 to 500 mg/dl; ↑↑↑, >500 mg/dl
§ Glucose content: N, CSF: serum ratio of >0.6; ↓, ratio < 0.4; ↓↓↓, ratio as low as zero

of raised ICP. Neuroimaging, EEG, and tests to demonstrate virus, its antigens or antibody are not needed in all cases.

Cerebrospinal fluid examination: Typically viral CNS disorders have lymphocytic pleocytosis (25-500 cells/μL), mildly elevated protein content (usually < 200 mg/dl), and a normal or slightly depressed glucose content (Table 21.4). Early in the course of viral CNS infections the CSF has predominance of neutrophils, mimicking bacterial meningitis, but typically shifts to lymphocytic pleocytosis over next 8 to 12 hours.[3,19] Virus associated reductions in CSF glucose content are usually modest. Hypoglycorrhachia (levels ranging from 25 to 50 mg/dl) is occasionally seen with herpes simplex, lymphocytic choriomeningitis (LCM), and mumps viruses. Some viruses (e.g. HSV) produce a hemorrhagic necrosis and the CSF exhibits this with moderately elevated proteins and evidence of red blood cells. Routine CSF culture for bacteria is sterile. Organisms are not seen on CSF Gram's stain, acid-fast stained smears or India-ink preparations.

Microbiologic evaluation: Viral identification is not always possible in the developing countries due to lack of facilities. However, all attempts to identify the etiologic agent should be done in cases of significant outbreaks or epidemics for prognostic and epidemiologic reasons. The diagnostic techniques available are serology, cell culture, immunohistology, and molecular methods such as polymerase chain reaction.[18] Serology provides indirect evidence of infection as it depends on antibody response by the host. Certain infections, such as those caused by arboviruses, EBV and LCM are usually identified by serologic studies. IgM antibody capture ELISA (MAC ELISA) is available for the diagnosis of Japanese encephalitis. Cell culture provides direct evidence of infection by demonstrating virus in CSF, blood (mumps) or other body fluids as urine (CMV), faeces (enteroviruses and adenoviruses), and throat swab (enteroviruses, mumps and adenoviruses). Viruses detected by this method include: CMV, HSV, enteroviruses, HIV and rabies virus. PCR is becoming the gold standard for evaluation of infants and children with HSV encephalitis or meningitis with a sensitivity of 75 to 95% and specificity upto 100%. PCR also affords rapid diagnosis of infections with CMV, enteroviruses, VZV and HIV. Immunohistological techniques for the detection of HSV and VZV infections are also available.

Electroencephalography: (EEG) has an important role in evaluating pediatric patients with suspected viral encephalitis. Usually focal or diffuse, epileptiform discharges with background slowing is seen; occasionally patients have normal EEG. HSV encephalitis frequently produces focal EEG slow sharp wave discharges usually localized to temporal lobe. However the sensitivity and specificity of EEG for HSV and other encephalitides is only modest; hence additional diagnostic studies would be required.

Neuroimaging: Patients should undergo imaging studies as computed tomography (CT) with contrast enhancement or magnetic resonance imaging (MRI) to exclude mass lesions as tumors and brain abscess. CT/MRI shows generalized cerebral swelling; focal findings especially involving temporal lobe suggests HSV encephalitis. Sensitivity of MRI exceeds CT in HSV encephalitis.[18]

Other laboratory tests: All patients should have a complete blood count, blood urea nitrogen, serum creatinine and electrolytes, blood glucose, liver function test and serum calcium. Other tests are done as needed to reject alternative diagnosis or monitor clinical progress.

APPROACH TO MANAGEMENT

Treatment depends on disease severity, suspected agent and availability of specific anti-viral medications. Distinction between meningitis and encephalitis is of little consequence. The first step in the management hinges on establishment of correct diagnosis which relies mainly on history, physical examination and investigations to exclude differential diagnosis. Definitive viral etiology is difficult to establish in all cases especially in resource constrained countries with limited lab facilities. In outbreak situations or in sporadic cases, only a representative number of samples should be tested to clinch the diagnosis. It is neither required nor is it feasible for laboratory to confirm all the cases. Potentially treatable diseases as bacterial meningitis, tuberculous meningitis, cerebral malaria, parameningeal infections, toxin ingestion, etc that can mimic viral CNS disease should be thoroughly and promptly investigated before the illness is attributed to viral etiology. In moderate to severely ill patients and where bacterial etiology cannot be confidently excluded, broad spectrum antibiotics may also be added, until culture reports are available.

Supportive Therapy

Treatment is generally supportive with the exception of acyclovir for HSV encephalitis. This is similar to the management of any unconscious patient. Fever and headache are managed with paracetamol. Fluid and electrolytes are carefully administered while monitoring serum sodium because of the possibility of associated syndrome of inappropriate anti-diuretic harmone (SIADH). Patient is admitted to PICU.

1. *Emergency management:* Ensure airway patency, breathing adequacy if required with ventilatory support and effective circulation.
2. *Fluid and electrolyte homeostasis:* Fluid therapy should be guided by the hydration status, electrolytes and osmolality with CVP monitoring in difficult cases. In cases with suspected SIADH, fluid input may be restricted to 2/3rd of the maintenance needs aiming normovolemia. Empiric fluid restriction is not justified as it may adversely effect circulating volume and result in hemodynamic instability. It is advisable therefore to give maintenance requirements plus replacement fluids aiming normovolemia and normal blood pressure. Shock is managed with appropriate fluids, dextran or vasopressors.
3. *Seizures:* Seizures may be generalized or focal and may progress to status epilepticus. Mostly they are due to the underlying inflammatory process but serum glucose, calcium, and sodium levels should be measured to rule out a metabolic etiology. Immediate therapy for seizure control includes diazepam (0.1-0.3 mg/kg/dose) or lorazepam (0.05 mg/kg/dose) slow I.V (repeated within 10-15 minutes if needed). Phenytoin (15-20 mg/kg loading followed by 5 mg/kg/day maintenance) should be added to prevent seizure recurrence. Avoid sedating antiepileptic drugs like phenobarbitone since sedation interferes with the assessment of sensorium. In cases with refractory status epilepticus, continuous diazepam infusion (0.01 mg/kg/min, increasing every 5 minutes followed by 0.01mg/kg/min, till seizures are controlled or till maximum dose of 0.08 mg/kg/min) may be used; alternatively, midazolam infusion may be used. After a seizure free period of 12 hours, the infusion is tapered over the next 12 hours.[20] High doses of these drugs are associated with risk of hypotension and respiratory depression requiring circulatory or ventilatory support.
4. *Management of elevated intracranial pressure:* Intracranial pressure is elevated to varying degrees in most patients with encephalitis. The aims of management of intracranial hypertension are reduction of ICP (to prevent herniation), maintenance of optimal cerebral blood flow (CBF) (to prevent further hypoxic ischemic injury), and reduction in cerebral metabolic rate (to prevent demand supply mismatch).
   i. *Positioning:* Head should be maintained in midline with moderate elevation of about 30°, to promote venous drainage and optimize cerebral perfusion pressure.[21]
   ii. *Hyperventilation:* Manual short-term hyperventilation with endotracheal tube in situ (maintaining $PaCO_2$ between 30-35 mmHg) has been shown to be the most effective way to decrease ICP in patients with signs of herniation or impending herniation[22] It is based on the cerebral vasoconstrictive effects of hypocapnia which results in decreased cerebral blood volume and ICP. However the modality is

effective only if the cerebral vasculature retains its responsiveness to hypocarbia which may be compromised once cerebral autoregulation is impaired.[22] Moreover, prolonged hyperventilation (>1 hour) causing decline in $PaCO_2 < 28$ mmHg is not recommended,[23] as it has been shown to decrease global CBF[24] and brain tissue oxygen pressure[25] below the threshold for ischemia.[26]

iii. *Prevent conditions that elevate ICP*: Minimal handling, anticonvulsants to control seizures, and control of fever. Prevent and treat pain as pain increases cerebral metabolism.

iv. *Mannitol:* is the most effective osmotic agent for reducing elevated ICP in a dose of 0.25-0.5 gm/kg/ dose of a 20% solution given as i.v bolus administration every 4-6 hourly avoiding dehydration and hypovolemia. Repeated higher doses are harmful due to severe hyperosmolality (> 340 mosm/l) and rebound intracranial hypertension. After adequate control of ICP, mannitol should always be tapered over next 24 hours to prevent rebound rise in ICP.[27]

v. *Steroids:* There is no consensus on the use of dexamethasone or other steroids to reduce cerebral edema.

5. *Vitals (pulse rate, respiratory rate, and blood pressure)* should be monitored regularly and supported as required. Cardiac arrhythmias can also develop in patients with viral encephalitis secondary to electrolyte abnormalities or brainstem involvement, and should be treated in the standard manner with antiarrythmic drugs.
6. *Frequent neurologic examinations* should be done in the first 48 to 72 hours to assess clinical progress and detect the development of complications.
7. *Feeding:* Initially unconscious patients are kept nil per orally. Nasogastric or oral feeding may be started once the general condition improves.
8. *Care of eyes, bowel, bladder, skin:* to prevent exposure keratitis, constipation, and decubitus ulcers.

Specific Therapy

Specific treatment for viral CNS infections is available for only a few infections. Acyclovir in a dose of 10-20 mg/kg every 8 hourly for 10-14 days has been used to treat suspected HSV infections and is effective especially if the treatment is initiated early. It is also useful for the treatment of VZV encephalitis.[2] Ganciclovir and foscarnet are of some use in cytomegalovirus infection.[18] Treatment of AIDS and its neurological complications involves the use of combination retroviral therapy (reverse transcriptase inhibitors and protease inhibitors) along with therapy for superadded and opportunistic infections like toxoplasmosis. There is no effective treatment for rabies.

PROGNOSIS

Prognosis depends on the causative organism, disease severity and host defenses. Overall the recovery from enteroviral aseptic meningitis is good. Rabies is universally fatal. Most other encephalitis are associated with varying degrees of morbidity and mortality.

Prevention

Vaccination against measles, mumps, and rubella has decreased the incidence of infections due to these agents in several countries in the west. China, Korea, Japan, Taiwan and Thailand faced major epidemics of Japanese encephalitis in the past but controlled it primarily with vaccination.[14] Indian JE vaccine is a formalin inactivated vaccine made from the brain of suckling mice inoculated with the Nakayama JE strain, produced at the Central Research Institute (CRI), Kasauli, Himachal Pradesh. Vector control measures are also important for the arboviral and other vector-borne diseases. Post-exposure prophylaxis with immunoglobulin and vaccine is effective in preventing rabies encephalitis.

Thus despite the limitations of non-availability of confirmatory laboratory tests, a high index of suspicion on clinical grounds, systematically excluding cases with different etiologies resembling viral encephalitis and planning early antiviral therapy in selected cases will help to reduce both mortality and morbidity associated with this potentially fatal disease.

REFERENCES

1. Rotbart HA. Viral meningitis and aseptic meningitis syndrome. In: Scheld WM, Whitley RJ, Durack DT (eds) *Infections of the Central Nervous System.* New York: Raven Press 1991;19-40.
2. Anderson M. Encephalitis and other brain infections. In: Donaghy M (ed) *Brain's Diseases of the Nervous System.* 11th edn. London: Oxford University Press 2001;1117-1131.
3. Prober CG. Central nervous system infections. In: Behrman RE, Kliegman RM, Jenson HB(eds) *Nelson Textbook of Pediatrics*, 17th edn. Philadelphia: WB Saunders 2004; 2038-2047.
4. Nicolsi A, Hausser WA, Beghi E, Kurland LT. Epidemiology of central nervous system infections in Olmstead County, Minnesota, 1950-1981. *J Infect Dis* 1986;154:399.
5. Johnson RT. Acute encephalitis. *Clin Infect Dis* 1996; 23:219.
6. Koskiniemi M, Rautonen J, Lehtokoski-Lehtiniemi, Vaheri A. Epidemiology of encephalitis in children: a 20 year survey. *Ann Neurol* 1991;29:492.
7. Cassady KA, Whitley RJ. Acute and chronic encephalitis. In: Armstrong D, Cohen J (eds) *Infectious Diseases*. Philadelphia: Mosby 1999;16.1-16.8.
8. Kumar R. Viral encephalitis of public health significance in India: current status. *Indian J Pediatr*. 1999;66:73-83.
9. Rodhain F. Recent data on the epidemiology of Japanese encephalitis. *Bull Acad Natl Med* 1996;180: 1325-1340.

10. Rojanosuphot S, Tsai TF. Regional Workshop on Control Strategies for Japanese Encephalitis. *Southeast Asian J Trop Med Pub Health* 1995;26: (S3):1-59.
11. Kar NJ, Bora D, Sharma RC, Bhattacharjee J, Datta KK, Sharma RS. Epidemiological profile of Japanese encephalitis in Gorakhpur district, Uttar Pradesh, 1982-1988. *J Commun Dis* 1992;24:145-149.
12. Mall MP, Kumar A, Malik SV. Seropositivity of domestic animals against Japanese encephalitis in Bareilly area, UP. *J Commun Dis* 1995;27:242-246.
13. Park K. Japanese encephalitis. In: *Park's Textbook of Preventive and Social Medicine*. 15th edn. Jabalpur: Banarsidas Bhanot Publishers 1997;217-216.
14. Rao PN. Japanese encephalitis. *Indian Pediatr* 2001; 38: 1252-1264.
15. Kumar R, Mathur A, Kumar A, Sharma S, Chakraborty S, Chaturvedi UC. Clinical features and prognostic indicators of Japanese encephalitis in children in Lucknow (India). *Indian J Med Res* 1990;91:321-327.
16. Chaudhuri N, Shaw BP, Mondal KC, Maity CR. Epidemiology of Japanese encephalitis. *Indian Pediatr* 1992;29:861-865.
17. Reuben R, Gajanana A. Japanese encephalitis in India. *Indian J Pediatr.* 1997;64:243-251.
18. Bale JF Jr. Viral infections of the nervous system. In: Swaimann KF, Ashwal S (eds) *Pediatric Neurology: Principles and Practice*, 3rd edn. St.Loius: Mosby, 1999;1001-1024.
19. Feigin RL, Shackelford PG. Value of repeat lumbar puncture in the diagnosis of meningitis. *N Engl J Med* 1973;289:571.
20. Singhi S, Banerjee S, Singhi P. Refractory status epilepticus–Role of continuous diazepam infusion. *J Child Neurol* 1998;13:23-26.
21. Durward QJ, Amacher AL, Del MR, Sibbald WJ. Cerebral and cardiovascular responses to changes in head elevation in patients with intracranial hypertension. *J Neurosurg* 1983;59:938.
22. Berkowitz ID, Berkowitz FE, Newton C, Willoughby R, Ackerman AD. Meningitis, Infectious encephalopathies, other central nervous system infections. In: Rogers MC (ed) *Textbook of Pediatric Intensive Care*, 3rd edn. Baltimore: William & Wilkins 1996;1039-1090.
23. Fazulin BR, Amcheslavskii VG, Iskhakov OS et al. Principles of intensive care during the acute period of craniocerebral trauma in children (Russian). *Anesteziol Reanimatol* 2000;4:57-59.
24. Moller K, Hogh P, Larsen FS, et al. Regional cerebral blood flow during hyperventilation in patients with acute bacterial meningitis. *Clin Physiol* 2000;20:399-410.
25. Carmona Suazo JA, Mass AI, van den Brink WA, van Santbrink H, Styerberg EW, Avezaat CJ. CO_2 reactivity and brain oxygen pressure monitoring in severe head injury. *Crit Care Med* 2000;28:3268-3274.
26. Ashwal S, Stringer W, Tomasi L, Schneider S, Thompson J, Perkin R. Cerebral blood flow and carbon dioxide reactivity in children with bacterial meningitis. *J Pediatr* 1990;117:523-530.
27. Singhi S, Singhi P, Baranwal AK. Bacterial meningitis in children: Critical care needs. *Indian J Pediatr* 2001;68:737-747.

Munni Ray

22 Bacterial Meningitis

INTRODUCTION

Bacterial meningitis is still a major cause of death and disability in children worldwide. With the advent of conjugate vaccines against the three major pathogens, the burden of disease is increasingly concentrated in developing countries that cannot afford the vaccines whereas antibiotic resistance is an increasing problem in developed countries. In developing countries, the problems are more fundamental like poor access to hospitals and late presentation with established brain injury.[1] Case fatality rates are as high as 50% and neurological sequelae occur in one- third of survivors. Hence, review of this topic is extremely important.

CAUSATIVE ORGANISMS

A wide range of bacteria cause purulent meningitis. In the neonatal period, which includes premature and term babies up to 3 months of life, group B streptococci cause most bacterial meningitis in developed countries usually of subtype III strains and the disease usually occurs after the first week of life. In the developing countries colliform organisms are the most important agents causing meningitis in this age group. They are especially strains of *Escherichia coli* possessing K1 antigen, *Klebsiella, Enterobacter* and *Salmonella.*[2] *Listeria monocytogenes,* particularly serotype IV b, is occasionally responsible for bacterial meningitis in newborns especially during zoonotic outbreaks. [3] Viridans streptococci, enterococci and staphylococci and non-typeable *H. influenzae* strains may also cause meningitis in this age group.

In infants and small children, *Streptococcus pneumoniae*, *Neisseria meningitidis*, and *Hemophilus influenzae* type b (rare in areas with routine Hemophilus vaccination) are the most common meningeal pathogens.

Children more than 5 years are almost exclusively infected by *Streptococcus pneumoniae* and *Neisseria meningitides*.[4-6]

Meningitis may be caused by various different bacteria such as Staphylococcus species, gram-negative enteric bacilli or *Pseudominas aeroginosa* in immunocompromised hosts and inpatients undergoing neurosugical procedures.[7]

EPIDEMIOLOGY

The frequency of neonatal meningitis varies greatly between different institutions and geographical areas with rates of about two to ten cases per 10000 live births.[8] Infections in neonates are mostly acquired by vertical transmission, but nosocomial transmission is also important, especially in preterm infants with low birthweight who required long-term intensive care. Although nearly all-newborn infants are colonized by many of the organisms with which they have contact, sepsis arises in fewer than 1% of these infants. About 25% of infants with septicemia develop meningitis.[9]

H influenzae type b meningitis is mainly a disease in infancy from 3 months to 3 years. During the first few months of life, passively acquired maternal antibodies protect most infants. Meningococcal and pneumococcal meningitis are at their highest rates in the first year of life, and rarely arise in infants younger than 3 months of age. These two organisms can cause systemic infection at any age both in children and adults unlike *H.influenzae* infections.

PATHOGENESIS

Meningitis usually follows invasion of the blood stream by organisms that have colonized mucosal surfaces. In the neonates these micro-organisms are acquired primarily during birth by contact with intestinal and genital tract secretions from the mother. In neonates who have prolonged intensive care in nurseries may also be exposed to various nosocomial infections.

In infants and children encapsulated organisms, which have colonized in the nasopharynx and thereafter, disseminated into the blood, cause meningitis. The organisms penetrate viable sites of the blood brain barrier and reach the subarachnoid space.

Direct extension of infection from a paranasal sinus or from the middle ear through the mastoid to the meninges can also result in meningitis. Severe head trauma with a skull fracture, cerebrospinal fluid rhinorrhea or both, can lead to meningitis caused by *Streptococcus pneumoniae*. Direct inoculation of bacteria into the cerebrospinal fluid can occur by congenital dural defects (dermal sinus or meningomyelocele), neurosurgical procedures (such as CSF shunts), penetrating wounds, or extension from a suppurative parameningeal focus.[10]

PATHOPHYSIOLOGY

The intense inflammation within the subarachnoid space noted in lumbar CSF, and the resulting neurological damage, are not the direct result of the pathogenic bacteria but rather of activation of the host's inflammatory pathways by the microorganisms of their products. Once the organisms enter the central nervous system, they replicate rapidly and liberate active cell wall or membrane associated components: lipoteichoic acid and peptidoglycan fragments of gram-positive organisms, and lipopolysaccharide of gram-negative bacteria. Antibiotics that act on cell walls cause rapid lysis of bacteria, which can initially cause enhanced release of these active bacterial products into the CSF. These potent inflammatory substances incite a cascade of events, which primarily lead to damage of the central nervous system[11,12] (Fig. 22.1). Genetic targeting of these molecular pathways, or both might prevent the irreversible focal or diffuse brain damage frequently associated with disease.

CLINICAL MANIFESTATIONS

Bacterial meningitis can be difficult to diagnose as the symptoms and signs are often nonspecific particularly in young children. The clinical picture mainly depends on the patient's age. The classic manifestations noted in older children are rarely present in the infants. In general, the younger the patient the more subtle and atypical are the signs and symptoms.[13]

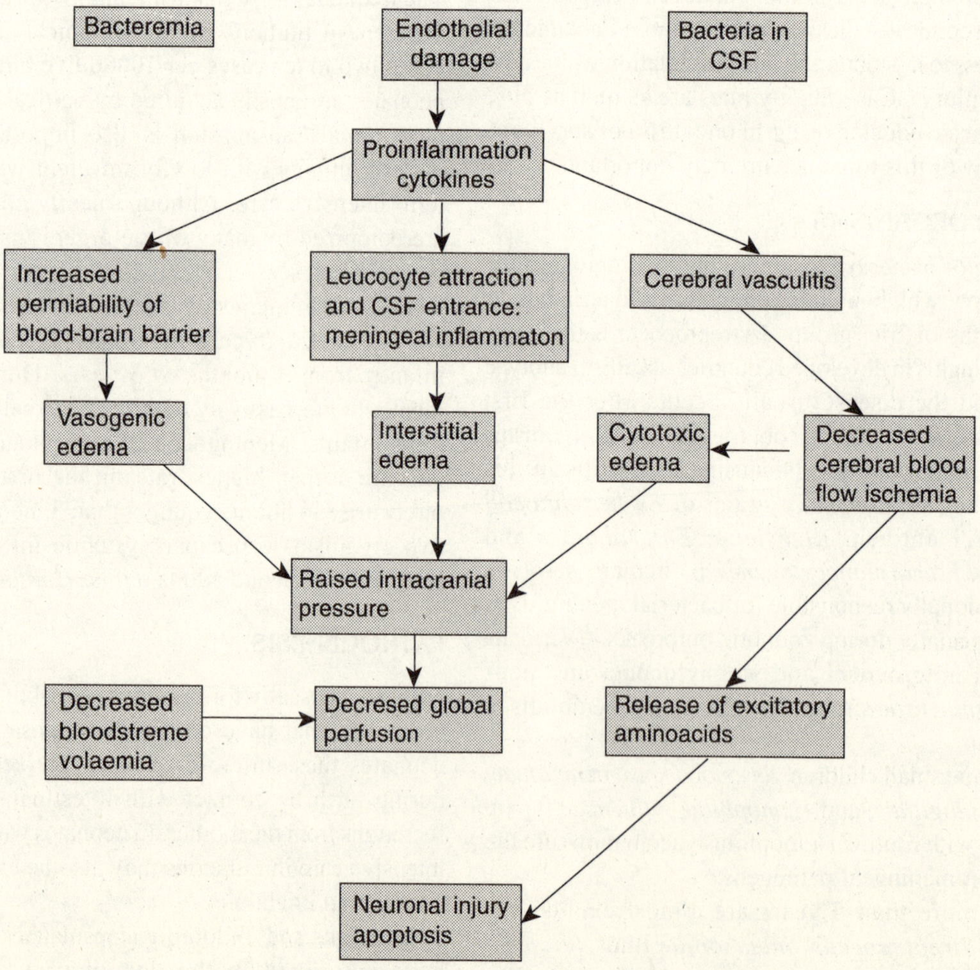

Fig. 22.1: Pahtogenesis of bacterial meningitis

The symptoms include high temperature, poor feeding, vomiting, lethargy and irritability.

The clinical signs include bulging fontanel, fever, drowsiness, apneas and convulsions. In older children the more classic signs of neck stiffness, headache and photophobia are more common. The specific signs of Kernig, Brudzinski and nuchal stiffness are often absent in children.[14] These signs are poorly sensitive in adults, let alone children. In one study in adults, both Kernig and Brudzinski signs had a sensitivity of only 5%, while sensitivity of nuchal rigidity was 30%.[15]

The nonspecific nature of the symptoms and clinical signs means that we often overtreat and look to other investigations to confirm diagnosis.

The signs and symptoms are common to all types of meningitis. However, there are certain manifestations, which are associated with specific infections. Petechial and purpuric eruptions with a shock-like state are almost pathognomonic of meningococcemia (Waterhouse Friderichsen syndrome). Rashes are very rarely seen in pneumococcal meningitis but may sometimes be seen in *H.influenzae* meningitis also. Joint involvement suggests infection with meningococci or *H. influenzae* either early as a part of suppurative arthritis or late as reactive arthritis. History of head trauma with or without fracture and a chronically draining ear are suggestive of meningitis due to pneumococci.

INVESTIGATIONS

CSF analysis and culture remains the definitive method for diagnosis of meningitis. Early diagnosis followed by appropriate management can have a favorable effect on outcome. If a child has focal neurological signs, especially pupillary signs or cardiovascular instability, whether accompanied by papilledema or not, the use of cranial CT or magnetic resonance imaging should be considered before lumbar puncture, to exclude a brain abscess or a generalized cerebral edema, to avoid danger of herniation. Lumbar puncture can be delayed till it is thought to be safe.[16] Regardless of the decision is to perform lumbar puncture or not, antibiotic treatment should not be delayed.

Acute bacterial meningitis characteristically reveals a cloudy CSF, consisting of raised white blood cell count and predominance of polymorphonuclear leukocytes, low glucose concentration in relation to serum value, a raised concentration of protein and a positive stained smear and culture of the causative micro-organism. A glucose concentration of less than 200 mg/L in CSF is associated with a higher rate of hearing impairment. The probability of visualizing bacteria on a gram-stained preparation of CSF is dependent on the number of organisms present. The lower limit of detection is about 10^5 colony forming units/ml in CSF, which equates to a positive stained smear in 70-80% cases. The introduction of molecular techniques has, however, meant that live organisms are not required for identification. So there is less need for an early CSF. Polymerase chain reaction (PCR) and rapid antigen latex agglutination test on CSF and on blood have been found to be useful for the diagnosis of meningitis.[13]

Cranial computed tomography is of limited use in acute bacterial meningitis. The main indication for a CT scan is when the diagnosis of meningitis is uncertain and other possible causes of meningism are being considered, e.g. posterior fossa tumors or if complications of meningitis are suspected. Any decision to perform a CT should not delay the use of antibiotics.

All children admitted to hospital with suspected meningitis should have a complete blood count (CBC), C-reactive protein, blood culture, clotting studies and electrolytes.

Aspiration of petechiae in meningococcal disease is a neglected investigation but in one study it was found that in two thirds of the patients it contained meningococci, which could be seen on Gram stain or cultured.[17] Antibiotics do not affect the visualization of meningococci in the skin aspirates.[18] Thus, this investigation is particularly useful in that a definitive diagnosis of meningococcal disease can be made when clinical signs preclude a lumbar puncture.

COMPLICATIONS

These can develop either before diagnosis or several days after starting treatment. Systemic circulatory problems usually arise during the first day in hospital with acute bacterial meningitis. Peripheral circulatory collapse is one of the most striking and serious complications of meningitis. This, complication is most frequently found in meningococcemia, but can accompany other types of infection also.[19] Disseminated intravascular coagulation (DIC) and gangrene of the distal extremities can occur in patients with fulminant hemorrhagic meningococcal meningitis. Treatment with antibiotics may initially worsen the picture because of release of active components such as endotoxin from the cell walls or membranes of rapidly lysed micro-organisms. In the past it was believed that these patients had inappropriate antidiuretic hormone secretion and hence, fluid restriction was advocated but recent studies have revealed that this raised concentration of the hormone in serum is an appropriate response to unrecognized hypovolemia and that liberal use of parenteral fluids can be beneficial.[20,21] This fact is important in the management of these cases because systemic blood pressure should be maintained at levels sufficient to prevent compromise of cerebral perfusion and fluid restriction may prove detrimental.

Focal neurological signs like hemiparesis, quadriparesis, facial palsy and visual field defects present in about 10-15% patients result from cortical necrosis, occlusive vasculitis or thrombosis of the cortical veins.[22] Second, third, sixth, seventh and eighth cranial nerves may be implicated while coursing through the subarachnoid space once the inflammation extends. Inflammation of the cochlear aqueduct and the auditory nerve can lead to reversible or permanent deafness in 5-30% cases.[23] Hydrocephalus either obstructive or communicating and brain abscesses may result as complications, particularly in younger infants. Subdural effusions are found in one third of patients particularly with H influenzae and pneumococcal meningitis and arise mainly in infants younger that 2 years of age. They are rarely responsible for long-term sequelae and should only be drained if there is a clinical suspicion of empyema, a rapidly enlarging head circumference in a child without hydrocephalus, focal neurological findings and evidence of raised intracranial pressure.[24]

Seizures (usually generalized) occur before, or during the first several days after admission to hospital in one third of the patients with meningitis. Seizures that are difficult to control or that persist beyond the fourth day in hospital, and seizures that arise for the first time late in the patient's hospital course have a greater chance of being associated with neurological sequelae.

Joint involvement may result early from direct extension of infection by *H.influenzae* or late as reactive arthritis due to meningococcal infections.[19]

TREATMENT

In a child with suspected meningitis, urgent transfer to hospital, followed by concurrent microbiological investigations and antibiotic treatment are the corner stones of management. The choice of antibiotic depends on the organism isolated but in most cases the initial treatment has to be empirical, but nonetheless based on epidemiological knowledge of the commonest organisms for each age group and local antibiotic resistance.[25]

In most cases of bacterial meningitis a broad spectrum cephalosporin (ceftriaxone or cefotaxime) is the most appropriate empirical choice in children over 3 months old.[26] In children younger than 3 months for gram-negative bacillary meningitis cefotaxime alone or combined with aminoglycosides are recommended.[25] Ceftriaxone is not recommended for use in neonatal period because of the potential for displacement of bilirubin from albumin binding sites and its profound inhibitory effect on growth or bacterial flora of the intestinal tract.[27] Using ceftriaxone as first line treatment is effective in dealing with the problem of poor outcomes from meningitis due to *Hemophilus influenzae* that is resistant to chloramphenicol, and a strategy of changing to chloramphenicol if *in vitro* susceptibility is shown will reduce the cost without comprising on clinical outcomes. For cases with suspected group B streptococcus or *Listeria monocytogenes* ampicillin has to be used along with an aminoglycoside.[3, 25] When the specific pathogen is identified and the results of susceptibilities are known, treatment can be modified. In children with resistant pneumococci vancomycin, carbapenems like meropenem or imipenem and fluroquinolones like gatifloxacin, trovafloxacin and moxifloxacin are potentially effective.[28, 29] (Table 22.1) For more complicated cases such as immunosuppressed patients or those with recent history of head trauma or neurosurgery, and those with cerebrospinal fluid shunts, a broad spectrum cover of both gram positive and negative organisms in the form of ceftazidine with vancomycin may be used.[30]

Duration of therapy in gram-negative meningitis in neonates is three weeks whereas in case of group b Streptococcus of Listeria 10-14 days of therapy may suffice. In older children 4-7 days of treatment is satisfactory for uncomplicated meningococcal meningitis, 7-10 days for Hemophilus disease, and 10days or longer for pneumococcal meningitis.

Apart from the definitive management, supportive and adjunctive treatment of these cases play a crucial role in the successful outcome. Adequate oxygenation, prevention of hypoglycemia and hyponatremia, anticonvulsant treatment, and measures designed to decrease intracranial hypertension and to prevent fluctuation in cerebral blood flow are extremely vital[31, 32] (Table 22.2).

PREVENTION

Vaccination

Immunization is the most effective means of prevention of bacterial meningitis in children. Universal immunization with conjugated vaccines has been associated with a reduction

Table 22.1: Dosage and frequency of the common antibiotics used in bacterial meningitis

Drug	*Dose*	*Frequency (times daily)*	*Maximum total daily dose*
Penicillin G	50 mg/kg	4-6	14.4gm
Cefotaxime	50 mg/kg	4	3 gm
Ceftriaxone	80-100 mg/kg	1	4 gm
Ampicillin	100 mg/kg	4	3 gm
Ceftazidime	50 mg/kg	3	6 gm
Vancomycin	15 mg/kg then 10 mg/kg	4	2 gm

Table 22.2: Commonly used supportive and adjunctive treatment in bacterial meningitis[25]

Rationale	*Strategies*	*Cautions*
Reduction of raised intracranial pressure	30° bed head elevation, antipyretic agents, avoidance of vigorous and frequent intra-tracheal suctioning and intubation, correction of hyponatremia, and SIADH, hyperventialation, use of mannitol, high dose barbiturate	Fluid restriction can be dangerous if patient has dehydration or hypovolemia, significant reduction of $PaCO_2$ (< 25 mm Hg) can affect cerebral blood flow; cardiac toxicity with pentobarbital
Control and prevention for seizures	Anticonvulsant drugs (lorazepam, diazepam phenytoin, Phenobarbital)	Respiratory depression and hypotension with benzodoazepines and phenobarbital, cardiac arrythmias with phenytoin
Amelioration of meningeal inflammation with reduced audiological & neurological sequelae	Dexamethasone administered before the first parenteral dose of antibiotic (0.4 mg/kg/dose every 12 hourly for 2 days)	Potential delayed eradication of highly resistant pneumococci from CSf; rare risk of GI bleeding; possibly, ling term cognitive impairment due to cell apoptosis in hippocampus

of more than 99% in invasive diseases caused by *H influenzae* type b in developed countries.[33] Appropriate vaccines against meningococcal and pneumococcal strains may be associated with a reduction of more than 90% of the invasive disease caused by these organisms.[34]

Chemoprophylaxis

The recommendations for chemoprophylaxis and prevention of secondary cases among contacts are shown in Table 22.3.[13]

Table 22.3: Recommendations for prevention for secondary cases among close contacts

H influenzae type b infection

- All home contacts should be given rifampicin 20 mg/kg/d for four days.
- Any unvaccinated children aged 12-48 months, should be given one dose of the vaccine.
- Unvaccinated children aged 2-11 months should be given three doses of the vaccine.

Meningococcal infection (should be given one of the following):

- Rifampicin 600 mg every 12 hours for 2 days for adults; for children dose is 10 mg/kg (under 1year, 5 mg/kg) every 12hours for 2 days orally.
- Ceftriaxone 250 mg in adults (child < 12 years, 125 mg) intramuscularly as a single dose.
- Ciprofloxacin 500 mg orally as a single dosein adults and children aged > 12 years.
- Unvaccinated children and close contacts age > 2 years and exposed to meningococcus A, C, Y or W 135 should be offered quadrivalent meningococcal vaccine (Where available).

Unless there has been mouth-to-mouth contact (or a direct exposure to infectious droplets from a patient with meningococcal disease) healthcare workers do not generally require chemoprophylaxis.

Pneumococcal meningitis

- Chemoprophylaxis not normally indicated for close contacts.

Other types of bacterial meningitis

- Secondary prevention not required.

PROGNOSIS

The outcome of these patients is dependent on many factors, including age of patient, time and clinical stability before effective antibiotic treatment is begun, type of microorganism, number of bacteria or quantity of active bacterial products in CSF at the time of diagnosis, intensity of the host's inflammatory response, and time elapsed to sterilize CSF culture.[35, 36] Extremes of age and infections caused by group B streptococci, gram-negative enteric bacilli and pneumococci are associated with poorest outcome.[25] The greater the host's inflammatory response in the subarachnoid space to the microorganism and its products the greater is the likelihood of permanent sequelae. The chances of survival today are excellent especially in infants and children and case fatality rates are as less as 10%, but the long-term sequelae have not been greatly reduced despite advances in treatment. Those who survive bacterial meningitis are more likely to have seizures, hearing deficits, learning and behavioral problems and lower intelligence. The rate of residual abnormalities after meningitis is about 15%.[19]

CONCLUSION

Over the course of the past decade, much has changed on the landscape of meningitis in children. The emergence of penicillin-resistant *Streptococcus pneumoniae* has complicated the treatment of bacterial meningitis, whereas the Haemophilus influenzae vaccine has fundamentally altered the disease's epidemiology. The recognition that much of the neuropathologic change induced by bacterial meningitis is inflammation mediated has paved the way to the demonstration that dexamethasone can substantially improve the outcome. Empirical antimicrobial therapy remains justifiable but periodic microbiological surveillance is essential. Using a third generation cephalosporin as first line treatment is effective in dealing with the problem of poor outcomes from meningitis but there is an urgent need to reduce their costs, to improve bacteriological services and to introduce effective and affordable vaccines against H influenzae and Streptococcus pneumoniae in the developing world.

REFERENCES

1. Duke T, Curtis N, Fuller DG. The management of bacterial meningitis in children. *Expert Opin Pharmacother* 2003;4: 1227-1240.
2. Moreno MT, Vargas S, Poveda R, Saez-Llorens Z. Neonatal sepsis and meningitis in a developing Latin American country. *J Med* 1994;13:516-520.
3. Kessler SL, Dajani AS. Listeria meningitis in infants and children. *Pediatr Infect Dis* 1990;9:61-63.
4. Diaz JM, Catalan L, Urrutia MT, Prado V, Ledermann W, Mendoza C, Topelberg S. Trends of etiology of acute bacterial meningitis in Chilean children from 1989 to 1998. Impact of the anti *H. influenzae* type b vaccine. *Rev Med Chil* 2001;129: 719-216.
5. Pallares R, Viladrich PF, Linares J, Cabellos C, Gudiol G. Impact of antibiotic resistance on chemotherapy for pneumococcal infections. *Micro Drug Resist* 1998;4:339-347.
6. Riedo FX, Plikaytis BD, Broome CV. Epidemiology and prevention of meningococcal disease. *Pediatr Infect Dis* 1995;14:643-657.
7. Nelson JD. Cerebrospinal fluid shunt infections. *Pediatr Infect Dis* 1984;3:530-532.
8. Klein JO, Feigin RD, Mc Cracken GH Jr. Report of the task force on diagnosis and management of meningitis. *Pediatrics* 1986;78:959-982.
9. Saez–Llorens X, McCracken GJ Jr. Antimicrobial and antiinflammatory treatment of bacterial meningitis. *Infect Dis Clin North Am* 1999;12:619-636.
10. Leib SL, Tauber MG. Pathogenesis of bacterial meningitis. *Infect Dis Clin North Am* 1999;13:527-548.
11. Pfister HW, Fontana A, Tauber MG, Tomasz A, Scheld WM. Mechanisms of brain injury in bacterial meningitis: workshop summary. *Clin Infect Dis* 1994;19:463-499.
12. Braun JS, Tuomanen EI. Molecular mechanisms of brain damage in bacterial meningitis. *Adv Pediatr Infect Dis* 1999;14:49-71.
13. Bashir H El, Laundy M, Booy R. Diagnosis and treatment of bacterial meningitis. *Arch Dis Child* 2003;88:615-620.
14. Radetsky M. Duration of symptoms and outcome in bacterial meningitis: an analysis of causation and the implications of a delay in diagnosis. *Pediatr Infect Dis 1*992;11:694-698.
15. Thomas KE, Hasbun R, Jekel J, Quagliarello VJ. The diagnostic accuracy of Kernig's sign, Brudzinski's sign, and nuchal rigidity in adults with suspected meningitis. *Clin Infect Dis* 2002;35: 46-52.
16. Riodan FAI, Cant AJ. When to do a lumbar puncture. *Arch Dis Child* 2002;87:235-237.
17. van Deuren M, van Dijke BJ, Koopman RJ, Horrevorts AM, Meis JF, Santman FW, van der Meer JW. Rapid diagnosis of acute meningococcal infections by needle aspiration or biopsy of skin lesions. *Brit Med J* 1993;306:1229-1232.
18. Taylor MR, Keane CT, Periappuram M. Skin scarping is a useful investigation in meningococcal disease. *Brit Med J* 1997;314:831-832.
19. Kaplan SL. Clinical manifestations, diagnosis and prognostic factors of bacterial meningitis. *Infect Dis Clin North Am* 1999;13:579-590.
20. Moller K, Larsen FS, Bie P, Skinhoj P. The syndrome of inappropriate secretion of antidiuretic hormone and fluid restriction in meningitis–how strong is the evidence? *Cand J Infect Dis* 2001;33:13-26.
21. Singhi SC, Singhi PD, Srinivas B, Narakesri HP, Ganguli NK, Sialy R, Walia BN. Fluid restriction does not improve the outcome of acute meningitis. *Pediatr Infect Dis J* 1995;14: 495-503.
22. Sell SH. Long term sequelae of bacterial meningitis in children. *Pediatr Infect Dis* 1983;2:90-93.
23. Auslander MC, Meskan ME. The pattern and stability of post-meningitic hearing loss in children. *Laryngoscope* 1988;98: 940-948.
24. Snedeker JD, Kaplan SL, Dodge PR, Holmes SJ, Feigin RD. Subdural effusion and its relationship with neurologic sequelae of bacterial meningitis in infancy: a prospective study. *Pediatrics* 1990;S6:162-170.
25. Saez–Llorens X, McCracken GJ Jr. Bacterial meningitis in children. *Lancet* 2003;361:2139-2148.
26. Frenkel LD. Once daily administration of ceftriaxone for the treatment of selected bacterial infections in children. *Pediatrics* 1988;82:486-491.
27. Fink S, Karp W, Robertson A. Ceftriaxone effect on bilirubin-albumin binding. *Pediatrics* 1987;80:873-875.
28. Mitchell L, Tuomanen EI. Vancomycin tolerant Streptococcus pneumoniae and its clinical significance. *Pediatr Infect Dis* J 2001;20:531-533.
29. Saez-Llorens X, McCoig C, Feris JM, Vargas SL, Klugman KP, Hussey GD, et al. Quinolone treatment for pediatric bacterial meningitis: a comparative study of trovafloxacin and ceftriaxone with or without vancomycin. *Pediatr Infect Dis J* 2002;21: 14-22.
30. Quagliarella VJ, Scheld WM. Treatment of bacterial meningitis. *N Engl J Med* 1997;336:708-716.
31. Kaplan SL. Adjunctive therapy in meningitis. *Adv Pediatr Infect Dis* 1995;10:167-186.
32. Ashwal S, Perkin RM, Thompson JR, Schneider S, Tomasi LG. Bacterial meningitis in children: current concepts of neurologic management. *Curr Prob Pediatr* 1994;24:267-284.
33. CDC. Progress toward elimination of Hemophilus influenzae type b invasive disease among infants and children: United States 1998-2000. *MMWR* 2002;51: 234-242.
34. Borges Laval CA, Pimenta FC, De Andrade JG, Andrade SS, Sgambatti De Andrade AL. Progress towards meningitis prevention in the conjugate vaccines era. *Braz J Infect Dis* 2003;7:315-324.
35. Saez-Llorens X, Ramilo O, Mustafa MM, Mertsola J, McCracken GH Jr. Molecular pathophysiology of bacterial meningitis: current concepts and therapeutic implications. *J Pediatr* 1990;116:671-684.
36. Feldman WE. Relation of concentrations of bacteria and bacterial antigen in cerebrospinal fluid to prognosis in patients with bacterial meningitis. *N Engl J Med* 1977;296:433-435.

Devendra Mishra

23 Guillain-Barré Syndrome (GBS)

INTRODUCTION

The term, *Guillain-Barré Syndrome (GBS)*, denotes a recognizable clinical entity characterized by rapidly evolving symmetrical limb weakness, loss of tendon reflexes, absent or mild sensory signs, and variable autonomic dysfunction.[1] Various distinct subtypes have been described and they differ in the degree of neurological deficit, which varies in terms of degree/distribution of weakness (cranial and limb distribution), respiratory compromise, sensory loss and autonomic dysfunction. First described by Landry in 1859 and further detailed by Guillain, Barré and Strohl in 1916, GBS is currently the leading cause of acute flaccid paralysis in western countries.[1] With the reducing number of poliomyelitis cases due to the success of the pulse polio campaign, GBS is gradually becoming an important component of AFP cases in our country also.

By convention, disease that reaches its nadir within 4 weeks is labeled GBS, whereas disease that continues to progress for at least 8 weeks is termed Chronic inflammatory demyelinating polyneuropathy (CIDP).[2] The classic pathology with demyelination and inflammatory infiltrate is usually known as acute inflammatory demyelinating polyradiculoneuropathy (AIDP). In addition to AIDP, the clinical spectrum of GBS has now been recognized to comprise a heterogeneous group of pathological entities with distinctive clinical features viz., Acute motor and sensory axonal neuropathy (AMSAN), Acute motor axonal neuropathy (AMAN), Miller-Fischer syndrome (MFS), and acute panautonomic/pandysautonomic neuropathy.[1] The pathogenesis is now becoming clearer and the disease is probably a result of aberrant organ-specific immune response. The prognosis in pediatric patients is favorable and, anticipating and preventing complications is the best strategy to improve outcome. Immunomodulatory therapy with intravenous immunoglobulin (IVIG) or plasma exchange is currently the accepted mode of therapy to foreshorten the disease course. Up to a third of GBS patients may require admission to intensive care unit (ICU) for intubation and assisted ventilation, and management of these patients is a challenge to the clinical acumen of the physician in charge and the adequacy of the supportive care provided in the unit.

This review emphasizes the treatment of GBS after discussing the pathogenesis and clinical features in short.

EPIDEMIOLOGY

All epidemiological studies are hampered by the lack of a reference diagnostic test. Although no population-based data are available from India, epidemiological studies in Europe, Australia and the North and Latin America have documented an annual incidence figure of 1-2 per 100,000 population, for those under forty.[1] These figures suggest that GBS occurs uniformly throughout the western hemisphere without geographical clustering and with only minor seasonal variations. The frequency of GBS is probably relatively stable over time. On the basis of these data, an estimated 20000 new cases of GBS would be encountered each year in India. GBS affects all age groups though it is rare in infancy and there is a slight increase in incidence in late adolescence and young adulthood, probably due to the increased risk of infection with C. jejuni and CMV (a second peak occurs in the elderly). The reported incidence for children under-15 years is similar to adults.[3] There is a slight male predominance with male to female ratio of 1.5:1. Occurrence of epidemic clusters has also been described specially for AMAN in China and other reports from Mexico, Columbia, Japan and India.[3]

PATHOGENESIS

Antecedent infections: Preceding acute infectious illness is reported in around two-third of patients, which is usually a respiratory or gastrointestinal infection and has resolved by the time the neurological symptoms appear. The interval between the prodormal infection and the onset of GBS symptoms varies between 1-3 weeks, occasionally longer; the average is around 11 days.[1] The pathogen causing the antecedent infection frequently remains unidentified. The antecedent pathogen identified most frequently with GBS (26-41% of the cases) has been *C. jejuni* in almost all the studies.[1,4] This infection is also strongly associated with the acute motor-axonal neuropathy and the Miller Fischer syndrome variants of GBS. The commonest viral trigger (10-22% of the cases) for the disease has been reported to be cytomegalovirus infection, which frequently presents as a respiratory tract illness. This association is particularly common in young female patients with GBS.[1,5]

Vaccines: Despite quite a few anecdotal case reports linking GBS to vaccines, no causal relation has been established for any of the currently used vaccines. Previously used rabies vaccine (prepared from animal brain tissue) and the swine influenza vaccine have been shown to carry an increased risk inducing GBS.[1] An association with oral polio vaccine was suggested but the causal relationship seems questionable.[1]

The close association between GBS and a preceding infectious agent strongly favours an immune basis to the syndrome in majority of the cases. The pathological changes seen in AIDP include mononuclear infilteration (mainly lymphocytic) and macrophage mediated demyelination in a patchy, multifocal distribution involving a fascicle or cluster of nerves. Macrophages are recognized as the principal cells producing demyelination in GBS. AIDP is viewed as a reactive, self-limited, autoimmune disease.[1]

CLINICAL FEATURES

Acute onset weakness in a child is a terrifying experience both for the child and the parents. History has to be obtained from anxious parents and repeat questioning is often necessary. However, the history and clinical examination usually suggest the correct diagnosis in majority of the patients. In about half the patients, an antecedent infection or other event is documented one to several weeks before the onset of the symptoms.

The classic presentation is with a very rapidly progressive paralysis associated with absent reflexes and distal numbness and tingling. The weakness can develop acutely (within a day) or subacutely (up to four weeks) and reach a plateau. About 50 to 75% of the patients reach their nadir with in 2 weeks and 90-98% within 4 weeks.[6] Although characteristically described as an 'ascending paralysis', the initial motor deficit may occur in the upper limbs or proximal muscles of the pelvic or shoulder girdle. Facial weakness, occasionally asymmetric, occurs in over 50% of patients. Bulbar muscles may also be involved, resulting in weakness of chewing, swallowing, and occasionally extraocular muscle paresis.

Sensory symptoms with paresthesia, pain and sensory impairment are usually present and occasionally sensory complaints may be the initial presentation, to be followed later by motor symptoms. However, as distinct from poliomyelitis, prominent myalgia and meningeal signs are less commonly seen in GBS. DTR are lost early, although preservation of DTR may be found in mildly affected patients. Bowel and bladder sphincter function must be specifically assessed, as prominent sphincteric disturbance is unusual and points to the diagnosis of a myelopathy (transverse myelitis). Minor sphincteric involvement is however, not uncommon in GBS. Papilledema is occasionally present but does not correlate with the severity of the neuropathy, and its cause is still not clear.[2]

DIFFERENTIAL DIAGNOSIS

Poliomyelitis is an important consideration in our country both from the epidemiological aspect and the prognostic aspect. Even a clear case of GBS needs to be reported as acute flaccid paralysis to the relevant authority.

Another important concern is the exclusion of a rapidly progressive spinal lesion. Other diagnoses should be specifically considered in the presence of significantly asymmetric muscle weakness, intact reflexes despite significant weakness, and in the absence of characteristic electrodiagnostic features.

A purely motor disorder may be confused with botulism and polymyositis, whereas an acute neuropathy in the context of disturbed mental function may suggest porphyria or toxin (lead, hydrocarbon) exposure.[2]

Tick paralysis, although not common in our country, requires removal of clothes and complete visual examination of the child. The differential diagnosis has been discussed in detail in many recent publications[7] and is detailed in Table 23.1.

DIAGNOSIS

The diagnosis of GBS is essentially clinical though laboratory studies like cerebrospinal fluid examination and electrophysiology help in confirming the diagnosis. The criteria required for and supportive of the diagnosis were defined in 1978 and later refined (Table 23.1 and 23.2).[8]

CSF examination Albuminocytologic dissociation is the characteristic finding required to make a diagnosis of GBS. This signifies an elevation of CSF protein without a proportionate increase in the CSF cell count. This protein rise usually takes a week to become apparent, thereby causin some diagnostic confusion in the first few days of the illness. Occasionally, it may not reach its peak until 4 to 6 weeks after onset of symptoms. CSF cell count is crucial to distinguish poliomyelitis from GBS. The CSF cell count is usually less than 10 mononuclear cells/ mm^2 in GBS and the presence of polymorphonuclear cells or >50 mono-

Table 23.1: Differential diagnosis of Guillain-Barré syndrome

Immediate consideration
Compressive myelopathy
Poliomyelitis
CNS
Bilateral strokes
Acute cerebellar ataxia,
Posterior fossa structural lesion
Transverse myelitis
Neuromuscular junction
Botulism
Neuromuscular blockers
Peripheral nerve
Diphtheria
Toxic neuropathy: Drugs (specially vincristine), toxins (specially lead and organophosphates)
Tick paralysis
Porphyria
Muscle Diseases
Acute viral myositis
Acute inflammatory myopathies (polymyositis, dermatomyositis)
Metabolic myopathies
Periodic paralysis
Miscellaneous
Critical illness neuropathy
Hysteria

nuclear cells/mm^2 does not support the diagnosis. The increase in CSF protein is usually between 80-200 mg/dl in children though the levels may be normal in up to 20% children early in the course.

Electrophysiology: Electrophysiological studies are needed for diagnostic confirmation and to demonstrate evidence of multifocal demyelination in sensory and motor peripheral nerves. Occasionally changes indicative of axonal involvement are present. The currently accepted electrophysiological criteria to support a diagnosis of GBS are listed in Table 23.3. The common findings in children are prolonged distal motor latencies and, reduced nerve conduction velocities and compound motor action potentials (with prolonged terminal dispersion). Children younger than 10 years of age have been reported to have a greater slowing of motor NCV than those older than 10 years. In a significant minority, electrophysiological evidence of nerve conduction slowing or conduction block may not be present early in the clinical course and the diagnosis may remain a clinical one through out the acute phase of the illness. Discordant sural and median sensory nerve conduction (normal sural conductions with abnormal median sensory conductions) has been reported to be suggestive of GBS in the appropriate clinical setting.[9]

Role of MRI: Due to the cost and availability constraints, the role of MRI is confined in children with an uncharacteristic clinical course or in those in whom the electrophysiological abnormalities are equivocal. Traverse myelitis is one condition in the differential diagnosis that may require a MRI study to exclude. Marked gandolinium enhancement of the cauda equina and lumbar nerves indicating an inflammatory process confined to dorsal and ventral roots is the characteristic MRI abnormality. Nerve root enhancement has been found to be 83% sensitive in the diagnosis of acute GBS and is present in 95% of typical cases.[6] A recent report has delineated the duration of contrast enhancement and its relation to clinical recovery in pediatric patients with GBS.[10]

Table 23.2: Clinical and laboratory features in the diagnosis of Guillain-Barré syndrome[8]

I. Required for diagnosis
- Progressive motor weakness of more than one limb
- Areflexia-Loss of ankle jerks and diminished knee and biceps reflexes will suffice if other features are consistent with the diagnosis

II. Strongly supportive of the diagnosis
- Progression–Weakness may develop rapidly but cease to progress after 4 weeks; roughly 50% will plateau within 2 weeks, 80% by 3 weeks and 90% after 4 weeks
- Relative symmetry
- Mild sensory symptoms or signs
- Cranial nerve involvement; facial weakness develops in approximately 50% of patients
- Autonomic dysfunction
- Absence of fever at the onset of neuralgic symptoms
- Recovery–Usually recovery begins 2 to 4 weeks after progression ceases; it may be delayed for months

Variants
- Fever at onset of symptoms
- Severe sensory loss with pain
- Progressive phase longer than 4 weeks
- Lack of recovery or major permanent residual deficit
- Sphincter dysfunction–Sphincters are usually spared, although transient bladder paralysis may occur
- CNS involvement

III. Features casting doubt on diagnosis
- Marked persistent asymmetry in motor function
- Persistent bowel or bladder dysfunction
- Bowel or bladder dysfunction at onset of symptoms
- Discrete sensory level

IV. Features that exclude the diagnosis
- History of recent hexacarbon abuse
- Evidence of porphyria
- Recent diphtheria
- Features consistent with lead neuropathy and evidence of lead intoxication
- A pure sensory syndrome
- Definite diagnosis of an alternate paralytic disorder

MANAGEMENT

Majority of patients with GBS undergo spontaneous recovery and for them, optimal therapy remains primarily supportive. However, it is a serious disorder for a significant

Table 23.3: Consensus electrophysiologic features supportive of a diagnosis of multifocal demyelinating neuropathy of Guillain-Barré syndrome[8]

Must demonstrate three of the following four features:
1. Reduction in conduction velocity in two or more motor nerves a. < 80% of LLN if CMAP amplitude is > 80% LLN b. < 70% of LLN if CAMP amplitude is < 80% LLN
2. Conduction block or excessive temporal dispersion of proximally evoked CAMPS in one or more motor nerves (peroneal, between ankle and below fibular head; median, between wrist and elbow; ulnar, between wrist and below elbow) a. Criteria for partial conduction block < 15% change in CAMP duration between proximal and distal sites and 20% drop in negative-peak area of peak-to-peak amplitude between proximal and distal sites b. Criteria for abnormal temporal dispersion and possible conduction block > 15% increase in CAMP duration between distal and proximal stimulation sites and > 20% decrease in negative-peak CMAP area or peak-to-peak amplitude between distal and proximal stimulation sites
3. Prolonged distal latencies in two or more nerves a. > 125% of ULN if amplitude > 80% of LLN b. > 150% of ULN if amplitude < 80% LLN
4. Absent F-waves or prolonged minimum F-wave latencies (10 to 15 trials) in two or more motor nerves a. > 120% of ULN if amplitude > 80% of LLN b. > 150% of ULN if amplitude < 80% of LLN

minority who develops respiratory failure and/or loses the ability to swallow and maintain nutrition. These are the patients who need intensive care and their outcome depends on close monitoring and excellent nursing care. With immune orchestrated macrophage-mediated demyelination of sensory and motor axons within the peripheral nervous being the currently accepted underlying pathogenesis of GBS, immunomodulating strategies remain the primary modality of specific therapy in this disorder. Plasmapheresis (PE) and high-dose intravenous immunoglobulin (IVIG) are the current specific treatment of choice. In contrast to other autoimmune disorders, glucocorticosteroids presently have no place in the treatment of GBS.[11] The management of GBS may be addressed under three separate heads-intensive care management, specific therapy, and supportive care.

INTENSIVE CARE MANAGEMENT

The key issue in the effective treatment of GBS remains intensive care unit (ICU) management, including respiratory care, monitoring and the early treatment of autonomic dysfunction, anticoagulation, and good nursing care.[1] Approximately 10-20% of children with GBS require ventilatory assistance. Respiratory failure and autonomic dysfunction are the common causes of death from GBS.[3]

The issues in the intensive care management of GBS are:

Intensive Care Unit Admission and Care

The decision whether to admit a child with acute GBS in the PICU or the general ward would depend on the resources available and also the policy of the individual PICU. Respiratory muscle paresis is almost never an initial manifestation but is a danger throughout the course. It is impossible to determine which patient may develop the potentially lethal complications of arrhythmia or respiratory collapse. Moreover, incipient respiratory failure can remain undetected until acute respiratory paralysis occurs. However, as a general guideline, all patients with newly diagnosed GBS should be admitted to the ICU, except for patients with very mild symptoms and signs, and constant cardiopulmonary monitoring carried out until clinical weakness and autonomic function are stable.[3] In case resources permit, all children with GBS must be admitted in the ICU, except those with a stable disease. ICU admission in GBS may be needed either because of the progression of the illness, its complications or complications of therapy. The commonest indication, however, remains overt or impending neuromuscular respiratory failure, which may occur in 10-20% of the children (33% of adult patients).[12] Autonomic dysfunction is also a quite frequent accompaniment of GBS (occurring in up to 65% patients) but is frequently missed unless the patient is being diligently monitored in the ICU. Various complications of the diseases that may require care in the ICU are listed in Table 23.4.

Airway Management and Respiratory Dysfunction

Ventilatory assistance in GBS may be required for three basic reasons viz., inadequate inspiratory effort, ineffective expiratory force and inability to protect the airway.[13] As soon as a diagnosis of GBS is entertained, assessment of the baseline cardiovascular and respiratory function should be done and then monitored for progression. The two important points to be considered when assessing the respiratory status of a patient with GBS are that the weakness in different respiratory muscles in the disease is not uniform and, peripheral muscle strength do not correlate strictly with diaphragmatic weakness.[12] Peak flow, which is a measure of airway diameter, is inappropriate for respiratory monitoring in GBS. Similarly, blood gases are very insensitive and do not predict impending respiratory catastrophe.[2] Although difficult to carry out in young children, forced vital capacity (FVC) and negative inspiratory force (NIF) need to be assessed at least every 8 hours, if possible. More frequent measurements may be required in case of rapid changes in the clinical condition.[3] Peak expiratory pressure and the ratio of VC in the supine and prone positions have been suggested as better indicators of evolving respiratory failure and diaphragmatic weakness, respectively.[12,13]

Table 23.4: Complications of Guillain-Barré syndrome that may require intensive care unit management

Complications of the disease	*Complications of critical illness*	*Complications of therapy*		
		IVIG	*PE*	*ICU care*
Hyponatremia	GI hemorrhage	Anaphylaxis	Pneumothorax	Barotrauma
Ileus	Sepsis	Aseptic meningitis	Sepsis	Pneumothorax
Paroxysmal hypertension	Sepsis thrombosis	Renal failure	Coagulopathy	Sepsis
		Thromboembolism	Symptomatic	Thrombocytopenia
Brady/tachyarrhythmias	Pulmonary embolism	Congestive heart failure	hypocalcemia	Drug reactions

Intubation and ventilatory assistance should be provided if FVC falls to below 10 cc/Kg or NIF falls below 30-cm water.[3] A decrease in VC of 50% or more over 48 hours is also a marker for impending respiratory failure.[12] Patients with VC > 15 ml/kg may also require postural drainage, supplemental oxygen, and even mechanical ventilation if there is impaired ability to clear the airway, atelectasis, and impaired sigh mechanism.[13] In younger children where these objective measures cannot be made, decisions for providing ventilatory support are usually based on the clinical condition. Even in the presence of a relatively normal vital capacity and normal gas exchange, children with marked bulbar weakness or those with poor cough effort will need intubation and respiratory support. The decision to intubate the patient is, therefore, based on the composite clinical picture and not on a single cutoff value of any particular measurement. Early predictors of mechanical ventilation in adult patients with GBS have recently been proposed and are enumerated below. It has been suggested that patients with at least one of these should be monitored in an ICU.[14]

- Time from onset to admission < 7 days
- Inability to cough
- Inability to stand
- Inability to lift elbows/head
- Increase in liver enzymes
- Vital capacity < 60%

Decision for intubation of a patient with GBS should always be a planned one as far as possible so as to avoid an emergency intubation. Airway management in GBS is more difficult compared to other acute neuromuscular emergencies because of the associated dysautonomia (exaggerating the hypotensive response associated with barbiturates, benzodiazepines, narcotics etc.) and the potential for lethal hyperkalemia with succinylcholine.[13] Vigorous suctioning of the airway may be associated with bradycardia or asystole because of vagal stimulation. Intubation is best performed using topical airway anesthesia, atropine and intravenous sedation with short-acting benzodiazepines.[13]

Tracheostomy

It should be performed in all patients who remain intubated for three weeks unless a rapid recovery is observed in the second week, as such a child may be successfully extubated. Tracheostomy may be performed early in patients with axonal forms of GBS or with acute motor-sensory axonal neuropathy in whom a rapid recovery is not anticipated.[13]

Table 23.5: Clinical grading scale from the United States Guillain-Barré syndrome plasmapheresis trial[15]

Score	*Clinical criteria*
0	Healthy
1	Minor signs or symptoms
2	Able to walk 5 m without a walker or equivalent support
3	Able to walk 5 m with a walker or support
4	Bed or chair bound (unable to walk 5 m with a 3 walker or support)
5	Requires assisted ventilation (for at least part of the day)
6	Dead

B. Specific Therapy

Plasmapheresis and high dose intravenous immunoglobulin are the only two modes of specific therapy for GBS that have been conclusively proven to be of benefit.[15-17] However, similar definitive, prospectively derived data in children with GBS is lacking.[6]

Plasmapheresis

Plasmapheresis is a technique that permits selective removal of plasma from circulation and separation either by a centrifugal cell separator or filtration across a semipermeable membrane. Plasma exchange (PE), although used inter changeably with plasmapheresis, includes the same process with replacement by fluids.[18] Although the mechanism of action of plasmapheresis in GBS is not entirely clear, the benefit most likely is due to the removal of circulating antibodies against peripheral nerve antigens and other potentially pathogenic soluble factors from the circulation.[19] By removal of cytokines, PE may also indirectly influence cellular immune reactions.[18] There are quite a few reports on plasmapheresis use among children with GBS but most are small, non-randomized studies using historical controls.[6]

The evidence for the efficacy of PE for treating GBS has recently been addressed in a Cochrane systematic review.[20] The reviewers identified six eligible trials (total

649 patients), and reported time to recover walking with aid, time to onset of motor recovery in mildly affected patients, and improvement in disability grade at four weeks to be significantly better in the plasma exchange group as compared to the control group (supportive therapy alone). Patients treated with PE also fared significantly better in the other outcome measures viz., time to recover walking without aid, percentage of patients requiring artificial ventilation, duration of ventilation, full muscle strength recovery after one year, and severe sequelae after one year.[20] Moreover, two PE sessions were superior to none and four sessions superior to two in mild and moderate GBS, respectively. In severe GBS, six sessions were not better than four.[17,20] Plasma exchange was found to be more beneficial when started within seven days after disease onset but was still beneficial when used up to 30 days after disease onset. Lesser patients in the PE group had infectious events and cardiac arrhythmias.[20] The reviewers concluded that the value of PE in children less than 12 years is not known.[20]

Most pediatric studies are in agreement that PE shortens the time required for non-ambulatory patients to regain independent ambulation, and therapy is more effective when started within 7 days of symptom onset.[6] Another recent study found PE to have a beneficial effect over and above all the poor prognostic factors. It was the only variable that the physician can influence for a better outcome.[18] Plasmapheresis is safe in children provided a well-trained technical team is available. There have been no reports of deaths due to the procedure in children and reported morbidity is also minimal.[21] Potential complications include hemorrhage, hypotension, pneumothorax related to central line placement, line related sepsis, transfusion reactions, transmitted infections, clotting abnormalities, symptomatic hypocalcemia, arrhythmias, cardiac arrest and local tissue injury.[22] Children as young as 8 months have undergone PE.[6]

Plasmapheresis in India: Within four years of the first report of the efficacy of PE in GBS, the first report of its use in India was published.[18] Soon after, beneficial effects were reported in the pediatric age group.[23] Many publications have subsequently reported PE use in Indian patients.

Method of PE: Procedural details are provided in most of the standard texts and also adequately described in a recent review.[18] PE can be done manually or by automated cell separators, although the latter method is being preferred. For use in children, continuous flow machines are preferred as it involves relatively smaller fluctuations in the blood volume of the patient. A recent meta-analysis also reported continuous flow plasma exchange to be superior to intermittent flow machines.[20] Ultrafiltration and centrifugation are the two continuous flow techniques and outcomes are reported to be similar with either of these.[3] The volume of PE in each session for optimal response still remains to be elucidated but 1.5 to 2 times the plasma volume has been used in various pediatric series. Small volume PE (10-15 ml/kg) has also been found to be effective by some authors.

Similarly, the number of PE required is also contentious but based on the findings of the meta-analysis.[20] It appears appropriate that at least two exchanges be done in all GBS patients and two more exchanges be done depending on the disease severity. Albumin has been shown to be a better replacement fluid as compared to fresh frozen plasma.[16,20] The cost of PE in the Indian setting is reported to be Rs. 10,000 per session on an intermittent flow machine.[18] The cost per patient for PE for treatment of acute GBS in the West is US $ 6204.[24]

Intravenous Immunoglobulin

The mode of action of IVIG is also unclear though it has rather broad potential immune modulatory effects. High-dose IVIG may act by binding anti-idiotype antibodies, absorbing complement, or down regulation of B-cell mediated antibody production.[6] Blockade of activated receptors, enhancement of suppressor cell activity, and interference with lymphocyte proliferation are some other likely mechanisms of action.[25]

A recent Cochrane meta-analysis concluded that there are no adequate trials to determine whether IVIG is more beneficial than placebo and, giving IVIG after PE is not significantly better than PE alone.[26, 27] However, IVIG and PE were shown to have similar ability to speed the recovery from GBS.[27] Further studies to determine the benefit of IVIG in mild GBS and to establish the optimal dose of IVIG in acute GBS were also stressed. Similar to the findings in adults, trials in children have also demonstrated efficacy equivalent to plasmapheresis.[6] A total dose of 2 g/kg/ IVIG on two consecutive days was found to cause improvement in the disability grade scales within 2 weeks of treatment in 25 children with GBS. Twenty patients were able to walk independently within 1 week and eighteen recovered by two weeks.[28] In a comparative study of PE and IVIG, Abd-Allah et al found IVIG to be equally effective to PE.[29]

Due to its ease of administration and relative safety, IVIG is currently considered the treatment of choice of GBS in children. Abd-Allah et al. also concluded that IVIG should be considered the initial treatment of choice in pediatric GBS.[29] However, the comparatively higher cost (Rs. 1000 per g IVIG or around Rs 20,000 for the total dose of a 10 kg child) is an important factor responsible for lesser use of this modality in our country. A recent cost effectiveness study also concluded that PE on an average was almost US $ 4000 cheaper per patient than IVIG.[24] No Indian data is currently available to compare this cost with the savings made by lesser duration of hospital stay and/or ventilation, which occurs with IVIG use.[18]

The main complications of IVIG are anaphylaxis related to IgA deficiency, acute renal failure, acute cardiogenic pulmonary edema, aseptic meningitis, hyperglycemia, and thrombotic complications related to transient hypercoagulability.[30]

IVIg in India. Due to the high cost of therapy, large case-series on IVIG use in GBS have not been forthcoming in India. However, Shanbag et al have recently reported on 25 children with severe GBS treated with IVIG in a dose of 2g/kg bodyweight over 2-5 days. Five patients died despite therapy. All were late referrals from other hospitals. The authors concluded that early use of IVIG could reduce mortality and the need for mechanical ventilation.[31]

Other Modalities

CSF filtration: It is a novel modality of therapy was recently proposed as an equivalent therapeutic strategy to PE in GBS. Patients were randomized to receive CSF filtration or plasma exchange during the acute phase of GBS. CSF filtration consists of the placement of a spinal catheter and the removal of 30-50 cc of CSF via a filter bypass designed for the elimination of cells, bacteria, endotoxins, immunoglobulins and inflammatory mediators. CSF filtration showed equal effectiveness compared with plasma exchange, with fewer complications.[32] However, further studies are warranted to establish its therapeutic utility and at the current point in time, this approach remains highly controversial.[33]

Interferons Treatment of acute GBS with interferon (IFN-b) with or without IVIG has also been reported. Theoretically it is possible that IFN-b and IVIG may act synergistically on the humoral and cellular immune response.[33] Larger prospective studies are needed to clarify the role of interferons in the therapy of GBS.

C. Supportive Therapy

Autonomic Dysfunction

It is common but usually benign. However, monitoring in an ICU setting, or at least continuous heart rate and frequent BP monitoring (4-hourly) in the general ward, is essential to detect any potential life-threatening autonomic dysfunction. Autonomic impairment is usually more prominent in patients with severe muscle weakness and respiratory failure. Autonomic dysfunction may manifest as hypertension/hypotension, bradycardia, bladder and bowel dysfunction, neurogenic pulmonary edema, pupillary and lens accommodation abnormalities, temperature and sweating alterations, lacrimal and salivary gland dysfunction, SIADH, bronchial smooth muscle dysfunction etc.[13]

Blood pressure abnormalities. Both paroxysmal hypertension and hypotension/orthostatic hypotension occur in around 10% of all GBS patients each. Short-acting antihypertensives (e.g., hydralazine or intravenous nitroprusside drip) should be used to treat hypertension.[3] Hypotension needs to be treated only if it is causing systemic hypoperfusion and the preferred mode of therapy is volume boluses rather than pressors. Elevation of the head-end of the bed and elastic compression stockings may also be used.

Cardiac arrhythmias are an ominous finding and may present as tachyrrhythmias or bradycardia and asystole. Abnormalities in the R-R interval and heart rate response to Valsalva maneuver precede other frank manifestations of dysautonomia.[13]

Urinary retention is best managed by intermittent bladder catheterization and, constipation with stool softeners. Fecal incontinence may require placement of a rectal tube. Hyponatremia is a well recognized complication but rarely requires any treatment other than fluid restriction.

Nutritional Support

Provision of adequate nutrition is a critical part of the supportive care. Severe GBS is a hypercatabolic state comparable to severe trauma or sepsis.[34] Moreover, many patients attending the hospital late or referred from smaller centers are often undernourished, as bulbar weakness precludes adequate oral intake. Nutritional status of the quadriplegic and/or ventilator-dependent children must therefore be monitored carefully with daily weighing and regular biochemistry (albumin, electrolytes). Inadequate nutritional support may lead to an undernourished patient more susceptible to pressure sores and infections, and a decreased ability for tissue repair. Nasogastric feeding should be instituted early and preferably be continuous rather than intermittent or bolus feeding. Contraindications to feeding are protracted vomiting, ileus, intestinal obstruction and hypotension (may lead to gut ischemia).[34] Parenteral nutrition may be used in the presence of intestinal obstruction, though it is infrequently required. Drugs like sucralfate, ranitidine, metoclopramide, stool softeners may be used as needed for various minor GI problems like erosive gastritis, stress ulcers, delayed gastric emptying and constipation.

Nursing Care

Careful nursing care is the cornerstone of the management of a child with GBS. Precautions for prevention of deep-vein thrombosis should be instituted early and may include subcutaneous heparin and/or leg compressive devices.[3]

Positioning: Patients with GBS are particularly prone to pressure palsies probably because of the unique susceptibility of inflamed nerves to pressure injury. Residual foot-drop, not due to GBS and severe enough to impede walking has been reported in 5-10% of adult patients, probably because of peroneal pressure palsy.[13] Patient position can be side-lying, supine 'frog-leg' or any other favored by the unit and cloth rolls/towels should be liberally used to maintain position and prevent pressure sores. Meticulous attention to skin care and frequent (hourly) repositioning to prevent decubitous ulcers in the plegic child are mandatory. Turning also helps prevent atelectasis in patients who are not connected to a ventilator.

Pain: Pain is common in patients with GBS (reported to occur in up to 50% of all patients) and therefore manipulations should be done only when necessary.[35] Analgesics may be used judiciously prior to physiotherapy if the pain is very severe. Various types of pain syndromes described in adult patients with GBS are deep muscle ache, neuropathic pain, joint pain and throat pain (due to intubation). Various measures including ice-packs, NSAIDS, narcotics and carbamazepine may be used for pain control.[13, 35]

Physical Therapy

Physical and occupational therapy should be started early. The physical therapist should maintain a program of passive range of motions and stretching to prevent contractures of heel cords, hips, knee and elbows. Occasionally splints and/or a footboard may be helpful. The initial physical therapy should be limited to maintaining the joint range of motion. However, once muscle groups attain antigravity strength, gait training can be started.

Psychological support: Acute neuromuscular paralysis is a terrifying experience for any patient but for the child admitted in the PICU, the psychological impact is compounded manifold. The inability to communicate further increases the anxiety. Attention must be paid to assisting communication in a ventilator-dependent, motorically compromised child. This is crucial to maintain the emotional health of a patient during what may be a prolonged, debilitating illness. Means to communicate should be discussed and used much before the peak disability is reached.[3] Allowing the parents to be present with the child during the waking hours further lowers the child's suffering. The nature of the illness and the good long-term prognosis should be discussed with the parents to reduce their anxiety. Particular attention needs to be paid to make the child comfortable by pain control, patient satiety, adequate sleep, comfortable positioning, patient hygiene, and ensuring prompt and delicate tracheal suctioning.[3]

PROGNOSIS

The clinical course of GBS across all age groups is usually favorable, with most cases showing a spontaneous and complete recovery. Despite there being some controversy regarding the prognosis of GBS in children vis-à-vis adults, the consensus in the literature is that children will do at least as well as older patients with GBS. In a group of 49 children with GBS, 80% were reported to achieve complete functional recovery within 6 months of onset of illness and around 20% had mild residual neurological deficits.[6] Another retrospective multicenter study of 175 children reported > 90% of 106 children to be free of symptoms at long-term follow-up.[36] A more recent cross-sectional study of long-term (at least 2 years) outcome in children with GBS treated with IVIG found 23% children with evidence of mild muscle weakness, though with minimal impact on function.[37] Factors known to be associated with a poor outcome in adults are advanced age, severely reduced muscle action potential amplitude on EMG, need for ventilatory support, and rapid progession of symptoms.[13] Recent diarrhea, recent CMV infection, inability to walk at 8 weeks, and MRC sum score less than 40 were found to be predictive of poor outcome in an analysis of a cohort of patients in the Dutch GBS trial.[38] Serum and CSF biochemical markers have also been reported to have prognostic value.[39]

REFERENCES

1. Hahn A. Guillain-Barré syndrome. *Lancet* 1998;352:635–41.
2. Winer JB. Guillain-Barré Syndrome. In: Miller DH, Raps EC (eds) *Critical Care Neurology*. Oxford: Butterworth Heinemann 1999;33–49.
3. Venkataraman VV, Chaudhry V. Guillain-Barré syndrome–recent advances. *Indian J Pediatr* 2000;67:635–646.
4. Rees JH, Soudain Se, Gregson NA, Hughes RAC. *Campylobacter jejuni* infection and Guillain-Barré syndrome. *N Engl J Med* 1995;333:1374–79.
5. Visser LH, van Der Meche FGA, Meulstee J, et al. Cytomegalovirus infection and Guillain-Barré syndrome: The clinical, electrophysiological and prognostic features. *Neurology* 1996;47:668–73.
6. Sladky JT, Ashwal S. Inflammatory neuropathies in childhood. In: Swaiman KF, Ashwal S (ed) *Pediatric Neurology*. Philadelphia: Mosby 1997;1202–1215.
7. Jones Jr. RH. Childhood Guillain Barré syndrome: Clinical presentation, diagnosis, and therapy. *J Child Neurol* 1996;11: 4–12.
8. Asbury AK, Cornblath DR. Assessment of current diagnostic criteria for Guillain Barré Syndrome. *Ann Neurol* 1990;27(Suppl):S21–S24.
9. Bansal R, Kalita J, Misra UK. Pattern of sensory conduction in Guillain-Barré Syndrome. *Electromyogr Clin Neurophysiol* 2001;41:433–37.
10. Coskun A, Kumandas S, Pac A, Karahan OI, Gulec M, Bay Kara M. Childhood Guillain-Barré Syndrome: MR imaging in diagnosis and follow-up. *Acta Radiologica* 2003;44:230–35.
11. Hughes RA, van Der Meche FG. Corticosteroids for treating Guillain-Barré Syndrome. *Cochrane Database Syst Rev* 2000;CD001446.
12. Borel CO, Guy J. Ventilatory management in critical neurologic illness. In: Jordan KG (ed) *Neurologic Clinics*. Philadelphia: WB Saunders 1995;627–644.
13. Chalela JA. Pearls and pitfalls in the management of Guillain-Barré syndrome. *Semin Neurol* 2001;21:399–405.
14. Sharshar T, Chevret S, Bourdain F, Raphael J-C. Early predictors of mechanical ventilation in Guillain-Barré syndrome. French Cooperative Group on Plasma exchange in Guillain-Barré syndrome. *Crit Care Med* 2003;31:278–283.

15. The Guillain-Barré Syndrome Study Group. Plasmapheresis and acute Guillain-Barré Syndrome. *Neurology* 1985;35: 1096–1104.
16. The French Cooperative Group on Plasma Exchange in Guillain-Barré Syndrome. Efficacy of plasma exchange in Guillain-Barré Syndrome–Role of replacement fluids. *Ann Neurol* 1987;22: 753–761.
17. The French Cooperative Group on Plasma Exchange in Guillain-Barré Syndrome. Appropriate number of plasma exchanges in Guillain-Barré syndrome. *Ann Neurol* 1997;41:298–306.
18. Mehndiratta MM, Chowdhury D, Goel V. Efficacy and cost–effectiveness of current therapies in Guillain Barré Syndrome. *J Assoc Phys India* 2001;49:459-469.
19. Rudnicki S, Vriesendrop F, Koski CL, et al. Electrophysiologic studies in the Guillain- Barré syndrome. Effects of plasma exchange and antibody rebound. *Muscle Nerve* 1992;15:57–62.
20. Raphael JC, Cherret S, Hughes RA, Anname D. Plasma exchange for Guillain-Barré Syndrome. *Cochrane Database Syst Rev* 2002;(2):CD001798.
21. Jansen PW, Perkin RM, Ashwal S. Guillain-Barré Syndrome in childhood-natural course and efficacy of plasmapheresis. *Pediatr Neurol* 1993;9:16–21.
22. Mahalati K, Dawson RB, Collins JO, Lietman S, Pearlman S, Golden D. Characteristics of 73 patients treated by plasma exchange for Guillain-Barré syndrome. *J Clin Apheresis* 1997;12: 116–121.
23. Kalra V, Dhar V, Haldar D. Plasmapheresis in acute Guillain-Barré syndrome. *Indian Pediatr* 1983;20: 867–869.
24. Nagpal S, Benstead T, Shumak K, Rock G, Brown M, Anderson DR. Treatment of Guillain-Barré Syndrome: A cost-effectiveness analysis. *J Clin Apheresis* 1999;4:107–113.
25. Thornton CA, Griggs RC. Plasma exchange and intravenous immunoglobulin treatment of neuromuscular disease. *Ann Neurol* 1994;35:260–263.
26. Plasma Exchange/Sandoglobulin Guillain-Barré Syndrome Trial Group. Randomised trial of plasma exchange, intravenous immunoglobulin, and combined treatment in Guillain-Barré Syndrome. *Lancet* 1997;349:225–230.
27. Hughes RA, Raphael JC, Swan AV, Van Doorn PA. Intravenous immunoglobulin for Guillain-Barré Syndrome. *Cochrame Database Syst Rev* 2001;(2): CD 002063.
28. Shahar E, Shorer Z, Roifman CM, et al. Immune globulins are effective in treatment of severe Guillain-Barré Syndrome. *Pediatr Neurol* 1997;16:32-36.
29. Abd – Allah SA, Jansen PW, Ashwal S, Perkin RM. Intravonous immunoglobulin as therapy for pediatric Guillain-Barré Syndrome. *J Child Neurol* 1997;12: 376–379.
30. Stangel M, Hartung H-P, Marx P, Gold R. Intravenous immunoglobulin treatment of neurological autoimmune diseases. *J Neurol Sci* 1998;153:203–214.
31. Shanbag P, Amirtharaj C, Pathak A. Intravenous immunoglobulin in severe Guillain-Barré Syndrome in childhood. *Indian J Pediatr* 2003;70:541–543.
32. Wollinsky KH, Hulser PJ, Brinkmeier H, et al. CSF filtration is an effective treatment of Guillain-Barré Syndrome: A randomized clinical trial. *Neurology* 2001;57:774–780.
33. Hartung H-P, Willison HJ, Kiedeier BC. Acute inflammatory neuropathy: Update on Guillain-Barré syndrome. *Curr Opin Neurol* 2002;15:571–577.
34. Roubenoff RA, Borel CO, Hanley DF. Hypermetabolism and hypercatabolism in Guillain-Barré syndrome. *J Parenter Enteral Nutr* 1992;16:464–472.
35. Moulin DE, Hagen N, Feasby TE, Amireh R, Hahn A. Pain in Guillain-Barré syndrome. *Neurology* 1997;48:328–331.
36. Korinthenberg R, Monting JS. Natural history and treatment effects in Guillain-Barré syndrome; a multicenter study. *Arch Dis Child* 1996;74:281–283.
37. Vajsar J, Fehlings D, Stephens D. Long-term outcome in children with Guillain-Barré syndrome. *J Pediatr* 2003;142:305–309.
38. Visser LH, Schmitz PIM, Van Doorn PA, Van der Meche FGA. Prognostic factors of Guillain-Barré syndrome after intravenous immunoglobulin or plasma exchange. Dutch Guillain-Barré syndrome Study Group. *Neurology* 1999;53:558–562.
39. Mokuno K, Kiyosawa K, Sugimura K, et al. Prognostic value of cerebrospinal fluid neuron-specific enolase and S-100b protein in Guillain-Barré syndrome. *Acta Neurol Scand* 1994;89:27–30.

Anju Kapoor

24 Coma

INTRODUCTION

Coma, a medical emergency par excellence, requires to be dealt with speedily and in an organized way.[1,2] According to a number of documentations, coma in children has a better prognosis than coma in adults.[3] In a majority of patients, a probable diagnosis can be arrived at bedside without much investigation if proper attention is given to both the history and physical examination. Simultaneously, it is important to provide the basic life-support.[4,5]

This chapter deals with general aspects of pediatric coma (nontraumatic).

PATHOPHYSIOLOGY

Altered level of consciousness may indicate a primary lesion in the brain or it may be secondary to other serious systemic illnesses such as septic shock. Alertness or arousal depends on an intact reticular activating system (RAS) running through the brainstem from where it projects to the thalami and on to both cortical cerebral hemispheres. Thus, alteration in the level of consciousness can be functionally localized to two areas, brainstem or bilateral cerebral hemisphere. Chemical or structural insult affecting one or both areas can result in altered level of consciousness. A unilateral cortical lesion by itself does not cause an alteration in the level of consciousness, unless it is associated with significant mass effect, causing distortion of the brainstem affecting the functioning of the RAS. For example, if patient is herniating and there is pressure on the 3rd cranial nerve adjacent to the brainstem, signs of brainstem coma, such as certain abnormal eye movements or a dilated pupil will be observed. If these brainstem signs are absent, then the coma is probably due to nonstructural effects on the RAS or bilateral hemisphere disease suggesting a totally different course of action for diagnosis and treatment.

STAGES OF ALTERED CONSCIOUSNESS[6]

Any pathologic process affecting the CNS is capable of producing a wide spectrum of changes ranging from irritability to coma.

State of Consciousness

It is a state of normal cerebral activity in which patient is aware of and able to respond to external and internal environment.

Sleep

Although a state of altered consciousness, is a normal variation of consciousness and patient can be aroused completely, both spontaneously and in response to external stimuli.

Acute Confusional State

It is a state of clouded alertness, associated with agitation, fright and confusion.

Drowsiness

It is a state before stupor and coma, where patient appears to be in normal sleep but cannot easily be wakened up and once awake, tends to fall asleep despite continuous effort to keep him awake. While awake these patients are disoriented and not able to perform higher functions.

Stupor

It is a state of altered consciousness, from which only vigorous stimuli can produce arousal, and that also is brief and incomplete. It is a non-quantitative state of altered consciousness that is very difficult to define.

Coma

It is a state in which the patient makes no physiologically meaningful response to external stimuli or to inner need.

Glasgow coma scale, now modified GCS for children (Table 24.1)[7] is being used as an objective tool to replace

Table 24.1: Modified glasgow coma scale

Eye opening to command			
Score	> 1 year age		< 1 year age
4	Spontaneously		Spontaneously
3	To verbal command		To shout
2	To pain		To pain
1	No response		No response
Best motor responses			
Score	> 1 year age		< 1 year age
6	Obeys		Spontaneous
5	Localizes pain		Localizes pain
4	Flexion withdrawal		Flexion withdrawal
3	Flexion abnormal (decorticate rigidity)		Flexion abnormal (decorticate rigidity)
2	Extension (decerebrate rigidity)		Extension (decerebrate rigidity)
1	No response		No response
Best verbal response			
Score	> 5 years	2-5 years	< 2 years
5	Oriented and converses	Appropriate words and phrases	Smile, coos appropriately
4	Disoriented and converses	Inappropriate words	Cries, consolable
3	Inappropriate words	Persistent cries and screams	Persistent inappropriate cry
2	Incomprehensible sounds	Grunts or restless	Grunts, agitated
1	No response	No response	No response

Score of 8 and less suggest coma. Score of 9 and more excludes coma.

all these ill-defined terms, with description of the state of consciousness confined to three categories of performance-eye opening to command, verbal responses and motor responses.

CAUSES OF COMA

Common causes of coma in pediatric age group are listed in Table 24.2.

CLINICAL APPROACH TO A COMATOSE CHILD

Attending a comatose child differs significantly than attending a conscious child. Here, the management starts simultaneously or even before proceeding for a detailed history and physical examination.

Immediate attention is given to the ABC (Airway, Breathing, Circulation) by checking the respiration, pulse and blood pressure. The first question to ask is "can the child protect his airway?" And if the answer is no, maintain the airway by putting either oropharyngeal airway or intubating the child. Oxygen therapy without or with ventilatory support should be started. Next is to check for vital signs. Presence of Cushing's triad (bradycardia, hypertension and irregular respiration) is an ominous sign of raised intra-cranial pressure (ICP) requiring immediate management (Table 24.3).

Take an intravenous (IV) line and preserve some blood samples, which may be needed later on for some laboratory investigations. If patient is in shock (septic/hypovolemic), give infusion of normal saline or Ringer's lactate 20 ml/kg to maintain blood pressure and peripheral perfusion. A seizing patient should be managed with IV diazepam (0.05-0.3 mg/kg/dose may be repeated every 30 minutes) or midazolam (0.15 mg/kg/dose). Possibility of hypoglycemic coma (blood glucose < 40 mg%) should be confirmed by Glucometer/Dextrostix test and promptly treated with 25% Dextrose given IV (2 ml/kg wt). In absence of bedside sugar testing, IV Dextrose may be given empirically without waiting for the laboratory report.

Hypertension may be the cause of encephalopathy that should be treated promptly with anti-hypertensive drugs (sublingual nifedipine, IV nitroprusside infusion 0.5–8.0 microgram/kg/minute, IV furosemide 1 mg/kg/dose). Heart rate > 200/minute suggest supra-ventricular tachycardia and treated accordingly either with IV adenosine (0.1 mg/kg given by *rapid push* followed by a 10 ml normal saline flush; dose may be doubled to a maximum of 12 mg) or synchronized cardioversion (0.5–2 joules/kg).

If there is history or suspicion of poisoning, gastric lavage (preserve contents for forensic test) along with specific antidote and supportive measures should be initiated.

Table 24.2: Common causes of coma

Metabolic
Hypoglycemia
Electrolyte imbalance like hypo/hypernatremia, hypercalcemia
Water intoxication
Diabetic ketoacidosis (DKA)
Hepatic encephalopathy and Reye's syndrome
Uremic encephalopathy
Acidosis/alkalosis
Drug overdose and toxins
Hypo/hyperthyroidism
Hypoxic encephalopathy
Hypo/hyperthermia
Lactic acidosis and Urea cycle disorder
Structural
Diffuse changes in CNS
CNS infection-meningitis, encephalitis, cerebral malaria
Epilepsy
Hypertensive encephalopathy
Sub-arachnoid hemorrhage
Focal changes in CNS
Head injury
Cerebrovascular accident (CVA) : Hemorrhage, thrombosis and embolism
Cerebritis, cerebral and cerebellar abscess
Subdural empyema
Tumor: Supra- and subtentorial
Vascular malformation
Postictal coma
Psychogenic (Rare)
Depression, hysteria
Popular mnemonic **TIPPS** on the **VOWELS** lists the frequent causes of coma.[3]
A–acidosis, alcohol, **E**–epilepsy, **I**–insulin, **O**–opiates, **U**–urea (metabolic) **T**–trauma, **I**–infection, **P**–poisoning, **P**–Psychogenic, **S**–shock, stroke
Note: Infection, hemorrhage and ICSOL associated with raised ICP (intracranial pressure) with brain herniation are most worrisome. Metabolic disturbances have multi- organ system involvement which may be life threatening other than their effects on CNS.

If psychogenic coma is suspected, inhalation of concentrated liquor ammonia can be tried.

Quick Clinical Examination

After stabilizing the patient with these emergency measures, do a quick clinical assessment to:

1. Determine the severity of neurologic injury and evidence of impending brain herniation or CNS infection.
2. Find out the base line status of the patient. Repeated assessment later on will tell the ongoing status of the condition.

Table 24.3: Management of raised ICP

A. Non-Pharmacological Measures
1. Head up by 30 degrees and in neutral position
2. Cold sponging to control hyperthermia
3. Restriction of fluid intake to 2/3rd of the requirement
4. Ensure adequate oxygenation
5. Hyperventilation to reduce PaCO2 below 25 mmHg
6. Avoid excessive stimulation like suctioning
B. Pharmacological Measures
1. Osmotic diuresis by mannitol 0.25-1 g/kg wt IV every 2-4 hourly
2. Injection furosemide 1-2 mg/kg
3. Injection dexamethasone-useful in cytotoxic edema
4. Tablet Acetazolamide (50-100 mg/kg/day) -decreases CSF production
5. In refractory cases thiopental or pentobarbital may be needed

General Examination

Respiratory Pattern (Table 24.4)[9]

Tachypnea is seen in pneumonia, metabolic acidosis (Kussumaul's breathing).

Pulse

It is very slow in complete heart block, very fast in tachyarrhythmias, and irregularly irregular in atrial fibrillation with cerebral embolism.

Blood Pressure

Hypertension may be a manifestation of raised ICP or hypertensive encephalopathy.

Temperature

Fever points to an infectious pathology, hypothermia can be an important clue to myxedema coma (though it is rare).

Breath Odor

Fruity odor in diabetic ketoacidosis (DKA), fetor hepaticus in hepatic coma, fishy smell of uremia. Typical odor is also found in organo-phosphorus (OP) compounds and aluminium phosphide poisonings and alcohol etc.

Cyanosis

Central cyanosis in respiratory failure and congenital cyanotic heart disease; peripheralcyanosis is seen in shock.

Head

Bruising over mastoid (Battle sign), depressed fracture of skull, bulging or depressed anterior fontanel.

Ear and Nose

CSF rhinorrhea or otorrhea, hemotympanum.

Table 24.4: Localization of cerebral dysfunction

Level of injury	*Breathing pattern*	*Pupils palsies*	*Ocular*	*Posturing*
Hemispheres/diencephalons	Cheyne-Stokes	Normal/dilated	Upward gaze difficulty	Decorticate
Midbrain	Central neurogenic hyper-ventilation	Dilated/palsy	III, IV nerve	Decerebrate
Pons	Apneustic	Normal/miotic	Loss of oculocephalic reflex	Flaccid
Medulla	Ataxic/Biot	Midposition	Loss of oculocephalic reflex	Flaccid

Cheyne-Stokes breathing: A phase of gradually deepening respiration is followed after a period of very deep rapid breaths, by a phase of slowly decreasing resp. excursion and rate. May be seen with large unilateral ICSOL with brain stem distortion.

Central neurogenic hyperventilation: Persistent tachypnea and hyperpnea.

Apneustic breathing: Similar to Cheyne-Stokes, but hyperpnea and apnea cycles at short interval.

Ataxic/Biot breathing: Irregularly irregular with respect to both rate and depth, due to damage of medullary respiratory neurons.Irregular, slow, deep and gasping resp. sometimes associated with hiccups suggest terminal medullary failure.

Oculocephalic reflex (doll's eye movement): Elicited by passively turning the head to one side and noting that the eyes move in the opposite direction. This means the function of the brain stem is intact. In most patients with drug-induced coma, doll's eye movements are normal.

Eye

- Pupil size and reaction–constricted in OP poisoning, pontine hemorrhage; dilated in hypoxic encephalopathy, unequal size in herniation.
- Fundus examination for papilledema (sign of raised ICP).
- Eye movements for cranial nerve palsy. Sixth nerve palsy is usually associated with raised ICP.
- Fluttering of eyelids, Bell's phenomenon with normal neurological assessment favors psychogenic coma.

Icterus

Hepatic coma, Reye's syndrome , cerebral malaria.

Tongue Bite

Seizure disorder.

Neck

Goitre in thyroid disorders. Do not move if injured.

Clothings

For identification, any drugs or prescriptions, suicidal note etc.

Systemic Examination

CVS

Arrhythmias (syncope, hypoxic encephalopathy), extreme bradycardia or tachycardia, murmurs, pericardial friction rub.

Chest

Air entry and crepitations (infection).

Abdomen

Hepatomegaly and splenomegaly (malaria, tuberculosis, liver pathology) ascites (chronic liver disease).

Neurological Examination

Important components of neurological assessment are given in Table 24.4.

Spotlight should be on

- Assessment of level of consciousness by GCS,
- Evidence of focal signs (asymmetry in tone, power and reflexes).
- Signs of meningeal irritation (neck rigidity, Kernig sign and Brudzinski sign) seen in meningitis, encephalitis, subarachnoid hemorrhage, intracerebral hemorrhage and rarely cerebral malaria.

Extremities Posturing (Table 24.4)

After initial examination and treatment, further detailed history can be obtained from the family members and patient should be re-evaluated thoroughly.

HISTORY

Onset

Acute onset of coma suggests cerebrovascular accident, rupture of abscess into ventricular system or hemorrhage is already existing intra-cerebral tumor. Gradual onset suggests slow growing tumors, inflammatory process or metabolic illness.

Seizures

History of similar episodes in past followed by recovery

favors grand-mal epilepsy, but 'syncope' should also be thought of. Seizures of recent onset associated with headache indicate cerebral disease like tumor, encephalitis, abscess or trauma.

Headache

History of headache before onset of coma is common in intracranial space occupying lesions (ICSOL).

Trauma

In head injury . in extra-dural hematoma a brief lucid interval follows the injury, followed by deep coma.

Fever

Presence of fever suggests infectious pathology like meningitis, encephalitis, cerebral malaria, enteric encephalopathy and cerebral abscess or heat stroke.

Underlying Medical Illness

Chronic pulmonary, cardiac, renal and liver disease, HIV infection or lupus may affect the CNS. History of diabetes or epilepsy will also give some clue to the diagnosis.

Drugs and Toxins Ingestion

Relatives might give the history of drug therapy with insulin, phenytoin, salicylate ingestion in viral illness or ingestion of some toxin.

INVESTIGATIONS

Initial Workup

- Complete blood count (CBC) including differential count
- Septic screen, blood culture
- Malarial parasite
- Blood glucose
- Serum electrolytes with calcium
- Renal function tests
- Liver function tests
- Bleeding and coagulation profile
- Arterial blood gases and pH
- Urine examination for color (cola colored in glomerulonephritis), odor, microscopic examination and presence of glucose and ketones (DKA).
- CSF examination, after exclusion of raised ICP.

Neuroimaging

- CT scan head, plain and contrast-should be done urgently if suspicion of raised ICP, ICSOL or trauma is there.
- Cerebral angiography- (arterio-venous malformation)
- MRI head and MR angiography.

Other Tests

- X-ray chest PA view (cardiac / respiratory failure)
- X-ray skull, cervical spine (trauma)
- ECG (arrhythmias)
- Echocardiography (look for congenital anomalies, right to left shunt, clot / vegetation)
- Thyroid profile
- Electroencephalography (EEG)-has diagnostic and prognostic role
- Evoked potentials-normal with intact brain stem function
- Toxicological studies
- Virological assay

Note: This is a comprehensive list of investigations; all tests are not required in every case. The selection and sequence for ordering of the laboratory tests will vary depending on the history and physical examination from case to case.

MANAGEMENT

After managing the ABC and other life-threatening complications like raised ICP, hypoglycemia and hypertension and ensuring that child is stabilized, he should be shifted to PICU.

Definitive treatment depends on the cause of altered sensorium.

Specific Management

Infection

If CNS infection is suspected and child is critically ill, especially with raised ICP, intravenous antibiotic is started within 15 minutes, before lumber puncture (LP) or CT scan of head is performed.[10] IV ceftriaxone 100 mg/kg/day divided into two doses is the empiric treatment of choice for suspected meningitis. Other antibiotics may be used as per the antibiotic policy of the hospital.

Cerebral Malaria

Antimalarial drug(s) should be started as early as possible. Choice of drug(s) will depend upon the sensitivity pattern in that area.

Metabolic Disturbances

DKA, hepatic and uremic encephalopathy are treated as per the protocol of the intensive care unit.

ICSOL/Head injury

A neurosurgeon should be consulted.

Poisoning

Activated charcoal, specific antidote if available.

Psychogenic

Psychiatric evaluation, counselling.

General Supportive Measures

Adequate airway and vascular access should be maintained all the time and if required central venous line and arterial line may be accessed. Fever is to be controlled with tepid sponging and paracetamol. Nutritional supplementation is done via enteral or parenteral route. Care of the back, eyes, skin and bladder is must to avoid decubitus ulcers and exposure keratitis. Continuous oxygen saturation monitoring by pulse oxymeter is helpful for the detection of hypoxia. All vital parameters (heart rate, respiratory rate, blood pressure and temperature) should be monitored frequently. Frequent and systematic neurological assessment is done for the assessment of response to therapy.

(Detailed management of individual conditions can be referred from a textbook of pediatrics/relevant chapters in this book).

PROGNOSIS

It depends on the etiology, depth and duration of coma. Most dramatic recovery occurs in hypoglycemic coma in response to intravenous dextrose. Patients with dilated fixed pupil, absent doll's eye reflex, irregular breathing, evidence of vasomotor center dysfunction, low score in GCS and who had cardio-respiratory arrest any time during the course will have a poor prognosis. To conclude, an organized approach will nearly always give the correct diagnosis and provide the proper management sequence with better chances of survival.

REFERENCES

1. Gupte S. Changing trends in pediatric coma. *Bull Emerg Med Sc* 2003;12:67-69.
2. Gupte S, Chowdhary B. Pediatric neurology. In: Gupte S (ed): *The Short Textbook of Pediatrics*, 10th edn New Delhi: Jaypee Brothers 2004;307-348.
3. World Health Organization. *The Child with Coma*. Geneva: WHO 1998.
4. Taylor DA. Coma in pediatric patients: Evaluation and management. *Indian J Pediatr* 1994;61:13-26.
5. Nair, RR. Coma. In: Gupte S (ed) *Recent Advances in Pediatrics (Special Vol 14: Criticare Pediatrics)*. New Delhi: Jaypee Brothers 2004;1-14.
6. Michael Swash. *Hutchison's Clinical Methods*, 21st edn. Philadelphia: WB Saunders 2002;337-345.
7. Singhi PD, Singhi SC. The comatose child. In: Singh M (ed) *Medical Emergencies in Children*. New Delhi:Sagar 2000; 208-218.
8. Starkman S, Fowler GC. Common neurologic emergencies. *http://www.aan.com/familypractice/pdf*.
9. David A. Lewis SDA, Nocton JJ.Altered mental status. In: *On Call Pediatrics*. Philadelphia: WB Saunders 1998;32-44.
10. Charles G. Prober CG. Central nervous system infection. In: Behrman RE, Kliegman RM, Jenson HB (eds) *Nelson Textbook of Pediatrics*, 17th edn. Philadelphia: Saunders 2004;2038-2044.

Section V

Respiratory Emergencies

Parang N Mehta

25 Acute Severe Pneumonia

INTRODUCTION

Sir William Osler described pneumonia as the "captain of the men of death" a hundred years ago. It remains the most frequent killer of children in India.[1] Every year, millions of children succumb to respiratory infections in our country and around the world. Considering that it is such a common and serious disease, it is not surprising that many children with pneumonia present to hospital in a critical condition. Quick evaluation and prompt, appropriate therapy can make the difference between life and death.

ETIOLOGY

Pneumonia is an inflammation of the lungs resulting most commonly from infection by bacteria, viruses, or fungi. Chemical exposure, radiation, smoke inhalation, reflux-aspiration of gastric contents, and some other causes can also give rise to pneumonia. In our country, bacterial infections are the most common cause of fatal pneumonia. This chapter will concentrate on these (Table 25.1).

Our understanding of the etiology of serious pneumonia has undergone a major change in recent years. We have always known that pneumococci, Hemophilus influenzae, and staphylococci are important causative organisms. Recent studies, both in India and elsewhere,[2-6] have shown that "atypical" organisms like Mycoplasma and Chlamydia species can also cause life-threatening pulmonary infections. Recent guidelines recommend that the term "atypical pneumonia" no longer be used.[7]

Table 25.1: Common bacteria responsible for pneumonia

Age	*Common organisms*
0 – 48 hours	Streptococcus group B.
1-14 days	E. coli, Group B streptococci, Klebsiella pneumoniae, Enterobacteriaceae, Legionella monocytogenes, Staphylococcus aureus, anaerobes.
14-60 days	Enterobacteriaceae, Group B streptococci, Haemophilus influenzae, Streptococcus pneumonia, S aureus, Staphylococcus epidermidis, Candida albicans, Chlamydia trachomatis.
2 months – 5 years	Hemophilus influenzae, Streptococcus pneumoniae.
5 years – 10 years	Streptococcus pneumoniae.
10 years – 21 years	Streptococcus pneumoniae, Mycoplasma pneumoniae

In the West, much pneumonia is caused by viruses. In tropical countries, most pneumonia is believed to be bacterial in origin. Though the clinical features and investigations do vary with the causative organism (Table 25.2), the degree of overlap is such that reliable differentiation is impossible.[7-9]

Fungal and tubercular pneumonias can be severe, but the clinical picture is not acute. Both these organisms cause disease gradually. Aspiration pneumonia is an acute event, and can be difficult to treat, because multiple organisms are usually involved.[10] Common pathogens include anaerobic Gram-positive cocci, Bacteroides melaninogenicus, Bacteroides fragilis, fuso-bacteria, alpha-hemolytic streptococci, Escherichia coli, Klebsiella pneumoniae, and Staphylococcus aureus.

DIAGNOSIS

Much of pneumonia diagnosis is clinical. A child with a history of fever and cough, with tachypnea and signs of respiratory distress, raises the suspicion of a pulmonary infection. It is important to look for signs of respiratory distress such as grunting, flaring, severe tachypnea, and retractions in every child with fever.

Good auscultation is very important to the diagnosis of pneumonia. In a seriously ill child, auscultation is relatively easier than in a struggling, crying child. A febrile child with localised crackles or crepitations usually has pneumonia and should be treated as such. Locally reduced breath sounds or bronchial breath sounds signify possible consolidation. Occasionally, auscultation is unproductive, but percussion reveals an area of consolidation. Oxygen saturation by pulse

Table 25.2: Differentiation of common etiologies of pneumonia

Viral pneumonia	*Bacterial pneumonia*	*Pneumonia caused by "atypical bacteria"*
Prodrome 2 or more days	Rapid onset.	Usually slow onset
Low fever, irritable, GI complaints, myalgia, photophobia.	Appear very sick, and have temperatures above 39°C.	Usually mild illness, but can cause severe and fatal disease. Conjunctivitis common with Chlamydia.
X-rays show hyper-expansion, parahilar peribronchial infiltrates, atelectasis, and hilar adenopathy.	X-rays show alveolar disease, consolidation, air bronchograms, and pleural effusions.	X-rays show diffuse interstitial infiltrates with hyperaeration, peribronchial thickening, and scattered areas of atelectasis.
	Pleural effusions are common.	Bedside cold agglutinin test is positive in Mycoplasma infection.
	Coexisting sepsis is almost diagnostic of bacterial pneumonia.	
Most cases occur in winter	No seasonal predilection	No seasonal predilection
Wheeze with pneumonia usually signifies a viral illness.	A wheeze almost never occurs with bacterial pneumonia	

oximetry is important in the evaluation of all children with respiratory symptoms, though it cannot be used to confirm the presence or absence of pneumonia.[11]

Clinical features and some laboratory tests can give information about the likely pathogen involved in pneumonia (Table 25.2). However, these clinical syndromes are well differentiated in adults and older children. In young children, it is almost impossible to reliably differentiate viral and bacterial pneumonias.

INVESTIGATIONS

Etiological investigation of pneumonia is difficult, because the seat of the infection, the lungs, is difficult to access. Since children do not often produce sputum, identifying the causative agent can be difficult. Older children should have a sputum Gram stain for identification of the involved organism.

A firm etiological diagnosis in young children requires a lung tap and culture, and this invasive procedure is not done routinely because of its invasiveness. It should be considered in:

- A critically ill child in whom a specific etiologic diagnosis might be of importance to guide antimicrobial therapy.
- A seriously ill child who has deteriorated while on therapy.
- A child with pneumonia complicated by underlying disease or drugs which compromise pulmonary defense mechanisms.

Leukocytosis, and elevated C-reactive protein (CRP) and ESR have always been considered a sign of bacterial infection, but are not dependable.[12,13] Adenoviral infections are sometimes associated with high leucocyte counts, and bacterial infections do not always cause an elevation in these acute phase reactants. Serial CRP estimations may be useful as a guide to effectiveness of therapy.[14]

Even research protocols, using lung taps, bronchoalveolar lavage, serology, PCR, and other sophisticated investigations, are able to identify the causative organism only in about half of cases. Besides, these investigations take several hours to days to perform, making them of little value in emergency situations. In a seriously ill child with pneumonia, the treatment of pneumonia is usually empiric.

Two view radiographs are often used for the evaluation of lung pathology. In most cases of pneumonia, they only confirm the clinical diagnosis. However, they should be done in all children hospitalized with pneumonia, even if only to serve as a baseline for follow up radiographs in children with progressive disease. Follow-up X-rays are not indicated in children who are responding to therapy, because radiological resolution takes weeks.

However, children who do not respond to initial antibiotic therapy should have repeat X-rays. These may show another diagnosis like empyema or lung abscess. Some infections cause lung tissue destruction, and the X-ray shows small cavities. This necrotizing pneumonia is caused by virulent organisms like Staphylococcus aureus, Klebsiella, Pseudomonas, Proteus mirabilis, Enterobacteriaceae, and anaerobes. Such an X-ray picture indicates management on different lines.

Blood cultures are positive in only 10-20% of cases of pneumonia. However, bacteremia is a sign of severe and potentially fatal disease.[15] CT and MRI scanning can provide accurate anatomical diagnosis of lung pathology, effusions, and empyemas. They are not indicated in the management of most cases.

A tuberculin test should also be performed if the family history suggests exposure, although it is uncommon for tubercular pneumonia to present as an acute disease.

APPROACH TO MANAGEMENT

Initial Assessment

The initial assessment should include the general condition of the child, and the respiration, mental status, and circulation. Malnutrition, age less than one year, diarrhea, inability to feed, altered mental status, short duration of fever, and bandemia are predictors of mortality in children with pneumonia.[16] Children with immunocompromise from any cause are also at risk for a poor outcome. Such children should be treated as having life-threatening disease.

Children with involvement of large areas of lung parenchyma are likely to be hypoxic. This manifests as tachypnea, intercostal retractions, cyanosis, anxiousness, and the use of accessory respiratory muscles. If a pulse oximeter is available, it should be used on all children with such signs. These children should receive oxygen support, and intubation if necessary.

Children with more severe lung involvement may have shallow breathing, altered sensorium, combativeness, obtundation, or frank coma. Such children need assisted ventilation. This should be started immediately by a bag and mask till intubation and a mechanical ventilator are available. The detailed management of acute respiratory failure is covered elsewhere in this book.

Children with bacteremia/toxemia may be in shock. Cold clammy skin, feeble pulses, hypotension, and stupor are important signs. These children need urgent fluid and inotrope resuscitation, and standard septic shock management. Time should not be wasted on investigating the pneumonia before starting resuscitation.

Indications for Admission

- In infants, respiratory rate > 70/min, dyspnea, intermittent apnea, grunting, and feeding difficulty.
- In older children, respiratory rate > 50/min, dyspnea, grunting, and signs of dehydration.
- Slow, irregular respiration, or signs of exhaustion.
- Hypoxia documented by pulse oximetry.
- Cyanosis.
- Refusal to feed.
- Inability to take or tolerate oral medicines.
- Suspected poor compliance, or inability of the family to care adequately.
- Age less than six months.

Indications for PICU Admission

- Failure to maintain SaO2 > 92% in $FiO_2 > 0.6$.
- Altered mental status.
- Shock.
- Rising respiratory and pulse rates with clinical evidence of severe respiratory distress and exhaustion with or without raised $PaCO_2$.
- Recurrent apnea or slow irregular breathing.

Supportive Therapy

- Oxygen, if the child is hypoxemic.
- Assisted ventilation, if indicated.
- Intravenous fluids, if the child is vomiting or unable to take fluids orally. Tachypnea is associated with increased insensible fluid loss, and dehydration should be looked for and corrected in these children. Children with significant distress should receive a little less fluid than calculated on the basis of age and weight.
- Parenteral nutrition is rarely required–pneumonia does not linger so long. If required, it must not be neglected.

Specific Therapy

Ideally, therapy should be based on etiology. However, an etiological diagnosis is rarely available in pneumonia, and waiting for one could be fatal. Empirical therapy is the rule in childhood pneumonia.

Most pneumonia in tropical countries is bacterial in origin, and antibiotics are indicated, especially in seriously ill children. Though viral and bacterial pneumonias usually present differently, it is not possible, on the basis of clinical features and commonly available investigations, to reliably differentiate between the two. In a child with severe pneumonia, which is a life-threatening situation, the prudent course would be to administer antibiotics.

Choosing Antibiotics

Though empiric treatment is the rule in the management of pneumonia, we need to know something about the pathogen we are aiming for. Since organisms vary with age, antibiotic recommendations are also based on age groups (Table 25.3). In addition, it is important to consider local bacterial prevalence and resistance data.

In children below 2 months, the common organisms are the group B streptococcus, Gram negative bacilli, and Chlamydia trachomatis. Bordetella pertussis is a rare cause, but the pneumonia it causes can be serious. The last two pathogens are macrolide sensitive, and one drug from this group should be used.

In children beyond infancy, the most common cause is still the pneumococcus. Most pneumococci in India are susceptible to amoxycillin,[17] and even pneumonia caused by penicillin resistant pneumococci can be successfully treated with beta lactam antibiotics.[18] When low or intermediate resistance is suspected, amoxicillin should be used in doses of 80-90 mg/kg/day.

However, when drug resistance is suspected in life-threatening disease, it is not justifiable to take risks with drugs that may not work. In such a situation, the drug of choice is vancomycin. Beta-lactamase inhibitors like clavulinic acid have no role, because pneumococci do not produce beta lactamases. They achieve resistance by alteration in penicillin binding proteins (PBP) in their cell walls.

Table 25.3: Antibiotic choices for pneumonia in children

Age	Non severe disease	Severe disease
Below 6 months	Parenteral ampicillin (100-200 mg/kg/day) and Gentamycin (5-7 mg/kg/day).	Cefotaxime (150-200 mg/kg/day) or Ceftriaxone (75-100 mg/kg/day) and a macrolide.
6 months to 5 years	Amoxycillin (50-90 mg/kg/day).	Ceftriaxone (75-100 mg/kg/day) or Cefotaxime (150-200 mg/kg/day), plus a macrolide.
5- 18 years	Azithromycin (10 mg/kg/day) or Clarithromycin (15 mg/kg/day)	IV Cefuroxime (100 mg/kg/day) or Cefotaxime (150-200 mg/kg/day), plus a macrolide

Hemophilus influenzae is another common cause of pneumonia in children. A high proportion of strains are beta-lactamase producers, and therapy should take this into account. In India, Gram negative bacteria are important causes of pneumonia, especially in young children.[19] Treatment of severe pneumonia in infancy should always include coverage for these organisms.

In children over five years of age, Mycoplasma pneumoniae and Chlamydia pneumoniae are common causes of pulmonary infection. Mycoplasma pneumoniae and Chlamydia species were earlier considered to cause only mild pneumonia. We now know that these "atypical" pathogens can cause severe pneumonia, and even death. The important thing to keep in mind is that these organisms do not respond to the beta lactam antibiotics that are generally used to treat pneumonia. The drugs of choice for these intracellular organisms are the macrolides. Since it is impossible to definitely diagnose the etiology of pneumonia, all children with severe pneumonia should receive initial coverage against these intracellular bacteria.

Staphylococci are not considered a common cause of pneumonia, but are important in India.[19,20] Staphylococcal pneumonia is often complicated by abscesses, empyema, pneumothorax, and cysts, and can be life threatening. This organism is often resistant to commonly used antibiotics, and special consideration is required. Staphylococcal pneumonia should be suspected in the presence of an abscess or multiple abscesses, infected scabies, and air leaks or breakdown seen on radiographs.

Antibiotic Considerations

The beta-lactam antibiotics are the most popular antibiotics for pneumonia. The most commonly used is amoxycillin. It is still an excellent drug, for adults, because most pneumococci are susceptible to it. However, most Hemophilus influenzae strains and other Gram negative bacilli are now resistant to amoxycillin, and it must not be used in severe pneumonia in children. When a child with serious pneumonia is admitted, the beta lactams recommended are cefotaxime and ceftriaxone.

Among the macrolides, we can choose between erythromycin, clarithromycin, and azithromycin. All three have been found to be equally effective. Azithromycin has the disadvantage of very low blood levels, which is an important consideration since many children with pneumonia have bacteremia as well. However, in children with serious pneumonia, macrolides are always used in combination with a beta lactam antibiotic. So this consideration may not be as important. One major problem with the macrolides is the nonavailability of parenteral formulations.

One group of drugs that is not often mentioned in pediatrics is the fluoroquinolones. These agents cover Gram positive and Gram negative bacteria, as well as anerobic and "atypical" pathogens. They are clinically effective, comparatively inexpensive, and available in both parenteral and oral forms. Various studies have found them to be as useful as the macrolides, cephalosporins, and amoxicillin in the treatment of pneumonia. However, they are considered unsafe for use in children.

Vancomycin is a valuable drug for pneumonia caused by penicillin resistant pneumococci (PRP) and methicillin resistant Staphylococcus aureus (MRSA). However, it is an expensive drug, and must not be started casually. Besides, it must be given as an intravenous infusion four times a day, so the child must stay in hospital till the course is completed.

Difficult Situations

Antibiotic therapy is a problem in necrotizing pneumonia. The organisms involved are Staphylococci, Pseudomonas aeruginosa, Klebsiella pneumoniae, Proteus mirabilis, other Enterobacteriaceae, and anaerobes. These pathogens are often multi-drug resistant, and knowledge of local resistance patterns is essential. A broad-spectrum penicillin and an aminoglycoside is a good starting point, to be modified in light of clinical response and microbiology reports. Necrotizing pneumonia is often fatal in spite of vigorous therapy.

Viral pneumonias are usually short lived and self-limiting, but can on occasion be severe. Respiratory syncytial virus (RSV) is the most common viral etiology; others are influenza A and B, cytomegalovirus, and adenoviruses. Varicella virus pneumonia is rare, but usually serious and often associated with a fatal outcome. Two antiviral drugs are available for use in children. Ribavirin (given as an aerosol) is mainly effective in RSV infections, but is also active against influenza, parainfluenza, and adenoviruses.

Amantadine is available for systemic use, but has a high incidence of adverse effects. At the present time, antiviral therapy available is neither dependable, nor easily available and affordable.

Followup Care

After initiating treatment, the child must be watched carefully for signs of progressive disease, development of complications like an effusion or empyema, or necrotizing pneumonia. Failure to respond or worsening pneumonia should lead to re-evaluation, further investigations, and a search for underlying factors like structural anomalies and immunodeficiencies (Table 25.4).

Table 25.4: Reasons for nonresponse to initial antibiotic therapy

Viral pneumonia
Inappropriate antibiotics
For example, beta lactam antibiotics for mycoplasma pneumoniae.
Bacterial drug resistance
Immunodeficiency
Severe combined immunodeficiency, hypogamma globulinemia, HIV disease, etc.
Anatomic abnormality
Sequestered pulmonary lobe, bronchogenic cyst, tracheo-esophageal fistula, etc.
Foreign body
Tuberculosis
Fungal infection
Histoplasmosis, blastomycosis, etc.

Once a child is improving, oral treatment should be substituted for parenteral as soon as it becomes feasible. Cefuroxime has both parenteral and oral forms; other parenteral cephalosporins should be replaced by oral co-amoxyclav. The total duration of therapy in severe childhood pneumonia should be at least 7-10 days. Some infections, like staphylococcus, require several weeks of therapy.

Pneumonia is one of the most common emergencies seen in pediatric practice. While much confusion exists about the diagnostic criteria, there are now good guidelines for the management of children with pneumonia. Early, appropriate therapy, both specific and supportive, is important for survival of these critically ill children.

REFERENCES

1. Indrayan A, Wysocki MJ, Kumar R, Chawla A. Estimates of the years-of-life-lost due to the top nine causes of death in rural areas of major states in India in 1995. *Nat Med J India* 2002;15:7-13.
2. Chaudhry R, Nazima N, Dhawan B, Kabra SK. Prevalence of Mycoplasma pneumoniae and Chlamydia pneumoniae in children with community acquired pneumonia. *Indian J Pediatr* 1998;65:717-721.
3. Dey AB, Chaudhry R, Kumar P, Nisar N. Mycoplasma pneumoniae and community-acquired pneumonia. *Nat Med J India* 2000;13:66-70.
4. Mathai E, Padmavathy K, Cherian T, Inbamalar U. Mycoplasma pneumoniae antibodies in children with acute respiratory infection. *Indian Pediatr* 2001;38: 157-160.
5. Lim WS, Macfarlane JT, Boswell TC, et al. Study of community acquired pneumonia aetiology (SCAPA) in adults admitted to hospital: implications for management guidelines. *Thorax* 2001;56:296-301.
6. Clements H, Stephenson T, Gabriel V, et al. Rationalized prescribing for community acquired pneumonia: a closed loop audit. *Arch Dis Child* 2000;83:320–324.
7. British Thoracic Society. Guidelines for the management of community acquired pneumonia in adults. *Thorax* 2001;56 (Suppl IV):1-64.
8. Esposito S, Blasi F, Bellini F, Allegra L, Principi N. Mycoplasma pneumoniae and Chlamydia pneumoniae infections in children with pneumonia. Mowgli Study Group. *Eur Respir* J 2001;17:241-245.
9. Virkki R, Juven T, Rikalainen H, Svedström E, Mertsola J, Ruuskanen O. Differentiation of bacterial and viral pneumonia in children. *Thorax* 2002;57:438-441.
10. I Brook and SM Finegold. Bacteriology of aspiration pneumonia in children. *Pediatrics* 1980;65:1115-1120.
11. Tanen DA, Trocinski DR. The use of pulse oximetry to exclude pneumonia in children. *Am J Emerg Med* 2002;20:521-523.
12. George Russell. Community acquired pneumonia. *Arch Dis Child* 2001;85:445-446.
13. Wubbel L, Muniz L, Ahmed A, et al. Etiology and treatment of community-acquired pneumonia in ambulatory children. *Pediatric Infect Dis J* 1999; 18:98-104.
14. RP Smith and BJ Lipworth. C-reactive protein in simple community-acquired pneumonia. *Chest* 1995;107:1028-1031.
15. Waterer GW, Wunderink RG. The influence of the severity of community-acquired pneumonia on the usefulness of blood cultures. *Respir Med* 2001;95:78-82.
16. Sehgal V, Sethi GR, Sachdev HPS, Satyanarayana L. Predictors of mortality in subjects hospitalized with acute lower respiratory tract infections. *Indian Pediatr* 1997;34:213-219.
17. Invasive Bacterial Infection Surveillance (IBIS) Group, International Clinical Epidemiology Network (INCLEN). Prospective multicentre hospital surveillance of Streptococcus pneumoniae disease in India. *Lancet* 1999;353:1216-1221.
18. Tina Q Tan, Edward O. Mason Jr, William J Barson, et al. Clinical Characteristics and Outcome of Children With Pneumonia Attributable to Penicillin-susceptible and Penicillin-nonsusceptible Streptococcus pneumoniae. *Pediatrics* 1998;102:1369-1375.
19. Patwari AK, Bisht S, Srinivasan A, Deb M, Chattopadhya D. Etiology of pneumonia in hospitalized children. *J Trop Pediatr* 1996;42:15-20.
20. John TJ, Cherian T, Steinhoff MC, Simoes EA, John M. Etiology of acute respiratory infections in children in tropical southern India. *Rev Infect Dis* 1991;13(Suppl 6):S463-469.

Akash Deep, Venkataraman and Radha Ghildiyal

26 Bronchiolitis

INTRODUCTION

Bronchiolitis is an acute, infectious, inflammatory disease of the lower respiratory tract that results in obstruction of the small airways. Symptoms are usually limited to young infants as the larger airways of older children and adults are usually able to cope with mucosal edema. This is one of the most common LRTI of infancy and is associated with significant morbidity and mortality.

ETIOLOGY

It is most commonly associated with viruses, the leading cause being the respiratory syncytial virus (RSV), which causes 20-40% of all cases and 44% of cases involving children younger than 2 years.[1,2] Other viruses include parainfluenza, adeno and influenza. *Mycoplasma pneumonia* accounts for 5-15% of cases of bronchiolitis, particularly among older children and adults.[3] Living in crowded conditions, cigarette smoking in the household, respiratory diseases in the newborn period, poor fetal nutrition all operate to increase the severity of the illness.

Abundant evidence reveals that complex immunological mechanism play a role in the pathogenesis of RSV bronchiolitis. Type 1 allergic reactions mediated by the immunoglobulin E (IgE) antibody may account for clinically significant bronchiolitis.[4] Babies who are nursed with colostrums rich in immunoglobulin A (Tg^A) appear relatively protected from bronchiolitis.[5]

PATHOPHYSIOLOGY

The earliest lesions in bronchiolitis is the necrosis of the respiratory epithelium. There is proliferation of goblet cells which results in excessive mucus production while epithelial regeneration with non-ciliated cells impairs elimination of secretions. The pathology results in obstruction of bronchioles by inflammation, edema and debris, leading to hyperinflation, increased airway resistance, atelectasis and ventilation-perfusion mismatching.

Bronchiolar obstruction→atelectasis of segmental areas of lung → V/Q mismatch → hypoxia → CO_2 retention → respiratory failure.

Infants are most affected as they have small airways, high closing volumes and insufficient collateral ventilation. Recovery begins with regeneration of bronchiolar epithelium after 3-4 days, but cilia do not appear for upto 2 weeks.[6] Risk factors include the following:[3]

- Low birth weight, particularly premature infants.
- Lower socioeconomic group.
- Crowded living conditions and/or day care.
- Bottle feeding leads to more severe bronchiolitis.
- Parental smoking.
- Chronic lung disease, particularly bronchopulmonary dysplasia.
- Severe congenital or acquired neurologic disease.
- Congenital heart disease with pulmonary hypertension.
- Congenital or acquired immune deficiency diseases.

CLINICAL FEATURES

As this disease primarily affects young infants, the clinical manifestations initially are subtle. Infants may become increasingly fussy and have difficulty feeding during the 2-5 days incubation period. A low grade fever, usually less than 101.5°F, and increasing coryza and congestion usually follow the incubation period.

As high as 60% of primary RSV infections are confined to the upper airway. During a period of 2-5 days, this may progress to lower respiratory tract involvement with the development of cough, dyspnea, wheezing and feeding difficulties. Infants younger than 1 month may present with hypothermia. Severe cases progress to respiratory distress with tachypnea, nasal flaring, retractions and irritability and possibly cyanosis.[6]

Physical examination often reveals tachypnea, tachycardia, fever (38-39°), retractions, fine rales and diffuse wheezing. Typical signs bear little relationship to the degree of hypoxia.

- Diagnosis is based on the age and seasonal occurrence, tachypnea and the presence of profuse coryza and fine rales and/or wheeze on auscultation of the lungs.
- Hypoxia is the best predictor of severe illness and correlates best with the degree of tachypnea. The degree of wheezing or retraction correlates poorly with hypoxia.
- First time infections usually are most severe. Subsequent attacks generally are milder, particularly in older children.
- Nonrespiratory manifestations of RSV infections include otitis media, myocarditis, supraventricular and ventricular dysrythmias, and inappropriate secretion of antidiuretic hormone.[7]
- Of infants hospitalized with RSV bronchiolitis, 18-20% develop apnea. Frequency of apnea increases among premature infants whose gestation was less than 32 weeks, infants who have not yet reached the age of 44 weeks from conception and especially among those who have neonatal apnea.[8]

RADIOLOGY

Chest radiography show hyperinflation and signs of segmental collapse and/or lobar infiltrates in 25% babies. Atelectasis is common and contributes to arterial desaturation. Because ciliated bronchial epithelium does not regernerate for 9-15 days, the atelectasis may be persistent and shifting. Chest X-rays are most useful in excluding unexpected congenital anomalies or other conditions.

DIFFERENTIAL DIAGNOSIS

Pneumonia, congestive cardiac failure, aspiration associated with reflux or tracheoesophageal fistula; foreign body in the trachea, tracheo- or bronchomalacia, vascular ring, cystic fibrosis or pertussis Sometimes viral myocarditis may mimick the clinical picture of acute bronchiolitis. A chest X-ray and ECG must be obtained as rarely both bronchiolitis and viral myocarditis may coexist.

TREATMENT

One of the biggest challenges in treating infants who present with wheezing is to differentiate RSV bronchiolitis from wheezing that is caused by early onset asthma Bronchodilators produce at the most only modest response in patients with bronchiolitis. In asthma they form the mainstay of therapy.

Medical Care

Treatment of bronchiolitis is mainly supportive. Despite the prominent role that inflammation plays in the pathogenesis of airway obstruction, corticosteroids have not proved beneficial in improving clinical status in a large, controlled multi-institutional study.[9-12]

- Indications for hospital admission include the following:
  - Oxygen saturation monitoring by pulse oximetry below 92% in room air.
  - Age less than 6 months and unable to maintain oral hydration.
  - Markedly elevated respiratory rate.
  - Desaturation in 40% oxygen ($SPO_2 < 92\%$), cyanosis.
  - History of chronic cardio-respiratory disease.
- Apnea and acidosis are indicators for pediatric intensive care referral.
- Hospital care
  - Administer supplemental humidified oxygen to maintain transcutaneous saturation above 92%.
  - Fluid replacement: These infants are mildly dehydrated because of decreased fluid intake and increased fluid losses from fever and tachypnea. The goal of fluid therapy is to replace deficits and provide maintenance requirements. Avoid excessive fluid administration because this may promote interstitial edema formation, particularly if a component of inappropriate antidiuretic hormone release exists.
  - Frequent nasal and oral suctioning.
  - Monitoring of patients carefully in order to detect apnea.
  - Attention to temperature regulation in every infant should be kept.
  - *Mechanical ventilation:* Infants with bronchiolitis occasionally require mechanical ventilation in cases of recurrent apnea or increased work of breathing with respiratory failure. The treatment of these patients is supportive, with provision of adequate oxygen, ventilation, and hydration. Continuous positive airway pressure (CPAP) and intermittent mandatory ventilation (IMV) with positive end-expiratory pressure (PEEP) have been used successfully in the treatment of these infants.[13]

The usual approach in patients requiring ventilation using IMV and PEEP[17] is to ventilate at rates slow enough to allow adequate emptying during exhalation. In addition, a short inspiratory time is used to optimize ventilation to more compliant lung units without over-distending more obstructed ones.[14] Aggressive weaning over the first 2 or 3 days is not warranted and is usually unsuccessful. Once the illness subsides, weaning can proceed quickly. Infants with progressive hypoxemia unresponsive to conventional ventilation may respond to high-frequency ventilation or extracorporeal membrane exygenation. Current experimental therapies for infants with pulmonary insufficiency from bronchiolitis include surfactant and nitric oxide.[15,16]

Diet

Although young infants have the unique ability to breathe and swallow simultaneously, risk of aspiration when the respiratory rate is above 60 breaths per minute is significant. Fever and hyperpnea may contribute to excessive fluid losses. For these reasons, infants who are hospitalized with bronchiolitis require careful fluid monitoring and provision of intravenous fluids when hyperpnea precludes safe oral feeding.[18]

Although a number of medications and interventions have been used to treat bronchiolitis, at present, only oxygen and racemic epinephrine have been shown to affect the condition of the young child with bronchiolitis appreciably.[19-22] Neither of these appreciably shortens the duration of the disease; however, each may prevent complications and improve comfort.

Therapeutic use of bronchodilators to treat bronchiolitis in infants and young children has been controversial. Efficacy in infants is complex because it can be a function of the pharmacologic agent, the route of administration, the clinical status of the patient, or the adequacy of the outcome measure used to demonstrate an effect.

A meta-analysis reviewed 15 randomized placebo-controlled trials of bronchodilator treatment in bronchiolitis. It concluded that bronchodilators produce modest short-term improvement in clinical features of mild or moderately severe bronchiolitis.[23]

A more recent meta-analysis of 8 clinical trials noted that conclusive analysis for the efficacy of beta 2-agonist therapy for bronchiolitis remains unavailable and that the routine use of beta 2-agonist therapy for bronchiolitis is not supported.[24]

Although evidence about the efficacy of bronchodilators in bronchiolitis is conflicting, administering a beta-agonist, such as albuterol (0.15 mg/kg/dose), on a trial basis to patients with bronchiolitis (particularly if a history of asthma exists) and assessing the clinical response in 10-15 minutes is reasonable. If improvement in retractions, respiratory rate and wheezing is noted, scheduled aerosol treatments may be continued, with additional treatments administered as needed.

Ribavirin, a nucleotide analog, may have a role in certain unique situations.

Ribavirin treatment for RSV infections has been controversial because of the aerosol route of administration, the variable course of RSV infection, drug cost, toxicity, and adverse effects.[26]

The current recommendations of the American Academy of Pediatrics are that ribavirin aerosol therapy may be considered in selected infants and young children at high risk for serious RSV disease.[27]

This includes patients with complicated congenital heart disease, including pulmonary hypertension; patients with bronchopylmonary dysplasia, cystic fibrosis, and other chronic lung disease; patients with underlying immunosuppressive disease; patients who are severely ill with or without mechanical ventilation; and hospitalized patients who are younger than 6 weeks or who have underlying conditions, such as multiple congenital anomalies or certain neurological and metabolic diseases.[27]

Subsequent studies have shown that ribavirin does not reduce mortality rate significantly or lower the probability of respiratory deterioration. Ribavirin treatment did not reduce the diagnosis of reactive airway disease, and pulmonary function test results did not show any differences when assessed 5-6 years after initial RSV infection.

PREVENTION

- Transmission of RSV probably occurs via contact with secretions of infected patients. Meticulous attention to hand washing between patient contacts should reduce the likelihood of hospital staff acquiring RSV infection from patients or of spreading infection by carrying RSV on their hands. Morbidity and death from RSV occurs predominately in children younger than 2 years. Other high-risk infants and children include premature infants younger than 6 months, infants and children with underlying pulmonary or cardiac disease, and those with immunodeficient states.[28]
- Active prophylaxis by the use of respiratory syncytial virus immunoglobulin intravenously (RSV-IGIV) at high doses (500-700 mg/kg) has been shown to prevent RSV in high-risk patients.[18]
- As with any disease, complications of the disease itself and complications of the therapy are present. In most cases, the disease is mild and self-limiting. In infants who are immunosuppressed and those with pre-existing heart or lung disease, RSV bronchiolitis can result in any of the following:
  - Acute respiratory distress syndrome (ARDS)
  - Bronchiolitis obliterans
  - Congestive heart failure
  - Secondary infection
  - Myocarditis
  - Arrhythmias
  - Chronic lung disease
- Complications of therapy include the following:
  - Ventilator-induced barotrauma
  - Nosocomial infections
  - Beta-agonist-induced arrhythmias
  - Nutritional and metabolic abnormalities
- Strict attention to fluid and nutritional therapy, avoidance of unnecessary invasive monitoring, infection control and judicious ventilator management, including the use of high-frequency oscillatory ventilation to avoid volutrauma/barotrauma may preclude many of these complications.

PROGNOSIS

RSV does evoke IgE elaboration. Recent studies suggest that IgE levels can be used as a marker of the severity of the acute disease.[4] Multiple small studies suggest that children who have been hospitalized with RSV bronchiolitis have a higher incidence of reactive airway disease and more abnormalities in their pulmonary function tests than children never hospitalized for RSV. These abnormalities may persist for as long as 5 years, though eventually normalizing. Wheezing and hypoxemia may last for as long as 3–4 weeks. Abnormal airway resistance is not uncommon on long-term follow-up.[29] Most babies have recurrent wheezing episodes. There is double the risk of developing asthmatic symptoms even 10 years after an attack of bronchiolitis Obliterative bronchiolitis, a chronic prognosive respiratory disorder, is a rare sequale of bronchiolitis due to adenoviral infection.

Conflicting small studies have failed to prove whether early treatment of acute RSV bronchiolitis with ribavirin reduces the persistence of pulmonary dysfunction.

REFERENCES

1. Klassen TP. Recent advances in the treatment of bronchiolitis and laryngitis. *Pediatr Clin North Am* 1997;44:249-261.
2. Everard ML. Bronchiolitis: Origins and optimal management. *Drugs*1995;49:885-896.
3. Henderson FW, Clydewa JR, Colier AM, et al. The etiologic and epidemiologic spectrum of bronchiolitis in pediatric practice. *J Pediatr* 1979;95:183-190.
4. Welliver RC, Wong DT, Sun M, et al. The development of respiratory syncytial virus specific IgE and the release of Histamine in nasopharyngeal secretions after infection. *N Engl J Med* 1981;305:841–846.
5. Downham MA, Scott R, Sims DG, et al. Breastfeeding protects against respiratory syncytial virus infections. *Br Med J* 1976;31:274-276.
6. La Via WV, Marks MI, Stutman HR. Respiratory Syncytial virus Puzzle: clinical features, pathophysiology, treatment and prevention. *J Pediatr* 1992;121: 503-510.
7. Njoku DB, Kliegman RM. Atypical intraputrionary presentations of severe respiratory synkytial virus infection requiring intensive care. *Clin Pediatr (Phila)* 1993;32:455-460.
8. Abreve Silva FA, Breyinoa V, Simpson H. Sleep apnea in acute bronchiolitis. *Arch Dis Child* 1982; 57:467-472.
9. Lugo RA, Nahata MC. Pathogenesis and treatment of bronchiolitis. *Clin Pharm* 1993;12:95-116.
10. Daugbjerg P, Brenoe E, Forchhammer H, et al. A comparison between nebulized terbutaline, nebulized corticosteroids and systemic corticosteroids for acute wheezing in children up to 18 months of age. *Acta Paedtr* 1993;82:547-551.
11. Leer JA Jr, Green JL, Heimlich EM, et al. Corticosteroid treatment in bronchiolitis. A controlled, collaborative study in 297 infants and children. *Am J Dis Child* 1969;117:495-503.
12. Springer C, Bar-Yishay E, Uwayyed K, et al. Corticosteroids do not affect the clinical or physiological status of infants with bronchiolitis. *Pediatr Pulmonol* 1990;5:181-185.
13. Arnold JH, Hanson JH, Toro-Figuero LO et al. Prospective, randomized comparison of high-frequency oscillatory ventilation and conventional mechanical ventilation in pediatric respiratory failure. *Crit Care Med* 1994;22:1530-1539.
14. Gavin R, Anderson B, Percival T. management of severe bronchiolitis: indications for ventilator support. *NZ Med J* 1996;109:137-139.
15. Leclerc F, Riou Y, Martinot A, et al. Inhaled nitric oxide for severe respiratory syncytial virus infection in an infant with bronchopulmonary dysplasia. *Intensive Care Med* 1994;20: 511-512.
16. Moller JC, Schaible TF, Reiss I, et al. Treatment of severe non-neonatal ARDS in children with surfactant and nitric oxide in a "pre-ECMO"-situation. *Int J Artif Organs* 1995;18:598-602.
17. Beasley JM, Jones SE. Continuous positive airway pressure in bronchiolitis. *Br Med J* 1981;283:1506-1508.
18. Wohl ME, Chernick V. Treatment of acute bronchiolitis. *N Engl J Med* 2003;349:82-83.
19. Sanchez I, De Koster J, Powell RE et al. Effect of racemic epinephrine and salbutamol on clinical score and pulmonary mechanics in infants with bronchiolitis. *J Pediatr* 1993;122: 145-151.
20. Menon K, Sutcliffe T, Klassen TP. A randomized trial comparing the efficacy of epinephrine with salbutamol in the treatment of acute bronchiolitis. *J Pediatr* 1995;126:1004-1007.
21. Lowell DI, Lister G, Von Koss H, McCarthy P. Wheezing in infants: the response to epinephrine. *Pediatrics* 1987;79: 939-945.
22. Kristjansson S, Lodrup Carlsen KC, Wennergren G et al. Nebulized racemic adrenaline in the treatment of acute bronchiolitis in infants and toddlers. *Arch Dis Child* 1993;69:650-654.
23. Kellner JD, Ohlsson A, Gadomski AM, Wang EE. Efficacy of bronchodilator therapy in bronchiolitis. A meta-analysis. *Arch Pediatr Adolesc Med* 1996;150:1166-1173.
24. Flores G, Horwitz RI. Efficacy of beta2-agonists in bronchiolitis; A reappraisal and meta-analysis. *Pediatrics* 1997;100: 233-239.
25. La Via WV, Marks MI, Stutman HR. Respiratory syncytial virus puzzle: Clinical features, pathophysiology, treatment and prevention. *J Pediatr* 1992;121:503-510.
26. Smith RA. Background and mechanism of action of rebavirin. In: Smith RA, Knight V, Smith JAD (eds) *Clinical Applications of Ribavirin*. Orlando: Academic Press 1984;18.
27. AAP. Reassessment of the indications for rebavirin therapy in respiratory syncytial virus infections. American Academy of Pediatrics Committee on Infectious Diseases. *Pediatrics* 1996;97:137-140.
28. Henderson FW, Collier AM, Clyde WA Jr, Denny FW. Respiratory-syncytial-virus infections, reinfections and immunity. A prospective, longitudinal study in young children. *N Engl J Med* 1979; 300:530-534.
29. Krilov LR, Mandel FS, Barone SR, Fagin JC. Follow-up of children with respiratory syncytial virus bronchiolitis in 1986 and 1987: potential effect of rebavirin on long term pulmonary function. The Bronchiolitis Study Group. *Pediatr Infect Dis* J 1997;16:273-276.

Rekha Harish

27 Acute Severe Asthma

INTRODUCTION

Asthma, also known as *hyperreactive airway disease,* is the most common chronic lung disease of childhood. Despite advances, asthma in general and acute severe asthma in particular continues to be surrounded by a plethora of controversies varying from etiology through pathogenesis to management.[1-4]

Around 10-15% of boys and 7-10% of girls in the west suffer from asthma as compared to 5-30% of Asian children. Deteriorating environmental scenario is reflected clearly by increasing prevalence of this illness in all age groups. As for instance, Bangalore, a metro, has shown three fold increase in asthma cases over the last 15 years.[5] Boys are twice more likely to be affected in prepubertal age but later on the sex incidence is equal. Around 80-90% of children have onset under 5 years of age. This age group not only has anatomical and physiological drawbacks but quite frequently is a a victim of indoor air pollution a well-recognized risk factor for childhood asthma.

Currently also labelled as a "diffuse obstructive lung disease", involving both large and small air passages in the lungs, asthma has two chief components, namely

- Hyperreactivity of airways.
- High degree of reversibility (spontaneous/following treatment).

A genetic predisposition coupled with environmental factors (triggering agents/allergens) explain most of the events. Various allergic stimuli/irritants in a genetically predisposed hyperreactive airway initiate bronchoconstriction and inflammatory response. Viral infections are the most common precipitating factor (40%). The common viruses implicated are respiratory syncytial virus, para influenza virus, corona virus and rhino virus. Other stimuli include inhaled allergens viz dust mites, pollens, molds, cockroach/pet's allergens, cigarette smoke, odors and drugs (NSAIDs, β-receptor antagonists, metabisulfite and benzalkonium chloride/edetate sodium present in some nebulization solutions).

ETIOPATHOGENESIS

The airway obstruction occurs not only because of broncho-constriction but other inflammatory mechanisms like hyper-secretion of mucus, mucosal edema, cellular infiltration, desquamation of epithelial and inflammatory cells also significantly contribute towards it. Therefore grossly there are two major components of airway obstruction (a) bronchoconstriction (b) Inflammation of which former occurs as an early immune response and latter in the late phase of immune response (Fig 27.1).[6] This process can initiate as a result of wide variety of autonomic, immunologic, infectious, endocrinal and even emotional factors.

The magnitude of bronchial obstruction is best evaluated by pulmonary function testing which is invaluable in screening suspects and monitoring an acute episode. An increase in at least 10% of PEFR/FEV1 after aerosol therapy is strongly suggestive of asthma. A fall in peak expiratory flow rate if monitored 2-3 times a day can predict exacerbation and encourage early intervention. An increase in diurnal variability of more than 30% indicates worsening of asthma.

CLINICAL FEATURES

History often reveals the diagnosis. Clues to diagnosis which may be present in history are:

- Onset triggered by exposure to an allergen/irritant/drug.
- Concomitant rhinitis/nasal polyp/sinusitis/atopy in 80%.
- Family history of asthma/allergy
- Artificially-fed baby
- Indoor environmental pollution e.g. biomass fuel/passive smoking/house-hold generator etc.

Symptoms may include cough (90%), chest discomfort,

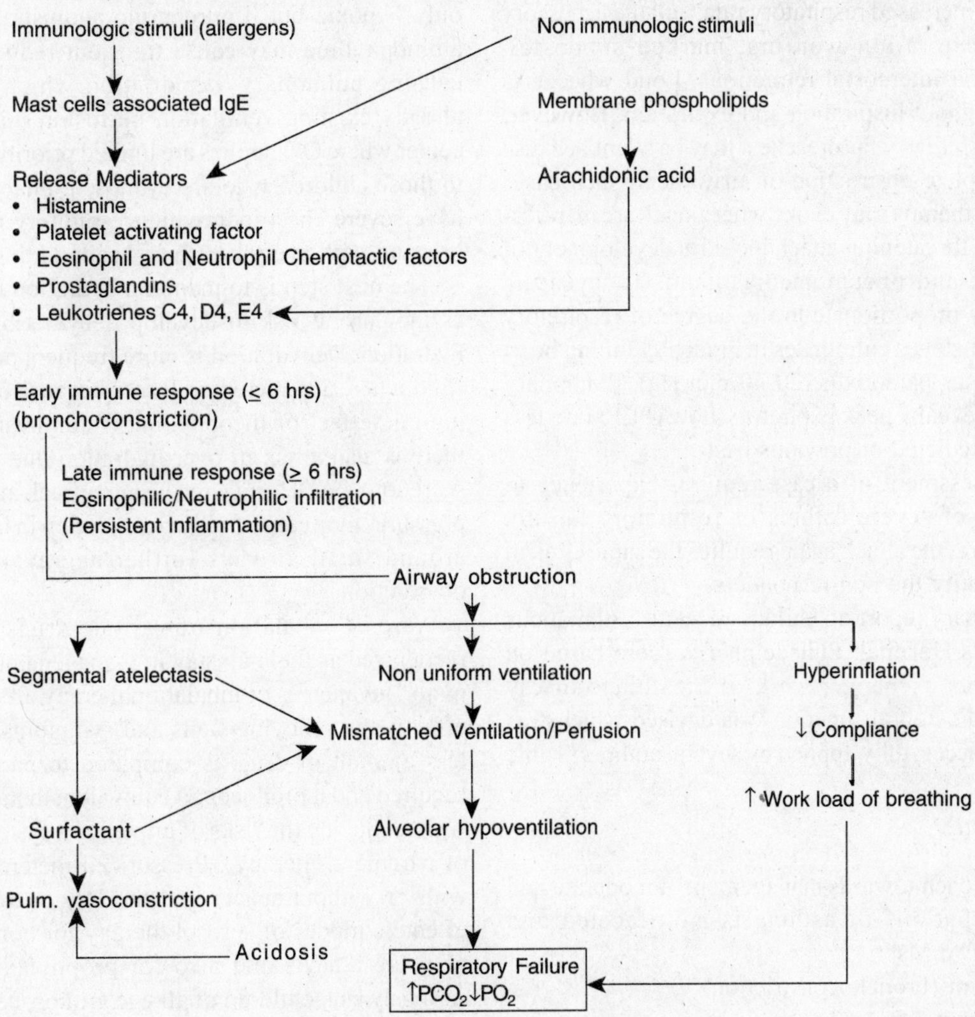

Fig 27.1: Pathophysiology of asthma

Table 27.1: Clinical asthma evaluation score

Score	*0*	*1*	*2*
PO_2 (mm Hg)/Cyanosis	70-100 in air/None	< 70 in air	< 70 in 40%O_2
Inspiratory breath sounds	Normal	Unequal	Decreased/absent
Use of accessory muscles	None	Moderate	Maximal
Expiratory wheezing	None	Moderate	Marked
Cerebral functions	Normal	Depressed/agitated	Coma

Score 5 or more indicates impending respiratory failure
Score 7 or more with $PCO_2 \geq 65$ mm Hg indicates existing respiratory failure.[8]

gagging or vomiting with cough (74%), breathlessness and wheezing, increasing difficulty in walking, talking and feeding, pain abdomen (3%), etc. As hypoxia increases there may be evident changes in sensorium. Initially the child is agitated but later on he becomes drowsy. Development of cyanosis is an ominous sign. While an older child with severe asthma is breathless even at rest, an infant stops feeding. Such children are restless in supine position and prefers an upright/tripod like position. Speech becomes fragmented and limited to words.

Children at high risk for asthma related deaths should receive immediate attention. High-risk factor include:

- History of severe episodes/prior intubation.
- Two or more hospitalizations for asthma in last year.
- Current use of systemic steroids/steroid dependence.
- Use of ≥ 2 canisters of β 2 agonist in last month.[6]

Examination reveals an anxious, irritable, sweating child with markedly increased respiratory rate,* all the accessory muscles of respiration working, marked subcostal, suprasternal and intercostal retractions. Loud wheeze is common throughout inspiration and expiration. However, in imminent respiratory failure, chest may be silent because of almost complete obstruction of airways. In such cases bronchodilator therapy may evoke wheezing. Rare manifestations of a life threatening attack includes development of pneumothorax and pneumomediastinum. Tachycardia though initially proportionate to the degree of respiratory distress, in later stages culminates in gradually falling heart rate** and pulsus paradoxus (20-40 mm Hg). Pulmonary function tests reveal a peak expiratory flow (PEF) rate less than 70% of predicted or previous best.

Clinical assessment of a case requires experience to identify cases of severe asthma or respiratory failure. Evolution of an acute attack again requires the same clinical acumen to identify the non-responders.

In a preliminary report on childhood status asthmaticus from Children's Hospital, Philadelphia, a score based on oxygenation gas exchange, work of breathing, airway obstruction and cerebral function was devised which was subsequently successfully applied by several authors (Table 27.1).

MANAGEMENT

The initial approach towards management of moderate and severe exacerbations of asthma is multifaceted and summarized by "6 Ms":[1]

1. Muscle spasm (bronchoconstriction)
2. Mucosal edema
3. Metabolic correction
4. Mucus secretion
5. Monitoring for infections, and
6. Mechanical ventilatory support.

All these children require hospitalization in a calm atmosphere. Installation of arterial catheter is required for arterial blood gas analysis (PO_2, PCO_2, and pH), complete blood count (CBC) and serum electrolytes. O_2 saturation should be assessed and cardiac monitoring be initiated as these children are predisposed to cardiac arrhythmias due to hypoxia, acid base disturbance and cardiotoxicity of bronchodilators.

O_2 administration by mask or nasal prongs is recommended at the flow rate of 2-3 litres/min to achieve PaO_2 of 70-90 mm Hg or O_2 saturation > 92%. Humidification is required if O_2 is administered by nasopharyngeal catheter but not if it is administered by nasal prongs/catheter. Not only hypoxia but β adrenergic agonists and intravenous aminophylline may cause transient reduction of PO_2 by causing pulmonary vasodilation which aggravates the already existing ventilation perfusion mismatching. In a center where O_2 supplies are limited priority should be given to those children who are cyanosed, unable to take feeds, have severe chest indrawing, respiratory rate of ≥ 70/min or grunt with every breath or headnodding.

The next step is to maintain hydration of these patients as they are at risk to develop dehydration or even over-hydration. Dehydration is more frequent due to inadequate fluid intake and increased losses because of tachypnea and diuretic effect of theophylline if administered. However, there is also a risk of over-hydration due to inappropriate secretion of ADH and large negative peak inspiratory pleural pressures may cause fluid accumulation in interstitial spaces around small airways further aggravating the airway obstruction.

Aerosol inhalation of various drugs has long been recognized as the mainstay in management of asthma. The major advantages of inhalation therapy are that it is rapidly effective in relieving signs and symptoms, a substantially less amount of drug as compared to parenteral route is required and it produces an equivalent therapeutic response while reducing the risks of unpleasant systemic side effects of parenteral therapy.[5] Pressurized metered dose inhalers with or without spacer and the Dry powder inhalers are effective modes of aerosol therapy for home management of acute attacks and also for prophylaxis. However in seriously sick children of all age groups, nebulizers are the preferred mode of drug delivery to the lungs. Despite airway obstruction which may limit aerosol delivery to the peripheral airways, aerosol therapy is probably more effective than traditional epinephrine. Commonly used inhaled β_2 agonists which can be administered by this route include salbutamol, albuterol and terbutaline. Anticholinergics like Ipratropium bromide are advocated as adjunct if the response to β_2 agonist is inadequate.[10]

In a primary care center where nebuliser is not available parenteral bronchodilator therapy is the option. After a trial of epinephrine 0.01 ml/kg (1:1000 dil.) subcutaneously in 2-3 doses at 15-20 min interval, a short burst of oral or parenteral steroids are recommended for those children anticipated in the late phase of inflammation. The other parenteral bronchodilators available are terbutaline and theophylline. Terbutaline is administered subcutaneously 0.01 mg/kg (maximum 0.3 mg) or intravenously (10 μg/kg bolus followed by 0.5 μg/kg/min increasing gradually by 0.2 μg/kg/min to 3-6 μg/kg/min. Theophylline does not score over b_2 agonists but is indicated in patients already on theophylline maintenance therapy or unable to tolerate β_2 agonists therapy. The dose

* Normal respratory rates/min ≤ 2 months ≤ 60, 2-12 months < 50, 1-5 years < 40, 6-8 years < 30

** Normal pulse/heart rates/min: – 2-12 months < 160, 1-2 years < 120/min, 2-8 years < 110/min.

recommended is 4-5 mg/kg IV over 20 min every 6 hours or 5 mg/kg loading followed by 0.75–1.25 mg/kg/hr constant infusion. Serum theophylline levels are indicated for monitoring these patients and aim should be to achieve a steady state concentration of 12-15 μg/ml.[11]

Oral or rarely intravenous (IV) or intramuscular (IM) corticosteroids should be given early to all patients with moderate to severe symptoms. There is probably no significant benefit of giving IV or IM steroids if patient is able to take medications orally. Inhaled or nebulised corticosteroids cannot be recommended as equivalent to systemic steroids till date.[8] Corticosteroid preferred is methyl prednisolone 1 mg/kg every 6 hours for first 48 hours followed by 1-2 mg/kg/day in two divided doses till 70% PEFR is attained. Methyl prednisolone scores over hydrocortisone as it has less mineralocorticoid activity when given in high doses. Steroids improve oxygenation, decrease airway obstruction and shorten the recovery time.[6]

If respiratory failure is impending mechanical ventilation should be anticipated. An elective intubation with diazepam, vecuronium and atropine premedication is preferred to emergency intubation. Important points in relation to intubation are given in Table 27.2.

Table 27.2: Intubation for acute severe asthma (refractory): Important points

- Rapid sequence induction is required for intubation in emergency department because of the likelihood of full stomach.
- Child should be preoxygenated and placed on respiratory and cardiac monitors with suction facilities.
- Ketamine (1-3 mg/kg) is recommended because of its bronchodilatory effect.
- Etomidate (0.2–0.4 mg/kg) may also be used for induction.
- Anticholinergic agents may also be added to reduce oral secretions.
- Midazolam, a benzodiazepine, 0.05 mg/kg is used to reduce the risk of an emergence reaction or dysphoria when awakening from sedation.
- Succinylcholine (2-4 mg/kg) or atracurium could be used as a rapidly-acting paralytic agent.
- Sellick maneuver (cricoid pressure) during intubation can decrease the aspiration risk.
- Correct placement of endotracheal tube is monitored by end-tidal CO_2 Monitor, equal bilateral breath sounds, visualization of chest movements and radiography.

A volume cycled ventilation with short inspiratory and long expiratory phase with 10-15 ml/kg tidal volume at 8-15 breaths/min and peak pressures of less than 60 cms H_2O is recommended. The goal is to maintain PCO_2 between 40–60 mm Hg by improving oxygenation but without barotrauma.

Breathing Heliox an 80: 20 mixture of helium to oxygen may reduce pulsus paradoxus, improve PEFR and avert mechanical ventilation in some patients.

In a refractory case, IV magnesium sulfate infusion may be resorted to. It has elicited improvement occasionally in children more than 6 years of age in a dose of 25 mg/kg (maximum of 2 gm) over 20 minutes.[13]

This agent acts by both antiinflammatory and bronchodilator effect. Minor adverse-effects include tingling, numbness, flushing, warmth, malaise, etc.[14]

Nebulized magnesium sulfate, though evaluated, is not quite effective.

Sedation of nonventilated agitated patients is best avoided as tranquilizers, morphine and other opiates are respiratory depressants. Even sedating medications present in cough suppressants can be detrimental.

Antibiotics given as a routine have neither shown to alter the course of status asthmaticus nor do they reduce the incidence of infectious complications.

Thus, the highlight of current strategies in management of childhood asthma include

- Prompt diagnosis
- Recognition of its severity
- Early identification of high risk factors for acute severe asthma, and
- Prompt institution of steroid therapy, as and when indicated, in addition to other measures.

REFERENCES

1. Bahrainwala AH. Medical treatment of acute asthma in the emergency department. *Synopsis* 2003;5:5-13.
2. Gupte S. Acute severe asthma: Role of prompt steroid therapy. *Eur Chron Emerg* Med 2002;23:65-66.
3. Lahiri K, Nadkarni UB. Childhood asthma: Targeting early diagnosis and effective therapy. In: Gupte S, Lahiri K (eds) *Recent Advances in Pediatrics (Special Vol 10: Pulmonology).* New Delhi: Jaypee Brothers 2002;41-58.
4. Gupta A, Gupta P. Controversies in childhood asthma. In: Gupte S, Lahiri K (eds) *Recent Advances in Pediatrics (Special Vol 10: Pulmonology*). New Delhi: Jaypee Brothers 2002;99-114.
5. Parmesh H, Subramanyam L, Somu N. Bronchial asthma. In: Parthasarthy A (ed) *IAP Text Book of Pediatrics* New Delhi: Jaypee Brothrs 2002;399-406.
6. Michael Sly R. Asthma. In: Behrman RE, Kliegman RM, Jenson HB (eds) *Nelson Textbook of Pediatrics*, 17th edn. Philadelphia: Saunder 2004;664-673.
7. Plotnick LH, Ducharme FM. Combined inhaled anticholinergics and b2-agonists for initial treatment of acute asthma in children. Cochrane Review. In: The Cochrane Library 2 Oxford: Update Software 2003.
8. David WW, Dowries JJ, Lecks HI. A Clinical scoring system for the diagnosis of respiratory failure: Preliminary report on childhood status asthmaticus. *Am J Dis Child* 1972;123: 227-228.

9. Sly PD. Current perspectives in management of chronic asthma in children. *Indian. Pediatr* 2002; 39:719-723.
10. Shuh S, Johnson DW, Callahan S, et al. Efficacy of frequent nebulized ipratorpium bromide added to frequent high dose albuterol therapy in severe childhood asthma. *J Pediatr* 1995;126:639-643.
11. Strauss RE, Westheim DL, Bonagura VR, et al. Controlled trial of oral prednisone in the emergency department of children hospitalized with acute asthmatic exacerbations. *Pediatrics* 1994; 93:205-208.
12. Scarfone RJ, Fuchs SM, Nages AL, et al. Controlled trial of oral prednisone in the emergency department treatment of children with acute asthma. *Pediatrics* 1993;92:513-519.
13. Rama Devi P, Kumar L, Singhi S, Prasad R, Singh M. Intravenous magnesium sulfate in acute severe asthma not responding to conventional therapy. *Indian Pediatr* 1997;34:389-397.
14. Singh D, Gupte S. Pediatric pulmonology. In: Gupte S (ed) *The Short Textbook of Pediatrics*, 10th edn. New Delhi: Jaypee Brothers 2004;247-279.

Akash Deep, Radha Ghildiyal and Shiv Sajan Saini

28 Pneumothorax

INTRODUCTION

Pneumothorax is defined as the presence of air or gas in the pleural cavity.[1] Primary spontaneous pneumothoraces occur in children without underlying lung disease or trauma to the thorax. Secondary spontaneous pneumothoraces occur in those with underlying parenchymal lung disease. Traumatic pneumothoraces result from injury, often secondary to medical intervention (i.e., iatrogenic pneumothorax). When air is trapped in the pleural cavity, resulting in positive pressure, a tension pneumothorax develops.

PATHOPHYSIOLOGY

Because of the inherent tendencies of the lungs to collapse and the chest wall to expand, the pleural space has a negative pressure compared with atmospheric pressure. Since the alveolar pressure is always greater than the pleural pressure (due to elastic recoil of the lung), a communication between an alveolus and the pleural space results in airflow down the pressure gradient until equilibrium occurs or until the communication is sealed. As the pneumothorax enlarges, the lung becomes smaller.

The main physiologic consequence of this process is a decrease in the vital capacity and a decrease in the partial pressure of oxygen. Healthy patients can tolerate these changes fairly well, with minimal changes in vital signs and symptoms, but those with underlying lung disease may have respiratory distress.

With pneumomediastinum, excessive intra-alveolar pressures lead to rupture of perivascular alveoli. Air escapes into the perivascular connective tissue, with subsequent dissection into the mediastinum. Air may then dissect superiorly into the visceral, retropharyngeal, and subcutaneous spaces of the neck. From the neck, the subcutaneous compartment is continuous throughout the body. Thus, air can diffuse widely. Mediastinal air can also pass inferiorly into the retroperitoneum and other extraperitoneal compartments. If the mediastinal pressure rises abruptly or if decom–pression is not sufficient, the mediastinal parietal pleura may rupture and cause a pneumothorax (in 10-18% of patients).[2]

Primary spontaneous pneumothoraces result from apical pleural blebs lying under the visceral pleura. Primary spontaneous pneumothoraces are typically observed in tall young people without parenchymal lung disease because of increased shear forces in the apex. These patients may have emphysema like changes on CT scan, particularly in upper lung zones.

Secondary spontaneous pneumothoraces occur in the presence of lung disease, primarily chronic obstructive pulmonary disease (COPD). Other diseases that may be present when secondary spontaneous pneumothoraces occur include tuberculosis, sarcoidosis, cystic fibrosis, malignancy, and idiopathic pulmonary fibrosis. Rates of secondary spontaneous pneumothoraces may be increasing because of rising incidence of *Pneumocystis carinii* pneumonia (PCP) in patients with AIDS.

Traumatic pneumothorax can result from both penetrating and nonpenetrating lung injuries. Complications include hemopneumothorax and bronchopleural fistula. Traumatic pneumothoraces can create a 1-way valve in the pleural space, only letting in air without escape, and can lead to a tension pneumothorax.

Iatrogenic pneumothorax is a complication of medical or surgical procedures. It most commonly results from transthoracic needle aspiration. Other procedures commonly causing iatrogenic pneumothorax are therapeutic thoracentesis, pleural biopsy, central venous catheter insertion, transbronchial biopsy, positive pressure mechanical ventilation, and inadvertent intubation of the right mainstem bronchus. Therapeutic thoracentesis is complicated by pneumothorax 30% of the time when performed by inexperienced operators in contrast to only 4% of the time when performed by experienced clinicians.

Tension pneumothorax typically occurs in the intensive care setting in patients who are ventilated. With air trapping in the pleural space, positive pressure rises. This pressure compresses the mediastinum, decreasing venous return to the heart and reducing cardiac output. In addition, owing to ipsilateral lung collapse and contralateral lung compression, gas exchange is compromised, leading to hypoxemia.[3]

MORTALITY/MORBIDITY

- *Spontaneous pneumothorax*:Although some view primary spontaneous pneumothorax as more of a nuisance than a major health threat, deaths have been reported. Secondary spontaneous pneumothoraces can be life-threatening, depending on the severity of the underlying disease and the size of the pneumothorax.
- *Iatrogenic pneumothorax* may cause substantial morbidity and, rarely, death.
  Recurrences usually strike within the first 6 months to 3 years. The overall recurrence rate is about 28% for primary spontaneous pneumothorax and 43% for secondary spontaneous pneumothorax over a period of 5 years.
- Recurrences are more common among patients with COPD and patients with AIDS. Predictors of recurrence include pulmonary fibrosis, younger age, and increased height-to-weight ratio.[4] Evidence of bullous lesions on CT scan or thoracoscopy is not predictive of recurrence.

HISTORY

Most episodes of spontaneous pneumothorax occur at rest. Spontaneous pneumothorax is not associated with trauma or stress.[5]

- Acute onset of chest pain—Severe and/or stabbing pain, radiating to ipsilateral shoulder and increasing with inspiration (pleuritic)
  - Sudden shortness of breath
- Anxiety, cough, and vague presenting symptoms (e.g., general malaise, fatigue) are less commonly observed.
- Dyspnea tends to be more severe with secondary spontaneous pneumothoraces because of decreased lung reserve.

PHYSICAL EXAMINATION

- General appearance
  - Diaphoretic
  - Splinting chest wall to relieve pleuritic pain
  - Cyanotic (with tension pneumothoraces)
- Vital signs
  - Tachypnea
  - Tachycardia (most common finding)—If faster than 135 beats per minute (bpm), tension pneumothorax is likely.
  - Pulsus paradoxus
  - Hypotension (often with tension pneumothorax)
  - Asymmetric lung expansion—Mediastinal and tracheal shift to the contralateral side with a large pneumothorax
  - Distant or absent breath sounds
  - Hyper-resonance on percussion
  - Decreased tactile fremitus
- Cardiovascular—Jugular venous distension (tension pneumothorax)
- Neurologic—Altered mental status
- Patients who are mechanically ventilated are difficult to ventilate during resuscitation. High peak airway pressures are a clue to an impending pneumothorax. A tension pneumothorax causes progressive difficulty with ventilation as the normal lung is compressed.

CAUSES

Causes of pneumothorax may include the following:

- Spontaneous pneumothorax [6]
  - Rupture of subpleural apical emphysematous blebs (accumulation of air between the layers of the visceral pleura that is not confined by connective tissue septa)
  - Physical height (Alveoli are subjected to a greater mean distending pressure over time, leading to subpleural bleb formation; since pleural pressure is more negative at the apex of the lung, blebs are more likely to rupture and cause pneumothorax)
  - Other (Contrary to popular belief, most spontaneous pneumothoraces occur while the patient is at rest)
- Iatrogenic pneumothorax
  - Transthoracic needle aspiration procedures (most common cause, accounting for 32-37% of cases)
  - Subclavian and supraclavicular needle sticks
  - Thoracentesis
  - Mechanical ventilation (directly related to peak airway pressures)
  - Pleural biopsy
  - Transbronchial lung biopsy
  - Cardiopulmonary resuscitation (consider the possibility of a pneumothorax if ventilation becomes progressively more difficult)
  - Tracheostomy

The following diseases can be associated with pneumothorax:

- Chronic obstructive lung disease
- Asthma
  - HIV infection
  - PCP
- Necrotizing pneumonia
- Bronchogenic carcinoma
- Sarcomas metastatic to the lungs
- Tuberculosis
- Cystic fibrosis

- Interstitial lung diseases associated with connective tissue diseases
- Idiopathic pulmonary fibrosis
- Sarcoidosis
- Lymphangioleiomyomatosis
- Langerhans cell histiocytosis
- Trauma—Penetrating and nonpenetrating injury
  - Rib fracture
  - Iatrogenic
- Transthoracic needle aspiration
- Transbronchial biopsy
- Thoracentesis
- Central venous catheter insertion
- Intercostal nerve block
- Tracheostomy
- Cardiopulmonary resuscitation
- Positive pressure ventilation
  - Acupuncture
  - Tall, thin stature in a healthy person or a person with Marfan syndrome.

Large bulla can simulate pneumothorax on chest radiographs, thus requiring CT scan to clarify the diagnosis.

Occasionally, skin folds on chest radiographs mimic the pleural line.

WORKUP

A strong clinical suspicion with a meticulous physical examination of the respiratory system (percussion and auscultation) can clinch the diagnosis. If a patient was doing fine on manual IPPR or ventilator and suddenly deteriorates, pneumothorax should be vigilantly ruled out while keeping in mind the other causes of such deterioration (displacement of endotracheal tube, obstruction of tube and equipment failure).

Imaging Studies

- A chest radiograph is required for confirmation of pneumothorax (Figs 28.1 to 28.4).
  - Although expiratory images are thought to better depicting subtle pneumothoraces (the volume of the pneumothorax is constant; hence, proportionally higher on expiratory images), a recent randomized controlled trial revealed no difference in the ability of radiologists to detect pneumothoraces on inspiratory and expiratory images.[7]
  - In patients with underlying pulmonary disease, the classic visceral pleural line may be harder to detect, because the lung is hyperlucent, and little difference exists in the radiographic density between the pneumothorax and the emphysematous lung.
  - Ratio of lung size to hemothorax size to estimate pneumothorax size.

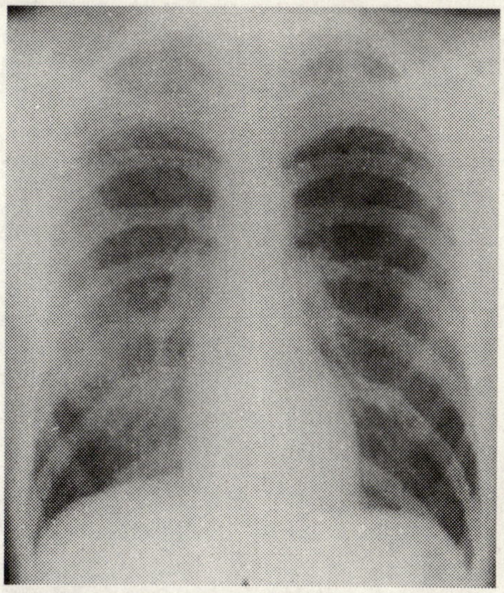

Fig 28.1: Small spontaneous primary pneumothorax

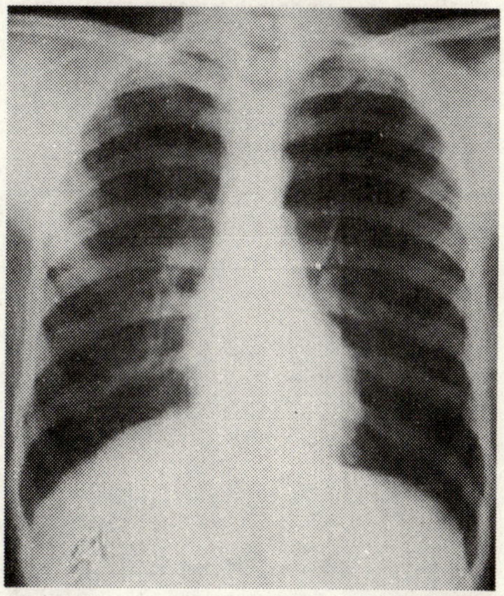

Fig 28.2: Spontaneous primary pneumothorax due to left upper lobe bleb

  - The size of a pneumothorax may be estimated by using the ratio of the lung diameter cubed to the hemithorax diameter cubed.
  - This formula assumes a constant shape of the lung when it collapses and is invalid if pleural adhesions are present.
  - The clinical status of the patient (not the size of the pneumothorax) should be emphasized when making therapeutic decisions.
- A supine chest radiograph may depict the deep sulcus sign (very wide and deep costophrenic angle). The anterior costophrenic recess becomes the highest point in the hemithorax, resulting in an unusually sharp definition of the anterior diaphragmatic surface or an increased lucency in the ipsilateral upper quadrant of the abdomen.

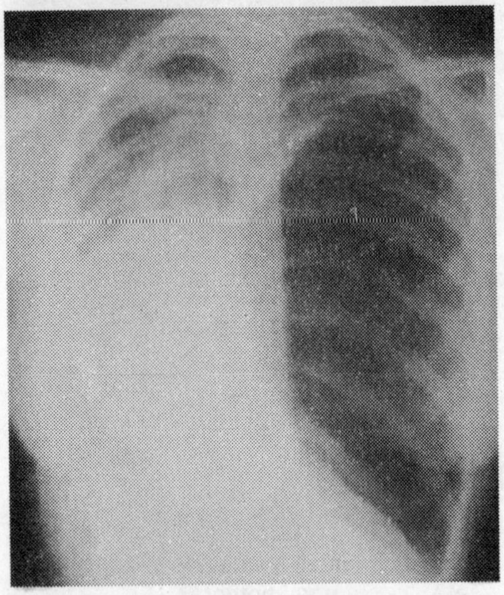

Fig 28.3: Large spontaneous tension pneumothorax

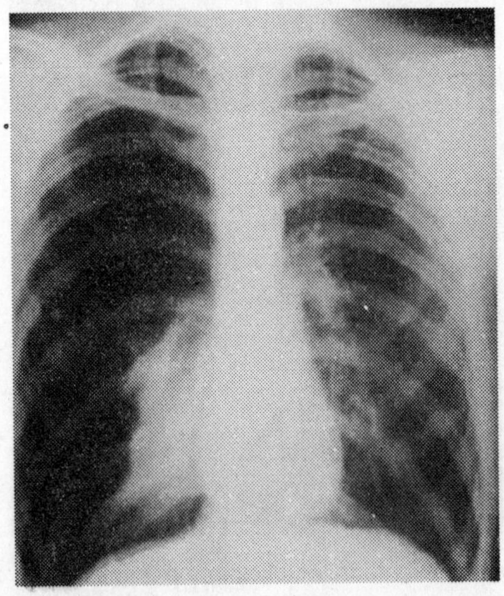

Fig 28.4: Right-sided pneumothorax due to a stab wound

- Confirmation of a suspected pneumothorax that is not readily observed on standard supine anteroposterior (AP) radiograph can be demonstrated by obtaining a lateral decubitus film with the involved hemithorax positioned uppermost.

- CT scan is not recommended for routine use[8] but can help to accomplish the following:
  - Distinguish between a large bulla and a pneumothorax
  - Indicate underlying emphysema or emphysemalike changes
  - Determine the exact size of the pneumothorax, especially if it is small
  - Confirm the diagnosis of pneumothorax in patients with head trauma who are mechanically ventilated

- Method to estimate the fractional size of pneumothorax:
  - Calculate the ratio of the transverse radius of the pneumothorax (cubed) to the transverse radius of the hemithorax (cubed).
  - To express the pneumothorax size as a percentage, multiply the fractional size by 100.

Laboratory Studies

- Arterial blood gas—In patients with severe underlying lung disease and in those with persistent respiratory distress despite treatment:
  - Hypoxemia occurs with increased alveolar-arterial oxygen tension gradient.
  - Hypoxemia tends to be more severe in patients with secondary spontaneous pneumothoraces.

MEDICAL CARE[9]

Treatment goals are air evacuation, lung re-expansion, and prevention of recurrence. Most patients are admitted to the hospital. Administer oxygen to all patients.

Treatment for primary spontaneous pneumothorax includes observation, simple aspiration, and chest tube placement.[10]

Secondary spontaneous pneumothorax usually requires chest tube placement, as does traumatic pneumothorax.[11]

Iatrogenic pneumothorax is frequently treated with observation or simple aspiration.

Tension pneumothorax is a medical emergency that requires immediate needle decompression and chest tube placement.

- Assess the ABCs, and evaluate the possibility of a tension pneumothorax. Assess the vital signs, and perform pulse oximetry. A tension pneumothorax is almost always associated with hypotension.
- Administer oxygen to the patient, and establish an intravenous line.
- Most paramedics are trained to perform needle decompression for immediate relief of a tension pneumothorax.

Recurrent spontaneous pneumothorax requires more definite treatment to prevent recurrence.

- Simple observation is appropriate for asymptomatic patients with a minimal pneumothorax (< 15% of the hemithorax) and without evidence of persistent air leak by radiographic assessment. Unrecognized air leaks can be fatal.[12]
- Oxygen administration at 3 L/min nasal canula or higher flow treats possible hypoxemia and is associated with a 4-fold increase in the rate of pleural air absorption over room air alone.
  - Monitoring pneumothorax size during this time is important.

– No protocols regarding serial radiography or imaging exist; the clinician typically reviews serial vital signs and clinical assessments, using the direction and rate of change in the clinical status to select imaging frequency.

- Simple aspiration (thoracentesis) is performed by placing a plastic catheter over the needle into the pleural space.
  – The puncture site is commonly in the second or third intercostal space in the midclavicular line or in the fourth or fifth intercostal space over the superior rib margin in the anterior axillary line.
  – The skin is prepared with Betadine solution and is covered with sterile drapes.
  – Local anesthesia is performed with 1% Xylocaine solution.
  – Use a 3-way stopcock and large syringe to evacuate air. When no more air can be aspirated or the patient suddenly coughs, the lung most likely has reexpanded.
  – Remove the catheter, and massage the insertion site with sterile gauze to seal the channel into the pleural space.
  – Most authorities consider this procedure to be the first-line treatment of pneumothorax, although the recurrence rate is high, particularly with secondary spontaneous pneumothoraces.
  – Studies show a 55-75% success rate, with a hospital stay of 2.3 days. A follow-up chest radiograph is required.
- Chest tube thoracostomy is usually reserved for patients with first-time secondary spontaneous pneumothoraces.
- Tube thoracostomy
  – If the patient is hemodynamically stable, consider conscious sedation with careful titration of a short-acting narcotic and benzodiazepine.
  – Place the patient in a 30-60° reverse Trendelenburg position. Scrub the site (centered around the fifth or sixth rib in the midaxillary line) with Betadine and/or alcohol.
  – Locally anesthetize site with lidocaine (Use a generous amount, and anesthetize all the way down to the pleura).
  – Make a 3 to 4 cm incision.
  – Use a curved hemostat, puncture (in a controlled manner) through the intercostal muscles and parietal pleura immediately superior to the rib border, avoiding damage to the underlying lung. Spread the hemostat wide to create an adequate opening.
  – Perform a digital examination to assess the presence and location of pulmonary adhesions. Sweep the finger in all directions, and feel for the diaphragm and possible intra-abdominal structures. To avoid losing the desired tract, some recommend keeping the finger in place until tube is inserted.
  – Insert the chest tube along the finger; use a clamp on the tube, if desired.
  – Direct the chest tube posteriorly, and insert it until it is at least 5 cm beyond the last hole in the tube.
  – Attach the tube to a water seal and vacuum device (e.g., Pleur-Evac). Look for respiratory variation of the water seal and bubbling of air through the water seal. Document the amount of blood or other fluids drained.
  – Suture the site, and secure the tube to the chest wall. Cover the site with Vaseline-impregnated gauze, and apply a suitable dressing. A variety of anchoring and closure techniques exist, all of which are probably equivalent.
  – Obtain a chest radiograph to confirm placement and lung re-expansion.
  – A small-bore catheter (e.g., 7-14°F) is safe to use in most patients. Use a larger tube (e.g., 28°F) to reduce resistance in patients who are ventilated and at greater risk for air leaks. Keep the tube in place for 24 hours after the air leak ceases.
  – Air leaks resolve within 7 days of treatment 80% of the time, with an average hospital stay of 5 days.

SURGICAL CARE

Indications for surgical assistance:[14]

- Persistent air leak for more than 7 days
- Recurrent ipsilateral pneumothorax
- Contralateral pneumothorax
- Bilateral pneumothorax.

Procedures that may prevent the recurrence of spontaneous pneumothoraces include the following:

- Chest tube with instillation of sclerosing agent (pleurodesis)
  – A patient treated with this procedure has a recurrence prevention rate of greater than 90%.
  – Talc is the preferred agent for pleurodesis. It can be administered by insufflation or as a slurry.
  – Video-assisted thoracoscopic surgery (VATS)with resection of large bullous lesions and/or insufflation of talc and thoracotomy are considered the most definitive treatment, with a recurrence rate of 2-14% and 0-7%, respectively. While VATS is used to prevent recurrence, not every patient with pneumothorax requires VATS.[14]
  – Indications include an unexpanded lung 5 days after tube thoracostomy, bronchopleural fistula persisting for 5 days or longer, recurrent pneumothorax after chemical pleurodesis, and occupational reasons.
- Complications of surgical procedures include the following:
  – Acute respiratory distress and/or failure
  – Infection of the pleural space

- Cutaneous or systemic infection
- Persistent air leak
- Reexpansion pulmonary edema
- Prolonged tube drainage and hospital stay.

COMPLICATIONS

- Respiratory or cardiac arrest
- Hemopneumothorax
- Bronchopulmonary fistula
- Pain at the site of chest tube insertion, infection, and hemorrhage.

PROGNOSIS

- Complete resolution of uncomplicated pneumothorax takes approximately 10 days.

PNEUMOTHORAX IN THE NEWBORN

Spontaneous pneumothorax usually occurs during the first few breaths soon after birth. The vast majority of infants are asymptomatic. Radiologic surveys have demonstrated an incidence of 1.0 to 20.% of all live births;[15] symptomatic pneumothorax, however, has been noted in only 0.05 to 0.07% of live births.[16,17-19] Most investigators have found a higher incidence of spontaneous pnuemothorax in full term infants. Postmature infants seem to be the most vulnerable.[16,20,21]

Distress is generally evident in the delivery room or soon after arrival in the nursery. Tachypnea (upto 130 breaths per minute) is a universal occurrence. Malan and Heese[17] stressed the frequency and prominence of chest bulge on the involved side.[19] Grunting, retractions, and cyanosis in room air have been noted in virtually all affected infants. As a rule, symptomatic infants have abnormal chest findings that are attributable to lung underexpansion and to displacement of the heart away from the affected hemothorax. Lubchenco was impressed with the frequency and degree of restlessness and irritability among affected neonates.[22] Spontaneous pneumothorax is sometimes a manifestation of serious lung disease. It has long been observed in association with meconium aspiration, RDS, transient tachypnea of the newborn, pneumonia, pulmonary hypo-plasia with renal anomalies, and diaphragmatic hernia. Although spontaneous alveolar rupture is sometimes a worrisome portent of serious underlying pulmonary disease, most infants have otherwise normal lungs. Approximately 80 to 90% are mildly ill and require no therapy other than O_2 supplementation.[16]

During ventilatory assistance, when pneumothorax occurs, tension pneumothorax is usual. Vigilance by expert personnel, particularly nurses, is effective for early detection a significant number of pneumothoraces can be predicted. Early gestational age, RDS, and high ventilatory pressures are the most significant risk factors. Their presence imposes a high risk for air leak. Predictions based on chest film review are more specific. Pneumomediastinum is another predictor that has long been identified as an occasional precursor of pneumothorax.

Identification and relief of pneumothorax can be accomplished within a few minutes by detection of abnormal signs. Tension pneumothorax produces abrupt duskiness or cyanosis. Ogata and colleagues[23] described significant declines of arterial blood pressure, heart rate, respiratory rate, and pulse pressure in 77% of their infants. They did not detect the expected abnormal chest signs. Detection of diminished breath sounds, bulging of the affected hemithorax, and mediastinal shift to the unaffected side are nevertheless valuable early indications.

The definitive treatment of tension pneumothorax is placement of a chest tube and application of continuous suction (–10 cm H_2O), particularly if PEEP is used for ventilatory assistance. Recurrence of pneumothorax during chest drainage is rather frequent. Yu and colleagues[24] described recurrence in 9 of 14 infants. In such circumstances, the existing tube must be replaced if it is demonstrably occluded; if the tube is not blocked, a second one must be inserted.

Pneumothorax as a result of certain procedures is rare. Leake and coworkers[25] reported a pnuemothorax that became evident 3 hours after birth in a term infant. The mother had an amniocentesis shortly before the onset of labor and several hours before the infant's birth. They also summarized three previous reports of pneumothorax, all attributable to entry of the amniocentesis needle into the fetal chest.

Important points for consideration are:

- Imaging studies should not delay the diagnosis of tension pneumothorax. Tension pneumothorax is a medical emergency and requires immediate treatment.
- Chest radiographs may fail to reveal pneumothorax. Radiologists or emergency physicians may fail to recognize the presence of the pneumothorax. A vertical skin line can be mistaken for a pneumothorax, leading to unnecessary and possibly harmful therapy.
- Expiratory chest radiographs do not improve detection of pneumothorax after procedures with the potential to cause a pneumothorax.
- A high index of suspicion for tension pneumothorax is recommended in patients on mechanical ventilation with acute onset of hemodynamic instability, difficult ventilation with high inspiratory pressures, and worsening hypoxemia and/or hypercapnia, even with a functioning chest tube in place.
- Always consider pneumothorax in the differential diagnosis of major trauma.
- Spontaneous pneumothorax is a life-threatening condition in patients with severe underlying lung disease.

REFERENCES

1. Paret G, Dekel B, Szeinberg A. Spontaneous pneumomediastinum in children: Clinical history. *Eur J Pediatr* 1997;156:582-585.
2. Tytherleigh MG, Connolly AA, Handa JL. Spontaneous pneumomediastinum. *J Accid Emerg Med* 1997;14:333-334.
3. Barton ED, Rhee P, Hutton KC. The pathophysiology of tension pneumothorax in ventilated swine. *J Emerg Med* 1997;15:147-153.
4. Lippert HL, Lund O, Blegvad S. Independent risk factors for cumulative recurrence rate after first spontaneous pneumothorax. *Eur Respir J* 1991;4:324-331.
5. Dekel B, Paret G, Szeinberg A. Spontaneous pneumomediastinum in children:clinical and natural history. *Eur J Pediatr* 1996;155:695-697.
6. Ba-Salamah A, Schima W, Umek W. Spontaneous pneumomediastinum. Eur Radiol 1999;9:724-727.
7. Seow A, Kazerooni EA, Pernicano PG. Comparison of upright inspiratory and expiratory chest radiographs for detecting pneumothoraces.*Am J Roentgenol* 1996;166:313-316.
8. Lesur O, Delorme N, Fromaget JM. Computed tomography in the etiologic assessment of idiopathic spontaneous pneumothorax. Chest 1990;98:341-347.
9. Baumann MH, Strange C. The clinician's perspective on pneumothorax management. *Chest* 1997;112:822-828.
10. Smith BA, Ferguson DB. Disposition of spontaneous pneumomediastinum. *Am J Emerg Med* 1991:9:256-259.
11. Baumann MH, Strange C. Treatment of spontaneous pneumothorax:a more aggressive approach? *Chest* 1997;112:789-804.
12. Miller AC, Harvey JE. Guidelines for the management of spontaneous pneumothorax. Standards of Care Committee, British Thoracic Society. *BMJ* 1993; 307:114-116.
13. Miller JD, Simone C, Kahnamoui K. Comparison of videothoracoscopy and axillary thoracotomy for the treatment of spontaneous pneumothorax. *Am Surg* 2000;66:1014-1015.
14. Schoenenberger RA, Haefeli WE, Weiss P. Timing of invasive procedures in therapy for primary and secondary spontaneous pneumothorax. *Arch Surg* 1991;126:764-766.
15. Davis CH, Stevens GW. Value of routine radiographic examinations of the newborn, based on a study of 702 consecutive babies. *Am J Obstet Gynecol* 1930;20:73.
16. Chernick V, Avery ME. Spontaneous alveolar rupture at birth. *Pediatrics* 1963;32:816.
17. Malan AF, Heese H de V. Spontaneous pneumothorax in the newborn. *Acta Paediatr Scand* 1966;55:224.
18. Harris LE, Steinberg AG. Abnormalities observed during the first six days of life in 8716 live-born infants. *Pediatrics* 1954;14:314.
19. Howie VM, Weed AS. Spontaneous pneumothorax in the first ten days of life. *J Pediatr* 1957;50:6.
20. Peterson HG, Pendleton ME. Contrasting roentgenographic patterns of the hyaline membrane and fetal aspiration syndromes. *Am J Roentgenol Radium Ther Nucl Med* 1955;74:800.
21. Emery JŁ. Interstital emphysema, pneumothorax and "airblock" in the newborn. *Lancet* 1956;1:405.
22. Lubchenco LO. Recognition of spontaneous pneumothorax in premature infants. *Pediatrics* 1959;24:996.
23. Ogata ES, Gregory GA, Kitterman JA, et al. Pneumothorax in the respiratory distress syndrome:incidence and effect on vital signs, blood gases and pH. *Pediatrics* 1976;58:177.
24. Yu VYH, Liew SW, Roberton NRC. Pneumothorax in the newborn:changing pattern. *Arch Dis Child* 1975;50:449.
25. Leake RD, Hobel CJ, Lachman RS. Neonatal pneumothorax and subcutaneous emphysema secondary to diagnostic amniocentesis. *Obstet Gynecol* 1974;43:884.

Section VI

Cardiovascular Emergencies

Snehal Kulkarni

29 Congestive Heart Failure

INTRODUCTION

Congestive cardiac failure (CCF) is a clinical syndrome that reflects the inability of myocardium to meet the metabolic requirements of the body including the needs incurred by growth process. It may be a consequence of excessive workload imposed on cardiac muscle (pressure and volume overload), primary alteration in myocardial function, metabolic derangements or a combination of these factors (Table 29.1).[1] Congenital cardiac defects are usually responsible for occurrence of heart failure in infancy and childhood.[2]

ETIOLOGY

Factors altering the workload (preload and afterload), the ionotropic state or the chronotropic state of the heart would result in CCF (Table 29.2).

SIGNS AND SYMPTOMS

Signs of Impaired Myocardial Performance

Excessive sweating and failure to thrive are predominant symptoms. Clinical evaluation reveals cardiomegaly, tachycardia, gallop rhythm, pulsus parodoxus or pulsus alternans. Cold extremities with weak peripheral pulsations are seen in very sick children.

Signs of Pulmonary Venous Congestion

Difficulty in feeding with interrupted feeds, chronic hacking cough, dyspnoea, tachypnoea and wheezing are common symptoms. Mild cyanosis and bilateral rales are found on clinical examination.

Signs of Systemic Venous Congestion

Tender hepatomegaly and neck vein distension occurs either with left ventricular failure or can occur in isolated right ventricular failure also. Facial edema is a common feature of congestive heart failure in children than peripheral edema.

INVESTIGATIONS

Laboratory Investigations

Hemoglobin and Red Blood Cell Count

Routine investigations like Hb% and RBC count are essential as severe anaemia accentuates the circulatory abnormalities associated with primary cardiac problem.

Table 29.1: Types of congestive cardiac failure

Physiological types of failure	*Underlying defect*
Type 1 Occurs with increase in volume or pressure loading	Volume overload : large left to right shunts, valvular regurgitation, arteriovenous fistula, anaemia Pressure overload: aortic stenosis, coarctation of aorta, systemic hypertension
Type 2 Conditions which impair the contractility of myocardium	Dilated cardiomyopathy, abnormal origin of left coronary artery from pulmonary artery(ALCAPA), postoperative systolic dysfunction
Type 3 Impaired ventricular filling leading to inadequate diastolic filling and reduced stroke volume	Tachycardia, myocardial fibrosis, hypertrophic cardiomyopathy

Table 29.2: Etiology of CCF

Age at presentation	*Causes (by descending order of occurrence)*
Infancy	LVOT Obstructions Large left to right shunts (PDA, VSD, Atrio-ventricular septal defects) Common mixing lesions Tachyarrhythmias ALCAPA Myocarditis (coxackie, adenovirous) Familial cardiomyopathy Metabolic disorders- Pompe's disease, Carnitnine deficiency Mitochondrial cardiomyopathy
More than 1 year old	Cardiomyopathy Rheumatic heart disease Congenital heart disease-Large left to right shunts, LVOT obstruction Postoperative-After open heart surgery Myocarditis, endocarditis Collagen vascular disease Kawasaki's disease Neuromuscular disorders Tachyarrhythmias Drug induced-e.g. anthracycline Anaemia

Blood Gas and Electrolytes

In acute CCF with low cardiac output metabolic acidosis and lactic acidemia is usually seen. In chronic CCF $PaCO_2$ is low and pH will be normal. Hyponatremia and hypochloremia caused by diuretic therapy needs to be detected by regular electrolyte monitoring. Hypokalemia and lactic acedemia can develop by reduced perfusion to tissues.[3]

Urine Analysis

Patients with CCF may have albuminuria, increased specific gravity and microscopic hematuria. Urinary sodium is usually less than 10 meq/L in CCF. Methylglutamic aciduria would suggest the metabolic cause for the failure.

Miscellaneous Tests

Hypoglycemia has been associated with CCF in infants and hypocalcemia noted with LV failure in neonates.[4] CPK MB and troponin T levels are supportive in detecting coronary insufficiency and asphyxia as a cause for CCF. Autoimmune disorders can be ruled out by RF, anti dsDNA and ANA assays. Blood levels of carnitine, lactate and glucose help to detect mitochondrial cardiomyopathies.

Radiography

Routine X-ray chest helps to assess cardiomegaly as it is a direct evidence of cardiac involvement. Pulmonary venous congestion, pulmonary blood flow and parenchymal diseases can be confirmed by chest radiography.

Electrocardiography

It often provides supportive data to define arrhythmias or heart block causing or complicating CCF. It also gives information regarding chamber enlargement and myocardial ischaemia.

Echocardiography

Two dimensional echocardiography helps to establish anatomic diagnosis, functional status and as a follow up assessment of response to therapy. Various indices can be used to differentiate abnormal loading conditions of heart from alteration in contractility. Antenatal echocardiography can diagnose fetal CCF which can manifest as fetal hydrops. Colour flow mapping and Doppler studies gives exact information about shunts and the gradients across the valves

Cardiac Catheterisation

It offers functional data of the failing myocardium and information regarding pulmonary artery pressure and resistance. Myocardial biopsy for histological and PCR testing may be helpful in diagnosing underlying cause like myocarditis.

APPROACH TO MANAGEMENT

Most desirable approach is to remove the underlying cause, recognize, manage and prevent the precipitating events and control of congestive heart failure.[5]

Goals in Controlling CCF

1. Relief of pulmonary and systemic congestion
2. Increase in myocardial performance
3. Reversal of underlying disease progression

Pharmacological Therapy

Diuretics

Major diuretics used are loop diuretics, thiazides and aldosterone antagonist. These act directly on kidneys to inhibit solute and water reabsorption thereby promoting excretion of excess salt and water.[6] Furosemide is the widely used drug for management of acute and chronic congestive heart failure. Thiazides are more commonly used for chronic CCF. Metolazone belongs to the same group, but needs effective monitoring due to the risk of excessive volume depletion and electrolyte imbalance. Common side effects are hypokalemia, metabolic alkalosis and hyperuricemia with chronic use. Ototoxicity has been reported very rarely in children and is usually reversible.

In acute situations furosemide is used at the dosage of 0.5 mg/kg/dose to a maximum of 2 mg/kg/dose intravenously. It can also be given as intravenous infusion at the dosage of 0.1 to 1 mg/kg/hour. For treatment of chronic congestive heart failure, oral furosemide is used at the dosage of 0.5 mg/kg/dose every 6-12 hourly. It can be increased upto 5 mg/kg/dose. Furosemide is usually combined with oral spironolactone at the dosage of 1-3.5 mg/kg/day given 2-4 times per day to compensate for potassium loss. Short term oral metolazone is used in resistant cases at the dosage of 0.1-0.5 mg/kg/day in 2-4 divided doses. Oral chlorthiazides are rarely used in children. The dosage is 20-40 mg/kg/day.

Ionotropes

Digoxin: It is still the most widely used and studied drug which is available in oral and parenteral form. Mechanism of action is inhibition of sarcollemal Na^+K^+-ATPase activity leading to increased intracellular calcium and hence increases ventricular contractility.[7] It also slows heart rate and conduction. Major indication in CCF is to improve myocardial contractility. The use of digoxin is controversial in congestive heart failure due to large left to right shunts.[8] It gives subjective benefit in those with systolic dysfunction due to neurohormonal modulating effect. It is also useful in treating fetal CCF induced by tachycardia.

For rapid digitalisation 1/2 of loading dose should to be given initially, 1/4th 6-12 hours later and remaining 1/4th 6-12 hours later. Half-life of digoxin is 20 hours in infants and 40 hours in older children. As loading dose is associated with side effects in infants and neonates, it is reasonable to give maintenance dose in majority of patients. Total digitalising dose in preterm neonates is 10-20 μg/kg, for term neonates and infants it is 20-30 μg/kg, for children between 1-5 years of age it is 30-40 μg/kg and above the age of 5 years the digitalising dose is 30 μg/kg. For maintenance, oral digoxin is used at the dosage of 5-10 μg/kg to be given 2-4 times per day. Anorexia, nausea, vomiting, visual, CNS disturbances, atrioventricular block and dysrrhythmias are the common side effects. Toxic level is above 4-5 ng/ml in infants and above 3 ng/ml in children.[9] In the presence of hypokalemia (diuretics induced) and renal dysfunction, dosage of digoxin should be adjusted. Likewise dosage should be reduced when combined with quinidine, verapamil and amiodarone. Toxicity can be treated with normalising potassium, antiarrhythmics, pacing and Fab fragments.[10]

Dopamine: It is useful in acute CCF and cardiogenic shock, especially in postoperative status with low cardiac output. It has α adrenergic and dopaminergic effects in lower doses and α adrenergic effects at higher doses. Monitoring of blood pressure, heart rate, urine output and ECG changes is needed during continuous intravenous infusion. Half life is 3-4 minutes. At 3-5 μg/kg it has best dopaminergic action which improves renal flow and naturesis. Hence it is very useful in acute CCF following cardiopulmonary bypass. At 5-15 μg/kg it has ionotropic effect. Dosage more than 20 μg/kg may compromise renal flow, increase pulmonary vascular resistance, oxygen demand and ventricular afterload.

Dobutamine: This differs from dopamine by its dominant action on β1 than β2 and α receptors and by not depending on norepinephrine stores to produce the desired effects.[11] It is used as continuous intravenous infusion at dosage of 2-20 μg/kg/min. It causes mild vasodilatation, increases the cardiac output, reduces the systemic vascular resistance with minimal alteration of blood pressure and heart rate. It's half life is 2-3 minutes and it does not alter renal flow. It is very useful in perioperative settings as it is less arrhythmogenic and increases cardiac output. Combination of 3-5 μg/kg of dopamine with dobutamine 5-10 μg/kg and after load reducing agents as milrinone is widely used for management of heart failure in postoperative period.

Epinephrine: It has mixed α and α effects. It may improve cardiac output in acute CCF and in postoperative situations with intense vasoconstriction by dilating vascular bed and by the ionotropic effect. Dosage used is 0.05-1 mg/kg/min. It's half-life is 2-3 minutes. It can be arrythmogenic by its excessive chronotropic action and causes downregulation of α receptors on long-term use. It should be strictly given through central catheter, as short term treatment for patients unresponsive to other drugs and to be tapered off as early as possible.

Norepinephrine: It is not widely used due to its deleterious effects on afterload, renal flow and myocardial demand.

Isoproterenol: It augments contractility and heart rate by its effects on β1 and β2 receptors. It is useful in CCF complicated by increased reactive pulmonary vascular resistance or complete heart block when used in dosage of 0.05-1 mg/kg/min. It is important to maintain adequate intravascular volume during its infusion.

Nonglycosidal, noncatecholamine agents: Phosphodiesterase III (PDEIII) inhibitors, routinely called as ionodilators, inhibit the breakdown of cyclic AMP in cardiac and peripheral vascular smooth muscle, which results in augmentation of myocardial contractility and peripheral arterial and venous vasodilatation.[12] Milrinone is the widely used drug amongst this group. It is used as slow intravenous injection (50 mg/kg slowly over 10 minutes) followed by intravenous infusion at a rate of 0.375-0.0750 mg/kg/min upto 48 hours. Milrinone can be combined with modest doses of dobutamine. It gives added benefits to patients already receiving ACE inhibitors. Milrinone is free of harmful side effects as compared to other drugs in this group like amrinone. Hypotension, ventricular arrhythmias and thrombocytopenia are the side effects noted with amrinone. Enoximone is an investigational drug in the same group which is still not approved for its use in clinical practice.

Vasodilators

Vasodilators play a vital role in the management of CCF secondary to left to right shunts, postoperative low cardiac output, severe atrioventricular valve regurgitation and dilated cardiomyopathy. They are also used with ionotropes and diuretics to augment function by altering afterload and preload. Long term use of vasodilators needs close monitoring of systolic blood pressure.

ACE Inhibitors (Captopril, Enalapril)

Angiotensin converting enzyme (ACE) inhibitors have become the cornerstone of treatment of heart failure. ACE inhibitors act on the crucial enzyme that generates angiotensin II, whereas newer angiotensin receptor blockers (ARB) act directly on the receptor subtype that responds to angiotensin II stimulation. It improves the hemodynamic status by altering ventricular modelling, reducing systemic vascular resistance and increasing venous capacitance.[13,14] Cough, hypotension, hyperkalemia, deterioration of renal function, neutropenia are major side effects and needs frequent monitoring. Use of ACE inhibitors is contraindicated in children with severe renal failure, bilateral renal artery stenosis, preexsting hypotension, severe aortic stenosis or hypertrophic cardiomyopathy. Captopril is given at a dose of 0.1-0.5 mg/kg/dose to be given 3 times per day. A test dose of captopril (0.1 mg/kg) is recommended before starting the drug in full dosage, as significant hypotension is known to occur after the first dose. Enalapril is another commonly used ACE inhibitor which is given at a dose of 0.1-0.4 mg/kg/day in 2 divided doses. Lisinopril, ramipril and perindopril are other ACE inhibitors in this group. There are no trials for use of angiotesin receptor blockers (ARB) in pediatric population.

Sodium Nitroprusside (SNP)

It is mostly used in acute CCF and in postoperative patients for after load reduction. It decreases filling pressures, systemic and pulmonary vascular resistance when used at a dosage of 0.5-5 mg/kg/min as continuous intravenous infusion. Thiocyanate toxicity and hypotension needs to be monitored if it is used for more than 48 hours.

Nitroglycerine (NTG)

It increases venous capacitance and reduces filling pressures. It is mainly used in conditions with increased preload and pulmonary venous congestion. Side effects are common when cardiac output is compromised.

Prazosin, hydralazine are not widely used in children

Beta-Blockers

Beta-blockers are increasingly added to ACE inhibitors and diuretics for treatment of heart failure in hemodynamically stable patients. Use of betablockers have shown to decrease the mortality upto 30% in many trials. It improves workload without increasing oxygen consumption and enhances ventricular relaxation. Increase in exercise capacity and upregulation of α receptors have been described in patients on beta blockers.[15,16] The starting dose should be low and the patients should be closely monitored during initial titration due to the risk of transient deterioration. Trial data favours the use of metoprolol, carvedilol and bisoprolol. Carvedilol is the most promising drug amongst this group because of its a mediated vasodilatory capacity. Recommended dosage of carvedilol is 0.05 mg/kg/dose orally to be given 2-3 times per day which can be increased upto 0.5 mg/kg/dose.

Management of Ventricular Arrhythmias in CCF

Incidence of ventricular arrhythmias is more in end stage CCF. It is essential to pinpoint the precipitating factor like hypokalemia, hypomagnesemia or use of sympathomimetics or digoxin. Amiodarone remains the drug of choice for symptomatic arrhythmias.

Mechanical Afterload Reduction

IABP (Intra aortic balloon pump)

It has not been used widely as analogous clinical settings are few in children unlike adults and due to technical problems related to catheter size. It is useful in CCF secondary to coronary artery involvement as in Kawasaki's or ALCAPA and in postoperative settings with reduced cardiac output to achieve diastolic augmentation of blood pressure. It remains a viable option for end stage failure.

ECMO (Extracorporal membrane oxygenation)

Pediatric experience is in infants for preoperative stabilisation and in postoperative state as a bridge before transplant.

VAD (Ventricular assist device)

It is in developmental stages in children. It can be used as a bridge to transplant or in difficulty in weaning from bypass.

Abdominal Compression Devices

Antistock trousers or ventilator reservoir bags are used to reduce right heart volume overload in children with right heart failure.

Adjunctive Therapy

Position

Keeping the child in semi-Fowler position either by keeping in modified cardiac chair or elevating head and shoulders to 45° angle. It improves the pulmonary function by easing respiration and reducing pulmonary pooling.

Table 29.3: Management of acute CCF

Digoxin		Ionotropic agent
Low dose dopamine		Increases cardiac output
Dobutamine		Less arrhythmogenic
Beta adrenergics	Epinephrine Norepinephrine	Increase contraction
Vasodilators	SNP, NTG	Reduce preload and afterload
	PDEIII inhibitors	Reduce afterload, ionotropic agent
	ACE inhibitors	
Diuretics	Loop Thiazides	Reduces pulmonary and systemic congestion
Positive pressure ventilation		Reduces afterload Increases cardiac output Reduces work of breathing and VO2

Oxygen

Severe CCF reduces arterial oxygen tension. Hence oxygen supplementation through mask or nasal prongs with adequate humidification helps to loosen secretions and improve oxygenation. Caution must be applied for duct dependent cardiac defects in neonatal period.

Positive Pressure Ventilation (PPV)

Intubation and PPV may normalise the blood gas tension and reduces the work of breathing in infants with severe CCF.

PGE1

It is useful for maintaining the ductal patency in duct dependent systemic circulation like HLHS to improve systemic perfusion and to reduce pulmonary congestion.

Bed Rest

Rest is advised as an attempt to reduce load on the compromised myocardium. Activity can be increased according to the response to treatment. It has to be a flexible and individualised programme for children.

Diet

Adequate calories and protein should be advised to meet the increased metabolic needs. Calorific requirement may be upto 130-170 Cal/kg/day in infants. Salt restriction will be necessary in the presence of severe systemic congestion or oedema. Low solute formula with 7-12 mEq/L may have to be used in infants. Diet has to be modified as per the child's response to salt restriction so that unnecessary weight loss can be prevented. Iron supplement of 2-3 mg/kg will benefit by improving anaemia. L Carnitine supplementation can be helpful in dilated cardiomyopathy. Nasogastric tube feeds can help to improve weight gain in severely symptomatic children.

Table 29.4: Management of cardiogenic shock

Increase stroke volume	Restore volume
Increase ventricular contractility	Correct underlying cause Treat hypoxia Correct acidosis Ionotropes-dopamine, dobutamine, epinephrine
Reduce afterload	SNP, NTG ACE inhibitors PDEIII inhibitors
Mechanical support	IABP, ECMO

*Digoxin to be used cautiously in shock as its effect is slower and chances of toxicity is more with reduced renal perfusion. If used, lower and less frequent dosage is preferable.

Treatment of Diastolic Failure

Diastolic dysfunction is defined as increase in end diastolic pressures in the presence of normal ventricular volume and systolic function. Therapy is of uncertain success.[17] Low dose diuretics, beta blockers, calcium channel blockers and ACE inhibitors are used with limited success. Constrictive pericarditis must be ruled out in such conditions.

Treatment of Underlying Condition

Transcatheter interventions may have to be carried out in patients with frank CCF to treat underlying defects like critical aortic stenosis or coarctation of aorta . Early surgical correction of large left to right shunts has to be planned after initial stabilisation. Procedures like dynamic cardiomyoplasty may help in few patients. Control of infection, anemia, arrhythmias, hypertension and metabolic deficiencies can help to control CCF early. Intravenous immunoglobulin has been proved to be useful in cardiomyopathy secondary to myocarditis. Role of steroids in rheumatic heart disease with CCF may be lifesaving but controversial. Treating the mother antenatally with digoxin helps to control supraventricular tachycardia causing failure in the foetus. The final option for end stage failure would be cardiac transplant.

Counseling

Frank discussion of the problem, genetic implications, treatment modalities and the prognosis with the parents is a must. Many authors suggest avoiding the term 'failure' when discussing with parents and terms like 'congestion' seem to be accepted more readily. The family will need continuous support by the primary pediatrician.

PREDICTORS OF MORTALITY

Degree of functional capacity, ventricular function, ventricular arrhythmias and neurohormonal activities has predictive value over 1-5years period. Most patients with clinically manifest failure progress to death within 10 years if the underlying condition is not treatable, despite the recent advances in the management.

FUTURE PERSPECTIVES

Improvement in therapy of cardiac failure is possible with increasing knowledge in mechanism of failure and newer therapeutic measures. Therapies like gene therapy and stem cell transfer are under trial and may give more promising results in future.

REFERENCES

1. Talner NS. Congestive heart failure in infant: Functional approach *Pediatr Clin N Am* 1971;18:1011-1029.
2. Fyler DC, Buckley LP, Hellenbrand WE, et al. Report of the New England Regional Infant Cardiac Program. *Pediatrics* 1980;65(Suppl 2):375-461.
3. Talner NS, Sanyal SK, Halloran KH, et al. Congestive heart failure in infancy: Abnormalities in blood gases and acid base equilibrium. *Pediatrics* 1965; 35:20-26.
4. Benzing GIII, Schubert W, Hug G, et al. Simultaneous hypoglycaemia and acute congestive heart failure. *Circulation* 1969;40:209-216.
5. Friedman WF, George BL. Treatment of cardiac failure in infants. *Compr Ther* 1986;12:8-14.
6. Thier SO. Diuretic mechanisms as a guide to therapy *Hospital Practice* 1987;22:61-78.
7. Soyka LL. Pediatric Clinical Pharmacology of digoxin. *Peditr Clin North Am* 1981;20:203-216.
8. Kimbalil TR, Daniels SR, Meyer RA, et al. Effect of digoxin on contractility and symptoms in infants with a large ventricular and septal defect *Am J Cardiol* 1991;68:1377-1382.
9. Hayes CJ, Butler VP Jr, Gersony WM. Serum digoxin studies in infants and children *Pediatrics* 1973;52:561-568.
10. Woolf AD, Wengek T, Smith TW, Lorejoy FH Jr. The use of digoxin-specific Fab Fragments for severe digitalis intoxication in children. *N Eng J Med* 1992;326:1739-1774.
11. Bhatt-Mehta V, Nahata MC. Dopamine and dobutamine in pediatric therapy. *Pharmacology* 1989; 9:303-314.
12. Marcus FL, Opie LH, Sonneneblick EH, et al. Digitalis and acute inotropes. In: Opic LH (ed) *Drugs for the Heart* 4th edn. Philadelphia Saunders 1994;83-103.
13. Davis R, Ribner HS, Keung E, et al. Treatment of chronic congestive heart failure with captopril, an oral inhibitors of angiotensin-converting enzyme. *N Engl J Med* 1979;301:117-121.
14. Stern H, Well J, Genz T, et al. Captopril in children with dilated cardiomyopathy: acute and long term effects in a prospective study of hemodynamic and hormonal effects. *Pediatr Cardiol* 1990;11:22-28.
15. Bristow MR, Port JD, Gilbert EM. The role of adrenergic receptor regulation in the treatment of heart failure. *Cardiovasc Drugs Ther* 1989;3:971-978.
16. Andenson JL, Gilbert EM, O'Connell JB, et al. Long term (2 yrs) beneficial effects of beta-adrenergic blockage with bucindoll in patients with dilated cardiomyopathy. *J Am Coll Cardiol* 1991;17:1373-1382.
17. Haber HL, Powers ER, Gimple LW, et al. Intracoronary angiotensin convecting enzyme inhibitors improves diastolic function in patients with hypertensive left ventricular hypertrophy. *Circulation* 1994;89:2616-2625.

Cardiovascular Emergencies

Poothirikovil Venugopalan

30 Acute Myocarditis

INTRODUCTION

Myocarditis refers to an inflammatory myocardial disease, most often viral in origin, that may present with a wide spectrum of manifestations ranging from asymptomatic rhythm disturbances to acute heart failure and shock.[1]

BACKGROUND

Table 30.1 lists the agents that can affect the heart and present a myocarditis-like picture.[2] Viral infections form the most common etiology, and Coxsackie B3 and Adeno viruses together account for almost 90% of cases. Experimental studies and clinical investigations have confirmed that the manifestations of myocarditis are immune mediated,[3] although there is an initial phase of active viral replication and myocyte damage. The immune and autoimmune responses that follow may persist even after the viral particles have been cleared. Cellular immune mechanisms mediated by both CD_4^+ and CD_8^+ lymphocytes form the major component of the immune response in myocarditis. They recognize viral proteins or specific class I or II major histocompatibility complex antigens present on the cell membrane surface, adhere to these cells and damage them. Macrophage infiltration and cytokine production [Interlukin (IL-1) and tumor necrosis factor (TNF)-a] follow and these promote leukocyte activation, local inflammation and fibrosis and the production of nitric oxide. Humoral antibodies in response to exposed antigens on the myocardial cell surface also play a role in the progressive myocardial damage. Besides injuring myocytes, the immune mediators also lead to coronary vascular injury with resulting myocardial edema and reduced ventricular compliance.

Table 30.1: Etiology of myocarditis-like presentation in infants and children

Infections	*Coxsackie B3 virus*
	Adenovirus
	Cytomegalovirus
	Herpes simplex virus
	Mumps virus
	Echovirus
	Epstein-Barr virus
	Parvovirus B19
	Hepatitis C virus
	Influenza A virus
	Respiratory syncytial virus
	Human immunodeficiency virus
	Rubella virus
	Measles virus
	Other non-viral infections
Immune mediated	Postinfectious
	Systemic disorders
	Drug hypersensitivity
Toxic	Drugs-anthracyclines
Other disorders	Idiopathic dilated cardiomyopathy
Kawasaki's disease	
	Anomalous coronary arteries
Other congenital heart diseases	

Myocyte loss and altered myocardial function decrease cardiac output and induce cardiac arrhythmias. When myocardial dysfunction persists, the neuro-humoral compensatory mechanisms of chronic heart failure set in, and a proportion of patients with myocarditis progress to a state of chronic dilated cardiomyopathy.

Clinical presentation depends on the age of the patient and severity of myocardial dysfunction. The main symptomatology is shown in Table 30.2. These symptoms are proceeded by a short period of fever, running nose, or cough in a majority of patients. Physical examination reveals features of heart failure. The older child shows tachypnea, tachycardia with a gallop rhythm, pedal edema, elevated jugular venous pressure and tender hepatomegaly. Blood pressure may be low and peripheral pulses weak. Rapid, slow or irregular pulses may point to a cardiac arrhythmia. Cardiomegaly, quiet precordium, accentuated pulmonary second heart sound, presence of a third heart sound, apical

Table 30.2: Clinical presentations of acute myocarditis

Mode of presentation	*Symptoms*
Heart failure	Infants
	Breathlessness
	Feeding difficulties
	Excessive sweating
	Wheezing
	Irritability
	Failure to thrive
	Shock or unresponsive state
	Cyanosis
	Children
	Effort intolerance
	Breathlessness
	Orthopnea
	Nocturnal dyspnea
	Fatiguability
	Malaise
	Cough
	Chest pain
	Pedal edema
	Abdominal pain
Cardiac arrhythmia	Infants
	As heart failure
	Children
	Palpitation
	Chest discomfort
	Fast pulse, slow pulse, irregular pulse
	Syncope
	Seizure like epidoses
Pericarditis	Chest pain
	Breathlessness
A systemic viral infection	Features of the systemic illness predominate (pneumonia, hepatitis, nephritis, encephalitis, gastroenteritis etc)
Asymptomatic	Detected during evaluation for unrelated problem

systolic murmur of mitral regurgitation are among the cardiac findings. Fine basal crepitations in both lung bases indicate pulmonary edema. In infants and neonates, tachypnea, tachycardia and hepatomegaly are the hallmarks of heart failure. Respiratory distress may take the form of nasal flaring, grunting and chest retractions. Poor capillary refill, cold and mottled skin are the other manifestations.

Diagnosis requires a high index of suspicion.[4,5] Myocarditis should be suspected in any older child with unexplained heart failure or cardiac arrhythmia and in neonates and infants with shock like state. Tachycardia out of proportion to the fever may be an early sign of myocarditis. In view of the poor contractility of the myocardium, cardiac findings may be minimal and in acute presentation cardiomegaly may not be prominent.

Chest radiograph or electrocardiogram often helps to suspect the diagnosis. Cardiomegaly and pulmonary congestion are common and occasionally pleural effusion and pneumonia may be present. Electrocardiogram shows nonspecific changes like low voltage QRS complexes, ST segment depression and T wave inversion. Nature of cardiac arrhythmia if any can be confirmed from the electrocardiogram. Echocardiogram forms the mainstay of the diagnosis in majority of patients, and shows dilated cardiac chambers especially the left-sided ones and global hypokinesia of the ventricles again more marked on the left. Other abnormalities include regional wall motion abnormalities, mitral regurgitation, elevated pulmonary artery pressures, restrictive mitral flow pattern and pericardial effusion. Congenital heart diseases with a similar presentation can be excluded from these studies.

Blood investigations like acute phase reactants, cardiac enzymes (creatine kinase-myocardial fraction, troponin T and I) and viral studies may contribute to the diagnosis in some patients. Nuclear imaging studies where available also reveal the patchy myocardial inflammatory process. Myocardial biopsy is the gold standard for diagnosis, however in view of the relative risks of such procedure in small babies in the acute stage of the illness, and the limited information available from such specimens, these are carried out only in selected centers. Tracheal aspirates have been shown to isolate the virus in intubated patients.[6]

APPROACH TO MANAGEMENT

Prompt institution of therapy is crucial to improve the outcome, and the treating physician has to recognize the presence of myocarditis and the possibility for rapid deterioration in the first few days of the illness. Poor myocardial contractility with reduced cardiac output and a high systemic vascular resistance are hallmarks of the hemodynamic state. Supportive therapy is the mainstay in therapy, with other options having an uncertain role.

Inotropic Support

Intravenous infusions of dobutamine, a sympathomimetic agent and milrinone, a phosphodiesterase inhibitor are the most widely used to maintain blood pressure and tissue perfusion in patients with severe myocardial dysfunction (Table 30.3). Both these should be administered only in a critical care unit with intensive monitoring facilities. However in severely hypotensive patients these agents are best used in conjunction with either dopamine or epinephrine until the tissue perfusion is at an acceptable level.

Digoxin has been documented to be harmful in the acute stage of myocarditis in adults, and in mouse models has been shown to mediate increased inflammation and mortality by inducing cytokines.[7] Hence, in children with acute

Table 30.3: Inotrope infusions useful in acute myocarditis

Drug	*Receptor/Mode of action*	*Cardiovascular effect*	*Dose range*
Dobutamine	α_1, β_1, β_2	Inotropy, vasodilatation	2-20 μg/kg/min
Milrinone	Phosphodiesterase inhibitor	Inotropy, vasodilation	0.25-1 μg/kg/min
Dopamine	α_1, β_1, D_1	Inotropy, vasocontriction, renal vasodilatation, tachycardia	2-20 μg/kg/min
Epinephrine	α_1, α_2, β_1, α_2	Inotropy, vasocontriction, tachycardia	0.05-1 μg/kg/min

myocarditis digoxin should not be given intravenously and loading doses should not be used, but oral maintenance doses (5 microgram/kg/dose po bd) can be initiated after the acute stage.

Diuretics

Removal of extracellular fluid with use of diuretics will help to improve cardiac function and reduce symptoms in patients with acute myocarditis, however when used alone these do not affect progression or improve survival in myocarditis. The dosages of common anti-heart failure medications useful in acute myocarditis is given in Table 30.4.[8] Higher doses of diuretics, used along with rigorous fluid restriction can lead to hypotension and renal dysfunction. Hyponatremia, hypokalemia, acidosis, hyperglycemia, hyperuricemia and hypercalciuria are other metabolic side effects of such therapy. Potassium supplements may be required in the presence of hypokalemia. Fursemide is the most widely used diuretic for immediate action, and can be given as intravenous boluses or infusion and in less severe situations by the oral route. Intravenous frusemide is a potent vasodilator and may worsen hypotension even before the diuretic action sets in. Spironolactone an aldosterone antagonist and amiloride are potassium sparing diuretics, usually used in combination with frusemide or thiazides for long term therapy.

Table 30.4: Maintenance oral doses of anti-heart failure medications in children

Medication	*Dose range*	*Maximum daily dose*
Digoxin	2-5 mcg/kg/dose bd	500 mcg
Frusemide	1-4 mg/kg/dose od-bd	160 mg
Spironolactone	0.5-1.5 mg/kg/dose bd	200 mg
Amiloride	0.2 mg/kg/dose bd	20 mg
Captopril	0.1-1 mg/kg/dose tid	150 mg
Enalapril	0.1-1 mg/kg/dose od	40 mg
Losarten	0.5–2 mg/kg/dose od	50 mg
Metolazone	0.1–0.2 mg/kg/dose od	20 mg
Carvedilol	0.07–0.1 mg/kg/dose bd*	25 mg*

*dosage still under evaluation

Afterload Reducing Agents

High vascular resistance is one of the characteristic features of acute myocarditis and hence afterload reducing agents have an important role in the acute and chronic stages of myocarditis. They relieve symptoms, decrease hospitalization, mortality and progression of the disease process. In the acute stage, infusion of milrinone has the additional benefit of afterload reduction in addition to it inotropic effect. Nitrosovasodilators like nitroprusside are at times useful, but it can worsen the hypotension and may necessitate discontinuation of the infusion. Once the child is more stable, usually within 24-48 hours, an angiotensin converting enzyme (ACE) inhibitors should be commenced, and this forms the mainstay of long term therapy. Captopril and enalapril have been the most extensively studied among this group of drugs. Better understanding of the Renin Angiotensin System (RAS) and of the myocardial remodeling form the basis for their use. Local RAS has been demonstrated in the myocardium and inhibition may explain the beneficial effect on myocardial remodeling.[9] Hypotension, the most serious side effect of ACEI is seen maximally after the first dose, particularly when used with high doses of diuretics.[10] It can be serious in children but can be minimized by ensuring adequate hydration and electrolytes, administering it preceding the dose of diuretic and closely monitoring the blood pressure. If moderate hypotension occurs but the child is asymptomatic the ACEI need not be discontinued; such patients often do well with maintenance therapy. Persistent dry cough, caused by increased concentrations of kinins in the pulmonary vasculature can be troublesome in some children (2-10%), and the drug has been known to exacerbate bronchial asthma. Angiotensin receptor blocking agent losarten can be used in such situations.[11]

Intravenous Immunoglobulin (IVIG) Therapy

Although the benefits of IVIG therapy in pediatric myocarditis remain unproven, this drug continues to be standard therapy in children suspected of being in the acute stage of viral myocarditis. It is usually administered in a dose of 400 mg/kg/day for 5 days (total dose of 2 g/kg) under careful monitoring for fluid overload and worsening cardiac output. It is believed that IVIG can temper the immune response in myocarditis, could help to clear the virus directly, to prevent it from entering the cells and harness the immune system's response to viral myocardial infection. Drucker et al used IVIG in 21 or 46 children with myocarditis, and showed improvement in 1-year survival and left ventricular cardiac function.[12] Murine studies with the drug also gave promising

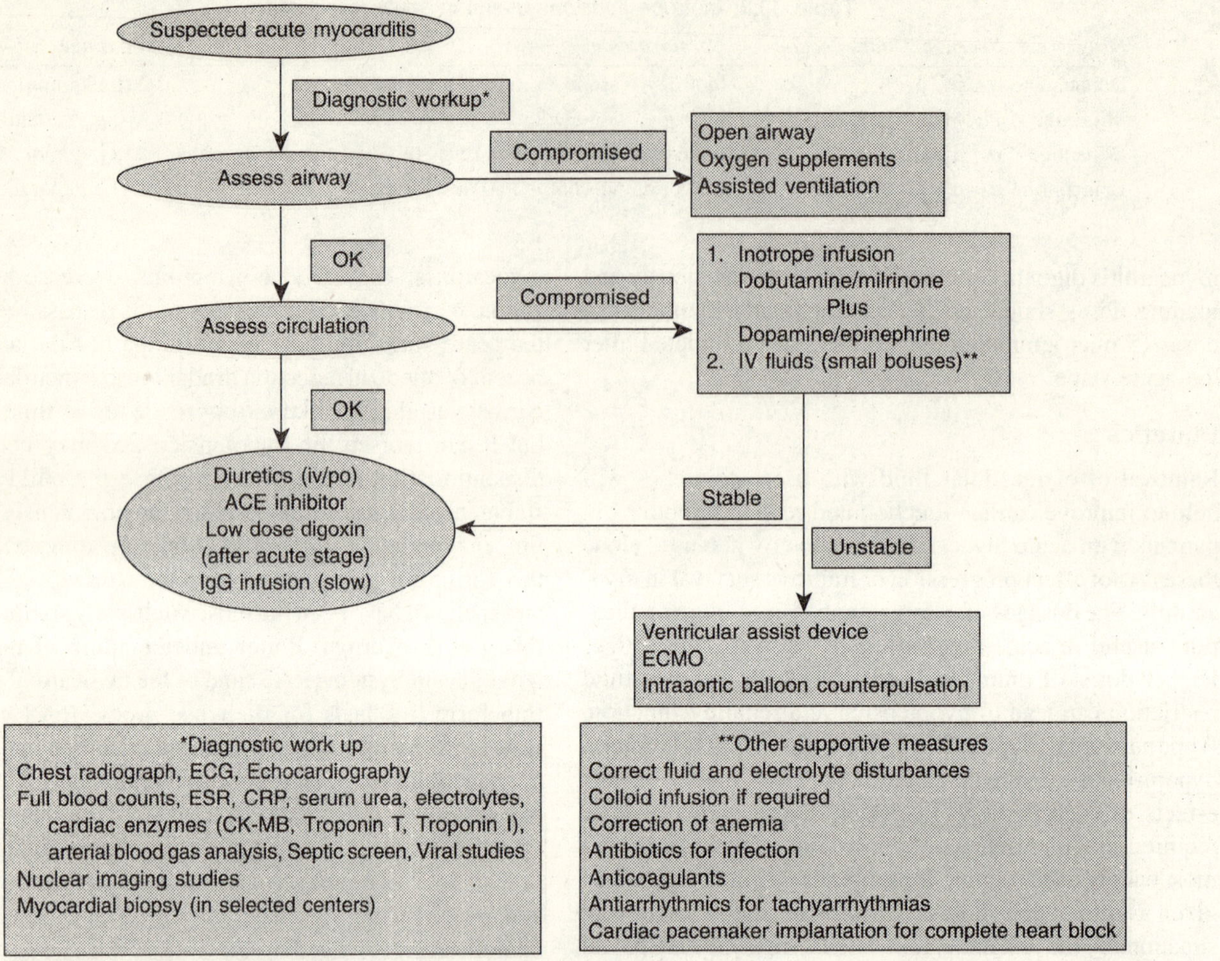

Fig. 30.1: Outline of management of acute myocarditis (ACE = angiotensin converting enzyme; IgG = immunoglobulin G; ECMO = extracorporeal membrane oxygenation; ECG = electrocardiogram; ESR = erythrocyte sedimentation rate; CRP = C-reactive proteins; CK-MB = creatine kinase–myocardial isoenzyme)

results. However a multicenter, randomized clinical trial in adults with acute myocarditis failed to substantiate these results.[13]

Immunosuppressants

Immunosuppressants should be avoided in the presence of active viral replication on account of the risk of promoting viral spread and interfering with the antiviral immune reaction. Patients with systemic autoimmune disorders, sarcoidosis, systemic lupus erythematosus, scleroderma etc do benefit from therapy. The Myocarditis Treatment Trial involving adults with histologically proven myocarditis did not show any benefit from use of prednisolone, azathioprime or cyclosporine over a study period of 6 months.[14] However a metaanalysis of seven other controlled studies also in adults showed that 60% of patients showed clinical improvement with or without therapy with prednisolone and either cyclosporine or azathioprine.[15] Antilymphocyte antibodies however have been shown to be beneficial in pediatric myocarditis patients in limited studies. This drug is very costly and larger studies are essential before any recommendations can be made.[16]

Mechanical Support Devices

Mechanical support devices are essential in patients with myocarditis who do not stabilize despite maximal medical therapy. These devices serve to prolong survival till recovery or until a suitable donor is available for cardiac transplantation. Pulsatile and nonpulsatile ventricular assist devices, as well as intraaotic ballon counterpulsation techniques are available for use in children and infants.[17] Extracorporeal membrane oxygenator circuits (ECMO) should be used in infants and smaller children in view of the physical limitations of VSDs presently available.[18] Recently small implantable mechanical support devices have been introduced to support the heart until a suitable donor is found for transplantation.[19] The Jarvik 2000 is an axial flow pump that can be placed inside the left ventricular apex and generates flow rates up to 10 litres per minute. Major limitations are risks of infection, thrombo-embolism, disturbance from the noise generated and the need to recharge batteries frequently. Prolonged support to left ventricular function with these devices has shown restoration of the native cardiac function, enabling removal of the device. This raises the possibility that mechanical intervention at an earlier stage in viral myocarditis might improve cardiac function.

Heart Transplantation

Heart transplantation represents a final treatment option for patients who do not recover from myocarditis and persist to have severe symptomatology. As recovery is possible even in the most severe cases of viral myocarditis, it is preferable to list children for heart transplantation only after they have progressed to the chronic stages of cardiomyopathy without improvement in their ventricular function. Five year survival for cardiac transplantation in children has gone up to almost 70-80%, rendering this form of therapy a viable option for children with resistant myocarditis.[20]

Other Supportive Measures

Antiarrhythmic agents (amiodarone), cardiac pacemaker implantation, anticoagulants, blood and blood product transfusions are essential in selected patients to support myocardial function and prolong survival.

REFERENCES

1. Venugopalan P, Houston AB, Agarwal AK. The outcome of idiopathic dilated cardiomyopathy and myocarditis in children from the west of Scotland. *Inter J Cardiol* 2001;78:135-141.
2. Levi D, Alejos J. An approach to the treatment of pediatric myocarditis. *Pediatr Drugs* 2002;4:637-647.
3. Henke A, Huber S, Stelzner A, et al. The role of CD8+ T lymphocytes in coxsackie B3-induced viral myocarditis. *J Virol* 1995;69:6720-6728.
4. Wiles HB, Gillette PC, Harley RA, et al. Cardiomyopathy and myocarditis in children with ventricular ectopic rhythm. *J Am Coll Cardiol* 1992;20:359-362.
5. Smith NM, Bourne AJ, Clapton WK, et al. The spectrum of presentation at autopsy of myocarditis in infancy and childhood. *Pathology* 1992;24:129-131.
6. Noorullah A, Jiyuan N, Stromberg D, et al. Tracheal aspirate as a substrate for polymerase chain reaction: Detection of viral genome in childhood pneumonia and myocarditis. *Circulation* 1999;99:2011-2018.
7. Matsumori A, Igata H, Ono K, et al. High doses of digitalis increase myocardial production of proinflammatory cytokines and worsen myocardial injury in viral myocarditis: a possible mechanism of digitalis toxicity. *Jpn Circ J* 1999;63:934-940.
8. Venugopalan P, Agarwal AK, Worthing EA. Chronic cardiac failure in children due to dilated cardiomyopathy: diagnostic approach, pathophysiology and management. *Eur J Pediatr* 2000;159:803-810.
9. Johnston CI, Fabris B, Yoshida K. The cardiac renin-angiotensin system in heart failure. *Am Heart J* 1993;126:756-760.
10. Reid JL, MacFadyen RJ, Squire IB, Lees KR. Angiotensin-converting enzyme inhibitors in heart failure: blood pressure changes after the first dose. *Am Heart J* 1993;126:794-797.
11. Pitt B, Segal R, Martinez FA, et al. on behalf of ELITE Study Investigators. Randomized trial of losarten versus captopril in patients over 65 with heart failure (Evaluation of Losarten in the Elderly Study, ELITE). *Lancet* 1997;349:747-752.
12. Drucker NA, Colan SD, Lewis AB, et al. Gamma-globulin treatment of acute myocarditis in the pediatric population. *Circulation* 1994;89:252-257.
13. McNamara DM, Rosenblum WD, Janosko KM, et al. Intravenous immune globulin in the therapy of myocarditis and acute cardiomyopathy. *Circulation* 1997;95:2476-2479.
14. Mason WJ, O'Connell JB, Herskowitz A, et al. A clinical trial of immunosuppressant therapy for myocarditis. *N Engl J Med* 1995;333:269-275.
15. Maisch B, Herzum M, Hufnagel G, et al. Immunosuppressive and immunomodulatory therapy for myocarditis. *Curr Opin Cardiol* 1996;11:310-324.
16. Ahdoot J, Galindo A, Alejos JC, et al. Use of OKT3 for acute myocarditis in infants and children. *J Heart Lung Transplant* 2000;19:1118-1121.
17. Farrar DJ, Hill JD. Recovery of major organ function in patients awaiting heart transplantation with thoracic ventricular assist devices. *J Heart Lung Transplant* 1994;13:1125-1132.
18. Levi D, Marelli D, Plunkett M, et al. The complementary use of ECMO and VSDs to support pediatric cardiomyopathy patients listed for transplantation. *J Heart Lung Transplant* 2002;21:760-770.
19. Costa RJ, Chard RB, Nunn GR, Cartinell TB. Ventricular assist devices in pediatric cardiac surgery. *Ann Thorac Surg* 1995;60:S536-S538.
20. Morrow RW. Cardiomyopathy and heart transplantation in children. *Curr Opin Cardiol* 2000;15:216-223.

Suraj Gupte and VS Puri

31 Paroxysmal Hypercyanotic Spells

INTRODUCTION

Infants and children suffering from tetralogy of Fallot (TOF) or Fallot's physiology run the risk of developing hypoxic bouts in which they become cyanotic, hyperpneic with gasping respiration and restless followed, in some instances, by syncope, seizures or hemiparesis. Such attacks have been referred to in the literature by such names *as paroxysmal hypercyanotic spells/attacks, hypoxic spells, blue spells* or *tet spells*.[1,2]

According to conservative data, incidence is around 70% in the target group of children.

ETIOPATHOGENESIS

Hypercyanotic spells are associated with a decrease in an already compromised pulmonary blood flow and increase in right-to-left shunt. When this compromised blood flow gets prolonged, result is hypoxia and metabolic acidosis.[1,2]

This state of affairs occurs in conditions in which there is a considerable mixing at ventricular level as also marked obstruction or atresia of the pulmonary outflow. These conditions are of two types, namely tetralogy of Fallot and physiology of Fallot which is a shield for a number of conditions (Table 31.1).

A number of factors are known to precipitate these spells (Table 31.2).[1,2,6]

Table 31.1: Etiology of hypercyanotoic attacks[1-4]

- Tetralogy of Fallot
- Physiology of Fallot which includes
  - tricuspid atresia,
  - double outlet right ventricle with pulmonary stenosis,
  - transposition of great arteries with ventricular septal defect and pulmonary stenosis, univentricular heart with pulmonary stenosis,
  - atrioventricular septal defect with pulmonary stenosis.

Table 31.2: Precipitating and aggravating factors for hypercyanotic spells[1,2,6]

- Fever
- Hypovolemia
- Anemia
- Excessive irritability
- Excessive crying
- Bowel movement
- Sudden waking up
- Feeding
- Exertion

MANIFESTATIONS[1-3,6]

A hypercyanotic spell usually occurs in the morning, is usually unpredictable and spontaneous and may last from a few minutes to a few hours. Manifestations include hyperpnea, restlessness, increasing cyanosis, gasping breathing, syncope, seizures, etc. Generalized weakness following a spell is usual. In some instances, hemiparesis may result.

During the attack, the heart murmur may become of poor intensity or may even disappear.

DIAGNOSIS

It is by and large clinical. In a known case of cyanotic congenital heart disease (both tetralogy of Fallot and physiology of Fallot), occurrence of blue spells with gasping breathing points to this diagnosis.

Breath-holding spells is an important differential diagnosis.

Investigations include echo-Doppler evaluation for establishing the diagnosis.

MANAGEMENT

The selective steps of treatment of a spell are outlined in Table 31.3.[3-6]

As a rule, beginning of spells is a strong indication for surgical correction of the underlying cardiac lesion. Pending

Table 31.3: Selective steps of treatment of hypercyanotic spells [3,6]

1. Comfort the infant/child and place him in knee-chest position.
2. Administer 100% oxygen by face-mask.
3. Administer morphine 0.1- 0.2 mg/kg (SC, IV) to reduce infundibular spasm and tachypnea.
4. Start IV line and administer fluid replacement and volume expansion, including blood transfusion in case of significant anemia.
5. Treat acidosis (arterial $PO_2 < 40$ mmHg) with IV sodium bicarbonate speedily within minutes if no response to foregoing therapy.
6. Administer a beta-blocker, preferably propranolol, 0.1 to 0.2 mg/kg (IV), to relieve infundibular obstruction that is precipitating the spell.
7. Increase systemic vascular resistance by IV administration of vasopressors like methoxamine or phenylephrine. Titrate dose to increase systemic blood pressure to 20%. In no case this step should be allowed to postpone surgical intervention.
8. If the spell fails to respond to medical treatment, do emergency surgery to repair the causative defect or to establish systemic-to-pulmonary artery anastomosis.

surgery, preventive measures should be resorted to, namely

- Long-term beta-blockers, say propranolol, for reducing infundibular hypercontractility, heart rate, hyperpneic reflex and systemic vascular resistance and, thereby, reducing the right-to-left shunt.
- Treatment of iron-deficiency anemia which usually accompanies the clinical spectrum in subjects in developing countries.

PROGNOSIS

As a rule, hypercyanotic spells are self-limiting. In most cases, the child comes out of a spell as such or following treatment. Occasionally, however, fatality may occur.

REFERENCES

1. Maiya PP, Karunakara BP, Gupte S. Pediatric cardiology. In: Gupte S (ed) *The Short Textbook of Pediatrics*, 10th edn. New Delhi: Jaypee 2004;270-306.
2. Gupta S. Cyanotic spell. In: Guha DK, Gupta S (ed) *Practical Critical Care Medicine*. New Delhi: Jaypee 2004;158-159.
3. Bernstein D. Congenital heart disease. In: Behram RE, Kliegman RM, Jenson HB (eds) *Nelson Textbook of Pediatrics*, 17th edn. Philadelphia: Saunders 2004; 1481-1551.
4. Hanley FL. Management of the congenitally abnormal right ventricular outflow tract–What is the right approach ? *J Thorac Cardiovasc Surg* 2000;119:1-3.
5. Godman MJ. Cyanotic congenital heart disease. In: Campbell AGM, McIntosh N (eds) *Forfar and Arneil's Textbook of Pediatrics*, 4th edn. London: ELBS with Churchill Livingstone 1992;685-696.
6. Gupte S. Experience with paroxysmal hypercyanotic spells. *Bull Pediatr Cardiol* 1999;2:54-57.

Poothirikovil Venugopalan

32 Hypertensive Emergencies

INTRODUCTION

Hypertensive emergency refers to severe hypertension with end-organ dysfunction. This may be in the form of hypertensive encephalopathy, bilateral retinal hemorrhages with or without papilledema (malignant hypertension), hypertensive cardiac failure or hypertensive renal failure.[1]

Background

The Second Task Force has defined severe hypertension as exceeding the 99th percentile for age, but have defined only the 90th and 95th centiles of blood pressure for various ages taking into account the height centile also (Table 32.1 and 32.2).[2] The urgency to initiate therapy depends mainly on the clinical presentation. Manifestations are related to effects on end-organs and these should be sought in every child who is noted to be hypertensive (Table 32.3). The major complications involve the central nervous system, eyes, heart and kidneys. Deal et al have reported hypertensive retinopathy in 27%, encephalopathy in 25%, convulsions in 25%, and left ventricular hypertrophy in 13% besides other manifestations like facial palsy, visual symptoms and hemiplegia.[3] Other rare manifestations include gastrointestinal hemorrhage, and microangiopathic hemolytic anemia. Heart failure is a common manifestation of severe hypertension in neonates, although some neonates remain asymptomatic even in the presence of severe hypertension. Along with the confirmation of significant hypertension every attempt should be made to identify the underlying cause. A significant number of children especially obese adolescents may have essential hypertension. However, younger children are more often found to have secondary hypertension (Table 32.4 and 32.5).

Certain pathophysiologic aspects are of importance when considering the acute management of hypertensive emergencies. Under normal conditions, blood flow to vital organs is controlled by an autoregulatory mechanism, which ensures adequate perfusion over a wide range of blood pressures. This is especially important in the cerebral circulation. In children with long-standing hypertension this autoregulation is disturbed so that sudden fall of blood pressure is not tolerated and lead to features of tissue hypoperfusion like cerebral infarction etc. Also subintimal cellular proliferation, which occurs in persistent hypertension can partially occlude arteries and arterioles, and sudden lowering of blood pressure may induce ischemic changes in the area of distribution of these vessels. Therefore, in long-standing hypertension sudden lowering of the blood pressure can be counterproductive.

Measurement of blood pressure should form routine part of examination of children, and special emphasis placed not to overlook this physical sign in children presenting with any of the suggestive signs and symptoms.[4] Children who present to the emergency services and are noted to have hypertension should receive special attention to confirm the suspicion and to assess the relationship to symptomatology. The blood pressure percentiles of the Task Force are based on pressures obtained using mercury sphygmomanometers. However, more hospitals now use aneroid sphygmomanometers or automated oscillometric devices such as the Dynamap. Too small a cuff can give a false high reading of blood pressure. The cuff should cover the whole circumference of the upper arm and the width should cover two-thirds the length of the upper arm. Sometimes in sick children, the recording may have to be done on the lower limb, and the cuff size has to be appropriate in such situations. Disappearance of the Korotkoff sounds (K5) in children of all ages should be the mark for diastolic blood pressure (not the muffling, as was previously recommended). Repeat examinations are recommended, and presence of features suggestive of end-organ damage may serve to confirm the diagnosis in emergency situations.

Table 32.1: The 90th and 95th percentiles of blood pressure for boys of different height percentiles*

Age	*Height percentile*	*Blood pressure percentile 90th centile*	*95th centile*
1 year	5th	94/50	98/55
	50th	98/53	102/57
	95th	102/55	106/59
2 years	5th	98/55	101/59
	50th	102/57	105/61
	95th	106/59	110/63
3 years	5th	100/59	104/63
	50th	105/61	109/65
	95th	109/63	113/67
4 years	5th	102/62	106/66
	50th	107/64	111/68
	95th	111/66	115/71
5 years	5th	104/65	108/69
	50th	108/67	112/77
	95th	112/69	116/74
6 years	5th	105/67	109/72
	50th	110/70	114/74
	95th	114/72	117/76
7 years	5th	106/69	110/74
	50th	111/72	115/76
	95th	115/74	119/78
8 years	5th	107/71	111/75
	50th	112/73	116/77
	95th	116/75	120/80
9 years	5th	109/72	113/76
	50th	113/74	117/79
	95th	117/77	121/81
10 years	5th	110/73	114/77
	50th	115/75	119/80
	95th	119/78	123/82
11 years	5th	112/74	116/78
	50th	117/76	121/80
	95th	121/78	125/83
12 years	5th	115/75	119/79
	50th	119/77	123/81
	95th	123/79	127/83

*Modified from Pediatrics 2

Table 32.2: The 90th and 95th percentiles of blood pressure for girls of different height percentiles*

Age	*Height percentile*	*Blood pressure percentile 90th centile*	*95th centile*
1 year	5th	97/53	101/57
	50th	100/54	104/58
	95th	104/56	107/60
2 years	5th	99/57	102/61
	50th	102/58	105/62
	95th	105/61	109/65
3 years	5th	100/61	104/65
	50th	103/62	107/66
	95th	106/64	110/68
4 years	5th	101/63	105/67
	50th	104/65	108/69
	95th	108/67	111/71
5 years	5th	103/65	107/69
	50th	106/67	110/71
	95th	109/69	113/73
6 years	5th	104/67	108/71
	50th	107/69	111/73
	95th	111/71	114/75
7 years	5th	106/69	110/73
	50th	109/70	113/74
	95th	112/72	116/76
8 years	5th	108/70	112/74
	50th	111/71	115/75
	95th	114/74	118/78
9 years	5th	110/71	114/75
	50th	113/73	117/77
	95th	116/75	120/79
10 years	5th	112/73	116/77
	50th	115/74	119/78
	95th	118/76	122/80
11 years	5th	114/74	118/78
	50th	117/75	121/79
	95th	120/77	124/81
12 years	5th	116/75	120/79
	50th	119/76	123/80
	95th	122/78	126/82

*Modified from Pediatrics 2

APPROACH TO MANAGEMENT

Prompt institution of therapy is crucial to improve the outcome, and the treating physician has to recognize the presence of hypertension and its significance in a particular situation.[5] The object of therapy should be to lower blood pressure in a controlled fashion, thus restoring target organ function without serious side effects of therapy. A rule of thumb is to reduce blood pressure by one-third of the amount in the first 24 hours, by a further third in the next 24-36 hours and to lower to the proposed maintenance levels during the next 48-72 hours. However more rapid reductions are feasible and sometimes advisable in patients with recent onset hypertension, especially in the presence of impending encephalopathy, heart failure, or renal failure. In such situations, it is possible to lower blood pressure to the 95th centile in a few hours, followed by further slower reduction. It is advisable to lower the blood pressure to below the 90th centile ultimately.

The initial drug used for the emergency management of hypertension varies with the center, and depends on the experience of the treating physician and availability of the medication. Drug therapy should be designed to maximize compliance and minimize adverse effects. Drugs with shorter duration of action and which can be titrated to achieve desired effects are ideal for immediate management, whereas those with longer duration of action for follow-up therapy. The initial agent chosen should be directed at the underlying pathophysiology of the child's hypertension. Thus, a vasodilator or diuretic would be more suitable for a child with acute glomerulonephritis, whereas an angiotensin-

Table 32.3: Manifestations of severe hypertension*

General	
	Headache, dizziness
	Epistaxis, anorexia
	Irritability, listlessness
	Features related to the etiology
Neurologic	
	Vomiting, ataxia, stupor
	Ataxia, seizures
	Visual disturbances
	Papilledema, retinal hemorrhage
	Intracranial hemorrhage
	Neurologic deficits
Renal	
	Oliguria, edema
	Failure to thrive
	Electrolyte disturbances and uremia
	Bleeding tendency
Cardiovascular	
	Chest pain, palpitation
	Dyspnea, feeding difficulties
	Breathlessness on exertion
	Pedal edema

*A number of children especially neonates may be asymptomatic

Table 32.4: Causes of acute/intermittent hypertension

Renal	
	Postinfectious glomerulonephritis
	Henoch-Schonlein nephritis
	Hemolytic uremic syndrome
	Acute tubular necrosis
	Post renal transplantation
	Acute pyelonephritis
Drug related	
	Corticosteroids
	Cyclosporine
	Sympathomimetic agents
	Lead, mercury poisoning
	Vitamin D toxicity
Neurologic diseases	
	Guillain-Barre syndrome
	Acute porphyria
	Raised intracranial pressure
	Encephalitis
Miscellaneous	
	Hypercalcemia
	Post coarctation repair
	Chronic upper airway obstruction

converting enzyme inhibitor or angiotensin-receptor blocker would be better for a child with diabetes and hypertension. Unlike in adults, no comparative studies have been conducted regarding the efficacy and safety of various antihypertensive medications in children, and the choice of the agent is mostly empirical, based on adult studies.

Table 32. 5: Causes of chronic hypertension

Renal	
	Chronic pyelonephritis
	Chronic glomerulonephritis
	Vasculitic syndromes
	Dysplastic kidneys
	Reflux nephropathy
	Polycystic kidney disease
Vascular	
	Coarctation of the aorta
	Renal artery stenosis
	Renal vein thrombosis
Endocrine	
	Congenital adrenal hyperplasia
	Hyperthyroidism
	Cushing's syndrome
	Pheochromocytoma
Miscellaneous	
	Essential hypertension
	Drug related (as above)
	Aldosterone responsive hypertension

Labetalol, sodium nitroprusside and more recently nicardipine have been used as initial therapy for life-threatening hypertension in children. Oral and sublingual nifedipine is another drug widely used in the emergency setting, but recent reports caution its use in this context. The absorption is erratic, possibly more by the oral route than sublingual, and there is risk of uncontrolled lowering of long-standing hypertension with intracranial complications. Other agents of use include pulsed intravenous diazoxide, hydralazine, clonidine, esmolol, enalaprilat, captopril and minoxidil.

A brief review of the main antihypertensive medications available for emergency situations follows:

Labetalol, often considered as the first line drug for emergency situations is a non-cardioselective alpha-blocker with additional beta-blocking properties. Loading dose is 250-500 mcg/kg over 1 minute followed by infusion 1-3 mg/kg/hr (500 mcg/kg/hr in neonates). Start at the low dose and titrate according to response, until the blood pressure has been reduced to an acceptable level. Maintenance oral dose is 1-2 mg/kg 3-4 times a day. Labetalol is best avoided in patients with bronchial asthma as it may precipitate an acute exacerbation. Liver damage has been reported, and the drug should be avoided in patients with liver disease, and liver function monitored during therapy, may cause hypoglycaemia in dialysis patients. Contraindications include bradycardia, cardiogenic shock, hypotension, metabolic acidosis, severe arterial circulatory disorders, second or third degree heart block, sick sinus rhythm, untreated pheochromocytoma, uncontrolled heart failure.

Sodium nitroprusside is a vasodilator of arterial and venous beds, and acts as an endogenous nitric oxide. Given as continuous infusion at 500 nanogram/kg/minute, and increase in dose in increments of 200 nanogram/kg/minute as necessary to a maximum of 8 microgram/kg/minute. The infusion is prepared in 5% dextrose and the bottle of medication should be protected from light. Terminate infusion slowly over 15-30 minutes to avoid any rebound effects. If treatment continues beyond 72 hours or patient is in renal failure, measure thiocyanate levels (maintain below 1.7 mmol/L). Contraindicated in the presence of severe hepatic impairment, severe vitamin B12 deficiency and Leber's optic atrophy. Use with caution in renal impairment, hypothermia, hypothyroidism and impaired cerebral circulation. Side effects include headache, dizziness, nausea, itching, abdominal pain, sweating, palpitation, apprehension, retrosternal discomfort secondary to rapid reduction in blood pressure. Excessive plasma concentrations of the cyanide metabolite include tachycardia, sweating, hyperventilation, arrhythmia, marked metabolic acidosis.

Nicardipine is a parenteral calcium channel blocker useful in hypertensive emergencies.[6] Initial dose is 500 nanogram/kg/minute, titrated according to the response and maintenance dose is 1-4 microgram/kg/minute. Limited information on the use in children. Contraindicated in aortic stenosis, calcium channel blocker hypersensitivity. Caution in liver impairment and in moderate to severe renal impairment.

Nifedipine is another calcium channel blocker extensively used in management of hypertension. It is given orally 200-300 microgram/kg upto 3 times a day depending on the preparation used. Older children are advised to crush the tablet in the mouth and then swallow it. Sublingual route widely used till recently is no longer advocated on account of the highly variable absorption and risk of sudden fall in blood pressure. The drug is available as a tablet, and if liquid preparation is required for young children, the liquid can be aspirated from the capsules using a syringe. The medication should be covered in foil and administered immediately as it is very light sensitive. Too rapid lowering of blood pressure may induce cerebral or coronary ischemia. It should be used with caution in patients whose cardiac reserve is poor.

Diazoxide is a directly acting arteriolar vasodilator, which can be administered as IV boluses in patients with severe hypertension. 1-3 mg/kg/dose is given as a bolus and repeated after 5-15 minutes if necessary. Close monitoring of blood pressure essential. Maximum 4 doses in 24 hours. This is not the drug of first choice in emergencies on account of the rapid fall in blood pressure that may lead to blindness, watershed cerebral infarction or death. Retention of sodium and water may necessitate therapy with diuretic. Caution in patients with severe renal impairment–maintain adequate urinary volumes and diuretic therapy. When used over a prolonged period monitor white cell counts and platelet counts regularly.. Enhanced hypotensive effect with ACE inhibitors, diuretics, calcium channel blockers etc. Side effects include nausea, extrapyramidal effects, sodium and water retention, tachycardia and hyperglycemia.

Hydralazine is another direct arteriolar vasodilator, and can be given as slow IV bolus 100-500 microgram/kg/dose over 20 minutes and repeated up to 4-6 times a day. It can also be administered as infusion at 12.5–50 microgram/kg/hour. Glucose solutions should not be used to dilute the medication. Contraindications include high output heart failure, porphyria, SLE, or known hypersensitivity. Side effects include fluid retention, headache, tachycardia, palpitations and blood disorders. Prolonged treatment may provoke a lupus erythematosus-like syndrome.

Captopril is an oral medication useful in the management of severe hypertension. It is an angiotensin converting enzyme inhibitor and hence is maximally effective in hyperreninemic states. Dose in neonates is 10-50 microgram/kg, given 3 times a day. For older children, a wide range of dosage have been employed ranging from 100 microgram to 2 mg/kg up to 3 times a day. The initial dose has to be low (test dose) with close monitoring of BP to detect first dose hypotension, and is better administered when the state of hydration is adequate. Contraindicated in renal artery stenosis and in the presence of left ventricular outflow obstruction. Monitor for worsening of renal function in patients with renal impairment. Side effects include hypotension, persistent dry cough, gastrointestinal upset, Hyperkalemia, angioedema and blood disorders.

Minoxidil, another direct acting vasodilator is at times helpful in the management of severe hypertension in renal disease. Given orally in a single daily dose of 200 microgram/kg, can be increased in steps of 100-300 microgram/kg/day to a maximum dose of 50 mg/kg/day. Higher doses are often given as two divided doses. Side effects include sodium and water retention, weight gain, tachycardia, hypertrichosis, rashes, etc.

Figure 32.1 gives an algorithm for management of pediatric hypertension.

During therapy, close monitoring for cerebral ischaemia and or renal impairment is essential. Ischemic neuropathy of the optic nerve with visual impairment and transverse ischemic myelopathy are less well known manifestations of neurologic ischaemia from sudden lowering of blood pressure.

Once emergency measures are instituted to bring down the high blood pressure, attention should focus on identification of the etiology, and interventions directed to cure the cause if feasible. Medications my be shifted to

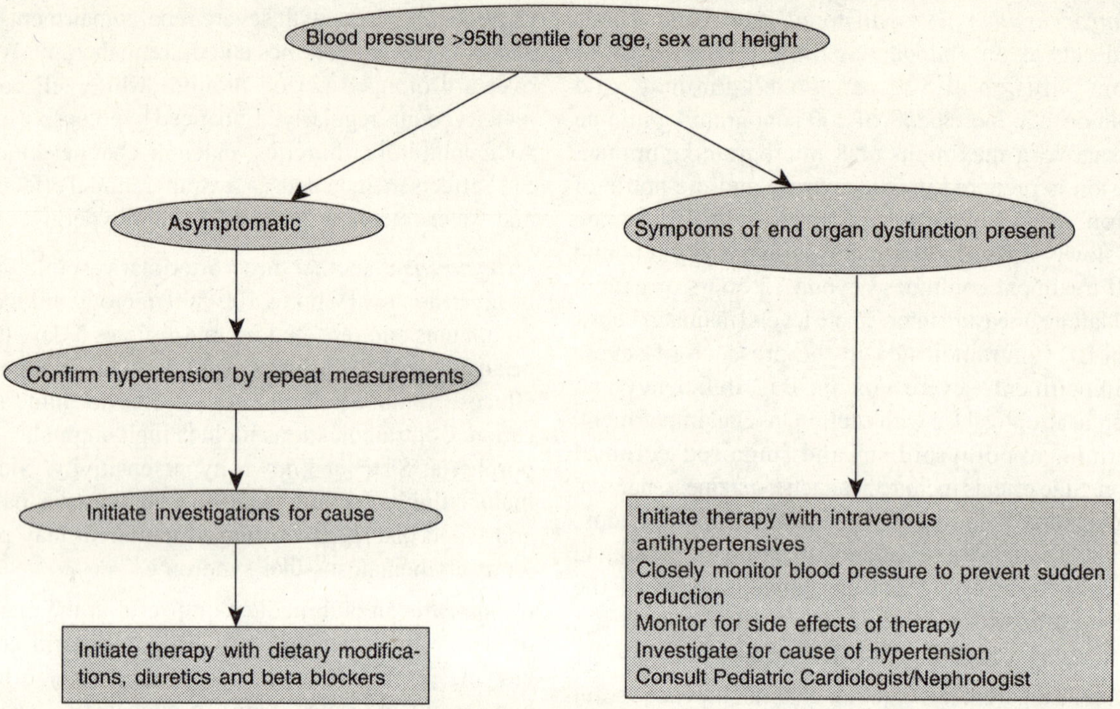

Drugs for management of hypertensive emergencies

1. Labetalol: Loading dose 250-500 mcg/kg over 1 minute followed by infusion 1-3 mg/kg/hr (500 mcg/kg/hr in neonates)
2. Sodium nitroprusside: Infusion at 500 nanogram/kg/minute, and increase dose in increments of 200 nanogram/kg/minute as necessary to a maximum of 8 microgram/kg/minute
3. Nicardipine: 500 nanogram/kg/minute, titrated according to the response and maintenance dose is 1-4 microgram/kg/minute
4. Diuretics, captopril, oral beta blockers, diazoxide, minoxidil etc are other options
5. Nifedepine oral may be tried in acute cases like acute glomerulonephritis, but with close monitoring of blood pressure to avoid sudden fall

Fig 32.1: Outline of management of hypertension in children

orally administered drugs once the child is stable for 48-72 hours.

The reader is referred to more detailed discussion on the long-term management of hypertension for further work-up and management.

REFERENCES

1. Adelman RD, Coppo R, Dillon MJ. The emergency management of severe hypertension. *Pediatr Nephrol* 2000;14:422-427.
2. Task Force on blood pressure control in children: Report of the second Task Force on Blood Pressure Control in Children-1987. *Pediatrics* 1987;79:1-15.
3. Deal JE, Barratt TM, Dillon MJ. Management of hypertensive emergencies. *Arch Dis Child* 1992;67: 1089-1092.
4. Flynn JT. Evaluation and management of hypertension in childhood. *Progress Pediatr Cardiol* 2001; 12:177-188.
5. Flynn JT. Recognizing and managing the hypertensive child. *Contemp Pediatr* 2003;20:3845.
6. Flynn JT, Mottes TA, Brophy PD, Kershaw DB, Smoyer WE, Buchman TE. Intravenous nicardipine for treatment of severe hypertension in children. *J Pediatr* 2001;139:38-43.

Daljit Singh and Vineet Arora

33 Shock

INTRODUCTION

Shock is defined as a clinical syndrome of acute disruption of both microcirculatory and microcirculatory function leading to a general insufficiency of tissue perfusion, oxygen utilization and cellular energy production that ultimately results in deranged homeostatic mechanisms and irreversible cellular damage.[1] It is a clinical state characterized by inadequate delivery of oxygen and metabolic substrates to meet the metabolic demands of tissues producing signs of inadequate organ and tissue perfusion and function, such as oliguria and lactic acidosis.[2]

Shock is not synonymous with hypotension. It may occur with a normal, increased or decreased blood pressure. Conversely, decrease in blood pressure may occur in absence of shock.[3,4]

PATHOPHYSIOLOGY

The cardiovascular system is under complex neuro-endocrinal control designed to maintain an adequate delivery of oxygen and substrates to the tissues. Delivery of oxygen is a direct function of the cardiac output and arterial oxygen content. Inadequate oxygen delivery can result from either limitation or maldistribution of blood flow.[5]

Cardiac output is the most important determinant of the tissue perfusion that depends on stroke volume and heart rate (Fig. 33.1). In young children and infants, heart rate is the main compensatory mechanism for increasing cardiac output.[2,5]

Blood pressure: Arterial pressure is the product of flow (cardiac output) and resistance (systemic vascular resistance).[2] Organ perfusion depends on both the cardiac output and perfusion pressure. Major factors that defend the blood pressure:

A. *Neuronal:* These include baroreceptors (carotid body, aortic arch), volume receptors (right atrium, pulmonary vessels), chemoreceptors (aortic and carotid, medullary) and cerebral response to ischemia.
B. *Humoral:* These include adrenal medulla (catecholamines) hypothalamo-pituitary response (ACTH and vasopressin) renin–angiotensin-aldosterone system.

Normal blood pressure can be maintained despite a fall in cardiac output only if compensatory vasoconstriction occurs. Tachycardia and increased cardiac contractility will also attempt to restore cardiac output. Hypotension is a late and often sudden sign of cardiovascular decompensation.[2]

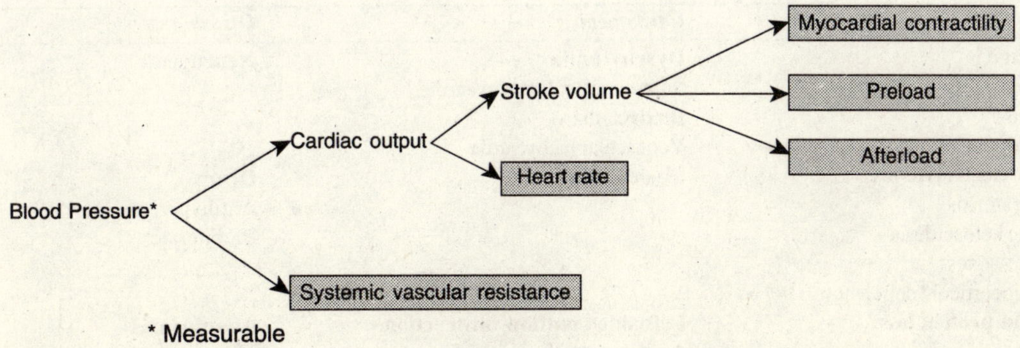

Fig. 33.1: Hemodynamic relations

Pathophysiological response to shock in newborn is blunted as compared to adults,[7-9] because of incomplete development of sympathetic nervous system, decreased myocardial contractility, decreased enzyme levels and decreased muscle fiber density.

Phases of Shock

Because of its progressive nature, shock can be divided into following stages:

I. *Early compensated*: It is characterized by maintenance of essential organ perfusion, with blood pressure, urine output and cardiac function remaining normal; early cellular metabolic alteration occurs.

II. *Decompensated:* As shock progresses, circulatory compensation fails due to ischemia, endothelial injury and effect of toxins. Cellular function deteriorates and disturbances in function become sequentially demonstrable in all organ systems.

III. *Irreversible shock: This* is the stage of terminal organ damage; cellular function deteriorates and death is inevitable.

CLASSIFICATION

There are many ways of classifying shock. Lack of a single universally accepted system indicates the complexity of underlying pathological processes and tremendous variability. Any classification must allow for various overlaps. For example, injury leading to hypovolemic shock due to hemorrhage and neurogenic shock resulting from associated intracranial injury may co-exist, while due to aspiration the patient may later develop septic shock.

An interesting way of looking at the definition and etiological classification of shock uses the mnemonic as follows[10]

S = Systemic impairment of oxygen consumption
H = Hypovolemia (Intrinsic and extrinsic)
O = Obstructive (cardiac temponade, massive pulmonary embolism, tension pneumothorax)
C = Cardiogenic (Primary pump failure)
K = Kinetic/distributive (sepsis, anaphylaxis)

Shock states may be broadly classified into four functional categories:[5]

a. Hypovolemic shock
b. Cardiogenic shock
c. Septic shock
d. Distributive shock

Hypovolemic Shock

Hypovolemic shock is the most common type of shock in pediatric patients.[3] It results from decreased intravascular volume and, therefore, decreased venous return and myocardial preload. Pathophysiology is shown in Figure 33.2.

Causes can be many as shown in Table 33.1.

The major cause of shock in the developing world is dehydration following diarrhea and vomiting. In developed countries, hemorrhage due to trauma is the leading cause.[11]

Cardiogenic Shock

It does not occur frequently in children but does account for a large number of admissions to a pediatric intensive care unit. It is the state in which an abnormality of cardiac function is responsible for the failure of the cardiovascular system to meet metabolic needs.[3,12] Causes include myocardial insufficiency due to CHF (congenital or acquired heart disease), cardiomyopathy (infectious or noninfectious), arrhythmia, hypothermia, drugs, toxins and obstructive causes like cardiac temponade and pneumopericardium. Hypoglycemia, acidosis and hypoxia, due to their myocardial depressant effect may also lead to cardiogenic shock.

Septic Shock

The incidence of septic shock is increasing world wide with a ten fold increase in past 20 years, the reason being that more patients are surviving with the diseases which are fatal previously like congenital heart disease, burns,

Table 33.1: Shock categories and common etiologies

Hypovolemic	*Cardiogenic*	*Distributive*
Hemorrhage	**Dysrhythmia**	**Neurogenic**
Trauma	Supraventricular tachycardia	
GI bleed	Bradycardia	
Coagulopathy	Ventricular tachycardia	
Fluid and electrolyte loss	**Myocarditis**	**Drugs**
Gastroenteritis		Antihypertensives
Diabetic ketoacidosis		Barbiturates
Polyuric states		
Mineralocorticoid deficiency		
Plasma and protein loss	**Left-sided outflow obstruction**	**Anaphylaxis**
Burns	Aortic stenosis	
Peritonitis	Hypoplastic left heart	
Bowel obstruction	Coarctation of aorta	

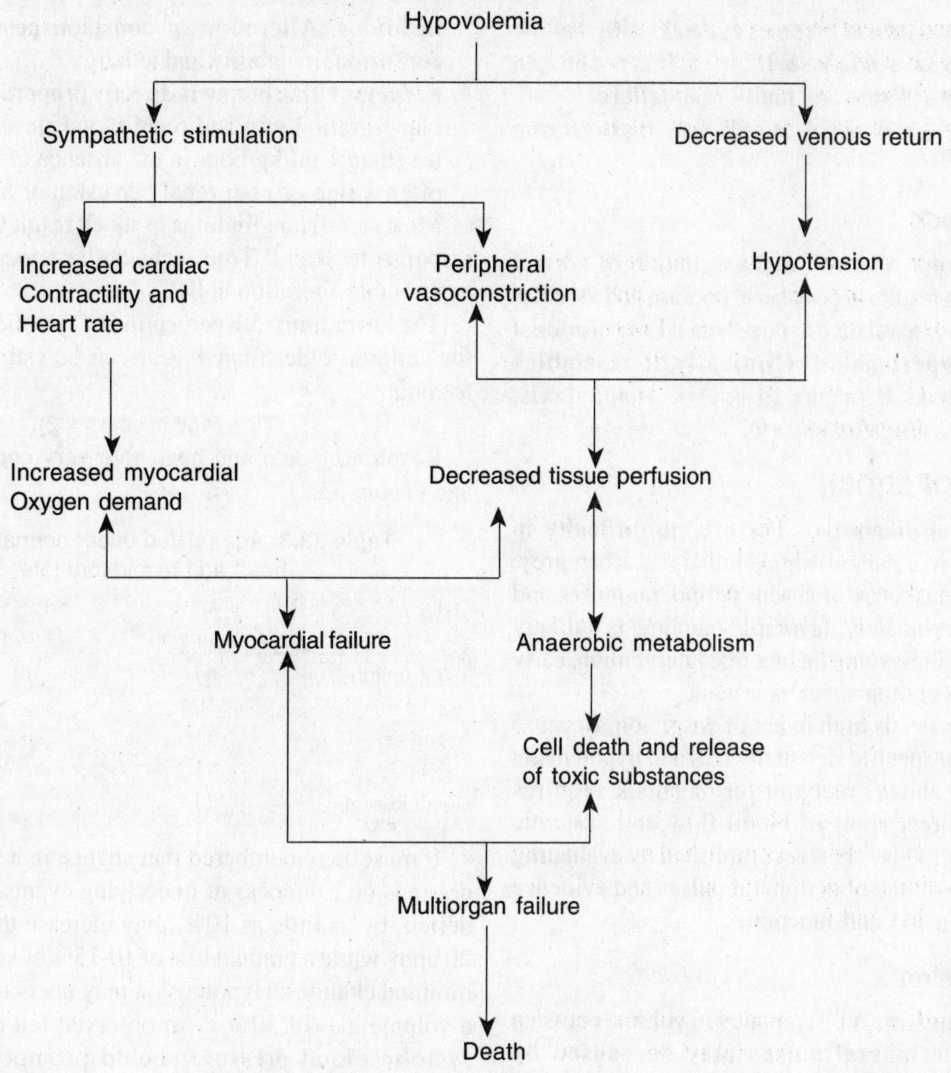

Fig. 33.2: Pathophysiology of hypovolemic shock

neoplasia, immunodeficiency, respiratory failure and trauma and due to increase in invasive procedures which constitute risk factors for developing sepsis. Diversity of pathophysiological deficits and marked early metabolic derangement justify a separate classification for septic shock.

Septic shock comprises a cascade of metabolic, hemodynamic and clinical changes resulting from the release of and the host response to the presence of microbial toxins (bacteria, virus, fungus, rickettsia) in the blood stream. Release of multiple vasoactive substances and endotoxins decrease the vascular resistance.[13-15]

Septic shock has two stages (Table 33.2). In early stage, also known as warm shock, the patient is warm, dry, well perfused, having bounding pulses and hyperdynamic metabolic state. Though cardiac output is increased, tissue injury is present with impaired cellular metabolism.[13]

Table 33.2: Stages of septic shock

Parameter	*Early (warm)*	*Late (cold)*
HR	↑	↑/↓
RR	↑ (tachypnea)	↓ (respiratory depression)
BP	N	↓
Pulse pressure	Wide	Narrow
Temp	Fever	Hypothermia
Pulses	Bounding	Thready
Skin	Warm	Cold, pale
Mental status	Anxious	Obtunded, Coma
Urine output	N/↑	↓

Subsequently due to increased capillary permeability, third space losses occur leading to hypovolemia with increase in peripheral resistance.[16-18] Blood pressure falls, pulse pressure narrows and patient becomes cyanotic with shallow laboured breathing i.e. cold shock. If the cycle is not broken it leads to vascular collapse and multiorgan failure.

Mortality from septic shock is still very high varying from 30-80%.[19-20]

Distributive Shock

Abnormal vasomotor tone and maldistribution of normal circulating volume results in peripheral pooling and vascular shunting which leads to relative hypovolemia. Loss of arterial tone leads to hypertension. Clinically it resembles hypovolemic shock. It occurs in sepsis, anaphylaxis, neurogenic shock, drugs/toxins, etc.

RECOGNITION OF SHOCK

Shock is a clinical diagnosis.[1] There is no difficulty in diagnosing shock in a patient who is lethargic, ashen grey, tachypneic, cold, has weak or absent peripheral pulses and hypotension. Unfortunately, favorable outcome is unlikely in such a case. For life-saving therapeutic intervention, early recognition of impending shock is crucial.

Early diagnosis needs high index of suspicion. Because tachycardia is a nonspecific sign of distress and hypotension is a late sign of shock, recognition of shock requires evaluation of indirect signs of blood flow and systemic vascular resistance. This is best accomplished by evaluating the presence and volume of peripheral pulses and evidence of end organ perfusion and function.[2]

Systemic Perfusion

1. ***Evaluation of pulses:*** A discrepancy in volume between central and peripheral pulses may be caused by vasoconstriction associated with a cold ambient temperature or may be an early sign of decreased cardiac output. When cardiac output decreases the pulse pressure narrows, making the pulse thready and finally impossible to feel. In contrast, early septic shock is a high-output state and is often characterized by a wide pulse pressure with bounding pulses. Loss of central pulses is a premorbid sign and should be treated as cardiac arrest.[2]
2. ***Skin:*** Decreased skin perfusion can be early sign of shock. When cardiac output decreases, cooling of the skin begins peripherally (in the fingers and toes) and extends proximally (towards the trunk).[21] Mottling, pallor, delayed capillary refill and peripheral cyanosis often indicate poor skin perfusion.
3. ***Brain:*** The clinical signs of brain perfusion are determined by the severity and duration of the ischemia.[22] When the ischemic insult is sudden, few signs of neurological compromise precede loss of consciousness. Muscular tone is lost and generalized seizures and pupillary dilatation may be observed. When the onset is more gradual, neurological symptoms are typically more insidious. Alteration of consciousness occurs, with confusion, irritability and lethargy.
4. ***Kidneys:*** Urine output is directly proportional to glomerular filtration rate and renal blood flow. Urine flow of less than 1 ml/kg/hour in the absence of renal disease is often a sign of poor renal perfusion or hypovolemia.[2]

Most significant findings in shock result from autonomic response to stress. True tachycardia appears well before any notable alteration in BP.

The lower limit (5th percentile) of systolic blood pressure for children older than 1 year can be estimated from the formula:[2]

$$70 + (\text{age in years} \times 2).$$

Respiratory rate and heart rate vary considerably with age (Table 33.3).

Table 33.3: Age related upper normal limit for heart and respiratory rate

Age	*RR (per minute)*	*HR (beats per minute)*
0-2 months	60	180
2-12 months	50	160
Toddler	30	140
School age	25	120
Adolescent	20	110

It must be remembered that change in heart rate and BP depends on acuteness of underlying events. Acute volume deficit, by as little as 10%, may increase the pulse rate by 20 bpm, while a gradual loss of 10-15% of volume produces minimal changes. Hypotension may not occur until there is a volume loss of 30%.[23] An observed fall of 10 mmHg in systolic blood pressure should prompt careful serial evaluations for additional signs of shock.

Assessment of Severity of Shock

The severity of shock can be assessed by careful recording of heart rate, respiratory rate, blood pressure and pulse pressure, skin colour, temperature and capillary filling time and urine output.

The shock may be categorized as compensated, decompensated or irreversible using the above parameters (Table 33.4).

A large number of laboratory measurements may be necessary in individual cases based on the clinical condition and underlying problem. However, investigations directly pertaining to shock which are usually necessary include: Complete hemogram, coagulation parameters blood urea, serum creatinine, calcium, electrolytes, RBS, urine routine examination and arterial blood gases. ABG is very important lab parameter but, unfortunately, restricted to few centers only.

Other investigations which may be required depending on specific indications include:

Table 33.4: Staging of shock

Stage	I	II	III
Parameter	Compensated	Decompensated	Irreversible
HR	↑	↑↑	↑↑↑
RR	N	↑	↑↑/0
BP	N	↓(low)	↓↓ (unrecordable)
Pulse pressure	N	↓	↓↓
Urine output	N	↓	0
Skin	Cool	Mottled	Cold, cyanotic
Mental status	Anxious	Obtunded	Coma

- Cultures: Blood, CSF, urine, stool, pus, etc.
- Chest X-ray, ECG, echocardiography
- LFT
- Stool for occult blood.

MONITORING

Clinical monitoring must include repeated and careful examination of the child's physiological status. The emphasis must be on continuing assessment of vital parameters and noninvasive monitoring of the child with cardiac monitor and pulse oxymeter (Table 33.5).

Table 33.5: Monitoring of shock

Clinical	Noninvasive	Invasive
Color	SpO_2	ABG
Temperature (skin, core)	ECG	CVP
Pulse rate and character	Chest Xray	RFT
CFT		Pulmonary arterial pressure
		Blood pressure
		Respiratory pattern
		Level of consciousness
		Intake/output

These simple parameters are generally adequate to make good assessment of response to therapy. In severe shock due to myocardial compromise, invasive venous and arterial pressure monitoring have been used in centres with such facilities. The role of CVP monitoring is more to avoid volume overload especially in patients with myocardial compromise or renal failure.

MANAGEMENT OF SHOCK

Shock must be identified at the earliest and corrective action taken immediately in the form of resuscitation, treatment of underlying cause and management of consequences and complications. The following interventions should be undertaken immediately for all cases.

Oxygen

The initial resuscitation involves securing a patent airway and administration of oxygen. In general, administer 100 % oxygen to all patients with shock in view of impaired peripheral oxygen delivery.[1,3,6] Maintain SpO_2 95-100% keeping $FiO_2 < 0.6$.

Venous Access

Intravenous access should be obtained within 5 minutes by any route.[24]

- *Route:* Within 90 seconds, do peripheral percutaneous IV cannulation. If unsuccessful, resort to intraosseous route while continuing attempt to cannulate peripheral veins. Do not waste time in performing cut-down. If the patient has cardiopulmonary arrest before IV access, intubate the child before IV access and give resuscitative drugs like epinephrine and atropine as indicated. Both can be given *via* endotracheal tube.
- *IV fluids:* Volume resuscitation is the first step in management of hypovolemic and distributive shock. Even if the precise etiology of shock or the volume status of the patient is not clear, fluid therapy should be initiated before establishing a line for monitoring the CVP, for example in a known case of CHD with vomiting or in unknown drug ingestion.
- *Type of fluid:* Initial fluid for all types of shock is crystalloid i.e. Ringers lactate or normal saline. Hypotonic fluids should be avoided as they diffuse rapidly from the vascular space.[25] Subsequently, in simple dehydration, crystalloids should be continued. However, in cases of sepsis or trauma, blood products to maintain hemoglobin and clotting factors, and/or maintain oncotic pressure should be used judiciously.
- *Amount of fluid:* Initial bolus of crystalloid 20 ml/kg should be given over 6-10 minutes.

Monitor response in the form of an improvement in capillary refill, an improvement in sensorium, a decrease in tachycardia, normalisation of blood pressure and an adequate urine output (1 ml/kg/hr).

On reassessment, if the BP and peripheral perfusion improves and urine is passed, IV fluids should be continued with further frequent assessment. If poor perfusion or hypotension persists after initial bolus, repeat 10-20 ml/kg of crystalloid and monitor urine output. A further bolus of 10 ml/kg is required if the urine output remains below 1ml/

kg/hr. If anuria is noted, 10-20 ml/kg should be administered before further interventions.

From the above steps it is clear that upto 60 ml/kg of fluid may be necessary while initially managing shock with hypotension and anuria. In spite of this, if improvement in these parameters does not occur, and is not explained by ongoing severe losses, CVP monitoring should be instituted and the cardiac status should be evaluated including chest X-ray and echocardiography. Further fluid therapy would then depend on CVP.

Specific Drugs

Whatever the etiology, the priority in treatment is the administration of oxygen and initial fluid bolus. During this period attempt should be made to determine the cause of shock. Specific management like administration of antibiotics in sepsis, or catecholamines and steroids in anaphylaxis, should be instituted as soon as possible after initiating the above.

Cardiovascular Support

All shock states can be characterized by some form of impairment of myocardial function. Whether this impairment is primary or secondary, therapeutic endeavours to optimize cardiac output should be the cornerstone of therapy.[1,6]

Management of Arrhythmia in Shock

The wide variation in heart rates associated with metabolic derangements may significantly impair cardiac performance. Treatment of arrhythmia includes correction of hypoxia, acidosis, hypocalcaemia, hypomagnesaemia, hypo/hyperkalemia.

Cardiotonic Drugs

Cardiotonic drugs increase the myocardial contractility. In hypotensive patients dopamine is the preferred drug in view of its inotropic and vasopressor effect. An infusion dose of 4-10 mg/kg/min is the usual initial dose. Infusion rate upto 20 mg/kg/min may be given as necessary.

Dobutamine is a good choice in patients with normal blood pressure and low cardiac output state, used in the dose of 5-20 mg/kg/min. However, it should be avoided in hypotensive patients because of its vasodilator effects.

In shock occurring after cardiorespiratory arrest and in patients where dose of more than 20 mg/kg/min of dopamine is required to maintain BP, epinephrine is the inotrope of choice. At low doses of 0.3 mg/kg/min, it has

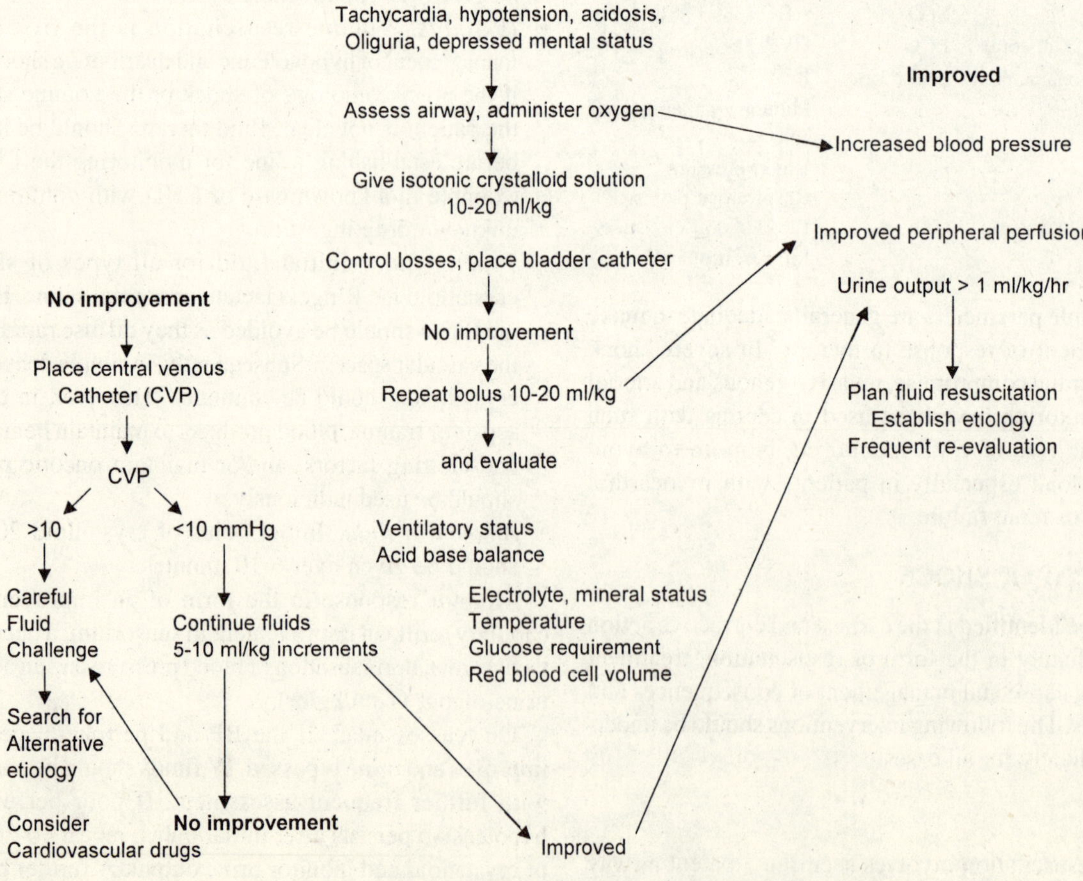

Fig. 33.3: Management of hypovolemic shock

primarily cardiac effects while at higher doses it is a potent vasoconstrictor.

Vasodilator Drugs

Drugs that improve cardiac performance by decreasing afterload are indicated in late stages of shock when vasoconstriction is severe. Sodium nitroprusside and nitroglycerine are the two main drugs in this category.

Correction of Acidosis

Metabolic correction of severe acidosis is important for improving cellular function and myocardial performance. Base deficit of > 10 mEq/L occurring in septic and cardiogenic shock is associated with poor outcome. Base deficit is better tolerated in hypovolemia and renal bicarbonate loss.

Indication for Use of Sodium Bicarbonate

Correction of acidosis is indicated when pH is less than 7.20.[1,6,26] The adverse effects of this degree of acidosis are impaired ventilatory response, depressed myocardial function, dysrhythmias and altered response of autonomic receptors to drugs.

A base deficit greater than 6 mEq/L in an acute shock state should be properly be treated. A dose of 1-2 mEq/kg of sodium bicarbonate given in slow bolus should be administered; subsequent dose is calculated using the formula: 0.3 × wt (kg) × base deficit = mEq of $NaHCO_3$.

This is given as continuous sodium bicarbonate infusion. Too rapid correction of pH with bicarbonate may result in paradoxical cerebrospinal fluid and brain cell acidosis and impaired delivery of oxygen to tissues.

Correction of Other Metabolic Abnormalities

While correcting acidosis with bicarbonate, other electrolyte abnormalities may occur, especially fall in serum ionized calcium. Sustained decreases in ionized calcium have been associated with depressed myocardial function, tachycardia, electrocardiographic changes, hypotension, acidosis, cyanosis, temperature instability, alterations in mental status and motor nerve excitability.

A level below 2.4 mg/dl justifies treatment. Intravenous infusion of 1-2 ml/kg of 10% calcium gluconate rapidly restores serum ionized calcium.[27]

Hypokalemia may occur as potassium re-enters the cells with return of pH towards normal. It can be corrected by using potassium concentration of 40-60 mEq/L.

Hyperglycemia, hypoglycemia and hypophosphataemia are other disturbances needing detection and appropriate intervention.

Table 33.6: Management of complications of shock

Organ system	*Complications*	*Management*
GIT	GI bleed Paralytic ileus	H_2 blockers NPO, NG aspiration
Renal	ARF	Diuretics, low dose dopamine, dialysis
Blood	DIC	Blood component transfusion
Lungs	Respiratory failure ARDS	Mechanical ventilation

Support for Renal, Gastrointestinal and Hematological Systems

Renal support for preventing failure is in the form of volume augmentation, use of diuretics and low dose dopamine.[28] If ARF is established early dialysis should be instituted.

Gastro-intestinal bleeding and ileus often occur in shock. Paralytic ileus is usually gastric in origin unless there is an associated peritonitis. Prevention and early management of dyselectrolytemia is important. The stomach should be emptied and kept empty with a nasogastric tube. Use of antacids and H_2 receptor blockers help in preventing stress ulceration.

Coagulation abnormalities are most striking in septic shock and also occur in terminal stages of other forms of shock. They can be corrected by giving blood transfusions, platelet transfusion or fresh frozen plasma as indicated.

Mechanical Ventilation

Shock is associated with increased work of breathing due to hyperventilation elicited by acidemia and hypoxia and alterations in pulmonary mechanics secondary to pulmonary vascular congestion. Respiratory muscle fatigue may occur leading to respiratory failure and circulatory collapse. Early institution of intubation and positive pressure ventilation are recommended.

Indications of Starting Mechanical Ventilation include:[1,6,29]

- Acute respiratory acidosis, resulting from ventilatory failure.
- Failure to adequately oxygenate with venturi mask, etc.
- Respiratory fatigue.

In some children, ARDS may develop. This may be managed with conventional mechanical ventilation with high PEEP. Use of nitric oxide for severe pulmonary hypertension or gross hypoxemia and of high frequency oscillation is restricted to few centres where facilities are available. In refractory septic shock, extracorporeal membrane oxygenation (ECMO) has been tried in the developed countries.[30]

Nutritional Support

Excessive catabolism with destruction of lean body mass is the most common nutritional abnormality in shock states. Utilization of aggressive nutritional support (both enteral and parenteral) in critically ill patients results in improved recovery from organ failure, improved immunological status, improved resistance to infection and reduced mortality.

Prevention and Control of Infection

Prevention of acquired infection in critically ill patients is of paramount importance. All catheters should be inserted using proper aseptic technique. Once infection is present every effort should be made to rapidly administer appropriate antimicrobial therapy. It is preferable to provide empirical broad spectrum antibiotic coverage taking into consideration the primary site of infection, local bacterial sensitivity pattern and immunocompetence of the host.[1,6,30]

Steroids

These are beneficial in adrenal failure associated with HIV or sepsis. Some publications recommend early use of steroids such as 30 mg/kg of methyl prednisolone initiated within 4 hours of septic shock followed by 3 or 4 doses 4-8 hours apart.[31,32]

Exchange Transfusion

Exchange transfusion has been used as a therapy for septic shock in newborns with an increase in survival rates.[30] Proposed benefits of exchange transfusion include removal of bacterial endotoxin and circulating inflammatory mediators, improved leukocyte lysing of organisms by mature functional granulocytes and increased opsonic activity, improved oxygen delivery of blood with adult hemoglobin, improved acidosis, coagulopathy and electrolyte abnormalities.

PROGNOSIS AND OUTCOME

Anticipation, early detection, immediate intervention, close monitoring and systemic approach to reverse the pathophysiological abnormalities are thus the key points in successful management of shock. The mortality depends upon the underlying etiology, being as high as 50% with septic shock. Low body temperature (< 37 °C), pulmonary disease, low cardiac index (< 3.3 L/min/m^2) and decreased oxygen utilization are all poor prognostic indicators in shock.[33]

REFERENCES

1. Joseph R, Randall T, Wetzel C. Shock and multiorgan system failure. In: Roger MC, Nichols DG (eds) *Textbook of Pediatric Intensive Care*, 3rd edn. Maryland: Williams and Wilkins 1996;589-605.
2. Chameides L, Hazinski MF (eds) Recognition of respiratory failure and shock. In: *Textbook of Pediatric Advanced Life support*. American Heart Association, 1997;2-10.
3. Perkin RM, Levin DL. Shock in the pediatric patient. Part I. *J Pediatr* 1982;101:163-169.
4. Perkin RM, Levin DL. Shock in the pediatric patient. Part II. *J Pediatr* 1982;101:319-332.
5. Uttam R. Shock in critically ill children. *Pediatrics Today* 1999;2:604-609.
6. Singhi S, Hiranandani M. Shock. In: Sachdev HPS, Puri RK, Bagga A, Choudhury P (eds) *Textbook of Principles of Pediatric and Neonatal Emergencies*.New Delhi: Jaypee Brothers 1994;23-44.
7. Friedman WF. The intrinsic physiological properties of the developing heart. *Progs Cardiovasc Dis* 1972;15:87-85.
8. O Brien WF, Golden SM, Davis SE. Endotoxemia in the neonatal lamb. *Am J Obstet Gynecol* 1985;151: 671.
9. McCartney FA. Heart and Circulation In: Godfrey S, Bower JD (eds) *Clinical PediatricPhysiology*. Oxford: Blackwell 1979;284.
10. Jerry J, Zimmerman, Kenneth A, Dietrich. Current perspectives on septic shock. *Pediatr Clin North Am* 1987;34:131.
11. National Safety Council. *Accident Facts. National Safety Council Annual Report*. Chicago: National Safety Council 1981.
12. Levin A. *Inotropic Agents in Pediatric Practice*. New York: US Sci Akad 1977.
13. Ellner JJ. Septic shock. *Pediatr Clin North Am* 1983;30:365.
14. Henrich WL, Hamasaki Y, Said SJ, et al. Dissociation of systemic and renal effects in endotoxemia. *J Clin Invest* 1983;71:351.
15. McCabe WR, Treadwell TL. Pathophysiology of bacteremia. *Am J Med* 1983;75:2.
16. Schumer W. Septic shock. *JAMA* 1979;242:1906.
17. Samuelson B. Leukotrienes. Mediators of immediate hypersensitivity reactions and inflammation. *Science* 1983;220:568.
18. Weissman G, Smolen JE. Release of inflammatory mediators from stimulated neutrophils. *N Engl J Med* 1980;303.
19. Parker MM, Parrillo JE, Septic shock hemodynamics and pathogenesis. *JAMA* 1983;250:3324.
20. Gaffin SL, Lachman E. The use of antilipophospholipids antibodies in the management of septic shock. *S Afric Med J* 1984;65:158.
21. Joly HR, Weil MH. Temperature of the great toe as an indication of the severity of shock. *Circulation* 1969;39:131-138.
22. Plum F, Posner JB. *The Diagnosis of Stupor and Coma*, 3rd edn. Philadelphia: FA Davis 1980.
23. Hauser CJ, Shoemaker WC. Volume therapy in diagnosis of hypovolemia. *Hosp Phys* 1980;16:38.
24. Zimmerman JJ, Streuss HH. History and current application of intravenous therapy in children. *Pediatr Emerg Care* 1989;5: 120-127.
25. Velanovich V. Crystalloid versus colloid fluid resuscitation: A meta-analysis of mortality. *Surgery* 1989:105:165.
26. Chameides L, Hazinski MF. Fluid therapy and medications. In: *Textbook of Pediatric Advanced Life Support*. New York: American Heart Association 1997;6:1-12.
27. Chernow B. Calcium: Does it have a therapeutic role in sepsis (ed). *Crit care Med* 1990;18:895.
28. Parker S, Carlon GC, Issacs M, Howland WS, Kahn RC. Dopamine administration in oliguria and oliguric renal failure *Crit Care Med* 1981;9:632.

29. Ward ME, Roussos C. The respiratory muscle in shock: service or disservice? *Intensive Crit Care Dig* 1985;4:3.
30. Butt W. Septic shock. *Pediatr Clin North Am* 2001;48: 601-625.
31. Bone RC, Fischer CJ, Ctemmer TP, et al. A controlled trial of high dose methylprednisolone in the treatment of severe sepsis and septic shock. *N Engl J Med* 1987;317:6653.
32. The veterens administration system sepsis cooperative study group. Effect of high dose glucocorticoid therapy on mortality in patients with clinical signs of systemic sepsis. *N Engl J Med* 1987;317:659.
33. Pollock MM, Fields AI, Ruttimann UE. Distribution of cardiopulmonary variables in pediatric survivors of septic shock. *Crit Care Med* 1985;13:454.

Poothirikovil Venugopalan

34 Cardiac Arrhythmias

INTRODUCTION

Cardiac arrhythmias especially bradyarrhythmias in children unlike in adults represent an end-result of systemic hypoperfusion and hypoxemia.[1,2] However, there are several instances of cardiac disorders presenting primarily as arrhythmias, e.g. supraventricular tachycardia and ventricular tachycardia secondary to congenital long QT syndromes. Moreover, cardiac arrhythmias may present with vague symptoms and even as neurologic problems, and seizure disorders may be associated with fatal cardiac events.[3,4] Hence, it is important to perform monitoring of cardiac rhythm in all at-risk patients.

This chapter focuses on the arrhythmias that need urgent attention, and once the condition is stabilized these children may be referred to a pediatric cardiologist for further evaluation and long-term therapy.

ETIOPATHOGENESIS

Table 34.1 lists the common types of cardiac arrhythmias. The etiological agents are enumerated in Table 34.2. Detailed discussions are available elsewhere.[5]

Table 34.1: Common cardiac arrhythmias in children

Benign arrhythmias
- Sinus arrhythmia
- Sinus tachycardia*
- Sinus bradycardia
- Premature atrial beats
- Premature junctional beats
- Premature ventricular beats
- First degree heart block
- Second degree heart block

Arrhythmias that may require intervention
- Supraventricular tachycardia
- Atrial flutter
- Atrial fibrillation
- Sustained ventricular tachycardia
- Ventricular fibrillation
- Pulseless electrical activity
- Cardiac asystole
- Complete heart block
- Sick sinus syndrome

*Usually requires investigation and treatment of the cause, which may be cardiac or noncardiac.

Cardiac arrhythmias may originate from either abnormalities in impulse formation or impulse propagation or abnormalities in autonomic influence. Often, more than one mechanism may operate to produce similar type of arrhythmia, and understanding the basic mechanism of arrhythmia is helpful in management of the patient.

Cardiac arrest refers to a state where there is no palpable pulse, and in a majority of instances is the end-result of respiratory or circulatory disorders like pneumonia, hypovolemic shock, etc.[2] Analysis of electrocardiogram in these situations may reveal one of the four types of rhythm disturbances–asystole (Fig. 34.1), pulseless electrical activity, ventricular fibrillation (Fig. 34.2) and, in some instances, ventricular tachycardia that has been persistent for sometime (Fig. 34.3). Occasionally, an older child with previously known cardiac disorder or a child with long QT syndrome or acute myocarditis may present with ventricular fibrillation or tachycardia without any of the systemic diseases mentioned above.

Supraventricular tachycardia (Fig. 34.4) is the most common primary cardiac arrhythmia that requires therapy in children.[6] Majority of these are the result of a re-entry mechanism, involving the normal atrioventricular conduction pathway and an accessory pathway (Fig. 34.5), and therefore a delay or transient block in the conduction will help to terminate the tachycardia and restore sinus rhythm (Fig. 34.6). Ventricular tachycardias are often due to ectopic activity in the ventricles but depolarization abnormalities form the basis in a subgroup of patients with long QT syndrome.

Clinical presentation depends on the age of the patient, duration of the arrhythmia and presence of any pre-existing

Table 34.2: Etiology of cardiac arrhythmias in children

- Accessory atrioventricular conduction pathways
  Manifest on electrocardiogram (WPW syndrome)
  Concealed pathway
- Hypoxemia, hypovolemia, hypothermia
- Electrolyte and acidbase disturbances
  Hypo/hyperkalemia, hypo/hypercalcemia, metabolic acidosis
- Myocardial disorders
  Myocarditis, cardiomyopathy
- Endocrine disturbances
  Hypo/hyperthyrodism
- Congenital heart diseases
  Corrected transposition of great arteries
  Ebstein's anomaly of tricuspid valve
  Single ventricle
  Ventricular septal defect
  Aortic stenosis
  Atrial septal defect
  Tetralogy of Fallot
  Tricuspid atresia
- Cardiac tumors
- Maternal disorders
  Maternal systemic lupus erythematosus
  Maternal diabetes mellitus
- Postoperative cardiac state
- Toxins/poisons/drugs
- Mitral valve prolapse
- Long QT syndromes
- Arrhythmogenic right ventricular dysplasia
- Tension pneumothorax
- Cardiac tamponade

cardiac disorder. Older children exhibit more specific symptoms like palpitation, chest pain, syncope, cardiac arrest and sudden death. Nonspecific symptoms include light headedness, tiredness, lethargy, nausea, and chest discomfort. Infants cannot verbalize their symptoms and, hence, often present late with nonspecific symptoms like irritability, lethargy, poor feeding, excessive crying, breathlessness or fast heart beats noted by parents. They may present in shock or manifest with cerebral hypoxemia in the form of seizures. Complete heart block may manifest effort intolerance or syncope or cardiac arrest due to the ventricular tachycardia secondary to the slow heart rate. Where the tachyarrhythmia is self limiting and recurrent, the symptoms are also paroxysmal and the heart rate and rhythm may be normal during the time of presentation to the physician. This does not exclude the presence of a serious cardiac arrhythmia. The clinical features of the underlying disease associated with the arrhythmia may be the prominent presenting feature in some patients.

Physical examination can help to identify the presence and rate of the pulse and to look for signs of poor systemic perfusion. In instances of bradyarrhythmias and cardiac arrest, it may give important clue as to the underlying disease process.

Investigations are directed to identify the cause and include blood and urine examinations and chest and skull radiographs, 12-lead ECG and in some instances echocardiography and EEG. Detailed electrophysiologic studies are indicated in resistant cases of tachyarrhythmias.

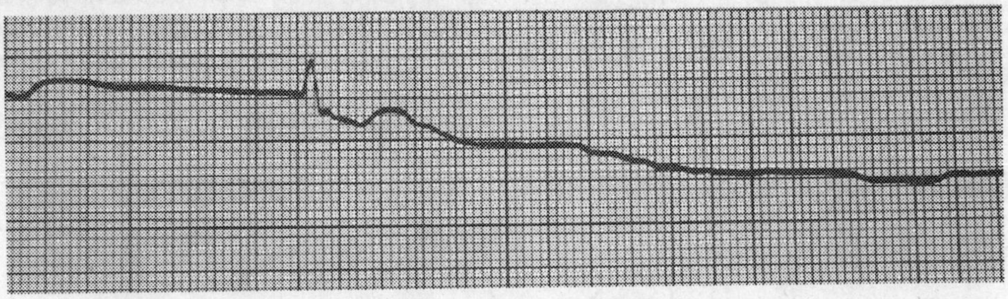

Fig. 34.1: Electrocardiogram showing cardiac asystole. This rhythm has to be confirmed by checking the pulse, checking the pulse, checking the leads and changing the leads

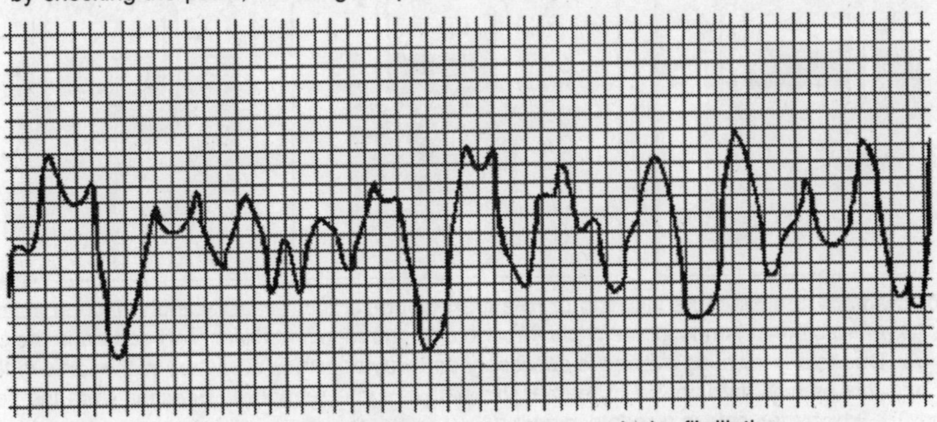

Fig. 34.2: Electrocardiogram showing ventricular fibrillation

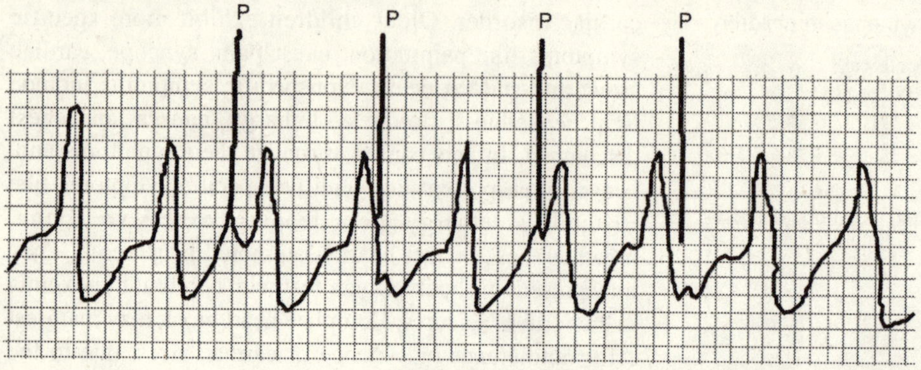

Fig. 34.3: Electrocardiogram showing broad complex tachycardia with atrioventricular dissociation, characteristic of ventricular tachycardia

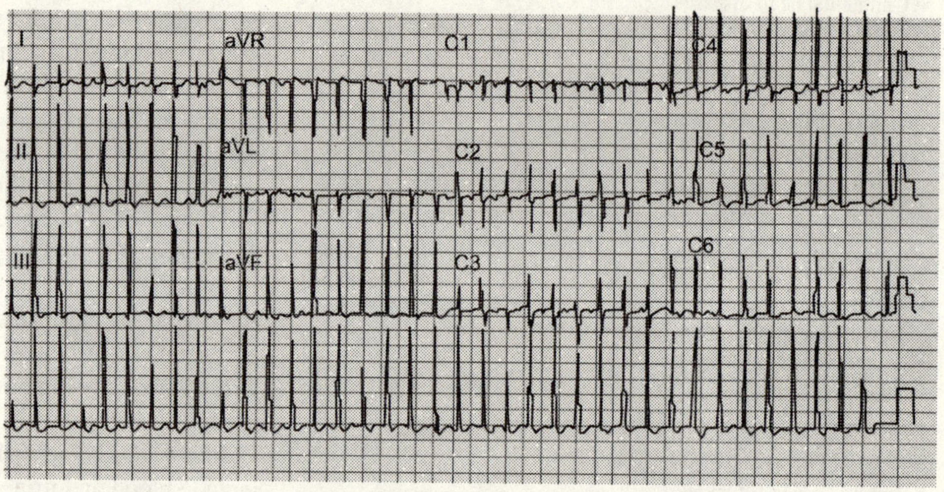

Fig. 34.4: 12-lead electrocardiogram from an 8-year old girl with supraventricular tachycardia

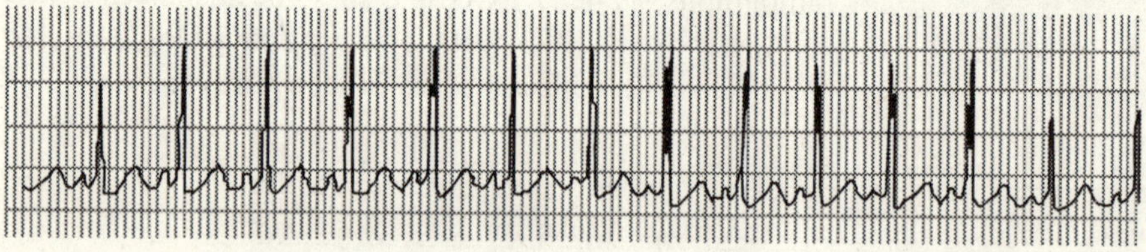

Fig. 34.5: Electrocardiogram showing the short PR interval, prolonged QRS interval, and the delta wave (representing forward conduction via accessory pathway). Wolff-Parkinson-White pattern refers to this ECG picture

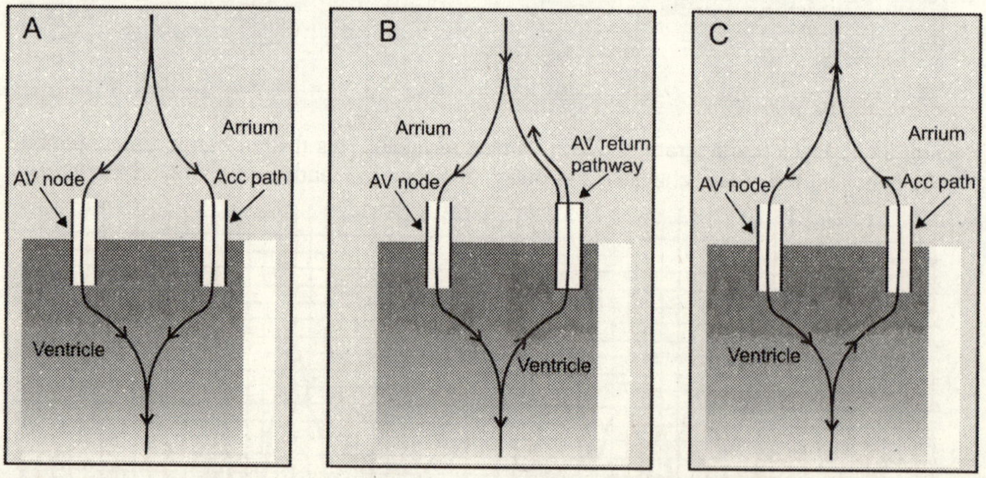

Fig. 34.6: Diagram to explain the initiation of re-entrant supraventricular tachycardia. During sinus rhythm, impulses travel from the atrium to the ventricle through both the atrioventricular (AV) node and the accessory pathway (A). Due to any initiating event, the accessory pathway beocmes refractory to the forward flow of the impulse, and this permits the impulse to reenter this pathway in a retrograde direction from the ventricle to the atrium (B), which then sets in a reentry circuit (C)

Seizure related cardiac arrhythmias are often unrecognized, although not uncommon, with an incidence ranging from 1:525 to 1:2100.[3] Associated bradycardia and asystole although rare could be life-threatening[7,8] and occur mostly in older children. Ictal arrhythmia should be considered in any patient who exhibits a dramatic loss of tone, or loss of consciousness associated with indeterminate events or seizures, especially in those who are not responding to antiepileptic medication. Autonomic response patterns have been implicated in the pathogenesis of seizure related arrhythmia.[9] Oppenheimer et al[10] have demonstrated asymmetric autonomic response patterns by intraoperative stimulation of insular cortex in patients undergoing surgery for intractable seizures. Tachycardia and pressor responses were more frequent with right anterior insular stimulation, while bradycardia and depressor responses were frequent with left anterior insular stimulation. Autonomic impulses (both sympathetic and parasympathetic) travelling to the cardiorespiratory system could cause not only sinus node dysfunction but also alterations in blood pressure, respiration and vasomotor tone.

The discussion on cardiac arrhythmias is incomplete without a mention of the congenital long QT syndromes. These are a group of disorders of ventricular repolarization, characterized by abnormally prolonged QT interval corrected for the heart rate (QTc), the upper limit of normal being considered as 0.45 seconds (Fig. 34.7). Other causes of prolongation of QT interval especially electrolyte abnormalities and myocarditis should be excluded before the diagnosis is made. These children often present with episodes of syncope, unconsciousness, seizures and apparent life-threatening episodes.[11]

APPROACH TO MANAGEMENT

Prompt institution of therapy is crucial to improve the outcome, and a certain degree of skill and experience on the part of the treating physician is essential. It is recommended that physicians involved in the management of sick children should undergo specially organized courses for basic life-support and advanced pediatric life-support.[12]

Table 34.3: Differential diagnosis of "narrow complex" tachycardia

	Sinus tachycardia	*Supraventricular tachycardia*
Heart rate	< 220 in infant < 180 in child	> 220 in infant > 180 in child
HR variability	Present	Absent
P Wave	Normal	Absent or abnormal if visible
Onset and termination	Gradual	Abrupt
Cause	Usually evident	Not obvious

Tachyarrhythmias (Fig. 34.8)

The history, physical examination and 12-lead ECG are very helpful in differentiating the three types of tachyarrhythmias i.e. sinus tachycardia, supraventricular tachycardia (Table 34.3) and ventricular tachycardia.

Sinus tachycardia requires attention to the cause of the tachycardia, and appropriate intervention.

In patients with SVT, vagal maneuvers have a role in the initial management. These include placing of ice-packs on the face (diving reflex), carotid sinus massage and stimulating throat with a tongue depressor. Do not press on the eyeball, as this has been shown to produce intraocular damage including hemorrhage. Older children can be asked to perform Valsalva maneuver, which involves closing the mouth and nose and breathing out against the closed mouth and nose. Blowing out through an obstructed straw is helpful in children who cannot perform the above technique. These vagal maneuvers may not produce remarkable effect on the heart rate. However, these should be attempted while waiting for the establishment of an IV access for adenosine administration or arranging for the cardioversion in an unstable patient. A continuous rhythm strip should be recorded during the procedure to review the changes.

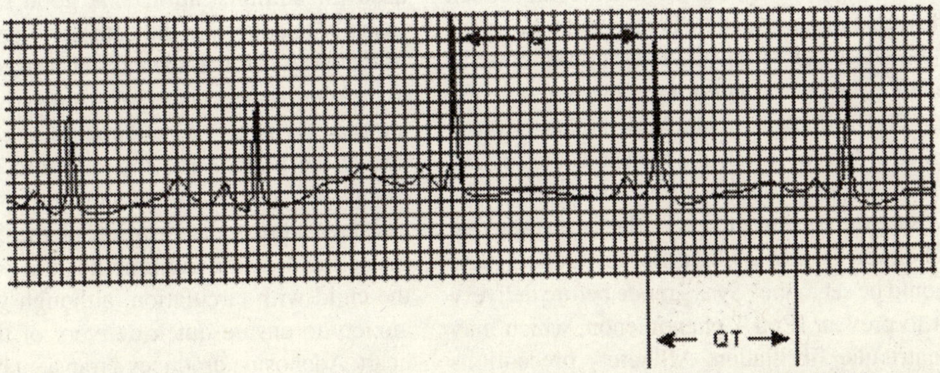

Fig. 34.7: Electrocardiogram from an infant with congenital long QT syndrome, demonstrating the measurement of QT and RR intervals. The corrected QT interval (QTc) is obtained by dividing the measured QT interval by the square root of RR interval

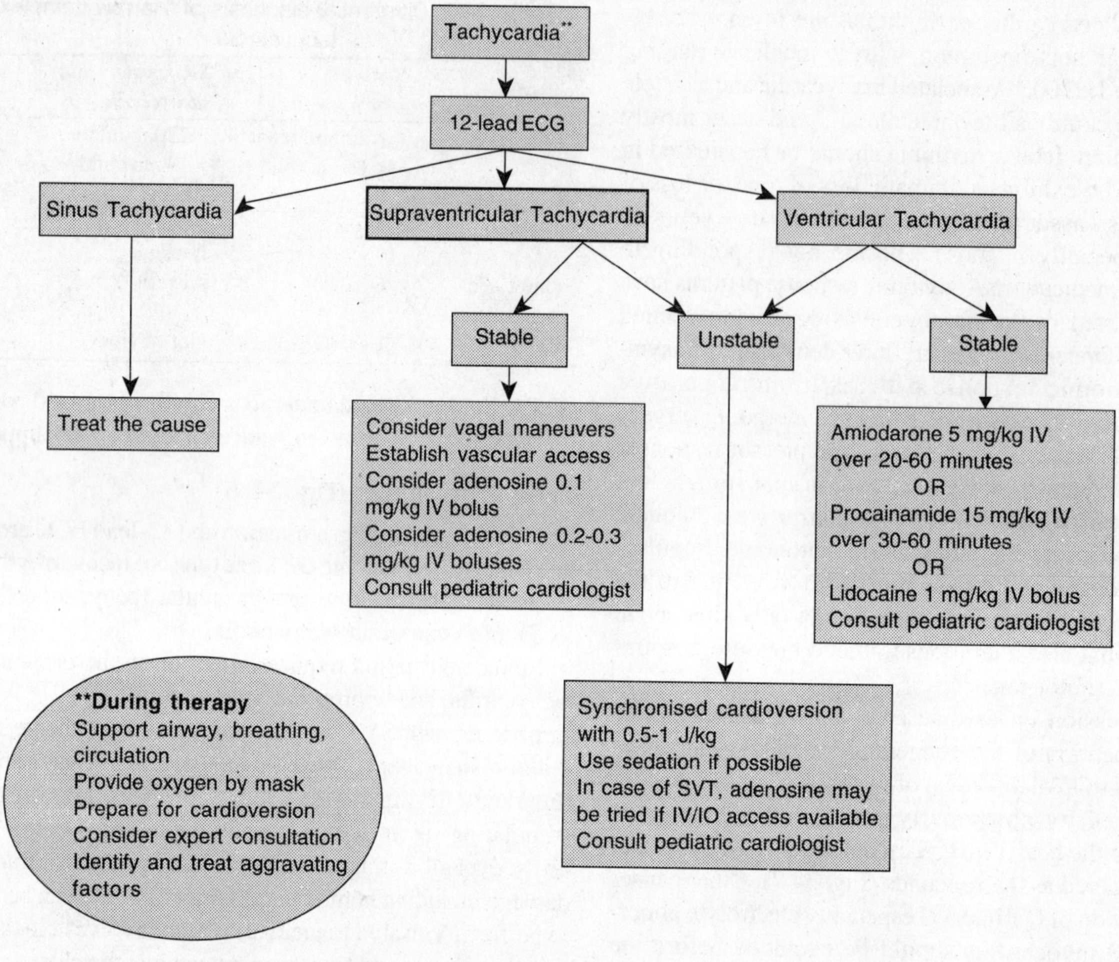

Fig. 34.8: Suggested algorithm for management of pediatric tachyarrhythmias

In the presence of poor perfusion (congestive heart failure with poor perfusion, breathlessness, altered sensorium, or shock with hypotension), synchronised electrical cardioversion is the treatment of choice. The health providers should be familiar with the type of cardiovertor/defibrillator available in the particular hospital. Larger size paddles should be used-infant paddles only for infants below age of 1 year, and the adult size paddles for all other ages.[13] The paddles should be placed in such a way that the heart is in between the two paddles. Usually, one paddle is placed on the upper right side of the chest below the clavicle and the other to the left of the left nipple in the anterior axillary line directly over the heart. Electrode pads or electrode cream or paste should be applied to the chest wall and firm pressure applied on to the paddles in order to reduce the impedance to the current flow. Electric current of 0.5-1 J/kg is the starting dose and can be increased to 2 J/kg if not responding. The instrument should be set to the "Sync" mode before delivery of the current to prevent R on T phenomenon, which may precipitate ventricular fibrillation. All safety precautions should be exercised to avoid accidental shocking of personnel involved in the resuscitation by speaking aloud and looking around to ensure all personnel are away from contact with the patient or the cot while discharging the paddles.

SVT patients who are stable can wait arrival of the pediatric cardiologist or be given intravenous bolus of adenosine depending on the experience of the physician. Adenosine is a very short acting drug (half life less than 20 seconds and the whole of the administered medication is inactivated in 30 seconds), and the rapid flush technique is used for administration.[14] A good sized venous catheter (usually needle over the catheter type) is inserted into one of the large veins in the cubital fossa and a 3-way attached to it. Adenosine is taken in a 1 ml syringe and 5 ml saline in another syringe. The adenosine is connected to the hub nearer the patient and the saline to the other hub of the 3-way. As soon as the adenosine is pushed in rapidly, the assistant adjusts the position of the 3-way and pushes in the saline. Raising the limb has not been shown to benefit the child with circulation, although we often do it in our anxiety to ensure quick delivery of the medication to the heart. Adenosine produces a transient block of the AV node, thereby breaking the vicious cycle or re-entry phenomenon that perpetuates the SVT. In a few seconds this action is reversed and sinus rhythm resumes. Again a continuous rhythm strip monitoring is essential during the procedure. Side effects to adenosine are rare and include vomiting, hot flushes, precipitation of bronchial asthma, prolonged asystole and other cardiac arrhythmias.

The most common cause of failure of adenosine in SVT is improper technique of administration, allowing the drug to be inactivated before it reaches the heart. A second dose of 0.2 and later 0.3 mg/kg can be administered. Maximum initial dose in a child is 6 mg and the second one 12 mg. Immediate recurrence of the SVT is another common problem. If this persists despite repeated doses, then an intravenous dose of digoxin 10 microgram/kg may be given over 3-5 minutes and the adenosine dose repeated. This is often found to produce sustained reversal to sinus rhythm. An important consideration in this situation is the accuracy of the diagnosis. One should reassess whether the child has sinus tachycardia or a primary *atrial* tachycardia both of which will not respond to adenosine. In the latter situation, the rhythm strip after adenosine assists in the diagnosis, as P waves at the high rate will persist even during the period of the AV block. Alternate medications that can be used include sotalol, flecainide and amiodarone,[15,16] but these are best administered under the supervision of a pediatric cardiologist in an intensive care set up.

Ventricular tachycardia in a stable child may be treated with IV amiodarone infusion or procainimide or lignocaine (Fig. 34.8). However, one should be on the look out for worsening of the circulation or onset of ventricular fibrillation and arrangements for cardioversion/defibrillation should proceed while waiting for the drug response. In the presence of hemodynamic compromise, VT should be treated as SVT with synchronized cardioversion. However, defibrillation is the preferred therapy for pulseless VT.

Whenever electrical shock is to be administered, if the child's condition permits, sedation should be used prior to the shock. This may require insertion of an IV access, and hence the potential for use of adenosine for SVT in circumstances other than the extreme emergency situations when the shock is applied without sedation. In the presence of hypoxemia, oxygenation and ventilation are to be ensured before definitive therapy for SVT is instituted. It is worth noting that current recommendations emphasise that adenosine can be effective even when administered by the intraosseous route.[17]

Bradyarrhythmias (Fig. 34.9)

Sinus bradycardia is the commonest type of bradycardia in children and is mostly secondary to systemic diseases.

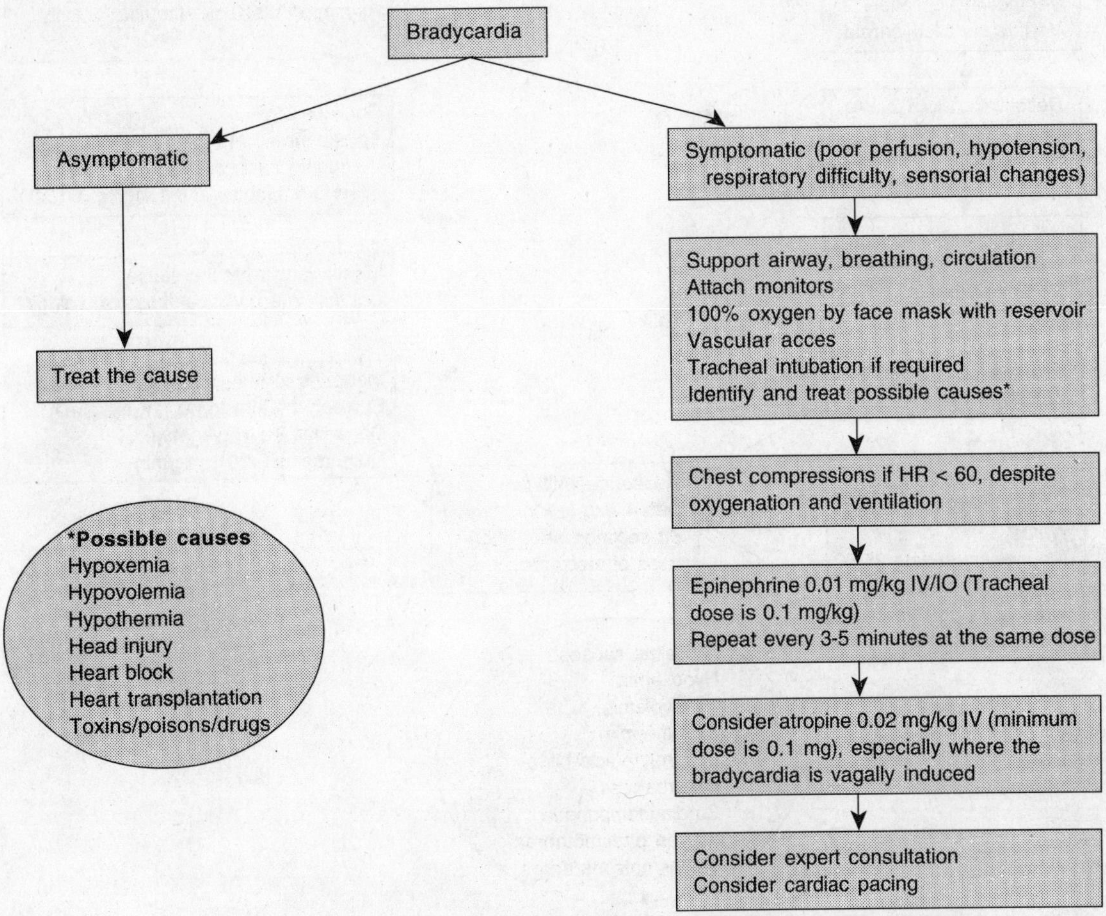

Fig. 34.9: Suggested algorithm for management of pediatric bradyarrhythmias

Immediate attention should be towards ensuring adequate oxygenation and ventilation. Meanwhile a rapid search should be initiated to find out the underlying cause. In the presence of poor perfusion, hypotension, respiratory difficulty or sensorial changes, more aggressive measures are required. External chest compressions are commenced if despite oxygenation and ventilation the heart rate remains below 60 per minute, with evidence of poor perfusion. The next step is the use of epinephrine in a dose of 0.01 mg/kg IV/IO, or 0.1 mg/kg by tracheal route if IV access is not available. The same dose can be repeated once in 3-5 minutes till improvement occurs. Selected patients may benefit from a dose of atropine 0.02 mg/Kg IV/IO. This drug is useful in patients in whom the bradycardia is in response to vagal stimulation as during tracheal intubation.

Temporary cardiac pacing and cardiology consultation are to be actively taken up in resistant patients.

Pulseless Rhythms (Fig. 34.10)

Ventricular fibrillation and pulseless ventricular tachycardia are treated by defibrillation.[18,19] A higher electrical energy is used compared to cardioversion, and no synchronization is possible. After the first 3 shocks, if the abnormal rhythm persists, airway is secured by tracheal intubation and IV access obtained. Epinephrine bolus is given and the shocks repeated. This can be done every 3-5 minutes. Alternate medications to be considered include amiodarone, lidocaine and magnesium (the latter only in Torsades de Pointes or documented hypomagnesemia).

Presence of organized electrical activity on the surface ECG without a palpable pulse and asystole are more often end result of a systemic cause, and require identification and treatment directed at the cause. However, cardiopulmonary resuscitation is essential to maintain circulation and epinephrine boluses or infusion are often used.

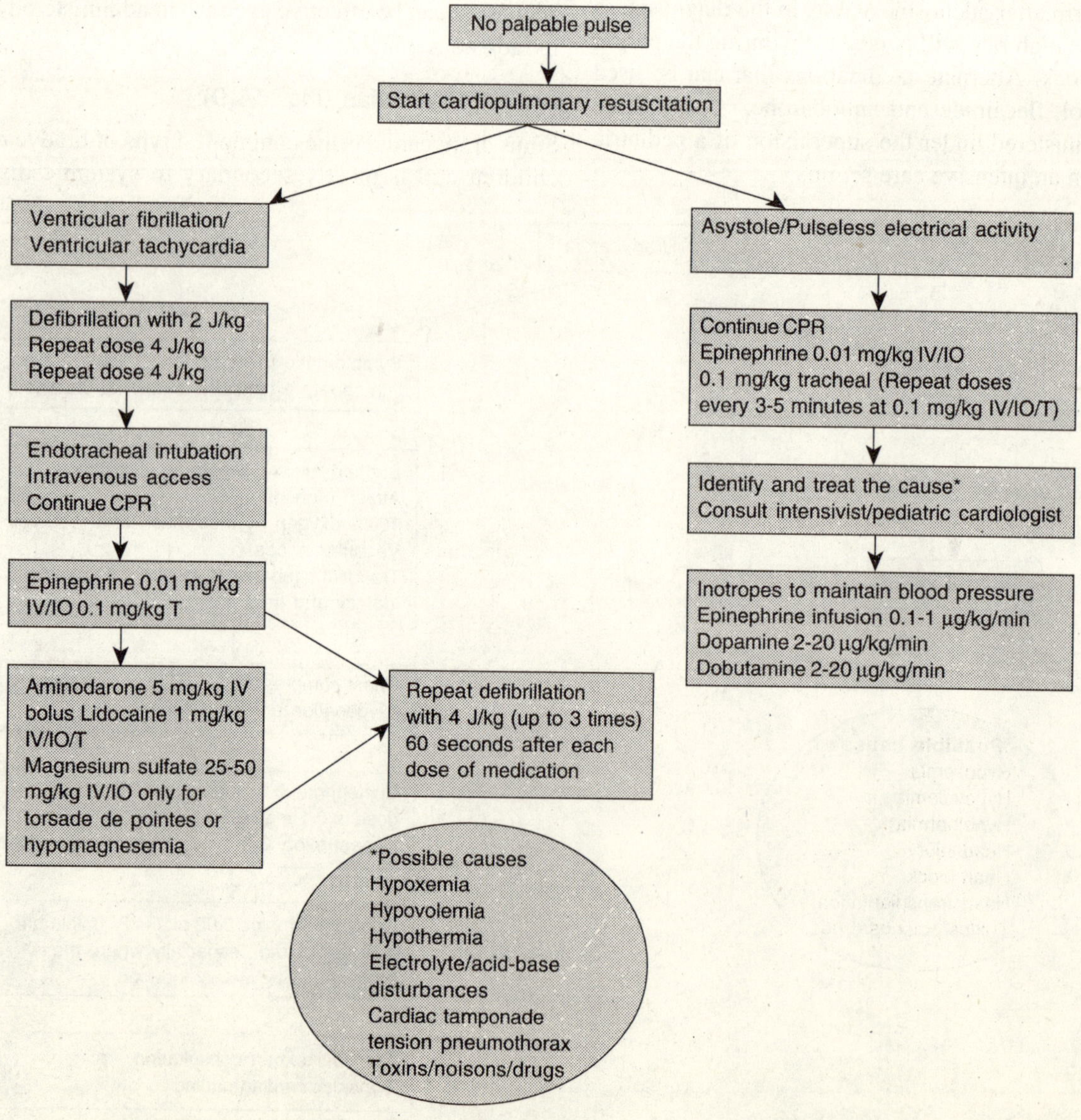

Fig. 34.10: Suggested algorithm for management of pediatric cardiac arrest rhythms

Seizure Related Cardiac Arrhythmia

The emergency management of these events is similar to other cardiac arrhythmias. However, these patients may require combination of antiarrhythmic and anticonvulsant therapy either during the acute stage or for prevention of similar episodes.[4]

REFERENCES

1. Young KD, Seidel JS. Pediatric cardiopulmonary resuscitation: Collective review. *Ann Emerg Med* 1999;33:195-205.
2. Richman PB, Nashed AH. The etiology of cardiac arrest in children and young adults: Special considerations for ED management. *Am J Emerg Med* 1999;17:264-270.
3. Earnest MP, Thomas GE, Eden RA, Hossack KF. The sudden unexplained death syndrome in epilepsy: demographic, clinical, and post mortem features. *Epilepsia* 1992;33:310-315.
4. Venugopalan P, Agarwal AK. Cardiac arrhythmia secondary to seizures in infancy. *Acta Paediatr* 2001;90:1208-1209.
5. Fish FA, Benson DW. Disorders of cardiac rhythm and conduction. In: Allen HD, Gutgesell HP, Clark EB, Driscoll DJ (eds) *Moss and Adam's Heart Disease in Infants, Children and Adolescents Including the Fetus and Young Adult*, 6th edn. Philadelphia: Lippincott Williams and Wilkins 2001;482-533.
6. Venugopalan P, Shakeel A, Al Amry A, Jaya S. Supraventricular tachycardia in children: a report of three cases, diagnosis and current management. *Medical Sciences* 2000;2:59-64.
7. Reeves AL, Nollet KE, Klass DW, Sharbrough FW, So EL. The ictal bradycardia syndrome. *Epilepsia* 1996;37:983-987.
8. Devinsky O, Pacia S, Tatambhotla G. Bradycardia and asystole induced by partial seizures: A case report and literature review. *Neurology* 1997;48:1712-1714.
9. Blumhardt LD, Smith PE, Owen L. Electrocardiographic accompaniments of temporal lobe epileptic seizures. *Lancet* 1986;1:1051-1056.
10. Oppenheimer SM, Gelb A, Girvin JP, Hachinski VC. Cardiovascular effects of human insular cortex stimulation. *Neurology* 1992;42:1727-1732.
11. Subramanyan R, Venugopalan P. Congenital long Q-T syndromes in children. *Indian Heart J* 2002;54: 152-158.
12. Cobb LA, Fahrenbruch CE, Walsh TR, et al. Influence of cardiopulmonary resuscitation prior to defibrillation in patients with out-of-hospital ventricular fibrillation. *JAMA* 1999;281: 1182-1188.
13. Atkins DL, Kerber RE. Pediatric defibrillation: current flow is improved by using "adult" electrode paddles. *Pediatrics* 1994;94:90-93.
14. Losec JD, Endom E, Dietrich A, et al. Adenosine and pediatric supraventricular tachycardia in the emergency department: multi-center study and review. *Ann Emerg Med* 1999;33:185-191.
15. Naccarelli GV, Wlbrette DL, Patel HM, et al. Amiodarone: clinical trials. *Curr Opin Cardiol* 2000;15: 64-72.
16. Perry JC, Garson A. Flecainide acetate for treatment of tachyarrhythmias in children. Review of world literature on efficacy, safety and dosing. *Am Heart J* 1992;123:1614-1621.
17. Friedman FD. Intraosseous adenosine for the termination of supraventricular tachycardia in an infant. *Ann Emerg Med* 1996;28:356-358.
18. Atkins DL, Hartley LL, York DK. Accurate recognition and effective treatment of ventricular fibrillation by automated external defibrillators in adolescents. *Pediatrics* 1998;101: 393-397.
19. Cecchin F, Perry JC, Berul CI, et al. Accuracy of automatic external defibrillator analysis algorithm in young children. *Circulation* 1999;100:I663-I664.

Section VII

Emergencies Related to Gastroenterology, Hepatology and Nutrition

Thapa BR and Anuj Walia

35 Acute Gastroenteritis

INTRODUCTION

The term, *acute gastroenteritis*, denotes acute infection of the gastrointestinal tract (GIT) due to infectious agents resulting in acute episode of vomiting and diarrhea. Diarrhea is one of the important symptoms of acute gastroenteritis, causing dehydration and dyselectrolytemia, a leading cause of death in infants and children.

Acute gastroenteritis is the most common cause of infectious diarrhea worldwide. Despite improvements in the sanitation, hygiene, public health and economic wealth, this remains the leading cause of morbidity and mortality in children in the developed world. It used to be number one killer disease of infancy and childhood. However, with the availability of oral rehydration therapy (ORT) the mortality has significantly decreased. Still this remains second top killer disease in children worldwide. At present about 3 million deaths occur each year due to gastroenteritis in children under 5 years of age i.e. one death every 10 seconds. There are an estimated 1.8 billion episodes of childhood diarrhea per year and virtually all these acute diarrheal episodes are related to infectious agents. On an average a child suffers from gastroenteritis 3 times annually. In Africa child suffers from 7 episodes of diarrhea annually.

Infections of GIT are caused by a wide variety of enteropathogens, including viruses, bacteria and parasites. The clinical manifestations and mechanism of diarrhea depend upon the underlying causative enteropathogens. There are basically two types of acute infectious diarrhea:

- Non-inflammatory diarrhea caused by enterotoxins of bacteria, destruction by viruses, enteroadherence by bacteria or parasite
- Inflammatory diarrhea is caused by direct invasion by bacteria.[1,2]

This chapter focuses on epidemiology, pathogenesis, clinical manifestations, diagnosis and therapy of acute gastroenteritis.

VIRAL GASTROENTERITIS

Viral gastroenteritis is a very important cause of diarrhea in children worldover. In developed world, rotavirus and other enteropathogen viruses are more common etiological agents for acute diarrhea than bacterial infections. In developing countries, viral infections of GIT are less frequently encountered in children.[1]

Rotavirus

Rotavirus was defined as a specific pathogen virus as a causative agent for diarrhea in children in 1973 by Bishop et al.[3] This is responsible for 20-70% of hospitalization of children with acute diarrhea worldover.

Rotavirus is a RNA virus belonging to Reoviridae family. Rotavirus consists of particle of 68 nm and has 2 capsids (shells). Rotavirus contains inner capsid of VP6 protein and outer capsid of VP4 and VP7. In human beings disease occurs due to group A virus whereas group B and C rarely cause disease. The serotypes are defined based upon the protein antigen, like VP7 are considered G type whereas VP4 positive are considered P type.

Rotavirus infection occurs throughout the world. The infection is more prevalent in winter months, whereas 2 peaks are observed during dry months of Winter and dry months of Summer. Spread is primarily through fecal contamination of water and virus may infect any age but diarrhea is more prevalent in 6 months to 2 years of age. Breast milk is protective. Very rarely outbreaks have occurred in neonates and infants in nursery and hospital settings.[4-7]

Clinical Manifestations

Incubation period varies from 2-3 days. The illness starts with sudden onset of diarrhea and vomiting. There is triad of symptoms like diarrhea, vomiting and fever. The diarrhea and vomiting result into dehydration. 25% patients may have upper respiratory treat infection like symptoms. The diarrhea lasts for 2-8 days. The sheeding of virus in the stool starts on day 3 of illness and continues for 3 weeks. The secondary lactose intolerance and persistent diarrhea develop in significant number of children.[4]

Pathophysiology

Rotavirus invades the mature epithelial lining of duodenum and jejunum lead to atrophy of villi. This leads into loss of brush border enzymes, results into poor absorption of nutrients and causes osmotic diarrhea. At the same time the undifferentiated cells in the crypts are also stimulated and lead to secretory diarrhea. Net result is profuse watery diarrhea and leads to dehydration.

Diagnosis

Diagnosis of rotavirus infection is made by demonstration of rotavirus antigen in the stools by immuno-assays and polymerase chain reaction (PCR). The sensitivity and specificity is 90%. On electron microscopy presence of viral particles in the biopsy specimen suggest rotavirus infection.[6,8]

Treatment

It is mainly supportive in the form of ORT to treat dehydration.[9] In case of severe dehydration shock state intravenous (IV) fluids may be required. Probiotics (Lactobacillus GG, Bifidobacterium bifidum, Streptococcus thermophilus and Saccharomyces boulardii) have been shown to decrease the duration of diarrhea and enhance the exertion of rota virus in the stool.[10,11]

Prevention

Natural infection with rotavirus provides protection against subsequent infection. The severity of new infection is less. Oral rotavirus vaccine is very effective to protect in a natural way but it is not available for use.[12] Probiotics have been shown to prevent the rota virus infection.[11]

Norwalk Virus

Norwalk virus belongs to calicivirus group and causes outbreaks of gastroenteritis, the so-called "Winter vomiting disease"[13] It is worldwide in distribution. Around 50% of the naturally infected individuals develop symptoms. The disease occurs in older children and adults.

In a study published from Finland, Norwalk virus antigen was demonstrated in the stool by enzyme-linked immunosorbent assay (ELISA) in 49% of infants in age group of 3-24 months.[14] This shows that the disease occurs in younger population also.

The transmission of the disease occurs by feco-oral route. The outbreaks of the disease have been documented in bakery employees and others, by ingestion of raw oysters and clams and due to the contaminated water supplies. The disease occurs throughout the year, despite the designation "Winter vomiting disease".

Norwalk virus causes the injury to the villous resulting in patchy atrophy and epithelial organization. The virus particles can be demonstrated in the stool by ELISA and polymerase chain reaction (PCR). The incubation period is 24 to 48 hours and symptoms persist for 24-48 hours. The disease is classically characterized by vomiting, nausea and cramping pain abdomen. Diarrhea occurs in 50% individuals.[15]

The treatment of Norwalk virus infection is supportive. Dehydration is uncommon and, when present, requires ORT.

Enteric Adenovirus

Enteric adenoviruses have recently been identified to cause gastroenteritis in younger children under 2 years age.[16] Largely, adenoviruses cause respiratory infection and keratoconjuctivitis. The infection occurs throughout the year though seasonal variations are known. The infection spreads by feco-oral route. Diarrhea is the dominant feature, causing dehydration in 50% patients. Vomiting is usually mild and lasts for shorter period. The enteric adenovirus diarrhea persists for 2 weeks; excretion of virus can be demonstrated for same period.[17] Diagnosis can be made by electron microscopy, ELISA or PCR of virus particles in the stool.

Treatment consists of supportive care and the ORT for the dehydration.

Astrovirus

Astrovirus is worldwide in distribution. It infects children in age group 1-3 years. This is the second most frequent viral cause of gastroenteritis in children (after rotavirus). Most of the children develop vomiting, diarrhea, abdominal pain and fever. Diarrhea persists for 1-4 days. The spread of infection occurs by feco-oral route.

Treatment is supportive, including ORT for dehydration.[18]

Other Viruses

The other viruses like pestivirus, coronavirus, torovirus and cytomegalovirus (CMV) can cause gastroenteritis. Coronavirus may cause outbreaks of necrotising enterocolitis. Cytomegalovirus causes enteritis and colitis in immunocompromised individuals.

Diagnosis is made by demonstration of cytomegalovirus inclusion bodies in biopsy. The virus can be detected in stool. CMV serology is also helpful.[19]

BACTERIAL GASTROENTERITIS

Infecting bacterial agents cause diarrhea by overpowering GIT defense factors like gastric acidity, intestinal motility, mucus secretion, normal intestinal bacterial flora and specific

Table 35.1: Bacterial pathogens depending upon the mechanisms of diarrhea

Invasive	*Cytotoxic*	*Toxigenic*	*Adherent*
Shigella	Shigella	Shigella	Enteropathogenic E. coli
Salmonella	Enteropathogenic E. coli	Enterotoxigenic E. coli	Enterohemorrhagic E. coli
Yersina enterocolitica	Enterohemorrhagic E. coli	Yersina enterocolitica	Enteroaggregate E. coli
Campylobacter jejuni	Clostridium difficile	Aeromonas	Diffuse adherent E. coli
Virbrio parahemolyticus		V Cholerae and non-O1 vibrios	

mucosal and systemic immune mechanisms. The bacteria reach the intestine. In the mucous layer, they proliferate and lead to diarrhea through various mechanisms like invasion of the mucosa, production of cytotoxins, production of entero-toxins and adherence to mucosal surface. Based upon this, the pathogenic bacteria can be grouped (Table 35.1).

Salmonella

Salmonella can cause various clinical syndromes in human being like gastroenteritis, focal non-intestinal infections, bacteremia, asymptomatic carrier state and enteric fever. Three distinct species of salmonella are recognized: *Salmonella enteriditis, Salmonella cholesesuis* and *Salmonella typhi*. Non-typhoidal salmonellosis occurs in any age. The disease spreads *via* contaminated water, food, meat, eggs, raw milk and other dairy products.

Incubation period is 12-72 hours. After ingestion, the bacteria reach the ileum and colon, invade the enterocyte, proliferate and enter lamina propria *via* lymphatics. They reach mesenteric lymph nodes and enter the circulation causing bacteremia. The organism is invasive, results in enteritis and manifests with watery diarrhea and colitis. Colitis is characterized by diarrhea with blood and mucus. Salmonella leads to fever, watery diarrhea as well as bloody diarrhea. The infection can spread to other systems of the body also. After the clearance of infection, the exertion of bacteria may remain for longer period.

Salmonella can be diagnosed by stool culture as well as blood culture. Salmonellosis in healthy or immunocompromised children requires antibiotics like cotrimoxazole, ciprofloxacin or third generation cephalosporins.[1,21-23]

Shigella

Shigella is common cause of bacillary dysentery in children. The organisms can be classified into 4 species: *Shigella dysenteriae, Shigella flexneri, Shigella Sonnei* and *Shigella boydii*. The pathogens, *Shigella dysenteriae* and *Shigella flexneri* are the most common organisms in the developing countries.[24,25]

Shigella is worldwide in distribution. Outbreaks of shigellosis have been reported. Shigella spreads by feco-oral route, contaminated food and water. Shigella mainly infects the colon. Bacteria attack the colonocytes and lead to cascade of events. The production of enzymes by the bacteria is responsible for epithelial injury and spreads to adjacent cells. Various toxins like neurotoxins, cytotoxins and enterotoxins are produced. Cytotoxins cause further injury to living epithelium. Hence, production of blood and mucus. The enterotoxins are responsible for the secretory type of watery diarrhea. In one third patients, watery diarrhea may precede the dysentery.

Clinically, shigella infection manifests with pain abdomen, fever and blood and mucus in the stools—the so-called *bacillary dysentery*. Initially the stools may be watery followed by bloody diarrhea by next day. There is very high frequency of stooling, invariably associated with tenesmus. Malnourished children may develop rectal prolapse.[25]

The other associations of shigella are hemolytic uremic syndrome (HUS), seizures, arthritis and purulent conjunctivitis. Shigellemia is very rare. The diagnosis is made by stool culture and sigmoidoscopy.

The treatment consists of supportive care and antibiotics. The most affective antibiotics are ciprofloxacin and norfloxacin. The shigella has already developed resistance to various commonly used antimicrobials for enteric infections in many areas.

Campylobacter

Campylobacter infection is worldwide in distribution. *Campylobacter jejnuni* is the commonly encountered organism responsible for sporadic infection and outbreaks. This infects mostly children under 2 years of age. Infection spreads by direct contact or contaminated water or food, under cooked meat, eggs, milk etc. The campylobacter produces disease by three potential mechanisms adherence to the mucosa and elaboration of toxins, invasion of mucosa in terminal ileum and colon and translocation. The organisms penetrate the mucosa and reach the lamina propria and mesenteric lymphnodes. Campylobacter may cause disease in form of watery diarrhea to frank dysentery. The disease starts with fever, malaise, nausea and abdominal pain. There may be blood and mucus in stools leading to dysentery.[26]

The other associations are Guillain-Barre' syndrome, Reiter's syndrome and Miller-Fisher syndrome. Campylobacter can cause infection in other systems of body *via* spread through blood.

The diagnosis of this infection is made by positive stool culture. Most of the times the supportive treatment is enough.

Severe disease may respond to erythromycin, chloramphenicol, gentamicin, ciprofloxacin, tetracycline, etc.

Yersinia

Yersinia infection is uncommon in our country. Yersinia enterocolitica is associated with gastroenteritis. Yersinia is worldwide in distribution but occurs more in cold climate. The disease occurs due to ingestion of contaminated food or water, refrigerated food items like bean sprouts, chocolate milk, pork, dairy products etc.

Yersinia is an invasive organism and involves terminal ileum and infection goes to Peyers patches and to mesenteric lymph nodes and bacteremia. The enterotoxins produced may cause watery diarrhea. The infection is characterized by fever, pain abdomen and diarrhea. Yersinia can give rise to appendicitis, erythema nodosum, reactive arthropathy and mesenteric lymphadenitis.

The organism is very difficult to grow and may require 4 weeks to grow.

Antibiotics can shortern the duration of diarrhea and infection. Almost all antibiotics effective in enteric infections can be used. These are cotrimoxazole, chloraimphenicol, aminoglycosides and third generation cephalosporin.[27,28]

Cholera

Cholera remains a grave public health problem in the developing world. The mechanism of diarrhea is well understood and based upon this the ORT was developed. Cholera affects children as well as adults and is responsible for high morbidity and mortality.[29] The disease occurs in sporadic, epidemic and epidemic forms. Until recently, all the epidemics were caused by V. cholerae O1 serotype. This has further 2 biotypes classic and EL for. Other serotypes are believed to cause sporadic disease. Another new serotype 0139 isolated from Bengal is identified to cause epidemic similar to O1 cholera.[30] *V. cholerae* is spread *via* contamination of water and food. Poor standards of hygiene and sanitation are responsible for the occurrence of the disease.

Pathogenesis

The organism after ingestion reach the small intestine and attach to mucosa. The process is aided by mucinase. V. cholerae produce toxin composed of central part A unit and surrounded by B toxin having five subunits. The B toxin attaches to the receptor site and allow the transfer of A unit to the cell membrane and gets elevated into A_1 and A_2. A_1 acts as a catalyst and leads to stimulation of adenylate cyclase and production of cyclic AMP. This leads to chloride secretion and net flux of fluid in the intestinal lumen. V. cholerae also contains other toxins like zonular occludens toxin and accessory cholera toxin which might be playing role in production of diarrhea.[1, 29]

Clinical Picture

The incubation period of cholera is 1 to 3 days. The symptoms start abruptly with vomiting and profuse watery diarrhea. The stools are clear with bits of mucus in it, called *rice water appearance.* There is sense of relief of discomfort after the defecation. The rate of fluid loss is tremendous and child develops shock state due to dehydration very fast. There is no fever.

The diagnosis is made by stool culture. Stool ganging drop preparation may be positive but confirmation comes with culture.

The mainstay of treatment of cholera revolves around dehydration. Oral dehydration therapy has revolutionized the treatment. But severe dehydration and shock state may require IV fluids. Antibiotics do not decrease the duration of diarrhea but are administered to decrease the exertion of bacteria in the stools. The drugs used are tetracycline, furazolidine, cotrimoxnzole, chloramphenicol and ciprofloxacin.[31]

Vaccine against cholera is available and is useful in epidemic situations. Adequate public health measures to provide safe water supply can control the occurrence of the disease effectively.

Other Vibrios

Gastroenteritis can occur following infections with non-cholera vibrios. Usually the disease is mild. V. parahemolyticus is capable of invasiveness as well as toxin production and results into dysentery.

Escherichia Coli

E. coli can be divided into pathogenic and non-pathogenic groups. The diarrheogenic E. coli can be classified depending upon the serotype and the mechanism of action. The five major group are:

i. Enteropthogenic E. coli (EPEC)
ii. Enterotoxigenic E. coli (ETEC)
iii. Enteroinvasive E. coli (EIEC)
iv. Enterohemorrhagic E. coli (EHEC)
v. Enteroaggregative E. coli (EAEC) and diffuse-adherent E. coli (DAEC)[32]

Enteropathogenic E. coli

EPEC is an important cause of diarrhea during infancy in developing countries. EPEC may exceed at times to that of rotavirus infection. This may be responsible for diarrhea in 30 to 40% infants.

The hallmark of EPEC infection is "attaching and effacing" lesions in the intestine. The bacteria adhere to the epithelial lining of small bowel lead to destruction of microvilli. At the same time, the cytoskeletal system of the enterocyte is also disturbed. EPEC pathogenesis consists of localized adherence which brings bacteria close to the enterocyte also called docking, signal transduction including increases in intracellular calcium and protein phosphorylation and intimate adherence a multigene process encoded in the bacterium by a locus of enterocyte effacement. The loss of microvilli is responsible for malabsorption.

The patients with EPEC infection develop diarrhea, vomiting, malaise and fever. The stool may contain mucus but no blood. The symptoms are more severe and may persist for 2 weeks or longer. EPEC causes protracted diarrhea, malnutrition and zinc deficiency. The diagnosis of EPEC can be made by stool culture and serotyping. The small intestine biopsy may show the EPEC attached to entrocytes. Cotrimoxazole is effective through oral neomycin and gentamicin have been tried shown to be effective.

Enterotoxigenic E. coli

ETEC is the common infection causing diarrhea in children during first few years of life. In adults it is responsible for travellers diarrhea. The transmission of infection is by feco-oral route.

The ETEC reach the small intestine and colonize on the mucosa. There is no destruction of villi. While sitting on the enterocyte certain enterotoxins are produced like heat labile (LT) and heat stable (ST). The LT stimulates guanylate cyclase, with the result there is increase of net secretion resulting into secretory diarrhea.[33]

ETEC leads to watery diarrhea, nausea and abdominal pain. The diagnosis of ETEC is made by bioassays, *immmoassays* gene probes specific for ST or LT; PCR assays are also available. The treatment of ETEC diarrhea is to treat the dehydration cotrimoxazole has been used to decrease the fecal excretion of organisms.

Enteroinvasive E. coli

EIEC cause invasive disease as disease similar to shigella infection. The organsims reach to the colon and invade colonic epithelium and lead to cell death. EIEC also elaborate enterotoxins to the diarrhea starts as watery contaminated food and water. The diagnosis is dependent upon the bioassay the (Sereny test), serotyping, ELISA or DNA probe techniques.

Treatment is supportive and the antibiotics like ampicillin, Chloroampenicol and Ciprofloxacin are effective to treat the infection.

Enterohemorrhagic E. coli

EHEC cause of 2 recognizable syndromes like hemorrhagic colitis and HUS. The diarrhegenic serotype is 0157 : H7 responsible for bloody diarrhea. There is little or no fever. There is cramping pain abdomen alongwith watery diarrhea followed by bloody diarrhea. HUS is characterised by bloody diarrhea followed by acute renal failure, microangiopathic anemia and thrombocytopenia.

The disease occurs in sporadic form and in form of outbreaks. The inadequately cooked hamburgers, apple juice, bean sprouts and contaminated water have been responsible for outbreaks. The cattles and other animals are the reservoir of infection and their droppings are responsible for spread of infection through water. The pathogenesis of this is not clear but follow the pathogenic mechanisms of attaching and effacing and infect the colon as in case of Shigella dysenterae infection. The cytotoxins produced are similar to shigella: Verotoxin called verotoxin E. coli (VTEC). Other name given is shigella like toxin producing E.Coli (SLTRC). The cytotoxins are also implicated in the pathogenesis of the disease.[34]

The diagnosis of this condition is based up stool culture, serotyping serum antibodies, cytotoxin broassays, DNA hybridization PCR based tests and cytotoxin detection by ELISA are also helpful.

The antibiotics have been found to be effective but prevention is very important. Proper cooking of food and hamburgers is going to kill the bacteria. Avoidance of contamination of drinking water with animal droppings. Attempts are being made to have exogenous source of receptor to absorb unbound toxins and to avoid subsequent injury to other systemic organs of body.

Enteroaggregative and Diffuse Adherent E. coli

Enteroaggregative and diffuse adherent E. coli (EAEC & DAEC) EAEC shows a pattern of aggregative or stack brick adherence and DAEC demonstrates a pattern of diffuse adherence.[35] The manner of adherence determines the pathogenic mechanisms. The EAEC enhances the mucus secretion and also elaborate enterotoxin and cytotoxins. They lead to watery diarrhea with mucus, fever and lead to persistent diarrhea . Less is known about DAEC to cause diarrhea. Electron microscopy can to demonstrate the EAEC in small bowel biopsy. DNA probes have been used to identify EAEC and DAEC.

Oral antimicrobials like gentamicin, neomycin and cotrimoxazole are effective with variable results.

Clostridium Difficile

C. difficile is a gram positive anaerobic bacillus. This organism is normally present in neonates—55% kept in the neonatal intensive care unit and 10% of term born babies. Children and adult (3%) may have asymptomatic infection. In neonates, it is believed that they don't have receptors to develop disease.

C. difficile elaborates two types of toxins. Toxin A is one that attaches to the receptors on the entercytes or colonocytes and lead to stimulation of intracelluar protein

G. Toxin B is thought to be important cytotoxin to lead to disease state.[36]

The administration of antimicrobials predispose to develop overgrowth of C.difficile. Around 20% cases develop diarrhea following administration of antimicrobials. The diarrhea, usually watery, is also called *antibiotics associated diarrhea (AAD)*. This is associated with cramping abdominal pain and fever. About 10% of the patients develop blood and mucus in the stool due to formation of pseudomembrane in the colon that is seen on sigmoidoscopy or colonscopy.

The diagnosis of C. difficile infection is made on demonstration of toxin assay and this is the gold standard. Psumdomenbrane due to C.difficile infection shows a classical feature like mushrooming lesion with lot of inflammatory tissue with entrapped fibrin in it and features of colitis.[37]

The treatment of C. difficile infection consists of metronidazole or vancomycin or cholestyramine.[38] Recently probiotics like Saccharomyces boulardii and Lactobacillus GG have been found to be effective in AAD.[39,40] Probiotics administration alongwith antimicobials has been shown to prevent the infection.

Aeromonas

These organisms were recognized to cause disease in immunocompromised individuals. A hydrophila and A. caviae infect children under 2 years of age.

The pathogenesis is not clear but it is known that Aeromonas produce cytotoxins and enterotoxins.

The clinical syndromes, produced by the Aeromonas infection are: acute watery diarrhea, the most common syndrome, the dysentery, self limited and persistent watery diarrhea. Cramping pain abdomen and fever may occur.

Antibiotics in form of tetracycline, chloramphenicol, aminoglycosides and cotrimoxazole are effective.[41]

Plesiomonas

P. shigelloides infect same way as Aeromonas but occurs as sporadic and epidemic form through contamination of water and seafood.

Pathogenesis is not known. Some strains produce cytotoxins. This has invasive property and results into colitis. In addition there is camping pain abdomen and fever. This leads to persistent diarrhea in majority Antimicrobials like cotrimoxazole and aminoglycosides are effective to control the infection.[41]

Other rare potential diarrheogenic micro-organisms include mycobacterium avium-intracellular infecting immunocompromised hosts, Entertoxigenic Bacteroides fragilis: mimicking ETEC,[43] Brachyspira aalgori: a spirochete produces dysentery, Hafnia alvei; like EPEC and Listeria monocytogenes: listeria gastroenteritis following ingestion of contaminated chocolate milk.[44]

PARASITIC GASTROENTERITIS

Giardia Lamblia

Giardiasis is a common protozoal infection in children in tropical countries. It infects the healthy as well as immunocompromised children. Giardia is found in 2 forms: the trophozoite and cyst form. The trophozoite form is motile form and attaches to the duodenal mucosal and upper part of jejunum. This is attached to the enterocytes with help of ventral disc and leads to effacement of microvilli. The mechanisms of diarrhea are multifactorial like atrophy of microvilli and villi, stunting of enterocytes, secondary lactose intolerance, bacterial overgrowth, malabsorption of nutrients and immunological injury. Giardiasis is characterized by acute watery diarrhea, persistent diarrhea and chronic malabsorptic diarrhea. There may be vomiting, discomfort, bloating sensation and pain abdomen. This can also cause traveller's diarrhea.

Diagnosis is made by demonstration of giardia cyst in stool (for three consecutive days)[46] giardia trophozoite in duodenal aspirate or biopsy and giardia antigen in the stool.

The treatment with metronidazole or furazolidine is effective.

Entameba Histolytica (EH)

This is not a common infection in children though 10% of general population is infected. Amebic infection occurs from the release of the trophozoite in the colon and by attachment to colonic epithelium. It leads to production of hemolysin and proteases. Hence, destruction of cells. There is production of proinflammatory cytokines. There is deep ulceration. The pathogens penetrate and can got to the portal circulation and get lodged in liver or other organs of the body. This involves the cecum, ascending colon and rectosigmoid region of large bowel.

There can be watery diarrhea or dysentery like illness. This could be acute in onset or may have chronic indolent course.

The diagnosis is made by demonstration of trophozoites of EH in the stool. ELISA and PCR and serology are very helpful in making the diagnosis of infection.

Treatment with metronidazole, tinidazole or ornidazole is effective.

Cryptosporidium

Cryptosporidium is now a well recognized organism to lead on to gastroenteritis in children in developing countries. It is responsible for 6-9% of cases of diarrhea. This can infect the healthy as well as immunocompromised hosts. There is attachment of the organisms to the enterocytes and lead to atrophy of microvilli. Clinically, it is characterized by watery diarrhea, pain abdomen and malaise. In immunosuppressed hosts the diarrhea is severe and losses may be equivalent to cholera. Diarrhea is self-limiting and may last for 3-30 days. The diagnosis is made by demonstration of oocyst in the stool.[47] Treatment is supportive care but immunocompromised individuals require spiromycin or paromomycin or azithromycin to reduce the shedding of oocyst and decrease the duration of diarrhea.[48]

Other parasitic infections like Dietameba fragilis, Blastocystis hominis, Balantidium coli, Coccidia, Sacrocystis, Cyclospora and Insospora belli may very rarely be responsible for acute diarrhea.[49]

SUMMARY AND CONCLUSION

To conclude, the acute diarrheal disorders are very important cause of high morbidity and mortality in children. Dehydration is the main killer. The mortality has come down significantly due to ORT. The WHO ORS has revolutionized the treatment of dehydration. Now this is replaced by hypotonic and rice-based ORS (Osmolality 245). In developing countries bacterial and parasitic infections dominate. They require antimicrobial agents to cut short the duration of diarrhea. The commonly used antimicrobials agents along with dosage and duration are given in Table 35.2.

Newer drugs like rececadotril, an encephalinase inhibitor, have been shown to be effective to reduce the duration of secretory diarrhea. There are many newer antimicrobial agents that have been found to be effective in gastroenteritis.

Role of probiotics in the rotavirus diarrhea and AAD is well documented.

In virtually 40% of cases of gastroenteritis it is difficult to ascertain the etiology in the best of hands though more and more newer pathogens are being recognized. Efforts must be made to develop advances in the prevention of infections by raising the standards of public health measures and development of newer vaccines to reduce the incidence of diarrheal disorders.

REFERENCES

1. Guerrant RL, Bobak DA. Bacterial and protozoal gastroenteritis. *N Engl J Med* 1991;325:327-340.
2. Blacklow NR,Cukor G. Viral gastroenteritis. *N Engl J Med* 1991;325:252-264.
3. Bishop RF, Davidson GP, Dolin R, et al. Virus like particles in epithelial cells of duodenal mucosa from children with acute nonbacterial gastroenteritis. *Lancet* 1973;2:1281-82.
4. Steinhoff MC. Rotavirus: The first five years. *J Pediatr* 1980;96: 611-622.

Table 35. 2: Antimicrobial therapy for acute infections diarrhea in children

Organisms bacteria	*Efficacy*	*Drug*		*Duration*
		I choice	*Alternative choice*	
V. cholerae	Proven	Tetracycline 25-50 mg/kg/day Ciprofloxacin 10-20 mg/kg/day	Doxicycline 2-5 mg/kg/day Cotrimoxazole TMP 5 mg/kg/day	3-5 days
ETEC	Proven	Ciprofloxacin Norfloxacin 4-12 mg/kg/day	Cotrimoxazole SMX 25 mg/kg/day Neomycin 50 mg/kg/day Gentamicin 5 mg/kg/day	5-7 days
EPEC	Possible	Cotrimoxazole	Neomycin,Gentamicin	5-7 days
EIEC	Possible	Cotrimoxazole	Ampicillin, Chloramphenicol	5-7 days
EHEC	Possible	Cotrimoxazole	Neomycin, Gentamicin	5-7 days
EAEC/DAEC	Possible	Cotrimoxazole	Neomycin, Gentamicin	5-7 days
Shigella sp.	Proven	Cotrimoxazole Norfloxacin Cinoxacin	Ciprofloxacin Fleroxacin	5-7 days
Salmonella sp.	Proven	Ciprofloxacin III generation cephalosporin Norfloxacin	Cotrimoxazole Ampicillin 50-100 mg/kg/day Amoxicillin 20-50 mg/kg/day	5-7 days
Campylobacter sp.	Proven	Erythromycin 20-40 mg/kg/day Ciprofloxacin	Azithromycin 10 mg/kg on day I 5 mg/kg/day on day II and III	5-7 days
Yersenia sp.	Proven	Ciprofloxacin	Tetracycline	5-7 days
Clostridium difficile	Proven	Metronidazole 10-20 mg/kg/day	Vancomycin 30-40 mg/kg/day	5-7 days
Protozoa				
Giardia lamblia	Proven	Metronidazole	Furazolidine 5-9 mg/kg/day	5-7 days
Cryptosporidium parvum	Possible	Paramomycin		5-7 days
Isospora belli	Proven	Cotrimoxazole		10 day
Cyclospora	Proven	Cotrimoxazole		5-7 days
Balantidium coli	Proven	Metronidazole	Tetracycline	5-7 days
Entameba histolytica	Proven	Metronidazole Dilaxanide furoate	Tinidazole 10-15 mg/kg/day	5-7 days

5. Santosham M, Yolken RH, Wyth RG, et al. Epidemiology of rotavirus diarrhea in a prospectively monitored American Indian Children. *J Infect Dis* 1985;152:778-783.
6. Yolken RH, Wyath RG, Zissis G, et al. Epidemiology of human rotavirus types 1 and 2 and as studied by enzyme-linked immunosorbent assay. *N Engl J Med* 1978;299:1156-1161.
7. Totterdell BM, Chrystie IL, Banatvala JE. Rotavirus infections in a maternity unit. *Arch Dis Child* 1976;51:924-928.
8. Wilde J, Yolken R, Willoughby R, et al. Improved detection of rotavirus shedding by polymerase chain reaction. *Lancet* 1991;337:323-326.
9. Nazarian LF, Berman JH, Brown G, et al. Practice parameter: The management of acute gastroenteritis in young children. *Pediatrics* 1996;97:424-435.
10. Saavedra JM, Bauman NA, Orung I, et al. Feeding Bifidobacterium bifidum and Streptococcus thermophiles in infants in hospital for prevention of diarrhea and shedding of rotavirus. *Lancet* 1994;334:1046-1049.
11. Huang JS, Boursvaros A, Lee JW, Diaz A, Davidson EJ. Efficacy of probiotic use in acute diarrhea in children: A meta-analysis. *Dig Dis Sci* 2002;47:2625-2634.
12. Glass RI, Compans R, Lang D. *Fifth Rotavirus Vaccine Workshop: Current Issues and Future Developments,* Atlanta, GA, October, 1995 *J Infect Dis* 1996;174:S1-S126.
13. Alder JL, Zickl R. Winter vomiting disease. *J Infect Dis* 1969;119:668-673.
14. Lew JF, Valdesus OJ, Vesikar T, et al. Detetction of Norwalk virus or Norwalk like infection in finish infants and young children. *J Infect Dis* 1994;169: 1364-1367.
15. Jiang X, Wang M, Wang K, Estes MK. Sequence and genomic organization of Norwalk virus. *Virology* 1993;195:51-61.
16. Kotloff KL, Losonsky GA, Morris JG Jr., et al. Enteric adenovirus infection and childhood diarrhea. An epidemiologic study in 3 clinical settings. *Pediatrics* 1989;84:219-225.
17. Wood D J. Adenovirus gastroenteritis. *Br Med J* 1988;296: 229-230.
18. Herrmann J, Taylor D, Echeversia P, et al. Astroviruses as a cause of gastroenteritis in children. 1991;324:1747-1760.
19. Pereira HG, Fireho AM, Flewett TH, et al. Novel viruses in human feces. *Lancet* 1988;2:103-104.
20. Bishop WP, Ulshen MH. Bacterial gastroenteritis. *Pediatr Clin North Am* 1988;35:69-87.
21. Pickering LK. Therapy for acute infectious diarrhea in children. *J Pediatr* 1991;118:S118-S128.
22. Casburn Jones AC, Farthing MJG. Management of infectious diarrhea. *Gut* 2004;53:296-305.
23. Guerrant RL, Van Gilder T, Steiner TS, et al. Practice guidelines for the management of infectious diarrhea. *Clin infect Dis* 2001;32:331-351.
24. Shears P. Shigella infectious. *Ann Trop Med Parasitol* 1996;90:104-114.
25. Thapa BR, Venkateswarlu K, Malik AK, Panigrahi D. Shigellosis in children from North India: Clinicopathological study. *J Trop Pediatr* 1995;41: 303-307.
26. Walker RI, Caldwell MB, Lee EC, et al. Pathophysiology of campylobacter enteritis. *Microbiol Rev* 1986;50:81-94.
27. Cover TL, Aber RC. Yersinia enterocolitica. *N Engl J Med* 1989;321:16-24.
28. Black RE, Jackson RJ, Tasai, et al. Epidemic yersinia enetrocolitica infection due to contaminated chocolate milk *N Engl J Med* 1978;298:76-79.
29. Kaper JB, Morris JG Jr., Levine MM. Cholera. *Clin Microbiol Rev* 1995;8:48-86.
30. Ramamurthy T, Garg S, Sharme R etal. Emergence of novel strain of vibrio cholera with epidemic potential in southern and eastern India. *Lancet* 1993;341: 703-704.
31. Khan WA, Bennish ML, Seas C et al. Randomized controlled comparison of single dose ciprofloxacin and doxycyline for cholera caused by Vibrio cholerae 01 or 0139. *Lancet* 1996;348:296-300.
32. Levine MM. Escherichia coli that cause diarrhea: enterotoxigenic enteropathogenic, enteroinvasive, enterohemorrhagic and entero-adherent. *J infect Dis* 1987;155:377-389.
33. Sears CL, Kaper JB, Enteric bacterial toxins mechanisms of actions and linkage to intestinal secretion. *Microbiol Rev* 1996;60:167-215.
34. Cohen MB. E.coli O 157: H7 infections: a frequent cause of bloody diarrhea and hemolytic uremic syndrome. *Adv Pediatr* 1996;43:177-207.
35. Bhan MK, Raj P. Levine MM, et al. Enteroaggregate Escherichia coli associated with persistent diarrhea in a cohort of rural children in India. *J Infect Dis* 1989;159:1061-1064.
36. Rolfe RD. Binding kinetics of Clostridium difficile toxin A & B to intestinal brush border membranes from infant and adult hamsters. *Infect Immun* 1991;59:1223-1230.
37. Fekety R, Shah AB. Diagnosis and treatment of clostridium difficile colitis. *JAMA* 1993;269:71-75.
38. Teasley DG, Gerding DN, Olson GM. Prospective randomized trial of metronidazole versus vancomycin for Clostridium difficile colitis. *JAMA* 1993;269:71-75.
39. Biller JA, Katz AJ, Flores AF, et al. Treatment of recurrent Clostridium difficile colitis with Lactobacillus GG. *J Pediatr Gastroenterol Nutr* 1995;21:224-226.
40. Cremonini F, DiCaro S, Nista EC, et al. Meta-analysis: The effect of probiotic administration on antibiotic associated diarrhea. *Aliment Pharmacol Therap* 2002;8:1461-1467.
41. Holmberg SD, Farmer JJ III. Eeromonas hydrophilia and Plesiomonas shigelloides as causes of intestinal infections. *Rev Infect Dis* 1984;4:663-669.
42. Sack RB, Albert MJ, Alan K, et al. Isolation of eterotoxigenic Bacteroides fragiles from Bangladeshi children with diarrhea: a controlled study. *J Clin Microbial* 1994;32:960-963.
43. Dacunha Ferreira RM, Phillip AD, Stevens CR, et al. Intestinal spirochaetosis in children. *J Pediatr Gastroenteral Nutr* 1993;17:333-336.
44. Balton CB, Austin CC, Sobel J, et al. An outbreak of gastroenteritis fever due to Listeria monocytogenes in milk. *N Engl J Med* 1997;336:100-105.
45. Pickering LK, Engel Kirk PG. Giardia lamblia. *Pediatr Clin North Am* 1988;35:565-577.
46. Hiatt RA, Markell EK, NgE. How many stool examination necessary to detect pathogenic intestinal protozoa? *Am J Trop Med Hyg* 1995;53:36-39.
47. Mackenzie WR. A Massive outbreak in Milwaukee of Cryptosporidium infection transmitted through the public water supply. *N Engl J Med* 1994;331:161-68.
48. Hicks P, Zwiener RJ, Squires J, Savell V. Azithromycin therapy for Cryptosporidium parvum infection in form children infected with human immunodeficiency virus. *J Pediatr* 1996;129: 297-300.
49. Ackers JP. Gut coccida-Isospora, Cryptosporidium, Cyclospora and Sacrocystis. *Semin Gastrointest Dis* 1997;8:33-34.

Suraj Gupte and Ghanshyam Saini

36 Diarrheal Dehydration

INTRODUCTION

Diarrheal dehydration as such and especially when complicated by dyselectrolytemia and acid-base imbalance is responsible for most of the morbidity and mortality associated with acute diarrheal disease.

MODUS OPERANDI OF DEVELOPMENT OF DIARRHEAL DEHYDRATION

It is important to appreciate that diarrheal losses are drawn from extracellular fluid (ECF) compartment constituted by circulating blood, interstitial fluid and secretions. Around 60% of the body weight of the child is accounted by this compartment. Loss of water from the body causes shrinkage in the volume of ECF compartment. In 50% cases with excessive sodium loss in stools, hyponatremia develops as result of fall in serum and ECF sodium levels, leading to fall in osmolality of ECF and movement of water from ECF to ICF compartment. This essentially causes further shrinkage of the already shrunk ECF compartment volume. This clinically manifests as loss of skin elasticity.

In case of a small proportion of dehydration cases who have received fluids containing very high amount of sodium, osmotic pressure of ECF becomes high, resulting in movement of water from ICF compartment to ECF compartment. This is likely to mask the existence of severe dehydration which may be wrongly interpreted as mild dehydration.

Depletion of ECF compartment causes reduction in blood volume and, consequent upon that, peripheral circulatory failure (PCF) and oliguria anuria.

Potassium loss in stools leads to hypokalemia which may manifest in the form of abdominal distention, hypotonia and ECG changes (ST depression and flat T wave).

Bicarbonate loss in stools causes acidemia manifesting with acidotic respiration i.e deep and rapid breathing (Kussmul breathing).

CLINICAL MANIFESTATIONS

These vary with the severity of dehydration (Table 36.1).

Table 36.1: Clinical manifestations of three grades of dehydration

Grade	*Clinical picture*
Mild (3–5% weight loss)	: Irritability/drowsiness : Pallor : Somewhat sunken eyes
Moderate (6–10% weight loss)	: Sick-looking child : Pallor : Depressed anterior fontanel : Sunken eyes : Dry mucous membrane : Dry and inelastic skin
Severe (over 10% weight loss)	: Signs of shock* : Metabolic acidosis : Oliguria/anuria : Moribund state

*Signs of hypovolemic shock: Limpness, pallor, cold and clammy skin, thin rapid or almost impalpable peripheral pulses.

Once dehydration is severe, it is bound to lead to CNS disturbances regardless whether it is isotonic, hypotonic or hypertonic. Of course, hypertonic dehydration is likely to have more of CNS manifestations (Table 36.2). Early irritability, alternating with mental apathy, may progress to restlessness, cloudiness of consciousness, delirium or stupor, lethargy and coma. Convulsions may occur at any stage.

On account of high viscosity of blood, cerebral thrombosis may occur.

Table 36.3 gives the clinical profile of dyselectroltemia and acid base disturbances.

Table 36.2: Clinical profile in different qualitative types of diarrheal dehydration

Parameter	Isotonic dehydration	Hypertonic dehydration	Hypotonic dehydration
Skin			
Color	Gray	Gray	Gray
Temperature	Cold	Cold or hot	Cold
Turgor	Poor	Fair	Very poor
Feel	Dry	Thickened	Clammy (moist)
Mucous membrane	Dry	Parched	Slightly moist
Eyes	Sunken and soft	Sunken	Sunken and soft
Anterior fontanel	Depressed	Depressed	Depressed
Sensorium	Drowsy	Very irritable	Comatose
Pulse	Rapid	Moderately rapid	Rapid
Blood pressure	Low	Moderately low	Very low

Table 36.3: Clinical profile of electrolyte and acid base disturbances in diarrheal dehydration

Disturbance	Clinical signs
Acidosis	Breathing increased in depth and rate
Alkalosis	Breathing decreased in depth and rate
Hypokalemia	Abdominal distention Paralytic ileus Hypotonia Hyporeflexia Mental apathy ECG changes
Hyperkalemia	Fibrillation/paralysis of skeletal muscles ECG changes
Hypocalcemia	Tetany Paralytic ileus
Hypercalcemia	Hypotonia Fecolith
Hypomagnesemia	Tetany Muscular twitching
Hypermagnesemia	CNS depression Hyporeflexia

MANAGEMENT

Management of Diarrheal Dehydration Without Significant Malnutrition

Oral Rehydration Therapy (ORT)

For mild-moderate dehydration, ORT is ideal, provided that persistent vomiting is not a handicap. One may use standard WHO ORS, one of its modifications or a home-made electrolyte solution (HES). There are advantages in using a cereal based solution (super ORS) such as rice-water electrolyte solution (RWES) in view of its better tolerance and capability to provide greater energy.

Generally speaking, each motion should be followed by replacement with an equal amount of ORS. Breastfeeding is known to potentiate the value of ORS and must not be discontinued.

Intravenous Fluid Therapy

Indications for IV fluid therapy are:

- Severe dehydration.
- Mild-moderate dehydration with persistent vomiting.

IV fluid therapy consists of two components, namely "deficit" and "maintenance".

Deficit Therapy

A. *Calculations Based on Dehydration Scoring System:* It consists in determining the severity of dehydration as per the scoring system given in Table 36.4. The deficit therapy is obtained by the following formula

$$\text{Deficit therapy} = \text{Score} \times \text{weight (kg)} \times 10$$

A 2-year-old child weighing 12 kg and scoring 11 points (11% dehydration or weight loss), therefore, shall need $11 \times 12 \times 10 = 1122$ ml fluids to make up the deficit as a result of dehydration.

B. *Calculations Based on Degree of Dehydration:* Here the degree of dehydration is assessed in terms of mild, moderate and severe dehydration as per Table 36.4.[4]

Table 36.4: Deficit fluid therapy in diarrheal dehydration

Grade of dehydration	Fluid deficit ml/kg	Deficit replacement in first 8 hours ml/kg
Mild (3-5%)	30–50	Nil
Moderate (6-10%)	60–90	50
Severe (>10%)	120–150	60-75

Maintenance Therapy: Calculations are based on the normal fluid requirements at different ages (Table 36.5). The child cited above shall need

$$125 \times 12 = 1500 \text{ ml of fluids in 24 hours}$$

Plan of Therapy

Initial Therapy: Out of the total fluids calculated for the first 24 hours, 1/5th is given rapidly in form of Ringer's

Table 36.5: Daily requirement of fluids (water)[2]

Age group	Requirement (ml/kg)
First 3 days	80-100
3-10 days	125-150
15 days-3 months	140-160
3-12 months	150
1-3 years	125
4-6 years	100
7-9 years	75
10-12 years and thereafter	50

lactate in 2.5% or 5% glucose during the first 1-2 hours. If oliguria/anuria persists despite rapid flushing in of the IV fluids, a bolus dose of frusemide may be administered . If the child passes urine, IV drip is continued. In case he fails to do so, he is managed as acute renal failure in which case fluid amount is considerably cut down.

Continuation Therapy: Rest of the 4/5th fluid is administered in the remaining 22-23 hours. The ideal fluid at this stage is half strength Darrow's solution.

This plan of therapy works well for most of the situations, taking care of potassium deficiency as well as metabolic acidosis, paralytic ileus and hypocalcemic tetany.

Maintenance of fluids and electrolytes should continue over the second 24 hours even if diarrhea has stopped in the very first 24 hours.

For ***severe acidosis*** ($CO_2 < 8$ mEq/L), additional alkali calculated as per the following formula should be infused:

$$\text{ml of NaHCO}_3\ (7.5\%) = \text{Bicarbonate deficit (mEq/L)} \times \text{body weight (kg)} \times 0.3$$

In situations where it is difficult to determine the base deficit, sodium bicarbonate may be given in the dose of 2-3 ml/kg. The calculated dose is administered in dilution of 1:1 with distilled water intravenously over 1-2 hours.

It is advisable to review the child after 2 hours to find if further correction is required.

For ***severe hypokalemia*** (serum potassium < 3.5 mEq/L), additional potassium in the dose of 1-3 mEq/kg may be administered to the infusion. It is not essential that the child passes urine freely before potassium is administered.

For ***hyperkalemia,*** exchange resins, digoxin, IV NaCl and Ca are of value.

For ***hyponatremia,*** full strength electrolyte solutions and even NaCl may be used.

For ***hypernatremia***, solutions with sodium content of around 30 mEq/L suffice. Highly diluted solutions run the risk of causing neurologic manifestations including seizures. Only very infrequently, peritoneal dialysis may be wanted in very serious cases of hypernatremia.

Plain solutions like 5% glucose should never be used for IV correction of dehydration.

Table 36.6 gives the composition of commonly employed intravenous fluids.

Table 36.6: Composition of commonly used intravenous solutions

Isolution	Na	K	Mg	Cl	HCO_3
Isotonic saline (0.9% NaCl)	154	–	–	154	–
Ringer's lactate	130	4	–	109	28
Half strength Darow's solution	61	18	3	52	27
Sodium bicarbonate (7.5%)	892	–	–	–	892
Sodium lactate (N/6)	167	–	–	–	167

Management of Diarrheal Dehydration Associated with Protein-energy Malnutrition

Assessment of Dehydration

Extreme caution needs to be exercised in evaluating a malnourished child for dehydration. Malnutrition causes certain signs that may be mistaken for dehydration (e.g. loss of skin elasticity, dry mucous membrane) which may contribute to overestimation of dehydration. On the other hand, certain signs of dehydration (e.g. poor skin turgor) are masked because of presence of nutritional edema. Thirdly, some signs of dehydration may be seen in septic shock which is not uncommon in advanced malnutrition.

World Health Organization (WHO)[5] has recommended use of 8 signs which are dependable in malnourished children:

- Watery diarrhea
- Excessive thirst
- Hypothermia
- Sunken eyes
- Weak or absent radial pulse
- Cold hand and feet
- Fall in urine output.

WHO has also put up some guidelines for interpreting the usefulness of these signs (Table 36.7).

Choice of Therapy: ORT or IV

The first choice should be ORT. IV fluids are indicated only in severe dehydration and shock associated with malnutrition.

ORT: In view of low potassium reserve and quite high sodium levels in malnutrition, the ORS should be such as provides high potassium and low sodium. It is available in two forms:

- WHO recommended special "rehydration solution for severely malnourished child" (ReSoMal) is available commercially. Table 36.8 shows its composition.
- ReSoMal can be prepared by diluting the standard WHO ORS in 2 liters of water rather than 1 liter, adding 50 g sucrose (in place of 25 g) and 40 ml of mineral mix (Table 36.9).

Table 36.7: Usefulness of WHO recommended signs for assessing dehydration and shock in malnourished children

Sign	*Some dehydration*	*Severe dehydration*	*Septic shock*	
			Incipient	*Overt*
Watery diarrhea	Yes	Yes	Yes or no	Yes or no
Thirst	Drinks eagerly	Drinks poorly	No	No
Hypothermia	No	No	Yes or no	Yes or no
Sunken eyes	Yes	Yes	No	No
Weak/absent radial pulse	No	Yes	Yes	Yes
Cold hand and feet	No	Yes	Yes	Yes
Urine output	Yes	No	Yes	No
Sensorium	Restless/Irritable	Lethargic, comatose	Apathetic	Lethargic
Hypoglycemia	Sometimes	Sometimes	Sometimes	Sometimes

Table 36.8: Composition of ReSoMal vis-a-vis standard WHO ORS

Ingredient	*ReSoMal*	*Standard WHO ORS*
Glucose	125 mmol/L	111
Sodium	45 mmol/L	90
Potassium	40 mmol/L	20
Chloride	70 mmol/L	80
Citrate	7 mmol/L	10
Magnesium	3 mmol/L	Nil
Zinc	0.3 mmol/L	Nil
Copper	0.045 mmol/L	Nil
Osmolarity	**300**	**311**

The ReSoMal is administered in a dose of 70–100 ml/kg body weight over 12 hours period, as shown in Table 36.10, for restoration of normal hydration.

Table 36.9: Composition of mineral mix required for making ReSoMal

Potassium chloride	89.5 g
Tripotassium citrate	32.4 g
Magnesium chloride	30.5 g
Zinc acetate	3.3 g
Copper sulfate	0.56 g
Sodium selenate	10 mg
Potassium iodide	5 mg
Water	1000 ml

IV Therapy: The fluid of first choice is half strength Darrow's solution or half strength Ringer's lactate with 5% dextrose. Alternatively, half normal saline with 5% dextrose may be employed.

- The fluid is given in a dose of 15 ml/kg over one hour. Simultaneously, ReSoMal is given in dose of 10 ml/kg/hour by nasogastric tube.
- If poor response after 1 hour of therapy, IV fluids are repeated and ReSOMal, 10 ml/kg/hour, is continued for the next 10 hours or so.

Table 36.10: Administration of ReSoMal in diarrheal dehydration associated with malnutrition

First 2 hours:	5 ml/kg every 30 minutes
Next 10 hours:	5–10 ml/kg/hour

Note: Ongoing losses in vomitus and stools should be considered for calculation of exact amounts of ReSoMal.

- Failure of the child to respond to this regimen denotes presence of septic shock (Table 36.11) which may need additional treatment with broadspectrum antibiotics, blood transfusion, and sympathomimetic agents such as dopamine and dobutamine.

Table 36.11: Points favoring diagnosis of septic shock in severe malnutrition

- Failure of the dehydration to respond to IV plus ReSoMal regimen of rehydration
- Such signs as limpness, apathy and anorexia without thirst or restlessness (incipient shock)
- Hypothermia
- Dilated superficial veins such as scalp veins
- Respiratory grunt or difficult breathing
- Gastrointestinal hemorrhage (coffee-ground vomitus, melena)
- Abdominal distention

REFERENCES

1. Gupte S, Anderson RA. Pediatric gastroenterology. In: Gupte S (ed): *The Short Textbook of Pediatrics*, 10th edn. New Delhi: Jaypee Brothers 2004;365-402.
2. Gupte S, Vani S. Pediatric nutritional requirements. In: Gupte S (ed) *The Short Textbook of Pediatrics*, 10th edn. New Delhi: Jaypee Brothers 2004;108-111.
3. Hahna, Kim Y, Garner P. Reduced osmolarity ORS for treating dehydration due to diarrhea in children. *Br Med J* 2001;323: 81-85.
4. Mittal SK, Agarwal A. Fluid and electrolytes management in acute diarrhea. *Indian J Pract Pediatr* 2004;6:131-138.
5. World Health Organization. *Management of Severe Malnutrition: A Manual for Physicians and Other Senior Health Workers.* Geneva: WHO 1999.
6. Gupte S, Pal M. Diarrheal dehydration in malnourished infants and children. *Asian Med Bull* 1999;6:56-39.

Suraj Gupte and Satish Gupte

37 Antibiotic-Induced Diarrhea (AID)

INTRODUCTION

Experience has established that practically each and every antibiotic has the inherent property of provoking diarrhea-like manifestations, usually by interference with the normal ecosystem of the gastrointestinal tract. The problem is more frequent in infancy and childhood. The incidence varies from 5 to as high as 25%. The patients administered an antibiotic for a short duration are less likely to develop AID as compared to those on longer duration. Every other pediatric subject put on an antibiotic, in our own experience, develops loose motions of variable magnitude. In a small proportion of the cases, these may well be severe enough to cause concern.[1]

To quote a Joint WHO/UNICEF Statement, there is hardly any known antibiotic that potentially is not diarrheagenic in pediatric practice[2] though some antibiotics are decidely high-risk *(vide infra)*. Nevertheless diarrheal manifestations are not always significant.

As a matter of fact, in most cases diarrhea resolves without any treatment whatsoever, without causing any noteworthy adverse effect on the health status of the child. In others, it may be fulminant and bloody, often refractory to discontinuation of the offending antibiotic and even other therapeutic and supportive measures. In between the two extremes, different grades of diarrhea with or without blood may be seen. According to one estimate, risk of AID varies from 5-25% with different antibiotics.[3] Pseudomembranous colitis associated with *C. difficile* occurs in 10-20% of all AID cases and most of the severe AID cases. It is termed *Clostredium difficile-associated diarrhea.*

TERMINOLOGY AND CONTEMPORARY DEFINITION

The plethora of sementics employed for *antibiotic-induced diarrhea (AID)* or colitis *(AIC),* also termed *antibiotic-associated diarrhea (AAD)* or colitis (AAC) and *antibiotic-related diarrhea (ARD)* or colitis (ARC) and the variable definitions used by different workers has led to much confusion in the literature. A research study from Italy[4] suggested that ARD should be restricted to diarrhea occurring only during the course of antibiotic administration. This has been challenged by other groups.[5-7] At present, the most widely accepted definition appears to be: "diarrhea that has no other known cause than antibiotic therapy given concurrently or discontinued at the most 4 weeks preceding it".

Let no mistake be made that the definition, contrary to the usual impression, does not stresses on the presence of blood in stools. The most plausible implication is that, in antibiotic-induced diarrhea, stools may be frequent, watery and voluminous with or without gross blood or mucus.

The term, *pseudomembranous colitis (PMC),* should be reserved for the advanced stage of the disease in which bloody stools, secondary to development of pseudomembrane, are characteristic.

FREQUENCY

In one multicentric prospective study from Sweden, incidence of antibiotic-induced diarrhea was found to be 4.9%. Fecal samples were positive for *C. difficile* cytotoxin B in 55.4%. Subjects treated with antibiotics for 3 days had a significantly (p value = 0.009) lower frequency of diarrhea than those treated for longer durations. Treatment with cephalosporins, clindamycin or broadspectrum penicillins was associated with an increased risk of diarrhea.

Table 37.1 highlights the high-risk antibiotics for antibiotic-induced diarrhea.[8]

Table 37.1: High-risk antibiotics for antibiotic-induced diarrhea

- Clindamycin
- Ampicillin
- Lincomycin
- Macrolides, especially azithromycin
- Cephalosporins

ETIOPATHOGENESIS

The most important point to remember is that any antibiotic is capable of causing diarrhea. Certain antibiotics, say clindamicin, ampicillin, amoxycillin, penicillin, cephalosporins, methotrexate, antiviral agents, etc, especially when administered orally, may particularly cause serious disease in the form of pseudomembranous colitis. Very rarely, even vancomycin and metronidazole, which are employed for treatment of PMC, may cause this condition.[1] Though clindamycin was the first antibiotic blamed for severe diarrhea (PMC), most cases appear to be secondary to ampicillin and cephalosporin administration because of a very extensive use of these agents in clinical practice.

The growth of a spore-forming gram-positive anaerobic bacillus, *Clostridium difficile*, which is ubiquitous in the environment in the soil, is responsible for the PMC. It is normally found in 70% neonates, 20-50% infants and only 3% of adolescents and adults. It is by no means invasive. you, overwhelming majority is Most of its strains are toxic, producing two toxins which disease through a plethora of effects (Table 37.2).

Table 37.2: Adverse effects produced by toxins of C. difficile

- Inflammation
- Loss of proteins
- Exaggerated peristalsis
- Hemorrhages
- Enhanced fluid and electrolyte secretions
- Cytotoxicity

Enterotoxin (toxin A) acts on the intestinal mucosa to produce diarrhea. Cytotoxin (toxin B) enhances vascular permeability in low doses but in higher doses it may prove lethal. What is remarkable toxin B is 1,000 times more powerful and have 100 fold greater enzymatic activity than toxin A.

Occasional strains of the pathogen may produce only one or neither toxin.

The significant mechanisms of production of diarrhea by C. difficile are listed in Table 37.3.

Table 37.3: Noteworthy mechanisms of production of diarrheal symptoms by *C. difficile*

- Overgrowth of the organisms with suppression of normal gut flora by antibiotics
- Interaction of the organisms with other flora of the gut
- Actual triggering of production of the toxin by organisms by the antibiotics
- Production of enzyme, *beta-lactamases,* by resistant organisms which inactivate antibiotics and facilitate growth *of C. difficile*

More recently, evidence has accumulated that *S. aureus* and *Clostridium perfringens*, when predominant in stool samples, should also be considered a possible etiologic agent for antibiotic-induced diarrhea.

PATHOPHYSIOLOGY

Among the several theories put forward to explain the pathophysiology of PMC, the following are significant:

- Changes in intestinal microbial flora
- Direct effects of antibiotics and their metabolites
- Localized Schwartzman reaction
- Hypersensitivity reaction
- Intravascular coagulopathy
- Elaboration of toxins by intestinal flora and production of enzyme, *beta lactamase, by* resistant organisms which inactivate antibiotics and facilitate growth of C. difficile.

As a rule, the so-called "pseudomembranous nodules" (also termed "plaques") develop in rectum, sigmoid colon or distal colon. In some cases, these may be noticed in cecum and transverse colon only. The lesions appear as greyish-white exudates that are surrounded by edematous and erythematous inflammatory response. These are only weakly adherent to the underlying tissue.

Generally speaking, the organism does not cause disease unless the subject is administered antibiotics.

However, recently, strains of *C. difficile* (around 8%) have been recognized that cause diarrhea even without preceding antibiotic administration.

Furthermore, evidence is available that any factor that disrupts the normal bowel flora (antibiotics) or bowel motility (bowel stasis, Hirschsprung disease, bowel surgery) predisposes to C difficile-associated diarrhea. Uremia, anesthesia and dietary changes also render the child vulnerable to pseudomembranous colitis.

Recently, increasing evidence has accumulated to the effect that, in addition to *C. difficile*, *Staphylococcus aureus* and *Clostridium perfinges* too are capable to cause diarrhea.

CLINICAL MANIFESTATIONS[9-13]

Manifestations are variable. These range from mild self-limited diarrhea without pseudomembrane through explosive watery diarrhea with occasional blood to severe hemorrhagic colitis with classic picture of blood and mucus accompanied by toxemia.

The toxemic patient may have pyrexia, cramps, crampy abdominal pain, nausea and vomiting, dehydration with dyselectrolytemia, protein-losing enteropathy, hypoalbuminemia.

Such serious complications as toxic megacolon, colonic perforation, peritonitis and shock my occur. Even death may result..

Manifestations do not necessarily occur during antibiotic therapy only. These may occur several days and even two or three (up to 4) weeks subsequent to discontinuation of therapy with offending antibiotic(s). Occasionally, manifestations may occur within hours of starting the implicated antibiotic. We have seen a few cases developing the entity just after a single dose of an antibiotic therapy.

DIAGNOSTIC CONSIDERATIONS[14-16]

High index of suspicion in a patient with significant diarrhea or colitis in the setting of prior or current antibiotic therapy constitutes the cornerstone of diagnosis of antibiotic-induced diarrhea.[2] It is established by demonstrating *C. difficile* or its toxins in the stools.

C. difficile and its cytotoxin B may be identified by tissue culture with appropriate neutralization by antitoxin or toxicity to cultured fibroblasts. It is advisable to inoculate stool specimens on cycloserine cetoxitin fructose agar. Following incubation anaerobically, *C. difficile* can be isolated. Unfortunately, diagnosis of *C. difficile* by culture is difficult and time-consuming because of strict anaerobic nature of the organism.

The application of enzyme immunoassay (EIA) for detection of *C. difficile* has turned out to be a highly sensitive and specific method for diagnosis of PMC, giving results in just 3 hours. This should be considered the method of choice, and, perhaps, as emphasized by the French workers (Sednaoui), the gold-standard test, for rapid diagnosis of *C. difficile*-induced diarrhea.

Toxin A can be identified by ELISA or latex agglutination assay.

On rectosigmoidoscopy/colonoscopy, the usual findings are mucosal edema, friability and ulceration of varying grades. Pseudomembranous nodules/plaques are seen in advanced cases only. Infrequently, these observations spare the rectum and the sigmoid colon but may be seen proximal colon.

However, this investigation should be reserved for atypical cases only.

Four stages of antibiotic-induced diarrhea may be recognized based on picture of the colonic mucosa (Table 37.4). Most children suffer from Stage II which is characterized by mild erythema and edema of the colonic mucosa.

Table 37.4: Four stages of antibiotic-induced diarrhea based on appearance of colon on rectosigmoidoscopy/ colonoscopy

Stage I	Normal appearance
Stage II	Mild erythema and edema
Stage III	Granular, friable or hemorrhagic mucosa
Stage IV	Pseudomembrane formation

Some fecal leukocytes can be detected in around half of the cases whereas a large number of red cells in feces are almost a rule. Histopathology of PMC nodules/plaques reveals mushroomy lesion with massive fibrin, red cells and leukocytes.

DIFFERENTIAL DIAGNOSIS[1,4,9,14]

Differential diagnosis of antibiotic-induced diarrhea is from diarrhea due to Shigella, Salmonella, inflammatory bowel disease, neutropenic colitis/typhlitis, malabsorption, and bloody diarrhea due to parasites such as *L. giardia, E. histolytica, H. nana, S. stercoralis and T. trichiura*. For dependable diagnosis of ARD, it is appropriate that these causes of diarrhea are excluded. Nevertheless, coexistence of one or more of these factors plus the AAD is not unusual in tropical and subtropical environs.

THERAPEUTIC APPROACH AND OUTCOME[1,12,19]

Immediate Measures

The cornerstone of treatment is immediate withdrawal of the antibiotic(s), provided that it is workable, and offering supportive treatment in the form of fluid and electrolyte replacement and adequate nutrition. If response is unsatisfactory within 48-72 hours and in case of a severe illness, oral metronidazole (20-50 mg/kg/day) or oral vancomycin (20-40 mg/kg/day) should be added for 7-10 days. Oral metronidazole should be the preferred agent since it is less expensive and yet very effective and cuts down the emergence of vancomycin-resistant enterococci which can become a trouble-shooter in hospitalized children. If the patient fails to respond to one, it may be substituted by the other. Evidence is now available to show that Ornidazole may be as effective as metronidazole and can easily be used as a substitute.

In yet more critical situations (toxic megacolon, adynamic ileus), the two drugs (metronidazole and vancomycin) may well be given simultaneously (intravenously).

Alternatively, vancomycin may well be substituted with a tetracycline in older children.

Response to treatment, as a rule is excellent, usually over 70-95%. However, a proportion of patients (say 5-30%) are likely to have a recurrence within 1-2 week. Another course of therapy usually resolves their problem.

Refractory Cases

In a small group of patients who continue to have further recurrence(s), it is advisable to give trials of oral cholestyramine, rifampicin (along with vancomycin), bacitracin, immune globulin, probiotics (lactobacilli and bifidobacterium species) for reconstitution of bowel flora, baker's yeast or instillation of fecal flora by tube feeding or enemas (Table 37.5).

Role of Probiotics[22,23]

A special word about the probiotics! These are friendly or health-enhancing microorganisms consumed as a food or dietary supplement Yoghurt and fermented milks are the most common foods that serve as probiotics. Dietary supplements serving as probiotics are available as powder, tablets and capsules.

Today, probiotics are beginning to emerge as the powerful armamentarium in the prevention and management of

Table 37.5: Salient details of drug treatment of antibiotic-induced diarrhea

Drug	Dosage	Side-effects	Special comments
Metronidazole	20-40 mg/kg/day (O) 21 mg/kg/day (IV)	Bad taste	Economical, effective
Vancomycin	40-50 mg/kg/day (O,IV) q6-8h	May per se cause diarrhea	expensive, effective, recommended in severe colitis not responding to metronidazole
Rifampicin	10-20 mg/kg/day(O) Q12-24h	Hepatotoxicity discoloration of urine	Caution against orange
Cholestyramine	240 mg/kg/day in 3	Hypercholeremic acidosis, divided doses vomiting, abdominal pain and distension, malabsorption	

diarrheal problems of infancy and childhood. Whereas their important role in rotaviral diarrhea stands by and large established,[26] their beneficial effect in AID is very likely. Their beneficial effect in AID appears to be related to the following two areas:

- Restoration of the normal gut flora
- Direct effect on the *C. difficile* colitis

In addition, probiotics have several other health-friendly benefits (Table 37.6).

Table 37.6: Examples of nonpathogenic organism employed in treatment of antibiotic-induced diarrhea

- Lactobacilli : L. acidophillus (readily available, economic though less potent), L. bulgaricus, L. GG (most potent but expensive)
- Bifidobacterium longum
- Enterococcus fecium
- Streptococcus thermophilus
- Sacchromyces boulardii

Role of Corticosteroids

Whether or not corticosteroids have a role in the management of severe ARD remains to be investigated (Table 37.7).

Table 37.7: Health-friendly benefits of probiotics

General
- Nutritional enhancement
- Promotion of weight gain
- Control of intestinal infections
- Control of lactose intolerance
- Control of hypercholesterolemia
- Control of colonic cancer
- Control of ethanol-induced liver damage
- Treatment of food allergies
- Immunomodulation

Specific in antibiotic-induced diarrhea
- Restoration of normal flora of the gut
- Inhibition of growth of *C. difficile*

PROGNOSIS

Early suspicion, identification, discontinuation of the suspected antibiotic and timely management are usually accompanied by a favorable outcome.[31,32] In one well-planned study comprising 125 infants and children in which 20% cases had presented with severe colitis, institution of vancomycin therapy was necessitated in only 4 instances. There was, however, one infant who succumbed to this complication despite all treatment, including three blood transfusions.

PREVENTIVE ASPECTS[34,35]

Prevention of ARD warrants the following measures:

- Good food and water hygiene
- Meticulous hand-washing
- Proper environmental cleaning
- Judicious use of antibiotics.
- Incorporation of probiotics in daily diet or as medicinal supplement, especially during the course of antibiotic administration. A recent study by Arvola, Laiho and Torrkeli[34] from Finland has confirmed the preventive potential of *Lactobacillus GG* in ARD.

In PICUs, prevention of AID revolves around avoidance of overuse of antibiotics. For prevention of *C. difficile* and other agents of AID, improved hygiene measures (single room, private bathrooms, use of gloves and handwashing for personnel)[8] are helpful.[12]

SUMMARY AND CONCLUSION

- All antibiotics, though some are high-risk, are capable of causing diarrhea.
- Though *C. difficile* is responsible for most cases of severe antibiotic-induced diarrhea (i.e. colitis), in some cases *S. aureus* and *C. perfringens* may well be the causative factor.
- The most important first-aid measure in antibiotic-induced diarrhea is withdrawal of the offending antibiotic and offering supportive measures to maintain fluid and electrolyte balance and nutrition.
- Probiotics may have both a preventive and therapeutic role in antibiotic-induced diarrhea.
- As a therapeutic measure (as and when considered warranted), metronidazole (preferably oral) should be considered the drug of choice. The superior though

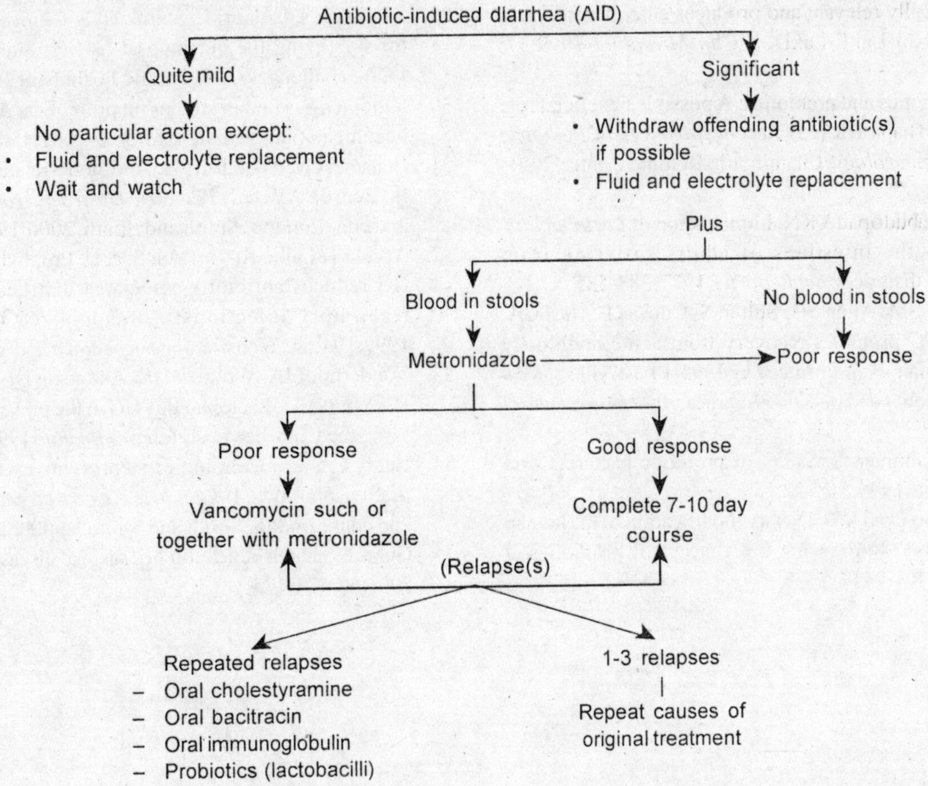

Fig. 37.1: Algorithmic approach for AID

expensive alternative is vancomycin. At times, the two drugs may be given simultaneously.

- Judious use of antibiotics is the most important preventive measure.

REFERENCES

1. Gupte S, Pal M. The problem of antibiotic-related diarrhea (colitis) in north Indian children. *Bull Trop Subtrop Med* 1997;7:123-129.
2. World Health Organization. *Diarrheal Disease*. Geneva: WHO 2000.
3. Wisham J, Norrby SR, Myhre CB, et al. Frequency of antibiotic associated diarrhea in 2462 antibiotic treated hospitalized patients: A prospective study. *J Antimicrob Chemotherap* 2000;47:43-50.
4. Ferguson AW. Antibiotic-related diarrhea/colitis in pediatric practice. *Eur Med Bull* 2001;7:123.
5. Smith E, Kennedy EA, June W. Antibiotic-related diarrheal illness. *Eur Med Bull* 2001;7:34-39.
6. Robert AS. Letter to the Editor: Antibiotic-related diarrheas. *Eur Med Bull* 2001;7:99-100.
7. Nord K, Wardhan R. Letter to the Editor: Antibiotic-related diarrheas. *Eur Med Bull* 2001;7:100-101.
8. Gorenek L, Dzer U, Besirbellioglu B, et al. The diagnosis and treatment of Clostridium difficile in antibiotic-associated diàrrhea. *Hepatogastroenterology* 1999;46:343-348.
9. Gupte S. Antibiotic-associated diarrhea in children. In: Thapa BR (ed) *Recent Advances in Pediatric Clinical Gastroenterology*. Chandigarh: Relume Printec 2001:42-47.
10. Gupte S: *The Short Textbook of Pediatrics*, 9th (millennium) edn. New Delhi: Jaypee Brothers, 2001.
11. Cleary RK: *Clostridium difficile*-associated diarrhea and colitis: Clinical manifestations, diagnosis and Treatment. *Dis Colon Rectum* 1998;41;1439-1445.
12. Bergogne-Berezin E. Treatment and prevention of antibiotic-associated diarrhea. *Int J Antimicrob Agents* 2001;16:521-526.
13. Tomar BS. Chronic diarrhea. In: Gupte (ed) *Recent Advances in Pediatrics*, Vol 10. New Delhi: Jaypee Brothers 2000;163-164.
14. Gupte S: *Differential Diagnosis in Pediatrics*, 4th edn. New Delhi: Jaypee, 2001.
15. Sutana Q, Chaudhary NA, Munir M, Anwar MS, Tayyab M. Diagnosis of *Clostridium difficile* antibiotic-associated culture versus toxin assay. *J Pak Med Ass* 2000;50:246-249.
16. Gupte S, Pal M: Perspectives in antibiotic-associated diarrhea in pediatric practice (Abstract of the invited lécture). *Proceedings of the International Conference on Pediatric Diarrheas*, Hong Kong: Biosci Publishers, 1999:56-57.
17. Gupte S. *Instructive Case Studies in Pediatrics*, 4th edn. New Delhi: Jaypee Brothers. 2002.
18. Sednaoui P, el Mantih B, Cauwell M. "Second look" at cytotoxic B of Clostridium difficile in the course of diarrhea associated with antibiotic therapy (original article in French). *Pathol Biol (Paris)* 1999;47:415-421.
19. Johnson S: Epidemics of diarrhea caused by a clindamycin-resistant strain of *Clostridium difficile* in four hospitals. *N Engl J Med* 1999;341:1645-1648.
20. Geridon DN: *Clostridium difficile*-associated diarrhea and colitis. *Infect Control Hosp Epidemiol* 1995;16: 459-463.
21. Gravet A, Rondeau M, Harif-Monteil C, et al. Predominant Staphylococcus aureus isolated from antibiotic-associated

diarrhea is clinically relevant and produces enterotoxin A and bicomponent toxin LukE-LukD. *J Clin Microbiol* 1999;37: 4012-4019.

22. Gopalan S. Prebiotics and probiotics: A possible beneficial role in diarrhea. In: Thapa BR (ed) *Recent Advances in Pediatric Clinical Gastroenterology*. Chandigarh: Relume Printec 2001: 48-54.
23. Gandhi DN, Nambudripad VKN. Implantation of *Lactobacillus acidophilus* in the intestines of adults suffering from gastrointwestnal disorders. *Sci Reporter* 1977;584-585.
24. Raza S, Graham SM, Allen SG, Sultan S, Cuevas L, Hart CA. *Lactobacillus GG* promotes recovery from acute nonbloody diarrhea in Pakistan. *Pediatr Infec Dis* 1995;14:107-111.
26. Saavedra J. Probiotics and infectious diarhea. *Am J Gastrornterol* 2000;95:S16-S18.
27. Donohue DC, Salminen S. Safety of probiotic bacteria. *Asia Pacific J Clin Nutr* 1996;5:25-28.
28. Gibsoin GR, Roberfroid MB. Dietary modification of the human colonic microbiota: Introducing the concept of probiotics. *J Nutr* 1995;125:1401-1412.
29. Salminen S, Isolauri E, Salminen E. Clinical uses of probiotics for stabilizing the gut muosal barrier: Successful strains and future challenges. Asia Pacific J Clin Nutr 1996;5:53-56.
30. Salminen S. Human studies on probiotics: Aspects of scientific documentation. *Scand J Clin Nutr* 2001;45:8-12.
31. Benson AW, Woodruff E: Antibiotic-related diarrheal colitis. In: Benson AW (ed) *Pediatric Gastroenterology and Nutrition*, 2nd edn. London: Smith and Smith, 2000;198-199.
32. Arvola T, Laiho K, Tarkkeli S, et al. Prophylactic Lactobacillus GG reduces antibiotic-associated diarrhea in children with respiratory infections: A randomized study. *Pediatrics* 1999;104:64. Website < *www.pediatrics.org*>.
33. Vanderhoof JA, Whitney DB, Antonson DL, Hanner TL, Lupo JV, Young RJ. Lactobacillus GG in the prevention of antibiotic-associated diarrhea in children. *J Pediatr* 1999;135:535-537.
34. Henry CA: Epidemiologic and preventive aspects of diarrheas. In: Benson AW (ed) *Pediatric Gastroenterology and Nutrition*, 2nd edn. London: Smith and Smith, 2000;222-231.
35. Gupte S. Health education in diarrheal disease. *Indian J Pediatr* 2001;68:474-475.

Emergencies Related to Gastroenterology, Hepatology and Nutrition

Suraj Gupte and CM Deshmukh

38 Acute Bacillary Dysentry

INTRODUCTION

By definition, it is a passage of loose stools containing mucus, pus and blood and accompanied by pyrexia, tenesmus and crampy abdominal pain as a result of acute bacillary enteritis (usually shigellosis).[1, 2]

Shigellosis occurs worldwide, usually toward late summer and rainy season when chances of contamination of food and water are considerably enhanced. It spreads primarily by oral-fecal route, the spread being higher in situations of low level of personal and food hygiene, environmental sanitation, causing breeding of flies, and contamination of water, ice, milk, salad and other food items needing much handling of the ingredients. Person-to-person transmission in families, custodial institutions and childcare centers appears to be the major modus operandi of infection wordwide.

Shigellosis most commonly occurs after 6 months of age when defense benefits of breastmilk are often taken away. Though no age is a bar, a large majority of the cases occur between 1-3 years of age.

Unlike *Vibrio cholerae*, shigella requires very low inoculum to cause disease.[1]

PATHOPHYSIOLOGY

The characteristic ability of shigella to invade intestine is encoded on a large plasmid. This plasmid is responsible for synthesis of a group of polypeptides involved in cell invasion and killing. The other important cause of bacillary dysentry, enteroinvasive *Eschericha. coli,* also harbor this plasmid and, therefore, behave like shigella.[1]

Over and above the plasmid-encoded virulence traits, chromosomally encoded factors such as toxins are also important for virulence. Interestingly the so-called *shiga toxin* is produced not only by *Shigella dysentria* serotype 1 but also by some *E. coli*, named Shige toxin-producing *E. coli* (STEC).

Following penetration of the epithelial cells of the intestine, invasive strains of Shigella multiply in the submucosa and lamina propria, causing local inflammation and superficial ulceration.

Shigellosis causes pathologic changes in colon, the most intense changes occurring in distal colon. The changes consist of localized or diffuse mucosal edema, ulcerations, friability of mucosa, bleeding and exudate.

ETIOLOGY

The causative pathogen, Shigella, is subdivided into 4 groups, A, B, C and D (Table 38.1).[2]

CLINICAL MANIFESTATIONS

Following an incubation period of 12 hours to several days, onset is with high pyrexia, prostration, vomiting, bloody diarrhea, vomiting, abdominal pain and tenesmus. Painful defecation is noteworthy.

Physical examination reveals abdominal distention with tenderness and exaggerated bowel sounds. On digital examination, rectum is tender.

Uncontrolled dysentry may cause considerable dehydration, electrolyte imbalance, hypovolemia and shock. Headache, drowsiness and even coma may follow.

DIAGNOSIS

Subsequent to the clinical lead, the following investigations should assist in confirming the diagnosis:

- Stools sample showing gross blood and mucus and on microscopy RBC and leukocytes (pus cells).
- Blood counts showing a marked leukocytosis (shift to the left) with rise of polymorphonuclear cells in a majority of the cases.
- Stool culture for isolating the pathogens. Though stool cultures are usually positive, they may be negative for two reasons: first, pathogens are somewhat fragile and

Table 38.1: Shigella groups responsible for acute dysentry

Group A	*Shigella shiga* (the most important of the 13 serotypes)
Group B	*Shigella flexneri or paradysenteriae* (the most important of the 6 serotypes and 15 subserotypes)
Group C	*Shigella boydii* (the most important of the 15 serotypes)
Group D	Shigella sonei (the only member of the group)

present only in small number late in the disease; second, laboratory techniques may well be suboptimal for the recovery of shigella.

- Blood culture in young and malnourished children who appear toxemic since they run the grave risk of septicemia.

When the child with bacillary dysentry is afebrile, the probability of enterohemorrhagic *E. coli (EHEC)* is high. The development of hemolytic-uremic syndrome following chemotherapy is enhanced in such cases.

DIFFERENTIAL DIAGNOSIS

All causes of acute bloody diarrhea should be considered, Differential diagnosis of bloody diarrhea is listed in Table 38.2.

Table 38.3 lists the differences between acute bacillar dysentry and amebic dysentry.[3]

Table 38.2: Major differential diagnosis of bloody diarrhea

Invasive bacteria	Shigella, E-coli (enteroinvasive, enterohemorrhagic), Compylocater jejuni, Salmonella (nontyphoidal), Clostridium difficile
Protozoa/helminths	E. histolytica (both luminal and invasive), L. giardia, hookworm, H. nana, S. stercoralis
Miscellaneous	Intussusception, vitamin K deficiency, inflammatory bowel disease (ulcerative/non-infectious colitis, Crohn's disease), leukemia, purpura (ITP, anaphylactoid purpura), antibiotic-induced pseudomembranous colitis

MANAGEMENT

General Measures/Symptomatic Treatment

These include correction of dehydration, dyselectrolytemia and acidosis, associated malnutrition including hypoproteinemia and anemia. Antimotility agents (diphenoxylate, loperamide) are best avoided in infants and young children. They, undoubtedly are likely to decrease frequency of stools but may not only cause complications but also reduce excretion of shigella through the colon.

Specific Treatment[2,4-6]

Choice of chemotherapy is dictated by the existing sensitivity pattern of the organisms in the community. Usually, ampicillin (injectable), cotrimoxazole and nalidixic acid are very effective. However, the problem of resistance to these drugs is becoming a bottleneck now. In resistant cases, parenteral ceftrioxone and oral cefixime are quite effective. Ciprofloxacin or ofloxacin may be used in older children and even in select younger ones in the event of multiple-resistant strains. Tetracyclines may be used in preadolescents and adolescents.

Table 38.4 gives pharmacotherapy and Figure 38.1 an algouthmic approach for acute bacillary dysentry.

Table 38.3: Differences between acute bacillary dysentry and amebic dysentry

Parameter	*Bacillary Dysentry*	*Amebic Dysentry*
Frequency of motions	Very frequent; over 10/day	Frequent , 6-8/day
Stool macroscopy		
Amount	Small	Relatively copious
Odor	Odorless	Offensive
Color	Bright red	Dark red
Nature	Blood and mucus with no or very little feces	Blood and mucus mixed with feces
Reaction	Alkaline	Acid
Consistency	Aherent to container	Nor adherent to container
Stool microscopy		
RBC	Bright red; discrete or in roleaux	Reddish-yellow; in clumps
Pus cells	Numerous	Scanty
Macrophages	Large and numerous;many engulf RBC Likely to be confused with E. histolytica	Very few
Eosinophils	Scarce	Present
Pyknotic bodies	Absent	Present
Ghost cells	Numerous	Absent
Parasites	Absent unless it is combined bacillary and parasite-induced dysentry	E. histolytica trophozoites
Bacteria	Absent	Many motile bacteria
Charcot-Leyden (CL)	Absent	Absent

Table 38.4: Recommended chemotherapy for acute bacillary dysentry

Agent	*Dose*	*Comments*
Cotrimoxazole	10 mg/kg/day (in terms of sulfamethoxazole) in 2-3 divided doses (O)	Contraindicated in G-6-PD deficient children
Ampicillin	100 mg/kg/day in 4 divided doses (IV, IM)	Avoid oral administration which is likely to cause further GI upset
Nalidixic acid	50-60 mg/kg/day in 4 divided doses (O)	Avoid in severely impaired renal function, liver disease and epilepsy
Ciprofloxacin	20 mg/kg/day in 2 divided doses (O) 10-15 mg/kg/day in 2 divided doses (IV)	Avoid in children < 12 years
Ofloxacin	10 mg/kg/day in 1 or 2 doses	Avoid in children < 12 years
Ceftrioxone	50-100 mg/kg/day in 1 or 2 divided doses (IM,IV)	Avoid in known penicillin allergy
Cefixime	8 mg/kg/day in 2 divided doses (O)	Avoid in known penicllin allergy

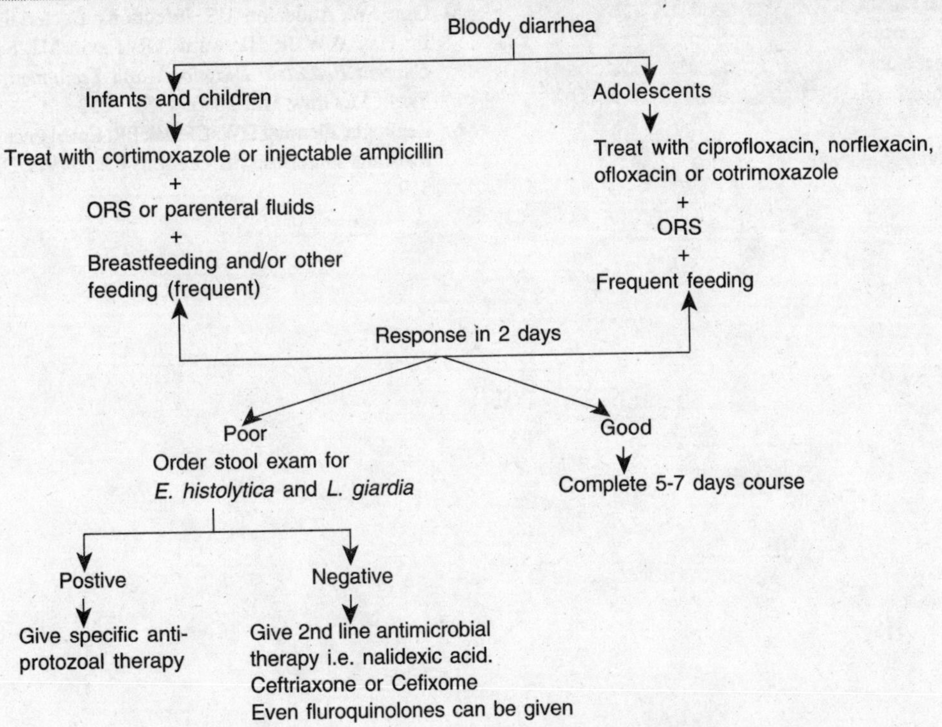

Fig. 38.1: An algorithmic approach to management of bloody diarrhea with special reference to acute bacillary dysentry

COMPLICATIONS

Major complications include dehydration, dyselectrolytemia, acidosis, anemia, shock and renal failure. Infrequently, bacteremia, metastatic infections, febrile seizures, hemolytic uremic syndrome and chronic dysentry with significant malnutrition and malabsorption may occur.

Occasionally, fulminant dysentry may prove fatal.[3]

Table 38.5 lists the complications likely to occur in cases in whom treatment is not instituted in time.

Rarely, Erkiri syndrome or lethal toxic encephalopathy may occur. It is characterized by toxemia, hyperpyrexia, seizures and headache. Terminally, cerebral edema with septicemia may occur.

PROGNOSIS

With provision of prompt therapy, especially appropriate rehydration and antibiotics, prognosis is excellent, except in malnourished children. Mortality in malnourished children who fail to receive appropriate fluid and antibiotic therapy, is particularly high.

PREVENTION

Since no vaccine is as yet available against shigellosis, prevention is mainly by:

- Control of carrier and active states and attention to personal, water and food hygiene, and
- Encouragement of breastfeeding which is known to not only cut down risk of symptomatic shigellosis but also

Table 38.5: Complications of shigellosis

Frequent
- Dehydrations and dyselectrolytemia
- Anemia with hypoproteinemia
- Malnutrition with malabsorption

Infrequent
- Rectal prolapse
- Arthritis
- Conjunctivitis
- Hepatitis
- Vaginitis.
- Myocarditis
- Reiter's syndrome
- Hemolytic uremic syndrome
- Acute renal failure
- Acute myocarditis
- Toxic megacolon
- Chronic shigellosis

Rare
Lethal toxic encephalopathy

reduce its severity who somehow get infected in spite of brastfeeding.

Work on candidate vaccines for *E. coli* is in progress.

REFERENCES

1. Cleary TG. Shigella. In: Behrman RE, Kliegman RM, Jenson HB (eds) *Nelson Textbook of Pediatrics*, 17th edn. Philadelphia: Saunders 2004: 919-921.
2. Gupte S, Anderson RA. Pediatric gastroenterology. In: Gupte S (ed) *The Short Textbook of Pediatrics*, 10th edn. New Delhi: Jaypee Brothers 2004:365-402.
3. Chatterjee KD. *Parasitology, Protozoology and Helminthology*, 12th edn. Calcutta: Chatterjee 1980.
4. Ozuah PO. Shigella update. *Pediatr Rev* 1998;19:100-103.
5. Ogie JW, Anderson MS. Infections: Bacterial and spirochetal. In: Hay WW Jr, Hayward AR, Levin MJ, Sondheimer (eds) *Current Pediatric Diagnosis and Treatment*, 16th edn. New York: McGraw-Hill 2003: 1151-1252.
6. Rephogle, Fleming DW, Cleslak PR. Emergence of antimicrobial-resistant shigellosis in Oregon. *Clin Infect Dis* 2000;30:515-519.

Suraj Gupte and RA Anderson

39 Gastrointestinal Hemorrhage

INTRODUCTION

Gastrointestinal hemorrhage is a leading pediatric emergency, often ending up with high morbidity and mortality if timely intervention is not available.[1-5] Despite adequate management, around 5% mortality is expected.

Depending on the location of bleed, it may be either upper or lower gastrointestinal hemorrhage.

Upper GI hemorrhage means bleed occurring above the ligament of Treitz.

Bleeding from the GI tract below this ligament is referred to as *lower GI hemorrhage*.

GI hemorrhage manifests as *hematemesis* or coffee-ground-colored emesis, or blood per rectum which may be fresh (*hematochezia*) or chemically-altered-black in color (*melena*).

GRADES OF GI HEMORRHAGE

GI hemorrhage may well be mild, moderate or severe (Table 39.1).

Table 39.1: Three grades of GI hemorrhage

Mild Vague symptoms of nausea, vomiting, abdominal discomfort and small amount of blood; no significant fall in hemoglobin; blood transfusion not required.
Moderate Significant blood loss, hypotension, tachycardia, cold sweats, pallor, altered sensorium, fall in hemoglobin, reduced central venous pressure; blood transfusion corrects the hypovolemic state.
Severe More pronounced features of shock which fails to quickly respond to volume replacement; significant fall in hemoglobin (<8 g%) requiring multiple blood transfusions, ongoing blood loss.

ETIOLOGY

Etiology depends on quite a few factors (Table 39.2).

Table 39.2: Factors having a bearing on etiology

- Age of the patient
- Whether bleeding is from upper or lower GIT
- Magnitude of bleeding
- Accompanying symptoms and signs
- General condition of the patient.

Table 39.3 gives the etiology of upper GI hemorrhage beyond neonatal period. By and large, the most frequent cause of upper GI hemorrhage in children is portal hypertension (usually extrahepatic obstruction), causing variceal bleed. Characteristically, variceal bleed is painless and massive and most often from esophagus, the other sites being stomach and duodenum. Factors responsible for hemorrhage are listed in Table 39.4.

Nonvariceal upper GI hemorrhage is more frequent than is usually believed. Many a times, it remains undetected. For instances, quite a proportion of infants and children with unexplained iron-deficiency anemia remain undiagnosed unless stools are tested for occult blood and/or upper GI endoscopy is carried out.[6]

Various factors contributing to acute hemorrhage in portal hypertension are listed in Table 39.4.

Table 39.5 lists causes of lower GI hemorrhage beyond neonatal period.

DIAGNOSIS

The first and foremost problem is confirmation if it indeed is blood coming from the GIT. Ingestion of iron or bismuth-containing preparations or eating clay or charcoal (pica), spinach may simulate melena. It is a healthy practice to establish the presence of occult blood by chemical testing. Not infrequently, we have come across parents insisting that the child's stools contain blood which, in actuality, is not blood.

Secondly, find the amount of blood loss, any previous history of bleeding, any constipation or diarrhea, abdominal or joint pain, epistaxis, surgery on tonsils, dental extraction, etc.

Determination of the location of bleeding is imperative. True hematemesis by and large always points to upper GI

Table 39.3: Etiology of upper GI hemorrhage according to age group

Infancy
- Stress ulcer
- Esophagitis
- Gastritis
- Malloy-Weiss tear
- Pyloric stenosis
- Vascular malformation
- Duplication

1-5 Years
- Stress ulcer
- Gastritis
- Mallory-Weiss tear
- Esophagitis
- Esophageal varices
- Foreign body
- Vascular malformation
- Hemobilia

6 Years and above
- Chronic peptic ulcer
- Stress ulcer
- Gastritis
- Mallory-Weiss tear
- Esophagitis
- Esophageal varices
- Inflammatory bowel disease
- Vascular malformation
- Hemobilia

Table 39.4: Factors contributing to acute hemorrhage in portal hypertension

- Rupture of varices
- Portal hypertensive gastropathy
- Coagulopathy

bleed. Hematochezia usually indicates lower GI hemorrhage (Table 39.6).

In case of lower GI bleeding, it is important to identify subjects with obstructive disorders (e.g. intussusception, midgut volvulus secondary to malrotation) and nonobstructive disorders.

Special efforts need to be made to look for evidence of portal hypertension, hemangioma, purpura, telangiectasia, intestinal obstruction and blood dyscrasia. Nasal passages should be carefully inspected for signs of epistaxis and anus and rectum for fissure, polyps or hemorrhoids. Proctosigmoidoscopy (preferably colonoscopy) is necessary in presence of evidence favoring polyps or colitis.

Investigations include:

- A complete blood count (CBC), BT, CT, PT, platelet count, blood group and cross-matching.
- Passage of nasogastric tube into the stomach may reveal if the source of blood is upper GIT. Presence of blood in gastric aspirate confirms that the bleeding site is proximal to the ligament of Treitz.

Table 39.5: Etiology of lower GI hemorrhage according to age group

Infancy
- Anal fissure
- Cow's milk allergy
- Infectious colitis
- Ischemic colitis
- Nonspecific colitis
- Pseudomembranous enterocolitis
- Juvenile polyp
- Intussusception
- Meckel's diverticulum
- Duplication
- Hemolytic-uremic syndrome
- Inflammatory bowel disease (Ulcerative colitis, Crohn's disease)

1-5 Years
- Infectious colitis
- Ischemic colitis
- Pseudomemranous colitis
- Juvenile polyp
- Anal fissure
- Meckel's diverticulum
- Angiodysplasia
- Henoch-Schoenlein purpura
- Hemolytic uremic syndrome
- Inflammatory bowel disease

6 Years and above
- Infectious colitis
- Ischemic colitis
- Inflammatory bowel disease
- Pseudomembranous colitis
- Polyps
- Hemolytic-uremic syndrome
- Hemorrhoids

Table 39.6: Pointers to lower GI hemorrhage

Blood profile in stools	*Condition(s)*
• Bloody diarrhea	Colitis (amebic, bacillary, antibiotic-induced/associated)
• Streaks of blood on outer stool	Rectal/perianal bleed (polyp, hemorrhoid, fissure)
• Current jelly stool	Intussusception

- *Upper GI endoscopy* is of great value to directly visualize lesions in esophagus, stomach and duoenum. Endoscopy, in addition to its diagnostic value, is useful from therapeutic angle as well. Table 39.7 gives indications of upper GI endoscopy. Elective endoscopy is usually done 12-24 hours following hospitalization.

Table 39.7: Indications of upper GI endoscopy in GI hemorrhage

Elective
• Situations warranting blood transfusion
• PCV < 30%
• Previous h/o unexplained upper GI hemorrhage
Emergency
• Life-threatening hemorrhage not responding to conservative measures
• Situation likely to benefit from specific endoscopic and/or surgical intervention

However, in the event of facility of pediatric endoscopy being not available, barium swallow/meal should be done.

- *Barium swallow* is good for pinpointing the lesions in the esophagus.
- *Barium meal* is good for defining the lesions in the stomach and duodenum.
- *Barium enema* is indicated in case of the lower GI bleeding. In suspected polyp, it is advisable to clean the bowel thoroughly. In intussusception or malrotation with volvulus, such a cleansing is contraindicated.
- Proctosigmoidoscopy is indicated in persistent lower GI bleeding, especially in a suspected polyp.
- *Angiography* is useful in detecting and defining vascular lesions in esophagus and stomach as also aneurysms in liver and pancreas.
- *Diagnostic exploratory laparotomy* may be required in case of significant bleeding defying a precise diagnosis.

MANAGEMENT

Management is mainly of the etiologic condition and the blood loss.

The essentials of management of this emergency are:

- Verification that the subject indeed has GI hemorrhage.
- Severity of hemorrhage.
- Identification of location of hemorrhage.
- Initial stabilization of heavy bleeding and side-by-side or followed by investigations to find the exact cause of bleeding.
- Definitive treatment of the cause of bleeding.

Stabilization

Massive bleeding, causing shock, regardless of the etiology, is an indication for IV fluids and blood transfusion. Caution should be exercised in case of massive transfusion that can complicate the management by causing hypercitremia, hyperlacticacidemia, hypocalcemia, thrombocytemia, etc.

Stepwise stabilizing approach is outlined in Table 39.8.

Table 39.8: Stepwise stabilizing approach in gross GI hemorrhage

• IV line.
• Blood for grouping, cross-matching and other investigations
• Oxygen in case of loss of one-fifth blood volume.
• Central venous line for maintaining pressure at 3–8 cm of water.
• IV infusion of bolus normal saline or Ringer lactate 10–20 ml/kg speedily.
• Whole blood or platelet cell transfusion.
• Monitor hematocrit (target at 30%) and urine output.

Therapeutic Options

A. Mucosal Lesions

In upper GI hemorrhage from mucosal erosion or ulceration, an appropriate-sized nosagastric tube should be introduced and repeated irrigation with tap water or normal saline (not ice-cold water which may cause vasoconstriction of gastric vessels and lead to stress ulcers) plus neutralization or prevention of release of gastric acid through medication (antacids, H_2 receptor antagonists like ranatidine, proton pump inhibitors like omeprazole, ulcer insulators like sucralfate) usually control it (Table 39.9). Make sure to avoid vigorous suction which can cause exacerbation of bleeding.

B. Persistent Hemorrhage from Esophageal Varices

Emergency sclerotherapy: In a hemodynamically stable subject, the treatment of choice is emergency sclerotherapy to immediately control life-threatening bleeding from esophageal varices. Endoscopic sclerotherapy consists in stopping variceal bleeding by causing thrombosis of the bleeding point(s) by submucosal injection of a sclerosing agent like hypertonic glucose, phenol, alcohol or ethanolamine directly into the varices or into paravariceal tissue).

Sclerotherapy has demonstrated a good control of acute bleeding and reduced recurrence rate. Nevertheless, it is not without side-effects (Table 39.10).[7,8]

Alternatives to sclerotherapy

These include:

- Sengstaken-Blackmore tube and balloon temponade
- Endoscopic measures other than sclerotherapy
- Variceal ligation
- Thermal coagulation
- Electrocoagulation
- Laser photocoagulation
- IV vasopressin, somastostatin or a somastostatin analogue (octreotide).

Balloon temponade: It is reserved for use when emergency sclerotherapy is not possible immediately or to buy time for endoscopic or surgical intervention (Table 39.11). It consists in introducing the Sengstaken-Blackmore tube so that gastric bulb reaches below the gastroesophageal junction. First the gastric balloon is inflated and then the esophageal balloon, maintaining a pressure of around 30 mmHg. The procedure reduces the gastroesophageal blood

Table 39.9: Recommended pharmacotherapy for mucosal lesions causing upper GI hemorrhage

Antacids for neutralizing the gastric acid	:	As high a dose as 0.5 ml/kg/dose every 1-2 hours
H_2 receptor antagonists	:	Ranitidine 2 mg/kg/dose (O or IV) 12 hourly
Proton pump inhibitors	:	Omeprazole 10-20 mg (O) 12 hourly (lower limit for infants and children under 3 years)
Ulcer insulators/protectors	:	Sucralfate 500 mg/dose every 6 hourly

Note: Usually, antacids are given in association with one or two of the other agents

Table 39.10: Side-effects of sclerotherapy in esophageal varices

- Esophageal ulceration
- Esophageal perforation
- Esophageal stricture formation
- Esophageal dysmotility
- Spinal cord paralysis
- Rebleeding

flow by compressing the esophageal varices. Despite availability of a pediatric Sengstaken and Blackmore tube, its use occasionally causes such serious complications as esophageal rupture, pulmonary aspiration and airway obstruction.

Table 39.11: Sengstaken-Blakemore tube and balloon temponade in esophageal varices

- The first lumen of the tube communicates with the stomach, second with stomach balloon, third with esophageal balloon and fourth for continuous aspiration of pharynx.
- The stomach ballon is filled with a radiopaque solution. A gentle suction is needed to retain it into the fundus of the stomach.
- Esophageal ballon is inflated with air to a pressure around 30 mm Hg.
- Pharyngeal balloon is deflated after 24 hours but left in situ for 12-24 hours before the tube is taken out.

Endoscopic measures other than sclerotherapy: A promising substitute for endoscopic sclerotherapy is band ligation of the variceal vein. Additional modalities include thermal coagulation, electrocoagulation and laser photo-coagulation. However, experience with these modalities in pediatric cases is as yet quite limited.

Pharmacotherapy: Precise recommendations are given in Table 39.12. Most frequently employed therapy is Vasopressin infusion which is of particular value in bleeding secondary to prehepatic portal hypertension, stress-induced gastritis and Mallory Weiss tear. Dose is 0.2-0.4 unit/1.73 sqm/minute. Side effects include arrhythmias, hypertension, oliguria and seizures secondary to water retention.

Propranolol therapy has been found to be of value in secondary prophylaxis of upper GI hemorrhage, especially in cases that have had sclerotherapy.[1,4,5] The beneficial effect is from reduced portal pressure secondary to decreased

Table 39.12: Pharmacotherapy of life-threatening bleed from esophageal varices

• Vasopressin	:	Dose 0.2-0.4 units/1.73 sqm/minute, diluted in 2 ml/kg of 5% dextroseinfusion, to be continued for 24-48 hours following stoppage of active bleeding in a tapering dose.
along with		
Nitroglycerin	:	Dose 0.25-0.50 mcg/kg/min IV
• Somatostatin	:	Dose 250 mcg/bolus, 1-3 bolus injections during first hour and then 250 mcg/hour continuous infusion for 2-5 days.
• Oteotide	:	Dose 1-2 mcg/kg with a miximum of 50 mcg and then a constant infusion of 0.4-2.0 mcg/kg/hour with a maximum of 50 mcg/hour.
• Glypressin	:	Dose 2mg IV every 4 hopurly until a bleedingfree interval of 24-48 hours is attained.

cardiac output. Propranolol is known to yield good results in primary prophylaxis of esophageal variceal hemorrhage. However, such a therapy is yet to be adequately studied in case of pediatric esophageal varices.

Shunt Surgery

It is indicated in certain situations (Table 39.13). Its objective is to divert the portal blood flow to reduce the portal pressure.

Table 39.13: Indications for surgery in esophageal varices [6,8,9]

Nondecompressive Surgery

- Failure of conventional medical therapy to control acute variceal bleeding
- Whole of splenoportal axis blocked in extrahepatic portal hypertension

Decompressive (Shunt) Surgery

- Post-sclerotherapy recurrent variceal bleeding
- Noncompliance to EST/EVL
- Failure of EST/EVL
- Rare blood group
- Overwhelming hypersplenism with platelet count under 50,000/mm^3
- Ectopic varices such as duodenal, small bowel or colonic
- Splenic infarcts
- Recurrent esophageal bleeding prior to liver transplantation
- Parent's option for only one time treatment.

C. GI Hemorrhage Related to Obstructive Lesions

Quite a few of the obstructive conditions responsible for life-threatening lower GI hemorrhage in particular need surgery (Table 39.14).

Table 39.14: Indications for surgical intervention in GI hemorrhage[9]

- Intussusception
- Volvulus
- Meckel's diverticulum
- Tumors
- Ongoing bleeding despite conservative measures in peptic or stress ulcer disease.

SUMMARY AND CONCLUSION

Gatrointestinal hemorrhage, a leading pediatric emergency contributing to considerable concern to the parents as well as the attending medical team, warrants careful evaluation (comprising a good history and physical examination, appropriate investigations) and prompt but planned therapeutic approach). It must be ascertained whether the subject in actuality has true bleed, its magnitude, whether it is upper or lower GI bleed and the specific location of bleed.

A speedy initial clinical workup should be accompanied by "initial stabilization". Meticulous diagnostic investigations aimed at determining the exact site and cause of bleeding and specific treatment of the cause of bleeding may be carried later. Stabilization of the subject is of great importance before resorting to an invasive procedure in the management.

Despite its limitations, sclerotherapy appears to be the best option in the treatment of esophageal varices at present. Alternative therapies are available and often prove of considerable value.

REFERENCES

1. Arora NK, Gaur M. Upper gastrointestinal bleeding. In: Gupte S (ed) *Recent Advances in Pediatrics (Special Vol 8: Emergency Pediatrics).* New Delhi: Jaypee Brothers 1998;191-229.
2. Yachha Sk, Khanduri A, Sharma BC, et al. Gastrointestinal bleeding in children. *J Gastroenterol Hepatol* 1996;11:903-907.
3. Sharara AI, Rockey DC. Gastroesophageal variceal hemorrhage. *N Engl J Med* 2001;345:669-681.
4. Gupte S, Anderson RA. Pediatric gastroenterology. In: Gupte S (ed) *The Short Textbook of Pediatrics,* 10th edn. New Delhi: Jaypee Brothers 2004;365-402.
5. Thapa BR. Upper gastrointestinal bleeding. In: Gupte S (ed) *Recent Advances in Pediatrics (Special Vol 14: Criticare Pediatrics).* New Delhi: Jaypee Brothers 2004;184-209.
6. Mittal SK. Nonvariceal upper GI bleeding in children. In: Thapa BR (ed) *Recent Advances in Pediatric Clinical Gastroenterology.* Chandigarh: Relume Printec 2001;19.
7. Donovan TJ, Ward M, Shepard RW. Evaluation of endoscopic sclerotherapy of esophageal varices in children. *J Pediatr Gastroenterol Nutr* 1986;5:696-700.
8. Dene E. Sclerotherapy in pediatric esophageal varices: Yes or no? *Eur Bull Hepatol* 2003;6:65-69.
9. Anderson. Gastrointestinal hemorrhage revisited. *Eur Chron Gastrenterol* 2003;6:124-129.

Subhash Singh Slathia

40 Liver Abscess

INTRODUCTION

Liver abscess, a life-threatening condition,[1] is generally regarded an infrequent condition in the Western world. However, it is, by no means, an uncommon problem in children residing in tropical countries. Bacterial and parasitic invasion of liver are the two common etiological factors. Clinical features are variable depending upon the cause, size of abscess, general health, the features of associated disease and complications.[2,3] Among investigations, role of ultrasound in diagnosing liver abscess and role of indirect haem agglutination in diagnosing cause of liver abscess are very important. Treatment of patient is either medical or surgical, depending upon the size, location, toxicity and response to antimicrobials. Surgical procedure depends upon surgeon's previous experience and facilities available. The best mode of management is controversial. The liver acts as the initial filter of absorbed contents of intestine and is thus at risk to contamination with microbial agents of all varieties.

Other than hepatotropic viruses, the liver can be affected by:

a. Spread of bacterial/parasitic infection from outside liver.
b. Primary infection by spirochaetes, protozoa, tubercular or fungal infections.
c. Systemic effects of bacterial or granulomatous infection.[4]

The various types of abscesses encountered in children are:

a. Amebic liver abscess (ALA)
b. Pyogenic liver abscess (PLA)
c. Fungal liver abscess
d. Tubercular liver abscess.

AMEBIC LIVER ABSCESS (ALA)

It is an inflammatory space-occupying lesion of the liver caused by *Entameba histolytica*. Amebic infection is common throughout the world; about 10% of the world's population is infected with *E. histiolytica*. Among all cases of amoebiasis, the incidence of ALA has been reported to vary between 3-9%.[5] ALA has highest rate of incidence in developing countries including India and Pakistan.[6] Surprisingly, there is paucity of literature on amoebic liver abscess in Indian children.

Age Incidence

Majority of ALA occur between the ages 21 and 50. Below 20 years of age, the incidence is less than 7% and above the age of 50, it is less than 21%. It must, therefore, be noted that no age is exempt and cases have been encountered in infants. The highest incidence between the ages of 1-3 years is perhaps because at this age children tend to swallow things indiscriminately.

Sex Incidence

Male predominance, as in adults, has not been observed in children.

Pathogenesis

Amebiasis is the third leading cause of death from parasitic disease[15] worldwide. *Entameba histolytica*, is a potent pathogen. Secretes proteinases that dissolve host tissues, and kill host cells on contact, engulf red blood cells, and invade the intestinal mucosa, causing amoebic colitis. In some cases amoebae reach liver via portal circulation after breaching the mucosal barrier and where they cause abscesses consisting of a few E histolytica trophozoites surrounding dead and dying hepatocyte and liquefied cellular debris.

Diagnosis

Amebic liver abscess is more common than pyogenic. The diagnosis of a liver abscess in children is often difficult. Therefore, awareness of the condition, especially in endemic areas, may aid in early detection. It depends on clinical findings, serology and hepatic imaging.

The complaints are often nonspecific, thus delaying the diagnosis. The most common symptoms are fever, abdominal discomfort or pain (more in the right upper quadrant of the abdomen). The child is very irritable and may present with vomiting. A preceding history of dysentery may be elicited in these children. On examination, a-slight fullness in the right hypochondrium may be detected. The right lobe of the liver is involved more often than the left.[7]

Elevated right dome of diaphragm is a common X-ray finding.

Investigations

Leukocytosis, moderate anemia, high ESR and raised liver enzymes particularly alkaline phosphatase, are common lab findings. E. histolytica trophozoites in stool are seen in <50% of ALA patients.[15]

Serum antibodies to amebae develop only during E. histolytica infection and not during E. dispar infection. Positive amebic serology like ELISA, indirect hemagglutination, counter current immunoelectrophoresis and latex fixation are helpful. PCR and detection of antigen by monoclonal antibodies are newer techniques. Indirect hemagglutination is highly sensitive and if it is negative ALA can be safely ruled out. However, 10% patients with acute ALA may have negative serology. Antibodies to E. histolytica become positive after one week of onset of symptoms and may remain positive upto 6 months.[5] Recently, Stanley et al[8] reported that serological test based on recombinant E.histolytica antigens may help in differentiating active infection from past exposure to parasite.

In most cases US, CT, MRI or isotope scans can localize and delineate the size of abscess. Aspiration of typical pus from the liver, its examination and amebic serology are often required to diagnose amebic etiology.

Management

Majority of the cases are treated conservatively. However, some advocate needle aspiration along with antiamebic drugs in management of ALA. Indication of aspiration of pus are given in Table 40.1.

Drugs

Nitroimidazoles, chloroquine, and dehydroemetine are effective drugs.

Metronidazole, a tissue amebicidal is given in a dose of 30-50 mg/kg/in three divided doses (maximum: 500-750 mg/dose) per day orally for 10 days. Other two nitroimidazoles, tinidazole and ornidazole are also effective.

Dehydroemetine 1-2 mg/kg. SC/IM (never IV) per day for ten days is preferred over emetine as it may be more effective and safer when administered in high doses. Development of tachycardia, T wave depression, arrhythmias, or proteinuria while giving drug warrants stoppage of drug.

Chloroquine may be useful but it is toxic to children if given in large doses.

Iodoquinol 30-40 mg/kg/24 hr orally divided in 3 doses for 20 days is drug of choice for a symptomatic cyst carriers. Paromomycin and diloxanide are also used.

Complications and Unusual Presentations

Pus can rupture into pleuro-pulmonary area, subphrenic space, peritoneal cavity, and pericardial space. The last is usually due to left ALA and may result in pericardial temponade. Other less common complications are rupture or compression or thrombosis of hepatic veins or inferior vena cava. In fact ALA has been reported as cause of Budd Chiari syndrome in few patients from Indian subcontinent.[5] ALA may coexist with hepatitis A and hepatitis E infection, or HbsAg carriers.[5]

PYOGENIC LIVER ABSCESS (PLA)

Bacterial abscess of the liver is relatively rare. Its incidence is not available. However, in one large study 25 per 100,000 hospital admission is recorded. The development of new radiologic techniques, the improvement in microbiologic identification, and the advancement of drainage techniques have decreased mortality rates to less than 15%.[9] Yet, the incidence has remained relatively unchanged. Untreated, this infection remains uniformly fatal.

Pathophysiology

The liver receives blood from both the systemic and portal circulations.

Increased susceptibility to infections would be expected given the increased exposure to bacteria. However, Kupffer cells lining the hepatic sinusoids clear bacteria so efficiently that infection rarely occurs. Biliary tract disease remains the most common source of pyogenic liver abscess (PLA) and accounts for 60% of cases in adults. Obstruction of bile flow allows for bacterial proliferation.

Though the portal venous system can be a source of abscess resulting from infections involving any organ drained by this system. Appendicitis was the leading source of PLA in the preantibiotic era, but it essentially has been eliminated in recent times.

The right hepatic lobe is affected more often than the left. Bilateral involvement is seen less often.[10] The predilection for the right lobe can be attributed to anatomic considerations.

Hepatic abscess formation in infants and children[7] can be seen in association with systemic bacteremia, umbilical

Table 40.1: Bacteriology of liver abscess[4]

Aerobes Gram –	Aerobes Gram +	Anaerobes	Others: candida albicans, tubercular
E. coli Kllebsiella	Enterococci	Bacteroid spp.	
Enterobacter spp.	StreptoPyogenes	Fusobact streptococci	
Pseudomonas spp.	Listeria monocytogenes (rare)	peptostreptococi peptococi	
Citrobacter spp	Strepto milleri.	actinomyces (rare)	
Morganella spp.			
Proteus spp.			
Salmonella spp.			
Staph. aureus			

vein infection, or vessel cannulation. In children liver abscess occurs mostly with underlying:

1. Defects in immunity, such as chronic granulomatous disease and leukemia.
2. From portal circulation the association through which this is thought to occur is pylephlebitis (septic thrombophlebitis) of any tributary of the portal venous system. Infections in organs in the portal bed (appendicitis, inflammatory bowel disease) can result in a localized septic thrombophlebitis. Septic emboli are released into the portal circulation, trapped by the hepatic sinusoids, and become the nidus for microabscess formation. Thus, abscesses initially are multiple but usually coalesce into a solitary lesion.
3. Generalized sepsis.
4. Cholangitis associated with biliary tract obstruction.
5. Systemic spread from intraabdominal infection or contiguous spread, and
6. Cryptogenic biliary tract infection.
7. Penetrating hepatic trauma can inoculate organisms directly into liver parenchyma, resulting in PLA. Nonpenetrating trauma results in localized hepatic necrosis, intrahepatic hemorrhage, and bile leakage due to disruption of canaliculi. The resulting tissue environment permits bacterial growth with resultant PLA. Lesions of this etiology typically are solitary.
8. Pyogenic liver abscess may occur in normal children and should be considered whenever fever of unknown origin is associated with abdominal complaints.[11]
9. PLA has been reported as a secondary infection of amebic abscess, hydatid cystic cavities, and metastatic and primary hepatic tumors. A unique case of sickle cell disease presenting as pyogenic hepatic abscess in a 4 year old boy has been reported. Streptococcus species was isolated from pus.[12]

A possible association between pyogenic liver abscess and intestinal nematodes, toxacara infection, has been also observed. Hemoglobinopathy as underlying disease, was frequently associated with PLA.[13] Multiple micro-abscesses have been found to be associated with catch-scratch disease.[14]

Sex

While abscesses once showed a predilection for males in earlier decades, no sexual predilection currently exists. However, in a study of 136 children of PLA 97 were male.

Age

Any age; in one of the studies mean age observed was 8.42 years with a range of 1-15 years.

Causes

These are listed in Table 40.2.

Mostly the organisms detected are staphylococcus aureus, klebsiella pneumoniae,[13,14] E. coli, almonella and anaerobic[9] organisms.

Fungal abscesses primarily are due to *Candida albicans* and occur in individuals with prolonged exposure to antimicrobials, hematologic malignancies, solid-organ transplants, and congenital and acquired immunodeficiency.

Diagnosis

The most frequent symptoms of hepatic abscess include the following:

- Fever (either continuous or spiking)
- Chills
- Malaise
- Anorexia
- Weight loss

Cough or hiccough (hiccup) due to diaphragmatic irritation may be reported. Pain referred pain to the right shoulder may be present in older children. Fever of unknown origin (FUO) frequently can be the only presentation. Multiple abscesses usually result in more acute presentations, with symptoms and signs of systemic toxicity.

Physical

Physical sequelae most commonly seen include fever and tender hepatomegaly, with point tenderness being highly specific. A palpable mass need not be present. Mid epigastric tenderness, with or without a palpable mass, is suggestive of left lobe involvement. Decreased breath sounds in the right basilar lung zones, with signs of atelectasis and effusion

Table 40.2: Differences between pyogenic and amebic liver abscess

Pyogenic liver abscess	*Amebic liver abscess*
May be solitary or multiple, either lobe.	Usually solitary, right hepatic lobe more often involved, secondary bacterial infection is common in multiple abscesses.
May arise from hematogenous spread or arise from contiguous spread of infection with in peritoneal cavity.	
Fever, abdominal pain seen in both. Fever with chills is more prominent.	
About 50% patients have right upper quadrant tenderness with hepatomegaly.	While 80% of patients with ALA has such symptoms.
Serum alkaline phosphatase ia raised in both but serum bilirubin is raised in about 50% of cases.	Serum bilirubin is raised in about 30% of cases. A high bilirubin (>3.5 mg/dl) level, encephalopathy, large volume of pus and low albumin (< 2.0 gm/dl) are bad progonostic signs of mortality independently.
Imaging studies show almost similar results.	
Microscopic examination reveals presence of neutrophils in aspirated pus and culture may yield bacterial flora.	Amoebic abscess does not show neutrophils, amoebae are rarely isolated. The yield is from the last few ml. of pus and from the walls of pus cavity.
Aspiration of pus and Gram's stain and culture of pus may be required to differentiate the two.	Amoebic serology is helpful. if negative diagnosis unlikely.
Treatment is iv drugs plus pus drainage.	Treatment is drugs and routine aspiration of pus is not indicated. Indication of aspiration are:lack of improvement in signs and symptoms with in 48 to 72 hrs, left lobe abscess, abscess size more than 10 cm, if suspected to be pressing inferior vena cava, multiple abscesses, presence of jaundice due to a large abscess or abscesses at porta hepatis and sero-negative abscesses.

on examination or radiologically, may be present. A pleural or hepatic friction rub can be associated with diaphragmatic irritation or inflammation of Glisson capsule. Jaundice may be present in as many as 25% of cases and usually is associated with biliary tract disease or the presence of multiple abscesses.

Radiologic Studies

Chest X-ray findings of basilar atelectasis, right hemidiaphragm elevation, and right pleural effusion are present in approximately 50% of cases; before advancements in radiologic technique, these served as diagnostic clues. Pneumonias or pleural diseases often are initially considered because of the radiographic findings.

Imaging Studies

The advancement in radiologic techniques has been credited with the improvement in mortality rates. CT evaluation with contrast and ultrasonography remain the radiologic modalities of choice as both screening procedures also can be used as techniques for guiding percutaneous aspiration and drainage.

CT Scan (Sensitivity 95-100%) is very useful. Lesions on CT evaluation are well-demarcated areas, hypodense to the surrounding hepatic parenchyma. Peripheral enhancement is seen when IV contrast is administered. Gas can be seen in as many as 20% of lesions. CT scan is superior in its ability to detect lesions less than 1 cm.

This technique also enables the evaluation for an underlying concurrent pathology throughout the abdomen and pelvis. Indium-labeled WBC scans are somewhat more sensitive in this regard.

Ultrasound (sensitivity 80-90%) Ultrasound evaluation reveals hypoechoic masses with irregularly shaped borders. Internal septations or cavity debris may be detected.

Gallium and technetium radionuclide scanning (sensitivity 50-90%) offer no benefit over other imaging.

Differentials

- Pneumonia, Bacterial
- Empyema (pleuropulmonary)
- Gastritis (acute)
- Hydatid cysts
- Hepatitis (nonviral)
- Hepatocellular carcinoma
- Metastatic disease of the liver
- Biliary disease
- Cholecystitis

MEDICATION

Until cultures are available, the choice of antimicrobial agents should be directed toward the most commonly involved pathogens. Regimens using beta-lactam/beta-lactamase inhibitor combinations, carbapenems, or second-generation cephalosporins with anaerobic are excellent empiric choices for the coverage of enteric bacilli and anaerobes. Metronidazole or clindamycin should be added for the coverage of Bacteroides fragilis if other employed antibiotics offer no anaerobic coverage. If fungal pathogens are a possibility, empiric anti-fungal therapy should be considered. Initial therapy for fungal abscess is currently amphotericin B. Lipid formulations may offer some benefit in that the complexing of drug to lipid moieties allows for concentration in hepatocytes. Further investigation is required for definitive proof. Cases of successful fluconazole treatment after amphotericin failure have been reported. However, its use as an initial agent is still being studied. Ultimately, the organisms isolated and antibiotic sensitivities should guide the final choice of antimicrobials.

Duration of treatment has always been debated. Short courses (2 weeks) of therapy after percutaneous drainage have been successful in a small series of patients. However, most series have reported recurrence of abscess even after more prolonged courses. Currently 4-6 weeks of therapy is recommended for solitary lesions that have been adequately drained. Multiple abscesses are more problematic and can require up to 12 weeks of therapy. Both the clinical and radiographic progress of the patient should guide the length of therapy.

The overall mortality (15%) has decreased considerably as compared for children with PLA before 1975. Prompt diagnosis of pyogenic liver abscess, its evacuation and antibiotic therapy has resulted in improved survival. Staph. Aureus was isolated in majority and anaerobes in 27% of children with PLA.[9]

TREATMENT

Medical Care

US or CT guided percutaneous aspiration with antimicrobial therapy is the first choice.[13, 15-16]

An untreated hepatic abscess is nearly uniformly fatal due to complications that include sepsis, empyema, or peritonitis from rupture into the pleural or peritoneal spaces, and retroperitoneal extension

Antibiotic therapy as a sole treatment modality is not routinely advocated, though it has been successful in a few reported cases. In 136 children of PLA 36.2% responded to antibiotics. It may be the only alternative in patients too ill to undergo invasive procedures or in those with multiple abscesses not amenable to either drainage technique.

Percutaneous catheter drainage with antimicrobial therapy:[17] This was introduced in the 1970s as an alternative to surgery.

Surgical Care

Surgical drainage was the standard of care until the introduction of percutaneous drainage techniques in the mid-1970s.

Current indications for surgical treatment of PLA include signs of peritonitis; existence of a known abdominal surgical pathology (such as diverticular abscess); failure of previous drainage attempts; and the presence of a complicated, multi-loculated, thick-walled abscess with viscid pus.

Antibiotics

Meropenem (Merrem): Bactericidal broadspectrum carbapenem antibiotic that inhibits cell-wall synthesis. Effective against most gram-positive and gram-negative bacteria. Has slightly increased activity against gram negatives and slightly decreased activity against staphylococci and streptococci species compared to imipenem.

Dose: 40 mg/kg IV q8h.

Imipenem and cilastatin (Primaxin): For treatment of multiple organism infections in which other agents do not have wide-spectrum coverage or are contraindicated due to potential for toxicity.

Dose: <12 years: Not established; 15-25 mg/kg/dose IV q6h suggested for >3 months.

Fully susceptible organisms: Not to exceed 2 g/d. Infections with moderately susceptible organisms: Not to exceed 4 g/d.

Cefuroxime (Ceftin): Second-generation cephalosporin maintains gram-positive activity that first-generation cephalosporins have; adds activity against Proteus mirabilis, Haemophilus influenzae, Escherichia coli, Klebsiella pneumoniae, and Moraxella catarrhalis.

Dose

Children : 250 mg PO bid for 20 d.
Adolescents : Administer as in adults.

Cefotetan (Cefotan): Second-generation cephalosporin indicated for infections caused by susceptible gram-positive cocci and gram-negative rods.

Dose: 20-40 mg/kg/dose IV/IM q12h for 5-10 d.

Cefoxitin (Mefoxin): Second-generation cephalosporin indicated for gram-positive cocci and gram-negative rod infections. Infections caused by cephalosporin-resistant or penicillin-resistant gram-negative bacteria may respond to cefoxitin.

Dose: 80-160 mg/kg/d IV divided q4-6h; higher doses for severe or serious infections; not to exceed 12 g/d.

Cefaclor (Ceclor): Second-generation cephalosporin indicated for infections caused by susceptible gram-positive cocci and gram-negative rods.

Dose: 20-40 mg/kg/d divided q8-12h; not to exceed 2 g/d.

Clindamycin (Cleocin): Lincosamide for treatment of serious skin and soft tissue staphylococcal infections. Also effective against aerobic and anaerobic streptococci (except enterococci). Inhibits bacterial growth, possibly by blocking dissociation of peptidyl t-RNA from ribosomes causing RNA-dependent protein synthesis to arrest.

Dose: 8-20 mg/kg/d PO as hydrochloride and 8-25 mg/kg/d as palmitate divided tid/qid 20-40 mg/kg/d IV/IM divided tid/qid.

Metronidazole (Flagy. Metrogyl, Aristgyl): Imidazole ring-based antibiotic active against various anaerobic bacteria and protozoa. Used in combination with other antimicrobial agents (except for Clostridium difficile enterocolitis).

Dose: 15-30 mg/kg/d PO divided bid/tid for 7 d, or 40 mg/kg once; do not exceed 2 g/d.

Antifungal agents: Their mechanism of action may involve an alteration of RNA and DNA metabolism or an intracellular accumulation of peroxide that is toxic to the fungal cell.

Amphotericin B (AmBisome): Produced by a strain of Streptomyces nodosus; can be fungistatic or fungicidal. Binds to sterols, such as ergosterol, in the fungal-cell membrane, causing intracellular components to leak with subsequent fungal-cell death.

Dose: 3-5 mg/kg/d IV of liposomal amphotericin B over approximately 120 min.

Precautions: Monitor renal function, serum electrolytes (e.g., magnesium and potassium) liver function, CBC, and hemoglobin concentrations; resume the therapy at the lowest level (e.g., 0.25 mg/kg) when the therapy is interrupted for more than 7 d; hypoxemia, acute dyspnea, and interstitial infiltrates may occur in patients who are neutropenic and receiving leukocyte transfusions (separate time of amphotericin infusion from time of leukocyte transfusion).

Fluconazole (Diflucan): Synthetic oral antifungal (broad-spectrum bistriazole) that selectively inhibits fungal cytochrome P-450 and sterol C-14 alpha-demethylation.

Dose: 3-6 mg/kg/d for 14-28 d or 6-12 mg/kg/d, depending on:

Precautions: Monitor closely if rashes develop and discontinue drug if lesions progress; may cause clinical hepatitis, cholestasis, and fulminant hepatic failure (including death), with underlying medical conditions, such as AIDS or a malignancy, and while taking multiple concomitant medications; not recommended for mothers who are nursing.

Many a times it is not possible to differentiate the ALA from PLA on clinical grounds, routine investigations and imaging techniques. Aspiration of pus, especially if the abscess was multiple, is most helpful in differentiating the two types of abscesses. Serological test of E. IHA was highly specific and sensitive for amebic liver abscess.[6]

Management of a Child with Suspected Liver Abscess

In addition to CBC, CXR, US and/or CT and amebic serology, start both anti-amebic and anti-pyogenic treatment. If amebic serology is positive give anti-amebic for 4 weeks and antipyogenic is stopped after 2 weeks. If amebic serology is negative give antipyogenic for 4-6 weeks and stop anti-amebic after 2 weeks.

If abscess size is < 5 cm, treat conservatively. If it is > 5 cm, drainage is required. Type of drainage depends upon merit of the case. However, US or CT-guided percutaneous needle aspiration is safe, cost-effective and is accompanied by least complications in majority of the cases.[16-18]

According to Thapa,[18] percutaneous catheter drainage (PCD) is preferred mode of treatment of liver abscess. The success rate is as high as 100%. Such complications as pain, pericatheter leak and bleeding are easily manageable. In an occasional case, there may be associated biliary communication of abscess which can be treated by putting stent in common bile duct (CBD), nasobiliary drain (NBD) or sphincterectomy.

REFERENCES

1. Parson E. Liver abscess in children. *Eur J Gastrenterol*, 2001;6:118-124.
2. Noons, Milar MW. Liver abscess in childhood. *Pediatr Surg Int*. 1988;3:27-32.
3. Ranairez CP, Hernandex H, Jauri H. Ameobic hepatic abscess in children. *J Pediatr Surg* 1995;30:662-664.
4. Raymond T, Chung, Lawrence S Friedman. Liver Abscess and Bacterial, Parasitic, Fungal and Granulomatous Liver Diseases.In: Mark Feldman, Lawrence S, Friedman, Marvin H, Sleisenger (eds) *Sleisenger and Fordtran's Gastrointestinal and Liver Diseases*. Philadelphia: WB Saunders 2002;1343-1346.
5. Mathur S, Gehbt RS, Mehta A, Bhargava N. *J Indian Acad Clin Med* 2002;3:212-216.
6. Ahsan T, Jehangir MU, Mahmood T, Ahmed N, Saleem M, Shahid M, Shaheer A, AnwerA. Amoebic versus pyogenic liver abscess *J Pak Med Assoc* 2002:52:497-501.
7. Sharon B, Weissman, Robert A, Salata Amebiasis. In: Behrman RE, Kliegman RM, Jenson HB (eds) *Nelson Textbook of Pediatrics*. Philadelphia: WB Saunders 2000;1035-1036.
8. Stanley Sl Jr, Jackson TF, Foster L, Singh S. Longitudinal study of the antibody response to recombinant Entamoeba histolytica

antigen in patient with amoebic liver abscess. *Am J Trop Med Hyg* 1998;58:414-416.

9. Pineiro-Carrero VM, Andres JM. Morbidity and mortality in children with pyogenic liver abscess. *Am J Dis Child* 1989;143:1424-1427.
10. Wang DS, Chen DS, Wang YZ, Li JS. Bacterial liver abscess in children. *J Singapore Pediatr Soc*. 1989;31:75-78.
11. Kaplan SL, Feigin RD. Experience and reason—briefly recorded. *Pediatrics* 1976;58:614-616.
12. Shulman ST, Beem MO. A unique presentation of sickle cell disease: Pyogenic hepatic absces. *Pediatrics*. 1971;47:1019-1022.
13. Ni YH, Chang MH, Hsu HY, Lee CY. Ultrasound-guided percutaneous drainage of liver abscess in children. *Zhonghua Min Guo Xiao Er Ke Yi Xue Hui Za Zhi*. 1995;36:336-341.
14. Stain SC, Yellin AE, Donovan AJ, Brien HW. Pyogenic liver abscess. Modern treatment. *Arch Surg* 1991;126:991-996.
15. Attar B, Levendoglu H, Cuasay NS. CT-guided percutaneous aspiration and catheter drainage of pyogenic liver abscesses. *Am J Gastroenterol* 1986;81:550-555.
16. Ch Yu S, Hg Lo R, Kan PS, Metreweli C.Clin pyogenic liver abscess: Treatment with needle aspiration. *Radiology* 1997;52:912-916.
17. Giorgio A, Tarantino L, Mariniello N, et al. Pyogenic liver abscesses: 13 years of experience in percutaneous needle aspiration with US guidance. *Radiology* 1995;195:122-124.
18. Thapa BR, Munish K. Liver abscess. In: Gupte S (ed) *Recent Advances in Pediatrics*, Vol 14. New Delhi: Jaypee Brothers 2004;110-118.

Suraj Gupte, Robin Abrams, Utpal Kant Singh and VS Puri

41 Hepatic Encephalopathy

INTRODUCTION

Hepatic encephalopathy (HE) is a complex neuropsychiatric syndrome resulting from accumulation of unmetabolized ammonia predominantly as a result of poor hepatic function of both acute and chronic types.[1-5]

The more or less alternative terms for the entity include *hepatic coma* (HC), *fulminant hepatic failure* (FHF) and *acute hepatic failure* (AHF). Acute liver necrosis with hepatic encephalopathy starting within 8 weeks of the first sign of liver disease is termed 'fulminant'.

Recent reviews have dubbed HE as "one of the most devastating pediatric emergencies that, if attended energetically, may have a gratifying outcome, especially following liver transplantation."[1,2] That sums up the importance of early recognition of the entity, its prompt workup to determine the exact cause and its aggressive management.

According to European Health Survey 2000-2001, some 8.5% infants and children admitted to hospitals for one or the other stage of coma suffer from HE.[1] At Government Medical College, Jammu, 10 to 12% pediatric subjects hospitalized for coma turn out to be cases of hepatic coma. Attempts to obtain figures in this field from certain other centres in the country have provided incidence varying from 9 to 20%.[3]

HE carries a very high mortality. Yet, the fact remains that it is a potentially treatable state. The availability of modern medical treatment together with liver transplantation in particular has considerably enhanced the survival rate.[4,6,8]

HYPOTHESES REGARDING PATHOGENESIS

The exact modus operandi of development of HE is yet not quite clear. Quite a few hypotheses have been put forward (Table 41.1).

Table 41.1: Some of the hypotheses postulated to explain pathogenesis of HE

- Accumulation of unmetabolized ammonia. Most popular; provides basis for most treatment measures of proven value
- Production of false neurotransmitters
- Activation of central c-aminobutyric acid-benzodiazepine receptors by ligands of endogenous origin
- Altered cerebral metabolism
- Disturbed activity of Na^+/K^+-ATPase
- Decreased activity of urea cycle enzymes due to zinc deficiency and the deposition of manganese in the basal ganglia

Seemingly, a multitude of factors noxious to CNS act in nexus to produce CNS changes since, for one or the other reason, liver becomes incapable of detoxifying them.

PATHOLOGY

It varies with the underlying etiologic disorder (Table 41.2).

Table 41.2: Major pathological findings in important conditions leading to HE

Conditions	*Major pathological findings*
Viral hepatitis, Wilson's disease, Toxin-induced HE	Massive confluent or multilobular liver necrosis
Reye's and Reye's-like syndromes	Diffuse hepatic steatosis
Inborn errors of metabolism	Swelling of hepatocytes with spotty necrosis

ETIOLOGY

As a rule, HE is considered either viral or nonviral in origin.

Viral

Hepatic coma is usually a complication of viral hepatitis (A,B,C,D,E,G); other infections like herpes simplex, EB virus, parvovirus B 19, varicella zoster, CMV, adenovirus, echovirus, and coxackie virus may also cause fulminant hepatitis and hepatic coma.

Nonviral

- *Hepatotoxicity*: A variety of hepatotoxic drugs and toxins (say paracetamol, NSAIDs, acetaminophen, isoniazid, halothane, sodium valproate, and phenytoin, antidepressants and toxins)
- *Ischemia and hypoxia:* Hepatic vascular obstruction
- Congestive heart failure (CHF)
- Circulatory shock
- *Metabolic disorders:* Wilson's disease, hemochromatosis, tyrosinemia
- *Mitochondrial disorders:* Fructose intolerance, a-1 antitrypsin deficiency, glycogen storage disease
- Indian childhood cirrhosis (ICC)
- Autoimmune hepatitis
- Idiopathic hepatitis.

It is also useful to consider etiology in relation to age (Table 41.3).

Table 41.3: Etiology of hepatic encephalopathy in relation to age

Early infancy (< 6 months): CMV, EBV, adenoviruses, hepatitis B, tyrosinemia
Late Infancy: Hepatitis A, B, C and D, EBV, Congenital biliary atresia, Allagile syndrome, alpha-1-antitrypsin deficiency, drugs (isoniazid, rifampicin, valproate, phenytoin, paracetamol, halotane, ketoconazole), ICC, Niemann-Pik disease
Childhood: Hepatitis A, B, C and D, Reye's syndrome, Rey's-like syndrome, Wilson's disease, drugs and toxins (vide above), cystic fibrosis, CSD type IV

CLINICAL MANIFESTATIONS

Clinical Presentation

In case of fulminant hepatic failure, the child is, as a rule, previously without liver disease and most often has no risk factors for liver disease. Initial manifestations include progressively increasing jaundice, a characteristic sweatish pungent breath odor *(fetor hepaticus),* fever, anorexia, vomiting, and abdominal pain. A hemorrhagic diathesis, ascites and impairment of renal function (manifested by oliguria/ anuria) may develop rapidly.

A rapid decrease in liver size without clinical improvement is an unfavourable sign. It is, therefore, important to measure the liver span at the outset of hospitalization and then every day.

Development of hepatic encephalopathy is initially characterized by minor disturbances of consciousness or motor function in the form of irritability, poor feeding, and a change in sleep rhythm (especially in the infants).

Older children may show asterixis in the form of abnormal muscle tremor consisting of involuntary jerking movements, more so in the hands, tongue and muscle groups of foot. This is termed "liver flap" or "liver tremor". In our experience with adolescent subjects, an important differential diagnosis of such asterixis is alcoholism or other substance abuse.

The patient may rapidly progress to deeper stages of coma in which extensor plantar responses and decerebrate and decorticate posturing appear.

Decerebrate posture results from elimination of cerebral function and consists of stiff and extended extremities and retracted head.

Decorticate posture results from elimination of a portion of cortex of brain from underlying white matter. The lesion is, therefore, at or above the upper brain stem. Here the patient is rigid with upper limbs flexed, fits clenched and legs extended.

Clinical Grading/Staging

Several grading systems have been proposed.

Grading System I (Conventional System)

The commonly employed conventional grading system is given in Table 41.4.

Table 41.4: Commonly employed conventional system

Grade I
Personality changes: Restlessness, irritability, violent behavior, confusion, loss of memory, disorientation
Grade II
Somnolence: All of above plus lethargy, brisk reflexes, easily arousable
Grade III
Stupor: Stuprose but arousable, hypertonia, hyperventilation, extensor planters
Grade IV
Coma: Comatose and unresponsive, decorticate /decerebrate rigidity on stimulus, irregular breathing, flaccidity, areflexia

Grading System II (More Elaborate New System)

This new grading system is more elaborate, taking into account the EEG changes in addition to the clinical features (Table 41.5).

DIAGNOSIS

Diagnosis is, by and large, clinical but needs to be supported by certain laboratory studies which are also important for following the progression of the disease. Nevertheless, practical bed-side tests are easily administered and provide useful information, especially in patients with subclinical hepatic encephalopathy that would otherwise be overlooked.

The level of ammonia in the arterial blood shows a tendency to be elevated in patients with more advanced hepatocellular dysfunction, especially when substantial

Table 41.5: Grading system for hepatic encephalopathy

Stage	Symptoms	Signs	EEG
I.	Spans of lethargy, euphoria; reversal of day-night sleeping; could be alert	Finds difficult to draw figures and perform mental tasks	Normal
II.	Drowsiness/agitatio, behavioral problems, wide swings in mood, disorientation	Asterix, inontinence, fetor hepaticus	Generalized slowing, q waves
III.	Stupor but arousable, confused, Incoherent speech	Asterix, hyperreflexia, rigidity, extensor reflexes	Remarkably abnormal Triphasic waves
IV.	Coma	No asterixis, flaccidity,	Remarkably abnormal bilateral slowing, D waves electric-cortical silence
IVa.	Response to noxious stimuli		
IV b.	No response to noxious stimuli		

portosystemic shunting is present. Yet, there is a poor correlation between ammonia level and grade of encephalopathy. Logically, therefore, this measurement is of little clinical value in establishing the diagnosis or following the progress of patients with hepatic coma.

Laboratory Investigations

- Serum aminotransferases i.e. aspartate aminotransferase (AST) or serum glutamic oxidase transaminase (SGOT) and alanine aminotransferase (ALT) or serum glutamic pyruvate transaminase (SGPT) levels are elevated. Elevated AST or SGPT is a very sensitive index of hepatic damage. Whereas its rise in HC following acute viral hepatitis is 10-100 times, it is 100 to 500 times in paracetamol-induced hepatic injury. As the patient deteriorates, these levels may demonstrate a fall.
- Serum bilirubin is high.
- Blood ammonia is increased.
- Prothrombin time is always prolonged.
- Hypoglycemia may occur.
- Dyselectrolytemia, metabolic acidosis, and respiratory alkalosis may develop.

Other investigations, needed depending on the merits of the situation, include:

- Sepsis screen
- Virologic markers and antibodies
- Blood grouping and cross matching
- Albumin:globulin (A : G) ratio
- ECG, EEG, and
- Radiological investigations.

DIFFERENTIAL DIAGNOSIS

Differential diagnosis of HE (Table 41.6) is in relation to metabolic, infective and toxic or drug-induced encephalopathies.[5] At times, intracranial lesions and neuropsychiatric disorders may cause confusion in arriving at the exact diagnosis.

None of the manifestations of HE are specific to this state. It is, therefore, mandatory to rule out alternative diagnoses.

PRECIPITATING/AGGRAVATING FACTORS

These include:

- Gastrointestinal hemorrhage (100 ml = 14 to 20 g protein)
- Constipation
- Infection
- Use of sedatives (diazepam and other benzodiazepines) and psychoactive drugs
- High animal protein diet
- Hypoglycemia
- Blood transfusion
- Azotemia
- Dehydration, dyselctrolytemia (especially hypokalemia) and systemic alkalosis
- Arterial hypotension
- Anemia
- Portosystemic shunts
- Rapid paracentesis
- Hypoxia.

IMPORTANT COMPLICATIONS

Superadded Sepsis

Superadded infections in the form of septicemia, pneumonia, peritonitis, and urinary tract infections are common in hepatic coma. Gram-positive microbes (*Staphylococcus aureus, Staphylococcus epidermidis*) are the most common pathogens; Gram-negative and fungal infections are also seen.

Table 41.7 lists important causes of infection in HE. Table 41.8 lists signals of infection.

Hepatorenal Syndrome

Acute renal failure manifested by oliguria and uremia. Tubular function is not significantly affected. The cause appears to be effective hypovolemia resulting from systemic vasodilatation and pooling of blood in portal circulation (Table 41.9). Mortality is high.

Table 41.6: Differential diagnosis of HE

- Infective Encephalopathies
- Meningitis
- Encephalitis
- Malaria
- Metabolic encephalopathies
- Hypoglycemia
- Electrolyte imbalance
- Hypoxia
- CO_2 narcosis
- Acidosis
- Ketoacidosis
- Toxic encephalopathies
- Alcohol
- Psychoactive drugs
- Salicylates
- Heavy metals
- Intracranial lesions
- Subarachnoid, subdural, intracerebral hemorrhage
- Cerebral infarction
- Cerebral tumor
- Cerebral abscess
- Epilepsy or postseizure encephalopathy
- Neuropsychiatric disorders
- Hysteria

Table 41.7: Factors that contribute to superadded infection in encephalopasthy

- Impaired opsonization of bacteria
- Reduced neutrophil adherence
- Chemotactic defects
- Inhibitors of leukocyte function
- Reduced host defenses from damage to reticuloendothelial system

Table 41.8: Signals of infection in HE

- Fall in blood pressure (not explained by other causes)
- Consistently reducing urine output
- Severe acidosis
- Worsening encephalopathy
- DIC

Table 41.9: Events precipitating hypovolemia and subsequent hepatorenal syndrome in HE

- Septicemia
- Excessive diuretic therapy
- Large volume paracentesis
- Gastrointestinal hemorrhage

Hepatopulmonary Syndrome

Impaired pulmonary may result from ventilation-perfusion inequality.

Coagulopathy

Injured and dysfunctional liver may:

- Impair synthesis of some coagulation factors (Factor II, V, VII, IX and X), and
- Reduce fibrinogen levels.

This leads to DIC, thrombocytopenia, and presence of fibrin degradation products in the blood. As a result, the child develops, bruising, gastrointestinal bleeding, intra-cerebral bleeding and profuse bleeding following procedures such as placement of an intravenous catheter.

Cerebral Edema

An important cause of mortality in HE, cerebral edema causes raised intracranial pressure (ICP). It usually results from:

- Vasogenic edema in which an insult to the blood-brain barrier (BBB) causes leakage of protein-rich edema fluid into extracellular space, and
- Cytotoxic edema in which edema is the result of cellular toxicity and is intracellular.

Factors precipitating cerebral edema are listed in Table 41.10.

Table 41.10: Factors precipitating cerebral edema in HE

- Sustained decubitus or horizontal position
- Body movements
- Frequent handling
- Frequent suctioning
- Noxious stimuli
- Excessive coughing, sneezing or vomiting
- Sustained sever hypoxia
- Sustained severe hypercapnia

Edema

Damaged liver may lead to poor synthesis of proteins (hypoproteinemia), resulting in fall in plasma oncotic pressure and, thereby contributing to development of edema.

MANAGEMENT

Aims of aggressive medical treatment are:

1. To achieve cure through supportive measures, if feasible.
2. To tide over the difficult period in preparing for the liver transplantation.

What follows relates to management of HC following acute hepatic failure rather than chronic hepatic failure.

I. GENERAL SUPPORTIVE MEASURES

General principles of management are those of most critically sick patients.

- Intravenous line: Energy supplementation in the range of 30 to 50 kcal/kg/day should be provided.
- Nasogastric tube.
- Administration of oxygen.
- Application of monitors and ventilators.

- Urinary catheters (preferably condom connection in males if there is no urinary retention) to measure urinary output.
- Facility for round-the-clock monitoring of vital parameters.
- Laboratory investigations.
- Endotracheal intubation may be required to prevent aspiration, to reduce cerebral edema, by hyperventilation, and to facilitate pulmonary toilet.
- Raise head end (30 to 45 degrees) and maintain head in neutral position.
- Input output balance chart should be properly maintained.

II. MEASURES DIRECTED AT COMPLICATIONS

Fluid and Electrolytes Imbalance

Electrolyte and glucose solutions should be administered intravenously to maintain urine output, to correct or prevent hypoglycemia, and to maintain normal serum potassium concentrations. Hyponatremia is common but is usually dilutional and not a result of sodium depletion. Parenteral supplementation with calcium, phosphorus, and magnesium may be required depending on clinical manifestations and laboratory results. Hypovolemia should be avoided and treated with cautious infusions of fluids and blood products.

Prevention and Control of Superadded Infection

Since at least one-half of the children with HC develop serious infection(s), it is mandatory to closely monitor the patient for a superadded infections such as septicemia, pneumonia, peritonitis, and urinary tract infections.

If an infection indeed develops, an intravenous antibiotics such as ampicillin or cephalosporin should be started till sensitivity pattern is available. Later, use of antibiotic would depend on antibiogram results.

Use of prophylactic antibiotics remains controversial.

Cerebral Edema

- *Mannitol* given by repeated bolus injections over a period 10 minutes remains the main pharmacologic treatment of cerebral edema.
- *Hyperventilation* ($PaCO_2$ 25-30 mm Hg) is frequently used to prevent or postpone the development of cerebral edema and intracranial hypertension in patients with FHF.[11]
- *Acetylcysteine* given by continuous infusion has been reported to improve cerebral blood flow and the cerebral metabolic rate for oxygen.
- Prostaglandin I_2 also improves the cerebral metabolic rate for oxygen.
- Elevation of bed by 30 degree.
- Fluid restriction.

Coagulopathy

- Coagulopathy should be treated with parenteral (IV) administration of vitamin K, 0.2 mg/kg (maximum of 10 mg).
- At times, fresh frozen plasma and blood may be needed, especially in the presence of DIC.
- Plasmapheresis may permit temporary correction of the bleeding diathesis without resulting in volume overload.[7,8]
- Prophylactic use of antacids or H_2 receptor blockers (antagonists) or both should be considered because of the high risk of gastrointestinal bleeding.

Renal Failure or Dysfunction

The cause may be hypovolemia from acute tubular necrosis or from functional renal failure (hepatorenal syndrome). It needs to be appropriately managed.

Respiratory Failure

Assisted ventilatory support.

Seizures

The recommended drug is diazepam. However, it should be administered in half of the dose recommended for controlling seizures routinely.

Gastrointestinal Bleeding

H_2 receptor antagonists, antacids, IV somatostatin or its analogue.

Hypotension

Dopamine infusion, colloids, epinephrine, etc.

Free Radicals

It is proposed that frequency and severity of multiorgan-failure (MOF) in FHF involves damage by free radicals. It is often caused by the presence of circulating iron and copper ions. Hence, the role of antioxidant therapy for beneficial effect.

III. MEASURES DIRECTED AT HEPATIC DYSFUNCTION

The fact remains that no known therapy is capable of reversing the hepatocyte injury or promoting hepatic regeneration. Management aimed at preventing and treating complications is essential until the liver function recovers or transplantations can be performed.

Reduction in Production and Absorption of Ammonia

- *Restriction of Dietary Protein*: Restricting the intake of dietary protein inhibits urease-producing colonic bacteria and intestinal production of ammonia. A minimal intake of 0.8 to 1.0 g per kg to maintain nitrogen balance is, however, in order. It is believed that the preferred source of protein should be vegetables.

- *Use of Nonabsorbable Disaccharides*: Non-absorbable disaccharides such as lactulose and lactitol are helpful in removing the dietary and endogenous ammoniagenic substances from the gut. The daily dose of lactulose, 1mg/kg/dose 6 hourly. This regimen results in two to four soft, acidic, stools daily. In addition to the cathartic effect, lactulose brings down the colonic pH as a result of production of organic acids by bacterial fermentation. Lowered pH antagonises the survival of urease-producing intestinal bacteria and may promote the growth of non-urease-producing lactobacilli. Thirdly, acidification of the colonic secretions also results in the net movement of ammonia from the blood into the bowel lumen.
  In case oral or nasogastric administration is not feasible, enemas containing lactulose or other carbohydrates may be employed.
- *Sterilization of the Gut:* Antibiotics with activity against urease-producing bacteria, such as neomycin, metronidazole, gentamicin or ampicillin also reduce the production of intestinal ammonia and have proved of value.
  Ours as also other workers experience spread over the recent past demonstrates that a combination therapy with neomycin and lactulose provides gratifying results. Understandably, administered together, lactulose and neomycin are likely to exert an additive effect in reducing the intestinal production of ammonia, eventually resulting in an enhanced clinical response in most of the subjects. *Lactobacillus acidophilus* alone has only limited beneficial effect.
- *Bowel wash:* It is recommended employing 5 ml vinegar in 500 ml plain water preferably every 6-8 hourly; else, at least twice a day. Its aim is to produce acidic colonic environments.
- *Helicobacter Pylori Eradication:* There is evidence that ammonia generated in the stomach by urease-producing *H. pylori* contributes to rise in blood ammonia levels, thereby precipitating or aggravating hepatic encephalopathy. Treatment of this infection is, therefore, likely to have beneficial effect.
- *Enhancing Metabolism of Ammonia in the Tissues*: Ornithine aspartate has been shown to have useful therapeutic effects in cirrhosis and mild hepatic encephalopathy. This is understandable since ornithine asparate is known to provide substrates for ammonia detoxification pathways.
- *Zinc Supplementation:* It is now well established that two of the five enzymes responsible for the metabolism of ammonia to urea in the urea cycle are zinc-dependent. Zinc deficiency reportedly precipitates and/or aggravates HC. It is also documented that reversal of encephalopathy may follow the supplementation with oral zinc. According to current recommendations, zinc deficient patients should , therefore, receive zinc supplementation.
- *Reduction of False Neurotransmitters:* Though levodopa and bromocriptine are employed in the treatment of HC, there is no convincing evidence that they have any beneficial effect.
- *Inhibition of c-aminobutyric acid:* It may be achieved following use of benzodiazepines. Until more evidence of its beneficial effect is available, this therapy should be considered controversial.
- *Benzodiazepine antagonists:* Flumazenil is claimed to reverse early hepatic encephalopathy. As a rule, it is safe and well tolerated. Infrequent side-effects include agitation, discomfort, anxiety, tearfulness, sense of coldness and withdrawl seizures.
- *Steroids:* Though frequently used in the past, Corticosteroids must be avoided since their use may in actuality be harmful..
- *Continuous venous-venous: dialysis* is helpful.
- *Artificial hepatic support devices:* These are in the process of development.

The dosage of various drugs/agents employed in hepatic coma is summarized in Table 41.11.[9]

Orthotopic Liver Transplantation[8-10]

Only a few centres in India are in a position to provide facility for the liver transplantation which should be considered life-saving in patients in advanced stage of hepatic coma. Now a live donated liver (right or left lobe) by a close relative is used rather than the whole liver from a cadaver. Reduced size allografts have been an important advances in the field. The patient's life-span becomes normal though he has to continue immunosuppressant medication throughout life.

In north India, Apollo Hospital, New Delhi, is doing commendable job in this behalf.

The approximate cost of live donor liver transplant in India is Rs. 2 million. Since the procedure is beyond the reach of most families and since 20 to 25% children with HE may recover with aggressive conservative medical measures alone, highly selective and sensitive criteria need to be applied for subjecting a patient to OLT (Table 41.12).

OLT may be accompanied by certain complications as given in Table 41.13.[10,12,16]

As a rule, outcome of survivors following OLT is gratifying with resumption of normal growth and normal

Table 41.11: Pharmacotherapy of HE

Drug/agent	*Dosage*	*Special Comments*
Mannitol	0.25-1.0 g/kg/dose as 15-25% soln over 30-60 min	Serum osmolality 300-310 mOsmol/L
Dextrose	10% drip throughout IV line period	Used as N/5 salie 10% D
Lactulose	Infants 2.5-10.0 mL/24 hrs, div 6-8 hrs orally Children 40-90 mL/24 hrs, div 6-8 hrs orally	Adjust dose 2-3 stools/day may be given as enema
Neomycin	50-100 mg/kg/24 hrs div, 6-8h	Monitor renal function
Bowel wash	5 ml vinegar in 500 ml plain water, every 6-8 hrs	Nil
Vitamin K	Infants 1 mg; Children 2-3 mg; adolescents 5-10 mg	I.V.
Fresh frozen plasma	10-15 mL/kg	For coagulopathy
Cryoprecipitate	4-5 bags/10 kg	For coagulopathy
Ranitidine	1-3 mg/kg 24 hrs, div 6-12 hrs i.v.; 2-6 mg/kg 24 hrs, 8-12 hrs, po	Also as 24 hours infusion
Sod bicabonate	mEq $NaHCO_3$= 0.3 × wt. (kg) × (12-serum $NaHCO_3$ mEq/L)	Diluted, give slowly
Calcium gluconate	1-2 mL/kg/dose IV	Under cardiac monitoring
Phenytoin	15-18 mg/kg loading then 5 mg/kg/day	8-12 hourly
Phenobarbitone	15-18 mg/kg loading then 5-8 mg/kg/day	12-24 hourly
Ampicillin	100-200 mg/kg 24 hrs po/IV	Every 6 hourly
Cloxacillin	50-100 mg/kg/day IV	Every 6-8 hourly
Cefotaxim	100-200 mg/kg/day IV	6-8 hourly
Ceftriaxone	75-100 mg/kg/day	12 hourly
Ceftazidime	100-150 mg/kg/day	8 hourly
Cefpodoxime	10 mg/kg/day po	12 hourly
Amikacin	15-25 mg/kg/day	12 hourly
Metronidazole	30 mg/kg/day po/IV	6 hourly
Antacids	15-30 mL	4 hourly after gastric lavage

Table 41.12: Criteria for subjecting a patient to OLT

Prothrombin time > 100 seconds or
Any 3 of these:
Age < 10 years
Drug induced or non-A non-B hepatitis
Encephalopathy after 7 days of jaundice
Serum bilirubin > 17.5 mg/dL
Prothrombin time > 50 seconds
Hypoalbuminemia

Table 41.13: Complications of ORT[10,12,16]

Very Early
Fluid and electrolyte balance, renal dysfunction, hypertension, thrombosis of graft vessels
Early
Bacterial infections, viral infection, fungal infection, parasitic infection; organ rejection
Late
Rejection, immunosuppressants-induced renal dysfunction, lymphoproliferative disease which may show progression to lymphoma

life. Occasionally, when chimersism exists between the host and the graft cells, it may become possible to withdraw immunosuppressive therapy. Experience with psychosocial issues in relation to OLT is yet limited.

PROGNOSIS AND PROGNOSTIC FACTORS[4,9,13-15]

Mortality without transplantation is around 75-80%. Following transplantations, it falls to 15-40%. Survivors without orthotopic liver transplantation run only very small risk of developing residual fibrosis, chronic liver disease or cirrhosis.

Factors that signify poor prognosis include:

- Stage IV coma
- non-A, non-B, non-C hepatitis: A frequent complication is bone marrow aplasia that may prove fatal
- Acute onset of Wilson's disease
- Major complications like septicemia, gastrointestinal and other bleeding, acute renal failure, ascites, etc.
- Prolonged prothrombin time over 50 sec
- Serum bilirubin over 17.5 mg/dl (300 mcmol/l)
- Jaundice for more than 7 days prior to onset of hepatic coma
- Hepatic necrosis
- Multiorgan failure

Factors that signify a favorable prognosis include:

- Presence of nests of liver cells amounting to more than 25% of the total cells in the liver biopsy
- Rising levels of serum a-1-fetoprotein
- HC following paracetamol overdose, HAV or HBV infection.

Hepatic coma carries grave prognosis without timely treatment, especially orthotic liver transplantation (OLT). Medical supportive therapy alone carries a high mortality rate. Its primary aim is to prepare the patient for liver transplantation which has revolutionized its outcome. Yet, when it is not feasible to go in for liver transplantation, the benefit of the energetic medical treatment must never be withheld. Undoubtedly, a proportion of subjects do respond to it.

Quality of life in a vast majority of the survivors following intensive medical care and/or liver transplantation is fair enough.[17,18] More studies are warranted on long-term survival and functional outcome. There is also need to determine the psychosocial issues related to liver transplantation.

REFERENCES

1. Douglas A, White AE. Fulminant hepatitis and hepatic encephalopathy. *Hepat Dis* 2004;3:32-39.
2. World Health Organization. *Liver Disease in the Developing World.* Geneva: WHO 1999.
3. Gupte S, Anderson RA. Pediatric hepatology. In: Gupte S (ed) *The Short Textbook of Pediatrics*, 10th (millennium) edn. New Delhi: Jaypee Brothers 2004; 387-410.
4. Gupte S. The Child with coma. In: Gardner WE (ed) *Tropical Health & Disease*. Johannesburg: Afr Scientific Publ 1999;234-239.
5. Gupte S. Coma. In: Gupte S (ed) *Differential Diagnosis in Pediatrics*, 4th edn. New Delhi: Jaypee Brothers 2002.
6. Sokal RJ, Narkewicz MR. Liver and pancreas. In: Hay WW Jr, Hayward AR, Levin MJ, Sondheimer JM (eds) *Current Pediatric Diagnosis and Treatment*, 16th edn. New York: Langel McGraw-Hill 2003;647-692.
7. Singer AL. Role of plasmapheresis in the management of acute hepatic failure in children. *Ann Surg* 2001;234:418-421.
8. Riordan SM, William R. Treatment of hepatic encephalopathy. *N Engl J Med* 1997;337:473-477.
9. Gupte S, Abrams R. Hepatic coma. In: Gupte S (ed) *Recent Advances in Pediatrics (Special Vol 14: Criticare Pediatrics).* New Delhi: Jaypee Brothers 2004;530-546.
10. Durand P, Debray D, Mandel R, Baujard C, Branchereau S, Gauthier F, Jacquemin E, Devictor D. Acute liver failure in infancy: A-14-year experience of a pediatric liver transplantation center. *J Pediatr* 2001;139:871-876.
11. Strauss GI, Hogh P, Moller K, et al. Regional cerebral blood flow during mechanical hyperventilation in patients with FHF. *Hepatology* 1999;30:1368-1373.
12. Riordan SM, Williams R. Treatment of hepatic encephalopathy. *N Engl J Med* 1997;337:473-479.
13. Srivastava KL, Mittal A, Kumar A, Gupta S, et al. Predictors of outcome in FHF in children. *Indian J Gastroenterol* 1998;17:43-45.
14. Suchy FJ. Fulminant hepatic failure. In: Behrman RE, Kliegman RM, Jenson HB (eds) *Nelson Textbook of Pediatrics*, 16th edn Philadelphia: WB Saunders 2000;1220-1222.
15. Sharda B: Acute hepatic failure and hepatic encephalopathy. In: Gupte S (ed) *Recent Advances in Pediatrics*, vol 13. New Delhi: Jaypee Brothers 2003.
16. Cox KL: Liver transplantation. In: Behrman RE, Kliegman RM, Jenson HB (eds) *Nelson Textbook of Pediatrics*, 16th edn. Philadelphia: WB Saunders 2000;1227-1228.
17. Woodworth ES, Robin E. Revisiting liver transplantation in hepatic encephalopathy. *Eur Bull Transplant* 2004;7:76-81.
18. Nelson A. Liver transplantation and ethical issues. *Eur Bull Transplant* 2004;3:123-124.

Suraj Gupte

42 Acute Severe Protein-Energy Malnutrition

INTRODUCTION

Acute severe protein-energy malnutrition (ASPEM), both primary and secondary, is still an important cause of mortality in India and other less developed countries.[1-5] Notably, it seldom exists in its pure form.[6] On the other hand, a multitude of conditions, particularly concomittant infections are, by and large, a rule. According to the World Health Organization,[5] no other condition qualifies for as holistic an approach as this state. The mortality rate in well-treated children with ASPEM is 8-10% compared to 50% in poorly managed children.[7,8]

This chapter deals primarily with management of acute severe PEM which should start off as soon as the child is brought to the hospital. Detailed clinical evaluation and investigations may be carried out simultaneously or later.

MANAGEMENT

Management of ASPEM is arbitrarily divided into three phases as shown in Table 42.1.[7,9]

Phase 1: Resuscitation/Stabilizing Phase (Admission to 24-48 hours)

During the first 6-24 hours, attempts are concentrated at stabilizing the acutely sick child through rehydration, thermoregulation, treatment of shock and treatment of severe anemia.

Rehydration

Immediately on hospitalization, IV line must be started. A caution needs to be exercised in assessing dehydration in the presence of edema since the former is most likely to be erroneously missed or underdiagnosed because of water-logging. In the presence of wasting, it is inclined to be overestimated.

Table 42.1: Three phases of management of acute severe PEM

Phase 1:	Resuscitation/stabilizing phase, extending from admission to 24-48 hours
Phase 2:	Acute phase, extending from stabilization to 7th day
Phase 3:	Rehabilitation phase, after 7th day

Most useful and dependable criteria for assessing dehydration in acute severe malnutrition include:

- Dryness of buccal mucosa
- Oliguria/anuria
- Acidotic respiration, absence of tears
- Shock (peripheral circulatory failure).

For initial correction of dehydration, only 75% of calculated fluid and sodium requirements need be administered. IV fluid employed for this purpose should be hypotonic rather than hypertonic in view of the diminished water and sodium excretion capacity of the kidneys.

Thermoregulation

Hypothermia is a known killer of malnourished children. It may well be secondary to starvation, infection or hypoglycemia and, not infrequently, all these factors working in nexus. It should, therefore, be mandatory to keep the child in a warm environment covered with a blanket in order to combat hypothermia.

Treatment of Shock

World Health Organization guidelines for treatment of shock in acute severe malnutrition are as follows:

- Infuse IV fluids at 15 ml/kg over 1 hour. Use half normal saline with 5% dextrose or Ringer's lactate with 5% dextrose or, if unavailable, Ringer's lactate alone. Reasses after this.

  If child in shock is severely dehydrated, there should be improvement with IV treatment, manifested by fall in respiratory and pulse rates. In such a case:
- Repeat IV fluids 15 ml/kg over 1 hour once more and then switch to oral or nasogastric rehydration up to 10 hours (leave IV line in place in case required again). Then, initiate refeeding.

If the subject fails to improve after 15 ml/kg/hour fluids, assume that he has septic shock. In this case:

- Maintenance IV fluids (4 ml/kg/hour) while waiting for blood. When blood is available, transfuse fresh whole blood at 10 ml/kg slowly over 3 hour. Then, initiate refeeding.

Treatment of Severe Anemia

According to the World Health Organization, for blood transfusion in severe anemia is indicated:

- When hemoglobin is < 4 g/dL.
- Respiratory distress with hemoglobin between 4–6 g/dL.

The WHO guidelines are as follows:

Administer whole blood 10 ml/kg slowly over 3 hours with frusemide 1 mg/kg IV at the start of transfusion. It is important that volume of 10 ml/kg is not exceeded. If the severely anemic child has signs of congestive cardiac failure (CCF), transfuse packed cells rather than whole blood.

Monitor for signs of transfusion reactions, namely fever, itchy rash, dark red urine, confusion and shock. In the presence of any of these signs, discontinue transfusion without loss of time.

While monitoring the respiratory rate and pulse rate every 15 minutes, if there is rise in any one, cut down the transfusion rate.

If, despite blood transfusion, hemoglobin remained under 4 g/dL with continuing respiratory distress, do not jump at repeating the transfusion.

Phase 2: Acute Phase (Second Day–7th Days)

Following stabilization of child's condition and his acceptance of oral feed in the stabilizing/resuscitation phase, nutritional rehabilitation should be initiated, preferably employing milk feeds.

Nutritional rehabilitation is given by providing high protein and high energy diet. To begin with, a daily intake of 100 Kcal/kg/day of expected weight or 150–200 Kcal /kg/day of actual weight and 3 g /kg of protein calculated with reference to the actual weight should be the goal in the very first week. At least 10% of total calories should come from proteins of high biological value. This is important for the catch-up growth.

Local resources should always be borne in mind while making a choice of the foodstuffs. It is advisable to feed small amounts of food at frequent intervals.

At times, it may become necessary to initiate nutritional therapy through Ryle's tube.

Phase 3: Rehabilitation Phase (After First Week)

Following the acute phase, the child usually accepts more and more food.[10-13] This, in fact, should be encouraged.

One factor that may become a bottleneck in initial management is lactose intolerance, In such a situation, it is advisable to use one of the lactose-free milks, soyabean milk or a vegetable-protein mixture. Subjects fed on soya-based preparations are better supplemented with zinc, 1mg/kg/day. Since zinc deficiency may accompany PEM otherwise too, such a supplementation is strongly recommended. In our and others' experience, zinc-supplemented malnourished children undergo faster disappearance in their dermatosis. In view of the fact that zinc supplementation may cause fall in plasma copper level, enough copper intake through diet should be ensured.

In our experience, highly concentrated milk with mashed banana and/or cereal syrup makes an excellent alternative to lactose-free preparations which are either expensive or poorly tolerated, often inducing vomiting. Such a mixture should contain 25 % milk and 75% banana and/or cereals. Addition of sugar and vegetable oil (high-energy milk formula) further improves its taste and nutritional value.

Administration of oral potassium, 5 mEq/kg/day (1 g-14 mEq) as potassium chloride solution is advisable.

In addition, it is of value to give magnesium sulfate, 0.5–1.5 ml/day (0.3 ml/kg/day with maximum of 2 ml) IM in 2 divided doses during the first one week or two. Thereafter, magnesium supplements should come from natural sources such as milk, groundnut, peas and grains.

Associated conditions need to be handled for optimal results following initiation of nutritional rehabilitation.[13-16]

Bleeding diathesis is an indication for vitamin K (IM) and/or platelet transfusion.

Dehydration and dyselectrolytemia complicating gross PEM needs correction at the very outset.

Superadded infection or infestation, if present or strongly suspected, should be treated with appropriate chemotherapy.

Factors contributing to poor response to treatment are listed in Table 42.3.

Administration of iron should be avoided in the first and the second phase and should instead be in the third phase for the following reasons:

- Free iron in the early phase may exacerbate oxidant damage, thereby precipitating development of edema in nutritional marasmus and thus leading to change over to kwashiorkor or marasmic kwashiorkor from the original nonedematous malnutrition.
- It is desirable to prevent binding of iron in already limited stores of transferrin. The transferrin may interfere with protein's host defense mechanisms.

TIME-TABLE OF FAVORABLE DEVELOPMENTS DURING NUTRITIONAL REHABILITATION

These are listed in Table 42.4. In addition, the child may develop certain unfavorable phenomena during nutritional rehabilitation, including the so-called "nutrition recovery syndrome."[17,18]

Table 42.2: Treatment of other conditions associated with acute severe PEM

Vitamin A Deficiency

In view of accompanying photophobia, it is important to examine the eyes essentially through though very gently.

- In case of any sign of vitamin A deficiency, administer vitamin A on day 1, 2 and 14 (200,000 IU for > 12 months age, 100,000 IU for 6-12 months age and 50,000 IU for < 6 months age).
- In case of inflammation or ulceration, instill antibiotic eye (gentamicin) drops for 7–10 days plus atropine eye drops thrice daily for 3-5 days and cover with a saline-soaked eye pad and bandage.

Skin Lesions

Dermatosis of malnutrition may be in the form of hypopigmentation or hyperpigmentation, desquamation, ulceration over limbs, thighs, genitalia, groin and behind ears.

- Give zinc supplementation, 1 mg/kg/day (O).
- Bathe or soak affected areas of skin for 10 minutes/day in 1% potassium permanganate solution.
- Apply a barrier cream (petroleum jelly or a zinc and castor oil ointment) to the raw areas.
- Avoid using a diaper to allow drying of the perineum.

Intestinal Parasites

Presence of one or the other intestinal parasitic infestation is, by and large, universal in malnourished children.

- In case of proved or highly suspected protozoa (*L. Giardia, E histolytica*), administer metronidazole or an alternative drug such as furazolidine, tinidazole, ornidazole or secnidazole.
- In case of a helminth (A Lumbricoides, A duodenale), administer albendazole or mebendazole.

Continuing Severe Diarrhea

If significant diarrhea interferes with the weight gain or feeding, consider lactose intolerance, osmotic diarrhea or superimposed giardiasis/ amebiasis.

- Carry out a meticulous examination of stools. Treat giardiasis/amebiasis, a common cause of protracted diarrhea.
- Suspect osmolar diarrhea in case diarrhea worsens with hyperosmolar load (say hyperosmolar starter F-75) and improve with reduction in sugar content of intake.
- Lactose intolerance needs treatment only when it is interfering with improvement. It usually responds to a low lactose feed. Only occasionally, elimination of lactose from diet is indicated.

Tuberculosis

History of a contact, poor growth in spite of a good intake, chronic cough and pneumonia not responding to adequate antibiotic therapy are indications for excluding tuberculosis. In fact, it is a sound policy in endemic areas to rule out tuberculosis in each and every case of significant malnutrition.

- Carry out sutable investigations (Mantoux test or BCG diagnostic test, X-ray chest) and treat with ATT if diagnosis gets confirmed.

Table 42.3: Factors responsible for unsatisfactory response to treatment in acute severe PEM

Factor	*Recommended action*
As a Group High mortality rate	*Within 24 hours*: Consider untreated or delayed hypoglycemia, hypothermia, septicemia, severe anemia, incorrect rehydration fluid or volume. *Within 72 hours:* Check whether refeeding with too high a volume/feed or wrong formula *At night:* Consider hypothermia from insufficient covers or missing night feeds. Transition to catchup formulation: Consider a sudden or far too rapid a change/transition.
As an individual inadequate feeding	Find out answers to the following questions: Does the child indeed receive the night feeds? Are the target energy and protein intakes achieved? Is the child fed frequently and offered unlimited amounts? Is the nursing staff caring, motivated, loving and patient? Is feed preparation correct? Is the child being given a catchup formulation? Ensure that it is modified.
Specific nutrient deficiencies	Adequacy of multivitamin composition, shelf-life. Preparation of electrolyte/mineral solution and whether correctly prescribed and administered.
Untreated infection(s)	For such hidden infections as UTI, AOM, giardiasis and tuberculosis • Re-examine carefully. • Repeat urine microscopy for pus cells. • Examine stool repeatedly • Take chest X-ray
HIV/AIDS	Tst for lactose intolerance and manage it on usual lines.
Psychological problems	Abnormal behavior e.g. rocking and other stereotyped movements, rumination and attention seeking; treatment is social love and attention. In case of rumination, firmness but without intimidation works

Table 42.4: Positive developments during nutritional rehabilitation

• Resumption of alertness as shown by a smile and interaction with the mother
• Initiation of gain in weight
• Regression of water-logging (edema) which usually disappears by 7-10th posttherapy day
• Disappearance of enteropathy and hepatomegaly
• Elevation in serum protein
• Attainment of normal weight for height in 1 to 3 months means "clinical recovery"

NUTRITION AND HEALTH EDUCATION DURING HOSPITAL STAY

The hospital stay needs to be utilized to educate the parents (mother, in particular) about the value of high protein and high calorie diet of the family type so that it becomes easy to achieve consolidation of cure at home.

At the same time, it is important to pay attention to child's immunization.

DISCHARGE CRITERIA

The best time to discharge the child is when he has gained weight that is in keeping with his actual height (not age). That usually takes on an average about 6-8 weeks. But, then retaining the child so long is, as a rule, not workable on account of the increasing pressure on hospital beds. An acceptable way out is to discharge the child when he has achieved a weight that is 85% of the weight for height. This usually happens in 2 to 4 weeks time.

NUTRITIONAL REHABILITATION AT HOME

For complete recovery, another 2-4 months nutritional rehabilitation at home may be needed.

FOLLOW-UP

Each follow-up visit should be utilized to record child's weight, for immunization, and for reinforcement of nutrition and health education.

PROGNOSIS

A number of factors point to bad prognosis (Table 42.5).[5,7-11]

Table 42.6 gives frequent causes of death in ASPEM.[12-18]

Table 42.5: Bad prognostic signs in acute severe PEM

• Severe dehydration, especially when accompanied by electrolyte and acid-base disturbances
• Hypoglycemia
• Hypothermia
• Fulminant infection
• Congestive cardiac failure
• Xerophthalmia
• Bleeding diathesis
• Grossly enlarged liver with deranged LFT
• Seizures
• Change in sensorium
• Cachexia
• Severe dermatosis

Table 42.6: Causes of death in acute severe malnutrition

• Severe dehydration and dyselectrolytemia
• Fulminant infections
• Hypothermia
• Hypoglycemia
• Severe anemia with CCF
Note: In a significant proortion of cases, more than one cause may well be contributing to mortality.

REFERENCES

1. Austin E. Management of severe undernutrition. *Hospital Rev* 2002;21:231-236.
2. Raju U. Nutritional management of the hospitalized ill child. In: Gupte S (ed) *Recent Advances in Pediatrics,* Vol 13. New Delhi: Jaypee Brothers 2004;51-62.
3. Elizabeth KE, George Jacob R. Nutritional support in the critically ill child. In: Gupte S (ed) *Recent Advances in Pediatrics (Special Vol 14: Criticare Pediatrics)*. New Delhi: Jaypee Brothers 2004;546-565.
4. Ashworth A. Treatment of severe malnutrition. *J Pediatr Gastroenterol Nutr* 2001;32:519-520.
5. World Health Organization. *Management of Severe Malnutrition: A Manual for Physicians and Other Senior Health Workers.* Geneva: WHO 1999.
6. Gupte S: Issues and controversies in rehabilitation of severely malnourished infants and children. *Hospital Rev* 2002;21: 112-115.
7. Gupte S. Acute severe protein-energy malnutrition (PEM). In: Gupte S (ed) *Recent Advances in Pediatrics (Special Vol 8: Emergency Pediatrics).* New Delhi: Jaypee 2001;172-179.
8. Gupte S, Gomez EM. Pediatric nutrition and nutritional deficiency states. In: Gupte S (ed) *The Short Textbook of Pediatrics.* 10th edn. New Delhi: Jaypee 2004;125-166.
9. World Health Organization: WHO Guidelines for inpatient treatment of severely malnourished children. *http:www.ishtm.ac.uk/eps/malnu,pdf*
10. Ghosh S. Current nutrition scenario. In: Gupte S (ed) *Recent Advances in Pediatrics (Special Vol 1: Nutrition, Growth and Development).* New Delhi: Jaypee 1997;1-14.
11. Gupte S. Chronic diarrhea and marasmus. *Lancet* 1970;20:725.
12. Gupte S, Padha V. Pitfalls in the treatment of advanced protein-energy malnutrition in a premier medical institute. *Int J Med Ped Pract* 1971;6:231-236.
13. Gupte S. Nutritional deficiency states in pediatric practice. *Quart Med Rev* 1983;34:1-45.
14. Gupte S. Nutritional rehabilitation. *Indian J Pediatr* 1983;50: 97-98.
15. Inamdar S. Changing trends in nutritional disorders. In: Gupte S (ed) *Recent Advances in Pediatrics.* New Delhi: Jaypee 1994;9: 34-47.
16. Mathur GP, Kushwaha KP, Mathur S. Protein-energy malnutrition (PEM) updated. In; Gupte S (ed) *Recent Advances in Pediatrics (Special Vol 6: Gastroenterology, Hepatology and Nutrition).* New Delhi: Jaypee 2000;479-506.
17. Gupte S. Nutrition recovery syndrome. *N Engl J Med* 1972; 291:501.
18. Gomez EM, Gupte S. Nutrition recovery syndrome: An obituary. *Bull Nutr Def* 2003;13:13-19.

Emergencies Related to Gastroenterology, Hepatology and Nutrition

43

Ajay Gaur

Management of Life-Threatening Complications in Severe Malnutrition

INTRODUCTION

Malnutrition remains one of the most common causes of morbidity and mortality among children throughout the world. Approximately 9% of children below 5 years of age suffer from wasting and are at risk of death or severe impairment of growth and psychological development.[1] Case fatality rates in these subjects have remained static at 20-30 percent over the past fifty years. According to the World Health Organization (WHO), a mortality of >20 percent in severely malnourished children is considered unacceptable: 11-20 percent is poor; 5-10 percent is moderate; 1-4 percent is good and < 1 percent is excellent.[2] Although the key to rapid recovery lies in the provision of an adequate nutrient intake, the reduction of mortality rates largely depend on the management of complications.[3] Thus, management of the child with severe malnutrition is divided into three phases. In the *Initial treatment life*-threatening problems are identified and treated in a hospital, specific deficiencies are corrected, metabolic abnormalities are reversed and feeding is begun. The second phase of *rehabilitation* intensive feeding is given to recover most of the lost weight, emotional and physical stimulation are increased, the mother or carer is trained to continue care at home, and preparations are made for discharge of the child. The last phase of *follow-up* after discharge, the child and the child's family are followed to prevent relapse and assure the continued physical, mental and emotional development of the child. A typical time-frame for the management of a child with severe malnutrition is shown in Table 43.1.[2,4]

Table 43.1: Time-frame for the management of severe malnutrition

Activity	*Initial treatment*		*Rehabilitation*
	Days 1–2	*Days 3–7*	*Weeks 2–6*
Treat or prevent:			
Hypoglycemia	→		
Hypothermia	→		
Dehydration	→		
Correct electrolyte imbalance	→	→	→
Treat infection	→	→	
Correct micronutrient deficiencies	Without iron	With iron →	→
Begin feeding	→	→	
Catch-up growth			→
Emotional and sensory stimulation	→	→	→
Prepare for discharge		→	→

Successful management of the severely malnourished child requires that each child be treated with proper care and affection, and that each phase of treatment be carried out as per the protocols. This chapter offers practical guidelines for emergency management of severely malnourished children, particularly on the basis of recent consensus guidelines.[2,4,5]

CRITERIA FOR HOSPITALIZATION

In majority of cases with malnutrition, hospitalization is not necessary. However, hospitalization becomes mandatory when these children develop acute complications. Any delay in such cases can result in rapid deterioration and death. Timely referral is, therefore, essential and crucial.

All children with a weight for height less than 70% of NCHS reference and edema should be referred to a tertiary referral center well equipped to handle such cases. Children with a weight for age < 60 percent (but weight for height > 70%) with any of the features listed in Table 43.2 should also be referred to a hospital.[2,4,5]

Table 43.2: Criteria for admission to a hospital

• Signs of circulatory collapse	• Persistent diarrhea (> 14 days)
• Convulsions, unconsciousness	• Bloody mucoid stools
• Cyanosis	• Persistent loss of appetite
• Inability to drink	• Severe vitamin A deficiency
• Chest in drawing	• Jaundice
• Fast breathing (60 breaths/min in <2 mo of age; >50/min in a child 2 months–1 year of age; >40/ min in child 1-5 yrs. old), or wheeze	• Purpura
• Hypothermia or high fever	• Distended tender abdomen
• Severe anemia	• Age less than 1 year

EVALUATION

When first seen, the child must be examined thoroughly, a history taken and a decision made on the treatment to be given. Treatment should be started as soon as these tasks have been completed. Details of the history and examination should be recorded later. A checklist of the important details of the history and physical examination is given in Table 43.3. Very sick children respond badly to frequent handling. They should not be taken away for the investigations initially and should remain in bed while clinical specimens are taken. After assessment of the child a decision should be made about the place and need of the treatment (Fig. 43.1).

Table 43.3: Checklist of history and physical examination

- Detailed feeding history including breastfeeding history
- Recent sinking of eyes
- Duration, frequency and appearance of vomiting or diarrhea
- Time when urine was last passed
- Contact with people with measles or tuberculosis
- Any deaths of siblings
- Birth weight
- Milestones reached (sitting up, standing, etc.)
- Immunization history

Physical examination:

- Weight and length/height
- Edema
- Enlargement or tenderness of liver, jaundice
- Abdominal distension, bowel sounds, ascites
- Severe pallor
- Signs of circulatory collapse and level of consciousness
- Temperature: hypothermia or fever
- Thirst: normal, eager or unable to drink
- Eyes: corneal lesions indicative of vitamin A deficiency
- Ears, mouth, throat: for any evidence of infection
- Skin: evidence of infection, skin changes or purpura
- Respiratory rate, type of respiration and chest indrawing
- Signs of CCF

LABORATORY TESTS

Laboratory investigations may help to diagnose certain specific problems but are not essential to monitor or guide the treatment of the child.[2,4] The interpretation of the results is frequently altered by malnutrition. It is important to remember that careful clinical assessment is the most important guide to treatment. The interpretation and importance of individual tests in severely malnourished subjects is given in Table 43.4.

MANAGEMENT OF LIFE-THREATENING CONDITIONS

All children with severe malnutrition are considered as severely ill at the time of hospitalization. They should be kept in intensive care area where constant monitoring is possible. The room temperature should be kept at 25°C-30°C. The common life-threatening conditions associated with malnutrition are:

a. Hypoglycemia

All severely malnourished children are at the risk of developing low blood sugar, especially with underlying serious systemic infection and infrequent feeding in the recent past. Hypoglycemia is defined as blood glucose of less than 54 mg/dl. Or 3 mmol/l[2]. Attention was directed to the prognostic significance of hypoglycemia in malnourished infants as early as 1932.[6] However; its clinical significance was realized much later.

Signs of hypoglycemia include hypothermia, lethargy, limpness and alterated sensorium. Malnourished children do not exhibit sweating or pallor, the typical features of hypoglycemia in well nourished children. Some time, the only presenting signs before death is drowsiness. Other clinical features include apneic spells and convulsions.

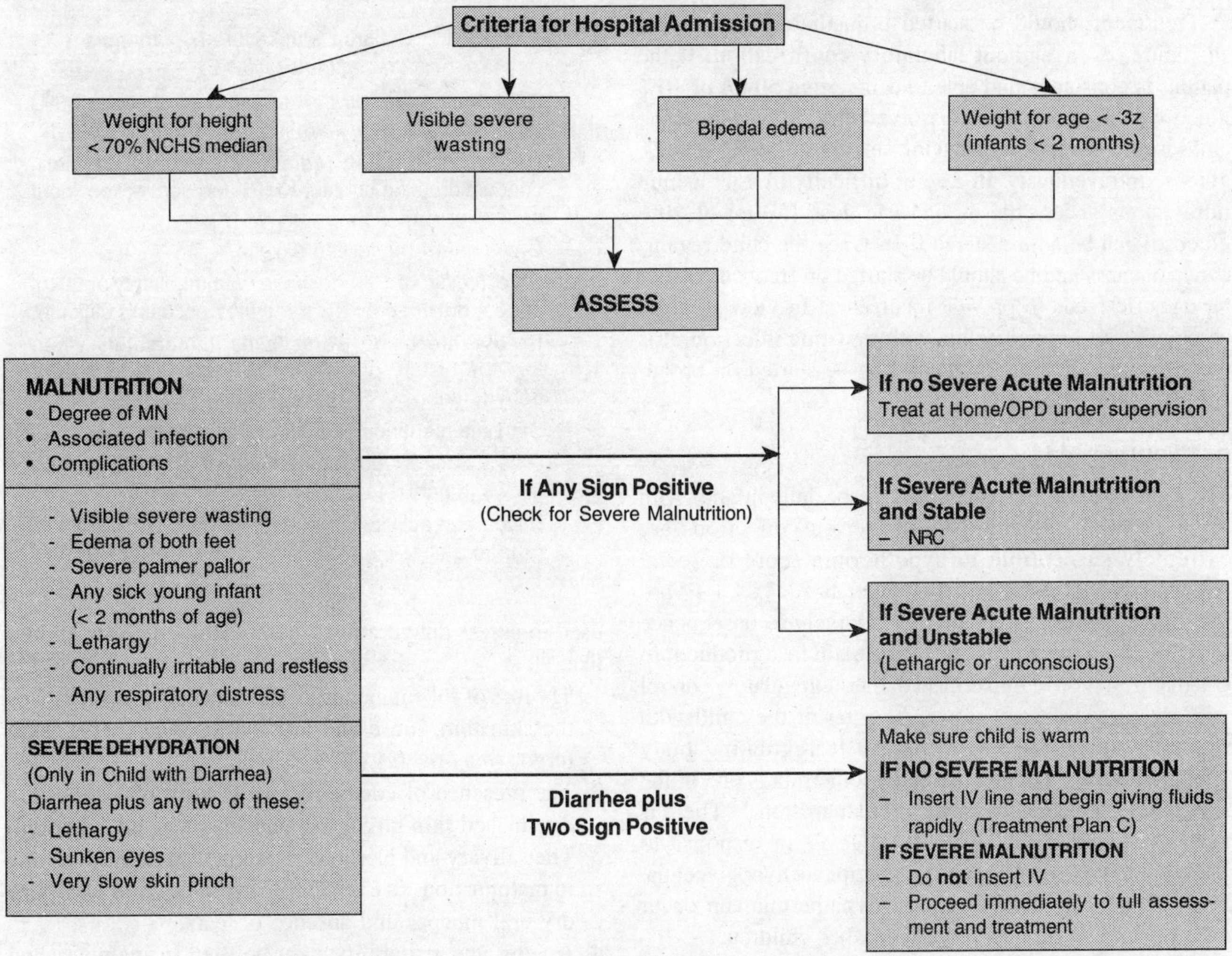

Fig. 43.1: Assessment and decision free for management of severe malnutrition

Table 43.4: Interpretation and importance of laboratory tests

Test	*Interpretation and significance*
Test that may be useful	
Blood glucose	<54 mg/dl indicative of hypoglycemia
Microscopic examination of blood smear	For presence of malarial parasite
Hemoglobin or PCV	Hemoglobin <4 g/dl or PCV <12% indicative of very severe anemia
Examination and culture of urine	Bacteruria or >10 leukocytes/hpf indicative of infection
Microscopic examination of stools	For presence of blood, Giardia cysts or trophozoites
Chest X-ray	1. Pneumonia: Malnourished children show less opacities in the lungs
	2. Vascular engorgement and cardiomegaly may indicate heart failure
	3. X-ray may also show features of rickets
Tuberculin test for tuberculosis	False-negative rates high
Tests that are of little value	
Serum proteins	Only guides the prognosis
Tests for HIV	Should not be done routinely and never without prior counseling
Serum electrolytes	Rarely helpful; may complicate therapy

Treatment should be started immediately on clinical suspicion, even without laboratory confirmation. If the patient is conscious and able to drink, give 50 ml of 10% glucose (or 5 g table sugar dissolved in 50 ml water). If the child is unconscious or is having seizures, 5 ml/kg of 10% glucose intravenously. In case of difficulty in establishing intravenous access the nasogastric dose (50 ml of 10% glucose) can be administered first. Once the child regains consciousness and he should be started on frequent oral or nasogastric feeds to prevent recurrence. In view of close association of hypoglycemia with systemic infection, it is recommended that all such children be started on broad-spectrum antibiotics.[2]

b. Hypothermia

Malnourished children (marasmic), especially infants, with large areas of damaged skin or serious infections are extremely susceptible to hypothermia (core or rectal temperature < 35.5°C; axillary temperature <35°C). Hypothermia in malnourished children is largely a consequence of reduction in the metabolic rate (i.e., in heat production) and manifestation of impairment of thermoregulatory control with decreased energy stores. As a result the child with severe malnutrition has difficulty in regulating body temperature. It is for this reason hypothermia is one of the causes for the cot death in severe malnutrition.[3,7] There is also a reduced ability to produce fever in response to infection.[8] Hypothermia can also precipitate hypoglycemia. It is important to remember that hypothermia can occur even in summer months in malnourished children.

A low reading thermometer should always be used to measure the temperature of malnourished children. Hypothermic children should either be warmed using the 'Kangaroo' technique (placing the child on the mother bare chest or abdomen "skin to skin" and covering both of them) or by clothing the child well including head and covering him with a blanket and placing an incandescent bulb close to the body but sufficiently away to avoid burns. Hot water bottles should be avoided as they are dangerous (can result in thermal injuries). It would be ideal to regulate the room temperature. The rectal temperature should be monitored every half hourly as the child may rapidly become hyperthermic. Children with severe hypothermia (rectal temp. <32°C) should be treated for hypoglycemia and systemic infections apart from marinating the temperature[2] (Chart. 43.1).

Box 43.1: Children with severe hypothermia *(rectal temp. < 32°C)*

- Rapidly re-warm till the temperature reaches 35°C after which slow re-warming should be continued.
- Provide heat using radiation (overhead warmer), conduction (skin contact-KMC) and convection (heat convector).
- Give (warm) humidified oxygen.
- Give 2 ml/kg of 10% dextrose IV immediately or 50 ml of 10% dextrose by NG route (if IV access is difficult).
- Re-hydrate using warm fluids immediately when there is history of diarrhea or there is evidence of dehydration.
- Start maintenance IV fluids (prewarmed).
- Give warmed feeds immediately if clinical condition allows the child to take orally.
- Encourage activity.
- Start IV antibiotics.

c. Diarrhea and Dehydration

Diarrhea with accompanying dehydration and electrolyte disturbances in severely malnourished children has been found to be the one of the worst prognostic indicator.[8] Evaluation of dehydration in a case of malnutrition is extremely difficult as many of the sign that are normally used to assess dehydration are unreliable in such children like:[9,10]

1. The loss of subcutaneous fat and supporting tissue makes the skin thin, loose and less elastic. The use of 'skin turgor' may overestimate dehydration.
2. The presence of edema in kwashiorkor may mask the diminished skin turgor and underestimate dehydration.
3. The salivary and lacrimal glands are severely atrophied in malnutrition, so even a well-hydrated child may have dry oral mucosa and absence of tears.
4. Apathy and irritability may be seen in malnourished children without any dehydration. Hypoglycemia, hypothermia and septic shock also altered consciousness.

Thus, it becomes difficult to detect dehydration reliably and to determine its severity. Furthermore, the clinical picture is confusing if septic shock is associated. Hence, it often becomes necessary to treat children for both. The signs of dehydration that remain reliable in malnourished children and can be used to assess its severity are:

i. History of diarrhea;
ii. Excessive thirst;
iii. Sunken eyes;
iv. Weak or absent peripheral pulses;
v. Cool extremities; and
vi. Decreased urine output.

Clinical signs, which are helpful to distinguish between dehydration and septic shock, are enumerated in Table 43.5.[2]

Treatment of Dehydration

In a dehydrated child with malnutrition, rehydration should be done orally as far as possible. Because of severe malnutrition these children are deficient in potassium and have abnormally high level of sodium though the total body

Table 43.5: Clinical signs of dehydration and septic shock in a malnourished child

Clinical sign	*Some dehydration*	*Severe dehydration*	*Incipient septic shock*	*Developed septic shock*
Watery diarrhea	Yes	Yes	Yes or No	Yes or No
Thirst	Drink eagerly	Drinks poorly	No*	No*
Hypothermia	No	No	Yes* or No*	Yes* or No*
Sunken eyes	Yes	Yes	No	No
Weak or absent radial pulse	No	Yes	Yes	Yes
Cold hands and feet	No	Yes	Yes	Yes
Urine flow	Yes	No	Yes	No
Mental state	Restless or irritable	Lethargic comatose	Apathetic	Lethargic
Hypoglycemia	Sometimes	Sometimes	Sometimes	Sometimes

* Signs that may be useful in diagnosing septic shock.

and cellular sodium may be normal. These children are more prone to develop fluid overload and heart failure. Therefore oral rehydration is performed gradually and intravenous are avoided as far as possible.[11]

In oral rehydration therapy (ORT) in place of standard ORS solution, WHO recommends the use of a special rehydration solution (ReSoMal) for the malnourished children. The composition of this solution is given in Table 43.6. When ReSoMal is not available, low osmolarity WHO-ORS may be employed. It canalso be made from the standard WHO-ORS solution by diluting it in 2 liters of water (instead of 1 liter), adding 50 g of sucrose (25 g/l) and 40 ml of mineral mix. The composition of the mineral mix is given in Table 43.7. Approximately 70 to 100 ml/kg body weight of this solution is given over 12 hours to restore hydration in the following manner:

i. 5 ml/kg every 30 min for the first 2 hours orally or by NG tube; and
ii. 5-10 ml/kg/hour thereafter. The child should be monitored at hourly intervals at least, for sign of under and/or over hydration. ORS should be stopped if:
   - The respiratory and pulse rate increase;
   - The jugular veins become engorged; or
   - There is increasing edema (puffy eyelids).

Table 43.6: Composition of oral rehydration salt solution for severely malnourished children

Component	*Concentration (mmol/l)*
Glucose	125
Sodium	45
Potassium	40
Chloride	70
Magnesium	3
Citrate	7
Zinc	0.3
Copper	0.045
Osmolarity	300

Rehydration is completed when the child is no longer thirsty, urine is passed adequately and other signs of dehydration have disappeared. In order to maintain hydration, as guide children less than two years of age are given 50-100 ml of ReSoMal after each loose stool; older children should be given 100-200 ml for each loose stool till diarrhea stops. Intravenous fluids are indicated only in the presence of severe dehydration or septic shock.

Table 43.7: Composition of mineral mix solution

Substance	*Amount*
Potassium chloride	89.5 g
Tripotassium citrate	32.4 g
Magnesium chloride	30.5 g
Zinc acetate	3.3 g
Copper sulfate	0.56 g
Sodium selenate	10 g
Potassium iodide	5 g
Water	1000 ml

The fluids used, in order of preference are:

i. Half strength Darrow's solution with 5% dextrose;
ii. Ringer's lactate solution with 5% dextrose;
iii. Half normal saline (0.45%) with 5% dextrose. The fluid is administered in the following manner[2,4] (Fig. 43.2): (i) 15 ml/kg is to be given over one hour, closely monitor for any signs of over hydration; (ii) Start ReSoMal simultaneously through NG tube at the rate of 10 ml/kg/hour; (iii) assess again after one hour and repeat the intravenous fluids in case of no improvement; (iv) Switch to ReSoMal (10 ml/kg/hour) for the next 10 hours; and (v) If the child fails to improve despite intravenous fluid therapy treat the child on the guidelines of septic shock (Fig. 43.3). As diarrhea in malnourished children is often multifactorial and may be complicated by mucosal malnutrition, early administration of oral fluids and feeds in such cases is beneficial.[12]

d. Septic Shock

Dehydration and septic shock are difficult to differentiate in children with severe malnutrition, as signs of hypovolemia

 # Ringers' Lactate at 15 ml/kg/hour for the first hour

Continue monitoring during the infusion.
Measure pulse, respiratory rates, capillary refill time
(at the beginning and then every 5-10 minutes)

Assess after 1 hour

If no improvement
(No change in pulse rate or capillary refill)
Or
Worsening
(Increase in pulse rate, slower capillary refill)

Consider septic shock
And treat accordingly

If improvement
(Pulse rate decreases/faster capillary refill/increase in blood pressure)

Consider severe dehydration with shock
Repeat Ringers' Lactate 15 ml/kg over 1 hour

Clinically better/no evidence of shock
Give IV fluids 10ml/kg/hour for next 8 hours and Substitute ORS for IV fluids when accepts child orally (Usually within 4-6 hours)

 # Add potassium to the IV fluids at the rate of 1.5 ml per 100 ml after the patient passes urine.

Fig. 43.2: Fluid management for severe dehydration

Septic shock

10 ml/kg bolus over 20-30 min with monitoring of vitals
Humidified oxygen
Packed RBC's 10 ml/kg over 4-6 hours if Hb < 10 g/dl or active bleeding

Improvement

Fluid responsive shock

Observe and continue maintenance fluids 2-4 ml/kg/hours.
Inj. Mag sulphate (50%) 2 ml.

No improvement

Repeat 10 ml/kg bolus over 20-30 min
(Upto 2 boluses)

No improvement

Fluid refractory shock

Start dopamine @10 µg/kg/min
Consider adding dobutamine @10 µg/kg/min
Check blood glucose.

Features of fluid overload

- Stop bolus
- Start dopamine
  @ 10 µg/kg/min dobutamine
  @ 10 µg/kg/min

Fig. 43.3: Treatment of septic shock

are present in both and progressively worsen if treatment is not given. Many cases of sepsis also have a history of diarrhea and dehydration, adding to the diagnostic dilemma. The comparison of clinical signs of dehydration and septic shock in the severely malnourished children are summarizing in Table 43.5. The important signs that help in establishing a diagnosis of septic shock are:[2] (i) Hypothermia; (ii) Incipient septic shock: The child is limp, apathetic, and anorexic without any thirst or restlessness; (iii) Developed septic shock: Superficial veins such as external jugular and scalp veins are dilated, rather than constricted; (iv) The child may groan, grunt or have difficult breathing; as veins in the lungs become engorged making lungs stiffer than normal; (v) Coffee ground vomitus, blood in stools and abdominal distension indicate worsening of shock and a grave prognosis.[2]

Treatment

All children with incipient or developed septic shock should be immediately started on broad-spectrum antibiotics. Hypothermia and hypoglycemia must be urgently managed as per standards protocol. Children with incipient shock are started on early nasogastric feeds. The algorithmic approach for developed septic shock is:[4,13] (Fig. 43.3)

1. Start intravenous rehydration immediately, using fluids mentioned for correction of dehydration. Fluids are given at 10 ml/kg/hour, with extreme care to avoid over hydration and congestive heart failure. As soon as peripheral circulation improves switch to oral rehydration.
2. If the child does not improve after one hour of therapy or develops features of congestive cardiac failure give a blood transfusion (10 ml/kg over 4-6 hours). Other fluids should be avoided during blood transfusions. If blood is not available plasma can be used.
3. If the child does not tolerate nasogastric feeds after completing transfusion (i.e., vomits or develops abdominal distension) intravenous infusion is continued at a rate of 2-4 ml/kg/hour. Such children should also receive 2 ml of 50% magnesium sulphate intramuscularly.
4. Add dopamine and dobutamine, at the rate of 10 ug/kg/min, if septic shock does not respond to intravenous fluids and child is unable to maintain normal blood pressure on fluid therapy alone. If hypotension remains refractory to this therapy as well, intravenous infusion of epinephrine or nor epinephrine, with or without sodium nitroprusside for reduction of after load, is indicated.
5. If there are signs of liver cell failure, such as tender hepatomegaly, jaundice, purpura, administer 1mg of Vitamin K intramuscularly.
6. At this stage iron supplements, steroids, epinephrine or nikethamide should not be used.

e. Metabolic Acidosis

Acidosis usually accompanies dehydration, and appropriate rehydration usually corrects the acidosis as well. In children with persistent clinical features of acidosis (i.e., rapid and deep breathing even after adequate rehydration, injection sodium bicarbonate (8.4%, 1 ml/kg) may be infused slowly.[14]

f. Hypokalemia

Malnourished children have severely depleted body stores of potassium, even though it may not manifest in the laboratory values. All hospitalized malnourished children should receive oral potassium supplement in a dose of 4 mmol/kg for a period of 5 days. If a child is requiring intravenous fluids or a very high purge rate that cannot be managed by ORS then potassium is to be added to the intravenous fluids in the following manner: (i) serum potassium< 2 mmol/L, add 40/mmol/L of KCl; and (ii) serum potassium is between 2 and 2.5 mmol/L , add 30 mmol/L of KCL.[15,16]

g. Infection

Bacterial infections are common in severely malnourished children, particularly pneumonia, diarrhea, skin and soft tissue and urinary tract infection. While majority of infections are bacterial, viral exanthematous infections like measles and chickenpox can be fatal. Signs of infection in these children are usually absent because of poor inflammatory response.[9,17] A high index of suspicion is therefore, required for early diagnosis. Early and effective treatment of bacterial infections helps in significant reduction in mortality otherwise child may develop septic shock. WHO recommends administration of broad-spectrum antimicrobials to all hospitalized malnourished children.[2,4] Choice of antibiotics also depends on the clinical condition, local sensitivity pattern, cost and availability of the drugs (Table 43.8).

Table 43.8: Choice of antibiotics as per clinical conditions

Clinical condition	*Antibiotics*
Infected child or complications present	• IV Ampicillin 50 mg/kg/dose q 6 hourly and IV Gentamicin 2.5 mg/kg/dose q 8 hourly. • Add IV Cloxacillin 100 mg/kg/day q 6 hourly if staphylococcal infection is suspected. • Revise therapy based on the culture sensitivity report.
For septic shock OR No improvement OR worsening in initial 48 hrs	• Add third generation cephalosporins i.e. IV cefotaxime 100 mg/kg/day q 8 hourly.

Contd...

Contd...

Clinical condition	*Antibiotics*
Meningitis	• IV Cefotaxime 200 mg/kg/day IV q 6 hourly with IV amikacin 15 mg/kg/day q 8 hourly.
Dysentery	• Nalidixic acid 55 mg/kg/day in 3 divided doses. • IV ceftriaxone 50 mg/kg/day in od or q 12 hourly if child is sick or has already received nalidixic acid.

Other infection like tuberculosis is quite common in malnourished children and an important cause for the failure to respond. It often presents diagnostic problems because the mantoux test is usually non-reactive due to phenomenon of energy, but may become positive as the child's nutritional status improves. In such cases supportive evidence such as gastric aspirate for acid-fast bacilli, chest X-ray of the child and screening of other family members must be done. In endemic areas malaria does not present with the typical signs of fever with rigors. In fact diarrhea has been mentioned as one of the presenting symptoms. Malnourished children with malaria should receive a full course of antimalarial therapy with the dosage based on body weight.[2,4,18]

h. Severe Anemia

Mild to moderate anemia is almost always present and is usually due to iron and folic acid deficiency. Many malnourished children are 'adapted' to anemia because of its chronicity and show relatively few functional effects. Children with kwashiorkor have an expanded blood volume which tends to exaggerate the severity of the apparent hemoglobin deficit.[3] Supplementation of oral iron is indicated but should be deferred in initial phase till infections are under control and diarrhea has subsided,[17] as it can have toxic effects and may reduce resistance to infection.[19] In cases of severe anemia (Hb <4.0 g/dl or PCV <12%) a blood transfusion is indicated (10 ml/kg of packed cells or whole blood) over 3 hours. In centers where adequate testing for HIV and Hepatitis B is not available, transfusion should be avoided until the hemoglobin is below 3.0 g/dl or the child develops heart failure.[20] In patients with impending heart failure, partial exchange transfusion may be beneficial.[21]

i. Congestive Cardiac Failure

Congestive cardiac failure in a malnourished child usually attributed to over hydration, impaired cardiac function, very severe anemia or blood transfusion, may combined with an expanded blood volume due to shift of edema fluid from the tissue which is not excreted satisfactorily.[3] In 1966, *alleyne* demonstrated that in malnutrition the heart does not escape the wasting that effects the other organs.[22] Studies have shown nearly 30 percent decrease in cardiac output in malnourished children in comparison to the recovered state.[20,23] Workers have attributed the decreased cardiac output to lower basal metabolic rate in these children.[3,24] The first sign of congestive cardiac failure usually is fast breathing. This is followed by development of chest indrawing, tachycardia, raised jugular venous pressure and peripheral circulatory failure. Cardiac failure must be differentiated from respiratory tract infections and septic shock, as latter two usually occur within the first 48 hours after presentation, cardiac failure occurs somewhat later.[20]

Once congestive cardiac failure is diagnosed the following steps should be taken: [2]

1. Stop all oral intake and intravenous fluids.
2. Furosemide (1 mg/kg/IV).
3. Digitalis should be avoided till the diagnosis of congestive cardiac failure is firmly established and the plasma potassium levels documented to be normal. In such children digoxin is administered in dose of 5 μg/kg intravenously or orally as a single dose.

j. Vitamin A Deficiency

Severely malnourished children are at high risk of developing blindness due to vitamin A deficiency. For this reason a large dose of vitamin A should be given routinely to all malnourished children on day 1, unless there is definitive evidence that a dose has been given during the past month.[4] The doses are designed as per the age of the child (Table 43.9). If there are any clinical signs of vitamin A deficiency (e.g. night blindness, conjunctival xerosis with Bitot's spots, corneal xerosis or ulceration, or keratomalacia), a large dose should be given on the first 2 days, followed by a third dose at least 2 weeks later.[2,5] Great care must be taken during examination of the eyes, as they easily rupture in children with vitamin A deficiency. If there is ocular inflammation or ulceration, protect the eyes with pads soaked in 0.9% saline. Tetracycline eye drops (1%) should be instilled four times daily until all signs of inflammation or ulceration resolve. Atropine eye drops (0.1%) should also be applied and the affected eye(s) should be bandaged, as scratching with a finger can cause rupture of an ulcerated cornea.[2,4]

Table 43.9: Treatment of clinical vitamin A deficiency

Timing	*Dosage*
Day 1	
< 6 months of age	50,000 IU
6-12 months	1,00,000 IU
>12 months	2,00,000 IU
Day 2	Same age specific
Two weeks later	Same age specific

To summarize, children with severe malnutrition is always 'at risk' because of altered physiologic and metabolic state who need to be managed diligently, comprehensively considering pathophysiology and handicaps present in severely malnourished child. Clinical judgment is always more reliable than laboratory investigation, some of which may be misleading the management process. The treating pediatrician/general physician should anticipate complications, monitor closely and manage associated metabolic disturbances like hypoglycemia, hypokalemia and metabolic acidosis. Maintenance of normal temperature is always beneficial. A high index of suspicion should be kept for infection, which should be empirically treated at the earliest with broad-spectrum antimicrobials. The objective of the management is to stabilise the child early and transfers for nutritional rehabilitation. Oral fluids and feeds need to be instituted as early as possible. Intravenous fluid should be used with great caution because of increased risk of developing sodium overload and congestive cardiac failure.[26] All the key elements in the emergency management of severely malnourished children are summarized in Figure 43.4. If the life-threatening complications are managed initially as an emergency process with standard guidelines and protocols, there will be decline in mortality because of malnutrition and a good progress towards recovery occurs.

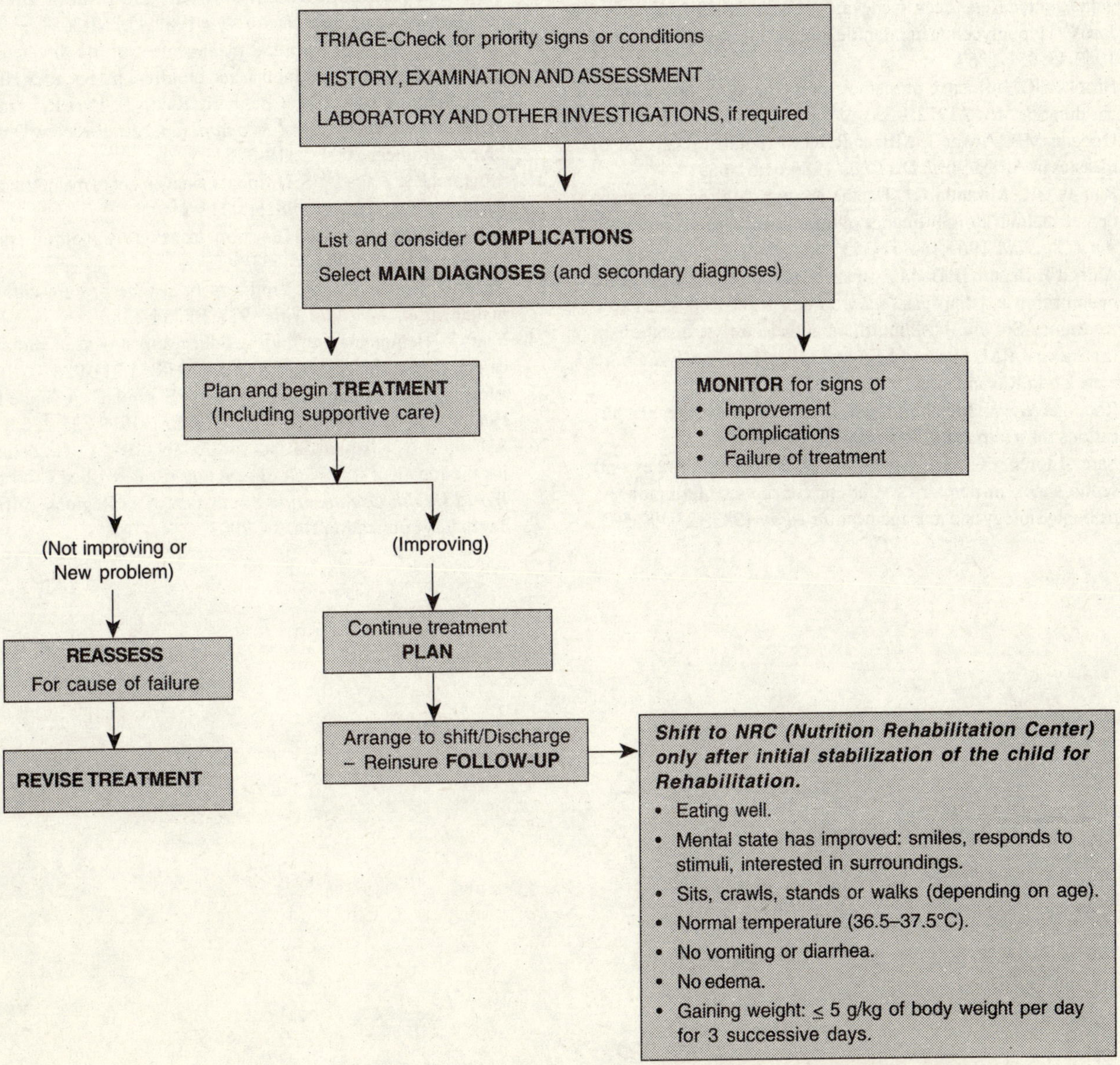

Fig. 43.4: Summary of key elements in the management of the malnourished child

REFERENCES

1. Schofield C, Ashworth A. Why have mortality rates for severe malnutrition remained so high? *Bull WHO* 1996;74:223-229.
2. World Health Organization. *Management of Severe Malnutrition: A Manual for physicians and other Senior Health Workers*. Geneva: WHO 1999.
3. Alleyne GAO, Hay RW, Picou DI, Stanfield JP, Whitehead RG. The treatment of severe protein-energy malnutrition. In: *Protein Energy Malnutrition*. New Delhi: Jaypee Brothers 1989:113-118.
4. World Health Organization. *Management of the Child with Serious Infection or Severe Malnutrition: Guidelines for care at the first referral level in developing countries*. Geneva: *WHO/* AITBS 2003;1:81-90.
5. World Health Organization. Pocket Book of Hospital Care for Children: Guidelines for the Management of Common Illnesses with Limited Resources. Geneva: WHO 2005;173-196.
6. Jaso E. Hypoglycemia in infantile malnutrition. *Am J Dis Child* 1932;43: 051-1067.
7. Brooke OG. Influence of malnutrition on body temperature of children. *Br Med J* 1972;1:331-333.
8. Duggan MB, Alwar J, Milner RDG. The nutritional cost of measles in Africa. *Arch Dis Child* 1986;61:61-66.
9. Ramos GR, Miranda CJ. Deaths among children with third degree malnutrition: Influence of the clinical type of condition. *Am J Clin Nutr* 1965;16:351-355.
10. Ahmed T, Begum B, Badiuzzaman, *et al.* Management of severe malnutrition and diarrhea. *Indian J Pediatr* 2001;68:45-51.
11. Rodriguez-Soriano J. Malnutrition and electrolyte metabolism In: Suskind RM, Suskind LL (eds): *The Malnourished Child.* New York: Ravan Press 1990;141-152.
12. Roediger WEW. Metabolic basis of starvation diarrhea: Implications for treatment. *Lancet* 1986;1:1082-1084.
13. Safez-Llorens X, McCracken GH Jr. Sepsis syndromes and septic shock in pediatrics: Current concepts of terminology, pathophysiology and management. *J Pediatr* 1983;123:497-505.
14. Brooke OG, Ashworth A. The influence of malnutrition on postprandial metabolic rate and respiratory quotient. *Br J Nutr* 1972;27:407-415.
15. Mann MD, Bowie MD, Hansen JDL. Total body potassium and serum electrolyte concentrations in protein-energy malnutrition. *S Afr Med J* 1975;49:76-78.
16. Smith R, Waterlow JC. Total exchangeable potassium in infantile malnutrition. *Lancet* 1963;1:147-149.
17. Tahmeed A, Ali M, Ullah M, Choudhary IA, Haque ME, Salam Ma, *et al.* Mortality in severely malnourished children with diarrhea and use of a standardized management protocol. *Lancet* 1999;353:1919-1922.
18. Singh S. Management of protein-energy malnutrition. In: Sachdev HPS, Choudhary P (eds): *Nutrition in Children: Developing Country Concerns*, New Delhi, Cambridge Press 1994;206-216.
19. Smith IF, Taiwo O, Golden MNH. Plant protein rehabilitation diets and iron supplementations of the protein energy malnourished child. *Eur J Clin Nutr* 1989;43:763-768.
20. Gera T, Sachdev HPS. Initial management of life-threatening problems in severely malnourished children. In: Sachdev HPS, Choudhary P, Bagga A, Chugh K, Ramji S, Puri RK (eds): *Principles of Pediatric and Neonatal Emergencies*, New Delhi: Jaypee Brothers 2004;2:319-325.
21. Rugmini PS, Walia BNS. Hospital management of malnutrition–part I. *Indian J Pediatr* 1981;48:211-216.
22. Alleyne GAO. Cardiac function in severely malnourished children. *Clin Sci* 1966;30:553-562.
23. Viart P. Hemodynamic findings in severe protein-calorie malnutrition. *Am J Clin Nutr* 1977;30:334-348.
24. Viart P. Hemodynamic findings during treatment of protein-calorie malnutrition. *Am J Clin Nutr* 1978;31:911-926.
25. World Health Organization. Nutrition Essentials: A Guide for Health Managers. Geneva: *WHO/UNICEF* 1999:225-235.
26. Ashworth A, Khanum S, Jackson A, Schofield C. Guidelines for the inpatient treatment of severely malnourished children. *World Health Organization* South East Asia Regional Office Technical Publication No. 24, 2003.

Section VIII

Hemato-Oncologic Emergencies

Sameer Bakhshi

44 Severe Anemia

INTRODUCTION

Anemia is defined as a reduction of the red cell volume or hemoglobin concentration below 2SD for age, race and sex. Physiologically, anemia is a condition in which reduced red cell mass leads to diminished oxygen-carrying capacity that does not optimally meet the metabolic demands of the body. Anemia is not a specific disease entity but a condition caused by a variety of underlying pathologic processes. It may be acute or chronic. The combination of anemia with leukopenia, neutropenia, and/or thrombocytopenia may suggest a more global failure of hematopoiesis.

In developing nations, the prevalence of anemia, particularly in preschool children, may be as high as 90%. Although iron deficiency is identified as the major factor,[1] the etiology is often multifactorial, including recurrent or chronic infections (bacteria, parasites), malnutrition, and reduced immunity. In addition, the prevalence of certain hereditary forms of anemia (e.g., thalassemia, sickle cell disease) varies with ethnicity and sex. For instance, certain hereditary X-linked red cell disorders (e.g., G-6-PD deficiency) are observed in males.

PATHOPHYSIOLOGY

The main physiologic role of red blood cells (RBCs) is to deliver oxygen to the tissues. Certain physiologic adjustments can occur in an individual with anemia to compensate for the lack of oxygen delivery. These include

1. Increased cardiac output;
2. Shunting of blood to vital organs;
3. Increased 2,3-diphosphoglycerate (DPG) in the RBCs, which causes reduced oxygen affinity, shifting the oxygen dissociation curve to the right and thereby enhancing oxygen release to the tissues; and
4. Increased erythropoietin to stimulate RBC production.

CLINICAL FEATURES

The clinical effects of anemia depend on its duration and severity. When anemia is acute, the body does not have enough time to make the necessary physiologic adjustments, and the symptoms are more likely to be pronounced and dramatic. They appear in distress with tachycardia, tachypnea, and hypovolemia. They may have signs of CHF (tachycardia, gallop rhythm, tachypnea, cardiomegaly, hepatomegaly). In contrast, when anemia develops gradually, the body is able to adjust, ameliorating the symptoms relative to the degree of the anemia.

CAUSES

The underlying pathologic processes that cause anemia can be categorized broadly as:

1. Decreased or ineffective red cell production;
2. Increased red cell destruction; or
3. Blood loss. Causes of anemia are either inherent in the RBCs or related to an external factor.

These can be simplified into 3 main categories, although more than one mechanism may be involved in some anemias (Table 44.1).

Severe Anemia accompanied by hemodynamic instability is usually due to acute and significant (5% of total blood volume) blood loss or pooling. Some causes include bleeding from traumatic injury, gastrointestinal hemorrhage, splenic sequestration in sickle cell disease, hemophilia with a bleeding episode in the retroperitoneum or thigh, DIC with uncontrollable bleeding, intra or postoperative blood loss.

APPROACH TO SEVERE ANEMIA

Diagnostic Approach

To evaluate anemia, obtain initial laboratory tests, including complete blood count (CBC) with red blood cell indices, reticulocyte count, and review of the peripheral smear.[2] Before any other tests, it is important to correctly ensure that the child is anemic looking at the hemoglobin and hematocrit levels on the reference range for the specific age group.

Table 44.1: Pathophysiological classification of anemia

A. Decreased red cell production
1. Marrow failure
   - Diamond-Blackfan anemia and aplastic anemia
   - Transient erythroblastopenia of childhood
2. Marrow infiltrative disorders
   - Leukemia
   - Solid tumor infiltration such as neuroblastoma, retinoblastoma
3. Impaired erythropoietin production
   - Anemia of chronic disease in renal failure
   - Hypothyroidism
4. Defect in red cell maturation
   - Nutritional anemia secondary to iron, folate, or vitamin B_{12} deficiency
   - Chronic inflammatory diseases
   - Congenital dyserythropoietic anemia
   - Sideroblastic anemias

B. Increased red cell destruction (hemolysis)
1. Extracellular causes
   - Mechanical injury (hemolytic-uremic syndrome, cardiac valvular defects)
   - Autoimmune hemolytic anemia
   - Infections, drugs, toxins
   - Hypersplenism
2. Intracellular causes
   - Red cell membrane defects (e.g., hereditary spherocytosis, elliptocytosis)
   - Enzyme defects (e.g., G-6-PD deficiency, pyruvate kinase deficiency)
   - Hemoglobinopathies (sickle cell disease, thalassemias, unstable hemoglobinopathies)

C. *Blood loss*
   - Obvious or occult site of blood loss either acute or chronic

Red Cell Indices

If the patient is anemic, look at the (mean corpuscular volume [MCV], mean corpuscular hemoglobin [MCH], and mean corpuscular hemoglobin concentration [MCHC]). Of these, the MCV is particularly helpful in classifying anemia, and most reliable as it is the only red cell index which is directly measured by the electronic cell counter. Note that normal ranges for these parameters also vary with age. In children less than 10 years, the lower limit for MCV is approximately 70 fl + age in years. After 6 months of age, the approximate upper limit of MCV is 84 + 0.6 fl per year until the upper limit of 96 fl is reached in adults. Based on the MCV, anemia is classified as microcytic, normocytic and macrocytic which is most evaluable in approaching any child with anemia (Table 44.2).

Another valuable parameter in classifying anemia is the RBC distribution width (RDW) which reflects the variability in cell size and is a measure of anisocytosis; it is increased with reticulocytosis.

Table 44.2: Classification of anemia based on MCV

A. Microcytic anemia
   - Iron deficiency anemia
   - Hemoglobinopathies
   - Sideroblastic anemia

B. Normocytic anemia
   - Bone marrow hypoplasia
   - Bone marrow infiltrative disorders
   - Chronic renal disease
   - Hemolytic anemia
   - Chronic inflammatory disease

C. Macrocytic anemia
   - Megaloblastic anemia
   - Myelodysplastic syndrome
   - Hemolytic anemia with profound reticulocytosis
   - Hypothyroidism

Reticulocytes

These are immature nonnucleated RBCs that indicate active erythropoiesis. The relative reticulocyte count is useful in differentiating whether decreased production, increased destruction, or loss of RBCs is causing the anemia. The term reticulocyte count is often used inaccurately to refer to the percentage of reticulocytes, a value that must be interpreted in light of the degree of anemia. Thus, a finding of 2-3% reticulocytes (*vs* the normal value of approximately 1%) in a patient whose hemoglobin is only 1/3rd to 1/2 of normal does not indicate a reticulocyte "response". Some clinicians prefer to use either the absolute number of reticulocytes per mm^3 of blood or a reticulocyte percentage "corrected" for the degree of anemia. (Corrected reticulocyte count = patient hematocrit/normal hematocrit X% reticulocyte count). During acute red blood cell destruction or loss, the reticulocyte response will not be evident until 3-5 days after the onset of the event. Maximal reticulocytosis is seen 7-10 days after the onset of hemolysis.

Examination of the Peripheral Smear

It helps identify the cause of the anemia by recognizing abnormal cell morphology such as schistocytes or fragmented cells (microangiopathic hemolytic anemia), spherocytes (hereditary spherocytosis, autoimmune hemolytic anemia), ghost or bite cells (G-6-PD deficiency), target cells (hemoglobin C) and stippled red blood cells (nonspecific but may suggest lead poisoning). It is important to recognize that normal red blood cell morphology does not rule out hemolysis.

THERAPEUTIC APPROACH

Acute anemia usually warrants immediate medical attention. Treatment depends on the severity and underlying cause of the anemia. Initial treatment begins with careful assessment of the signs and symptoms of the anemia that indicate therapy. Guidelines for the treatment of patients with critical illness apply to children with severe anemia who are in acute distress and unstable (Fig. 44.1). Samples for further testing should be collected before the blood transfusion.

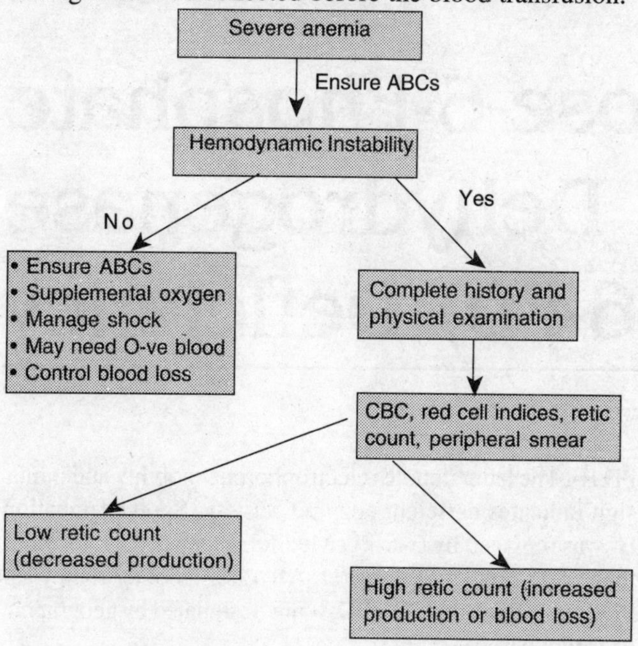

Fig. 44.1: Algorithm for management of severe anemia

Supportive measures such as supplemental oxygen for decreased oxygen-carrying capacity, fluid resuscitation for hypovolemia, and bed rest or activity restriction for fatigue, may be required.

Transfusion with packed RBCs (PRBC) is the universal treatment for most individuals with acute anemia. The indication to transfuse should not be based solely on the hemoglobin or hematocrit levels; more importantly, one must consider the clinical effects or signs and symptoms of the individual with anemia. PRBC dose is 10-15 mL/kg over 3-4 hours. Rate of transfusion can be modified according to the clinical situation. Transfusion can be administered faster in individuals with acute blood loss or slower or in smaller aliquots in persons with CHF. Occasionally, in severe anemia, a partial exchange transfusion may have to be done. In individuals with autoimmune hemolytic anemia, blood must be given with extreme caution, using the blood unit that is least reactive on crossmatching.

When Not to Transfuse

It must, however, be remembered that transfusion does not solely depend on the level of hemoglobin.[3] Physiologic adaptations to anemia, including elevated 2,3-DPG content and increased cardiac output, compensate to a significant extent for chronic anemia. Perhaps, the only situation wherein a transfusion needs to be done rapidly without looking at the type of anemia is a patient in shock due to blood loss.

Otherwise, one should repeat the CBC in the hospital before transfusion for two reasons. First, to make sure that the first reading was correct. This is particularly important if the reading is the basis for transfusion. Second, to provide some information about the course of the condition. For example, if the patient's hemoglobin level had fallen from 5.4 to 4.4 g/dL during the hour or two that it took to travel from the office to the hospital, it suggests rapid progression. Look at the red cell indices and peripheral smear before transfusion. Many types of anemia can be treated with medical therapy. For example, hemoglobin of 6 g/dL due to iron deficiency anemia may be treated with iron supplementation rather than a transfusion, thereby avoiding the hazards of transfusion.

Selection of blood for Emergency Transfusion[4,5]

Occasionally, in patients with hemorrhagic shock, it is necessary to transfuse blood without a cross match. In such a situation, a specimen of the patient's blood and a segment from the donor blood bag should be sent to the blood bank for an antibody screen and cross-match, as the transfusion is proceeding. If the patient's blood group is known, then unmatched blood of the same group may be used; otherwise group O RBCs should be chosen. Patients of blood group AB may be given either blood group A or B cells. Such unmatched blood should be Rh (D) negative in female children in whom sensitization to D would be undesirable. As Rh-negative blood is in short supply, Rh-positive blood is used for the emergent transfusion of males. Despite the lack of cross-match, transfusion of group O blood under emergency situation is safe. The incidence of red cell all antibodies in healthy people is low, and most such antibodies do not cause dangerous hemolytic transfusion reactions even if incompatible blood is given. However, the decision to use unmatched blood is the responsibility of the attending physician, who must weigh against the expected benefits and document in the patient's record the need for the unmatched blood.

REFERENCES

1. Kapur D, Agarwal KN, Agarwal DK. Nutritional anemia and its control. *Indian J Pediatr*. 2002;69:607-616.
2. Hermiston ML, Mentzer WC. A practical approach to the evaluation of the anemic child. *Pediatr Clin North Am* 2002;49:877-891.
3. Carmel R. A focused approach to anemia. *Hosp Prac* 1999;34:71-78.
4. Klein HG. Standards for Blood Banks and Transfusion Services, 17th edn. Bethesda: American Association of Blood Banks 1996.
5. Gupte S. Pediatric hematology. In: Gupte S (ed) *The Short Textbook of Pediatrics*, 9th edn. New Delhi: Jaypee Brothers 2001;409-437.

Pankaj Abrol

45 Glucose-6-Phosphate Dehydrogenase (G-6-PD) Deficiency

INTRODUCTION

Glucose-6-Phosphate dehydrogenase (G-6-PD) deficiency is a hereditary, sex-linked enzyme defect that results in the breakdown of red blood cells when the person is exposed to the stress of infection or certain drugs.

The incidence of G-6-PD deficiency is estimated to be 2.6% in India.[1] It has been demonstrated that in vitro growth of malarial parasites is inhibited by G-6-PD deficient RBCs. Inhibition of parasitic growth in G-6-PD deficient red blood cells has been attributed to overwhelming oxidant stress and GSH instability, both of which can destroy the host cell and its parasite.

ETIOLOGY

G-6-PD deficiency is an inheritable x-linked recessive disorder whose primary effect is the reduction of G-6-PD in the red blood cells, with resultant hemolysis of the cell. The ultimate effect of the disease is to produce anemia, either acute hemolytic or chronic non-spherocytic type.

GENETICS

The gene for G-6-PD is located on the X chromosome (band X q28).[2] The gene lies in juxtaposition to the genes of color blindness. Consequently enzyme deficiency manifests completely in males, carrying a variant gene, whereas heterozygous females are clinically normal. The G-6-PD activity of red blood cells of females with a single variant gene is usually intermediate between that of affected males and normal subjects. Some obligate heterozygotes have normal enzyme level whereas some others no more than hemizygous males. Beutler had tried to explain this by X-chromosome inactivation.[3]

ENZYME AND ITS VARIANTS

The normal enzyme is designated as G-6-PD B, the black variant G-6-PD A-, and the Mediterranean variant as G-6-PD B-. The letter denotes electrophoretic mobility and minus sign indicates deficient enzyme activity. Soon designation B- was replaced by G-6-PD Mediterranean. There are more than 380 variants of G-6-PD. All variants other than G-6-PDB, G-6-PDA and G-6-PDA- are designated by geographic or trivial names.

Leukocyte and platelet G-6-PD is regulated by same gene as red blood cells. Hence, detection of decreased activity of the enzyme in leukocytes and platelets of G-6-PD deficient individuals is not surprising. These cells do not show functional impairment, as their normal life span is short. Functional abnormality of G-6-PD deficient platelets have been described,[4] but it does not lead to any bleeding tendency.

PATHOPHYSIOLOGY

Young red blood cells have higher G-6-PD activity, declining exponentially with cell age. The normal enzyme (G-6-PD B) has in vivo half-life of 62 days.[5] The activity is twice in reticulocytes and half in aged cells, when compared to mixed population. The activity of G-6-PD A- in reticulocytes is normal but declines rapidly to half-life of only 13 days.[5] The activity of G-6-PD Mediterranean is more decreased and its half-life is measured in hours only. Thus the red cells with unstable variants undergo premature metabolic aging.

The precise mechanism of premature destruction of G-6-PD deficient red cells is not yet clear. Probably the enzyme deficient red cells have limited ability to generate NADPH and therefore, GSH. Hydrogen peroxide and free radicals are generated in small amounts during normal red cell metabolism, and in large amounts due to metabolism of certain drugs.[6] GSH required to reduce hydrogen peroxide and free radicals, gets oxidized itself. In G-6-PD deficient cells, there is inefficient NADPH generating system and therefore conversion of oxidized glutathione to GSH is limited. Heme is liberated from globin and latter gets denatured. Denatured globins get attached to red cell membrane possibly by disulphide bridges. These denatured proteins, also called Heinz bodies impair the red cell shape in such a manner that, they get trapped while passing through liver and spleen. The macrophages remove Heinz bodies along with the adherent cell membrane. In G-6-PD variants associated with chronic hemolytic anemia, the shortened red cell survival appears to be mediated by oxidant induced membrane injury rather than by Heinz body formation.[7]

CLINICAL FEATURES

Clinical expression of G-6-PD variants consists of a continuous spectrum of hemolytic syndromes. The deficiency state may remain undetected in the individual. On the other hand, it may present as a major problem in the neonatal period or later. Anemia may present as acute and episodic, or chronic and lifelong.

Acute and Acquired Hemolytic Anemia

In usual G-6-PD variants (G-6-PD A- and G-6-PD Mediterranean), the patient presents with acute severe hemolysis, when exposed to certain offending agents or drugs. Otherwise the individual presents with no anemia or altered blood morphology. Nevertheless, by using isotopic techniques, some shortening of red cell survival can be shown. Sudden hemolysis can be precipitated by drugs having high redox potential, some infections, certain metabolic disturbances and surgery.[8]

Clinical and laboratory features acute hemolytic episode are best illustrated by primaquine-induced hemolysis in individuals with G-6-PD A- variant. After 2 to 4 days of primaquine ingestion, clinical and laboratory picture of an acute hemolytic episode appears. Patient develops jaundice, pallor and high colored urine. He may have acute abdominal and/or backache. Hemoglobin may abruptly fall by 3 to 4 g/dl. Peripheral smear may show fragmented red cells, micro-spherocytes and Heinz bodies. Heinz bodies disappear as hemoglobin reaches its nadir. Body produces more red cells and reticulocytosis appears within 5 days. Reticulocytosis peaks by 7 to 10 days after onset of hemolysis. Plasma hemoglobin is raised and hemoglobinuria may be positive during acute hemolysis. Acute hemolysis stops abruptly after about one week, even if offending drug is continued. Hemoglobin returns to normal level thereafter. Self-limiting nature of the episode can be explained by higher concentration of G-6-PD level in young red cells. Although red cell survival remains shortened as long as use of the drug continues, compensation by erythroid marrow is complete and anemia is abolished.

In G-6-PD Mediterranean variants anemia is more severe as G-6-PD Mediterranean has shorter half-life. Less amount of drug can cause more hemolysis and sharper fall in hemoglobin.

Drug-Induced Hemolysis

Primaquine is only one of the drugs incriminated for drug-induced hemolysis in G-6-PD variants. These have been listed in Table 45.1. Some drugs like phenacetin can be given safely in usual therapeutic doses. Ascorbic acid can be given in usual therapeutic doses but large amounts may cause problems.[9] Chloramphenicol, quinacrine (Atabrine), sulphamethoxypyridazine and sulphone (Dapsone) do not cause significant hemolysis. Aspirin at the dosage of 50 mg/kg/day does not cause detectable hemolysis in G-6-PD deficient subjects. Similarly acetaminophen, aminopyrine, sulfisoxazole and vitamin K can be given in usual therapeutic doses.

Table 45.1: Agents precipitating hemolysis in glucose-6-phosphate dehydrogenase (G-6-PD) deficiency

Antimalarials	*Miscellaneous*
Primaquine	Phenacetin
Pamaquine	Aspirin
Pentaquine	Vitamin K analogues
Chloroquine	Methylene blue
Quinacrine	Probenecid
Antibacterials	Thiazides
Sulfonamides	Phenothiazine
Trimethoprimsulfamethoxazole	Dimercaprol
Chloramphenicol	Phenazopyridine
Nalidixic acid	Orinase
Nitrofurantoin	Naphthalene (moth balls)
Furazolidone	Phenylhydrazine
Dapsone	Toluidine blue
Nitrofurazone	Trinitrotoluene
	Fava beans
Anthelmintics	*Illness*
B-Naphthol	Diabetic acidosis
Stibophen	Hepatitis
Niridazole	

Infection-Induced Hemolysis

Infection is probably a more common cause of hemolysis in G-6-PD deficient subjects than drug exposure.[10] Approximately 20% of G-6-PD deficient subjects having pneumonia show sudden loss of hemoglobin. Many infectious agents like salmonella, escherichia coli, b-hemolytic streptococci, rickettsiae and hepatitis virus have been implicated for hemolysis and sudden fail in hemoglobin. The exact mechanism of hemolysis in such individuals is not known.

Favism

In some patients, ingestion of fava beans, a Mediterranean dietary staple, may also cause an acute and severe hemolytic syndrome called *favism*. This results from oxidative products derived from two glucosidic compounds, vicine and convicine. These are hydrolyzed to divicine and isouramil, ultimately producing hydrogen peroxide and other reactive oxygen products.

Hemolysis-Induced by Diabetic Acidosis

Diabetic ketoacidosis is also known to cause hemolysis in G-6-PD deficient subjects. Correction of acidosis and restoration of glucose homeostasis stalls the hemolytic process.

Neonatal Jaundice

G-6-PD deficiency is also implicated in causation of neonatal hyperbilirubinemia. The reason is not yet clear. However, the suggested mechanisms are–environmental variables, herbs used in traditional medicines, drugs and chemicals used by mother in late gestation.

Chronic Nonspherocytic Hemolytic Anemia

In some G-6-PD variants, there is such profound deficiency of enzyme activity, that life long hemolysis occurs in the absence of any infection or drug exposure. These variants have quantitative as well as qualitative deficiency. The anemia in these subjects clinically and hematologically indistinguishable from the congenital nonspherocytic hemolytic syndromes related to other glycolytic enzyme deficiencies. These variants have been identified in black Americans, as well as in Caucasians. These include the Loma Linda, Tomah, Iowa, Beverly Hills, Riverside, Santiago de Cuba and Andalus variants. Usually associated with intermittent hemolysis, G-6-PD Mediterranean rarely is the cause of life-long hemolytic disease.

Anemia and Jaundice are often noted in neonatal period, requiring exchange transfusion at times. Hemolysis may occur in absence of a recognized trigger factor. Beyond infancy the manifestations of hemolysis may be subtle. Pallor and jaundice may be intermittent. No specific hematological alterations are there but mild to moderate anemia is the rule. Leukocyte dysfunction has also been observed in some of severely deficient patients.[11] This results in decreased bactericidal activity and recurrent infections with catalase-positive organisms.

DIAGNOSIS

The G-6-PD deficiency is an important cause of non-immune hemolytic anemia. Usually it presents after exposure to certain drugs/chemicals, or during/after an infection. Less commonly, it may present as anemia or hemolysis-an incidental finding.

Individual with G-6-PD deficiency usually present as sudden appearance of jaundice and anemia following intake of a precipitating drug or presence of some infection. Less commonly, they may also present as incidental anemia or jaundice. Clinical and hematological features reflect the severity of hemolysis. Proper diagnosis can be made only after the assessment of G-6-PD activity of red cells. When hemolytic episode occurs, the old red cells get destroyed and are soon replaced by reticulocytes and young red cells. These younger cells are richer in G-6-PD enzyme, and therefore assessment of their G-6-PD status will not help us, till reticulocytosis resolves. This may take a few weeks. The diagnosis can be suspected when the G-6-PD activity is within the low normal range in the presence of a high reticulocytes count. By direct measurement, enzyme activity in affected persons is 10% of normal or less.

Several simple screening tests are available. The fluorescent spot test is the simplest, most reliable and most sensitive of screening tests.[12] This test is based on the fluorescence of NADPH. This test is suitable for mass screening but does not reliably identify the heterozygous state. In the methemoglobin reduction test, methylene blue is used for transfer of hydrogen from NADPH to methemoglobin.

APPROACH TO MANAGEMENT

Prevention forms an important component of management of G-6-PD variants. Individuals with any known predisposition or earlier diagnosis should avoid exposure to oxidizing drugs known to trigger hemolysis (Table 44.1). Pregnant and nursing mothers known to be heterozygous also should avoid such drugs. If unavoidable, such drugs may be given cautiously. For example, primaquine can be safely given to individuals with G-6-PD A- variants, provided it is started cautiously in the dose of 15 mg/day or 45 mg once or twice a week and the blood counts are monitored. The usual doses of aspirin and co-trimoxazole do not cause significant hemolysis but aspirin in dose administered for acute rheumatic fever (75-100 mg/kg/24 hr) may produce severe hemolytic episode.

When hemolysis has occurred, blood transfusion can be given as a part of supportive therapy. Severe hemoglobinuria should be treated as an emergency with sodium bicarbonate sufficient to alkalinize the urine to prevent the precipitation of acid hematin in the renal tubules and consequent development of renal failure. Usually the oxidizing drug is stopped and any other possible cause is treated. Recovery is the rule even if the offending drug is not stopped as new and young red cells have higher G-6-PD level.

Nonspherocytic hemolytic anemia due to G-6-PD deficiency requires more active intervention. In a neonate with jaundice, exchange transfusion may be required to prevent kernicterus. Regular transfusions may be required after neonatal period. At times the patient may have aplastic crisis requiring blood transfusion as life-saving measure.

Splenectomy usually is without any benefit. Vitamin E is an oxidant but is also of little value.

Screening

It is not usually of any help as variants of G-6-PD responsible for acute hemolytic anemia pose little health hazard. Even chronic/congenital hemolytic anemia is very rare, rendering screening an impractical option. Blood bank screening also appears to be unwarranted as there are no deleterious consequences and it will unnecessarily impair the supply of a valuable resource.

REFERENCES

1. Panich V. Glucose-6-phosphate dehydrogenase deficiency: Tropical Asia. *Clin Hematol* 1981;10:800-814.
2. Kirkman HN, Hendrickson EM. Sex-linked electrophoretic difference in glucose-6-phosphate dehydrogenase. *Am J Hum Genet* 1963;15:241-258.
3. Beutler E, Yeh M, Fairbans VF. The normal human female as a mosaic of X-chromosome activity: Studies using the gene for G-6-PD deficiency as a marker. *Proc Natl Acad Sci USA* 1962;48: 9-16.
4. Schwartz JP, Cooperberg AA, Rosenberg A. Platelet function studies in patients with glucose-6-phosphate dehydrogenase deficiency. *Br J Hematol* 1974;27: 273-280.
5. Piomeli S, Gorash LM, Davenport DD, Miraglia J. In vivo lability of glucose-6-phosphate dehydrogenase in Gd A- and Gd Mediterranean deficiency. *J Clin Invest* 1968;47:940-948.
6. Kosower NS, Vanderhoff GA, London IM. The regeneration of reduced glutathione in normal and glucose-6-phosphate dehydrogenase deficient human red blood cells. *Blood* 1967;29:313-319.
7. Alhanty E, Snyder M, Sheetz MP. Glucose-6-phosphate deficient erythrocytes have an impaired shape recovery mechanism. *Blood* 1984;63:1198-1202.
8. Sazama K, Klein HG, Davey RJ, Corash L. Intra-operative hemolysis. *Arch Intern Med* 1980;140:845-846.
9. Udomratn T, Steinberg MH, Campbell GD, Oelshlegel FN. Effects of ascorbic acid on glucose-6-phosphate dehydrogenase-deficient erythrocytes: Studies in an animal model. *Blood* 1977;49:471-475.
10. Shannon K, Buchanan GR. Severe hemolytic anemia in black children with glucose-6-phosphate dehydrogenase deficiency. *Pediatrics* 1982;70:364-369.
11. Mamlok RJ, Mamlok V, Mills GC, Daeschner CW, Schwalstring FC, Anderson DC. Glucose-6-phosphate dehydrogenase deficiency, neutrophil dysfunction and Chromobacterium violaceum sepsis. *J Pediatr* 1987;111:852-854.
12. Beutler E, Mitchell M. Special modifications of the fluorescent screening methods for glucose-6-phosphate dehydrogenase deficiency. *Blood* 1968;32:816-818.

Sameer Bakhshi

46 Hemolytic Crisis

INTRODUCTION

The term, *hemolysis*, is employed to denote the destruction of red cells. Normal red cells have a life-span of 120 days, at which time they are destroyed primarily by the spleen.

Hemolytic anemia is defined as the premature destruction of red cells either within the bloodstream or in organs such as the spleen. Mild hemolysis is compensated for by increased production of red cells by the marrow (up to eight-fold). Since it takes several days for the marrow to upregulate production of red cells, sudden, massive hemolysis is life threatening.

Severe chronic hemolysis can outstrip the marrow's ability to compensate, resulting in persistent anemia and even death from cardiac failure or side effects of repeated transfusion (infections, iron overload).

Hemolytic crisis is the rapid destruction of red blood cells beyond the point at which the body can compensate by increasing blood cell production.

CLINICAL FEATURES OF HEMOLYTIC ANEMIA

The clinical features are those of anemia, which include malaise, fatigue, pallor and weakness. In addition. chronic hemolyis produces splenomegaly, bone deformities, iron overload, and gallstones. Death can ensue from congestive heart failure.

The clinical signs and laboratory findings depend on the rate of hemolysis and the site of red cell destruction. If red cells are destroyed extravascularly in the reticuloendothelial system, which is the normal site of red cell catabolism, then the hemoglobin is degraded into iron, bilirubin metabolites and amino acids. Since the hepatic clearance of bilirubin may exceed several times, a normal bilirubin value does not exclude the presence of hemolysis. However, patients with severe hemolytic anemia have jaundice.

Acute intravascular hemolysis releases free hemoglobin in the plasma where it is bound to haptoglobin and subsequently cleared in the liver or lost in urine. Thus, hemoglobinemia and hemoglobinuria, and decrease in plasma haptoglobin are features of intravascular hemolysis. In severe cases this is followed by shock, DIC, hypotension, renal failure, and death.

HEMOLYTIC CRISIS

This may be precipitated in any of the congenital or acquired forms of hemolytic anemias (Table 46.1) due to an intercurrent infection, and in some enzymopathies such as G-6-PD deficiency due to exposure to certain drugs or toxins. Often, the warm antibody type of autoimmune hemolytic anemia results in a sudden drop in hemoglobin due to hemolysis.

Hemolytic reactions due to blood *transfusions usually involve the destruction of transfused blood cells by the recipient's antibodies. Less commonly, the transfused antibodies can cause hemolysis of the recipient's blood cells.*

Table 46.1: Etiology of hemolytic anemias

A. *Inherited Causes of Hemolytic Anemia*
1. **Membrane defects**
   Hereditary spherocytosis
2. **Enzyme defects**
   G-6-PD deficiency, Pyruvate kinase deficiency
3. **Hb defects**
   Amino acid substitutions (Sickle cell anemia, HbC, HbE)
   Production defects (alpha or beta thalassemia)

B. *Acquired Causes of Hemolytic Anemia*
1. **Mechanical** Shear stress to circulating red cells (Disseminated intravascular coagulation, microangiopathic hemolytic anemia).
2. **Immune** *Warm antibody, cold antibody*
3. **Infection** Malaria, Mycoplasma, EBV
4. **Membrane defect** Paroxysmal nocturnal hemoglobinuria

There are acute (also known as intravascular) hemolytic reactions and delayed (also known as extravascular) hemolytic reactions.[1]

Acute hemolytic reactions are usually due to ABO blood type incompatibility—in other words, human error plays a large part in these reactions. This type of reaction has been reported to occur approximately 1 in 25,000 transfusions but it is often very severe and accounts for over 50% of reported deaths related to transfusion. The severity of the reaction often depends in the amount of blood given. Symptoms of acute hemolytic reactions include chills, fever, nausea, chest pain and flank pain in awake patients. In anesthetized patients, one should look for rise in temperature, unexplained tachycardia, hypotension, hemoglobinuria, oozing in the surgical field, DIC, shock and renal shutdown.

Delayed hemolytic reactions are generally mild in comparison. These are caused by antibodies to non-D antigens of the Rh system or to foreign alleles in other systems such as the Kell, Duffy or Kidd antigens. Following a normal, compatible transfusion there is a 1-1.6% chance of developing antibodies to these foreign antibodies. This takes weeks or months to happen and by that time, the original transfused cells have already been cleared. Re-exposure to the same foreign antigen can then cause an immune response. Thus, the reaction is typically delayed from two to twenty-one days after transfusion. Symptoms are generally mild and include malaise, jaundice, fever, a fall in hematocrit despite transfusion, and an increase in unconjugated bilirubin.

DIAGNOSIS

The diagnostic workup (Table 46.2) aims to determine:

1. Presence of hemolysis.
2. Site of hemolysis (intravascular or extravascular).
3. Immune *versus nonimmune* hemolysis.
4. Specific underlying defect of nonimmune hemolysis.

Table 46.2: Laboratory tests for hemolysis

1. *Presence of hemolysis*
Reticulocytosis, polychromasia
Immature (nucleated) red cells
Erythroid hyperplasia in bone marrow
Thinning of bones (in chronic cases)
Increased indirect bilirubin
2. *Signs of intravascular hemolysis*
Plasma free hemoglobin
Urine hemoglobin and hemosiderin
Haptoglobin (a serum molecule that binds is decreased Hb)
3. *Immune versus non immune hemolysis*
Coombs test
Differentiate between warm and cold antibody type immune hemolysis depending on the temperature at which antibodies are active
4. Specific tests for nonimmune hemolysis
Enzyme estimation e.g. G-6-PD
Osmotic fragility
Hemoglobin electrophoresis

TREATMENT GUIDELINES

General

A patient having an acute attack of hemolysis should be treated with appropriate measures to relieve shock, maintain fluid balance and to allow renal repair if kidneys have been damaged. Remove any predisposing drug or toxin; treat any intercurrent infection aggressively. Management of acute hemolytic reactions mandates that the transfusion be stopped immediately. The unit should be re-checked. Blood from the recipient patient should be drawn to test for hemoglobin in plasma, repeat compatibility testing and coagulation tests. A Foley catheter should be placed to check for hemoglobin in the urine. Osmotic diuresis with mannitol and fluids should be utilized (low-dose dopamine may help renal function and support blood pressure). With rapid blood loss, platelets and fresh frozen plasma may be indicated.

Blood Transfusion

This has to be judiciously used in immune hemolytic anemias because it is difficult to find a compatible donor; often the antibody is a panagglutinin. Therefore, one may use the "least incompatible" donor. Inspite of this incompatibility, the transfused red cells have a life-span as long as the existing red cells in the body which are being destroyed by the antibodies. Occasionally, destruction of the transfused red cells occurs with an increase in the burden on the kidneys. Thus, one should start this transfusion slowly and carefully observe plasma and urine for signs of intravascular hemolysis.

Specific Treatment

The specific treatment for the acute hemolytic crisis depends on the underlying cause. For example, in warm antibody type immune hemolytic anemia,[2] steroids have to be started immediately, and one may expect a response in 24-48 hours due to their property of Fc receptor blockage of the splenic macrophages and also by reducing the production of auto-antibodies. Very high doses of intravenous immunoglobulin have been used in refractory immune hemolytic crisis[3] but routine use is not advocated. In some refractory cases, splenectomy may be effective not only because spleen is a site of erythrocyte destruction, but also because it may be a source of antibody.[4] In general, patients with warm antibodies are more likely to respond than those with cold antibodies; patients with splenomegaly respond better than those without a palpable spleen. Those with incomplete antibodies (warm antibody type), especially if present in small amounts, are more likely to respond favorably to splenectomy than those with complete agglutinins or complement-fixing antibodies (cold antibody type). Plasmaphereis on the other hand is likely to work better for IgM antibody-mediated hemolysis because the IgG antibodies diffuse out of the vascular system and so may not be effectively removed by plasmapheresis.

REFERENCES

1. Beuregard P, Blajchman MA. Hemolytic and pseudohemolytic transfusion reactions: An overview of the hemolytic transfusion reactions and the clinical conditions that mimic them. *Transfus Med Rev* 1994;8:184-199.
2. Petz LD. Treatment of autoimmune hemolytic anemias. *Curr Opin Hematol*. 2001;8:411-416.
3. Majer RV, Hyde RD. High-dose intravenous immunoglobulin in the treatment of autoimmune haemolytic anaemia. Clin Lab Haematol. 1988;10:391-395.
4. Heisel MA, Ortega JA. Factors influencing prognosis in childhood autoimmune hemolytic anemia. *Am J Pediatr Hematol Oncol* 1983;5:147-152.

Pankaj Abrol

47 The Bleeding Child

INTRODUCTION

Bleeding child is an emergency for the anxious parents as well as the pediatrician. The parents want the immediate relief and the treating physician aims at proper work-up and the appropriate management. It has varied etiology. Physician should, therefore, aim at providing appropriate emergency management, keeping in mind the clinical differential diagnosis, without affecting the specific therapy adversely.

PHYSIOLOGY OF HEMOSTASIS

Whenever there is trauma to blood vessels, the bleeding stops after some time due to following mechanisms:

1. *Vascular spasm:* The spasm lasts for 20-30 minutes.
2. *Platelet phase:* Platelet adhesion, aggregation and plug formation. von Willebrand factor (vWf) is synthesized in platelets and endothelial matrix. Platelet binding to sub-endothelium (adhesion) is mediated by the platelet surface glycoprotein Ib and von Willebrand factor (vWf).[1]
3. Coagulation cascade (Fig. 47.1). Factor X gets activated by intrinsic as well as extrinsic pathway. Extrinsic pathway gets activated by tissue thromboplastin following tissue injury. Tissue factor activates factor X to Xa after forming a complex with factor VIIa. Intrinsic system gets activated by activation of factor XII to XIIa, which then activates factor XI and IX. Factor IXa activates factor X in presence of factor VIII. After activation of factor Xa, factor V is activated. Factor V converts prothrombin to thrombin. Thrombin activates fibrinogen to fibrin monomers which then forms fibrin polymers in presence of factor XIII and calcium. Thrombin also potentiates activation of factor VII and V. It also releases platelet factor-3 from platelets.

MEDICAL HISTORY AND CLINICAL EXAMINATION

There are certain pointers to likelihood of underlying bleeding disorders, in which the bleeding may be prolonged or excessive.

1. Epistaxis not relieved by 15 minutes of pressure.
2. Menstrual periods lasting for longer than 7 days, associated with passage of clots or frequently stained clothing.
3. Excessive bleeding from dental procedures, lasting for more than a day or even requiring blood transfusion.
4. Ecchymosis of a size not consistent with degree and size of trauma.

When there is history of surgery or dental extraction without any bleeding complication, it is unlikely that there is an underlying congenital hemorrhagic disorder.

In a similar manner, one needs to probe the family history of the patient. Inherited hemorrhagic disorders (especially if mild) in the family may have been undiagnosed or misdiagnosed for many generations. The history should cover all the family members, regardless of any suspicion. Hemophilia, an X-linked disorder usually involves males, but may also result in excessive bleeding in female carriers.[2,3] Make objective assessment of menstrual periods by asking certain direct questions. Up to 20% of girls with menorrhagia beginning at menarche have an underlying bleeding disorder.[4]

The type of bleeding is also important. Mucosal membrane bleeding (gum bleeding, epistaxis, menorrhagia), petechiae, and bruising are more typical of quantitative and qualitative platelet disorders and von Willebrand disease (vWD). Spontaneous deep muscle bleeding and joint bleeding (hemorthrosis) suggest deficiency of coagulation factor like hemophilia. Table 47.1 provides a list of causes of bleeding in a child.

Acute onset over a period of days to weeks suggests an acquired disorder like idiopathic thrombocytopenic purpura (ITP) or vitamin K deficiency. Long history of bleeding suggests disorders like hemophilia or vWD. In congenital

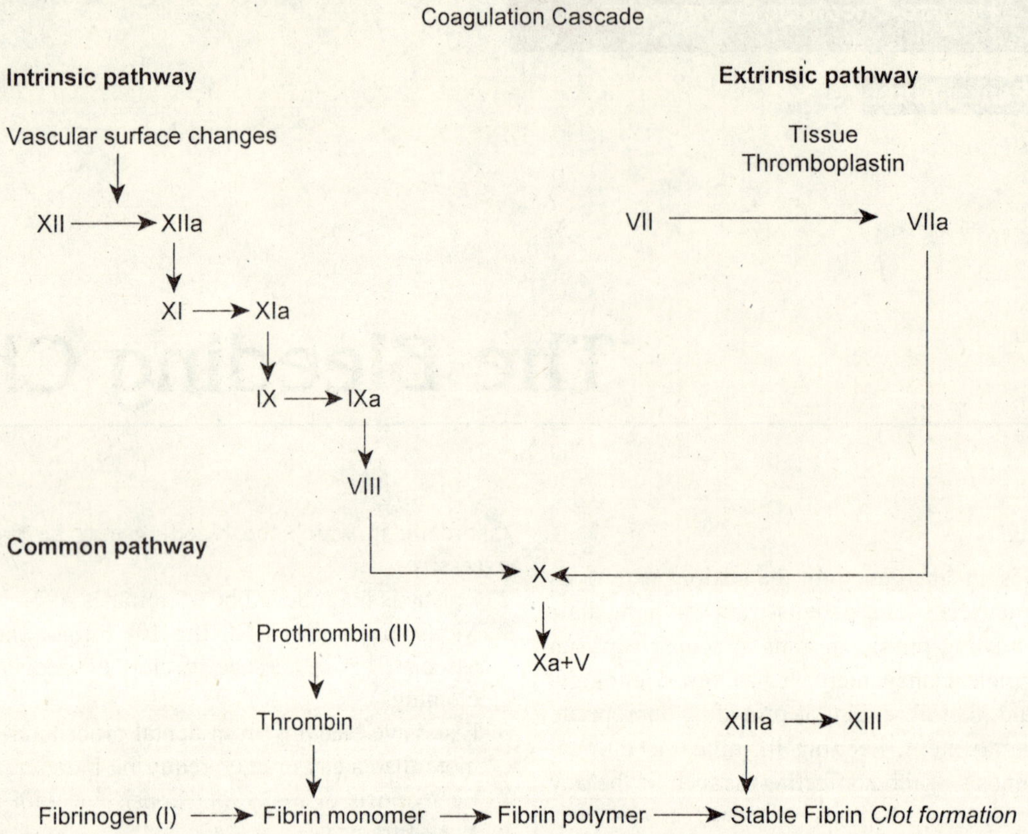

Fig. 47 1: A simplified version of the coagulation "cascade". An abnormality in the extrinsic pathway results in a prolonged prothrombin time (PT). An abnormality in the intrinsic pathway results in a prolonged activated partial thromboplastin time (aPTT). An abnormality in the common pathway results in prolongation of PT and aPTT.

bleeding disorders, an infant may also present after circumcision or immunization but he usually manifests after he gets mobile and experiences mild trauma. Mild bleeding disorders may present with bleeding only after getting sufficient hemostatic challenge following trauma, surgery, dental extraction or menstruation. In some children, there is good initial hemostasis, followed by persistent oozing due to failure to form a good clot. This type of bleeding may present in factor XIII deficiency or disorder of fibrinolytic pathway.

General condition and overall health of patient may also give good clue to etiology. Congenital bleeding disorders and ITP are usually seen in the children who are otherwise well. Disseminated intravascular coagulation (DIC) usually occurs in sick children. Liver disease often associated with deficiency of coagulation factors, will also have associated clinical features and complications. Persistent diarrhea and malabsorption may lead to bleeding due to vitamin K deficiency. Renal disease may lead to bleeding due to abnormality of platelet functions.

Physical examination of the patient may also give further clues to diagnosis. Platelet related bleeding presents with purpura, petechiae and bleeding from mucous membranes. A child who has severe anemia without any liver or spleen enlargement is likely to have aplastic anemia, whereas a child with enlarged lymph nodes and significantly enlarged liver and spleen is likely to have acute leukemia. In Ehlers-Danlos syndrome, patient has skin hyperelasticity, joint hypermobility and fragility of skin and blood vessels.[5] In Henoch-Schönlein purpura, there is IgA-mediated systemic vasculitis. The patient has non-thrombocytopenic purpura, abdominal pain, arthritis and nephritis. The purpura is palpable. Patient with bleeding diathesis may bleed in flanks, abdomen or back. Such patients may have bruises and hemarthrosis. The possibility of child abuse must be excluded in any child presenting with large hematomas and bruises. Platelet count and coagulation studies are normal in these cases.

Mild transient nonthrombocytopenic purpura may result from measles, scarlet fever or typhoid. Meningococcaemia and rickettsial diseases may cause direct damage to blood vessels causing purpura. Violent coughing, vomiting or strangling may cause petechiae in the head and neck area. Psychogenic purpura (Gardner-Diamond syndrome) is

Table 47.1: Causes of bleeding in a child (Post-neonatal)

Thrombocytopenia

1. *Increased platelet destruction.*
   Immune thrombocytopenic purpura (ITP),
   Drug induced immune thrombocytopenia–valproic acid, quinidine, sulfonamide
   Viruses- AIDS, CMV, herpesvirus
   Post-transfusion purpura, Hemolytic-uremic syndrome
   DIC- sepsis, snakebite, giant hemangioma, malignancy, purpura fulminans
2. *Decreased platelet production.*
   Thrombocytopenia absent radii (TAR) syndrome, Fanconi anemia, Wiscott-Aldrich syndrome, Infections,
   Drug reactions (alkylating agents, antimetabolites, anticonvulsants, diuretics),
   Bone marrow infiltration (leukemia, histiocytosis, myelofibrosis, storage disorder, Neuroblastoma, granulomatosis)
3. *Sequestration of platelets.* Splenomegaly, giant hemangioma (Kasabach-Merritt)

Platelet Dysfunction

1. *Congenital*
   Glanzmann's thrombasthenia, Bernard-Soulier syndrome
2. *Acquired.*
   Drugs (Aspirin, furosemide, nitrofurantoin, some NSAID, heparin)
   Uremia, chronic liver disease, FDPs

Coagulation Factor Deficiencies

1. Hereditary
   Hemophilia (factor VIII, IX, XI), von-Willebrand disease
2. Acquired
   DIC, Circulating anticoagulants, Liver disease, Vitamin K deficiency, Uremia

Vascular Factors

1. *Congenital*
   Hereditary telangiectasia, Ehlers-Danlos syndrome
2. *Acquired*
   Henoch-Schoenlein purpura, Infection, Mechanical causes

characterized by spontaneous painful ecchymoses in patients having psychological instability.[6]

Acute ITP is usually preceded by viral infection and occurs in age group of 2 to 4 years. Chronic ITP is more likely to occur in teenage females and has more insidious onset. Post-transfusion purpura is characterized by onset about five to fourteen days after a transfusion.[7] In hemolytic-uremic syndrome there is thrombocytopenia as well as impaired aggregation of platelets. TAR syndrome is an autosomal recessive trait. It may present in first few days of life. Wiscott-Aldrich syndrome is characterized by thrombocytopenia, eczema and recurrent infections. It is transmitted as X-linked recessive trait.

In Glanzmann's disease there is defective platelet aggregation. It is an autosomal recessive disorder. Bernard-Soulier disease is an autosomal recessive trait caused by deficiency of platelet membrane protein Ib and factor X and V.[5]

LABORATORY DIAGNOSIS

The initial workup must include CBC, peripheral blood smear, prothrombin time (PT) and activated partial thromboplastin time (aPTT). Subsequent tests can be decided later.

CBC

Rapid determination can exclude thrombocytopenia. Degree of anemia can give the idea of duration of blood loss. Patients with chronic bleeding disorder may have severe anemia. Anemia, thrombocytopenia and leucocyte abnormalities may indicate aplastic anemia, leukemia etc.

Peripheral Blood Smear

Low platelet count may be confirmed. Clumping of platelets may cause falsely low automated counts, which can be excluded by smear examination. Platelet morphology can also be seen in a smear. On a well-prepared slide, each platelet in a 100´ field contributes approximately 15000/mL to the platelet count.[8] In Bernard-Soulier syndrome, majority of platelets are of size similar or larger than the erythrocytes. In ITP, both small and large platelets can be seen. In Wiscott-Aldrich syndrome, platelets are smaller than normal.

PT and aPTT

PT evaluates extrinsic and common pathways of coagulation whereas aPTT evaluates intrinsic and common pathways. PT is prolonged in vitamin K deficiency. Prolongation of aPTT indicates circulating anticoagulant, presence of inhibitor or factor deficiency. The factor level at which either PT or aPTT gets prolonged is usually around 40% of normal pooled plasma levels for any given factor.[9]

aPTT and PT Mixing Studies

By mixing equal volumes of a patients plasma with normal plasma, any factor deficiency can be corrected to minimum of 50% level. In a factor deficiency, PT and aPTT can become normal after mixing studies. Persistent prolonged tests indicate presence of inhibitors (antibodies against one or more coagulation factors).[10] Most of inhibitors are transient in nature and return to normal level after viral infection subsides.

Coagulation Factor Assays

This is done by modifying PT or aPTT, depending on factor being investigated. The result is expressed as a percentage of activity seen in normal plasma.

Thrombin Time

It is time required to form a clot when thrombin is added to plasma. It is a measure of fibrin formation. Its prolongation suggests low fibrinogen activity, presence of fibrin degradation/split products or heparin contamination.

APPROACH TO MANAGEMENT

Appropriate management of a bleeding child consists of the following:

Proper Diagnosis

The diagnosis is likely to influence the treatment. In ITP there is thrombocytopenia but physician may prefer to wait for evaluation before rushing for specific therapy, whereas, in hemophilia, one may have to transfuse fresh frozen plasma (FFP)/cryoprecipitate/factor VIII at the earliest.

Emergency Measures

A bleeding patient is usually brought in casualty and may require emergency management.

Anemia and shock: Patient with severe anemia and hypovolemic shock will require packed cells or whole blood transfusion to tide over the crisis. If severe anemia is present, the child may be transfused packed cell transfusion (about 5-10 ml/kg), otherwise whole blood may be transfused. A partial exchange transfusion may be done if patient is having incipient or overt presentation of congestive heart failure. Whole blood is transfused when patient requires red blood cells, as well as restoration of blood volume. The so-called "fresh whole blood"(<24 hrs old) does not provide sufficient platelets and clotting factor to the recipient. Almost 90% of platelets and 40 percent of activity of factor VIII are lost within 24 hours of storage at 4°C. Specific components of blood should be used as per the requirement in different etiologies.

Thrombocytopenia: Patients with platelet (PLT) counts less than 50×10^9/L are given platelet transfusion, when they are bleeding. It is observed that chances of spontaneous bleeding increase markedly in patients with thrombocytopenia and bone marrow failure, when platelet level falls below 20×10^9/L. For this reason, many pediatricians give PLT transfusion, when PLT count falls below 20×10^9/L. Some favor PLT transfusion when count falls to 5-10 $\times$ 10^9/L.

In qualitative platelet disorders, PLT transfusions are justified only if significant bleeding is there. Repeated PLT transfusions may lead to alloimmunization and refractoriness. Prophylactic PLT transfusions are justified only if some invasive procedure is planned. Desmopressin acetate may be used as alternative therapy.

The goal of most of platelet transfusions in a child (post-neonatal) is to raise PLT count to greater than 50×10^9/L. This can be achieved by transfusing 10 ml/kg of standard platelet concentrates in children weighing 30 kg. In larger children, 4-6 pooled concentrates from whole blood units may be transfused. Platelets must be transfused as rapidly as possible and certainly within 2 hrs.

Treatment of complications: Some of patients may have complications like intra-cranial hemorrhage or renal failure, which are to be managed accordingly.

Specific Treatment

Patient is given specific therapy depending on the diagnosis.

Thrombocytopenia

ITP: In idiopathic thrombocytopenic purpura (ITP), patients may require observation before being administered specific therapy. Patient of acute ITP with severe bleeding episodes are given steroids or intravenous gammaglobulins. Oral prednisolone in the dose of 1-4 mg/kg has been used for years. It is used for 2-3 weeks are till the platelet count improves. Rapid tapering is done to avoid long-term side effects. Alternatively patient may be administered intravenous immunoglobulin (IVGG) in a dose of 0.8 to 1 g/kg/day × 1-2 day. IVGG induces rapid rise in platelet count to $>20 \times 10^9$/L in 95% of patients within 48 hrs. In non-responders to steroids or IVGG therapy, patients with uncontrolled bleeding and chronic ITP patients; splenectomy is indicated.

In other causes of thrombocytopenia, the causative drug has to be stopped or the primary cause has to be treated.

Platelet Functional Disorders

Management is supportive. Drugs, which impair the platelet functions are avoided. Hormonal therapy may be used to control menorrhagia. Platelet transfusions are indicated to control the bleeding.

Coagulation Factor Deficiencies

Hemophilia A and B are the most common inherited bleeding disorders. These account for 80-90 % of coagulation disorders. Though they require very comprehensive management, prompt replacement therapy is urgently required in a bleeding child in hospital casualty. It controls bleeding and prevents musculo-skeletal deformities. Patient requires either cryoprecipitate or factor VIII concentrate. As factor VIII concentrate is expensive in India, patient may be given fresh frozen plasma (FFP) or cryoprecipitate. FFP is useful in mild bleeding episodes. One unit of FFP provides one unit of factor VIII and IX along with other plasma factors. FFP usually alone is not helpful in intra-cranial bleeding, hemarthrosis or large intra-muscular hemorrhages. Cryoprecipitate contains factor VIII-C, von Willebrand factor activity, fibrinogen and factor XIII. Single bag of cryoprecipitate contains approximately 100 units of F VIII-C. Cryoprecipitate is prepared from single units and is therefore more safe from blood transmitted infections. In developed countries, factor VIII and IX are the mainstay of treatment in severe hemophilia A and B, as these are easily available, and are not very expensive. When bleeding occurs, factor VIII level must be raised to hemostatic levels (35-40%) or for major bleeds to 100% (100 U/dl). Mild to moderate hemophilia A and von Willebrand's disease can be controlled with desmopressin acetate (DDAVP).

Acquired causes of coagulation factor deficiencies like DIC, liver disease, uremia, vitamin K deficiency can be managed by treating the precipitating/underlying cause and providing the supportive therapy.

Vascular Factors

Hereditary hemorrhagic telangiectasia may require surgical management in addition to management of anemia. Ehlers-Danlos may require supportive therapy and platelet transfusion. Intestinal hemorrhage in Henoch-Schoenlein purpura may show dramatic response to corticosteroids. Patients with infection should be managed with appropriate antibiotics.

REFERENCES

1. Duerst RE. Petechiae and purpura. In: Hockelman RA, Friedman SB, Nelson NM, Seidel HM (eds) *Primary Pediatric Care,* 2nd edn. St. Louis: Mosby Year Book, 1992;1023-1027.
2. Lee CA. Women and inherited bleeding disorders: menstrual issues. *Semin Hematol* 1999;36(Suppl 4): 21-27.
3. Kadir R. Women and inherited bleeding disorders: pregnancy and delivery. *Semin Hematol* 1999;36 (Suppl 4):28-35.
4. Kadir RA, Economides DL, Sabin CA, et al. Frequency of inherited bleeding disorders in women with menorrhagia. *Lancet* 1998;351:485-489.
5. Karayalcin G, Paley C, Redner A, Shende A. Disorders of platelets. In: Lanzkowski P (ed) *Manual of Pediatric Hematology and Oncology,* 2nd edn. New York: Churchill Livingstone 1995;185-238.
6. Moll S. Psychogenic purpura. *Am J Hematol* 1997; 55:146-147.
7. McCrae KR, Herman JH. Post-transfusion purpura: Two unusual cases and a literature review. *Am J Hematol* 1996;52:205-211.
8. Buchanan GR. Quantitative and qualitative platelet disorders. *Clin Lab Med* 1999;5:40-48.
9. Cook CS. Routine and special laboratory evaluation of coagulation. In: Stiene-Martin EA, Lotspeich-Steininger CA, Koepke JA (eds) *Clinical Hematology: Principles, Procedures, Correlations.* Philadelphia: Lippincott-Raven 1998;635-649.
10. Geoffrey AA, Glader B. Approach to the bleeding child. *Pediatr Clin North Am* 2002;49:1239-1256.

Shailesh A Kanvinde

48 Idiopathic Thrombocytopenic Purpura (ITP)

INTRODUCTION

Idiopathic thrombocytopenic purpura (ITP), also referred to as primary immune thrombocytopenic purpura, is a disorder characterized by destruction of platelets *via* an immune process directed against variable platelet antigens. ITP is one of the most common causes of thrombocytopenia in pediatric practice. It is referred to as "acute" if the episode resolves within 6 months, and "chronic" if it persists beyond this period. The episodes may also be "recurrent".

ETIOPATHOGENESIS

ITP results due to platelet destruction by an immune process.[1,2] Antibodies to various platelet antigens (GP IIb/IIIa, Ib/IX, Ia/IIa, V, IV, etc.) have been identified. The primary site of antibody production is the spleen, with some contribution from the bone marrow. The platelet-antibody complex is cleared by tissue macrophages. In compensation for the reduced platelet life-span, there is an increase in platelet production, as evidenced by increased bone marrow megakaryocytes. The residual platelets in ITP are larger and younger, with preserved function, resulting in better hemostatic control, compared with patients of aplastic anemia for equivalent platelet counts.[1] However, in some cases, thrombocytopenia may occur due to impaired platelet production, destruction of antibody coated platelets by intramedullary macrophages, or as a result of antibodies directed against later stages of differentiation of megakaryocytes.[3]

In most cases, it is not possible to identify a specific cause for the immunological disturbance (hence "idiopathic"). It is not clear whether this is an abnormal host response to normal platelet antigens, a normal immune response to altered platelet antigens or deposition of antigen-antibody complexes on the platelet surface (as in drug-related ITP).

History of systemic viral infection in the preceeding weeks is often present, but as such infections are common in childhood, it is difficult to attribute a causal relationship. Typical ITP has been described following common viral illnesses of childhood, like varicella, CMV, EBV, hepatitis A, B or C, parvovirus and rubella infections, as well as following use of live attenuated vaccines.[1,2] HIV infection is also an important association.[4]

ITP may also occur in association with other disorders (secondary ITP) such as systemic lupus erythrematosus (SLE), autoimmune thyroiditis, and IgA deficiency.[1,2] These secondary causes account for only about 3-5 % of all cases. H. pylori infection has also been postulated to contribute to development and/or persistence of ITP in infected individuals.[5,6] However, the data in this regard is still conflicting. Table 48.1 lists some of the associations of ITP.

Table 48.1: ITP: Etiological factors/associations

Idiopathic

Secondary (4-5% of all cases)

- Systemic Lupus erythrematosus
- Infections: HIV, hepatitis A, B, C, parvovirus, varicella, rubella, H. pylori
- Malignancies: Hodgkin's disease
- Drugs: vaccines, penicillin, sulphonamides
- IgA deficiency
- Other autoimmune disorders: thyroiditis, myasthenia gravis
- Chronic graft versus host disease

CLINICAL FEATURES

A typical case of acute ITP presents with sudden onset of purpura in a previously healthy child. History should include the type, severity and duration of bleeding, hemostasis with prior invasive procedures, occurrence of systemic viral infection in recent past and recent vaccination or drug ingestion. Risk factors for HIV status should be assessed. Family history of thrombocytopenia or other hematological disorders should be assessed. Clinical examination should be normal, except for the bleeding manifestations.

Lymphadenopathy and hepatomegaly are absent. Presence of a palpable splenic tip (seen in 10% of normal children) does not go against the diagnosis of ITP. However, larger splenomegaly should be viewed with suspicion and would point towards a diagnosis other than ITP. One should also look for skeletal anomalies and auditory acuity to detect specific congenital syndromes such as Fanconi anemia, Thrombocytopenia–absent radius, Alports syndrome, etc.

In addition to purpura, the child may have gum bleeding, oral mucosal blisters (hemorrhagic), epistaxis, malena (usually secondary to epistaxis) and hematuria. Intracranial bleeding is a feared complication, occurring in about 0.5-1% cases (vide infra). Retinal hemorrhages are a strong predictor of subsequent intracranial bleeds, and should be routinely looked for. Subconjunctival hemorrhages and skin/palatal petechiae are not predictive of intracranial bleeds. Menorrhagia is rarely a problem in acute ITP, but could pose significant problems in chronic ITP.

INVESTIGATIONS

As there is no "gold standard" test for diagnosis of ITP, diagnosis is based on history, physical examination and complete blood count, to exclude other causes of thrombocytopenia. Except for thrombocytopenia, the complete hemogram is essentially normal. Peripheral blood smear usually shows large platelets. Giant platelets (almost the size of RBCs) are not a feature of ITP and their presence should indicate other disorders like Bernard Soulier syndrome. In a typical case, bone marrow evaluation is not considered necessary (provided IVIg and not steroids are first line of therapy).[7] The risk of acute leukemia presenting as isolated thrombocytopenia (rest of the hemogram normal, no lymphadenopathy or hepatosplenomegaly) is < 0.1%.[1] Bone marrow evaluation should be done if the clinical presentation is atypical, if the non-platelet lineages of the hemogram are abnormal, or if the patient fails to respond to initial treatment.[7,8] Bone marrow examination will show normal cellularity, with normal or increased number of megakaryocytes.

Table 48.2: Diagnosis of ITP

Features consistent	*Features not consistent*
Clinical	
Skin and mucous membrane bleeding	Delayed bleeding Following trauma
Absence of lymphadenopathy and hepatosplenomegaly	Joint bleeding Lymphadenopathy, hepatosplenomegaly Sick look, fatigue, lassitude Congenital skeletal anomalies
Laboratory	
Thrombocytopenia	Giant platelets
Large platelets	Leukopenia, blasts
Normal RBC morphology	Schistocytes, nucleated RBCs, macrocytes.
Normal WBC counts and morphology	

Patients having thrombocytopenia as the sole manifestation of SLE behave as and are to be treated as any other case of ITP. Hence, routine testing for SLE is not warranted unless there are additional clinical evidences of SLE.[1,7]

Testing for HIV should be done in patients who are considered "at risk". Coagulation function tests like prothrombin time and activated partial thromboplastin time are not indicated. Although anti-platelet antibodies are detectable in 80% cases, lack of specificity makes testing unreliable.[1,9]

MANAGEMENT

Management of ITP is primarily directed towards prevention and treatment of hemorrhage. Significant bleeding rarely occurs with platelet counts > 20,000/cmm. As there is no conclusive evidence that pharmacological treatment of ITP changes the natural history of the disease or hastens remission, treatment is directed towards maintaining a platelet count of > 20,000-30,000/cmm ("safe limit"). A critical issue is determining which patients of ITP require treatment, either at diagnosis or later. Selection of an appropriate treatment option will depend on the risk of hemorrhage at any given point of time, the toxicity and cost of treatment, comorbid conditions (HIV, SLE, etc.), as well as parental anxiety.

General Measures

Hospitalization is indicated with initial platelet counts < 20,000/cmm, even if there is no bleeding. Patients may be discharged once there is evidence of recovery of platelet counts to the "safe limit". Drugs such as NSAIDs, which affect platelet function, should be avoided. Measures to avoid trauma must be adopted. Contact sports should be avoided if platelet counts are less than 50,000/cmm.

Non Interventional Approach

Observation alone would be appropriate for a child with minimal or no bleeding and platelet counts > 20,000/cmm, whereas treatment should be advocated for a child with mucous membrane bleeding, or platelet count < 10,000/cmm. Children with ITP who are managed with observation alone show a spontaneous rise in platelet count to > 20,000/cmm by a median time of 4 days and > 50,000/cmm by a median time 16 days.[7,10-12] Risk of intracranial bleeding in this group is < 0.9%.

Steroids

Glucocorticoids impair clearance of antibody coated platelets by tissue macrophages, inhibit antibody production and increase platelet production by inhibiting phagocytosis of platelets by bone marrow macrophages.[1] Various treatment schedules have been used:[7,10,13,14]

Prednisolone 2 mg/kg/day for 21 days.

Prednisolone 4 mg/kg/day for 7 days, taper over next 14 days (total 21 days).

Methylprednisolone 10-30 mg/kg/day for 3 days.

The potential adverse effects of glucocorticoid therapy include weight gain, hyperglycemia, hypertension and seizures. The toxicities of glucocorticoids are dose and duration dependent. Long-term use is associated with growth retardation, cataracts and osteoporosis. Short courses of steroids are usually well tolerated and are inexpensive, compared to the other agents. The mean time to reduce platelet count > 20,000/cmm is 48 hours, marginally longer than that obtained with IVIg (24 hours).[10,15] Higher doses of steroids produce faster platelet increments almost equivalent to those produced with IVIg.[13,16]

Immunoglobulins (IVIg)

IVIg impairs clearance of IgG coated platelets by competing for FcRIIa receptors of tissue macrophages and by upregulating FcRIIb, the inhibitory Fc receptor.[1] Single dose of 0.8 g/kg is as effective as 2 g/kg given over 5 days.[7,14] Rapid platelet increments are usually seen (within 24 hours). IVIg can produce platelet responses even in splenectomized patients. Toxicity is usually mild. Headache, aseptic meningitis, direct antiglobulin test positive hemolytic anemia, thrombosis and anaphylaxis (especially in IgA deficient individuals) have been reported following IVIg administration.[1,7]

The major limitation of IVIg therapy is exorbitant cost.

Anti-D

Administration of anti-D to Rh (D) positive individuals results in a mild hemolytic anemia. These anti-D coated RBCs compete with antibody coated platelets for FcRIII receptor of tissue macrophages (distinct from site of action of IVIg), thereby preventing/reducing platelet destruction. As evident from the mechanism of action, anti-D therapy will not be useful for Rh (D) negative patients. Response rates with 50 mg/kg are slower (72 hours to platelet counts > 20,000/cmm) than IVIg or steroids,[14,17] but use of higher doses of 75 mg/kg produces equivalent response rates as IVIg.[18] Anti-D is more convenient to administer (over 5-10 min.) than IVIg, and is less expensive. It is especially useful in HIV positive individuals.

Limitations of treatment include occurrence of hemolytic anemia (mean drop in Hb 1-2 gm%) and ineffectiveness in splenectomized patients.[17] Rare cases of intravascular hemolysis with hemoglobinuria have been described.[19]

Splenectomy

Splenectomy is an effective treatment for ITP, producing remissions in approximately 75% cases (children and adults).[1,7,20,21] It is a common procedure for steroid/IVIG failures in adults, but its use in the pediatric population is quite restricted, for 2 reasons. First, unlike adults where spontaneous remissions are infrequent, about 70-80% of children will achieve complete remission by 1 year after diagnosis.[1,2,22] Hence, provided that the clinical situation permits, it is worthwhile to wait for spontaneous remission to occur rather than subject the child to early splenectomy. Secondly, there is a risk of mortality (1-2%) due to fulminant post-splenectomy sepsis, especially in children less than 5 years of age.[2,20] The benefit of splenectomy (avoiding the 1% risk of death due to intracranial bleed) has to be weighed against this risk of sepsis. Patients with persistent bleeding problems 12 months after diagnosis would be reasonable candidates for the procedure. Very rarely, splenectomy may be required for management of acute ITP not responding to initial treatment (steroids, IVIg) and having life-threatening bleeding problem. Children undergoing splenectomy should receive prophylactic polyvalent pneumococcal, H.influenzae and meningococcal vaccines, as well as lifelong antimicrobial prophylaxis with penicillin.[1,8]

Splenectomy may be done by an open or laproscopic approach. Advantages of the latter include shorter hospital stay and lesser bleeding complications.[20,23]

Role of Platelet Transfusions

Transfused platelets have a very short *in vivo* life-span in patients with ITP and are not very useful in routine cases. Their use is restricted for the emergency situation like intracranial bleeding, where they are given along with IVIg and steroids.[1] An initial bolus of 5-10 units/m2 BSA, followed by a continuous infusion, is recommended.

Selection of Therapy

As stated above, children with minimal bleeding and platelet counts more than 20,000/cmm may be safely observed without any pharmacological therapy. Those with mucous membrane bleeding or counts less than 10,000/cmm should receive therapy. IVIg has generally been considered the drug of choice as it produces overnight platelet increments in the majority.[7,10,13,15] However, IV methylprednisolone (10-30 mg/kg) and anti-D (75 microgram/kg) have also been shown to produce similar results at a lesser cost.[7,13,24] Lower doses of steroids (prednisolone 4 mg/kg/day) are also useful agents, especially in developing countries where cost of therapy is a major concern, producing platelet increments within 48 hours to "safe limits". In emergency situations like intracranial bleeding, it is judicious to use more than 1 agent (IVIg plus IV methylpred dnisolone), in combination with platelet transfusions.[1,24] If there is an unsatisfactory response, emergency splenectomy may be required, especially if craniotomy becomes necessary.[24] Table 48.3 compares the efficacy of the various treatment options.

Table 48.3: Comparative efficacy of treatment options in acute ITP

Treatment Option	Median time (days) to achieve platelet count	
	> 20,000/cmm	> 50,000/cmm
Noninterventional approach[7,10-12]	4	16
Prednisolone 4 mg/kg/day for 7 days, taper and omit over next 14 days[7,10,14,15]	2	4
IV Methylprednisolone[7,16] 10-30 mg/kg/day for 3 days	1-2	3-4
IVIg 0.8 gm/kg single dose[7,14]	1	2
Anti-D 50 microgram/kg[7,14,17,18]	4	7
Anti-D 75 microgram/kg[18]	1	—

Management of Patients with Persistent Bleeding

Children who do not respond to initial "standard" treatment, or those who relapse after an initial response, would need additional therapy. Various treatment options are available, used either to defer splenectomy, or to salvage post splenectomy failures. Splenectomy should be done if bleeding symptoms persist for more than 12 months after diagnosis, or if the quality of life is affected as a result of the thrombocytopenia.

Intermittent Doses of "Standard" Therapy

Intermittent doses of IVIG, anti-D or steroids once every 3-4 weeks are useful to achieve remission or maintain platelet counts > 20-30,000/cmm. Anti-D is especially useful in HIV positive patients, where steroids and splenectomy are to be avoided as much as possible. Pulse dexamethasone (40 mg/kg/day for 4 days, 6 such cycles) has been shown to achieve durable platelet counts > 1,00,000/cmm.[7,25,26]

Azathioprine

It is an immunosuppressive agent, used in the dose 1-2 mg/kg/day. Response rates of 30-50% are reported, but it may take 4-8 months to achieve maximum effect. Hematological and liver dysfunction are important acute toxicities. Long- term use may have carcinogenic or teratogenic effects.

Rituximab (Anti CD 20 Monoclonal Antibody)

Recent reports indicate a very promising role for this agent in management of resistant cases of ITP.[27,28] It is administered in the dose of 375 mg/m2 IV weekly for 4 doses. About 50% of cases show a durable response. Toxicity is mild (infusional side-effects). It is useful in both splenectomized and non-splenectomized patients. Cost of treatment with this drug is a major limiting factor for its use.

Cyclosporine

There is still limited data regarding its efficacy in management of resistant ITP. Response rates appear to be high, but relapses are common once the drug is omitted. Toxicities such as hypertension, renal dysfunction and bodyache occur in about 30% cases. It may be useful to postpone splenectomy.[29-31]

Danazol

Danazol, a weak androgen, acts by impairing macrophage mediated clearance of antibody coated platelets, as well as inhibition of antibody production. It is given in the dose of 10-15 mg/kg/day for atleast 6 months. Remissions usually require continuing drug administration, with relapses occurring weeks to months after it is omitted. It is useful mainly to postpone splenectomy. Toxicity is mainly hepatic (hepatitis, peliosis and neoplasia).

Cyclophosphamide

Cyclophosphamide may be used alone or in combination with other agents like prednisolone and vincristine. Although it produces responses in 80% cases, with over half of them being durable, use of this agent is restricted in view of its potential toxicity (bone marrow suppression, infertility, predisposition for malignancies, etc.)[32]

Vinca Alkaloids

These agents bind to platelets, which get delivered to the macrophages. Inhibition of phagocytic capabilities of the macrophages is believed to be the mechanism of action of these agents in ITP. Responses are seen in only about 20% cases. Treatment is necessary every 2-4 weeks for an indefinite period. Toxicity is mainly neurological (vincristine) or hematological (vinblastine).[1]

Intracranial Bleeding

Intra-cranial bleeding is a devastating complication of ITP, occurring in 0.1-0.5% cases, with approximately 50% mortality. About 40-50% cases occur within the first 4 weeks, but may occur at any time during the course of acute or chronic ITP, whenever the platelet count drops below 10,000-15,000/cmm.[24,33,34] In addition to low platelet counts, head injury, AV malformations and NSAID usage predispose to its development.[24,33]

The location and extent of bleeding influences subsequent management. Supratentorial bleeds are associated with gradually progressive deterioration in consciousness and neurodeficits, while infratentorial bleeding causes catastrophic deterioration with cerebellar herniation and brainstem compression. Management is directed towards assessing location and extent of bleeding (CT scan) and rapidly increasing the platelet count. Platelet transfusions, IVIg and IV methylprednisolone are used in combination for additive effect.[8] Emergency craniotomy (with splenectomy) is indicated in all patients with progressive neurological deterioration or with posterior fossa bleeding.[24,35]

The outcome is not always hopeless, with about 50% patients surviving with minimal neurodeficit.

PROGNOSIS

About 70-80 % of children < 16 years of age recover completely within the first 6 months.. Features of the presenting illness that are associated with an increased risk of chronic persistent thrombocytopenia include

- A history of purpura for more than 2 to 4 weeks before diagnosis,
- Female sex,
- Age over 10 years, and
- A higher platelet count at presentation.[7]

Amongst the patients who develop chronic ITP, more than two-thirds eventually recover over the next few months or years, either spontaneously or after splenectomy. Mortality rates are low (1-2%) and are, either due to intracranial bleeding or post-splenectomy sepsis. Overall, only about 5% of children presenting with ITP have persistent bleeding symptoms, even after splenectomy.

REFERENCES

1. Bussel J, Cines D. Immune thrombocytopenic purpura, neonatal alloimmune thrombocytopenia, and posttransfusion purpura. In: Hoffman R, Benz EJ, Shattil SJ, Furie B, Cohen HJ, Silberstein LE, McGlave P (eds) *Hematology: Basic Principles and Practice*, 3rd edn. Philadelphia: Churchill Livingstone 2000;2096-2114.
2. Di Paola JA, Buchanan GR. Immune thrombocytopenic purpura. In: Vichinsky E, Walters M, Feusner J (eds) *Pediatr Clin North Am* 2002;49:911-928.
3. Ballem PJ, Segal GM, Stratton JR, et al. Mechanisms of thrombocytopenia in chronic autoimmune thrombocytopenic purpura. Evidence of both impaired production and increased platelet clearance. *J Clin Invest* 1987;80:33-40.
4. Murphy M F, Metcalfe P, Waters A H, et al. Incidence and mechanism of neutropenia and thrombocytopenia in patients with human immunodeficiency virus infection. *Br J Hemat* 1987;66:337-340.
5. Gasbarrini A, Francechi F, Tartaglione R, Landolfi R, Pola P, Gasbarrini G. Regression of autoimmune thrombocytopenia after eradication of Helicobacter pylori. *Lancet* 1998;352:878.
6. Emilia G, Longo G, Lippi M, et al. Helicobacter pylori eradication can induce platelet recovery in idiopathic thrombocytopenic purpura. *Blood* 2001;97:812-814.
7. George J, Woolf S, Raskob G, et al. Idiopathic thrombocytopenic purpura: Practice guideline developed by explicit methods for the American Society of Hematology. *Blood* 1996;88:3-40.
8. Eden OB, Lilleyman JS, on behalf of the British Pediatric Hematology Group. Guidelines for management of idiopathic thrombocytopenic purpura. *Arch Dis Child* 1992;67:1056-1058.
9. Mueller-Eckhardt C, Mueller-Eckhardt G, Kayser W, Voss RM, Wegner J, Kuenzlen E. Platelet associated IgG, platelet survival and platelet sequestration in thrombocytopenic states. *Br J Hemat* 1982;52:49-58.
10. Blanchette VS, Luke B, Andrew M, et al. A prospective, randomized trial of high dose intravenous immune globulin G therapy, oral prednisolone therapy and no therapy in childhood acute immune thrombocytopenic purpura. *J Pediatr* 1993:123:984-995.
11. Dickerhoff R, von Ruecker A. The clinical course of immune thrombocytopenic purpura in children who did not receive intravenous immunoglobulins or sustained prednisolone treatment. *J Pediatr* 2000;137:629-632.
12. George JN. Initial management of immune thrombocytopenic purpura in children: Is supportive counseling without therapeutic intervention sufficient? *J Pediatr* 2000;137:598-600.
13. Albayrak D, Islek I, Kalayu A G, Gurses N. Acute immune thrombocytopenic purpura: A comparative study of very high oral doses of methylprednisolone and intravenously administered immune globulin. *J Pediatr* 1994;125:1004-1007.
14. Blanchette VS, Imbach P, Andrew M, et al. Randomized trial of intravenous immunoglobulin G, intravenous anti-D, and oral prednisolone in childhood acute immune thrombocytopenic purpura. *Lancet* 1994;344:703-707.
15. Imbach P, Berchtold W, Hirt A, et al. Intravenous immunoglobulin versus oral corticosteroids in acute immune thrombocytopenic purpura in childhood. *Lancet* 1985;2:464-68.
16. Ancona KG, Parker RI, Atlas MP, Prakash D. Randomized trial of high-dose methylprednisolone versus intravenous immunoglobulin for the treatment of acute idiopathic thrombocytopenic purpura in children. *J Pediatr Hematol Oncol* 2002;24:540-544.
17. Scaradavou A, Woo B, Woloski BMR, et al. Intravenous anti-D treatment of immune thrombocytopenic purpura: experience in 272 patients. *Blood* 1997; 89:2689-2700.
18. Newman GC, Novoa MV, Fodero EM, Lesser ML, Woloski BMR, Bussel JB. A dose of 75 microgram/kg of i.v. anti-D increases the platelet count more rapidly and for a longer period of time than 50 microgram/kg in adults with immune thrombocytopenic purpura. Br J Hemat 2001;112:1076-1078.
19. Gaines AR. Acute onset hemoglobinemia and/or hemoglobinuria and sequelae following Rh(o)(D) immune globulin intravenous administration in immune thrombocytopenic purpura patients. *Blood* 2000;95:2523-2529.
20. Mantadakis E, Buchanan GR. Elective splenectomy in children with idiopathic thrombocytopenic purpura. *J Pediatr Hematol Oncol* 2000;22:148-153.
21. El-Alfy MS, El-Tawil MM, Shahein N. 5- to 16-year follow-up following splenectomy in chronic immune thrombocytopenic purpura in children. *Acta Haematol* 2003;110:20-4.
22. Tamary H, Kaplinsky C, Levy I, et al. Chronic childhood idiopathic thrombocytopenic purpura: Long term follow-up. *Acta Pediatr* 1994;83:931-934.

23. Cordera F, Long KH, Nagorney DM, et al. Open versus laparoscopic splenectomy for idiopathic thrombocytopenic purpura: clinical and economic analysis. *Surgery* 2003;134:45-52.
24. Medeiros D, Buchanan GR. Current controversies in the management of idiopathic thrombocytopenic purpura during childhood. *Pediatr Clin North Am* 1996;43:759-769.
25. Borgna-Pignatti C, Ruogolotto S, Nobili B, et al. A trial of high-dose dexamethasone therapy for chronic idiopathic thrombocytopenic purpura in childhood. *J Pediatr* 1997;130:13-16.
26. Andersen JC. Response of resistant idiopathic thrombocytopenic purpura to pulsed high-dose dexamethasone therapy. *N Engl J Med* 1994:30:1560-1564.
27. Stasi R, Pagano A, Stipa E, Amadori S. Rituximab chimeric anti-CD 20 monoclonal antibody treatment for adults with chronic idiopathic thrombocytopenic purpura. *Blood* 2001;98:952-2007.
28. Shanafelt TD, Madueme HL, Wolf RC, Tefferi A. Rituximab for immune cytopenia in adults: idiopathic thrombocytopenic purpura, autoimmune hemolytic anemia, and Evans syndrome. *Mayo Clin Proc* 2003; 78:1340-1346.
29. Kappers-Klunne MC, van't Veer MB. Cyclosporin A for the treatment of patients with chronic idiopathic thrombocytopenic purpura refractory to corticosteroids or splenectomy. *Br J Hemat* 2001;114:121-125.
30. Emilia G, Messora C, Longo G, Bertesi M. Long-term salvage treatment by cyclosporin in refractory autoimmune hematological disorders. *Br J Hemat* 1996;93:341-344.
31. Gesundheit B, Cividalli G, Freeman A, Yatziv S, Koren G, Baruchel S. Cyclosporin A in the treatment of refractory immune thrombocytopenia purpura in children. *Eur J Hemat* 2001; 66:347-351.
32. Reiner A, Gernsheimer T, Slichter SJ. Pulse cyclophosphamide therapy for refractory autoimmune thrombocytopenic purpura. *Blood* 1995;85:351-358.
33. Lilleyman JS, on behalf of the Pediatric Hematology Forum of the British Society of Hematology. Intracranial hemorrhage in idiopathic thrombocytopenic purpura. *Arch Dis Child* 1994;71:251-253.
34. Butros LJ, Bussel JB. Intracranial hemorrhage in immune thrombocytopenic purpura: a retrospective analysis. *J Pediatr Hematol Oncol* 2003;25:660-664.
35. Woerner SJ, Abildgaard CF, French BN. Intracranial hemorrhage in children with idiopathic thrombocytopenic purpura. *Pediatrics* 1981:67:453-460.

Ravinder K Gupta and Ritu Gupta

49 Disseminated Intravascular Coagulation (DIC)

INTRODUCTION

Disseminated intravascular coagulation (DIC) is defined as a systemic thrombo-hemorrhagic disorder which is characterized by increased intravascular coagulation with consumption of platelets and plasma clotting factors. Features of intravascular thrombosis and hemorrhagic manifestations are present.

The diagnosis and treatment of this syndrome requires an understanding of its pathogenesis and the precipitating causes and its early recognition for effective management.

PATHOPHYSIOLOGY

DIC occurs following the exaggeration of normal coagulation process. The coagulation system may be triggered by one of the following three major mechanisms:

- Direct activation of factor X by proteolytic enzymes,
- Activation of factor XII, and
- Activation of extrinsic pathway by release of tissue thromboplastin.

Once the clotting system is stimulated, the continuation of clotting mechanism is dependent upon the following three factors viz.:

- Consumption of clotting factors and platelets,
- Thrombin generation, and
- Activation of fibrinolytic system.

Thrombin generation plays the key role in the continuation of coagulation and initiation of fibrinolytic processes leading to DIC. Thrombin itself activates the fibrinolytic system. Fibrin monomers and polymers along with fibrin are degraded to fibrin degradation products and D-dimers. Increased levels of fibrin degradation products (FDP) are highly suggestive of DIC while raised levels of D-dimers are diagnostic of DIC.

Accelerated intravascular coagulation results in diffuse deposition of fibrin and thrombin in the microvasculature. The FDP and fibrin complexes are cleared from the circulation. The FDP has an anticoagulant activity. Process of increased intravascular coagulation results in:

- Increased thromboembolic phenomenon resulting in tissue ischemia and necrosis in multiple organs,
- Depletion of clotting factors and fibrinolysis manifesting widespread bleeding and hemorrhage, and
- Red cell fragmentation resulting in microangiopathic hemolytic anemia.

PREVALENCE AND ETIOLOGY

In the pediatric age group over 50% of cases with DIC occur during the neonatal period. The neonate is more susceptible to develop DIC because of:

a. Frequent occurrence of conditions leading to DIC, and
b. Immaturity of defense mechanism against excessive thrombosis.

The causes of DIC are depicted in Table 49.1.

CLINICAL FEATURES

Types of DIC

The underlying disease that triggers DIC determines the clinical presentation in two aspects. First, the clinical manifestations of the triggering disease itself and second, the magnitude and rate of exposure of the triggering factor depends on the disease. This determines the acuteness of clinical presentation of DIC *per se.* In severe head trauma, burns or sepsis where there is a sudden massive exposure of tissue factor over a brief time period, the control mechanisms are overwhelmed and there is no time for regeneration of coagulation factors. This is referred to as *acute or decompensated* DIC wherein there would be profound bleeding due to consumption of coagulation factors of diffuse microvascular thrombosis with resultant end organ damage or a combination of the two. If, however, the triggering factor is exposed slowly and in small amounts such as in malignancies and vasculitides, the control mechanisms in the body replenish the factors by augmented production. This is referred to as *chronic or compensated DIC* wherein there may be very minimal or no clinical features or there may be

Table 49.1: Etiology of DIC

Infection	
Bacterial	Meningococcus, S. aureus, Pseudomonas, E.coli, Klebsiella, Proteus, H.influenzae, Salmonella.
Viral	Disseminated varicella, measles, cytomegalovirus, acute hepatitis.
Fungal	Candida, histoplasmosis, aspergillus.
Others	Malaria, Rickettsial.
Trauma	Head injury, multiple fractures, crush injury, burns, hypo or hyperthermia.
Hematological disorders	Incompatible blood transfusion, paroxysmal nocturnal hemoglobinuria, sickle cell anemia.
Venoms or toxins	Snake bites, insect bites.
Malignancies	Acute Leukemia (mainly promyelocytic) Neuroblastoma, Histocystosis-X.
Neonatal	Septicemia, birth asphyxia, RDS, hypothermia, necrotising enterocolitis.
Collangen vascular	JRA, acute vasculitis, SLE.
Miscellaneous	Purpura fulminans, congenital malformations giant hemangioma, heat stroke, graft reactions.

only laboratory evidence of DIC. The clinical signs and symptoms in DIC are highly variable in patients with acute DIC. Hemorrhage from multiple sites is the common clinical presentation and is seen in nearly 90% of the cases. It is caused by the generation of free plasmin and depletion of coagulation factors and plasmin. Predominantly microvascular thrombosis is seen in nearly 25% of cases. Clinical manifestations include localized hemorrhages, such as purpura, ecchymosis, easy bruising, bleeding from puncture sites, mucous membrane bleeding, gangrenous skin lesions, renal failure, diarrhea, abdominal distention, ileus, vomiting, respiratory distress, deterioration of consciousness, coma, convulsions, hematuria and oliguria leading to acute renal failure. Pallor or jaundice may occur as a result of hemolytic anemia. Hypotension leading to vascular collapse and shock may manifest in serious cases.

Sudden onset of bleeding from multiple sites associated with thrombocytopenia should suggest DIC. Hypotension is often associated with DIC when it occurs following the activation of factor XII. Clinical manifestations of the underlying conditions and sudden worsening of the child are evident. Diagnosis of DIC requires s high index of suspicion in the above clinical setting and detailed laboratory investigation.

LABORATORY DIAGNOSIS (Table 49.2 and 49.3)

Diagnosis of DIC is based on:

- Platelet utilization;
- Consumption of coagulation factors such as fibrinogen, factor II, V, VIII and XIII;
- Secondary fibrinolysis leading to production of FDP and D-dimers; and
- Microangiopathic hemolytic anemia.

Peripheral blood film in DIC shows fragmented, distorted and contracted red cells along with the presence of schistocytes. Consumption of fibrinogen and various clotting factors (II, V, VIII and XIII) and fibrinolysis results in prolongations of thrombin time, prothrombin time (PT) and partial thromboplastin time (PTT). Fibrinogen levels are reduced and its levels are usually less than 150 mg/dl in 70-80% of patients. Partial thromboplastin time (PTT) and prothrombin time are prolonged while FDP and D-dimers levels are increased.

All children with suspicion of DIC should be screened for DIC through:

Table 49.2: Laboratory profile in DIC

A. Global laboratory tests
   1. Prolongation of PT, aPTT, TT.
   2. Hypofibrinogenemia.
   3. Elevated FDPs.
   4. Peripheral smear: Schistocytes and thrombocytopenia with large platelets.

B. Tests for procoagulant activation
   1. Elevated prothrombin fragment 1 + 2.
   2. Elevated fibrinopeptide A & fibrinopeptide B.
   3. Elevated thrombin–antithrombin (TAT) complex.
   4. Elevated D-dimer and soluble fibrin monomer (sFM).

C. Tests for plasmin activation
   1. Elevated D-dimer & sFM (soluble fibrin monomer).
   2. Elevated fibrinogen degradation products (FDPs).
   3. Elevated plasmin.
   4. Elevated plasmin-anti plasmin complex (PAP).

D. Tests for inhibitor consumption
   1. Decreased antithrombin.
   2. Decreased antiplasmin.
   3. Decreased protein C and S.
   4. Elevated TAT complex.
   5. Elevated PAP complex.

E. Tests for end organ damage
   1. Elevated LDH.
   2. Elevated creatinine.
   3. Decreased pH.
   4. Decreased paO_2.

Table 49.3: Laboratory features of chronic DIC

- Platelet count: Usually normal or borderline.
- Fibrinogen: Normal/increased.
- PT: Normal/supernormal.
- PTT: Normal/supernormal.
- Schistocytes: 90% patients.
- FDP: Usually increased.
- Fibrinopeptide A: Usually increased.
- D-dimer: Usually increased.

a. Detailed clinical examination.
b. Platelet count.
c. Estimation of fibrinogen level and measurement of thrombin time, PT and PTT, and
d. Estimation of FDP and D-dimers levels.

TREATMENT

The most important guiding principle for therapy of DIC in to identify the triggering disease and manage it aggressively. Restoration of fluid balance and reversal of shock, acidosis, electrolyte disturbance, and hypoxia, are important in the management of DIC syndromes.

General measures include:

- All medication should be administered IV.
- Administration of vitamin K (10 mg per day for 3 days) to correct vitamin K dependent factors.

Specific treatment includes:

- Drug therapy to interrupt the clotting process.
- Replacement of coagulation factors and platelets.
- Exchange transfusion to remove the potential triggers and to replace the coagulation factors.

Heparin

Heparin inhibits thrombin formation. It is therefore, more effective in cases with prominent thrombotic manifestations. Heparin therapy is indicated for purpura fulminans, severe DIC with giant hemangioma and promyelocytic leukemia. It is administered in loading dose of 50 units/kg followed by 50-100 units/kg every four hourly. Coagulation factors should become normal if heparin therapy is effective. Heparin therapy should be continued until fibrinogen levels increase over 150 mg/dl and platelet count increases to more than 100,000/ul.

Replacement Therapy

Platelet concentrate along with coagulation factors have been used to replenish the platelets, coagulation factors and antithrombin III levels. Children may be given 10-15 ml/kg of fresh frozen plasma along with 1/2 to 1 unit of platelet concentrates for every 10 kg body weight every 12-24 hourly. Fresh frozen plasma contains fibrinogen and other coagulation factors along with the natural anticoagulants such as antithrombin III and protein C. Platelet counts should be maintained above 50,000/cumm while fibrinogen levels should be maintained above 100 mg/dl. Blood should be administered to correct the anemia. Replacement therapy should be monitored by clinical assessment of bleeding status and laboratory evaluation of DIC. Currently, it forms the mainstay of treatment and it should be continued. Antithrombim III concentrates have been found to be beneficial in treatment of acute DIC if its levels are low. The dose of antithrombin III is calculated every 8 hourly prior to its administration by the formula: (desired level-initial level) × 0.6 × total body weight in kg.

Exchange Transfusion

Exchange transfusion not only provides the factors needed for coagulation but has the added advantage of removing the: (a) circulating FDP (b) activated procoagulants, and (c) toxins. All these factors aggravate bleeding. Double volume exchange transfusion should be performed with fresh blood or with packed red cells suspended in fresh frozen plasma. Platelet concentrates should be administered after the exchange transfusion.

Inhibitors of Excess Fibrinolysis

Inhibitors of fibrinolytic system have been used at times for the management of DIC. Antifibrinolytic drugs (e.g. episilon, aminocaproic acid, aprotinin) may be indicated, if hemorrhage is a major problem. E-aminocaproic acid may be given orally or IV in the doses of 200-300 mg/kg body weight daily every 6-8 hours. Aprotinin may be given in the dose of 500,000 kallikrein inactivator units (KIU) intravenously over 10-15 min initially followed by 200,000 KIU every four hourly.

Gabexate is a synthetic serine protease inhibitor that has an inhibitory effect on several coagulation and fibrinolytic proteases including thrombin and plasmin.

MORTALITY

The prognosis of patient with severe DIC is grave and mortality rates vary between 50-85%. In most patients death occurs secondary to the underlying disease process. Early diagnosis of DIC and identification of its causative factors, along with its prompt treatment are essential for the successful treatment.

REFERENCES

1. Choudhry VP, Thavaraj V, Saraya AK. Disseminated intravascular coagulation: Diagnostic and current therapy. *Indian Pediatr* 1990;27:280-288.
2. Bick R. Disseminated intravascular coagulation and related syndrome: A clinical review. *Thromb Hemost* 1988:14: 299-315.
3. Whaun JM, Oski F. Experience with disseminated intravascular coagulation in a children's hospital. *JAMA* 1972;107:963-967.
5. Miner ME, Graham SH, Cildrnberg PL. Disseminated intravascular coagulation fibrinolytic syndrome following head injury in children: Frequency and prognostic implications. *J Pediatr* 1982;100:687-691.
6. Bakhshi S, Arya LS. Diagnosis and treatment of Disseminated intravascular coagulation. *Indian Pediatr* 2003:8:721-730.
7. Gupte S. Pediatric Hematology. In: Gupte S (ed) *The Short Text book of Pediatrics*, 9th edn. New Delhi: Jaypee Brothers 2001;425-427.
8. Marwaha N, Marwaha RK. Disseminated intravascular coagulation. In: Gupte S (ed) *Recent Advances in Pediatrics (Special Vol. 7: Hematology)* New Delhi: Jaypee Brothers, 2000: 206-216.

AM Graham and Suraj Gupte

50 Oncologic Emergencies

INTRODUCTION

With advances in management of pediatric oncologic disorders, resulting in increasing survival rate, anticipation. Recognition and treatment of complications in such subjects has assumed special significance.

Else, quite a proportion of oncologic pediatric subjects may become victims of such life-threatening emergencies and urgencies, thereby negating the gains of modern treatment.

DEFINITION

By definition, an oncologic emergency is an acute potentially life-threatening event, directly or indirectly related to a patient's neoplasm or its treatment and, left untreated, may cause considerable morbidity and mortality.[1,2] It is likely to be confused with nonneoplastic condition(s) from which differentiation becomes important. Furthermore, it should not only be anticipated but also identified and aggressively treated.

COMMON ONCOLOGIC EMERGENCIES

These may be in relation to space-occupying lesions, abnormalities of blood vessels and metabolic problems.

Superior Vena Cava Syndrome (SVCS)[4-6]

On account of its location in a tight compartment in the right superior mediastinum surrounded by chains of lymph nodes and thymus plus its thin vessel wall and low intravascular pressure, superior vena cava is susceptible to compression, obstruction and thrombosis.

SVCS is an infrequent but serious emergency associated with non-Hodgkin lymphoma (NHL), acute lymphoblastic leukemia (ALL), Hodgkin lymphoma, Ewing sarcoma, rhabdomyosarcoma and germ-cell tumor.

SVCS is characterized by manifestations of compression/obstruction to the superior vena cava in the form of cough, hoarseness, dyspnea, orthopnea, stridor, anxiety, confusion, drowsiness and, at times, unconsciousness. Clinical findings include facial edema including edema of conjunctiva, plethora, cyanosis, engorged veins over neck, chest and arms with collateral vessels. Signs of pleural or pericardial effusion may be present.

Manifestations become worse in supine position or on flexion of the body (as during lumbar puncture). Often, progression of these manifestations is in a matter of hours or days.

Diagnosis is by chest X-rays, CT scan and MRI. Chest X-rays reveal an anterior superior mediastinal mass with or without pleural/pericardial effusion. For finding the extent of compression, CT scan and/or MRI may be needed. Echocardiography demonstrates pericardial effusion.

Treatment is aimed at tiding over the emergency pending histologic confirmation of the diagnosis by biopsy at a later stage. Radiotherapy (with or without steroids) together with chemotherapy is often of value. Else, assuming that the cause may be intracaval thrombosis, urgent throractomy is indicated.

Spinal Cord Compression

Acute spinal cord compression, including compression of cauda equina, may result from local extension or metastasis in such tumors as Ewing sarcoma, neuroblastoma, lymphoma, leukemias, osteogenic sarcoma, soft tissue sarcoma, Wilms tumor, hepatoblastoma, etc. Most often it is seen in terminal stage of the metastatic disease. Yet, it can occur even early.

Manifestations include backache (local or radicular) with localized tenderness, limp secondary to motor weakness, sensory disturbances (including bladder and bowel dysfunction).

Investigations include spinal X-rays, lumbar myelography and MRI.

Treatment consists in prompt IV administration of dexamethasone, 1-2 mg/kg, local radiotherapy, surgical decompression and chemotherapy which is most effective in such chemosensitive malignancies as neuroblastoma, non-Hodgkin's lymphoma, Hodgkin's lymphoma, acute leukemias and Ewing's sarcoma.

Early institution of therapy is the key to prevent permanent neurologic sequelae.

Cardiac Temponade

A proportion of subjects with oncologic disease (especially leukemias and non-Hodgkin lymphoma) develop elevated intraperitoneal pressure to the extent that it interferes with adequate diastolic filling of the heart and, as a consequence, fall in cardiac output.

Manifestations are in the form of cardiovascular involvement, particularly pericardial effusion.

Diagnosis is by high index of suspicion supported by physical examination, X-ray chest, ECG and echocardiography and CT scan of chest. A diagnostic and therapeutic percardiocentesis is an important modality.

Treatment options include pericardiocentesis, surgical decompression, radiotherapy, and chemotherapy. In addition supportive measures such as oxygen administration, maintenance of fluid and electrolyte balance and positioning of the subject to maximize cardiac output are important.

Hyperleukocytosis

In a proportion of children with leukemias, peripheral total leukocyte count may jump to > 100,000/cumm, sometime even 300,000/cumm when risk of morbidity and mortality further increases (Table 50.1).

Table 50.1: Signals of hyperleukocytosis

Intracerebral	Frontal headache
	Convulsions
	Papilledema
	Retinal venous distention
Pulmonary	Dyspnea
	Right ventricular failure
Others	Priapism

Management consists in giving attention to fluid and electrolytes, allopurinal to prevent uric acid nephropathy, cytorduction with exchange transfusion and leukopheresis. Following these measures, specific chemotherapy should be instituted without delay.

Neutropenia

Febrile Neutropenia

Cancer chemotherapy as well as certain hematologic malignancies cause bonemarrow suppression, thereby considerably reducing number of leukocytes (neutropenia), RBCs and platelets. This makes the subject vulnerable to life-threatening superadded infections (Table 50.2) and hemorrhages.

Table 50.2: Superadded infections in oncologic patients

Gram negative	E. coli
	Klebsiella
	Pseudomonas
	Enterobacter spp
Gram positive	Staphylococcus aureus
	Coagulase negative staphylococci
	Streptococcus pneumoniae
Fungi	Candida albicans
	Aspergillus spp
	Mucor

Febrile neutropenia is the most common complication. The count falls below 500/cumm. Once it is under 100/cumm, the risk of sepsis (including fungal infection) becomes very high. Diagnosis is established by blood cultures from both central and peripheral lines, cultures of other body fluids (throat, urine, wound, etc) and chest X-rays.

Early institution of IV broadspectrum antibiotics is recommended. In case of poor response to such a treatment given over 7 days, an antifungal agent needs to be incorporated. The use of hematopoietic growth factors (G-CSF, GM-CSF) in prolonged neutropenia is now gaining popularity.

Typhilitis (Neutropenic Enterocolitis)[7,8]

During course of chemotherapy for hematologic malignancies, severe neutropenia may damage to the small as well as large gut, the so-called *neutropenic enterocolitis or typhilitis*. The intestinal lesions are in the form of mucosal ulceration and full thickness necrosis and perforation.

Manifestations in the beginning are nonspecific but rapidly advance to those of perforation.

A high index of suspicion is the key to recognition of the condition. X-ray and CT scan assist in ruling out the close differential diagnoses such as necrotizing enterocolitis.

Treatment consists in providing best possible supportive care with broadspectrum antibiotics to cover gram negative pathogens as well as clostridia, bowel rest, blood component therapy and a vigilance for surgical intervention.

Table 50.3: Indications for surgery in typhilitis

- Intestinal perforation
- Persistent nonthrombocytopenic gastrointestinal bleeding
- Uncontrolled septicemia.

Prognosis in early diagnosed and adequately treated cases is fairly good. Unfortunately, most cases are detected late, ending up in high mortality varying from 50 to 100%.

Myelosuppression

The term refers to bone marrow suppression by lymphoma, leukemia and other malignancies as also antimalignant chemotherapy, resulting in fall in fall in number of RBCs, leukocytes and platelets. Infections in such children worsen the state of myelosuppression and may contribute to life-threatening complications, delay chemotherapy, hike in treatment cost and poor quality of life.

Metabolic Emergencies

Acute tumor lysis syndrome, characterized by hyper-uricemia, hyperkalemia and hyperphosphatemia, is the result of rapid release of intracellular metabolites at a rate that is far more than the excretory capacity of the kidneys. The rapid release of intracellular metabolites is secondary to spontaneous or treatment-related tumor necrosis or apoptosis. The syndrome may develop prior to or during the course of chemotherapy.

This syndrome can be prevented by measures directed at:

- Reducing uric acid production.
- Increasing uric acid solubility.
- Reducing concentration of uric acid in urine.

Syndrome of inappropriate secretion of ADH and hyper-calcemia are other metabolic emergencies seen in children suffering from oncologic disease.

REFERENCES

1. Jones A. Emergencies in oncologic settings. *Pediatr Cancer* 2003;4:213-214.
2. Kelly KM, Lange B. Oncologic emergencies. *Pediatr Clin North India* 1997;44:809-830.
3. Graham AM. Experience with pediatric oncologic emergencies. *Pediatr Cancer* 2003;4:215-219.
4. Arya LS. Oncologic emergencies. In: Gupte S (ed) *Recent Advances in Pediatrics (Special Vol 14: Criticare Pediatrics)*. New Delhi: Jaypee Brothers 2004;520-530.
5. Arya LS, Narain S, Tomar S, Thavaraj V, Dawar R, Bhargava M. Superior vena cava syndrome. *Indian J Pediatr* 2002;69: 293-297.
6. Ingram I, Rivera GK, Shapiro DN. Superior vena cava syndrome associated with childhood malignancy: Analysis of 24 cases. *Med Pediatr Oncol* 1990; 18:476-481.
7. Shamberger RC, Weinstein HJ, Deloney MJ, Levey RH. The medical and surgical management of typhilitis in children with acute nonlymphocytic (myeloenous) leukemia. *Cancer* 1986;57:603-609.
8. Moir CR, Scudamore CH, Benny WB. Typhilitis: Selective surgical management. *Am J Surg* 1986;151: 563-566.

Section IX

Endocrinal and Metabolic Emergencies

Endocrinal and Metabolic Emergencies

Tapabrata Chatterjee

51 Diabetic Ketoacidosis

INTRODUCTION

There is unfortunately very little evidence to support the current guidelines for the management of diabetic ketoacidosis. An example of this is that much of the information about specific fluid and electrolyte deficit was obtained in the 1930s from the work of two young men with diabetes, whose fluid and electrolyte balance was studied in great detail before, while, and after they were allowed experimentally to become ill with DKA.[1] The reported fluid deficit appeared to be approximately equally divided between intra and extra-cellular compartments, forming the basis for most of the DKA management protocol in existence.[2,3] For obvious reasons these studies have never been repeated in children although their body composition and fluid requirements are very different from those of adults. There is also substantial difference in the management of paediatric DKA among physicians of different specialities presumably due to differences in speciality training. Differences in surveyed management show that 59% of the endocrinologist as opposed to 11% of general emergency physicians could give a fluid bolus of 20 ml/kg; 83.5% of general emergency physicians compared to 42.5% of the intensivist could administer an initial insulin bolus; 58.2% paediatric intensivist versus 9% of the general emergency physicians would replace fluids over a period of greater than 24 hrs and 54.3% of the general physicians versus 7.3% of the pediatric intensivist would use potassium chloride alone for potassium replacement.[4]

FLUID MANAGEMENT AND RISK OF CEREBRAL EDEMA

The aim of management of DKA is to restore metabolic homoeostasis, while minimizing the risk of complications including hypoglycemia, hypokalemia, cardiac failure and cerebral edema. There is clear evidence that volume depletion in DKA leads to the release of counter regulatory hormones including catacolamines, growth hormones and cortisol as well as rennin, aldosterone and vasopressin.[5,6] These hormones whose combine action is directed towards preserving intravascular volume, also cause insulin resistance. An important effect of fluid administration is therefore reducing the stimulus for counter regulatory hormones. Indeed it has been shown that plasma glucose starts to fall following fluid administration prior to giving insulin, although insulin is required for the correction of the metabolic acidosis.[7]

Thus, the importance of prompt restoration of circulating volume for patients presenting with DKA is clear. However, the observation that symptomatic cerebral edema often occurs several hours after treatment has began, usually at a time, plasma glucose has started to fall and metabolic acidosis to improve, has led to concern that treatment itself may contribute to development of cerebral edema. We know that part of physiologic disturbance is hyperosmolality due to hyperglycaemia. When hyperosmolality occurs cells especially brain cells accumulates osmoprotective molecules (osmolytes) as a defense against cell shrinkage;[8] these consist largely of taurine and myoinositol. It is also known that most intracranial capillaries are joined by tight junctions, forming the anatomical basis of blood brain barrier. This barrier permits virtually instantaneous diffusion of water but retards the rate of solute (e.g. sodium and chloride) diffusion in both directions up to 6 hrs.[9] When sodium chloride concentration is lower in plasma, than in the cerebrospinal fluid, water pours into the brain. Cells with added osmolytes, which do not diffuse easily, rapidly absorb water. The result is not a primary increase in interstitial fluid (i.e. edema) but an increase in cell volume, similar to that seen in cerebral hypoxia and lead encephalopathy. The osmolytes will continue to pull water from the interstitium to cells, so that rapid administration of osmotic "free" water will result in rapid cell swelling. Finally, we know that brain is encased in a rigid box, the skull, so that when a fluid volume continuous to increase, the intra-cranial pressure rises gradually at first; then, at a critical point the pressure raises expodentially for each added unit volume. This combination explains the phenomenon of CNS damage during treatment of DKA.

Notably, the first episode of DKA is more likely than a recurrent episode to go unrecognized for a long time. Thus, there is a greater accumulation of osmolytes and sometimes cell swelling before therapy in patients with newly diagnosed Diabetes. If the intravenous therapeutic solution, and thus the plasma, has a lower osmolarity than CSF, water will enter the brain space disproportionately to other tissues. The brain cells and the interstitial fluid will increase in volume, in contrast to other tissues where, as the cell volume rises the interstitial fluid will diminish proportionately. If this process continues, the critical point in the brain volume to pressure relationship will be reached, and a sudden increase in intracranial pressure occurs with consequences including herniation or cerebral vessel constriction with thrombosis and infarct. A rapid fall in the glucose concentration due to aggressive insulin administration further worsens the process because the end point of glucose metabolism is more free water.[10] There have been few case controlled studies of cerebral oedema complicating DKA and there is conflicting evidence as to role of iartrogenic factor in fatal cases.[11, 12] However, excessive rates of fluid administration, particularly in early resuscitation,[13] and failure of serum sodium to rise, as the plasma glucose declines have been identified as risk factors. Clinicians have been consistently shown to overestimate the degree of dehydration, in this condition[14,15] Nevertheless, the assumption underlying most DKA protocols is that rehydration is desirable and achievable in 24 hrs, using a volume calculated by "maintenance plus deficit". From a renal perspective, the term maintenance fluid is a misnomer. True maintenance fluid volume in children is the sum of insensible loss + the obligate urine production and are probably only 40% of recommended amounts.[16] In non-diabetic dehydration, it is customary to assess if the dehydration is hyper tonic, hypo tonic or isotonic. It is accepted that the safe therapy of hypertonic dehydration should be both prolonged and cautious rehydration over at least 48 hrs.[17] There is no evidence that the use of modest fluid regime is harmful.[18,19] Harris and colleagues[14,20] have shown that in 149 episodes of childhood DKA, rehydration over 48 hrs was associated with "no deaths or near death episodes" and Johnson reported that in adults, a regimen of 2-3 ml/kg/hour, which means rehydration over 72 hrs was safe.[21] It is prudent to avoid the use of the term bolus with respect of fluid resuscitation. One approach may be to use no more than 7.5-10 ml/kg of normal saline in the first hour followed by 3.5–5 ml/kg in the next hour. Osmolality is calculated by the formula 2 (Na + K) + Urea + Glucose. Urea is not an effective osmol because it moves freely across the membrane and therefore may not be included in the calculation.[22] As the glucose comes down during the treatment of DKA, the concentration of Na needs to be kept high to prevent sudden fall of osmolality. Patients treated with a revised protocol of more sodium in their IV fluid, needed fewer intravenous fluid changes, were treated at lower cost and resolved their acidosis more rapidly than patients treated under original protocol using lower salt concentrations in their intravenous regime. The rate of development of cerebral edema, however, did not show any statistically significant difference.[23]

BICARBONATE THERAPY: YES OR NO

There is a temptation of using sodium bicarbonate when the pH is less than 7.10. This is because of the fear that severe metabolic acidosis associated with DKA may diminish minute volume, cause hypotension, impaired myocardial function and promote insulin resistance. However, bicarbonate therapy is associated with a left shift of the oxygen dissociation curve resulting in deterioration of tissue hypoxia, hypokalemia and paradoxical cerebral acidosis.[24] In a recently published retrospective multicentre analysis of children with DKA, bicarbonate therapy together with low PCO_2 level and high serum sodium concentration at presentation were identified as particular risk factors for development of cerebral edema. Around 90% of physicians in all specialities stated that they would not use bicarbonate in DKA management. Pediatric intensivists were more likely (25%) and pediatric emergency physicians are less likely (8%) to state that they would never use bicarbonate in any patient.[4] In one study two groups of patients with severe DKA (pH between 6.83 and 7.08), who were treated with and without bicarbonate, it was found out that there was no advantage of use of bicarbonate with regard to clinical or biochemical recovery. However, the group treated with bicarbonate required more potassium supplementation.[25] One may speculate that bicarbonate is indicated if the pH is less than 6.9. However, there appears to be no place for it if the pH is higher than this.

POTASSIUM PHOSPHATE IN MANAGEMENT OF DKA

It is almost inevitable that patients with DKA receive excess of chloride, which aggravates acidosis. The extent of acidosis, however, can be reduced by substitution of phosphate, which is also significantly depleted in DKA. Moreover, phosphate in conjuncture with glycolysis is essential for formation of 2,3 DPG, which governs the oxygen dissociation curve. During deficiency of 2,3 DPG the oxygen dissociation curve is shifted to the left, i.e. more oxygen is retained by haemoglobin and less is available to the tissues, a situation that predisposes towards lactic acidosis. Acidosis per se tends to shift the oxygen dissociation curve towards the right and thus partially compensates for 2,3 DPG deficiency but as any acidosis resulting from accumulation of ketones is corrected by provision of insulin, the effect of 2,3 DPG deficiency may no longer be compensated and release of oxygen to the tissues may again be impaired. Exogenous phosphate, by contributing to the formation of 2,3 DPG permits the oxygen dissociation curve to the right and thus facilitates release of oxygen to the tissues and aids in the correction of acidosis. Furthermore, resistance to insulin action is associated with hypophosphataemia; hence replacing potassium using potassium phosphate is a logical solution. Overuse of phosphate may result in hypocalcemia; hence, serum calcium should be measured periodically.[24]

RECURRENT DIABETIC KETOACIDOSIS

Recurrent ketoacidosis is often related to omitting insulin and major psychosocial turmoil in the family, such as depression, substance abuse, physical and or sexual abuse. Prevention of recurrent DKA remains a major challenge to the diabetologists and involves detailed assessment of family psychodynamics.[26]

The relationship between psychiatric disorders and poorly controlled diabetes may be reciprocal and interactive. Psychopathology could be a consequence of poorly controlled diabetes. Repeated episodes of severe DKA increase stress as a result of repeated hospital admission. However, in a study in which patients' plasma glucose levels was fixed by overnight insulin infusion at either hyperglycaemic and normoglycaemic levels, it was found that sustained high plasma glucose values induced psychological changes characteristic of a stress like CNS arousal pattern, which would increase susceptibility to environmental stress and could lead to a variety of psychiatric symptoms.[27] Psychiatric illness can influence blood glucose control indirectly by poor compliance with treatment and directly by emotional arousal contributing to ketoacidosis by way of sympathochromaffin activation and attendant catecholamine and corticosteroid release.[28] Similar reciprocal mechanisms, account for recently described relationships between psychiatric illness and diabetic complication of retinopathy.[29]

In families of recurrent DKA, subjects were less effective in problem solving and more poorly defined family rules and roles were demonstrated. Both children and parents in these families reported less diabetic specific family support and less support specially in the area of diabetes related empathy. It was noted "that a parenting style of affection less control might be a consequence of chronic disorder in a child."[30] However, the finding may be exaggerated in this study because the assessment was done when the parent may have been reacting strongly to the current DKA episodes. Repeated illnesses may also be a consequence of parenting styles. The DKA subjects has lower self esteem, where described by their parents as having less social competence, and reported more non compliance which may reflect difficulties with parenting style that emphasises behavioural control at the expense of emphatic responses.[31]

Subjects with DKA reported more noncompliance with diabetes treatment than it controls in 3 of the 4 areas assessed; this findings suggest non-compliance may have a path by which psychiatric disorder and family dysfunction affected metabolic control. Diet compliance was found to be most likely associated variable with the assignment of the control group. For children, " the diet component of diabetic regime is perhaps the most complex and has been rated by youngsters as the most difficult aspect of diabetic treatment."[32] Because the DKA children require hospitalisation, it seems likely that their reports, which describes more areas of noncompliance, were closer to truth than those of their parents, which differ only on diet compliance. This suggests the parents of children with poorer metabolic control were not sufficiently aware of how much their children were failing to comply with the insulin injection and testing components of medical regime.

Parents in DKA group differed from controlled parents only in having more somatisation symptoms; this finding suggest parental psychopathology was not a significant confounding factor for parental assessment of their children. Although, parents of children who have psychiatric disorder tend to have a higher rates of psychiatric disorder,[33] it may be that psychiatric disorders in DKA children are more directly related to the course of the diabetes than to parental hereditary or environmental influences.

Thus, children hospitalized for DKA have higher rates of psychopathology than children with diabetes who have no history of DKA. Since symptoms of anxiety and depression in this population may be confused with symptoms related to abnormal glycemia,[34] systemic psychiatric diagnostic interviews may be critical. Attention should also be focused on DKA children's reports of noncompliance, as they may be more sensitive than their parents' report. Families of children with poor metabolic control appear less organized and less efficient at problem solving, have less well defined family roles and rules, and demonstrate a diabetes related parenting style that emphasises control but at the expense of empathy. Diagnosis and treatment of specific psychiatric disorder in children, hospitalised with recurrent DKA combined with attempt to optimise warm, caring, diabetic specific family support, may improve compliance and metabolic control, and thereby helping to reduce later complications.[35,36]

SUMMARY

An evidence based appraisal of childhood Diabetic ketoacidosis is difficult as there is inadequate knowledge of fluid compartment and electrolyte balance during the episodes in a child. Slow rehydration, maintaining adequate sodium concentration and avoidance of sodium bicarbonate are logical approaches towards prevention of cerebral edema. The use of potassium phosphate instead of potassium chloride as a form of potassium supplement should be considered. The steady glycemic state towards optimal blood sugar level should be aimed in all diabetic as abnormal glycemic control leads to neuropsychiatric manifestations which in turn lead to noncompliance and recurrent diabetic ketoacidosis.

REFERENCES

1. Kennedy EL. Issues in diabetic ketosis. *Eur Bull Diab* 2002; 13:112-120.
2. Harrison E, Kennedy EL. Pitfalls in management of pediatric diabetic ketoacidosis. *Eur Bull Diab* 2003;14:61-63.
3. Waldhausi W, Kleinberger G, Korn A, et al. Severe hyperglycemia: Effects of rehydration on endocrine derangements and blood glucose concentration. *Diabetes* 1979;28:577-584.
4. Glaser NS, Kuppermann N, Yee CK, Swartz DL, Styne DM. Variation in the management of pediatric diabetic ketoacidosis by speciality training. *Arch Pediatr Adolesc Med* 1997;151:1125-1132.
5. Tulassay T, Rascher W, Korner A, et al. Atrial natriuretic peptide and other vasoactive hormones during treatment of severe diabetic ketoacidosis in children. *J Pediatr* 1987;111:329-334.
6. Luzi L, Barrett EJ, Groop LC, et al. Metabolic effects of low-dose insulin therapy on glucose metabolism in diabetic ketoacidosis. *Diabetes* 1988;37:1470-1477.
7. Owen OE, Licht JH, Sapir DG. Renal function and effects of partial rehydration during diabetic ketoacidosis. *Diabetes* 1981;30:510-518.
8. Finberg L, Luttrell C, Redd H. Pathogenesis of leis ions in the nervous system in hypernatremic states, II: experimental studies of gross anatomic changes and alterations of chemical composition of the tissues. *Pediatrics*. 1959;23:46-52.
9. Finberg L. Why Do Patients With Diabetes Ketoacidosis Have Cerebral Swelling And Why Does Treatment Sometimes Makes It Worse. *Arch Pediatr Adolesc Med* 1996;150:785-786.
10. Glaser N, Barnett P, McCaslin I, Nelson D, Trainor J, Louie J, Kauffman F, Quayle K, Roback M, Malley R, Kuppermann N. Risk factors for cerebral edema in children with Diabetes ketoacidosis. *N Engl Med* 2001;344:264-269.
11. Dunger DB, Edge JA. Predicting cerebral oedema during diabetic ketoacidosis. *N Engl J Med* 2001;344:302-303.
12. Mahoney CP, Vleck BW, Del Aguila M. Risk factors for developing brain herniation during diabetic ketoacidosis. *Pediatr Neural* 1999;21:721-727.
13. Rosenbloom AL, Schatz DA, Krischer JP, et al. Therapeutic-controversy: prevention and treatment of diabetes in children. *J Clin Endocrinal Metab* 2000;85:494-522.
14. Harris GD, Fiordalisi I, Harris WL, et al. Minimizing the risk of brain herniation during treatment of diabetic ketoacidemia: a retrospective and prospective study. *J Pediatr* 1990;117:22-31.
15. Grove LM, Nobel-Jamieson CM, Barnes ND, et al. Assessment of dehydration, fluid balance and insulin requirements in diabetic ketoacidosis. *Proc Br Paediatr Assoc Annu Meet* 1995;67:26.
16. Molteni KH. Initial management of hypernatraemic dehydration in the breastfed infant. *Clin Pediatr* 1994;33:731-740.
17. Oddie S, Richmond S, Coultard M. Hypernatraemic dehydration and breastfeeding: A population study. *Arch Dis Child* 2001; 85:318-320.
18. Lebovitz HA. Diabetic ketoacidosis. *Lancet* 1995;345:767-771.
19. Adrogue H, Barrero J, Eknoyan G. Salutary effects of modest fluid replacement in the treatment of adults with ketoacidosis. *JAMA* 1989;262:2108-2113.
20. Harris GD, Fiordalisi I. Physiologic management of diabetic ketoacidemia. A 5-year prospective pediatric experience in 231 episodes. *Arch Pediatr Adolesc Med* 1994;148:1046-1052.
21. Johnston C. Fluid management in diabetic ketoacidosis. *BMJ* 1992;305:522.
22. Bohn D, Daneman D. Diabetic ketoacidosis and cerebral edema. *Curr Opin Pediatr* 2002;14:287-291.
23. Felner EI, White P. *Improving Management of Diabetic Ketoacidosis in Children*. American Academy of Pediatrics 2002: 735-740.
24. Alemzadeh R, Wyatt DT, Diabetes mellitus in chikldren. In: Behrman RE, Kliegman RM, Jenson HB (eds) *Nelson Textbook of Pediatrics*, 17th edn. Philadelphia: Saunders 2004;1947-1972.
25. Glaser N, Barnett P, Mc Caslin I, et al. Risk factors for cerebral edema in children with diabetic ketoacidosis. *N Engl J Med* 2001;344:264-269.
26. Brink SJ. Diabetic ketoacidosis. *Acta Pediatrica* 1999;(Suppl 88):14-24.
27. Lustman PJ, Skor DA, Carney RM, Santiago JV, Cryer PE. Stress and diabetic control. *Lancet* 1993; 1:588.
28. Lustman PJ, Harper GW, Griffith LS, Clouse RE. Use of the Diagnostic Interview Schedule in patients with diabetes mellitus. *J Nerv Ment Dis* 2995;174:743-746.
29. Kovacs M, Mukherji P, Drash A, Iyengar S. Biomedical and psychiatric risk factors for retinopathy among children with IDDM. *Diabetes Care* 1995; 18:1592-1599.
30. Parker G. *Parental Overprotection: A Risk factor in psychological Development*. New York: Grune and Stratton 1993.
31. Fairburn CG, Peveler RC, Davies B, Mann JI, Mayou RA. Eating disorders in young adults with insulin dependant diabetes mellitus: a controlled study. *BMJ* 1991;303:17-20.
32. Reid GJ, Dubow EF, Carey TC, Dura JR. Contribution of coping to medical adjustment and treatment responsibility among children and adolescents with diabetes. *J Dev Behav Pediatr* 1994;15:327-355.
33. Offord DR, Fleming JE. Epidemology. In: Lewis M (ed): *Child and Adolescent Psychiatry: A Comprehensive Textbook*. Baltimore: Williams and Wilkins 1996;1166-1178.
34. Jacobson AM. The psychological care of patients with insulin dependant diabetes mellitus. *N Engl J Med* 1996;334:1249-1253.
35. Gupta N, Midha P, Singh G. Psychiatric aspects of endocrine disorders. In: Gupte S (ed) *Recent Advances in Pediatrics (Special Vol 13: Pediatric Endocunlogy*. New Delhi: Jaypee Brothers 2004;309-326.
36. Gupte S, Smith R, Choudhary RK. Childhood endocrinepathies and psychiatric problems. *Br J Pedict Psychal* 1993;3:118-123.

Suraj Gupte and Javed Chowdhary

52 Hyperthyroid Crisis

INTRODUCTION

Hyperthyroid crisis or storm is defined as a form of hyperthyroidism manifested by an acute onset of hyperthermia, severe tachycardia and restlessness.[1-3] It is, by all means, quite an infrequent condition in pediatric practice. Nevertheless, as and when it occurs, it needs to be handled immediately. Else, it may prove a killer.

ETIOLOGY

Invariably, the underlying cause is Graves disease which is hyperthyroidism due to diffuse toxic goiter during childhood. Graves disease occurs in around 0.02% of children (1 in 5000), predominantly in females (male to female ratio 1 : 5). The disease has autoimmune origin. Hence, the sementic "autoimmune thyrotoxicosis".

Hyperthyroid crisis is precipitated by stress and/or such intercurrent problems as sepsis, trauma, surgical emergency, etc.

CLINICAL MANIFESTATIONS

These include hyperthermia (fever), gross tachycardia, sweating and restlessness. Table 52.1 lists the manifestations in relation to different systems. If not immediately attended to, the condition may progress to delirium and coma, usually ending up fatally.[2-5]

Table 52.1: Systemic manifestations of hyperthyroid crisis

CNS	• Restlessness
	• Tremor
	• Psychosis
	• Delirium
	• Coma
GIT	• Nausea, vomiting and diarrhea
	• Abdominal pain
CVS	• Severe tachycardia
	• Arrhythmias
	• CCF
	• Hepatic failure
Endocrinal	• Adrenal failure

DIAGNOSIS

It is primarily clinical. In a suspected situation, the following investigations need to be carried out for confirmation of the diagnosis:

- Serum thyroxine (T_4), triiodothyronine (T_3), free T_4 and T_3 all of which are raised and serum thyroid stimulating hormone (TSH) which is lower than normal.
- Thyroid peroxidase antibodies which are often present.
- ECG revealing arrhythmias.
- Skeletal X-rays showing advanced skeletal maturation and craniosynostosis and reduction in bone density.

MANAGEMENT

For controlling an acute crisis, a beta-blocker like propranolol in a dose of 0.1-0.2 mg/kg (IV) may be required.[3-5] In a less sever case it may be given orally in a dose of 0.5-2.0 mg/kg/24 hours. The modus operandi of action is through resolution of action of catecholamines potentiated by thyroid hormones. Mind you such symptoms in hyperthyroid crisis as tachycardia, tremor, sweating, lid lag and stare are due to catecholamines rather than excessive thyroid hormone as such. While treating with propranolol, one should watch for such side effects as hypotension, bronchospasm. Hypoglycemia and heart block.

The most widely employed antithyroid agents are propylthiouracil (PTU) and methimazole. Dose of PTU is 5-10 mg/kg/24 hours in 3 divided doses and that of methimazole 0.25-1.0 mg/kg/24 hours in a single dose or in two divided doses.

Supportive measures include:

- Reduction in body temperature with tepid sponging; at times chlorpromazine, 25-50 mg (IV) may be employed for this purpose.

- Adequate hydration.
- Treatment of such precipitating factors as infection.
- Treatment of such complications as CCF.
- Adequate cover with steroids for "stress" cover.

REFERENCES

1. Franchi S. Disorders of the thyroid gland. In: Behrman RE, Kliegman RM, Jensom HB (eds) *Nelson Textbook of Pediatrics*, 17th edn. Philadelphia: Saunders 2004; 1870-1890.
2. Burrow PA. Hyperthyroid crisis in childhood. *Pediatr Endocr Chron* 2003;20;23-24.
3. Zimmerman D, Latif AN. Thyrotoxicosis in children. *Endocr Clin North Am* 1998;27:109-126.
4. Dallas JS, Foley TP Jr. Hyperthyroidism. In: Lifshtz F (ed) *Clinical Pediatric Endocrinology*, 3rd edn. New York: Marcel Dekker 1996;401-414.
5. Gupte S, Koff AW. Pediatric endocrinology. In: Gupte S (ed) *The Short Textbook of Pediatrics*, 10th edn. New Delhi: Jaypee Brothers 2004;534-552.

Suraj Gupte, AW Koff and VS Puri

53 Adrenal Crisis

INTRODUCTION

This is a life-threatening situation associated with adrenal failure precipitated by stress and/or intercurrent illness.

ETIOLOGY

It may follow primary adrenal insufficiency or secondary adrenal insufficiency (Table 53.1). Primary adrenal insufficiency is either congenital (usually genetic) or acquired (usually autoimmune). Secondary adrenal insufficiency results from damage to anterior pituitary or hypothalmus. This damage causes a deficiency of adrenocorticotropin hormone that ends up leading to hypofunctioning of the adrenal cortex.[1,2]

Table 53.1: Etiology of adrenal crisis

Primary	
Congenital	
• Congenital adrenal hyperplasia	
• Adrenal hypoplasia/aplasia	
• Congenital unresponsiveness to ACTH	
Acquired	
• Adrenal hemorrhage	
• Fulminant infections	: Waterhouse-Friderichsen syndrome
• Addison's disease	
• Tuberculosis	
• AIDS	
• Adrenal leukodystrophy	
• Drugs	: Ketoconazole, rifampicin, anticonvulsants like phenytoin, phenobarbital
Secondary (Central)	
• Congenital hypopituitarism	
• Long-term glucocorticoid administration	
• Hypopituitarism	
– Tumor	: Craniopharyngioma
– Trauma	: Hemorrhage
– Surgery	
– Irradiation	

It is important to bear in mind that in primary adrenal insufficiency, adrenal cortex undergoes atrophy with involvement of all hormones. In secondary adrenal insufficiency, on the other hand, secretion of mineralocorticoids is spared. The reason for this is that it is not under control of the ACTH.

Table 53.2 lists the mechanism of production of adrenal insufficiency by certain pharmacologic agents.

Table 53.2: Modus operandi of production of adrenal insufficiency by certain pharmacologic agents

Pharmacologic agent	*Mechanism* responsible for adrenal insufficiency
Ketoconazole	Inhibition of adrenal enzymes
Mitotane	Toxic damage to adrenal cortex and alteration of extra-adrenal cortisol metabolism
Rifampicin	Induction of steroid metabolizing enzymes in liver
Phenobarbital	Induction of steroid metabolizing enzymes in liver
Phenytoin	Induction of steroid metabolizing enzymes in liver

CLINICAL MANIFESTATIONS

In adrenal crisis related to glucocorticoid deficiency, manifestations include change in sensorium, vomiting, diarrhea, fever, hypoglycemia and low cardiac output.

In adrenal crisis related to mineralocorticoid deficiency, manifestations include dyselectrolytemia, metabolic acidosis, dehydration and shock. Advanced cases develop irreversible shock which usually ends up fatally.

The term, *Addisonian crisis*, denotes presenting features in a so-far unsuspected case precipitated by severe stress or intercurrent illness. Clinical manifestations include hypotension, dehydration, prostration, collapse, hypoglycemia and dyselectrolytemia in the form of hyponatremia, hyperkalemia and high blood urea.[2]

DIAGNOSIS

In a suspected case, certain investigations (Table 53.3) should be carried out without loss of time.

Table 53.3: Investigations in a child with suspected adrenal crisis

Specific
- Cortisol levels.
- ACTH levels which help in differentiating between primary and secondary adrenal insufficiency. In primary adrenal failure, levels are high. These are low in secondary adrenal failure.
- ACTH stimulation test: A stimulated cortisol level (above 15 mcg/dl) following 0.25 mg bolus IV ACTH at 0 and 60 minutes is a sensitive index of adrenal insufficiency.

Supportive
- Blood counts for eosinophilia with relative neutropenia.
- Serum electrolytes for hyponatremia and hyperkalemia.
- Acid-base studies for hypochloremic acidosis.
- Blood sugar for hypoglycemia.
- Urinary electrolytes for high urinary sodium and low urinary potassium.
- Noninvasive imaging (ultrasonography, CT scan, MRI) may be of assistance in delineating the actual size of the adrenal glands after the acute crisis has been tided over.

MANAGEMENT

Therapy of acute adrenal insufficiency has got to be immediate and aggressive. An IV line must be started immediately, employing 5% glucose in 0.9% saline solution to correct hypoglycemia, hypovolemia and hyponatremia.

Specific

Without loss of time, the patient should be administered hydrocortisone sodium succinate, 50-100 mg (IV) stat followed by 100 mg/msq/day as IV infusion or in divided doses. Later, dose is slowly reduced to 10–20 mg/msq/day (maintenance dose) over 5 days. Tapering off is by 1/3rd reduction every day until maintenance dose is reached.

Alternatively, dexamethasone (0.2 mg/kg) may be employed initially and later substituted with hydrocortisone after completion of the stimulation test.

Supportive

It comprises correction of:
- Shock, dehydration
- Dyselectrolytemia
- Acidosis, and
- Hypoglycemia.

Rapid volume expansion is achieved by 20 ml/kg of normal saline. Thereafter, degree of dehydration is determined and deficit is replaced over next 24 hours on top of the maintenance fluids.

For treating hypoglycemia, IV infusion of 0.5 g/kg dextrose over 5-10 minutes is followed by 0.5 g/kg/hour.

For resistant hypokalemia, give sodium polysterene sulfonate enema.

Sodium deficit is also corrected. It is important to closely monitor hemodynamic status and laboratory values, say glucose, sodium, potassium, acid-base.

Subsequent Treatment

Hydrocortisone, 10-20 mg/msq/day in divided doses (larger dose in the morning) and fludrocortisone, 0.05-0.3 mg/day with salt at lib, esp during summer. At times of stress, dose of hydrocortisone should be made double. In case of difficulty in obtaining hydrocortisone, prednisolone may be given.

PREVENTION

It is important to remember that dose of steroid has got to be stepped up 2 to 3 fold in children who are on replacement therapy with steroids as and when they suffer from conditions of stress.[3] If it is not possible to give high doses orally, parenteral dosing may be resorted to.

Secondly, as and when high dose steroid therapy is given for a prolonged period (say over 2 weeks), it must never be suddenly withdrawn. On the other hand, it should be slowly tapered off.

REFERENCES

1. Levine LS, White PC. Disorders of the adrenal glands. In: Behrman RE, Kliegman, RM, Jenson HB (eds) *Nelson Textbook of Pediatrics*, 17th edn. Philadelphia: Saunders 2004; 1898-1923.
2. Gupte S, Anderson AE, Chowdhary J. Adrenal insufficiency. In: Gupte S (ed) *Recent Advances in Pediatrics (Special Vol 13: Pediatric Endocrinology)*. New Delhi: Jaypee Brothers 2004;147-152.
3. Koff AW. Endocrinal crises in pediatric practice. *Eur Endocr News Letter* 2002;3:7-8.

Suraj Gupte and Javed Chowdhary

54 Acute Hypercalcemia

INTRODUCTION

Hypercalcemia is defined as a serum level of > 11 mg/dl with or without signs and symptoms. In practice, manifestations are encountered only when serum calcium level > 12 mg/dL. It is an uncommon emergency.

ETIOLOGY

Table 54.1 gives the detailed list of causes of hypercalcemia though, admittedly, common causes are immobilization, iatrogenic and neoplasia.[1-3]

Table 54.1: Etiology of hypercalcemia as such

Parathyroid Hormone Related
Adenoma, hyperplasia
Calcium-sensing defects

Vitamin D Related
Iatrogenic (toxicity)
- Excessively fortified milk

Ectopic production
- Sarcoidosis
- Tuberculosis
- Subcutaneous fat necrosis
- Willims syndrome (7q11.23 deletion)
- Granulomatous lesions

Drug related
- Theophylline
- Lithium
- Thiazide

Miscellaneous
- Hyperphosphatasia
- Hyperthyroidism
- Malignancy/leukemia
- Immobilization
- McCune Albright syndrome

Immobilization

Prolonged immobilization is known to cause hypercalcemia in addition to poor renal function, hypertension and encephalopathy.

Iatrogenic

Excessive intake of calcium-containing foodstuffs (excessively fortified milk), especially in a subject suffering from a malignancy and undergoing prolonged immobilization, excess of vitamin D (from intake or ectopic productions as in sarcoidosis, tuberculosis).

Neoplasia

The most common neoplasm causing hypercalcemia is a parathyroid adenoma.

Undoubtedly, primary hyperparathyroidism due to a primary defect of the parathyroid gland may cause hypercalcemia. In practice, however, hypercalcemia usually is due to secondary hyperparathyroidism which is a compensatory mechanism for correction of hypocalcemic states.

CLINICAL MANIFESTATIONS[1,2]

At lower blood calcium level, manifestations include anorexia, nausea, vomiting, constipation, muscular weakness, polyuria, polydipsia, weight loss, fever, abdominal pain and hypertension. Any immobilized child with unexplained hypertension needs to have hypercalcemia excluded actively.

At higher blood calcium level, ventricular ectopics and altered sensorium are the important manifestations.

ECG changes include shortening of QT interval, lowering of ST-T wave.

MANAGEMENT

The crux of treatment is lowering the serum calcium level by reducing the calcium intake and by enhancing calcium excretion. This is achieved by the following measures.

General Measures

- Discontinue high calcium-containing foods.
- Discontinue calcium-containing fluids.
- Mobilize the subject.

Specific Measures

- *Hydration with Diuretic Therapy:* It is good to use normal saline (4-10 ml/kg/hour) with potassium supplementation. Frusemide is given in a dose of 1 mg/kg/day IV every 4 hourly.
- *Calcitonin:* 1 mg/kg SC every 12 hourly.
- Hemodialysis.
- *Glucocorticoids:* Hydrocortisone 10 mg/kg/day or prednisolone 1-2 mg/kg/day for 2 weeks.[3]

Once the acute phase is controlled, treatment of the underlying cause is needed. For example, malignancy requires resection along with chemotherapy.

REFERENCES

1. Bajpai, A, Sharma J, Menon PSN. Hypercalcemia. In: *Practical Pediatric Endocrinology*. New Delhi: Jaypee 2003;43-46.
2. Gupte S, Koff AK: Pediatric endocrinology. In: Gupte S (ed) *The Short Textbook of Pediatrics*, 10th edn. New Delhi: Jaypee 2004:534-552.
3. Rivkees SA. Hyperparathyroidism in children. In: Lifshitz F (ed) *Pediatric Endocrinology*, 3rd edn. New York: Marcel Dekker 1996;497-505.

Endocrinal and Metabolic Emergencies

Suraj Gupte and Utpal Kant Singh

55 Acute Hypocalcemia

INTRODUCTION

Acute hypocalcemia is defined as a state in which serum calcium is < 7 mg/dL in association with normal or low ionized calcium with or without symptoms and signs. It is a common complication in PICU, warranting immediate action.[1]

ETIOLOGY

Table 55.1 lists the various causes of acute hypocalcemia.

Table 55.1: Various causes of acute hypocalcemia

Parathyroid hormone deficiency
DiGeorge syndrome
Velocardiofacial syndrome
Conotruncal-face syndrome
Autoimmunedestruction of parathyroids
Iatrogenic
Use of citrated preserved blood
Drugs like aminoglycosides, steroids, frusemide, albumin, etc.
Infections
Septicemia
Acute pancreatitis
Surgery
Thyroidectomy
Parathyroidectomy T
Tracheal reconstruction
Cardiopulmonary bypass
Infiltrative diseases
Wilson's diseases
Thalassemia
Hemochromatosis
Magnesium deficiency
Aminoglycoside therapy
Magnesium malabsorption
Renal magnesium loss
Vitamin D deficiency
Nutritional
Vitamin D dependency
Malabsorption
Renal failure
Liver disease
Drugs: Phenobarbital, phenytoin

CLINICAL MANIFESTATIONS

Early and mild deficiency causes only neuromuscular manifestations such as muscular pain and cramps which may progress to numbness, stiffness and tingling of hands and feet. Later, there may develop positive Chvostek sign or Trosseau sign or even frank carpopedal spasm and laryngospasm leading to stridor.

CNS manifestations include tremors, seizures, tonic rigidity, head retraction and cyanosis. An intracranial space-occupying lesion (ICSOL) may be suspected in the presence of a combination of such manifestations as headache, vomiting, raised intracranial pressure (RICP), papilledema and seizures.

Cardiovascular manifestations include hypotension, poor myocardial contractility, bradycardia, other dysarhythmias, and ECG changes in the form of prolongation of P-R interval and T wave inversion

DIAGNOSIS

Serum calcium level is low, usually between 5-7 mg/dL, whereas phosphorus level is high i.e. 7-12 mg/dL.

Serum ionized calcium level too is low.

Alkaline phosphatase is within normal limits or low.

Serum magnesium is normal.

Serum PTH level is low.

ECG shows prolongation of QT interval.

EEG shows widespread slow activity.

MANAGEMENT

Emergency therapy consists in administering 10% calcium gluconate, 1-2 ml i.e. 10-20 mg (1 ml = 9.3 mg elemenal calcium)/kg, diluted 1:1, infused intravenously over 10-20 minutes period while the heart rate is monitored carefully in view of the risk of bradycardia. If feasible, ECG monitoring should be preferred. One should avoid concomitant administration of bicarbonate or phosphate-containing solutions.[2]

An appropriate intake of calcium (around 800 mg/day of elemental calcium) in diet should be ensured. Else, medicinal calcium may be given orally.

Dietary intake of high phosphorus-containing foods (milk, cheese, eggs) should be cut down. If hypocalcemia remains unresponsive, the possibility of hypomagnesemia (serum magnesium < 1.5 mg/dL) as the impeding factor should be considered. There is evidence that hypomagnesemia impairs release of parathyroid hormone, leading to resistance to the effects of hormone. In such a situation, it is advisable to give 50% magnesium sulfate, 0.1 ml/kg (IM) 6 hourly over a period of 4 days.[1,2]

REFERENCES

1. Donald A, Henry AM. Pediatric hypocalcemia. In: Donald A (ed) *Pediatric Metabolic Disorders,* 2nd edn. London: Smith and Smith 2003;211-219.
2. Henry AM. Managing unresponsive hypocalcemia. *Bull Endocr Metab* 2003;7:327-329.

Section X

Renovascular Emergencies

Pankaj Abrol

56 Acute Glomerulonephritis

INTRODUCTION

Bright had described acute glomerulonephritis in 1927. Acute post-streptococcal glomerulonephritis is archetype of acute glomerulonephritis. It is the most common cause of acute nephritis in children. It is characterized by the abrupt onset of hematuria and proteinuria, often accompanied by azotemia, edema, hypertension and water retention. Acute nephritic syndrome can be most serious and potentially devastating form of renal diseases. The clinical and histological severity may vary. A patient may have mild disease which may go undetected but classical clinical picture is severe.

ETIOLOGY

Post-streptococcal glomerulonephritis follows infection of the throat or skin, by certain nephritogenic strains of group A beta-hemolytic streptococci. The nephritogenic strains involved are type 12 and 4 in pharyngitis and type 49 in skin infections.[1] Immunity to these strains is type-specific and long-lasting.[2] The streptococcal antigen–antibody complexes are trapped in glomerular capillaries where they activate complement and initiate inflammatory changes. Recurrent infections and nephritis are rare. Due to more widespread use of antibiotics, this entity is decreasing in frequency.

Other postinfectitious causes (Table 56.1) include staphylococcus, hepatitis-B and other viruses, bacterial endocarditis and infected ventriculo-atrial shunts.[3,4,5]

Table 56.1: Differential diagnosis of acute glomerulonephtritis

1. *Postinfectious:* Streptococcus, coagulase positive and negative staphylococcus, streptococcus pneumoniae, gram-negative bacteria, hepatitis-B, other viruses, bacterial endocarditis, infected ventriculo-atrial shunts, prosthesis, certain fungi and rickettsial diseases.
2. *Systemic vasculitis:* Systemic lupus erythematosus, Henoch-Schoenlein purpura, polyarteritis nodosa, Wegener's granulomatosus.
3. *Membranoproliferative glomerulonephritis.*
4. IgA nephropathy

PATHOLOGY

The kidneys are enlarged. On light microscopy, all glomeruli are enlarged, relatively bloodless and show diffuse mesangial proliferation with increase in mesangial matrix. Leukocyte proliferation along with cellular proliferation is seen in glomeruli. Crescents and interstitial inflammation may be seen in severe cases. Electron microscopy may reveal electron dense deposits on the epithelial side of glomerular basement membrane (GBM).[1]

CLINICAL PROFILE

Post-streptococcal glomerulonephritis is most common in children. Mean age is 7 years and is rare below 3 years of age. It is twice more common in males than females. The severity may vary from asymptomatic microscopic hematuria with normal renal function to acute renal failure. The patient develops acute nephritic syndrome 1-2 weeks after the preceding streptococcal infection. The onset is rapid with oliguria, puffiness around eyes, hypertension and pedal edema. Periorbital edema may precede onset of hematuria. The degree of oliguria usually correlates with the severity of disease. Urine is cola colored. Edema is usually because of salt and water retention. Patient may have nonspecific symptoms like lethargy, abdominal pain and fever. He may be brought to casualty with hypertensive encephalopathy with convulsions, left ventricular failure with hypertension and acute renal failure. The acute phase usually recovers in 2 months after onset but urinary findings may persist for as long as one year.[6,7]

DIAGNOSIS

Urine shows hematuria. It contains red blood cells and red cell and granular casts. There is 1+ to 2+ proteinuria. Presence of white blood cells indicates glomerular inflammation and should not be taken as indicator of urinary tract infection. Mild normochromic anemia may be present due to hemodilution and low-grade hemolysis. ESR may be a little elevated. The serum C3 level is usually reduced. Blood urea and serum creatinine are elevated and their level reflect the degree of renal impairment.

Confirmation of diagnosis requires evidence in favor of streptococcal infection. Throat culture may grow streptococcus that could even be due to carrier state. Serological tests may show raised antibody titers to streptococcal antigens. ASLO titer may be raised in 80% of cases. Anti-DNase B is elevated in streptococcal skin infections. These titers decrease in 4-6 weeks. Serum C3 also normalizes by 5-6 weeks. Its persistence may indicate other forms of glomerulonephritis. Streptozyme test, a slide agglutination procedure, detects antibodies to streptolysin O, DNase B, hyaluronidase, streptokinase and nicotinamide-adenine dinucleotidase.

Usually in such children, renal biopsy is not indicated. However, it is indicated in following conditions:

1. Age less than 2 years.
2. Development of renal failure or nephritic syndrome.
3. Presence of systemic features–arthritis, skin rash and hepatosplenomegaly.
4. Absence of evidence of streptococcal infection.
5. No hypocomplementemia.
6. Persistence of hematuria or proteinuria or both.
7. Low C3 level for beyond 3 months.

COURSE

Diuresis begins spontaneously in 4 to 7 days after onset resulting in prompt resolution of hypertension and edema. Microscopic hematuria and proteinuria may persist for much longer. Most of patients recover completely with excellent prognosis. Infrequently, the acute phase may lead to glomerular hyalinization and chronic renal failure. Less than 5% patients will require dialysis. Recurrences are extremely rare.[2]

APPROACH TO MANAGEMENT

A 10-day course of systemic antibiotic therapy usually with penicillin is recommended to eradicate nephritogenic group A streptococcus. However, there is no evidence to suggest its effect on natural course of glomerulonephritis. The patient needs supportive care till resolution of glomerular inflammation. Patients with mild oliguria and normal blood pressure can be managed at home. Others require hospital admission, as close observation is necessary.

1. *Rest:* Activity is restricted in acute phase of disease. When complications of acute phase are present, patient may be confined to bed. Activity as such has no adverse effect on healing.
2. *Diet:* Patient requires restricted intake of protein, sodium and potassium till oliguria and blood urea improve. Protein intake is restricted to 0.6 to 0.8 mg/kg/day. Sugar is allowed freely.
3. *Fluid restriction:* It is mandatory as overhydration can lead to hypertension and left ventricular failure. Strict intake and output charting of fluids is required. Intake of fluid should be restricted to an amount equal to insensible loss, 24-hour urine output and extrarenal fluid losses (vomit, stools). The daily insensible water loss is approximately 300 ml/m^2. The insensible losses should be replaced by 5% dextrose without any electrolytes.
4. *Weight:* Child should be weighed daily. Gain in weight suggests over hydration, and requires fluid restriction. The patient should lose 0.5-1% of his weight daily, because of tissue catabolism. Serum sodium level should also be monitored. More rapid weight loss and rising serum sodium suggests inadequate fluid replacement, whereas absence of weight loss and hyponatremia indicates fluid excess.
5. *Diuretics:* Usually not indicated as edema resolves following return of renal function. However, intravenous furosemide (4-6 mg/kg) may be given if pulmonary edema is there.
6. *Hypertension:* Mild hypertension can be controlled with restriction of activity, and salt and water intake. Drugs like hydralazine, beta-blockers (atenolol), ACE-inhibitors (captopril, enalapril) or calcium channel blockers (nifedipine) may be used. Malignant hypertension may require drugs like intravenous nitroprusside or labetalol.
7. *Left ventricular failure:* Hypertension is managed. Intravenous furosemide is administered. Onset of diuresis leads to improvement of heart failure. Venesection with removal of 100-200 ml of blood may be life-saving. Rotating tourniquet may be tied to reduce the venous return. Respiratory support with positive end-expiratory pressure may be required.
8. *Dialysis:* It is required in patients with severe renal failure, prolonged uremia, fluid overload and life-threatening dyselectrolytemia.

REFERENCES

1. Bergstein JM. Gross or microscopic hematuria. In: Behrman RE, Kliegman RM, Jenson HB (eds) *Nelson Textbook of Pediatrics* 16th edn. Philadelphia: WB Saunders: 2000;1581-1582.
2. Brady HR, O'Meara YM, Brenner BM. Acute nephritic syndrome and rapidly progressive glomerulonephritis. In: Braunwald E, Fauci AS, Kasper DL, Hauser SL, Longo DL, Jameson JL (eds) *Harrison's Principles of Internal Medicine* 15th edn 2001;1580-1584.
3. Arze RS, Rashid H, Morley R. Shunt nephritis: Report of two cases and review of the literature. *Clin Nephrol* 1983;19: 48-53.

4. Neugarten J, Gallo GR, Baldwin DS. Glomerulonephritis in bacterial endocarditis. *Am J Kidney Dis* 1984;3:371-379.
5. Ronco P, Verroust P, Morel-Maroger L. Viruses and Glomerulonephritis. *Nephron* 1982;31:97-102.
6. Baldwin S, Gluck MC, Schacht RG. The long-term course of poststreptococcal glomerulonephritis. *Ann Intern Med* 1974;80:342-358.
7. Dodge WF, Spargo BH, Travis LB. Poststreptococcal glomerulonephritis: A prospective study in children. *N Engl J Med* 1972;286:273-278.

Preeti Shanbag and Vaishali More

57 Hemolytic Uremic Syndrome

INTRODUCTION

Hemolytic uremic syndrome (HUS) consists of a triad of hemolytic anemia, thrombocytopenia and acute renal failure and was first described in 1955.[1] It is one of the most common causes of acute renal failure in children. The clinical course of HUS can vary from subclinical to life-threatening. Studies have revealed distinct subgroups of the disease and have identified several etiologies.

HUS and thrombotic thrombocytopenic purpura (TTP) seen in adults are considered two ends of the spectrum of the same disease with severe renal failure in the former and multiorgan involvement in the latter as the main differentiating feature.

Major epidemiological studies conducted throughout the world have shown a variety of etiological factors.[2] E.coli diarrhea was postulated to be a predisposing factor in 1968.[2] Karmali et al later discovered that 85% of patients of HUS have evidence of exposure to verotoxin (shiga toxin)-producing *E. coli* 0157:H7.[3] Shiga-toxin associated HUS occurs mainly in childhood. HUS is classified in a variety of ways which are not mutually exclusive: diarrhea-associated (D+ HUS) or atypical or sporadic (D- HUS);[4] an etiological classification such as Shiga toxin-associated HUS (Stx HUS); clinical classifications of severity such as mildly affected or severely affected; and a histological classification of the renal involvement as predominantly glomerular, predominantly arteriolar or cortical necrosis.[5]

EPIDEMIOLOGY

The incidence of HUS is 0.3-10% per 100,000 population. It is seen less commonly in blacks than in whites.[6] Males and females are affected in equal numbers, though the disease may affect females more severely. Diarrhea-associated HUS usually occurs in children aged 7 months to 6 years. No age predilection exists for D-HUS. Major epidemiological studies conducted throughout the world have shown a variety of etiological factors.[2] Epidemics of HUS are reported from all parts of the world, including India.[7] The incidence increases after the diarrhea season and also after consumption of contaminated or under-cooked beef, raw milk, fruits, vegetables soiled by manure, or swimming in contaminated water.[8] Person-to-person infection can occur due to poor hygienic practices.[9] Seasonal variation is not observed in D-HUS.

In the developed world, mortality rates have decreased from near universal fatality in 1955 to 3-5% during the 1990s. This is attributed to better management of renal failure with preemptive dialysis and management of hypertension. However mortality in India remains high.[7] Patients with hereditary HUS have a worse prognosis.[10]

ETIOLOGY

The etiological classification of HUS is given in Table 57.1.[5] HUS has several genetic forms. Genetically induced cases are usually not preceded by diarrheal disease, often manifest a recurrent course and are associated with a more guarded long-term prognosis as regards maintenance of normal kidney function.[10] The best studied genetic variant of HUS involves mutations in one of the short consensus repeat segments of the gene for factor H, a protein that regulates complement.[11]

PATHOPHYSIOLOGY

The disease process begins with the systemic absorption from the gastrointestinal tract of a toxin that causes endothelial damage. The major toxins that cause HUS, Shiga toxin1 (Stx1) and Shiga toxin2 (Stx2) are similar in structure to the classic Shiga toxin (Stx). Organ injury occurs after binding of the toxin to globotriocylceramide (Gb3), a glycolipid receptor molecule present on the endothelial cells. Damage primarily occurs in the kidney but may occur in the other organs. The predominance of renal injury may be caused by differential expression of GB3 on the glomerular capillaries versus other endothelial cells.[12, 13]

In populations expressing the P1 blood, the P1 blood group antigens have a terminal disaccharide, galactose (alpha-

Table 57.1: Etiological classification of HUS[5]

Infections
• E. coli O157:H7
• Shigella dysenteriae
• Streptococcus pneumoniae
Inherited forms of HUS
• Autosomal-recessive HUS
• Autosomal-dominant HUS
• Inborn error of cobalamin metabolism
Drug-associated HUS
• Cyclosporine
• FK-506
• OKT3
• Mitomycin-C
• Oral contraceptives
• Crack cocaine
Thrombotic Microangiopathy
• BMT-associated HUS
• Cancer-associated HUS
• Systemic lupus
• Systemic sclerosis
• Pregnancy-associated HUS
Rare HUS Associations
• Poststreptococcal glomerulonephritis
• Nail-patella syndrome

4)–galactose. These antigens can bind Stx and provide protection to these individuals from developing HUS. Hence, in populations with a greater expression of the P1 blood group the incidence of the disease is very low.[14,15]

The damaged endothelial cells lead to release of vasoactive and platelet-aggregating substances which cause deposition of fibrin on the damaged endothelial wall. Microthrombi formation within the glomerular capillaries leads to a localized intravascular coagulopathy. This in turn causes a fall in the glomerular filtration rate and renal insufficiency. Erythrocytes are damaged and fragmented as they traverse the narrowed glomerular capillaries. This leads to the characteristic microangiopathic hemolytic anemia. Also, pathogenic VTEC release a lipopolysaccharide which after gastrointestinal absorption causes release of inflammatory mediators like TNFα, interleukins and elastase. These add further to endothelial cell damage and free radical release leading to oxidative cell membrane injury.[13] In cases of HUS caused by Streptococcus pneumoniae, the bacteria produce neuraminidase which damages endothelial cells.[16] The Gb3 receptors are present in greater numbers in the cortex as compared to the medulla in the kidney which co-relates with the lesions found in patients of HUS.[17]

In spite of localized intravascular coagulopathy, there is no evidence of disseminated intravascular coagulation. Coagulation studies reveal a normal prothrombin time (PT), partial thromboplastin time (PTT) and fibrinogen with normal or elevated factors V and VIII. Serum levels of prothrombotic substances are increased. These include tissue factor, platelet activating factor, tissue plasminogen activator inhibitor, von Willebrand factor and thromboxane A2.[18] Thrombocytopenia is believed to result from a combination of platelet destruction, increased consumption, sequestration in the liver and spleen, and intrarenal aggregation.

CLINICAL FEATURES[5]

Patients usually have a history of diarrhea with or without vomiting followed by pallor and irritability. Usually the diarrhea is bloody. Patients may present with restlessness, oliguria and macroscopic hematuria. In patients with STEC infection, the incidence of developing HUS is 5-15%. This incidence increases with use of antibiotics and antimotility drugs especially in very young or elderly patients. Extrarenal involvement of D+ HUS has been described in the gastrointestinal tract, pancreas, liver, gall bladder, central nervous system, heart and lung.

Gastrointestinal

The most affected organ is the colon with 100% involvement.[19] The colonic involvement may be misdiagnosed as ulcerative colitis, acute appendicitis, intussusception, rectal prolapse or gastroenteritis. Rectal prolapse, toxic megacolon and bowel wall necrosis may occur as a complication.[20] Increased liver size along with increase in serum transaminases due to hypoxia or hepatitis is seen. Rarely, pancreatic involvement also occurs in less than 10% of patients. This manifests as glucose intolerance, IDDM and elevated serum amylase and lipase.[21,22] Late complications of pancreatic insufficiency may be seen in patients who have recovered from the acute episode. Decreased serum albumin results due to gastrointestinal loss.[23]

Renal

Renal manifestations are severe in patients with HUS presenting as oliguria or anuria. Occassionally increased urinary volumes have been reported.[24] Hematuria can be either microscopic or macroscopic. Blood pressure may be normal or elevated. Sometimes patients present with signs of fluid overload like edema, hypertension or congestive cardiac failure. Renal functions show an elevation of serum creatinine and blood urea nitrogen. Serum potassium, phosphorus and uric acid are elevated but serum concentrations of bicarbonate, sodium and albumin may be low.

Hematological

Hemolysis occurs in all patients with HUS and can proceed rapidly resulting in a fall of hematocrit. Hemolysis may occur repeatedly over a prolonged period. Platelet counts fall usually below 40,000/mm^3. However, the degree of thrombocytopenia does not correlate with the renal function, some children maintaining relatively normal renal function despite severe hematological abnormalities. Patients may have petechiae, purpura and oozing from venepuncture sites but overt bleeding is less common.[25]

Neurological

Patients are usually irritable, have behavioral changes, restlessness, ataxia, dizziness, tremors and twitching.[26] Severe neurological involvement may occur either as seizures or focal neurological deficits e.g. hemiparesis, stupor, coma, decerebrate rigidity and blindness. Neurological involvement may occur during the recovery also.[27] Usually the outcome from these deficits is good. Magnetic resonance imaging (MRI) is the modality of choice for early detection of structural lesions, especially for basal ganglia involvement.[28]

Cardiorespiratory

Most cardiovascular manifestations are caused by volume overload. Myocarditis has been reported occasionally in patients of HUS.[29] Some patients may develop the adult respiratory distress syndrome.

INVESTIGATIONS[5]

1. Complete blood count reveals an increase in the leukocyte count with the differential showing a shift to the left with immature WBCs including band forms, myelocytes and metamyelocytes. There is anemia and thrombocytopenia. Fragmented RBCs are seen on the peripheral smear. The reticulocyte count is increased. Coombs test is positive only in patients with HUS following S. pneumoniae infection.
2. Prothrombin time and partial thromboplastin time are normal but fibrin degradation products are elevated. Serum fibrinogen may be normal or elevated.
3. Renal function tests show an elevated blood urea nitrogen (BUN) and serum creatinine. Serum sodium may be low due to fluid overload. Serum potassium may be initially low due to potassium losses during the diarrheal prodrome but are later elevated because of renal failure and hemolysis. Serum phosphorus and uric acid are elevated. The arterial blood gases show metabolic acidosis.
4. Liver function tests show elevated transaminases and lactate dehydrogenase. Serum triglycerides and cholesterol may be elevated.
5. Urinalysis usually reveals dysmorphic red blood cells and red blood cell casts. Proteinuria and microscopic hematuria are invariably present unless patient is anuric.
6. Stool culture has a poor yield if done after 7 days of diarrhea.
7. A chest X-ray may show evidence of congestion.
8. An ECG may show changes of hyperkalemia.
9. Shiga toxin may be detected using specific antibody testing, genetic studies or enzyme-linked immunosorbent assay (ELISA).
10. Renal biopsy is rarely indicated in patients with D+ HUS.

Histopathology[5]: The characteristic histopathologic lesion is thrombotic microangiopathy (TMA) which consists of thrombi in the glomeruli and small arterioles. The glomerular lesion is often focal and consists of endothelial cell swelling and widened subendothelial space. This results in a thickened capillary wall and reduced capillary lumen. Fibrin-like substances and lipids are present in the sub-endothelial space. The glomerular basement is intact. Thrombi may occlude arteriolar lumens. Tubulointerstitial disease may be present and in some cases widespread cortical necrosis.

Immunofluorescent microscopy may show deposits of fibrin, fibronectin, IgM and C3 along capillary walls, in the mesangium, and in the sub-endothelial spaces of capillaries and arterioles.

Electron Microscopy: Ultrastructural changes are normal laminae densa and rara externa, swollen endothelial cells with prominent nuclei and damaged membrane fenestrata; detachment of endothelial cells from the basement with the formation of a sub-endothelial space; deposition of fibrin, cellular fragments, lipids and occasional platelets in this space and swollen endothelial cells with effacement of foot processes.

TREATMENT[5]

Successful management begins with early recognition of the disease and supportive care. Management includes good control of volume status, electrolyte abnormalities, hypertension and anemia. Hydration status should be monitored closely with frequent measurements of body weight, fluid intake and output, heart rate and blood pressure.

Fluid and Electrolyte

In the acute phase, patients may be dehydrated due to the loose motions and require repletion but over hydration should be avoided. In patients who are euvolemic the fluids should be limited to urine output plus insensible water losses. In the patients of HUS intravascular fluid volume could be best monitored using a central venous pressure line. Electrolyte and arterial blood gases require frequent monitoring in the early stages of the disease or while patient is on dialysis. In children in whom renal function is stable, testing may be performed daily.

A diuretic such as furosemide may be administered if fluid overload is present.

Potassium should not be added to replacement fluids unless the child is hypokalemic. Hyperkalemia may be treated with oral or rectal Kayexalate. Severe hyperkalemia may be treated with intravenous bicarbonate, glucose and insulin and calcium (if ECG changes are present).

Dialysis

Nonoliguric patients generally need dialysis. Early dialysis should be considered if the patient develops severe fluid overload, severe hyperkalemia, severe acidosis, hyponatremia or oliguria unresponsive to diuretics. The dialysis techniques may be peritoneal dialysis, hemodialysis or continuous arteriovenous hemodiafiltration. Hemodialysis is indicated in cases of abdominal surgery or circulatory imbalance. It otherwise has no added advantage over peritoneal dialysis. Peritoneal dialysis is well-tolerated in young infants and is technically easier. Some data indicate that peritoneal dialysis may be preferred because it facilitates the clearance of plasminogen activator inhibitor-1 (PAI-1).

Anemia and Thrombocytopenia

If the hemoglobin falls below 6 mg/dl patients should receive packed cell transfusions of 5-10 ml/kg. Blood transfusions require close monitoring as they may be followed by hypertension.

Platelet transfusions are not routinely indicated since further platelet aggregation may increase thrombus formation. They are indicated only if the platelet count falls below 10,000/cumm, patient has active bleeding or an invasive procedure is to be undertaken.

Hypertension

ACE-inhibitors should be used with caution in patients with a decreased glomerular filtration rate and hyperkalemia. For hypertension, calcium channel blockers or hydralazine usually suffice though in some cases, sodium nitroprusside may be required.

Convulsions

Convulsions are treated with intravenous diazepam or phenytoin. If status epilepticus develops, treatment may include a continuous infusion of midazolam or pentobarbital and mechanical ventilatory support. In the absence of recurrent seizures or structural neurological damage, anticonvulsants may be discontinued before discharge from hospital.

Nutrition

Maintaining adequate energy intake enterally or parenterally is important. Patients may require total parenteral nutrition because of continued diarrhea, colitis, ileus or abdominal pain.

Specific Therapy

Plasma exchange has been found to be beneficial in patients with D-HUS and prolonged or recurrent HUS.[30] It should be avoided in patients with HUS following pneumococcal infections since plasma contains antibodies to the T antigen which can worsen the hemolysis.[31]

Antithrombotic therapy and fresh frozen plasma infusions have been tried without much success especially in D+ HUS.[32,33] Corticosteroids, Vitamin E, furosemide and captopril do not affect the outcome though diuretics may help in controlling hypertension.

Oral therapy with Synsorb PK developed from chromosorb, a silicon dioxide which adsorbs the toxin has been tried but failed to diminish the severity of disease in pediatric patients with diarrhea-associated HUS.[34]

Follow-up

Patients should be monitored for arterial hypertension and proteinuria. Persistence of proteinuria or hypertension 1 year after an episode of HUS indicates an increased risk of progression to chronic renal failure.

Renal Transplant in HUS[5]

Patients with D+HUS rarely require renal transplant.

Patients respond well to renal transplant in cases of D+HUS. In cases of D-HUS or HUS secondary to drugs, there may be a recurrence in the transplanted kidney.

PROGNOSIS[5]

Prognosis depends on the nature of the HUS. In general, patients with D+HUS have a better outcome than patients with D- HUS. Most patients with D+ HUS who receive appropriate therapy have a good recovery.

Poor prognostic indicators are:

- Elevated WBC count at diagnosis.
- Prolonged anuria.
- Severe prodromal illness.
- Severe hemorrhagic colitis with rectal prolapse or colonic gangrene.
- Severe multisystem involvement.
- Persistent proteinuria.

ATYPICAL HUS

Atypical/D-HUS has an insidious onset with a rapid progression. These may be inherited with relapses and remissions. These cases have a poor outcome,[35] especially when hypertension is a feature at presentation. Histopathologically, they show arteriolar lesions predominantly with intimal cell proliferation, thickening and necrosis of the wall and narrowed lumen. Plasmapheresis and plasma infusions may be helpful in these cases.

REFERENCES

1. Gasser C, Gautier C, Steck R, et al. Hamolytisch– uramische syndrome: Bilaterle Niennindennekrosen bie akuten erwobenen Hamolytischen Anamien. *Schweiz Med Wochenschr* (Abstract) 1955;85:905-909.

2. Kibel M, Barnard P. The hemolytic uremic syndrome: a survey in Southern Africa. *S Afr Med J* 1968;42:692-698.
3. Karmali M, Steele B, Petric M, et al. Sporadic cases of haemolytic-uremic syndrome associated with fecal cytotoxin and cytotoxin-producing E.coli in stools. *Lancet* 1983;619-620.
4. Trompeter R, Schwartz R, Chantier C, et al. Hemolytic-uremic syndrome: an analysis of prognostic features. *Arch Dis Child* 1983;58:101-105.
5. Meyers KEC, Kaplan BS. Hemolytic-Uremic Syndromes. In:Barratt TM, Avner ED, Harmon W, eds. *Pediatric Nephrology.* Baltimore: Lippincott, Williams and Wilkins 1999;811-822.
6. Jernigan SM, Waldo FB. Racial incidence of hemolytic uremic syndrome. *Pediatr Nephrol* 1994;8:545-547.
7. Srivastava R, Moudgil A, Bagga A, et al. Hemolytic uremic syndrome in northern India. *Pediatr Nephrol* 1991;5:284-288.
8. Su BL. Escherichia coli O157:H7 infection in humans. *Ann Intern Med* 1995;123:698-714.
9. Parry SM, Palmer SR. The public health significance of VTEC 0157. *Symp Ser Soc Appl Microbiol* 2000; 29:1S-9S.
10. Siegler R, Pavia A, Hansen F, et al. Atypical hemolytic uremic syndrome: a comparison with post-diarrheal disease. *J Pediatr* 1996;128:505-511.
11. Neumann HP, Salzmann M, Bohnert-Iwan B, et al. Hemolytic uremic syndrome and mutations of the factor H gene: a registry-based study of German speaking countries. *J Med Genet* 2003;40:676-681.
12. Obrig T, Moran T, Brown J. The mode of action of Shiga toxin o peptide elongation of eukaryocytic protein synthesis. *Biochem J* 1987;244:287-294.
13. Taylor C. Verocytotoxin-producing Escherichia coli and the haemolytic uremic syndrome. *J Infect* 1995; 30:189-192.
14. Newburg D, Chaturvedi P, Lopez E, et al. Susceptibility to hemolytic uremic syndrome relates to erythrocyte glycosphingolipid patterns. *J Infect Dis* 1993;168:476-479.
15. Orrr P, Dong V, Schroeder M, et al. P1 blood group antigen expression and epjdemic hemolytic uremic syndrome. *Pediatr Nephrol* 1995;9:612-613.
16. Novak R, Martin C, Orsini E. Hemolytic uremic syndrome and T-crypt-antigen exposure by neuraminidase-producing pneumococci: an emerging problem. *Pediatr Pathol* 1983;1: 409-413.
17. Boyd B, Lingwood C. verotoxin receptor glycolipid in human renal tissue. *Nephron* 1989;51:207-210.
18. Leonard M, Ruchelli E, Kaplan B. The pathogenesis of typical diarrhea-associated hemolytic uremic syndrome. In: Andreucci V, Fine L (eds) *International Yearbook of Nephrology.* London: Springer-Verlag 1993;199-216.
19. Gallo G, Gianantonio C. Extrarenal involvement in diarrhea-associated hemolytic-uremic syndrome. *Pediatr Nephrol* 1994;9:117-119.
20. Siegler RJ. Spectrum of extra-renal involvement in post-diarrheal hemolytic-uremic syndrome. *J Pediatr* 1994;125:511-518.
21. Grodinsky S, Telmesani A, Robson W, et al. Gastrointestinal manifestations of hemolytic uremic syndrome: recognition of pancreatitis. *J Pediatr Gastroenterol Nutr* 1990;11:518-524.
22. Andreoli S, Bergstein J. Development of insulin-dependent diabetes mellitus during the hemolytic uremic syndrome. *J Pediatr* 1982;100:541-545.
23. Goos G, Declereq P, Proesmans W. Serum proteins in the haemolytic uraemic syndrome. *Pediatr Nephrol* 1995;9:292-294.
24. Schulman S, Kaplan BS. Management of patients with hemolytic uremic syndrome demonstrating severe azotemia but no anuria. *Pediatr Nephrol* 1996;10:671-674.
25. Fong J, Kaplan BS. Impairment of platelet aggregation in hemolytic uremic syndrome: evidence for platelet exhaustion. *Blood* 1982;60:564-570.
26. Hahn J, Havens P, Higgens J, et al. Neurological complications of the hemolytic-uremic syndrome. *J Child Neurol* 1989;4:108-113.
27. Rasoulpour M, Leichtner A, Jorge MS, et al. Cerebral vascular accident during the recovery phase of hemolytic uremic syndrome. *Int J Pediatr Nephrol* 1985;6:287-288.
28. Dimario F, Bronte-Stewart H, Sherbotie J, et al. Lacunar infarction of the basal ganglia as a complication of the hemolytic uremic syndrome. *Clin Pediatr* 1987;26:586-590.
29. Ray C, Portman J, Stamm S, et al. Hemolytic uremic syndrome and myocarditis. Association with coxsackie B infection. *Am J Dis Child* 1971;122:418-420.
30. Kaplan B. Recurrent hemolytic uremic syndrome. In: Kaplan BS, Trompeter RS, Moake JL (eds) *Hemolytic Uremic Syndrome/Thrombotic Thrombocytopenic purpura.* New York: Marcel Dekker 1992;151-162.
31. McGraw M, Lendon M, Stevens R, et al. Hemolytic uraemic syndrome and the Thomson-Friedenreich antigen. *Pediatr Nephrol* 1989;3:135-139.
32. Loriat S, Sonsino E, Hinglais N, et al. Treatment of childhood haemolytic uraemic syndrome with plasma. A multicenter randomized controlled trial. *Pediatr Nephrol* 1988;2:279-285.
33. Rizzoni G, Claris-Appiani A, Edefonti A, et al. Plasma infusion for hemolytic-uremic syndrome in children: results of a multicenter controlled trial. *J Pediatr* 1988;112:284-290.
34. Trachtman H, Cnaan A, Christen E, et al. Effect of an oral Shiga toxin-binding agent on diarrhea-associated hemolytic uremic syndrome in children: A randomized controlled trial. *JAMA* 2003;290:1337-44.
35. Neuhans TJ, Calonder S, Leumann EP. Heterogeneity of a typical hemolytic uremic syndromes. *Arch Dis Child* 1997;76: 518-521.

Pankaj Hari and Mukta Mantan

58 Acute Renal Failure

INTRODUCTION

Acute renal failure (ARF) is characterized by an abrupt decline in renal function, resulting in a rise in levels of blood urea and creatinine. Mortality due to ARF in intensive care setting continues to be high. However, on most other occasions the decline in renal function may be reversible, especially for prerenal causes. In children, acute renal failure may be associated with anuria, oliguria or normal urine output. Oliguria is defined in infants and young children as urine output less than 0.5-1.0 ml/kg/hour. In older children, an output less than 400 ml/day is termed oliguria. Urine output less than 1 ml/kg/day is labeled as anuria. ARF is frequently associated with abnormalities of fluid and electrolyte homeostasis.[1]

The reported incidence of ARF in neonatal units is 1-3%.[2] In older children, it is estimated roughly at 4 per lakh child population. The etiology of ARF may be prerenal, intrinsic renal or postrenal.[1,3] Prerenal failure is renal insufficiency due to inadequate systemic and/or renal circulation. It can be caused by either systemic hypovolemia or renal hypoperfusion. 'Postrenal' failure occurs as a consequence of mechanical obstruction in the urinary collecting system. Both pre- and post-renal categories can, if prolonged, lead to parenchymal injury to the kidneys (intrinsic renal failure). ARF related to overwhelming sepsis or following major surgery (especially cardiac) is common in hospitalized children. Children with ARF due to acute interstitial nephritis, aminoglycoside toxicity and neonatal hypoxia may have normal urine output *(nonoliguric renal failure)*. Nonoliguric ARF may remain subclinical and is often missed if renal functions are not performed.

The important causes of ARF are listed in Table 58.1. The most common cause of ARF in developing countries is acute tubular necrosis (ATN) due to dehydration. Diarrhea-associated hemolytic uremic syndrome (HUS) is an important cause of intrinsic renal failure in preschool children. Glomerulonephritis is more common in older children.

Table 58.1: Important causes of ARF

Prerenal failure
- Hypovolemia (dehydration, diabetic ketoacidosis, hemorrhages)
- Third space losses (sepsis, nephrotic syndrome)

Congestive heart failure
- Bilateral renal vessel occlusion (arterial or venous)
- Drugs (diuretics, ACE inhibitors, prostaglandin synthetase inhibitors)

Intrinsic renal failure
- Acute tubular necrosis
- Ischemic: hypoxic insult
- Drug-induced: Aminoglycoside, radiocontrast, ifosphamide, NSAID
- Toxin mediated: Exogenous (diethylene glycol, methanol), endogenous (hemoglobinuria, myoglobinuria)
- Tumor lysis syndrome
- Interstitial nephritis (drug-induced, idiopathic)
- Hemolytic uremic syndrome
- Glomerulonephritis (GN)
- Pos tinfectious GN, lupus nephritis, microscopic polyangiitis, Henoch Schonlein nephritis, membranoproliferative GN

Obstructive uropathy
- Obstruction in solitary kidney
- Bilateral pelviureteric junction obstruction, ureteral obstruction (stenosis, stone)
- Posterior urethral valves
- Neurogenic bladder
- Ureterocele
- Urethral stricture

DIAGNOSIS

A carefully-recorded history provides useful clues to the diagnosis of the underlying cause of ARF. A history of preceding diarrhea and features of dehydration indicate ATN. Presence of gross hematuria with hypertension suggests glomerulonephritis. History of intake of nephrotoxic drug may point towards drug-induced ATN. The presence of rash, arthropathy, fever may indicate a diagnosis of glomerulonephritis, vasculitis or interstitial nephritis.

Palpable flank masses or bladder indicate postrenal obstruction.

Conditions that result in decreased intravascular volume result in oliguria and prerenal failure. Prerenal failure is reversible if treated promptly. If the hypovolemia persists, sustained renal hypoperfusion results in ATN. Almost 10% of the patients presenting with ARF have chronic renal disease.[1] A careful history and examination are often useful to identify these cases. A history of growth failure and recurrent urinary tract infections is suggestive of reflux nephropathy. A history of polyuria, polydipsia, and nocturnal enuresis may indicate concentration defects. Poor growth, bony abnormalities, anemia, hypertension, retinopathy, left ventricular hypertrophy are markers of chronic renal disease. Small kidneys with increased echogenicity on ultrasonography, radiological evidence of osteodystrophy and elevated parathormone levels are suggestive of chronic or acute on chronic renal disease.

Role of Urinary Indices

Urinary osmolality, urine sodium and fractional excretion of sodium (FeNa) have been used to differentiate prerenal failure from ATN (Table 58.3). In ATN, tubular dysfunction manifests as failure to concentrate urine (osmolality < 400 m Osm/kg), failure to reabsorb sodium (urine sodium > 40 mEq/l or FeNa > 3%). However, the utility of these indices in clinical practice is limited.[3] These can be used if the patient seeks medical attention early and has not been given fluid challenge or diuretics.

A more practical approach to differentiate prerenal failure from ATN is as follows. The hydration status of the patient should be assessed. If dehydration is present, intravenous fluids should be given to correct dehydration, which should be followed by administration of frusemide. Patients with normal hydration may be given a fluid bolus of 10-20 ml/kg (normal saline) over 30 minutes, followed by frusemide (2 mg/kg). Edematous patients should be given diuretics straightaway. There is no need to give additional fluids in overhydrated patients as it may worsen fluid overload and precipitate congestive heart failure. If clinical assessment of volume status is difficult, central venous pressure monitoring may be indicated. Patients who fail to pass urine after these measures should be considered to have intrinsic ARF or ATN.[4,5] If diuretic administration improves the urine output, further doses can be given on regular basis.

Investigations

Relevant investigations in a case of ARF are listed in Table 58.2. A kidney biopsy is not needed in all cases of ARF and is probably unnecessary in the first 2 weeks of illness. It is required in patients with rapidly progressive renal failure, nonresolving acute glomerulonephritis where specific therapy may be needed. In patients with ATN and HUS renal biopsy may be indicated later for prognostication if the patient fails to improve after 4 weeks of supportive management. A patient with severe azotemia (blood urea > 180 mg/dl, creatinine >3-4 mg/dl) is at risk of bleeding from a renal biopsy. A bleeding, clotting time, prothrombin time and platelet count should always be done before planning for biopsy. Patients with severe azotemia should be dialyzed (hemodialysis or peritoneal dialysis) prior to biopsy to reduce the risk of bleeding. Intranasal administration of desmopressin 30 minutes prior to the procedure improves the bleeding time. Desmopressin is given in doses of 2-3 µgm/kg.[6] Stringent monitoring should be done after the procedure.

Table 58.2: Investigations in ARF

- Complete blood count, peripheral smear, reticulocyte count
- Blood urea, creatinine, calcium, phosphate, bicarbonate, sodium, potassium, albumin, cholesterol
- Urine routine and microscopy, urine sodium
- Stool culture- diarrhea, HUS
- Chest X-ray (rule out fluid overload, cardiomegaly)
- Renal ultrasound (kidney, bladder)
- Doppler ultrasonography (suspected arterial or venous thrombosis)
- (Suspected rapidly progressive glomerulonephritis)
- Antistreptolysin O titre, C3 level
- Antinuclear antibody, antineutrophil cytoplasmic antibody
- Kidney biopsy

MANAGEMENT

The management of ARF is largely supportive. The aim of therapy is to maintain fluid and electrolyte balance and treat the underlying cause wherever possible.

Specific Therapy

Intensive immunosuppression with methylprednisolone and cyclophosphamide is indicated in patients with rapidly progressive glomerulonephritis due to lupus nephritis, vasculitis with crescent formation. Oral corticosteroids may be useful in acute interstitial nephritis. In diethylene glycol poisoning, early dialysis and intravenous ethanol administration may prevent further renal damage.[7] In HUS, the treatment is mainly supportive and there is no role of antibiotics, steroids and plasmapheresis. In drug induced ATN, the offending drug should be discontinued.

Table 58.3: Indices to differentiate prerenal from established (intrinsic) ARF

	Prerenal	*Intrinsic renal*
Urinary sodium (mEq/l)	< 20	> 40
Urinary osmolality (mOsm/kg)	> 500	< 300
Fractional excretion of sodium*	< 1	> 3

$$\text{*FeNa}(\%) = \frac{\text{urine sodium} \times \text{serum creatinine}}{\text{serum sodium} \times \text{urine creatinine}} \times 100$$

Table 58.4: Management of complications

Problem	*Treatment*
Fluid overload	Fluid restriction
Pulmonary edema	Oxygen; frusemide 2-4 mg/kg IV, dialysis in resistant cases
Hypertension	*Symptomatic* Sodium nitroprusside 0.5-8 mg/kg per minute infusion; frusemide 2-4 mg/kg IV *Asymptomatic* Nifedipine 0.3-0.5 mg/kg oral, atenolol 1-2 mg/kg/day
Metabolic acidosis	Sodium bicarbonate (IV or oral) depending on severity
Hyperkalemia	*Emergency* Calcium gluconate (10%) 0.5-1 ml/kg over 5-10 minutes iv (stabilizes the myocardium)
Salbutamol	5-10 mg nebulized (shifts potassium from extracellular to intracellular compartment) Less urgent Sodium bicarbonate (8.4%) 1-2 ml/kg over 15 minutes Glucose (50%) 0.5-1 g/kg and insulin 0.1-0.2 U/kg Calcium or sodium resonium (kayexalate) 1g/kg per day (removes potassium from the body)
Hyponatremia	Fluid restriction; if sensorial alteration or seizures, 3% saline 6-12 ml/kg over 30-90 minutes. If resistant consider dialysis
High serum phosphate	Phosphate binders (calcium carbonate, acetate); dietary phosphorus restriction

Supportive Treatment

Role of Mannitol, Frusemide and Dopamine

Although, improving the urine output and converting oliguric to nonoliguric renal failure eases the management of ARF, it does not alter the course of renal failure. Mannitol has been used in the past but no clear benefit has been demonstrated. Moreover, in patients with volume overload and oliguria, mannitol may cause congestive heart failure. Recent studies and a meta-analysis have shown that low dose dopamine (0.5-5 µg/kg/min) does not offer any benefit and the need for dialysis and mortality remain unchanged.[8,9] Frusemide should be tried initially; if there is no change in urine output its further administration should be abandoned

Fluid and Electrolyte Balance

Fluids should be restricted to less than 400 ml/m^2/d (insensible losses) plus the urine output and other significant losses in an oliguric patient. Fluid restriction is often difficult to achieve in children. It requires stringent monitoring of intake and output. Preferably the child should be catheterized initially. For effective fluid restriction parents should be counseled repeatedly, drinking water should be removed from the vicinity of the child and free water should be allowed for consuming oral medications only.

In order to restrict potassium intake fruits (especially citrus) and fruit juices should be avoided. In addition potassium-binding resin (kayexalate) may be used. Acute rise in serum potassium can be managed by giving intravenous sodium bicarbonate, calcium, and glucose with neutralizing drip of insulin. Nebulized salbutamol has also been shown to reduce serum potassium in some studies.

Patients with ARF may have hypocalcemia and hyperphosphatemia. The administration of sodium bicarbonate for the correction of acidosis reduces the levels of ionized calcium and can precipitate tetany. It is better to administer intravenous calcium before sodium bicarbonate is given for correction of acidosis. The patient should also receive oral calcium supplements and phosphate binders such as calcium carbonate.

The doses of the drugs administered to patients with ARF should be modified according to the creatinine clearance. Oral anti hypertensive drugs of choice are nifedipine and beta-blockers.

The management of complications of ARF is listed in Table 58.4.

Nutrition

Protein and calorie intake: Nutrition is one of the most difficult issues in the management of ARF. Children with ARF are in a hypercatabolic state. The aim of nutritional support is to provide adequate calories, avoid catabolism and minimize the production of nitrogenous waste. Initially proteins may be restricted to 0.5 g/kg/day to minimize urea generation. However in prolonged renal failure, 100% of the RDA for proteins should be given to prevent malnutrition. Similarly, 100% of the RDA for calories should be given.

In infants, it is aimed to provide 120 Kcal/kg/day. Carbohydrates should provide majority of these calories. Sometimes, it may be difficult to achieve the intended caloric intake in a child who is primarily on semisolid or liquid feeds. Feed fortification can be done in such patients. An anorexic patient can be fed by nasogastric tube. Also, an early institution of dialysis can ease the restrictions on liquids.[10,11]

Monitoring

It is extremely important to record the fluid intake, output and weight daily. On fluid restriction, and inadequate calorie intake the patient should lose weight by 0.5-1% daily. Often the course of ARF is complicated by infections; hence these patients should be examined for infections periodically.

Renal Replacement Therapy

Acute renal failure in children requiring dialysis can be managed with a variety of modalities, including peritoneal dialysis, intermittent hemodialysis, and continuous hemofiltration or hemodiafiltration. The choice of dialysis modality to be used is influenced by several factors, including the goals of dialysis, patient parameters, the unique advantages and disadvantages of each modality, and institutional resources.[12] Common indications of instituting dialysis in ARF are listed in Table 58.5. A comparison of different modes of dialysis is given in Table 58.6.

Table 58.5: Indications for renal replacement therapy

Persistent hyperkalemia
Refractory acidosis
Uremic encephalopathy
Pulmonary edema
Resistant hypo or hypernatremia
Hyperuricemia*
Tumor lysis syndrome
Hyperammonemia and inborn errors of metabolism

Intermittent Peritoneal Dialysis (IPD)

The initial renal replacement therapy of choice in sick and unstable patient is peritoneal dialysis (PD).[13] It is usually done by using a rigid catheter and trocar. It is desirable to use a soft peritoneal dialysis catheter such as Tenckhoff or Cook's catheter if prolonged dialysis is anticipated. Tenckhoff catheter has to be placed surgically but the Cook's catheter can be inserted using a guide wire by Seldinger technique. The risk of infection is decreased with the use of soft catheters. Rigid peritoneal dialysis catheter should be removed after 48-72 hours, beyond which the risk of peritonitis is high. Most studies have shown the incidence of peritonitis with acute PD to be as high as 35-75%.[14,15]

The dialysis prescription would depend upon the clinical condition of the patient. Commercially manufactured solutions are available in dextrose concentrations of 1.5%, 2.25%, and 4.25%. Dialysate volumes of 20-50 ml/kg/cycle are used with dwell times varying between 15-60 minutes. In patients with fluid overload, peritoneal dialysis solution containing high glucose concentration (up to 4.25%) may be used. The dialysis cycles should be of shorter duration (20 minutes) and gradual fluid deficit should be aimed over 30-40 cycles. After 10 cycles if the potassium levels are normal potassium chloride (2 ml to a litre) may be added in the dialysis fluid. Patients who are sick and have severe lactic acidosis should be dialyzed using bicarbonate dialysis fluid.

Hemodialysis (HD)

It is effective in correction of electrolytic abnormalities and hypervolemia rapidly. However it is expensive, requires expertise, skilled nursing and is not available at most centers in our country. It is not suitable for patients with hemodynamic instability, bleeding tendency (as it requires anticoagulation) and in infants and young children where vascular access is difficult to obtain. The equipment required is the HD machine, pediatric dialyzer with tubings and dialysate fluid. An appropriate vascular access in the patient completes the circuit. The dialysis circuit is given in Figure 58.1.

The most common type of vascular access for children is a double lumen venous catheter inserted into femoral vein, subclavian or internal jugular. The dialysis machine has a blood pump, which regulates the outflow of blood from the child and delivers it to the dialyzer. In children the rate of blood flow is adjusted between 100-200 ml/min depending upon the size of the patient. Younger children (< 15 kg body weight) may be dialyzed with flow rates of 50-

Table 58.6: A comparison of different dialysis modalities

	Hemodialysis	*Peritoneal*
Advantages	Good for toxin or drug removal	Simple procedure Can be done easily in small children, especially in emergency situations
	Electrolytic abnormalities and fluid overload corrected more rapidly	Better metabolic control due to continuous nature
Disadvantages	Requires vascular access Access difficult in small children Need for technical skills and trained personnel Requires dialysis machine, Difficult in hemodynamically unstable patients	Not effective for drug, toxin removal Peritoneal infections common

* Modalities like CAVHD (continuous arterio-venous hemodiafiltration), CVVHD (continuous venovenous hemodiafiltration) are useful in management of ARF in intensive care setup. They require sophisticated machines(expensive) and advanced technical skills and are not easily available.

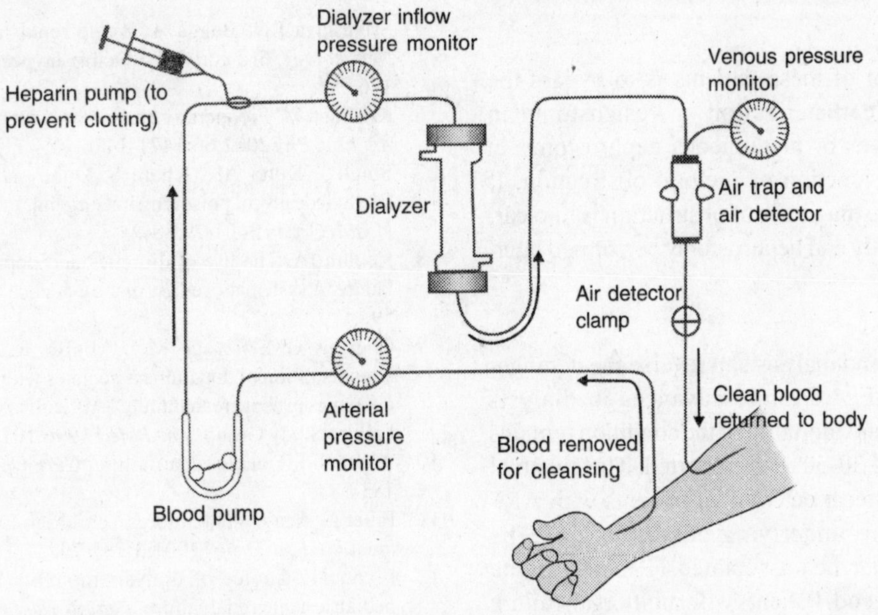

Fig. 58.1: Showing hemodialysis circuit (patient end, machine end and the monitors). The vascular access for most pediatric patients is through femoral vein for acute dialysis

75 ml/min (about 5 ml/kg/min). Heparin is commonly used for anticoagulation during the procedure. The blood flows on one side of the semipermeable membrane of the dialyzer while a concentrate of dialysate, mixed in a fixed proportion with pretreated water, flows at a rate of at least 1.5 times the blood pump rate on the other side. After dialysis the blood is returned back to the patient's circulation. Tap water is pretreated using different methods like activated carbon, ion exchange deionization and reverse osmosis. *Reverse osmosis* is the primary water purification process of choice. It effectively reduces the level of inorganic contaminants and any bacteria in the water. Activated carbon removes chloramines from the water, which are used as an alternative to chlorine in water supplies. Deionization removes extra calcium and magnesium from the water.

Common complications of acute hemodialysis include vomiting and headaches. Rapid ultrafiltration may result in hypotension. Hemodialysis is, however, useful in patients who require prolonged dialysis support. Studies have shown that daily hemodialysis of patients with ARF improves the eventual outcome compared to intermittent HD.[16]

Continuous Renal Replacement Therapy (CRRT)

CRRT is gradually replacing PD and conventional HD as the procedure of choice for treatment of *acute renal failure* in intensive care units.[17] The technique involves the removal of solutes and water by hemofiltration (convection) or dialysis (diffusion) in a continuous mode. These include CAVH (continuous arteriovenous hemofiltration), CVVH (continuous venovenous hemofiltration).

Continuous arteriovenous hemofiltration (CAVH) is an extracorporeal method for the management of hypervolemia and electrolyte disorders in patients with oliguria. It is a useful modality in critically ill patients who have multiorgan failure.

The circuit consists of an arterial access, a hemofilter and a venous access for the return of blood. The blood pressure of the patient provides the driving force while the hemofilter removes ultrafiltrate. Blood pumps are not required though heparinization of blood is essential. The indications for CAVH are primarily unstable, sick patients with fluid overload. It is useful in neonates and infants with cardiovascular and abdominal surgery, trauma, shock and multiorgan failure. It has also been used to treat acute metabolic derangements.

Continuous venovenous hemofiltration (CVVH) involves the addition of blood pump, which improves the ultrafiltration of the system. Use of high flux dialyzers converts the system to hemodiafiltration (CAVHD), in which solute clearance is much better. The circuit is similar to CAVH with addition of constant inflow of dialysate through the filter.

The advantages of CRRT are that it avoids rapid fluid and electrolyte shifts, provides hemodynamic stability, improves the adequacy of hemodialysis and allows unlimited fluid administration during the therapy. However it requires more experienced personnel, large amounts of dialysate and stringent patient monitoring and is expensive.

Postrenal ARF

The ideal management of these patients is to bypass the obstruction for e.g., catheterization or vesicostomy in posterior urethral valves or percutneous nephrostomy in bilateral pelviureteric junction or urethral obstruction. If the patient is sick or the diagnosis of obstruction is unclear, IPD may be done initially and nephrostomy performed later.

PROGNOSIS

Optimal management and dialysis can reverse the derangements caused by ARF.[18] Despite advances in dialysis techniques, morbidity and mortality of the condition remains high; mortality rates of 30-50% are reported. The eventual recovery and the long-term outcome of patients with ARF chiefly depend on the underlying condition.[19,20] The prognosis in ATN, diarrhea-associated HUS and acute interstitial nephritis is good. Patients with multiorgan failure and cortical necrosis have poor prognosis. Patients with rapidly progressive glomerulonephritis if treated late, are less likely to recover. Patients with persistent ARF should be dialyzed for at least 2-3 months. Those in whom recovery of renal function is incomplete by this duration are likely to develop chronic renal failure. Dialysis-dependent patients should be managed as end-stage renal disease.

REFERENCES

1. Andreoli SP. Management of acute renal failure. In: Barratt TM, Avner ED, Harmon (eds) *Pediatric Nephrology*, 4th edn Baltimore: William and Willkins 1999;1119-1134.
2. Stapleton FB, Jones DB, Green RS. Acute renal failure in neonates: Incidence, etiology and outcome. *Pediatr Nephrol* 1987;1: 314-320.
3. Moghal NE, Brocklebank JT, Meadow SR. A review of acute renal failure in children: Incidence, etiology and outcome. *Clin Nephrol* 1998;49:91-95.
4. Srivastava RN, Bagga A, Moudgil A. Acute renal failure in north Indian children. *Indian J Med Res* 1990;92:404-408.
5. Srivastava RN, Bagga A. Acute renal failure. In: *Pediatric Nephrology*, 3rd edn. New Delhi: Jaypee Brothers 2001;158-176.
6. Krishnan M. Preoperative care of patients with kidney disease. *Am Fam Phy* 2002;66:1471-1476.
7. Singh J, Dutta AK, Khare S, Dubey NK, Harit AK, et al. Diethylene glycol poisoning in Gurgaon, India, 1998. *Bull World Health Organ* 2001;79:88-95.
8. Kellum JA. The use of diuretics and dopamine in acute renal failure: A systematic review of the evidence. *Crit Care* 1997;1:53-59.
9. Chertow GM, Sayegh MH, Allgren R, Lazarus JM. Is the administration of dopamine associates with adverse or favorable outcomes in acute renal failure? Auriculin Anaritide Acute Renal Failure Study Group. *Am J Med* 1996;101:49-53.
10. Andreoli SP, acute renal failure. *Curr Opin Pediatr* 2002;14: 183-188.
11. Filler G. Acute renal failure in children: Etiology and management. *Pediatr Drugs* 2001;3:783-792.
12. Flynn JT. Choice of dialysis modality for management of pediatric acute renal failure. *Pediatr Nephrol* 2002; 17:61-69.
13. Flynn JT, Kershaw DB, Smoyer WE, Brophy PD, Mc Bryde KD, Bunchman TE. Peritoneal dialysis for management of pediatric acute renal failure. *Perit Dial Int* 2001;21:390-394.
14. Dandecha P, Sangthawan P. Peritonitis in acute peritoneal dialysis in a university hospital. *J Med Assoc Thai* 2002;85: 477-481.
15. Kim PK, Kim JH. Pediatric peritoneal dialysis in Korea: Practical solutions to the problems of peritoneal dialysis for children. *Perit Dial Int* 1999; 19(Suppl 2):S489-S492.
16. Sciffl H, Lang SM, Fischer R. Daily Hemodialysis and the outcome of acute renal failure. *N Engl J Med* 2002:346: 305-315.
17. Ronco C, Bellomo R, Ricci Z. Continous renal replacement therapy in critically ill patients. *Nephrol Dial Transplant* 2001;16(Suppl 5): 67-72.
18. Flynn JT. Causes, management approaches, and outcome of acute renal failure in children. *Curr Opin Pediatr* 1998;10: 184-189.
19. Barretti P, Soares VA. Acute renal failure: Clinical outcome and cause of death. *Ren Fail* 1997;19:253-257.
20. Hari P, Srivastava RN. Acute renal failure. In: Gupta RP, Maheshwari RK (eds) *Recent Trènds in Pediatrics*. New Delhi: BI Churchill Livingstone: 1998;324-337.

Section XI

Rheumatological Emergencies

Rheumatological Emergencies

Surjit Singh and Sonal Kansra

59 Emergencies in Pediatric Rheumatology

INTRODUCTION

Pediatric rheumatology is now a recognized speciality at many centers. Nevertheless, most practicing pediatricians may still be unfamiliar with the clinical presentation of children with rheumatological disorders.[1-4] In the outpatient clinic, most of these disorders are seen to have a chronic course with exacerbations and remissions. The morbidity is significantly high though the risk of mortality is low.[2-4] Under these circumstances, the treating pediatrician has to use his clinical skills and marshal his therapeutic resources to prevent or minimize disability. Contrary to common belief there is a lot that one can do to help out these patients. With the advent of newer biologicals (especially anti-TNF agents), disease limitation in pediatric rheumatology now seems like a distinct possibility.[3,4]

A significant proportion of children with rheumatological disorders, however, may present acutely, often as an emergency. In these circumstances it is incumbent upon the treating pediatrician to recognize the condition and initiate a line of management, frequently before any laboratory tests have trickled in. Timely recognition of these conditions and institution of appropriate action is crucial if unnecessary complications have to be avoided. Some rheumatological emergencies (e.g. lupus involving the central nervous system, acute arthritis, Kawasaki disease) may give only a rather narrow window period for the physician to intervene. Decision-making in such cases has to be based on clinical grounds alone. Delays can be rapidly fatal.

This review attempts to highlight some of the common rheumatological disorders that can present acutely.

ACUTE ARTHRITIS

Arthritis is said to be present when there is swelling or effusion in a joint or when there are any two of the following four clinical features: limitation of the range of motion, tenderness, pain and increased heat. Arthritis can be said to be acute when the duration of symptoms is less than two weeks. Acute arthritis is by far the most common rheumatological emergency. The diagnosis is based primarily on a detailed clinical assessment (Table 59.1). One should avoid the temptation of sending unnecessary tests, as some of these can be misleading.

Common clinical conditions that need to be considered in the differential diagnosis of acute arthritis are:

- Septic arthritis.
- Acute osteomyelitis.
- Rheumatic arthritis.
- Transient synovitis.
- Juvenile rheumatoid arthritis.

Septic Arthritis

Septic arthritis is usually a monoarthritis and more commonly occurs in the lower extremity, most of the cases being under 2 years of age (approx 50%). In pediatric age group it arises mainly by hematogenous spread.[5,6] The usual causative organisms are Staphylococcus aureus and Hemophilus influenzae.[1,2]

Table 59.1: Acute arthritis

	Etiology	*Treatment*	*Comments*
Septic arthritis	Staphylococcus aureus, Hemophilus influenzae	Surgical drainage and appropriate antimicrobials	Monoarthritis with systemic toxicity
Acute osteomyelitis	Staphylococcus aureus, GroupA streptococci, Psuedomonas sp.	Appropriate antimicrobials, surgery	
Transient synovitis	—	Conservative	Hip joint inolvement, no systemic features
Rheumatic arthritis	Antecedent infection with Group A α-hemolytic streptoccous	Aspirin	Migratory polyarthritis of large joints; response to aspirin within 24 hours

Diagnosis

Usually the child is sick and toxic looking and the joint is exquisitely tender, painful and red. Aspiration reveals fluid with a neutrophilic leukocytosis, increased protein and decreased glucose. Gram staining may be of help but cultures are frequently unrewarding. Blood cultures may occasionally be positive. X-rays may be completely normal in the initial stages but may later reveal joint space widening and some soft tissue swelling. Ultrasound examination may show presence of effusions and can guide aspiration of fluid. Radio nuclear scans can be done to look for areas of increased uptake.

Treatment

Treatment is with drainage and appropriate antimicrobials.

Pitfalls

It should be noted that a synovial fluid specimen with high protein and low glucose should not be always taken to be synonymous with septic arthritis as similar findings can also be seen in children with juvenile rheumatoid arthritis. Decision making in such a situation should be guided by the clinical presentation of the child i.e. a sick looking child with a single tender, red hot joint).

Acute Osteomyelitis

Acute osteomyelitis presents with swelling and pain at the site of infection. The swelling may take some time to manifest due to the deep placement of bone as compared to the joint synovium. Staphylococcus aureus is the commonest organism. Streptococci are the other important organisms, especially in neonates.[5,6]

Diagnosis

X-rays may be unrewarding in the initial few days as they show only soft tissue swelling, with the other destructive changes appearing late. Aspiration needs to be done from the metaphysis. Radio nuclide technetium scans help delineate joint from bone swelling.[6]

Treatment

Treatment is with long-term antimicrobials administered parenterally for atleast 4-6 weeks. Surgical decompression may be needed to drain subperiosteal or intramedullary pus.

Pitfalls

Transient synovitis of the hip may have overlapping clinical features.

Rheumatic Arthritis

Rheumatic arthritis is classically a fleeting migratory polyarthritis involving large joints, especially knees, ankles and wrists. Arthritis serves as one of the major criteria for diagnosis of acute rheumatic fever. The joints are red, warm and tender and respond quite dramatically (often within 24 hrs) to salicylate administration.[3,7]

Diagnosis

Diagnosis is mainly clinical but may be guided by the other major or minor manifestations of rheumatic fever in the same child. Response to salicylates is quite characteristic

Pitfalls

Diagnosis may be a problem if either there is no response to salicylates or there is predominant small joint involvement. The entity of post-streptococcal reactive arthritis is another source of confusion.

Transient Synovitis of the Hip Joint

This is a rather common condition and, in our experience, is often misdiagnosed as septic arthritis. It usually occurs in younger children (the mean age being 6 years) and is generally preceded by an upper respiratory illness one to two weeks earlier. The child presents with pain and limitation of movement but these patients may continue to be ambulatory and fever is not marked. Children characteristically appear well and lack of systemic toxicity is a clinical clue, which helps to differentiate the condition from septic arthritis.

Diagnosis

There may be some amount of joint effusion but it does not require to be tapped for diagnosis and the laboratory examination is non-contributory. Technetium bone scans may be done to rule out infection but are usually not required.

Treatment

Conservative management with skin traction and bed rest is all that is necessary Analgesics may be useful.

Pitfalls

It is not difficult to misdiagnose this condition as septic arthritis. From the epidemiological point of view transient synovitis is far more common than septic arthritis.

Juvenile Rheumatoid Arthritis

The term juvenile rheumatoid arthritis (JRA) should be used only for arthritides lasting more than six weeks.[8,9] In the initial stages, however, this arthritis may be difficult to differentiate from the aforementioned conditions.

Diagnosis

Clinical features, pattern of joint involvement, eye involvement, presence of systemic features aided by laboratory investigations (like erythrocyte sedimentation rate, platelet counts, C-reactive protein, rheumatoid factor, anti-nuclear antibody) help in the diagnosis of this condition. It should be noted, however, that none of these tests are pathognomic of the disease and the diagnosis remains essentially clinical. Investigations like X-rays, ultrasound, MRI and synovial biopsy may be occasionally required but rarely contribute to establishment of the diagnosis.

Treatment

The aim of treatment is to suppress the disease activity rather than cure. For pauciarticular disease, nonsteroidal anti-inflammatory drugs (like naproxen or ibuprofen) may be used initially. Involvement of a single large joint is best managed with intra-articular steroids (usually triamcinolone). For polyarticular JRA methotrexate is the therapy of choice. Response to therapy in JRA is often unpredictable and idiosyncratic responses are well known.

Pitfalls

It needs to be emphasized that synovial fluid characteristics of JRA may be quite similar to those of septic arthritis.

SYSTEMIC ONSET JRA

Systemic onset JRA is always a challenging diagnosis and may test the acumen of even experienced clinicians. Fever may be the only clinical finding. It is often quotidian (ie two peaks every day) and may be accompanied by a rash, which may only be discernible in fair skinned individuals. Children appear to be sick and toxic and may have associated features like hepatosplenomegaly, evanescent rash and joint symptoms, lymphadenopathy and pericardial effusion. It may be noted that overt arthritis need not always accompany the fever in a child with systemic onset JRA. The differential diagnosis includes conditions like infections and acute leukemia. Pericardial effusion may be a potential life threatening complication.[8,9]

Diagnosis

The most important factor in arriving at a diagnosis is a high index of suspicion. Laboratory investigations (including rheumatoid factor and antinuclear factor) are usually unrewarding. Other common causes of fever (infections and acute leukemia) should be ruled out, as the diagnosis of systemic onset JRA is essentially clinical.

Treatment

NSAIDs in appropriate doses should be started. Most children, however, need corticosteroids. Parentral steroids (e.g. methylprednisolone 30 mg/kg/day or dexamethasone 3-5 mg/kg/day) may hasten recovery. These are usually followed by oral steroids which need to be continued for many weeks/months.

Pitfalls

Occult tuberculosis may need exclusion.

MACROPHAGE ACTIVATION SYNDROME

Patients with systemic onset JRA may sometimes present with rapidly deteriorating liver functions, encephalopathy and evidence of systemic coagulation abnormalities-the macrophage activation syndrome.[7,8]

Diagnosis

Laboratory investigations may show thrombocytopenia, deranged coagulogram, elevated transaminases and raised bilirubin. The erythrocyte sedimentation rate is usually normal. There may be evidence of hemophagocytosis in the cerebrospinal fluid, bone marrow or liver.

Treatment

Macrophage activation syndrome needs to be treated aggressively with intravenous methyl prednisolone. Cyclosporin is also effective. Delays can be fatal.

Pitfalls

Viral hepatitis may be a close mimic. The diagnosis should be suspected if a child with JRA suddenly becomes sick and has features of acute liver dysfunction with the viral markers being negative.

VASCULITIDES

The common vasculitides encountered in pediatric practice are as follows:[10-14]

Large vessel: Takayasu arteritis.

Medium vessel: Polyarteritis nodosa, Kawasaki Disease.

Small vessel: Henoch-Schoenlein purpura.

In many cases the clinical presentation may be rather abrupt and timely intervention is critical.

Kawasaki Disease

Kawasaki disease is a common vasculitic disorder of children.[10] Some epidemiologic surveys have suggested that the condition is even more common than Henoch Schonlein Purpura. The diagnosis of Kawasaki disease can be made only on the recognition of a constellation of clinical findings, none of which are by themselves pathognomonic. The difficulty is further compounded by the fact that these clinical features appear sequentially and all need not be present at a given point of time. KD should be considered in the differential diagnosis of any febrile child (especially below 5 years of age) whose fever persists beyond 5 days.

KD is a clinical diagnosis, there being no confirmatory laboratory test. It is our belief that the condition remains grossly under diagnosed in our country. It is perhaps the most important and most common rheumatological emergency almost exclusive to the pediatric age group.

Diagnosis

A high grade fever often in the range of 39-40°C which is unresponsive to antimicrobials with a characteristic irritability, associated cervical lymphadenopathy (usually unilateral) and an erythematous oral mucosa (strawberry tongue and vertically fissured lips) are pointers to the diagnosis in most of the children who present in the early phase. Children may also have erythema and edema of hands and feet. Tachycardia is common.[10,12]

Characteristic periungual desquamation in fingers and toes and the back, arthritis of joints, elevated ESR and high platelet counts help identify patients presenting late in the convalescent phase. Platelet counts may often exceed 10^5/cu.mm; we have occasionally seen counts as high as 14×10^5/cu.mm. The desquamation may sometimes involve the entire area of the palms and soles. It is said that a combination of desquamation and thrombocytosis is virtually diagnostic of KD.

Treatment

Patients with a strong clinical suspicion of KD need close clinical supervision on a day-to-day basis. It is our practice to hospitalize all children in whom a diagnosis of KD is suspected so that the patient can be kept under close supervision. Investigations are then carried out to exclude other common causes of fever (e.g. typhoid, malaria and urinary infections). If the diagnosis is strongly suspected, treatment with intravenous immunoglobbulin[10] (IVIG 2 gms/kg stat) and aspirin (initially 80 mg/kg/day) should be expeditiously started. Almost all patients demonstrate an increase in well being and decreased fever in the subsequent 24 hours.

Pitfalls

Diagnosis of KD is primarily clinical and there are no specific laboratory tests. It is imperative to treat early to prevent the cardiac morbidity. Delays in treatment can have serious long-term cardiac sequelae. In our experience many children with KD are being incorrectly diagnosed as having measles, drug reactions or even Stevens Johnson Syndrome.

Henoch-Schönlein Purpura (HSP)

Is the most commonly diagnosed vasculitis of childhood. It is characterized by palpable purpura, arthralgia/arthritis, abdominal pain and variable renal involvement. While short-term morbidity in most patients of HSP is due to gastrointestinal problems, renal involvement is responsible for long term morbidity/mortality.

Diagnosis

Diagnosis of HSP again is based on clinical features rather than on any specific laboratory investigations. The characteristic palpable purpura, arthralgia/arthritis, abdominal pain, gastrointestinal bleeding and subcutaneous edema may suggest the diagnosis. Ultrasound examination is the investigation of choice for follow-up of children with significant gastrointestinal involvement, especially intussusception.

Treatment

Treatment is generally supportive and conservative. Steroids can be used for severe abdominal symptoms like bleeding and intussusception. Renal involvement may sometimes be very severe and mandate treatment with methylprednisolone followed by long-term prednisolone and azathioprine.[13]

Pitfalls

The diagnosis of HSP can be missed if the rash is not prominent or typical. We have had patients in whom laparotomies have been erroneously performed for a suspected "acute abdomen" when the correct diagnosis was in fact HSP.

Polyarteritis Nodosa

Polyarteritis nodosa is uncommon in children and there is no specific pattern of presentation.The manifestations are protean reflecting the various organs affected by the vasculitic process. Unexplained fever weight loss, abdominal pain, skin lesions, musculoskeletal pain and arthritis may be present.

Diagnosis

Ozen[11] proposed the following criteria for diagnosis of PAN in children:

Major Findings: Renal involvement, musculoskeletal involvement

Minor Findings: Cutaneous findings, gastrointestinal involvement, peripheral neuropathy, CNS disease, hypertension, cardiac involvement, lung involvement, constitutional symptoms, acute phase reactants, presence of HbSAg.

The diagnosis can be reasonably suspected by these diagnostic criteria but can be confirmed only by pathologic demonstration of lesions or by radiographic demonstration of aneurysms. The latter are characteristically located at bifurcation of arteries.

Treatment

Gucocorticoids need to be given in high doses and for prolonged periods. Cyclophosphamide or azathioprine may need to be added if there is no response.

Pitfalls

PAN can mimic many other medical conditions and is always a very difficult clinical diagnosis to establish, especially in children. Investigations may not always be contributory and treatment may sometimes have to be started based on a high index of suspicion.

Takayasu Arteritis

Takayasu arteritis is a large vessel arteritis with a predilection for the aorta and its branches. It is more common in females as compared to males. The usual presenting feature is hypertension and congestive cardiac failure. Dilated cardiomyopathy, myocarditis and aneurysmal dilatation are other presentations.[14,15]

Diagnosis

The most important clue to diagnosis is asymmetry of pulses/blood pressure on clinical examination in a hypertensive child. An elevated ESR, cardiomegaly on chest X-ray and evidence of left ventricular hypertrophy on ECG, raised complement levels and nonspecific hypergammaglobinemia may be present. Arteriography is essential for confirmation of diagnosis and may reveal stenoses/anuerysmal dilatations of various vessels viz. subclavian, carotid, renal and occasionally coronary arteries. Descending aorta is said to be most commonly involved in Indian patients.

Treatment

Treatment is by high dose steroids (prednisolone 1-2 mg/kg) for 4-8 weeks followed by tapering and low dose maintenance therapy. Cyclophosphamide and methotrexate are other therapeutic options in cases with more severe disease, especially those with myocarditis. Angioplasty and stenting are valid therapeutic options and have been successfully carried out in some of our patients. Early identification and surgical removal of anuersymal lesions may be required. Surgical intervention for renal hypertension and cerebral hypoperfusion have been tried with varying success.

Pitfalls

Measurement of four-limb blood pressure is mandatory in all children with hypertension. Control of hypertension should be done under close supervision as a sudden fall may cause ischemic effects in the eyes and brain. Blindness and cortical infarcts have been known to result from such measures. Use of angiotensin convertase enzyme inhibitors for hypertension should be withheld until renal artery stenosis has been ruled out.

SYSTEMIC LUPUS ERYTHEMATOSUS

Systemic lupus erythematosus is a prototype autoimmune disorder and is defined by its clinical features and presence of antibodies directed against one or more components of the nucleus.[16-20] The criteria used for classification of SLE were laid down by the American College of Rheumatology in 1982 and subsequently modified in 1997 (Table 59.2). Although these were originally given as classification criteria, they are widely used for diagnosis also.

Table 59.2: Criteria For classification of SLE (ACR 1997 criteria)[16]

Malar rash
Discoid lupus rash
Photosensitivity
Oral or nasal mucocutneous ulcerations
Nonerosive arthritis
Nephritis
Proteinuria > 0.5 gm/day
Cellular casts
Encephalopathy
Seizures
Psychosis
Pleuritis or pericarditis
Cytopenia
Positive immunoserology
Antibodies to dsDNA
Antibodies to Sm nuclear antigen
Positive finding of antiphospholipid antibodies based on
1. IgG or IgM anticardiolipin antibodies
2. lupus anticoagulant
3. false positive serologic test for syphilis for at least six months, confirmed by *Treponema pallidum* immobilization or fluorescent treponemal antibody.
Positive antinuclear antibody test

Diagnosis

Presence of four of the aforementioned criteria, either concurrently or sequentially, has high sensitivity and specificity for a diagnosis of SLE but one does not have to wait for fulfilment of these criteria beforee therapy is started. Less than one-fourth of children will meet four at the time of their initial diagnosis.[16-18]

Pitfalls

There are a few important points that need to be borne in mind. Although SLE is a multisystem disease, symptoms of a particular organ system may be more prominent at presentation as compared to others. Further, these criteria have not yet been validated in pediatric patients.

Systemic lupus erythematosus may present with renal, hematological, cardiac, nervous system or pulmonary involvement requiring emergency attention (Table 59.3).

Lupus Nephritis

Evidence of lupus nephritis is said to be present at the time of diagnosis in most patients of SLE. Acute renal insufficiency may supervene at presentation or during the course of the illness. Renal involvement is lupus is graded histologically according to WHO criteria (Table 59.4). Though the classification is pathological, clinical clues generally point towards the type of renal lesion. Progression of nephritis may occur during the course of the disease. In

Table 59.3: Emergency complications/presentation of SLE

Renal Complications
Acute renal failure
Pulmonary Complications
Pleural effusion
Lupus pneumonitis
Alveolar hemorrhage
Shrinking lung syndrpme
Upper airway obstruction
Infections
Neuropsychiatric Complications
Seizures
Stroke
Aseptic meningitis
Transverse myelitis
Cardiovascular Complications
Coronary artery disease
Vasculitis
Myocarditis
Pericarditis
Hematologic Complications
Anemia: Hemolytic, anemia of chronic disease, pure red cell aplasia
Thrombocytopenia
Leukopenia
Infectious Complications
Infections by viruses, bacteria, fungi, mycobacteria

WHO Class 1 and Class 2 nephritis there may be no or only minimal proteinuria and/or hematuria. Most of these patients do not develop renal insufficiency. In WHO Class 3, 4 and 5 (focal/diffuse proliferative lupus glomerulonephritis and membranous lupus nephritis reespectively) there would be significant hematuria and/or proteinuria. A large majority would develop nephrotic syndrome and renal insufficiency and only a small percentage will show remission without aggressive therapy.

Treatment

Treatment of lupus nephritis involves aggressive and sustained treatment with steroids. Diffuse glomerulonephritis may require treatment with cyclophosphamide in addition to prednisolone. Intravenous pulses of methylprednisolone and cyclophospamide can be life saving in such situations.

Neuropsychiatric Manifestations of Lupus

Acute SLE may present with lupus cerebritis, cerebovascular accidents, aseptic meningitis, seizures and transverse myelitis.

i. *Stroke:* Patients with SLE ae 8 times more prone to have stroke as compared to general population. They may present with transient ischemic attacks, hemiplegia or aphasia. These symptoms may arise due to thrombotic or embolic strokes or vasculitis.
ii. *Seizures:* Any kind of seizures, focal or generalized, may occur in patients with SLE.
iii. *Aseptic meningitis:* This is usually characterized by headache and meningeal signs.The cerebrospinal fluid shows pleocytosis, predominantly lymphocytic.

Diagnosis

Oligoclonal bands may be present in the cerebrospinal fluid. MRI is the neuroimaging of choice.

Treatment

Unlike lupus nephritis, where one can predict the severity of renal involvement based on the clinical and urinary findings, CNS involvement in lupus may be more difficult to categorize. There may be little or no correlation between the clinical and radiological findings. Infections need to be vigorously ruled out. Aggressive immunosuppressive therapy with steroids and cyclophosphamide/azathioprine is the treatment of choice. Patients with the antiphospholipid syndrome require prolonged anticoagulation.

Pitfalls

CNS lupus is a difficult condition to manage. Decisions must be based on clinical rather than radiological findings.

Pulmonary Complications of SLE

Pulmonary complications in lupus may cause significant mortality and morbidity. Infections remain the most common cause for pulmonary deterioration in these patients.

Table 59.4: WHO classification of lupus nephritis

CLASS I	Normal	No proteinuria
CLASS IIA	Minimal change	Low grade proteinuria or hematuria
CLASS IIB	Mesangial glomerulitis	Low grade proteinuria and hematuria
CLASS III	Focal and segmental proliferative glomerulonephritis	Minimal proteinuria, microscopic hematuria Nephrotic syndrome in 20%
CLASS IV	Diffuse proliferative glomerulonephritis	Proteinuria and hematuria, nephrotic syndrome Renal insufficiency in 60%
CLASS V	Membranous glomerulonephritis	Persistent nephrotic syndrome, renal insufficiency in majority

The other causes may be lupus pneumonitis, alveolar hemorrhage and shrinking lung syndrome.

i. *Lupus pnuemonitis:* presents with clinical features of pneumonia, bilateral infiltrates on X-rays and hypoxemia. It may be difficult to differentiate this condition from a bacterial pneumonia.

ii. *Alveolar hemorrhage:* is a serious pulmonary complication with high morbidity and mortality. Diagnosis is suggested by presence of cough, hemoptysis, and pulmonary infiltrates on X-rays associated with a sudden fall in hematocrit.

iii. *Infections:* Children with lupus are prone to develop pulmonary infections. SLE should be viewed as an immunodeficiency state in which there is phagocytic dysfunction, lymphopenia, CD4 lymphocytopenia, decreased cytokine production, reduced immunoglobulin and complement levels and also a functional asplenia. Moreover therapy with steroids and immunosuppressive agents further predisposes them to infections which may be fungal, bacterial or viral.

Treatment

Pulmonary complications of lupus need to be managed promptly and aggressively, as the mortality is high. Emperic therapy with parenteral high dose corticosteroids should be initiated. Antimicrobials also need to be given. Ventilation may be required.

Pitfalls

Clinically it may be very difficult to distinguish between a bacterial pneumonia and other pulmonary manifestations of lupus. The two may also not be mutually exclusive and may need to be tackled simultaneously.

ANTIPHOSPHOLIPID ANTIBODY SYNDROME

The antiphosholipid antibody syndrome (APLS) is a syndrome of hypercoagulability characterized by widespread venous and arterial thrombosis associated with antibodies directed against phospholipids.[21,22] It may be primary (idiopathic) or secondary (when it is seen in association with a rheumatological disorder). The clinical spectrum of antiphospholipid syndrome varies from subacute presentation (with recurrent migraine, visual disturbances and occasional dysarthria) to the catastrophic APLS characterized by severe multiple organ dysfunction and rapid diffuse small vessel ischemia predominantly affecting the parenchymal organs.

Diagnosis

The preliminary criteria for classification of the antiphosholipid syndrome are based on clinical and laboratory findings. Clinical criteria include vascular thrombosis i.e. one or more clinical episodes of arterial, venous or small vessel thrombosis, occurring within any tissue or organ. Laboratory criteria include detection of the lupus anticoagulant or anticardiolipin antibodies. The classification criteria for CAPS are given in Table 59.5.

Table 59.5: Classification of CAPS

1. Evidence of involvement of > 3 organs, systems and/or tissues$^{\Psi}$
2. Development of manifestations simultaneously or in < 1 week
3. Confirmation by histopathology of small vessel occlusion in at least 1 organ/tissue$^{\Phi}$
4. Laboratory confirmation of the presence of APLA (LAC and/or Acl and/or anti -b_2 GPI antibodies)$^{\xi}$

Definite CAPS

All 4 criteria

Probable CAPS

All 4 criteria, except for involvement of only 2 organ systems and/or tissues

All 4 criteria, except for absence of laboratory confirmation of the presence of aPL at least 6 weeks after a first positive test(due to early death of patient never tested for aPL before onset of CAPS)

1, 2 and 4

1, 3 and 4,plus development of a third event in > 1 week but < 1 month,despite anticoagulation treatment

$^{\Psi}$ Usually clinical evidence of vessel occlusions, confirmed by imaging techniques when appropriate. Renal involvement is defined by a 50% rise in serum creatinine, severe systemic hypertension (>180/100 mmHg),and/or proteinuria (> 500 mg/24 hrs).

$^{\Phi}$ For histopathologic confirmation,significant evidence of thrombosis must be present, although vasculitis may coexist occasionally.

$^{\xi}$ If the patient had not been previously diagnosed as having APS, the laboratory confirmation requires detection of the presence of aPL on > 2 occasions atleast 6 weeks apart (not necessarily at the time of event) according to the proposed preliminary criteria for classification of definite APS.

Treatment

Prolonged anticoagulation (intravenous heparin followed by warfarin) is required for children with APLS. Corticosteroids are necessary for secondary forms of the syndrome and also for the CAPS. Adequate intensive care backup, hemodialysis for renal failure and ventilation for pulmonary failure may all be necessary in seriously ill patients. Mortality rates are high in patients with CAPS.

Pitfalls

APLS may need to be differentiated from other hypercoagulable states.

REFERENCES

1. Lampe RM. Osteomyelitis and suppurative arthritis. In: Behrman RE, Kliegman RM, Jenson HB (eds) *Nelson Textbook of Pediatrics*, 17th edn. New Delhi: Elsevier 2004;2297-2302.

2. Singh S. Rheumatic disorders. In: Ghai OP, Gupta P, Paul VK (eds) *Essential Pediatrics*, 5th edn. New Delhi: Interprint 2000;428-433.
3. Singh S, Khubchandani R. Pediatric rheumatology in India: In need of a joint effort. *Indian J Pediatr* 2002;69:873-874.
4. Cassidy JT, Petty RE. Infectious arthritis and osteomyelitis.In: Cassidy JT, Petty RE (eds) *Textbook of Pediatric Rheumatology*, 4th edn. Philadelphia: WB Saunders 2001;640-665.
5. Knudsen CJM, Hoffman EB. Neonatal Osteomyelitis. *J Bone Joint Surg* 1990;72:846-851.
6. Lew DP, Waldvogel FA. Osteomyelitis. *N Engl J Med* 1997;336:999-1006.
7. Special Writing Group of the Committee on Rheumatic fever, Endocarditis and Kawasaki disease of the Council on Cardiovascular Disease in the Young of the American Heart Association. Guidelines for the diagnosis of rheumatic fever: Jones Criteria, 1992 Update. *JAMA* 1992;268:2069-2073.
8. Schneider R, Passo MH. Juvenile Rheumatoid Arthritis. *Rheum Dis Clin North Am* 2002;28:503-530.
9. Singh S. Chronic arthritis: Current perspectives. *Indian Pediatr* 2003;40:393-397.
10. Oates-Whitehead RM, Baumer JH, Haines L, Love S, Macono. Intravenous immunoglobulin for the treatment of Kawasaki disease in children (Cochrane Review).http://www.cochrane.org/cochrane/revabstr/ab004000.htm
11. Ozen S, Besbas N, Bakkaloglu A. Diagnostic criteria for polyarteritis nodosa in childhood. *J Pediatr* 1992;120:206-209.
12. Singh S, Das R. Clinical approach to vasculitis in children. *Indian J Pediatr* 2002;69:27-34.
13. Singh S, Dayal D, Minz RW, Joshi K, Datta U, Kumar L. Severe Henoch-Schonlein nephritis: treatment with azathioprin and steroids. *Rheum Int* 2002;22:133-137.
14. Jain S, Sharma N, Singh S, Bali HK, Kumar L, Sharma BK. Takayasu arteritis in children and young Indians. *Int J Cardiol* 2000;75(Suppl 1):S153-157.
15. Panja M, Kar AK, Dutta AL, Chhetri M, Kumar S, Panja S. Cardiac involvement in nonspecific aortoarteritis. *Int J Cardiol* 1992;34:289-295.
16. Hochberg MC. Updating the American College of Rheumatology revised criteria for the classification of systemic lupus erythematosus. *Arthritis Rheum* 1997;40:17-25.
17. Raj R, Murin S, Matthay RA, Wiedemann HP. Systemic lupus erythematosus in the intensive care unit. *Crit Care Clin* 2002;18:781-803.
18. Petty RE, Cassidy JT. Systemic lupus erythematosus. In: Cassidy JT, Petty RE (eds) *Textbook of Pediatric Rheumatology*, 4th edn. Philadelphia: WB. Saunders. 2001;396-449.
19. Gupta A, Singh S, Minz RW, Radotra BD, Ahluwalia J, Grover A. Lupus myocarditis in children. *Ann Rheum Dis* (In Press).
20. Singh S, Dayal D, Kumar L, Joshi K. Mortality patterns in childhood lupus-10 years experience in a developing country. *Clin Rheum* 2002;21:462-465.
21. Erkan D, Cervera R, Asherson RA. Catastrophic antiphospholipid syndrome: Where do we stand? *Arthritis Rheum* 2003; 12:3320-3327.
22. Levine JS, Branch DWA, Rauch J. The Antiphospholipid syndrome. *N Engl J Med* 2002;346:752-763.

Section XII

Environmental Emergencies

Akash Deep and Anupam Gupta

60 Scorpion Sting

INTRODUCTION

Scorpion stings are a major public health problem in many underdeveloped tropical countries. Case fatality rates of 3-22% were reported among children hospitalized for scorpion stings in India, Saudi Arabia and South Africa.[1-4] Children represent about half of all envenomations, and the vast majority of serious reactions occur in children 10 years of age or younger.

SCORPIONS

Scorpion bodies can be divided into three main sections: cephalothorax, abdomen, and tail. The six-segmented tail extends from the posterior section, with the last segment terminating in the venom apparatus or telson containing a stinger at the tip. Scorpion venom is produced in two glands in the telson and injected through the stinger into the victim by contraction of gland muscles. The tail thrusts over the back of the scorpion, striking the victim held in its pincers as venom is injected.

Some 1500 species of scorpion have been identified worldwide. Of these, only 25 species have medical importance to humans, most of which are members of the Buthidae.[8-10] Among the 86 species of scorpions in India, *Mesobuthus tamulus* and *Palamneus swammer-dami* are of medical importance.[11]

Properties

Geographical distribution: Warm dry regions, regions with abundant red soil.[12]

Common sites of habitat: The crevices of dwellings, underground burrows, under logs or debris, paddy husk, sugarcane fields, coconut and banana plantations.

May be found outside their natural range of distribution when inadvertently transported with other items such as luggage.

Diurnal variation: Scorpions are nocturnal creatures. Scorpions retreat in the crevices of dwellings during the day only to emerge at night to avoid the light; thus most stings are reported at night.

Nature: Scorpions are not aggressive. They do not hunt for prey; they wait for it. Thus, accidental human stinging occurs when scorpions are inadvertently touched while in their hiding places.

Venom

The scorpion can voluntarily regulate the amount of venom to be injected with each sting. The striated muscles in the stinger allow regulation of the amount of venom ejected, which is usually 0.1-0.6 mg. If the entire supply of venom is used, several days must elapse before the supply is replenished. Furthermore, scorpions with large venom sacs, such as the *Parabuthus* species, can even squirt their venom.

The venom glands are located on the tail lateral to the tip of the stinger and are composed of 2 types of tall columnar cells. One type produces the toxins, while the other produces mucus. The potency of the venom varies with the species, with some producing only a mild flu and others producing death within an hour. Generally, the venom is distributed rapidly into the tissue if it is deposited into a venous structure. Venom deposited *via* the intravenous route can cause symptoms only 4-7 minutes after the injection, with a peak tissue concentration in 30 minutes and an overall toxin elimination half-life of 4.2-13.4 hours through the urine. The more rapidly the venom enters the bloodstream, the higher the venom concentration in the blood and the more rapid the onset of systemic symptoms.

The venom is composed of varying concentrations of neurotoxin, cardiotoxin, nephrotoxin, hemolytic toxin, phosphodiesterases, phospholipases, hyaluronidases, glycosaminoglycans, histamine, serotonin, tryptophan, and cytokine releasers.[13] The most potent toxin is the neurotoxin, of which 2 classes exist. Both of these classes are heat-stable, have low molecular weight, and are responsible for causing cell impairment in nerves, muscles, and the heart by altering ion channel permeability.

The long-chain polypeptide neurotoxin causes stabilization of voltage-dependent sodium channels in the open position, leading to continuous, prolonged, repetitive firing of the somatic, sympathetic, and parasympathetic neurons. This repetitive firing results in autonomic and neuromuscular overexcitation symptoms, and it prevents normal nerve impulse transmissions. Furthermore, it results in release of excessive neurotransmitters such as epinephrine, norepinephrine, acetylcholine, glutamate, and aspartate. Meanwhile, the short polypeptide neurotoxin blocks the potassium channels.

PATHOPHYSIOLOGY

1. **Effect of Venom on Ion Channels and ANS**[14,15]
   Scorpion venoms are species-specific complex mixtures of short neurotoxic proteins (31-64 aminoacid sequences).
   Voltage dependant ion channels are altered by the venom. The side chains of scorpion venom are positively charged. This is important in their ability to bind to specific membrane channels. Alpha (of *Buthus* sp.) and beta (of *Centruoides* sp.) toxins act on sodium channel. Scyllatoxin, charybdotoxin of *Leiurus* species and *Tityus* toxin act primary on potassium channels. The toxin acts by opening sodium channel at presynaptic nerve terminals and inhibiting calcium dependant potassium channels. Autonomic storm is thus initiated.
2. **Effect of Venom on Cardiovascular System**[16-19]
   Hypertension and Tachycardia, Myocardial Dysfunction.
   Mechanism-Autonomic storm
   - Suppression of insulin secretion leading to hyperglycemia, hyperkalemia, free fatty acids and free radicals accumulation injuring myocardium.
   - Direct toxic effects of cardiac sarcolemmal defects, depletion of glycogen content of heart-coronary spasm as a result of circulating catecholamines.
3. **Effect on Hemopoitic System**[20]
   Acute DIC.
4. **Effect on Central Nervous System**[21,22]
   Seizures and encephalopathy, hemiplegia.
   Mechanism-Fibrin deposition resulting from DIC
   - Acute rise in blood pressure leading to hypertensive encephalopathy
   - Rupture of unprotected perforating arteries
   - Intracerebral hemorrhage
   - Cerebral infarction due to DIC.
5. **Effect of Venom on Lungs**[23]
   Pulmonary Edema
   Mechanism: Both cardiogenic and non cardiogenic—abundant microthrombi, increased alveocapillary membrane permeability.
6. **Effect of Venom on Kidney**[24]
   Acute Renal Failure.
7. **Effect of Venom on Skin**[25]
   Unusual in Indian Red Scorpion envenomation but seen in yellow scorpion (Buthus cosmobuthus and Hemiscorpus) seen in Iran produce varied skin reaction viz. Erythema, edema, lymphangitis, and severe necrosis.
8. **Effect of Venom on Pancreas**[26]
   Case reports of scorpion bites causing acute pancreatitis have been seen from Trinidad.
9. **Effect of Venom on Liver**
   Although no report of overt liver failure seen so far but could lead to rise of liver enzymes, necrosis of liver at autopsy.
10. **Systematic Inflamation Response Syndrome (SIRS)**
    Systematic
    Inflamation Response like Syndrome is triggered by species *Tityus serrulatus.* Increased levels of IL-6, IL-1a and IFN-gamma has been documented.

CLINICAL PRESENTATION

The toxicity, variation, and duration of the symptoms depend on the following factors:

a. *Related to scorpion*
   - Scorpion species.
   - Scorpion age, size, and nutritional status.
   - Healthiness of the scorpion's stinging apparatus (telson).
   - Number of stings and quantity of venom injected.
   - Depth of the sting penetration.
   - Composition of the venom.

b. *Related to victim*
   - Site of envenomation: Closer proximity of the sting to the head and torso results in quicker venom absorption into the central circulation and a quicker onset of symptoms.
   - Age of the victim.
   - Health of the victim.
   - Weight of the victim relative to amount of venom.
   - Presence of co-morbidities.
   - Body Temperature.

   The duration to progress to systemic symptoms ranges from 5 minutes to 4 hours after the sting. The symptoms generally persist for 10-48 hours.

c. *Related to Geographical region*
   - In India, Israel, Brazil and Mexico, cardiac manifestations are common.
   - In Iran—tissue necrosis and hemolysis.
   - In South Africa and USA—neurological features and in Trinidad acute pancreatitis dominate the picture.

d. *Related to specific scorpion species*
   - Mesobuthus, Tityus, *and* Leiurus-*Tend to cause severe cardiovascular symptoms.*

- Centruroides—*Tend to cause neurological symptoms*
- Hemiscorpius—*Tend to cause tissue necrosis.*

SYMPTOMS

1. *Local:* Nonlethal scorpion species tend to produce local reactions similar to a hymenopteran sting, while lethal scorpion species tend to produce systemic symptoms.
2. *Pain:* Screaming within seconds to minutes due to pain after the sting, children appear irritable, at times excitable. Random movements of head, eye and neck are seen.
3. Symptoms suggestive of autonomic storm[5,6,9,12]
   a. Cholinergic storm:vomiting, salivation, sweating, priaprism.
   b. Adrenergic storm: diaphoresis, palpitation, blurred vision due to mydriasis.
4. *CNS manifestation*
   Cranial nerve dysfunction e.g. blurred vision, slurred speech, tongue fasciculations, drooling, and poor airway control (especially in infants). Abnormal eye movements, Somatic neuromuscular dysfunction may begin as restlessness, with the victim unable to lie still, and progress to uncontrollable fasciculations and jerking of the extremities that resembles a seizure. Opisthotonos and hemiballistic movements can occur.
5. Acute onset of breathlessness.
   It may develop within 30 min to 3 hours due to pulmonary edema.

APPROACH TO A PATIENT WITH SCORPION ENVENOMATION

History

For patients presenting with scorpion stings, ascertaining the following is essential:

- Time of envenomation
- Nature of the incident
- Description of the scorpion
- Local and systemic symptoms.

Physical Examination

The signs of the envenomation are determined by the scorpion species, venom composition, and the victim's physiological reaction to the venom. The signs occur within a few minutes after the sting and usually progress to a maximum severity within 5 hours. The signs last for 24-72 hours and do not have an apparent sequence. Thus, predicting the evolution of signs over time is difficult. Furthermore, a false recovery followed by a total relapse is common.

The grading of these scorpion envenomations depends on whether or not neurological signs predominate and is as follows:

- *Nonneurological predominance*
  - Mild—Local signs
  - Moderate—Ascending local signs or mild systemic signs
  - Severe—Life-threatening systemic signs.
- *Neurologic predominance*[5]
  - Grade I-Local pain or paresthesia at the sting site
  - Grade II-Pain or paresthesia that has traveled from the sting site
  - Grade III-Either cranial nerve or somatic neuromuscular dysfunction
  - Cranial nerve dysfunction such as blurred vision, irregular eye movements, difficulty swallowing, tongue fasciculations, slurred speech, and occasional upper airway incoordination
  - Peripheral skeletal neuromuscular dysfunction such as jerking of extremities, restlessness, severe involuntary shaking, and jerking that may be mistaken for seizures
  - Grade IV-Both cranial nerve and somatic neuromuscular dysfunction Local signs.
- *Neurotoxic local effects*
  - Local evidence of a sting may be minimal or absent in as many as 50% of cases of neurotoxic scorpion stings. In fact, tissue necrosis rarely is found.
  - A sharp burning pain sensation at the sting site, followed by pruritus, erythema, local tissue swelling, and ascending hyperesthesia, may be reported. This paresthesia feels like an electric current, persists for several weeks, and is the last symptom to resolve before the victim recovers.
  - The **tap test** is administered by tapping at the sting site. A positive result is when the paresthesia worsens with the tapping because the site is hypersensitive to touch and temperature. In fact, wearing clothing over the area and sudden changes in temperature exacerbate the symptoms. This test is usually not positive in Indian children.[12]
- *Cytotoxic local effects*
  - A macule or papule appears initially at the sting site, occurring within the first hour of the sting.
  - The diameter of the lesion is dependent on the quantity of venom injected.
  - The lesion progresses to a purpuric plague that will necrose and ulcerate.
  - Lymphangitis results from the transfer of the venom through the lymphatic vessels.
- *Nonlethal local effects*
  - Pain, erythema, induration, and wheal may be present.
  - These are secondary to venom activation of kinins and slow-releasing substances.
- *Neurologic signs.*

Central Nervous System Signs

- Thalamus-induced systemic paresthesia occurs in all 4 limbs.
- Patients experience venom-induced cerebral thrombosis strokes.
- The level of consciousness is altered, especially with restlessness, confusion, or delirium.
- Patients have abnormal behavior.
- Ataxia is also a sign.

Autonomic nervous system signs—Predominately sympathetic signs, parasympathetic signs, or a combination of signs

Sympathetic signs
- Hyperthermia
- Tachypnea
- Tachycardia
- Hypertension
- Arrhythmia
- Hyperkinetic pulmonary edema
- Hyperglycemia
- Diaphoresis
- Piloerection
- Restlessness and apprehension
- Hyperexcitability and convulsions

Parasympathetic signs
- Bronchoconstriction
- Bradycardia
- Hypotension
- Salivation, lacrimation, urination, diarrhea, and gastric emesis (SLUDGE)
- Rhinorrhea and bronchorrhea
- Goose pimple skin
- Loss of bowel and bladder control
- Priapism
- Dysphagia
- Miosis
- Generalized weakness

Somatic signs
- Rigid spastic muscle of the limbs and torso
- Involuntary muscle spasm, twitching, clonus, and contractures
- Alternating episthotonos and opisthotonus from inactivation of sodium channels, leading to increased sodium and calcium uptake
- Increased tendon reflexes, especially prolongation of the relaxation phase
- Piloerection accompanied by goose pimples

Cranial nerve signs
- Classic rotary eye movement may result in ptosis, nystagmus, and blurred vision.
- Mydriasis is a sign.
- Patients may have tongue fasciculations.
- Dysphagia, dysarthria, and stridor occur secondary to pharyngeal reflex loss or muscle spasm.
- Patients may present with excessive salivation and drooling.

Peripheral nervous system signs: Intense local burning pain with minimal swelling at sting site, followed by ascending numbness and tingling, then paralysis and convulsions.

Nonneurologic Systemic Signs

Cardiovascular signs—Usually follow a pattern of a hyperdynamic phase followed by a hypodynamic phase
- Hypertension is described as follows:
- Secondary to catecholamine and renin stimulation.
- Observed as early as within 4 minutes after the sting
- Lasts a few hours.
- High enough to produce hypertensive encephalopathy
- Hypotension-Less common and occurs secondary to excess acetylcholamine or catecholamine depletion.
- Tachycardia is usually present, although bradycardia can be observed.
- Transient apical pansystolic murmur is consistent with papillary muscle damage.
- Cardiovascular collapse occurs secondary to biventricular dysfunction and profuse loss of fluids from sweating, vomiting, diarrhea, and hypersalivation.
- Observed in 7-38% of cardiovascular cases.
- Mild envenomation–Vascular effect with vasoconstriction hypertension.
- Moderate envenomation–Left ventricular failure hypotension with and without an elevated pulmonary artery wedge pressure, depending on fluid status of the patient.
- Severe envenomation–Biventricular cardiogenic shock.
- Cardiac dysfunctions attributed to catecholamine-induced increases in myocardial metabolism oxygen demand (leading to myocardial ischemia) and to the direct effects of the toxin (leading to myocarditis).

Respiratory signs
- Tachypnea may be present.
- Pulmonary edema with hemoptysis and a normal-sized heart is observed in 7-32% of respiratory cases. This is secondary to a direct toxin-induced increased pulmonary vessel permeability effect and is also secondary to catecholamine-induced effects of hypoxia and intracellular calcium accumulation, which leads to a decrease in left ventricular compliance with resultant ventricular dilation and diastolic dysfunction.
- Respiratory failure may occur secondary to diaphragm paralysis, alveolar hypoventilation, and bronchorrhea.

Allergic signs
- Patients may have urticaria.
- Angioedema is reported.

– Patients may present with bronchospasm.
– Anaphylaxis is possible.

Gastrointestinal signs

– Patients may present with excessive salivation.
– Dysphagia is possible.
– Nausea and vomiting are reported.
– Gastric hyperdistention occurs secondary to vagal stimulation.
– Increased gastric acid output may lead to gastric ulcers.
– Acute pancreatitis may lead to hyperglycemia.
– Liver glycogenolysis may occur from catecholamine stimulation.

Genitourinary signs

– Patients have decreased renal plasma flow.
– Toxin-induced acute tubular necrosis renal failure may occur.
– Rhabdomyolysis renal failure may result from venom-induced excessive motor activity.
– Priapism may occur secondary to cholinergic stimulation. One small study by Bawaskar found a positive prognostic correlation to the development of cardiac manifestations following scorpion stings.

Hematological signs

– Platelet aggregation may occur because of catecholamine stimulation.
– Disseminated intravascular coagulation with massive hemorrhage may result from venom-induced defibrination.

Metabolic signs

– Hyperglycemia may occur from catecholamine-induced hepatic glycogenolysis, pancreatitis, and insulin inhibition.
– Increased lactic acidosis may occur from hypoxia and venom-induced increased lactase dehydrogenase activity.
– Patients may have an electrolyte imbalance and dehydration from hypersalivation, vomiting, diaphoresis, and diarrhea.

DIFFERENTIAL DIAGNOSIS:

a. *Toxins/Drugs*
   Dystonic reaction to medication
   Hymenoptera envenomation
   Lactrodectus envenomation
   Sympathomimetic (e.g., cocaine, amphetamine) poisoning
   Phencyclidine
   Organophosphates/carbamates
   Strychnine
   Withdrawal sedative/hypnotic or ethanol

b. *Other Disorders*
   Seizures of other etiology
   Pulmonary edema of other etiology
   Pancreatitis of other etiology
   Cerebrovascular accident
   Diseases with cranial nerve dysfunction (multiple sclerosis, myasthenia gravis, botulism)
   Infections
   Sepsis
   Tetanus
   Meningitis
   Encephalitis.

LABORATORY STUDIES

Basic

1. Perform a CBC count for leukocytosis and hemolysis in patients with stings from the *Hemiscorpius* species.
2. Electrolyte evaluation is warranted in patients with venom-induced salivation, vomiting, and diarrhea.
3. Coagulation parameters should be measured for venom-induced defibrination because, at high concentrations, the venom is an anticoagulant.
4. Glucose levels should be measured to evaluate for hyperglycemia from liver and pancreas dysfunction.
5. Creatine kinase and urinalysis help evaluate for venom-induced excessive motor rhabdomyolysis.
6. Obtain amylase/lipase values to assess for pancreatitis from *Tityus trinitatis* stings.
7. Patients may have increased aspartate aminotransferase and alanine aminotransferase levels from venom-induced liver cell destruction.
8. Arterial blood gas determinations show a decrease in arterial oxygenation tension and an increase in PCO_2 within 15 minutes of the envenomation, findings consistent with mild metabolic acidosis.
9. Unilateral pulmonary edema may be seen on chest X-ray films because of the venom effect on pulmonary vascular permeability.
10. Electrocardiogram
    - ECG changes persist for 10-12 days before normalizing.
    - ECG changes are observed in approximately two-thirds of children who have been envenomated.
    - Rhythm disturbances are not dose-dependent but are related to the venom composition.
      – Sinus tachycardia is the most common rhythm
      – QTc prolongation
      – ST changes
      – T-wave inversion
      – Ventricular re-polarization abnormalities
      – Bundle-branch block
      – First-degree block
    - A possible sequence of ECG changes has been noted. This sequence starts with bizarre, broad-notched,

biphasic, peaked T waves with a beat-to-beat variation. This bizarre T wave is followed by the appearance of tiny Q waves and then atrioventricular dissociation with an accelerated junctional rhythm.

HIGHER INVESTIGATIONS

1. *Echocardiography* findings are discussed as follows:
   Echocardiography is more sensitive than electrocardiography and creatine kinase assays for assessing myocardial compromise after a scorpion sting.
   Findings show a diffuse global biventricular hypokinesis with a decreased left and right ventricular ejection fraction of approximately 0.14-0.38. This dysfunction can appear just a few hours after the sting and usually normalizes within 4-8 days.
   Serial echocardiography findings show that the return of left ventricular function to a normal state correlates to clinical cardiorespiratory improvement.
2. *Color-flow Doppler* study findings show mitral incompetence, probably secondary to venom-induced dilated cardiomyopathy.
3. *Pulmonary artery catheterization* findings may include the following:
   - Elevated systemic vascular resistance occurs up to 4 times the normal level, with elevated mean arterial pressure (MAP) of 203 mm Hg.
   - Left ventricular failure produces a MAP of 57-69 mm Hg.
   - Biventricular failure produces a MAP of 47 mm Hg.
   - Low cardiac index occurs with elevated filling pressures.
   - Perform serial spirometry measurements to help detect impending venom-induced diaphragmatic failure.
4. *Histologic Findings*
   The local sting site shows mixed inflammatory cell infiltrates with eosinophils scattered among collagen bundles in an edematous dermis. Myocardial changes, which are most prominent at the papillary muscle and subendocardial region, include focal myocardial necrosis; myofibril destruction, especially at the I band; fine fatty deposits in the cardiac muscle fibers; interstitial edema; and increased cellularity, mainly lymphocytes and monocytes. Changes resemble interstitial hypoxia-induced myocarditis caused by large doses of catecholamines.

TREATMENT

General

Local treatment is discussed as follows:

1. A negative-pressure extraction device (i.e., the extractor) may be useful, although the benefit is unproven. The extractor creates a negative pressure of 1 atm. Apply it to the sting site after incision. Oral extraction is contraindicated.
2. Use ice bags to reduce pain and to slow the absorption of venom *via* vasoconstriction. This is most effective during the first 2 hours following the sting.
3. Immobilize the affected part in a functional position below the level of the heart to delay venom absorption.
4. Calm the patient to lower the heart rate and blood pressure, thus limiting the spread of the venom.
5. For medical delay secondary to remoteness, consider applying a lymphatic-venous compression wrap 1 inch proximal to the sting site to reduce superficial venous and lymphatic flow of the venom but not to stop the arterial flow. Only remove this wrap when the provider is ready to administer systemic support. The drawback of this wrap is that it may intensify the local effects of the venom.
6. Apply a topical or local anesthetic agent to the wound to decrease paresthesia; this tends to be more effective than opiates.
7. Administer local wound care and topical antibiotic to the wound.
8. Administer tetanus prophylaxis.

Systemic

It is instituted by directing supportive care toward the organ specifically affected by the venom.

Admit to hospital for most severe envenomations in a monitored setting for at least 24 hours of observation because symptoms can be delayed.

- Establish airway, breathing, and circulation (i.e., ABCs) to provide adequate airway, ventilation, and perfusion.
- Monitor vital signs (e.g., pulse oximetry heart rate, blood pressure, and respiratory rate monitor). Use invasive monitoring for patients who are unstable and hemodynamic.
- Administer oxygen.
- Administer intravenous fluids to help prevent hypovolemia from vomiting, diarrhea, sweating, hypersalivation, and insensible water loss from a tropical environment.
- Perform intubation and institute mechanical ventilation with end-tidal carbon dioxide monitoring for patients in respiratory distress.
- Administer systemic antibiotics if signs of secondary infection occur.
- Administer muscle relaxants for severe muscle spasms (i.e., benzodiazepines).
  - Insulin administration in scorpion envenomation animal experiments has helped the vital organs to use metabolic substrates more efficiently, thus preventing venom-induced multiorgan failure, especially cardiopulmonary failure.[28]

– Administer barbiturates and/or a benzodiazepine continuous infusion for severe excessive motor activity.

Specific Management

Prazosin

A competitive post-synaptic alpha1, adreno-receptor antagonist, it should be the first line of management, since alpha receptors stimulation plays a major role in the evoluation of clinical spectrum.[29,30]

Mechanism of action:

- Prazosin suppresses sympathetic outflow and activates venom-inhibited potassium channels.
- It decreases the preload, afterload and blood pressure without increasing the heart rate.
- Prazosin counters vasoconstriction induced by endothelins through accumulation of cyclic GMP (cGMP). Thus prazosin is a cellular and pharmacologic antidote to the actions of scorpion venom and it is also cardioprotective.

Dosage: 30 microgram/kg/dose.
Prazosin is available as 1 mg tablet. Sustained release tablets are not recommended in this condition. In case of vomiting, it can be administered through nasogastric tube.

Monitoring and precautions: Blood pressure, pulse rate and respiration must be monitored every 30 minutes for 3 hours, every hour for next 6 hours and later every 4 hours till improvement. Prazosin should be repeated in the same dose at the end of 3 hours according to clinical response and later every 6 hours till extremities are warm, dry and peripheral veins are visible easily.

- It should not be given as prophylaxis in children when pain is the only symptom.
- After giving prazosin, mother should be advised not to lift the child to prevent the effects of 'First dose phenomenon' due to prazosin.
- Prazosin can be given irrespective of blood pressure provided there is no hypovolemia.

Scorpion Antivenom

Scorpion venoms reach their target too rapidly to be neutralized and anti-venom within 30 minutes of sting may reverse their effect. Usefulness of scorpion anti-venom varies between countries. Doctors from Brazil, Mexico and Saudi Arabia report benefit.[31-33] Systematic administration of scorpion antivenin did not alter the clinical course of scorpion sting in a matched pair study undertaken at some places.[34,35]

Dosage: 1 vial (5 mL) in 50 mL saline IV over 30 min; if severe symptoms still persist after 1 h, repeat once prn

Perform a skin test prior to administering the antivenom. First, dilute 0.1 mL of antivenom in a 1:10 ratio with isotonic sodium chloride solution. Second, administer 0.2 mL intradermally. A positive test result is if a wheal develops within 10 minutes. The skin test has a sensitivity of 96% and a specificity of 68%.

The best result occurs when antivenom is administered as early as possible (preferably within the first 2 hours after the sting) and with adequate quantities to neutralize the venom (usually 50-100 times the LD 50 amount). A decrease in curative effects occurs with longer sting-serotherapy delay and administration of insufficient amounts of antivenom.

Treatment of Pulmonary Edema

Principle

Management should be directed towards relieving afterload without compromising preload.

- The use of diuretics to minimize or reduce fluid overload seems a reasonable measure but only when renal water excretion is impaired. Otherwise the best way to prevent fluid overload is to maintain an adequate cardiac output.
- Thus, dobutamine support (5-15 mg/kg/min) with vasodilatation through sodium nitroprusside (0.3-5 mg/kg/min) or nitroglycerine (5 mg/min) infusate is preferred in this situation.
- Prazosin is to be given one hour before termination of sodium nitroprusside (SNP) drip. If SNP is not available, one can use isosorbide dinitrate 10 mg every 10 minutes sublingually as an emergency measure.
- Morphine, a standard therapy in pulmonary edema, should be avoided in scorpion sting, since narcotics worsen dysrythmias in these children.

Pain and Fluid Management

Local ice packs, xylocaine (local anesthetic), dehydroemetine (counter irritant) and streptomycin (neuromuscular blockade) are useful.

The loss of fluid due to profuse sweating and vomiting is usually overlooked. So oral fluids whenever feasible must be encouraged. When children present with tachypnea and altered sensorium, parenteral fluids (N/5 saline) are required. Fluid requirements need to be balanced carefully. In children with pulmonary edema, CVP monitoring is essential.

UNHELPFUL TREATMENTS

Standard therapy was not clearly defined in earlier days; many therapies were in vogue without experimental justification.

Lytic Cocktail (Pethidine + Promethazine + Chlorpromazine) pethidine may convert sublethal dose of scorpion venom into a lethal one.

It also interferes with protective respiratory reflexes.[2]

Morphine: worsens dysrythmias.[3]

Steroids: In randomized case controlled studies no significant difference was found in steroids and placebo groups.[35]

Steroids might enhance the necrotizing effects of excessive catecholamines on myocardium.[12]

Atropine: Complete abolition of parasympathetic effects may permit the domination of the overstimulated sympathetic system. Atropine potentiates tachycardia and sustains hypertension.[36]

Nifidepine: Reflex tachycardia and negative inotropic effect argues against its use.[26]

Despite its antihypertensive and vasodilator effect, it could lead to myocardial failure and pulmonary edema.[37]

Ace Inhibitors: (Captopril) aggrevate hyperkalemia and inhibit breakdown of bradykinin, which is implicated in experimental pulmonary edema due to scorpion sting. It does not correct hemodynamics and does not prevent cardiac arrythmias.[38]

COMPLICATIONS

- Dilated cardiomyopathy
- Ankylosis of small joints if the sting occurs at a joint
- Rhabdomyolysis
- Persistent paresthesias
- Antivenom anaphylaxis and serum sickness
- Latrogenic, high-dose, sedative-hypnotic respiratory arrest.

PROGNOSIS MORTALITY/MORBIDITY

Underreporting of scorpion stings is frequent because most envenomations occur in desert and jungle areas that do not have large medical facilities. Furthermore, reporting is not required.

- Most deaths occur during the first 24 hours after the sting and are secondary to respiratory or cardiovascular failure.
- Children as a group are at a greater risk for morbidity and mortality. A smaller child, a lower body weight, and a larger ratio of venom to body weight lead to a more severe reaction.
- Furthermore, patients in rural areas tend to fare worse than patients in urban areas because of the delay in getting medical help due to a longer travel time to medical centers.
- Symptoms generally persist for 10-48 hours. If the victim survives the first few hours without severe cardiorespiratory or neurologic symptoms, the prognosis is usually good. Furthermore, surviving the first 24 hours after a scorpion sting also carries a good prognosis.
- A worse prognosis can be expected with the presence of systemic symptoms such as cardiovascular collapse, respiratory failure, seizures, and coma.
- Since the use of prazosin (1984 onwards), the mortality in these victims is reduced to less than 1%.[3,30]

REFERENCES

1. Rajarajeswari G, Sivaprakasam S, Viswanathan J. Morbidity and mortality pattern in scorpion sting–A review of 68 cases. *J Indian Med Assoc* 1979;73:123-126.
2. Mahadevan S, Choudhury P, Puri RK, Srinivasan S. Scorpion envenomation and the role of lytic cocktail in its management. *Indian J Pediatr* 1981;48:757-761.
3. Biswal N, Charan MV, Betsy M, Nalini P, Srinivasan S, Mahadevan S. Management of scorpion envenomation. *Pediatr Today* 1999;2:420-426.
4. Ismail M. The scorpion envenoming syndrome. *Toxicon* 1995;33:825-828.
5. Curry SC, Vance MV, Ryan PJ, et al. Envenomation by the scorpion *Centruroides sculpturatus. J Toxicol Clin Toxicol* 1983;21:417–449.
6. Likes K, Banner W, Chavez M. *Centruroides exilicauda* envenomation in Arizona. *West J Med* 1984;141:634–637.
7. Sofer S, Gueron M. Vasodilators and hypertensive encephalopathy following scorpion envenomation in children. *Chest* 1990;97:118–120.
8. Minton SA. *Venom Diseases.* Springfield, IL: Charles C Thomas 1974.
9. Peters W. *A Color Atlas of Arthropods in Medicine.* London: Wolfe 1992.
10. Polis GA. *The Biology of Scorpions.* Stanford Stanford University Press 1990.
11. Erfati P. Epidemiology, symptomatology and treatment of buthinae stings. In: Bettini S (ed) *Arthopod Venoms. Handbook of Experimental Pharmacology.* New York: Springer-Verlag 1978; 312-315.
12. Mahadevan S.Scorpion Sting. *Indian Pediatr* 2000;37:504-514.
13. Basu A, Gomes A, Dasgupta SC, Lahiri SC. Histamine, 5-HT and Hyalouronidase in the venom of scorpion Lychas laevifrons (Pock). *Indian J Med Res* 1990;92:371-373.
14. Zlotkin E, Miranda F, Lissitszky S. Proteins in scorpion venoms toxic to mammals and insects. *Toxicon* 1972;10:207-209.
15. Zlotkin E, Shulov AS. Studies on the mode of scorpion neurotoxins–A review. *Toxicon* 1969;7:217-221.
16. Bawaskar HS, Bawaskar PH. Management of cardiovascular manifestations of poisoning by the Indian red scorpion (Mesobuthus tamulus). *Brit Heart J* 1992;68:478-480.
17. Hagag M, Tua T, EI-Asmar F. Isolation of minax toxins from the venom of the scorpion *Buthus minax* and their metabolic effects. *Arch Biochem Biophys* 1983;220:459-466.
19. Murthy KRK, Billimora FR, Khopkar M, Dave KN. Acute hyperglycemia and hyperkalemia in acute myocarditis produced by scorpion (*Buthus tamulus*) venom injection in dogs. *Indian Heart J* 1986;38:71-76.
20. Murthy KRK, Zolfagharian H, Medh JD, Kudalkar JA, Yeolekar ME, Pandit SP, *et al.* Disseminated intravascular coagulation and disturbances in carbohydrate and fat metabolism in acute myocarditis produced by scorpion (*Buthus tamulus*) venom. *Indian J Med Res* 1988;87:318-325.
21. Reddy CRRM, Suvarnakumari G, Devi CS, Reddy CN. Pathology of scorpion venom poisoning. *J Trop Med Hyg* 1972;75:98-102.

22. Devi CS, Reddy NC, Lakshmidevi S, Subramaniyam YR, Reddy CRRM. Defibrina-tion syndrome due to scorpion venom poisoning. *Brit Med J* 1970;1:345-346.
23. D'Suze G, Comellas A, Pesce L, Sevci KC, Sanchez-de-Leon R. *Tityus discrepans* venom produces a respiratory distress syndrome in rabbits through an indirect mechanism. *Toxicon* 1999;37:173-180.
24. Chadha JS, Leviav A. Hemolysis, renal failure and local necrosis following scorpion sting. *JAMA* 1979;241:1038.
25. Bawaskar HS, Bawaskar PH. Indian red scorpion envenoming. *Indian J Pediatr* 1998;65:383-391.
26. Bartholomew C. Acute scorpion pancreatitis in Trinidad. *Brit Med J* 1970;1:666-668.
27. Bawaskar HS. Diagnostic cardiac premonitory signs and symptoms of red scorpion sting. *Lancet* 1982; 1(8271): 552-554.
28. Murthy KR Hase NK. Scorpium envenoming and the role of Insulin. *Toxicon*. 1994;32:1041-1044.
29. Bawaskar HS, Bawaskar PH. Prazosin in the management of cardiovascular manifestations of scorpion sting. *Lancet* 1986; 1:510-511.
30. Bawaskar HS, Bawaskar PH. Severe envenoming by Indian red scorpion *M. tamulus*–the use of Prazosin therapy. *Quart J Med* 1996;89:701-704.
31. Freire-Maia L, Campos JA, Amaralk CF. Approaches to the treatment of scorpion envenoming. *Toxicon* 1994;32:1009-1014.
32. EI-Amin EO, Sultan OM, al-Magamci MS, Elidrissy A. Serotherapy in the management of scorpion sting in children in Saudi Arabia. *Ann Trop Pediatr* 1994;14:21-24.
33. Sofer M, Shahak E, Gueron M. Scorpion envenomation and antivenom therapy. *J Pediatr* 1994;124: 973-978.
34. Belghith M, Boussarsar M, Haguiga H, Abroug F. Efficacy of serotherapy in scorpion sting: A matched pair study. *J Toxicol Clin Toxicol* 1999;37:51-57.
35. Abroug F, Elatrous S, Nouria S, Haguiga, Touzi N, Bouchoucha S. Serothgerapy in Scorpiun Envenomation: a randomized controlled trial. *Lancet* 1999;354:906-909.
36. Bawaskar HS, Bawaskar PH. Role of atropine in management of cardiovascular manifestations of scorpion envenoming in humans. *J Trop Med Hyg* 1992;95:30-35.
37. Bawaskar HS, Bawaskar PH. Vasodilators, scorpion envenoming and the heart (an Indian experience). *Toxicon* 1994;32:1031-1040.
38. Karnad DR. Hemodynamic pattern in patients with scorpion envenomation. *Heart* 1998;79:485-489.

Suraj Gupte and Arun Bansal

61 Snakebite

INTRODUCTION

Snakebite is a common pediatric emergency, especially in slums, villages and forests in tropical and subtropical countries where it is a frequent cause of morbidity and mortality. Population of sea snakes is far more than that of land snakes.[1-4] The former are, however, only rarely responsible for snakebite in children.

Though the very sight of a snake is terrifying, a large majority of snakes neither are proactive in attacking a host (in fact, they are rather defensive and scared of the man) nor are poisonous. In India, there are around 240 species. Only a little over 50 of these are known to be poisonous. According to conservative estimates, only 20% snakes are poisonous.

Snakebite is not the only mode of causing morbidity or mortality in the host. Some snakes constrict and suffocate the prey. Another category just grabs the prey with teeth and then swallows it in totality.

TYPES OF POISONOUS SNAKES[4-7]

Three types of poisonous snakes are encountered in India, namely neurotoxic cobra, hemorrhagic hemotoxic viper and neuro-hemotoxic krait. Russell viper is the deadliest snake in Indian subcontinent.

Neurotoxic Cobra

It causes paralysis of muscles of eyes (ptosis in particular), palate, jaws, tongue, larynx, neck, deglutition and chest. Respiratory failure may prove fatal. Cardiotoxicity (hypotension, tachycardia, ECG changes) and hemolysis may also occur. Onset of manifestations is very rapid, local pain beginning within 10 minutes.

Hemorrhagic-Hemotoxic Viper

It causes tissue destruction and hemorrhage by affecting the clotting mechanism of blood. Onset of manifestations is relatively slow. Local symptoms include swelling, skin discoloration, edema, pain, ecchymosis and even bleeding from the bite site. Generalized bleeding is usually a signal that disseminated intravascular coagulation (DIC) has developed.

Neuro-Hemotoxic Krait

It contains both neurotoxins and hemotoxins. It is the most common as well as dangerous variety in India. Manifestations are by and large similar to that of cobra bite. However, local pain is less but there is a severe abdominal pain.

Table 61.1 lists the major differences between poisonous and nonpoisonous snakes.

Table 61.1: Major differences between poisonous and nonpoisonous snakes[5, 6]

Feature	*Poisonous*	*Nonpoisonous*
Belly scales	Large, covering entire breadth of the belly	Small or moderately large but never covering the entire breadth of the belly
Head scales	Small	Usually large
Fangs	Long and canalized just as in case of Hypodermic needle	Short and solid
Tail	Compressed	Only modestly compressed
Habits	Generally nocturnal	Not so
Bite	Two fangmarks with or without small teeth marks	Small teeth marks in a row

PATHOGENESIS

Snake venom (toxin) is just a modified form of saliva which is stored in the sort of modified salivary glands. During snakebite, the venom passes from the snake's venom gland through a duct into the snake's fangs (two maxillary teeth lying apart, the interfag distance varying proportionally with size of the snake) and then into the host.

Snake venom is a mixture of toxins, polypeptides and proteolytic enzymes. These are species specific. For instance, in case of crotalidae, venom is cytolytic. It causes tissue necrosis, vascular leak and coagulopathy. It kills the victim by hemorrhagic shock, acute renal failure (ARF) and adult respiratory distress syndrome (ARDS). Snake venom from Elipidae and Hydrophidae is predominantly neurotoxic. It exerts curare-like effect by blocking neurotransmission at neuromuscular junction. It causes death from respiratory depression.

The fresh snake venom is a clear, transparent fluid which contains toxalbumins and several toxic principles e.g. fibrinolysins, proteolysins, neurotoxins, cholinestrase, hemolysins, thromboplastin, agglutinins, cardiotoxins, coagulase, hyaluronidase, lecithinase, etc.[6] Neurotoxins are predominant in elapid venom, cholinestrase in elapid venom, hemolysins in viper venom and thromboplastin in viper venom.

Table 61.2 lists the precise toxic effects of different proteins present in the snake venom.

Table 61.2: Different snake venom proteins and their adverse effects in the human prey

Protein	*Adverse effect in the victim*
Cytotoxin	Local tissue damage
Hemotoxin	Internal bleeding
Neurotoxin	Neurotoxicity
Cardiotoxin	Direct damage to heart

CLINICAL MANIFESTATIONS[5-9]

The term, *ophitoxemia,* is applied to the symptom complex produced by snakebite.

Irrespective whether it is poisonous or nonpoisonous snake, the very sight of a snake may be frightening, causing shock in some subjects.

Local manifestations of snakebite include fang marks, bruises, lacerations, oozing of serosanguinous fluid, painful swelling, redness and numbness at the location of bite.

Constitutional symptoms appear 15-30 minutes after the bite and include headache, dizziness, vomiting, convulsions and CNS stimulation. Then there occur CNS depression, respiratory difficulty and various paralyses. Hemorrhage from various sites and circulatory collapse may occur. Hemorrhagic sing is the most dreaded manifestation. It include bleeding from fang punctures, venepuncture sites, ecchymosis, epistaxis, bleeding gums, and subconjunctival and intracranial bleeding. Intracranial hemorrhage is the usual cause of death within 24-48 hours.

LABORATORY INVESTIGATIONS

Laboratory investigations are useful only for monitoring the patient.

Baseline tests should include:

- Complete blood count, including hemoglobin and hematocrit
- Platelet count
- Clotting time
- Bleeding time
- Prothrombin time
- Partial thromboplastin time
- Fibrinogen
- Fibrin products
- Blood urea nitrogen
- Creatinine
- CPK
- ECG

Immunodiagnosis by ELISA is useful in detecting specific snake venom in wound aspirate, serum or other body fluids.

GRADING OF ENVENOMATION

Table 61.3 gives classification of envenomation severity.

Table 61.3: Four-point scale for grading envenomation severity

Grade	*Features*
Grade 0	No envenomation
Grade 1	Minimal envenomation in the form of local swelling and pain without progression
Grade 2	Moderate envenomation in the form of swelling, pain or ecchymosis progressing beyond the site of injury; mild systemic or laboratory manifestations
Grade 3	Severe envenomation in the form of marked local response, severe systemic findings and significant alteration in laboratory findings

MANAGEMENT

Immediate (Prehospital) Measures

These should primarily be directed at allaying fear, and treating shock and respiratory failure with all available means.

The child should be kept recumbent, quiet and reassured.

Wound should be cleaned with saline water.

The bitten part should be immobilized and placed in a dependent position.

During transportation to the hospital, in order to prevent absorption of the venom by lymphatics, a tourniquet is applied proximal to the bite site about 5 cm above the upper limit of swelling that allows one finger beneath so that lymphatic drainage is occluded but arterial blood flow is not hampered causing ischemia and aggravating local tissue damage. It should be left in situ as long as antivenin serum (AVS) is not administered. Many authorities have discouraged this maneuver on the plea that tightly applied tourniquet is likely to impede arterial circulation and loose tourniquet turns out to be ineffective, especially in case of coral snake venom that may have hematogenous spread.

The application of ice locally and incision and sucking of the venom from the bite site are best avoided. There is evidence that ice application may cause cold-induced injury that means more tissue damage than the benefit.

Incision and sucking, at best, can remove only a marginal amount of venom. Instead, the manipulation may contribute to enhanced absorption.

Specific Measures[2,5-8]

Grade 0 envenomation needs no particular treatment. Grade 1 envenomation needs only pain control and careful observation. For Grade 3 and Grade 4 envenomation, AVS is definitely needed.

In practice, in India in particular, around 70-80% children suffer from moderate to severe envenomation, requiring administration of AVS.

Ideally, antivenom serum (AVS) should be snake species-specific i.e monovalent. However, in India and other less developed countries, such an AVS is usually not available and we have got to content with the polyvalent lympholized AVS. It is effective against Indian cobra, Indian krait and Russell's viper. It is manufactured by the Central Research Institute, Kasauli, and Haffkine Biopharmaceutical Corporation Ltd, Mumbai. AVS is of equine origin since it is derived from immunization of horses and, therefore, capable of causing type 1 and type 3 hypersensitivity reactions.

For best results, AVS should be administered intravenously. Local infiltration and intramuscular administration are not dependable.

Definite indications for administration of AVS are:

- Systemic envenomation as manifested by bleeding, DIC, shock, ARF, neurotoxicity, etc.
- Progressively spreading swelling over site of snakebite.

Presence of fangmarks, local pain, edema, swelling, numbness and weakness indicate envenomation. AVS should be administered in such a case without any loss of time.

Once a decision to administer AVS has been arrived at, attempts should be made to find out if the individual is hypersensitive to it (Table 61.4) before its administration.

Table 61.4: Evidence of hypersensitivity to AVS

- History of allergy to AVS or some other horse serum in the past.
- Skin test by intradermal injection of 0.1 ml of 1:100 saline dilution of AVS. Hypersensitivity is indicated by appearance of a wheal of over 10 mm in 10-30 minutes.
- Conjunctival test by instilling one drop of 1:10 dilution in saline in lower conjunctival sac. Hypersensitivity is indicated by development of conjunctivitis and tears in 10–30 minutes.

If required desensitization is carried out by intradermal injection of 0.1 ml of 1 : 100 saline dilution of AVS. Every minute the injection is repeated with a gradually increased dose of AVS until dose of 1 ml is given. This is followed by administration of 0.1 ml of undiluted AVS which again is built up to 1 ml gradually. If all goes well, 10 ml AVS diluted in 500 ml of normal saline is infused IV by slow drip. Subsequently, total calculated dose is administered carefully (vide infra).

Children require a much larger dose on account of higher concentration of venom in terms of body weight. The dose varies from 50–200 ml or even more in select cases. AVS is given as an IV infusion by reconstituting with distilled water or normal saline and diluted with 3 volumes of glucose saline, beginning at the rate of 1 ml/minute and increased slowly as tolerated, usually 20 ml/kg/hour. Ideally, AVS should be given as early as possible. Nevertheless, it may still remain useful even upto 1 week after the snakebite.[5]

Concurrent administration of steroids and antihistaminics cuts down the risk of anaphylaxis due to AVS.

Nevertheless, one should remain vigilant to manage anaphylaxis. The availability of epinephrine and antihistamines should be ensured

Supportive Measures

In addition to clinical and laboratory monitoring, the following measures are warranted:

- Prophylaxis against tetanus should be provided.
- Antibiotics are needed in the presence of superadded sepsis.
- Fresh blood or frozen plasma for bleeding manifestations.
- Restriction of fluids and electrolytes in ARF.
- Respiratory support.
- Surgical debridement in case of gangrene.

COMPLICATIONS

From Snakebite

- Compartment syndrome characterized by 6 Ps
  Pain out of proportion to injury
  Pressure symptoms in the form of swollen part
  Paresthesia
  Absent pulses
  Pain with passive stretch
  Paress/paralysis
- Tissue necrosis
- Bleeding diathesis.

From AVS

- Immediate hypersensitivity reactions which are duly preventable if appropriate sensitivity testing/desensitization is done.
- Serum sickness within 3 weeks: urticaria, malaise, arthralgia, lymphadenopathy, fever. Usually, it responds to antihistamines and oral steroids.

PROGNOSIS

Poisonous snakes are known for potentials to cause severe mobility and mortality. Nevertheless, timely institution of adequate treatment, especially administration of AVS, both morbidity and mortality are remarkably cut down.

Overall mortality due to snakebite is about 10%.

PREVENTION

As eminently put forward by Henry,[9] "snakebite is potentionally a preventable state".

- In snake-infested areas, use of boots, socks, trousers and torch plays an important role in preventing snakebites.
- People should be discouraged from playing with snakes. Often, snake-charmers are on record falling prey to snakebite.
- Often, the tendency in case of a snakebite is to carry the said snake, dead or alive, to the health center for identification. Extreme caution needs to be exercised in handling even a dead snake. Cases are on record where even a decapitated snake caused envenomation through reflex bite.
- Time must not be wasted in indulging in "useless endeavors" (say witchcraft) in case of a snakebite. Instead, the subject must be immediately transported to a nearby health center where suitable facilities for treatment, including AVS, are readily available. Such a transportation is, as a matter of fact, the best guarantee for the victim's correct treatment and probable recovery.

REFERENCES

1. Holve S. Envenomations. In: Behrman RE, Kliegman, RM. Jenson HB (eds) *Nelson Textbook of Pediatrics,* 17th edn. Philadelphia: Saunders 2004;2387-2392.
2. Kaushal RK, Gupte S. Pediatric envenomations. In: Gupte S (ed) *The Short Textbook of Pediatrics*, 10th edn. New Delhi: Jaypee Brothers 2004;531-534.
3. Arora A. Snakebite. In: Gupte S (ed) *Recent Advances in Pediatrics* (Special Vol 14: Criticare Pediatrics). New Delhi: Jaypee Brothers 2004;480-501.
4. Goodyear AE, Nair PVC, Mathai MKC. *Tropical Envenomation*, 3rd edn London: Smith and Smith 2004.
5. Gupte S, Pal M. Snakebite: Experience in north Indian children. *International Workshop on Tropical and Subtropical Diseases,* Johannesburg, 1995. Abstract IWTSD-PL6:21-22.
6. Parikh CK. *Parikh's Textbook of Medical Jurisprudence, Forensi Medicine and Toxicology*, 6th edn New Delhi: CBS 1999.
7. Dart R, McNally J. Efficacy, safety and use of snake antivenoms in the United States. *Ann Emerg Med* 2001;37:181-188.
8. McKinney P. Out of hospital and hospital management of crotaline snakebite. *Ann Emerg Med* 2001;37: 168-174.
9. Henry E. Safeguarding against snakebite. *Bull Trop Med* 2004;21:23-29.

Kamran Afzal and Shazia Afzal

62 Heat Stroke

INTRODUCTION

Despite accumulated knowledge and experience, deaths during heat waves are not uncommon[1,2] even among children.[3] Of the environmental heat illnesses, heat stroke is the most important because of its potential for high morbidity and mortality, especially during hot and humid weather.[4,5] Children are more susceptible to heat illness than adults for many reasons, including greater absorbance of ambient heat secondary to a greater surface area to body mass ratio, lower rate of sweating, slower rate of acclimatization and also generation of higher metabolic heat per mass unit.[6, 7]

There is a wide spectrum of disorders resulting from exposure to high environmental temperature ranging from the relatively benign muscular cramps to the potentially fatal heat stroke with serious CNS dysfunction.

Heat cramps are brief, intermittent and often severe muscular cramps that frequently occur in muscles fatigued by heavy work or exercise, particularly the calf and hamstring muscles. They are believed to be caused by a rapid change in the extracellular fluid osmolarity resulting from sodium and water loss.[7] Treatment consists of rest in cool environment and fluid and salt replacement.

Heat exhaustion is a more severe form of heat illness due to water or salt depletion results from exposure to high environmental temperature or strenuous physical exercise. It is characterized by dizziness, fainting, nausea, weakness, headache, profuse sweating and intense thirst. It is distinguished from heat stroke by having essentially intact mental functions and a temperature that is normal/below normal/ slightly elevated (less than 39°C).[8] Removing the patient from the hot environment and administering fluids will usually result in a rapid recovery. Left untreated, heat exhaustion may progress to heatstroke.

Heat stroke is defined clinically as a core body temperature that rises above 40°C[9] (or 40.6°C)[10] and that is accompanied by hot, dry skin and central nervous system abnormalities such as delirium, convulsions, or coma. However, heat stroke should be suspected in any patient with abnormal mentation during heat stress even if the core temperature is below 40°C.[11] Heat stroke results from either exposure to a high environmental temperature (classic, or non-exertional, heat stroke) or from strenuous exercise (exertional heat stroke). The hypothalamic set-point remains unchanged (normothermic) and the uncontrolled increase in body temperature results from overwhelming of the body's capacity to lose heat.[12] Based on its pathophysiology, heat stroke has been alternatively defined as a form of hyperthermia associated with a systemic inflammatory response leading to a syndrome of multiorgan dysfunction in which encephalopathy predominates.[9] Severe cases result in death.

THERMOREGULATION

Normal body function depends upon a relatively constant body temperature. In man, as in other warm blooded animals, a group of reflexes that are primarily integrated in the hypothalamus operate to maintain body temperature within a narrow range despite the wide fluctuations in environmental temperature.[13] Body heat is produced by metabolism, muscular activity (shivering), and non-shivering thermogenesis (heat production in certain organs and brown fat). When the ambient temperature approaches body temperature, heat is also gained from the environment. This overall heat load must be dissipated depending on the body-to-environment temperature gradient by radiation (60% heat transfer to the air), vaporization of water in the respiratory passages and on the skin (20-25%), convection (15%) and conduction.[7]

The hypothalamus maintains body temperature by balancing heat loss and heat production and coordinates these responses with regulation of thyroid and adrenal harmones, by induction of behavioral changes (e.g. seeking cooler or warmer environments) and by caloric adaptation.[14] This process is called thermoregulation (Fig. 62.1). A rise in the temperature of circulating blood by less than 1°C activates peripheral and hypothalamic heat receptors that signal the hypothalamic thermoregulatory center (thermosensitive neurons in the preoptic anterior hypothalamus).[14] The anterior hypothalamus sends signals to neuronal effectors of heat dissipation and generation predominantly located in the posterior hypothalamus. Heat dissipation is accomplished by cutaneous vasodilatation (resulting in the delivery of heated blood to the surface of the body) and increased sweating. The evaporation of 1.7 ml of sweat consumes 1 kcal of heat energy and at maximal efficiency in a dry environment, sweating can dissipate about 600 kcal per hour in adults.[15] Losses of salt and water by sweating must be balanced by generous salt supplementation to facilitate thermoregulation. Dehydration and salt depletion impair thermoregulation.[9]

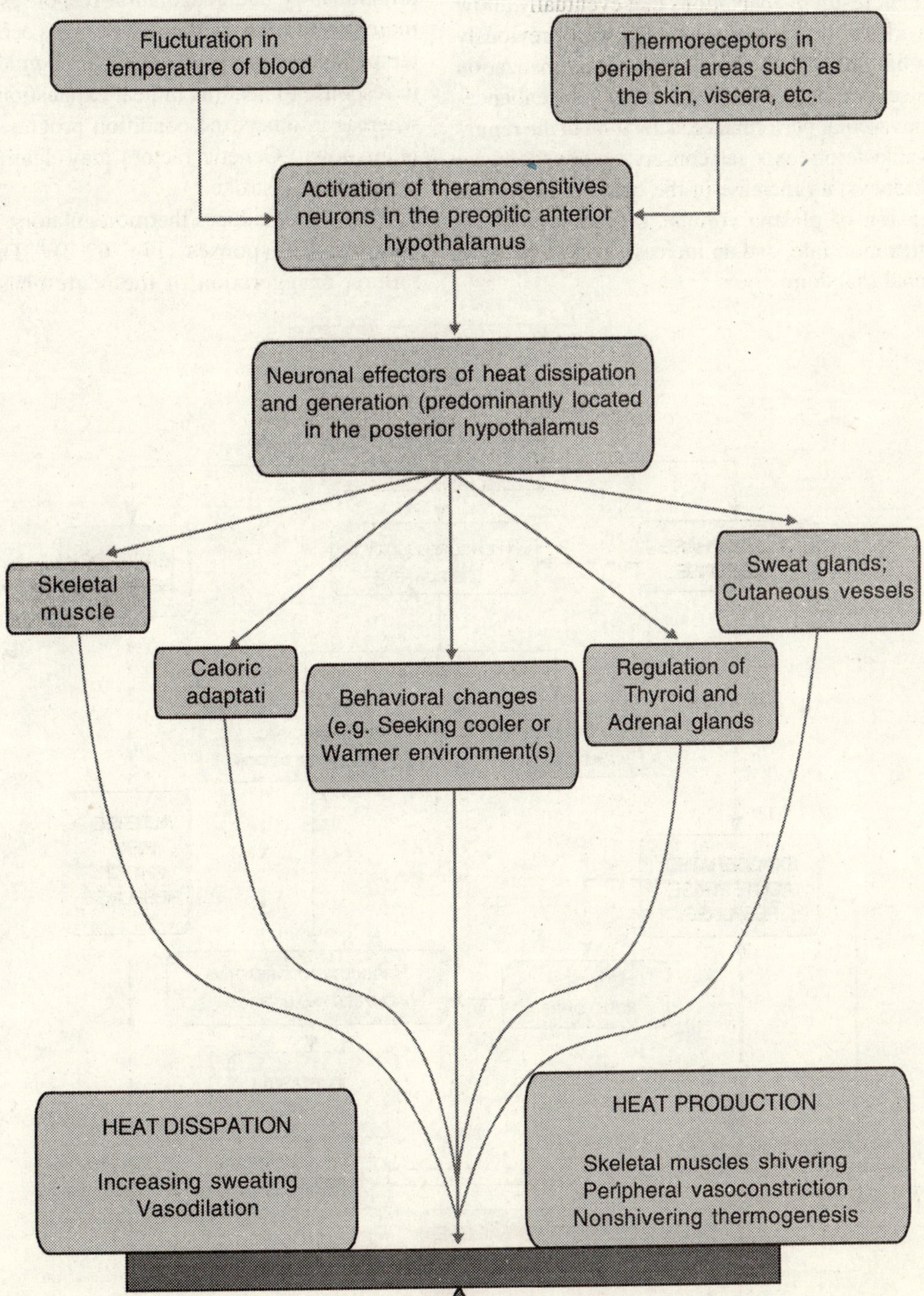

Fig. 62.1: Thermoregulation

The hyperthermic response in heat stroke probably results from interference with the normal heat dissipating mechanisms of the anterior hypothalamus. Heat stroke also leads to anhydrosis as part of the hypothalamic dysfunction.

ACCLIMATIZATION

Successive increments in the level of work performed in a hot environment result in adaptations that eventually allow a person to work safely at levels of heat that were previously intolerable or life-threatening. The process of acclimatization to heat takes several days to weeks and involves enhancement of cardiovascular performance, activation of the renin–angiotensin–aldosterone axis, salt conservation by the sweat glands and kidneys, an increase in the capacity to secrete sweat, expansion of plasma volume, an increase in the glomerular filtration rate, and an increase in the ability to resist exertional rhabdomyolysis.[9]

PATHOPHYSIOLOGY AND PATHOGENESIS

Heat stroke and its progression to multiorgan dysfunction syndrome (MODS) are due to a complex interplay among the acute physiological alterations associated with hyperthermia (e.g. circulatory failure, hypoxia, and increased metabolic demand), the direct cytotoxicity of heat, and the inflammatory and coagulation responses of the host. The more severe neuropathologic changes occur when the body temperature exceeds 40.5°C. Why a mild illness develops in response to heat (as in heat exhaustion) in some people whereas in others the condition progresses to heat stroke is unknown. Genetic factors may determine the susceptibility to heat stroke.[9]

Heat stress induces thermoregulatory, acute-phase, and heat-shock responses (Fig. 62.2).[9] Thermoregulatory failure, exaggeration of the acute-phase response, and

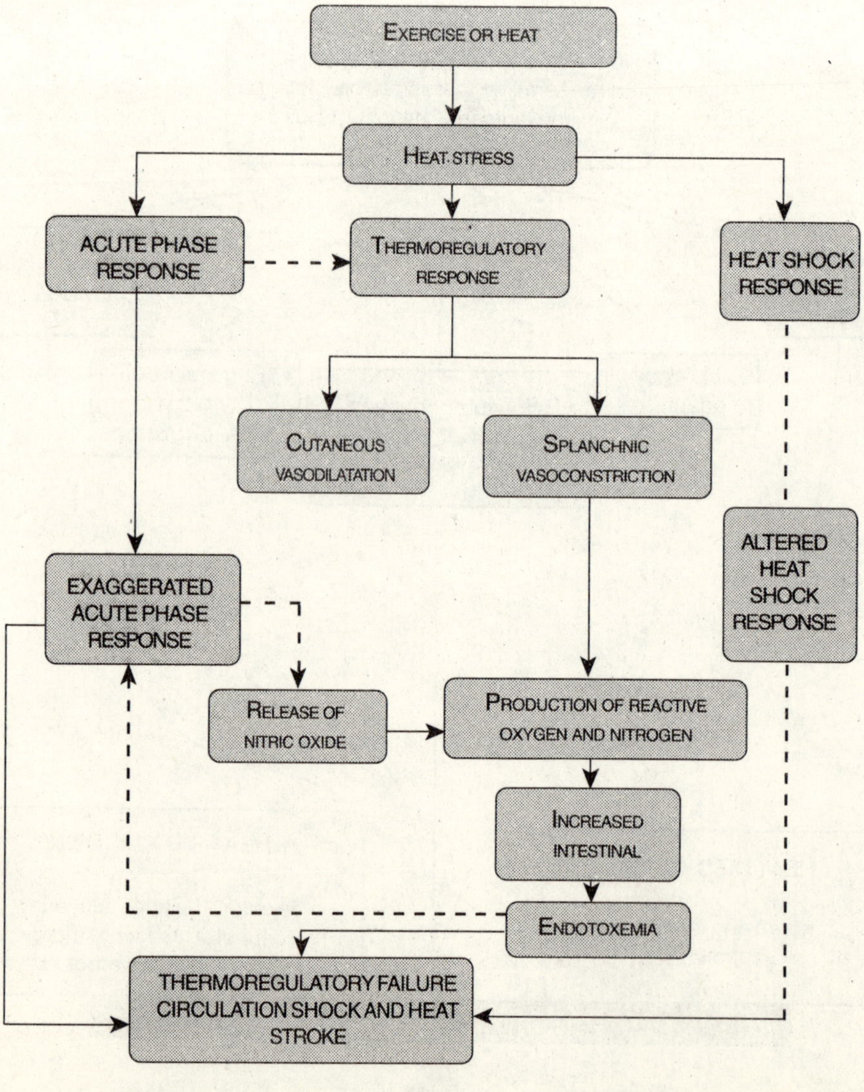

Fig. 62.2: Sequence of events in the progression of heat stress to heat stroke[9]
*Solid arrows indicate pathways for which there is clinical or experimental evidence, and the broken arrows indicate putative pathways

alteration in the expression of heat-shock proteins, individually or collectively, may contribute to the development of heat stroke. Active cutaneous vasodilatation and splanchnic vasoconstriction permit the shift of heated blood from the central organs to the periphery, from which heat is then dissipated to the environment. This change may also lead to splanchnic hypoperfusion and ischemia, resulting in increased production of reactive oxygen and nitrogen species, which may in turn induce intestinal mucosal injury and hyperpermeability. This constellation of events also leads to alterations in blood flow in the microcirculation and results in injury to the vascular endothelium and tissues. Endotoxins may then leak into the circulation and enhance the acute-phase response, leading to increased production of pyrogenic cytokines and nitric oxide. Both cytokines and nitric oxide can interfere with thermoregulation and precipitate hyperthermia, hypotension, and heat stroke.

CLINICAL FEATURES

Hyperthermia and CNS dysfunction are essential for the diagnosis of heat stroke. Tachycardia with wide pulse pressure and severe tachypnea are universally present. Cardiovascular system is usually hyperdynamic. Hypotension and shock may complicate the picture due to myocardial injury and peripheral vasodilatation combined with microvascular leakage secondary to endothelial damage.

Initial temperature generally exceeds 40.6°C but may be lower if cooling had already been initiated. Although sweating is usually absent in the classic form of heatstroke, 50% of exertional heatstroke cases have persistent sweating as a result of catecholamine release. The presence of sweating does not preclude the diagnosis of heatstroke.[8] The severity and domains of cognitive function affected can vary from mild deficits in attention and memory to severe global dementia.[16] More often, however, patients have delirium or frank coma with seizures in upto 50% cases, especially during cooling.[8] Opisthotons, hallucinations, decerebrate rigidity, cerebellar dysfunction, dystonia and tremors along with pupillary abnormalities may occur.

Several complications may appear either acutely or during the course of illness (Table 62.1). Acute renal failure occurs in upto 35% of patients with heat stroke and is caused by a combination of direct thermal injury, hypotension and shock from cardiovascular collapse and rhabdomyolysis.[10,17] Electrolyte abnormalities, coagulopathy and liver function derangements may occur. Most changes are potentially reversible but permanent neurological sequelae may be observed in up to 20% of the severe cases.[18,19]

DIFFERENTIAL DIAGNOSIS

It is crucial to begin treatment for heat stroke even while considering alternative diagnosis, since cooling does not harm any hyperthermic patient and is life-saving in heat stroke.

Table 62.1: Complications of heat stroke

Early	*Late*
Seizures	Persistent neurological deficit
Coma, Cerebral edema	Liver failure
Hypothermia (by overzealous cooling)	Disseminated intravascular coagulation (DIC)
Rhabdomyolysis	Adult respiratory distress syndrome
Hypokalemia, hyponatremia	Renal failure
Hypotension, shock	Hyperkalemia
Arrythmias, ECG abnormalities	Hypocalcaemia

1. Meningitis, encephalitis and other CNS infections are suggested by the history and presence of meningeal signs. Antibiotic therapy may be started pending lumbar puncture/CT report in doubtful cases.
2. Complicated malaria especially blackwater fever and cerebral malaria should be considered in residents of endemic area or those with recent visit to such areas.
3. History rules out the association of toxic agents as sympathomimetics, anticholinergics, antidopaminergics, cyclic antidepressants, lithium, etc. Various agents may cause neuroleptic malignant syndrome and malignant hyperthermia but these are differentiated from heat stroke by the presence of muscular rigidity.
4. Thyroid storm, pheochromocytoma and diabetic ketoacidosis with concomitant sepsis are some of the endocrinological conditions to be considered in the differential diagnosis.
5. Hemorrhagic shock encephalopathy: This is an idiopathic syndrome of infants characterized by sudden onset encephalopathy, profound shock, coagulopathy and diarrhea with rectal temperature above 39°C.[20]

APPROACH TO MANAGEMENT

Heat stroke is a major life threatening emergency and prompt and appropriate management may help reduce the mortality. When faced with any patient with hyperpyrexia and evidence of CNS dysfunction especially in a hot and humid weather, a high index of suspicion should be kept for the possible diagnosis of heat stroke. If the core temperature exceeds 40°C, move the patient to a cooler place, remove his/her clothings, and initiate external cooling while en route to a medical facility. Obtain history focusing on the activity immediately preceding symptoms, predisposing factors (Table 62.2), and prehospital cooling measures. Consider sepsis, cerebral malaria, meningoencephalitis and neuroleptic malignant syndrome in the differential diagnosis. Assess for the presence of complications. Investigations are done to exclude other diagnosis and to screen for complications, while the treatment is already in progress (Table 62.3).

Table 62.2: Risk factors of heat stroke

Predisposing factors	*Remarks*
1. *High ambient temperature and high humidity*	Heat waves (i.e., = 3 consecutive days of air temperatures = 90°F [= 32.2°C]) contribute significantly to heat-related deaths.[21] High humidity and decreased air current are also significant. Heat loss is limited to evaporation as ambient temperature approaches body temperature.
2. *Extremes of age, poor nutritional status and general state of health.*	Children (=4 years) and the elderly (=70 years) irrespective of gender are at high risk.[22]
3. *Strenuous outdoor activity*	Athletes and manual workers with inadequate or poor acclimatization are especially predisposed at lower ambient temperatures.
4. *Overbundling*	Overclothing especially of neonates and infants with clothing made of tight and impervious fabric in warm and humid weather decreases heat loss by conduction, convection and evaporation.
5. *Persons with chronic mental disorders or cardiopulmonary disease*	Usually they are receiving medications that interfere with salt and water balance, such as diuretics, anticholinergic agents, and tranquilizers that impair sweating.[9,10]
6. *Endocrine disorders*	Hyperthyroidism, uncontrolled diabetes mellitus.
7. *Autonomic dysfunction*	Children with familial dysautonomia and other neurologic disorders with impaired autonomic regulation are more susceptible because of, altered thirst mechanism/s, and inability to obtain enough water.[23]
8. *Toxins/Medications*	Anticholinergics, phenothiazines, antihistamines, diuretics, sympathomimetics, cyclic antidepressants, calcium channel blockers, amphetamines, inhaled anaesthetics, cocaine, heroin, etc.

Table 62.3: Investigations in a case of heat stroke

Test	*Remarks*
1. Complete blood counts and peripheral smear	Rule out sepsis, malaria; Total leukocyte count often increased in heat stroke to as high as 30,000-40,000/mL.[30]
2. Liver function test	Liver enzymes are universally elevated; extreme elevations of SGOT signify adverse outcome.[10]
3. Electrocardiogram	Non-specific ST-T changes may precede arrhythmias and conduction abnormalities.
4. Arterial blood gases	In non-exertional heat stroke respiratory alkalosis is common; exertional heat stroke is usually associated with respiratory alkalosis and lactic acidosis. In both varieties, the arterial carbon dioxide tension is often less than 20 mm Hg.[9]
5. Serum electrolytes, blood urea nitrogen, serum creatinine and urinalysis	Screen for acute renal failure and myoglobinuria (rhabdomyolysis); Hypo/hypernatremia and hypokalemia are common. Hypophosphatemia, hypomagnesaemia and hypocalcaemia may be present.
6. Blood glucose	Hyperglycemia is classic heat stroke; hypoglycemia is rare.[9] In exertional type hypoglycemia common.[30]
7. Coagulation studies	Rule out DIC.
8. CSF examination	To exclude CNS infections. In heat stroke: clear CSF, normal pressure, occasional pleocytosis and mild protein elevation (upto 150 mg/dl).[28]

The most important guiding principle in the management of heat-stroke is cooling of the patient with simultaneous maintenance of airway, breathing and circulation and monitoring for secondary complications.[24] However, it may be emphasized here that since the condition involves acute phase reactants and multiple inflammatory mediators, normalizing the body temperature may not prevent the cascade of inflammation, coagulation, and progression to multiorgan dysfunction triggered by the onset of heat stroke.[10] Thus patients with prolonged hyperpyrexia due to heat stroke have a poor outcome.

Following are the essential steps in the management: Admit the patient to a pediatric intensive care unit.

1. *Ensure ABC:* Rapidly evaluate and ensure airway patency, breathing adequacy and circulation integrity. If the patient is comatose protect the airway and use 100% oxygen and endotracheal intubation if necessary. Support circulation if required with the judicious use of fluids and inotropes like dopamine and dobutamine (see below). Establish secure intravenous line.
2. *Immediate and effective cooling:* Effective cooling brings down the rectal temperature below 39°C within one

Table 62.4: Methods of cooling[9,10]

Techniques for conductive cooling	*Techniques for evaporative or convective cooling*
• *External cooling** – Cold water immersion – Application of cold packs or ice slush over whole or part of the body – Use of cooling blankets • *Internal cooling* (mostly experimental but may be used if other measures fail) – Iced gastric lavage – Iced peritoneal lavage	• Fanning the undressed patient at room temperature (20 to 22°C) • Wetting of the body surface during continuous fanning‡ • Use of body cooling units§

* Massage skin to prevent cutaneous vasoconstriction induced by external cooling.
‡ Skin covered with fine gauze soaked in water at 20°C and patient is fanned till core temperature decreases to <39.4°C.
§ A special bed that sprays atomized water at 15°C and warm air at 45°C over the whole body surface.

hour.[25] Cooling rates should generally exceed 0.1-0.2°C/min with aggressive treatment.[10] There is no evidence that one cooling technique is superior to other and more than one technique may be used simultaneously (Table 62.4). Non-invasive techniques that are easy to apply, well tolerated, and not likely to cause cutaneous vasoconstriction are generally preferred.[9]

a. In persons with hyperthermia, transfer of heat from the core to the skin is facilitated by active cutaneous vasodilatation. Therapeutic cooling techniques are therefore aimed at accelerating the transfer of heat from the skin to the environment without compromising the flow of blood to the skin.[9] This is accomplished by increasing the temperature gradient between the skin and the environment (for cooling by conduction) or by increasing the gradient of water-vapor pressure between the skin and the environment (for cooling by evaporation), as well as by increasing the velocity of air adjacent to the skin (for cooling by convection). In practice, cold water or ice is applied to the skin, which is also fanned. Lowering of skin temperature to below 30°C triggers cutaneous vasoconstriction and shivering which can be overcome by vigorous massaging, spraying tepid water (40°C), or exposure to hot moving air (45°C), either at the same time as cooling methods are applied or in an alternating fashion.[3,9,10]
b. No pharmacologic agents that accelerate cooling are helpful in the treatment of heat stroke. Dantrolene sodium has been found ineffective in a double-blind, randomized study.[26] An increased hypothalamic set point is not the etiology of the increased body temperature. Thus, antipyretics do not help decrease body temperature. Moreover, salicylates can worsen coagulopathies, and acetaminophen in large doses can worsen hepatic damage and hence should not be used.[9] Several other drugs, including anticholinergics (decrease sweating) and alpha-adrenergic agonists (increase peripheral vascular resistance without increasing cardiac output) should also be avoided.
c. *Monitor temperature:* Regularly every 5 minutes initially and cooling may be stopped once the rectal temperature goes below 39.4°C. Measure rectal temperature (not skin/oral temperature) to ensure response to therapy and to avoid hypothermia by overzealous treatment.

3. *Fluids:* Although hypotension is common in heat stroke, majority of the patients are relatively normovolemic, peripherally vasodilated, and suffer from distributive shock and severe dehydration. Cooling will redistribute volume from the periphery to the core. Aggressive fluid administration can contribute to significant pulmonary edema. Hence cautious administration of boluses of isotonic cryatalloids (0.9% normal saline) allowing the body's natural compensatory response to regain function will normalize blood pressure and prevent fluid overload. Inotropes (dopamine) may be used if hypotension persists.
4. *Convulsions:* Prompt control of seizures is achieved with intravenous (or per rectal if i.v access is not available) diazepam (0.2 -0.3 mg/kg slow i.v over 2 minutes; maximum dose 10mg). If the seizures persist, phenytoin (15-20 mg/kg loading dose i.v. not faster than 25 mg/min; followed by maintenance 5-8 mg/kg in two divided doses) may be given.
5. *Monitor urine output and renal functions:* If the patient presents with anuria give normal saline bolus (20 ml/kg over ½ to 1 hour) to establish urine flow. Bladder may be catheterized to monitor urinary output. Manage on the lines of acute renal failure using careful balance of fluid and mannitol/furosemide to ensure urine flow. Exertional heat stroke may produce myoglobinuria and result in acute tubular necrosis. Alkalization of urine by giving intravenous sodium bicarbonate prevents renal shutdown.
6. *Cardiac monitoring:* Since cardiac arrhythmias are quite common, continuous cardiac monitoring or if this is not

available frequent ECG monitoring should be done and arrhythmias treated using appropriate drugs. ECG abnormalities may precede dysrhythmias.[10]

7. *Electrolyte abnormalities:* Alterations in sodium, potassium, phosphate and calcium levels may occur.[9] Serum potassium may be decreased in the initial stages and in the presence of acidosis represent true deficit requiring correction. Hyperkalemia secondary to muscle damage, rhabdomyolysis and renal failure is managed in the standard manner.
8. *Coagulopathy:* Nasogastric tube is put to check for gastrointestinal hemorrhages. Transfuse fresh blood if necessary. Prothrombin time, partial thromboplastin time, platelet count and fibrin degradation product should be closely followed. DIC is managed on the usual lines. Role of heparin in DIC occurring in patients of heat stroke is controversial.[9]
9. *Liver enzymes:* Should be monitored as required. All patients with heat stroke have some degree of liver enzyme elevation;[10] progression to fulminant hepatic failure following heat stroke has also been reported.[27] Treatment is mainly supportive.

PROGNOSTIC FACTORS

Morbidity and mortality are directly related to the peak temperature and to the duration of time the elevated temperature persists. Mortality may be as high as 70% if treatment is delayed by 2 hours.[10] Rapid improvement in sensorium with effective cooling is a good sign.

Other adverse prognostic indicators are presence of:

1. Prolonged coma of more than 4 hours.[28]
2. Prolonged hyperthermia and rectal temperature more than 42.2°C at admission.
3. Coagulopathy.
4. SGOT more than 1000 IU/L.[29]
5. Acute renal failure, hyperkalemia, lactic acidosis or myoglobinuria.
6. Presence of multiorgan dysfunction.

PREVENTION

Heat stroke is a preventable illness, and thorough knowledge of the disorder can help to reduce mortality and morbidity. Following steps may be helpful in this regard:

1. Acclimatize to heat. Unacclimatized persons are more prone to heat stroke.[28,30]
2. Drink additional water and consume salty foods, especially while going outdoors in hot and humid weather. Dehydration and salt depletion impair thermoregulation.[31] When fluid losses approach 6-10% of body weight, heat stroke and heat exhaustion become life-threatening.[32]
3. Reduce the level of physical activity and schedule outdoor activities during cooler times of the day.
4. Wear light, loose-fitting, and light-colored clothing during hot weather and increase the amount of time spent in cooler environments.
5. Identify at-risk individuals and conduct patient and family teaching. Public education about the signs, symptoms, and risks of heatstroke may facilitate early diagnosis and treatment.
6. Children should never be left unattended in closed automobiles during hot weather because deaths from heat stroke have been reported in such situations.[33,34]
7. Improved weather forecasting, alerting those at risk, and providing readily accessible shelters during extreme weather may decrease morbidity and mortality during heat waves.

REFERENCES

1. Kalkstein LS. Saving lives during extreme weather in summer. *BMJ* 2000;321:650-651.
2. Kellerman AL, Todd KH. Killing heat. *N Engl J Med* 1996;335:126-127.
3. Mittal SK. Heat illness in children. *Indian Pediatr* 1981;18:401-404.
4. Kilbourne EM, Choi K, Jones TS, Thacker SB. Risk factors for heat stroke: a case control study. *JAMA* 1982;247:3332-3336.
5. Ghaznawi HI, Ibrahim MA. Heat stroke and heat exhaustion in pilgrims performing the Hajj (annual pilgrimage) in Saudi Arabia. *Ann Saudi Med* 1987;7:323-326.
6. Bytomski JR, Squire DL. Heat illness in children. *Curr Sports Med Rep* 2003;2:320-324.
7. Hergenreader AC, Chorley JN. Sports medicine. In: Behrman RE, Kliegman RM, Jenson HB (eds) *Nelson Textbook of Pediatrics.* 17th edn Philadelphia: WB Saunders 2004;2302-2320.
8. Weinmann M. Hot on the inside. *Emerg Med Serv* 2003;32:34.
9. Bouchama A, Knochel JP. Heat Stroke. *N Engl J Med* 2002;346:1978-1988.
10. Tek D, Olschaker JS. Heat illness. *Emerg Med Clin North Am* 1990;10:299-309.
11. Bhargav SK, Mittal SK, Kumari S, Kumar A, Ghosh S. Heat injury in the newborn. *Indian J Med Res* 1977;65:688-695.
12. Dinarrelo CA, Gelfand JA. Fever versus hyperthermia. In Braunwald E, Hauser S, Fauci AS, Longo DL, Kasper LD, Jameson JL (eds) *Harrison's Principles of Internal Medicine*, 15th edn. New York: McGraw-Hill 2001;91.
13. Ganong WF. Thermoregulation. In: Ganong WF (ed) *Review of Medical Physiology*, 20th edn. New York: Lange/McGraw-Hill, 2001;242-247.
14. Disorders of thermoregulation. In: Swaimann KF, Ashwal S, (eds) *Pediatric Neurology*, 3rd edn. St Louis: Mosby 1999;1329.
15. Adams WC, Fox RH, Fry AJ, MacDonald IC. Thermoregulation during marathon running in cool, moderate, and hot environments. *J Appl Physiol* 1975;38:1030-1037.
16. Romero JJ, Clement PF, Belden C. Neuropsychological sequelae of heat stroke: report of three cases and discussion. *Mil Med.* 2000;165:500-503.
17. Wang AY, Li PK, Lui SF, Lai KN. Renal failure and heatstroke. *Ren Fail* 1995;17:171-179.

18. Dematte JE, O'Mara K, Buescher J, et al. Near-fatal heat stroke during the 1995 heat wave in Chicago. *Ann Intern Med* 1998;129:173-181
19. Knochel JP, Reed G. Disorders of heat regulation. In: Narins RG(ed) *Maxwell & Kleeman's Clinical Disorders of Fluid and Electrolyte Metabolis,* 5th edn. New York: McGraw-Hill, 1994;1549-1590.
20. Tobin JR, Watzel RC. Heat Stroke. In Rogers MC (ed) *Textbook of Pediatric Intensive Care*, 3rd edn Baltimore: William and Wilkins 1996;605-655.
21. Anonymous. Heat-related deaths—Chicago, Illinois, 1996-2001, and United States, 1979-1999. *MMWR* 2003;52:610-613.
22. Nakai S, Itoh T, Morimoto T. Deaths from heat-stroke in Japan: 1968-1994. *Int J Biometeorl* 1999;43:124-127.
23. Tirosh I, Hoffer V, Finkelstein Y, Garty BZ. Heat stroke in familial dysautonomia. *Pediatr Neurol* 2003;29:164-166.
24. Bouchama A. Heatstroke: a new look at an ancient disease. *Intensive Care Med.* 1995;21:623-625.
25. O'Donell TF, Clowes GHA. The circulatory abnormalities of heat stroke. *N Engl J Med* 1972;287:734-737.
26. Bouchama A, Cafege A, Devol EB, Labdi O, el-Assil K, Seraj M. Ineffectiveness of dantrolene sodium in the treatment of heatstroke. *Crit Care Med* 1991;19: 176-180.
27. Berger J, Hart J, Millis M, Baker AL. Fulminant hepatic failure from heat stroke requiring liver transplantation. *J Clin Gastroenterol* 2000;30:429-431.
28. Shibolet S, Lancaster MC, Danon Y Heat stroke: a review. *Aviat Space Environ Med.* 1976;47:280-301.
29. Kew M, Bershas I, Sefteh H. The diagnostic and prognostic significance of the serum enzyme changes in heat stroke. *Trans R Soc Trop Med Hyg* 1971;63: 325.
30. Khosla R, Guntupalli KK. Heat-related illnesses. *Crit Care Clin* 1999;15:251-263.
31. Deschamps A, Levy RD, Cosio MG, Marliss EB, Magder S. Effect of saline infusion on body temperature and endurance during heavy exercise. *J Appl Physiol* 1989;66:2799-2804.
32. Naghii MR. The significance of water in sport and weight control. *Nutr Health* 2000;14:127-132.
33. King K, Negus K, Vance JC. Heat stress in motor vehicles: A problem in infancy. *Pediatrics* 1981;68: 579-582.
34. Krous HF, Nadeau JM, Fukumoto RI, Blackbourne BD, Byard RW. Environmental hyperthermic infant and early childhood death: circumstances, pathologic changes, and manner of death. *Am J Forensic Med Pathol* 2001;22:374-382.

Suraj Gupte and Javed Chowdhary

63 Electric Shock

INTRODUCTION

The term, *electric shock,* denotes an accidental physical injury as a result of flow of electricity through the body, varying from trivial skin burns to complete charring and destruction of skin or unconsciousness from paralysis of the respiratory centers, fibrillation of the heart or both.[1-3]

If the individual succumbs to electric shock, the term, *electrocution,* is employed.[3]

With increasing use of electricity, the incidence of electric shock is on the increase. The factors contributing to this unfortunate state of affairs include[4-10]

- Low-lying power points in the household
- Naked (exposed) wiring at places
- Short circuit
- Greater dependence on electrical appliances without attention to rectification of defects
- Poorly disciplined child.

According to the World Health Organization, 4000 people suffer from electric shock and 1000 people get electrocuted every year in USA only. Around 5-6% admissions to burn centers are on account of electric shock.[2, 3]

A special type of burns, the so-called *lightning burns* result from passage of a high-voltage current directly or when it strikes the ground or an adjacent object. The burns are dependent on

- Current path
- Type of clothing
- Presence of metal
- Presence of cutaneous moisture.

ETIOPATHOLOGY[3-7]

The passage of electric current causes thermal injury to tissues. There results electrical disruption of cell membrane, causing cell death. When the current passes directly through such organs as heart, pathologic changes are imminent.

The magnitude of the injury an electric current causes depends on the following factors:

- *Pathway* adopted by the current through the body. Electrical current taking a vertical pathway is more likely to be dangerous, causing myocardial damage.
- *Amount of current.* High voltage causes most extensive burns with damage to muscles, blood vessels, nerves and bones.
- *Type of current.* Direct current (DC) is likely to produce prolonged muscular contraction, paralyzing the involved muscles. Low frequency AC is more dangerous than high frequency AC. The former stops electrical impulses from brain and produces ventricular fibrillation. High AC of several thousand volts with 0.5 million cycles/second, used in physiotherapy, is safe.
- *Duration of contact.* Dry battery current (as in mobile phone) in contact with chest for prolonged periods may cause ventricular fibrillation.
- *Skin resistance.* Dry callosed skin is a bad conductor and wet moist skin is a better conductor.

Understandably, even a very small amount of electric current applied directly to the heart may be severe enough to stop the heart. As small as 1 milliampere of 60 cycle current applied directly to the ventricle is capable of causing fibrillation.

On the other hand, a very large amount of electric current may fail to penetrate the dry calloused skin of the fingers and hands, thereby causing no harm.

It is known that an effective current > 15 milliamperes for direct current causes muscle tissue to contract. Thus, the hand exposed to a sufficient electric current is unable to release its grip.

Chest muscle get paralyzed and respiration ceases if sufficient current passes across thorax.

CLINICAL MANIFESTATIONS

Local Manifestations

The following developments occur at the point where the electric current makes its entry:

1. The so-called "Joule burn" is an electric mark produced at the site of entry of electric current, usually hands and finger tips. It is yellow-brown in color and of variable size depending on area of contact. To start with, it is dry and bloodless, However, in due course (say 36 hours), it develops considerable edema and hyperemia.
2. Shallow depression, ulcer or a raised mark.
3. Blackening of the skin at the location of contact with formation of blisters and charred area.

Over and above this, there is a secondary mark over another part of the body, usually thorax which is in contact with extremities.

In addition, there is a burn mark at the exit point (usually soles and legs) which resembles Joule burn though it is larger in area.

Table 63.1 gives the classification of cutaneous electrical burns.

Table 63.1: Classification of cutaneous electrical burns

Category I
Low voltage current (< 220 V) producing first and second degree burns
Category II
High voltage circuit causing electrothermal injuries which may be to the extent of involvement of the underlying bone.
Category III
Arcing current producing a mixture of flame and electrical burns

Systemic Manifestations

Coagulation necrosis in muscles and vasculature by transverse current may cause widespread thrombosis, resulting in much more extensive tissue destruction than one expects on first examination.

Miscellaneous Manifestations

These include unconsciousness, rigors, seizures, deafness, visual disturbances, apnea, anoxia, psychiatric symptoms, neurobehavioral disorders, brain hemorrhage, cardiac asystole, fibrillation, bundle branch block, nodal block, cataract, pleural effusion and acute renal failure (Table 63.2).

COMPLICATIONS

These, usually encountered in electric shock secondary to high tension current, include

- Ventricular fibrillation
- Respiratory muscle spasm
- Respiratory failure
- Sepsis
- Hemorrhage
- Acute renal failure

Any of these complications may end up fatally.

Table 63.2: Manifestations of electric burns[5-8]

System	*Manifestations*
Respiratory	Respiratory arrest (apnea)
	Acute respiratory distress
	Aspiration syndrome
Cardiac	Dysrhythmias
	Asystole
	Fibrillation (both ventricular and atrial)
	Sinus tachycardia
	Sinus bradycardia
	Conduction defects
	PVC
	PAC
	ST-T wave changes
Neurologic	*Immediate*
	Unconsciousness
	Agitation
	Amnesia
	Motor paralysis
	Visual disturbances
	Intracranial hematoma
	Secondary
	Pain
	Paraplegia
	Brachial plexus injury
	SIADH
	Autonomic disturbances
	Cerebral edema
Renal	Acute renal failure
	Myoglobinuria
Cutaneous	Oral commissure burns
	Tongue and dental injuries
	Skin burns, including entrance and exit burns
	Arc burns
Abdominal	Perforation of viscera
	Solid organ damage
	Paralytic ileus
Musculoskeletal	Compartment syndrome
	Long bone fractures
	Spine injuries
Ocular	Visual disturbances
	Extraocular muscle paralysis
	Optic neuritis
	Cataracts

DIAGNOSIS/INVESTIGATIONS

PCV high because of accompanying dehydration with hyopkalemia

Reticulocyte count raised in presence of hemolysis

Blood urea high

Creatinine high

Urine positive for myoglobin

ECG heart block and/or ventricular fibrillation; tachycardia and minor ST segment changes

Lumbar puncture high pressure, blood-stained CSF

MANAGEMENT

Immediate First Aid

- While taking due self-protection and, if possible, cutting off the electric circuit (by switching off or cutting the wire with a poor conductor), the victim should be rescued. He needs to be immediately separated from the electric line employing a dry wooden stick, rubber gloves or dry thick cloth (folded).
- Respiration should be revived by mouth-to-mouth breathing.
- External cardiac massage should be given for cardiac asystole.
- Burn area should be cleaned aseptically.
- The patient should be carefully examined for any other injuries, including fractures. The fractured limb should be immobilized.

Transportation to Hospital

While shifting the child to hospital, make sure that he receives cardiorespiratory support.

Management in Hospital

On arrival in the hospital, a thorough physical examination should be conducted with special reference to the points listed in Table 63.3.

Table 63.3: Special examination of a child with electric shock

- General condition, including rehydration status
- Cardiorespiratory status
- Renal status
- Amount of fluid administered before arrival
- Degree of burns
- Injuries, including fractures, spinal and cranial trauma

Fluid Resuscitation

It should be initiated immediately guided by urine output, hematocrit, osmolality, CVP and arterial blood gases. Instead of following the principles employed in treating burn cases, one should count on the ones used for crush injuries in calculating fluids. In other words, more than 1–2 ml/kg of urine output needs to be the aim, especially in the presence of myoglobinuria. In the later situation, it is important to achieve urine alkalization and osmotic diuresis through mannitol and/or frusemide.

Feeding

In order to prevent gastric dilatation and vomiting, nasogastric tube is passed. Through this tube a small amount of an antacid is introduced. This assists to prevent development of stress ulcer. After 24 hours, milk feed is started in small increments, simultaneously cutting down at the IV fluids. By second or third day, a soft diet may be initiated.

Tetanus Prophylaxis

All cases of electric injuries need to be given tetanus prophylaxis.

Antibiotic Prophylaxis

The choice of antibiotic(s) depends on the merits of the case. However, in most cases, it is advisable to give injectable penicillin, say procaine penicillin 50,000 units/kg (IM) daily for 10 days or benzathine penicillin 12,00,000 units (IM) as a single dose. The aim is to safeguard from beta-hemolytcus streptococcal infection.

Attention to Local Wounds

Burns are cleaned and debrided under aseptic conditions. Daily irrigation, debridement, and topical and systemic antimicrobial therapy, splinting of affected parts and other surgical interventions may be needed.

Blood Transfusion

A blood transfusion may be in order during the course of treatment to replace the blood loss.

Treatment of Complications

Complications are usually a feature of cases hit by a high tension electric current.

Cardiopulmonary Complications: Such complications as congestive cardiac failure, pulmonary edema, ventricular fibrillation, ventricular tachycardia, supraventricular tachycardia, sinus tachycardia and heart block as also pneumonia and pleural effusion should be anticipated and appropriately handled.

Renal Complications: Renal insult from electric shock may cause ARF. It usually responds to conservative measures. A small proportion of cases may need dialysis.

Neurologic Complications: Such complications as seizures, coma, amnesia, spinal cord injury, paralysis and transversemyelitis should be suitably treated.

Miscellaneous Complications: Gastrointestinal hemorrhage, ocular hemorrhage, thromboses and orthopedic problems need to be properly treated.

Rehabilitation

Medical, nursing, surgical and orthopedic team work is required to counter the potentially crippling effects of electric shock.

PROGNOSIS

An overwhelming proportion of children who survive electric shock show full and fast recovery. In a small proportion complete though delayed recovery, taking several weeks, is seen. Causes of death are listed in Table 63.4.

Table 63.4: Causes of mortality in electric shock

- Ventricular fibrillation
- Respiratory muscle spasm
- Mechanical asphyxia
- Respiratory failure
- Superadded sepsis/septicemia
- Severe bleed
- Acute renal failure

PREVENTION

The following preventive measures are of value in cutting down the incidence of electrical shock/injuries:

- Appropriate wiring, using safe, good-quality material.
- Using electric appliances of safe design and in good working condition.
- Not fixing electric switches and sockets at floor level or on beds and bathtubs.
- Replacing loose sockets.
- Placement of electric and water supplies fairly apart.
- Never leave electric appliances within children's reach.
- Medicolegal/Forensic Aspects.

REFERENCES

1. Whitehead E, Smith AE, Solomon A. Electrical shock and burn injuries. *Eur Bull Trauma* 2003;19:1232-1235.
2. Anderson AA. Electrical injuries: Natural history, pathophysiology and treatment. *Eur Bull Trauma* 2001;17:134-141.
3. Lee A, Gee AE. Electrocution revisited. Br Trauma Bull 1999;3:62-64.
4. Hall ML, Sills RM. Electrical and lightning injuries. In: Barkin RM (ed) *Pediatric Emergency Medicine*. St Louis: CV Mosby 1997;484-495.
5. Hunt JL, Sato RM, Baxter CR. Acute electrical burns. *Arch Surg* 1980;115:434-439.
6. Antoon AY, Donovan MK. Burn injuries. In: Behrman RE, Kliegman RM, Jenson HB (eds) *Nelson Textbook of Pediatrics*, 17th edn Philadelphia: Saunders 2004;330-337.
7. Wilkinson C, Wood H. High voltage electrical injury. *Am J Surg* 1978;136:693-695.
8. Remensnyder JP. Acute electrical injuries. In: Martyrn JAJ (ed) *Acute Management of the Burned Patient*. Philadelphia: WB Saunders 1990;66-86.
9. Parikh CK. Thermal injuries. In: *Parikh's Textbook of Medical Jurisprudence*, Forensic Medicine and Toxicology, 6th edn New Delhi: CBS 1999;4.151-4.183.
10. Franklin Ca. Electricity. In: *Modi's Medical Jurisprudence and Toxicology*, 21st edn. Mumbai: Tripathi 1988;243-249.

Ajay Gaur

64 Drowning

INTRODUCTION

Drowning, defined as death within 24 hours of a submersion incident, and near-drowning defined as survived for at least 24 hours following in submersion incident, result in substantial morbidity and mortality in children. Death from submersion incident is the leading cause of accidental death in children[1] with nearly one third of survivors sustaining significant neurologic damage due to anoxic encephalopathy.[2]

Most pediatric drowning victims are toddlers. Drowning rates peak at 0–4 years and again at 16–18 years of age. Risk factors for drowning relate to gender, age, race, and season. The male to female ratio of 3:1 among young children increases to 6:1 among late adolescents. Most drowning and near drowning occur during the summer months. The adolescent peak is seen only in boys. Children with epilepsy and those with long QT syndrome are at increased risk of drowning.

PATHOPHYSIOLOGY

The Drowning Episode

The major consequence of the submersion is global hypoxia. While aspiration of water and hypothermia may add to the injury, hypoxia-induced cell death in multiple organs is the main injury. Each organ system's response to hypoxic injury follows a relatively predictable timetable. Central nervous system and myocardium manifest the most acute responses. Unresponsiveness and apnea may develop in 1 to 3 minutes; ventricular dysrhythmias and asystole may develop within 3 to 4 minutes.

Several pathogenic mechanism of death can occur while a drowning victim is submerged. Cerebral hypoxia, carbon dioxide narcosis, laryngospasm, pulmonary reflexes, or vagally mediated cardiac arrest may cause brain death the common final pathway (Fig. 64.1).

The volume of water aspirated or swallowed may be large or small, and the depth of water may be shallow. Laryngospasm may occur, and hypoxia may follow without

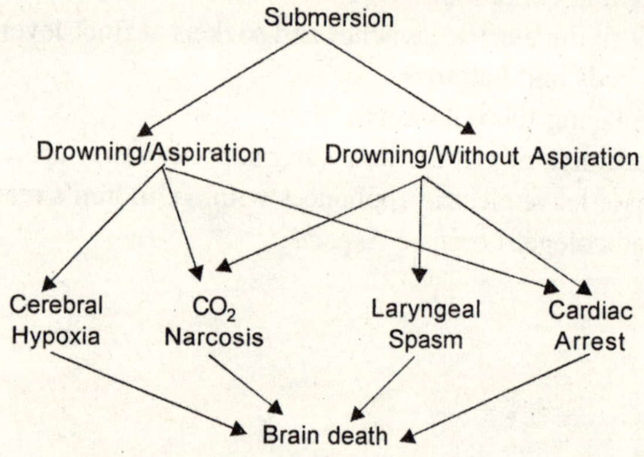

Fig. 64.1: Pathophysiology leading to brain death in drowning victims

the active aspiration of water in as many as 10% of victims. This is probably caused by a small amount of water entering the larynx or trachea and provoking a reflex causing spasm.

When a child is first submerged, a period of initial voluntary apnea occurs (Fig. 64.2). There may not be a struggle, but swimming movements occur. In the younger age group (< 5 years), the diving reflex may be stimulated and make a significant difference in survival. Within seconds of the victim's face touching cold water and before consciousness is lost, a reflex mediated by the trigeminal nerve sends sensory afferent impulses to the central nervous system (CNS) medullary respiratory center, which causes bradycardia and shunting of blood from cutaneous and splanchnic vascular beds to the cerebral and coronary circulations (i.e. the diving reflex) (Fig. 64.3). These reflex changes are independent of peripheral chemoreceptors and baroreceptors and are augmented by progressively colder water temperatures and the startle response. Infants who are taught to swim at a young age ("waterproofing") and who are not afraid of the water may lack a startle response and may be at greater risk for near drowning. The victim can hold his or her breath voluntarily until the break point is reached, as determined by the oxygen and carbon dioxide levels (peripheral and central chemo receptors respectively).

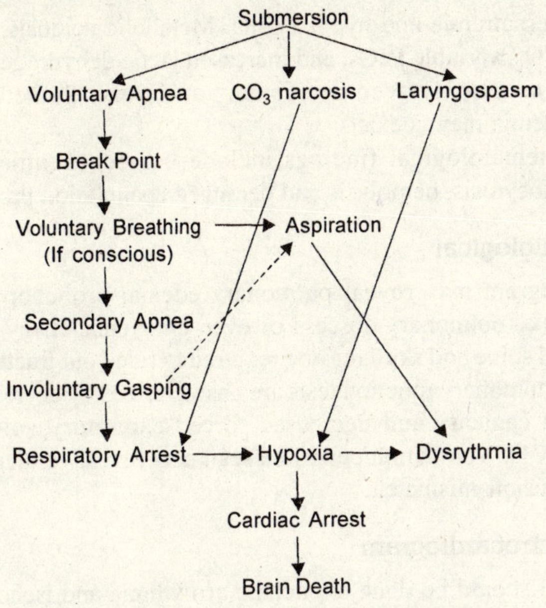

Fig. 64.2: Sequence of respiratory reflexes occurring in drowning

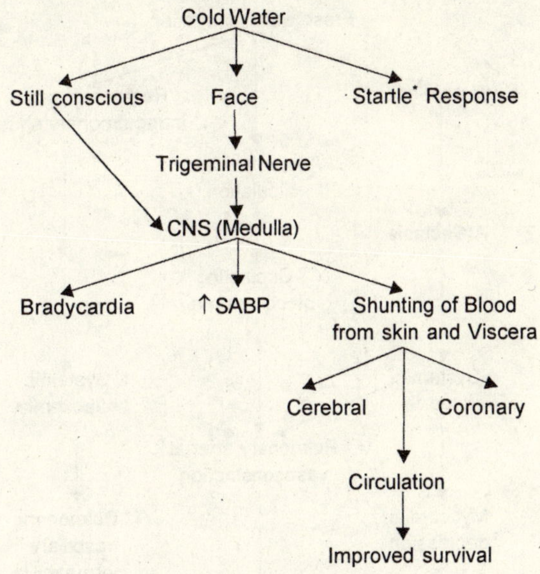

Fig. 64.3: The diving reflex

The break point is when an individual takes an involuntary breath, which occurs at $PaCO_2$ levels of 51 mmHg and PaO_2 of 73 mmHg after 87 seconds at rest.

After voluntary hyperventilation the break point can be prolonged to 140 seconds ($PaCO_2$ 46 mmHg and PaO_2 mmHg) at rest and 85 seconds ($PaCO_2$ 49 mmHg and PaO_2 43 mmHg) with exercise. The break point may not occur while the victim is conscious if he or she has voluntarily hyperventilated to low $PaCO_2$ values before submersion and hyperventilation is followed by exercise (underwater swimming). Hypoxia may cause loss of consciousness before activation of carbon dioxide receptors causes voluntary breathing movements.

Within seconds of the first submerged breaths, secondary apnea occurs and, if followed by involuntary gasping under the water lasting for several minutes, respiratory arrest follows. Dysrhythmias occur due to hypoxia, and eventually cardiac arrest and brain death occur. Once aspiration of fluid takes place, metabolic acidosis and systemic arterial hypertension persist even if the victim is saved or pulled from the water.

How long an individual can tolerate hypoxia is depends on many factors, including the age of the victim, previous health, water temperature and promptness and effectiveness of the rescue efforts. Young victims usually survive if submersion is less than 3 minutes and upto 10 minutes in water 10° to 15°C.

Systemic Complications

A. *Neurological*

Hypoxemia and metabolic acidosis alter the blood brain barrier and cerebral edema occurs. Edema causes hemispheric swelling and shifts of brain across compartments (herniation). If hypoxia is severe enough, brain death may occurs.[10, 17-20]

Neurological residual effects include blindness, electroencephalographic changes, dilation of ventricles due to brain atrophy and persistent coma.

B. *Pulmonary*

The cornerstone is the development of pulmonary edema which is caused by the increased peripheral airway resistance; variable degrees of laryngospasm; reflex pulmonary vasoconstriction, leading to pulmonary hypertension, decreased lung compliance; fall in ventilation–perfusion ratios; fluid shifts across the alveolar membrane; surfactant loss (salt water) or alteration in its properties (fresh water); foam and froth production; and anatomic changes in alveolar epithelial cells (Fig. 64.4).

C. *Cardiovascular*

Electrocardiographic (ECG) changes, bradycardia or asystole and ventricular fibrillation can occur. Systemic arterial blood pressure may be normal, high or low, depending on oxygenation, acid-base balance, cardiac function, peripheral vascular resistance, the level of circulatory catecholamines and elevated intracranial pressure (ICP).

D. *Hypothermia*

Hypothermia (Core temperature < 35°C) after submersion is common due to their high body surface area, low amount of subcutaneous fat and compromised thermogenic capacity. Hypothermia develops in two ways first, as a result of contact with water and aspirating cold water and secondly when child is removed from the water and exposed to air,

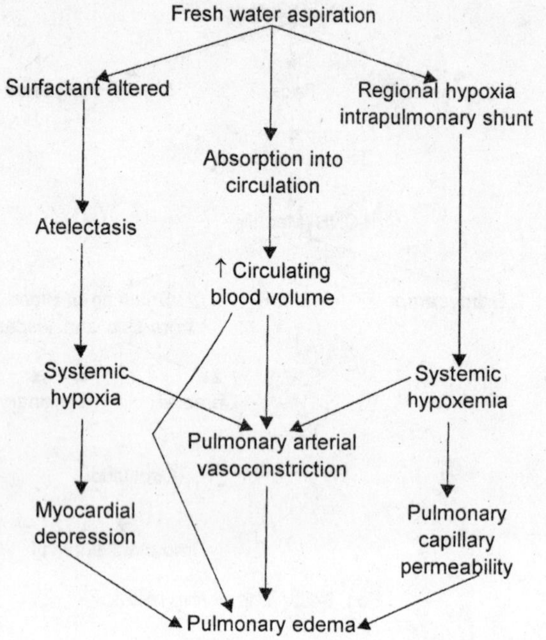

Fig. 64.4: Pathophysiology of pulmonary edema

wet clothes and during transport to the hospital in same condition. In moderate hypothermia (Core temperature 32°-35°C) compensatory mechanisms will usually attempt to restore normal temperature but in severe hypothermia (core temperature < 32°) the process of thermoregulation fails, shivering ceases and the cellular metabolic rate decreases. In cases where temperature drops down to 28°C, extreme bradycardia and asystole are common. The depression of respiratory centers results in hypoventilation and apnea. Temperature between 25°-29°C with deep coma, fixed and dilated pupils and absent reflexes may give the false appearance of death. The secondary systemic effects of hypothermia persist even after temperature comes to the normal.

E. *Renal*

Renal function is usually normal, but albuminuria, hemoglobinuria, oliguria, and anuria can occur. This is probably due to ischemia.

CLINICAL MANIFESTATIONS

Clinical manifestations are mainly associated with neurological and respiratory consequences. They depend upon the duration of submersion and effectiveness of the first aid resuscitation efforts. In majority of the children respiratory distress, pulmonary edema and cyanosis are present. On auscultation crepitations may be found. Sometimes features of cardiogenic shock, acute renal failure and disseminated intravascular coagulation (DIC) coexist.

LABORATORY INVESTIGATIONS

Biochemical and Hematological

Electrolyte abnormalities occur the form of hyponatremia, hypernatremia and hypokalemia. Metabolic acidosis, low $PaCO_2$, variable PaO_2, and increased lactic dehydrogenase are commonly seen in submersion injury. Sometimes azotemia may coexist.

Hematological findings include hemoconcentration, leukocytosis, hemolysis and deranged coagulation profile.

Radiological

Skiagram may reveal pulmonary edema, bronchopneumonia, pulmonary abscess or even empyema. X-ray cervical spine and skull may be required to ruled out fractures.

Pulmonary function tests are characterized by decreased vital capacity and decreased forced expiratory volume (FEV1). Ventilation perfusion scan may reveal ventilation perfusion mismatch.

Electrocardiogram

ECG should be done to exclude arrhythmia and ischemic changes.

Hepatorenal Functions

There is a need to monitor hepatic and renal functions.

Bacteriological Examination

Throat swab and tracheal swab should be sent for culture and sensitivity especially in contaminated water to identify the presence of any pathogenic organisms.

APPROACH TO MANAGEMENT

The ultimate aim of the management is to prevent the target organs from hypoxic–ischemic insult. The management is summarized in Fig. 64.5.

Spot management

The most devastating aspect of the drowning episode is hypoxemia. Mouth-to-mouth or mouth-to-nose breathing must be given promptly, even in the water if necessary. Supplemental oxygen must be given to all victims as soon as possible until it is proved that they no longer need it. All parents, childcare personnel and pool owners or supervisor should be trained in CPR.

In the Emergency Department

All patients must be given oxygen and have their stomach contents removed, particularly if they are not completely awake or lack intact protective airway reflexes. They need to have their head and neck assessed for concomitant trauma. In children where extremities are cool and mottled and weak peripheral pulses, with > 3 second capillary refill time there is a need to continue CPR maneuver, ventilatory assistance and use of inotropic and vasoactive agents along with isotonic intravenous fluids are recommended.

Neurological Management

Neurological complications occur in 35 to 40% of young

victims. One should measure ICP and calculate CPP. Progressive use of measures, including positioning (head elevation to 30 degree), hyperventilation and mechanical ventilation, osmotic and loop diuretics is indicated to maintain an ICP less than 20 mm Hg and CPP greater than 50 mmHg. Seizures must be controlled with routine use of anticonvulsants. The use of phenobarbitone should be avoided as it interferes with the white blood cell functions and increases the risk of secondary infections. Similarly, the steroids have not proved beneficial to decrease the elevated ICP. Hypovolemia can be corrected by use of colloid–crystalloid solutions.

Pulmonary Management

Pulmonary management is started with the supply of the oxygen at a rate to maintain $SaO_2 > 90\%$, as most of the children are at risk to develop pulmonary edema. For the severely involved, positive end expiratory pressure is helpful in increasing lung volumes, decreasing oxygen requirements, and improving systemic oxygenation. The use of mechanical ventilation will be beneficial in patients with severe pulmonary edema, respiratory failure, aspiration pneumonia, profound anoxic injury (GCS <8). When conventional ventilation fails to respond to hypoxemia, extracorporeal membrane oxygenation (ECMO) and high frequency jet ventilation become the treatment of choice.

Routine use of antibiotics should be avoided until there is a history of drowning in polluted water. Prophylactic use of corticosteroids for treatment of pulmonary complications has no justified support from the studies.

Cardiovascular Management

Because of global hypoxia there is a stage of persistent cardiac dysfunction. To overcome these, inotropic agents like dopamine and dobutamine along with intravenous colloids facilitate the end-organ perfusion.

Rewarming Measures

Rewarming measures are definitely helpful in preventing mortality because of drowning related hypothermia. In the triage area itself removal of the wet clothes along with rewarming with radiant warmers, warmed blankets in a warm room will be useful to combat hypothermia.

In several hypothermia (core temperature < 30°C) these measures may be ineffective. In such circumstances administration of prewarmed intravenous fluids (37°–40°C) and heated humidified inspired oxygen (40°–44°C) is recommended. The gastric bladder and peritoneal lavage with warm fluid may be effective to raise the core temperature. The recent modalities include hemodialysis, extracorporeal rewarming and cardiopulmonary bypass.

In the process of rewarming the child, the phenomenon of "afterdrop" of the temperature is seen as a result of cooler blood from the extremities to the relatively warmer central core.

As a rule, all submersed children should be critically reviewed and monitored for at least 6–24 hours. For any sign of respiratory distress and early features of shock.

PROGNOSIS

The over all mortality rates are 40–60% for near drowning in children and adolescents. Accurate neurological prognostication is important because of anoxic–ischemic injury, but certain individual predictors[23,24,26] are of practical help. These includes:

1. Cold water (< 5°C) submersion has better prognosis.
2. Submersion of < 5 minutes generally has good prognosis.
3. Resuscitation time <10 minutes.
4. Age > 3 years.
5. PRISM score < 25 and hemodynamic stability at admission.
6. Glasgow coma score (GCS) of > 5.
7. Neurological responsive at the scene of drowning.
8. Improvement in GCS in first 24 hours.
9. Children with normal brain stem functions 24 hours after drowning.
10. ABG analysis of pH >7.1

Bad prognosis is likely in the following situations:

1. Hyperglycemia (glucose > 300 mg/dl).
2. Warm water submersion.
3. Pupils that remained dilated after 6 hours admission and seizures continuing 24 hours after admission predicted a poor out come.

It is wise to consider each child on his individual merits and demerits. Neurological examination and progression during the first 24–72 hours is still the key for prognostication although some new laboratory methods have been investigated in prognosis of drowning. They include CT scans, brain stem auditory evoked response, EEG, somatosensory evoked responses, cerebral spinal fluid creatine kinase and lactate assays, measurement of cerebral blood flow, position emission tomography, and magnetic resonance spectroscopy.

PREVENTION

Preventing the child from drowning and near drowning should be the message to parents, swimming pool owners and health care providers. They should be educated and made aware of the various aspects of submersion, use of effective barriers in the form of pool safety measures, rescue and CPR training to staff is advocated. Parents are advised not to leave small children alone near the pooled water especially during the rainy seasons and picnics.

Majority of the children can be saved if effective preventive strategies is taken on the spot in the community.

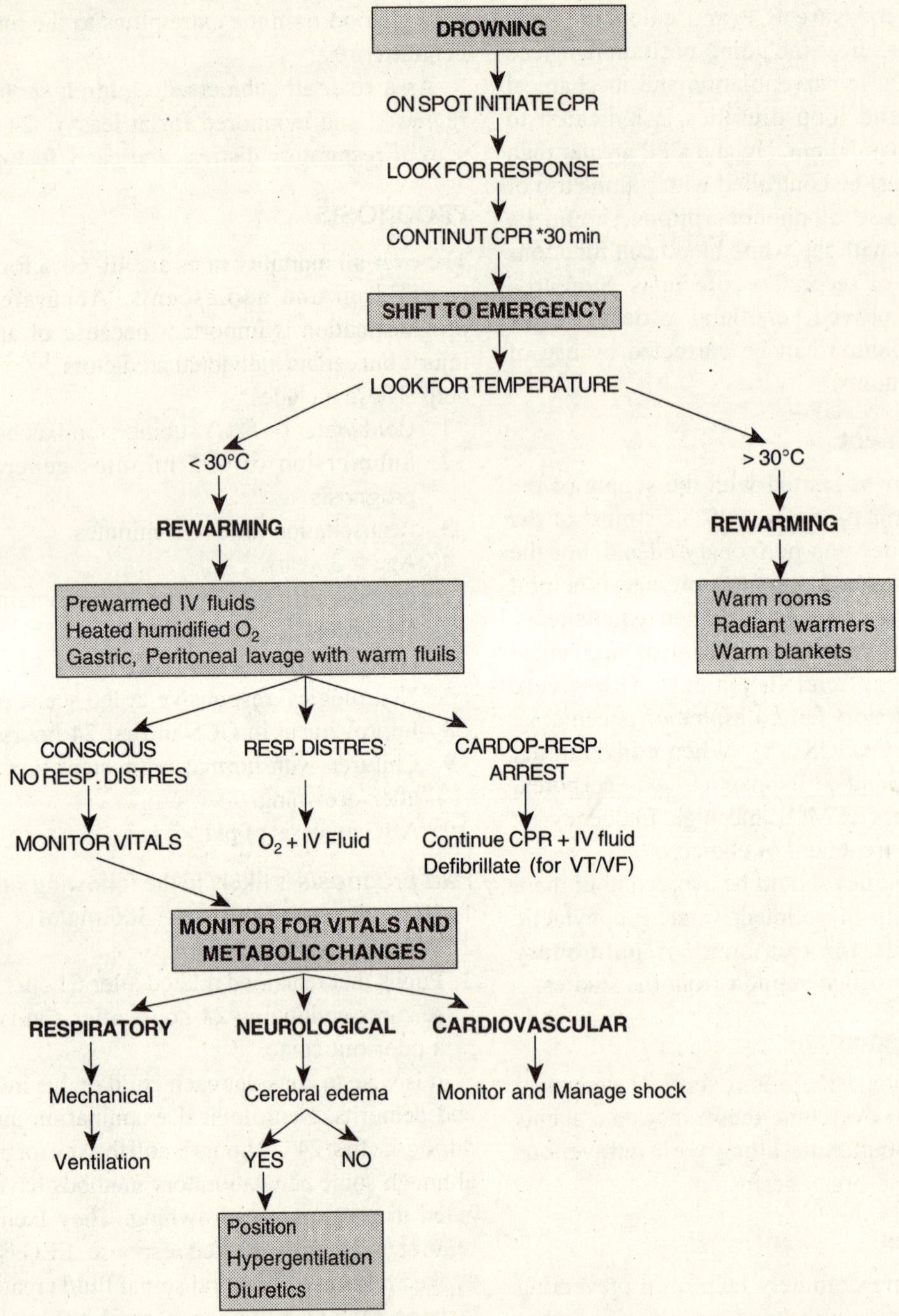

Fig. 64.5: Management protocol

REFERENCES

1. Ortowski JP. Drowning, near–drowning and ice–water drowning. *JAMA* 1988;280:390-391.
2. Peterson B. Morbidity of childhood near drowning. *Pediatrics* 1977;59:364-376.
3. Spyker DA. Submersion injury. Epidemiology, prevention and Management. *Pediatr Clin North Am* 1985;32:113.
4. Beyda DH. Pathophysiology of near drowning and treatment of the child with a submersion incident. *Crit Care Nurs Clin North Am* 1991;3:273-280.
5. Levin DL: Near–drowning. *Crit Care Med* 1980;8:590-595.
6. Modell JH. Treatment of near drowning: Is there a role for HYPER therapy? *Crit Care Med* 1986;14: 593-594.
7. Pearn JH. Pathophysiology of drowning *Med J Aust* 1985; 142:586-588.
8. Biggart MJ, Bohn DJ. Effect of hypothermia and cardiac arrest on outcome of near–drowning accidents in children. *J Pediatr* 1990;117:179-183.
9. Bohn DJ, Biggar WD, Smith CR, et al. Influence of hypothermia, barbiturate therapy, and intracranial pressure monitoring on morbidity and mortality after near–drowning. *Crit Care Med* 1986;14:529-533.
10. Jacobsen JB, Nielsen H, Andersen PK. Resuscitation from drowning in cold water. *N Engl J Med* 1981; 305:580-581.
11. Rogers MC. Near–drowning: Cold water on a hot topic? *J Pediatr* 1985;106:603-604.

12. Skarpnes S. Near drowning in children, Axone 1989;11:20-21.
13. Beyda DH. prehospital care of the child with a submersion incident. *Crit Care Nurs Clin North Am* 1991;3:281-285.
14. Bierens JJLM, van der Velde EA, van Berkel M. Submersion cases in the Netherlands. *Ann Emerg Med* 1989;18:366-373.
15. Hopkins RS, Writer JV, Mortensen BK, et al. Childhood injury mortality in Ohio, 1979 to 1986, Setting priorities for prevention. *Am J Dis Child* 1990;144:79-82.
16. Nagel FO, Kibel SM, Beatty DW. Childhood near drowning: Factors associated with poor outcome. *S Afr Med J* 1990;78: 422-425.
17. Nichter MA, Everett PB. Childhood near drowning: Is cardiopulmonary resuscitation always indicated: *Crit Care Med* 1989;17:993-995.
18. O'Rourke PP. Outcome of children who are apneic and pulse less in the emergency room. *Crit Care Med* 1986;14:466-468.
19. Jacobsen WK, Mason LJ, Briggs BA. Correlation of spontaneous respiration and neuralgic damage in near drowning. *Crit Care Med* 1983;11:487-489.
20. Taylor MJ, Houston BD, Lowry NJ. Recovery of auditory brain–stem responses after a severe hypoxic ischemic insult. *Med Intelligence* 1983;309:1169-1170.
21. Effmann EL, Merten DF, Kirks Dr. Adult respiratory distress syndrome in children. *Radiology* 1985;157:69-74.
22. Bonis S, Heaton JFG, Fajardo EM. Extracorporeal membrane oxygenation in pediatric patients. Fourth Annual children's hospital National Medical Centre ECMO Symposium, February 1988.
23. Beyda DH. Childhood submersion injuries. *J Emerg Nurs* 1998; 24:140.
24. Bratton SL. Jardine DS. Morray JP. Serial neurologic examinations after near drowning and outcome. *Arch Pediatr Adolesc Med* 1994;148:167.
25. Zuckerman GB, Gregory PM, Santos–Damiani SM. Predictors of death and Neurologic Impairment in pediatric submersion injuries. *Arch Pediatr Adolesc Med* 1998;152:134.
26. Orlowski JP. Drowning, near drowning and ice water submersions. *Pediatr Clin North Am* 1987;34:75.

Section XIII

Accidental Poisoning

Shabina Ahmed

65 Accidental Poisoning: General Management

INTRODUCTION

Accidental ingestion of poisons and household products is a potential source of morbidity and mortality in children of all ages, especially in the developing world.

National Poison Information Centre (India) reported 30.6% of poisoning in children. The most vulnerable age include children in the 1-6 year range, with males outnumbering females.[1]

Although the accidental mode was the most common (79.7%), intentional attempts were also noticed (20.2%) in the under-12 to 16 year and over 16-18 year age groups. In the majority of cases, the route was oral (96.8%) followed by dermal exposure (3.2%) comprising bites and stings. These conform to other studies in the world.

Studies carried out in Singapore[2] showed 54% of admissions to be boys. Majority of them were toddlers between the ages of 1-3 year, 30% of them being accidental poisoning. This ingestion may be accidental, non-accidental or iatrogenic. A study from Saudi Arabia shows that 1.7% of all child admissions are for accidental poisoning.[3]

FACTORS INFLUENCING POISONING IN CHILDREN BETWEEN 0-5 YEARS

Biological Variables

Childhood poisoning is correlated with biological variables, such as skeletal anomalies, language disorders, number of recent infections and complications of pregnancy.

Social Factors

Social factors, such as parental educational level, socio-economic status, overcrowding, place of stay, carelessness of caretakers and keeping medicines in non-labeled, non-pilferproof containers, have a strong correlation.

Packaging

Attractive packaging, colors and fruity tastes entice children.[4]

HOME POISONING

This is a major concern for parents specially those who have young children. According to the US Center for Disease Control and Prevention, about 90% of poisoning occurs at home, and common household items are often the cause. As many as 2000 poison control centers in the US reported approximately 2.2 million poison exposures; of these, 52.7% occurred among children younger than 6 years.[3]

US poison control centers handle an average of one poison exposure every 75 seconds. The most common poison exposures for children are ingestion of household products, such as cosmetics, personal care products, cleaning substances, pain relievers, foreign bodies and plants. Vitamins are another potential source of accidental poisoning in very young children.

PATTERN OF POISONING IN CHILDREN

Poisoning agents involved are drugs in three-fifth of cases, while the rest comprise household products. Ingested items may be classified as drugs (prescribed and OTC), household items and plants.

A. Drugs

- Analgesics and anti-inflammatory
- Antiemetics, laxatives
- Vitamins, appetizers
- Contraceptives
- Antibiotics
- Antileptics
- Cardiovascular
- Unidentified, thyroid hormones, benzodiazepines.

B. Household Products and Plants

- Chorine bleach
- Petroleum products–kerosene
- Pesticides–organophosphorus compounds Disinfectants
- Washing lotions
- Super glue
- Lubricating lotions

- Paint thinner
- Unidentified
- Plants, like *dhatura*.

Methanol is one of the most commonly used organic solvents and is accessible to the public in a variety of products. Ethylene glycol is a solvent found in products ranging from antifreeze fluid and de-icing solutions to carpet and fabric cleansers.[1,5]

PRINCIPLES OF MANAGEMENT

1. History and physical examination
2. Appropriate supportive care
3. Prevention of further absorption
4. Enhancing product elimination
5. Treatment with specific antidote
6. Discharge from the emergency department.

Physician in contact must anticipate cardiovascular and pulmonary instability and rapid changes in central nervous system functioning. Definitive emergency care is completed only after the provision of a developmentally-oriented preventive strategy.[6]

The importance of local poison centres must be emphasized.

History

A. History is taken from different family members to help identify type and dose of ingestion. One must keep in mind that 50% of histories are incorrect as to the substance, quantity and even actual exposure. It is easier for a doctor to treat the patient if the poison and the circumstances of the poisoning are known.

B. Attempts are to be made to try to get the bottle, tablet strip, any container of the ingestant and remnants of the ingestant to ascertain evidence.

C. The following points are noted in the history sheet:
   1. Name of the drug.
   2. Concentration of the drug.
   3. Weight of the child.
   4. Amount of intake should be ascertained to help in decision-making; as in case of ingestion of diluted bleach, hospitalisation is not recommend if the amount is < 100 ml. In cases of concentrated bleach, any amount of intake demands hospitalisation.[7]
   5. Any medication that is being used by family members.
   6. Probable toxicity of the agent.
   7. The time lapsed between time of ingestion and reporting to doctor.
   8. Complaints of the patient.
   9. Any pertinent medical history, such as age, and history of drug allergy. One may not be able to tell if the patient is poisoned just by examining the patient, because many poisons cause symptoms and signs that are similar to those of other diseases or even injury.

Physical Examination

A thorough physical examination helps in the differential diagnosis and treatment planning.

I. General Appearance

The general appearance gives us a lot of information. One has to look for pallor or flushed face, or whether apprehensive or relaxed, or anxious. Flushed face may be due to atropinics and anti-histaminics, alcohol, carbon monoxide, cyanide and boric acid. Absence of sweating and a dry skin is seen with anticholinergics.

One must look for bleeding especially from the nasal and oral orifices, seen in late cases of acetominophen and brodifacoum poisoning (rodenticide).[8] Signs of corrosives and blistering must be looked for. Inside of the mouth should be looked for burns and stains, pieces of tablet, coloured tongue, pieces of leaves and berries.

Cyanosis is seen with aniline dyes, nitrites, benzamine, phenecetin nitrobenzene, phenazopyridine; all of these lead to methaemaglobinemia.

Jaundice is a presentation in poisoning by naphthalene, acetaminophen, carbon tetrachloride plants (mushrooms, fava beans) and heavy metals (iron, phosphorus and organic).

Clothing should be observed for signs of corrosion, and how the person is clad.

Odour gives interesting leads. A sweet smelling odour may be due to acetone, methyl or propyl alcohol, phenol and salicylates. Bitter almond smell is noted in cyanide poisoning, garlic smell is observed in heavy metal poisoning (arsenic, phosphorus and thallium) and oil of winter green with methyl salicylates.

II. Measurement of Vital Signs

Baseline measurements of Pulse, Blood pressure, Temperature, Respiration are taken.

Pulse

The rate, rhythm and volume are noted. Bradycardia indicates ingestion of digoxin, narcotics, organophosphorus compounds, petroleum products, cyanide, clonidine and beta-blockers. Tachycardia is noted in conditions where there is ingestion of alcohol, amphetamine, sympathomimetics, substances containing atropine, tricyclic antidepressants, theophylline, salicylates and cocaine.

Respiration

It is important to note the rate of breathing, depth and the rhythm. If the respiration is slow and depressed probable cause may be due to alcohol, barbiturates at their late stage, narcotics, clonidine, sedatives and hypnotics.

Tachypnoea is noted with early barbiturate poisoning, methanol, salicylates, carbon monoxide and amphetamines

Blood Pressure

While measuring blood pressure the age of the child is to be taken under consideration. If the blood pressure is found to be low, poisoning by antihypertensives, narcotics, barbiturates, iron, theophylline, antidepressants, phenothiazines, carbon monoxide, cyanide methaemoglobinemia (nitrites, nitrates) should be suspected while high blood pressure leads us to suspected agents like phenylpropanolamine (ingredient of cough syrup), antihistaminics, atropines and amphetamines.

Temperature

A record of the basal temperature gives us clue to the ingested agent. If there is hypothermia, substances under suspicion should be ethanol, barbiturates, sedatives, hypnotics, narcotics, phenothiazines, tricyclic antidepressants, clonidine and carbon monoxide.

Hyperpyrexia is noted in conditions where there is an intake of atropine, quinine, salicylates, amphetamines, phenothiazines, tricyclic antidepressants, theophylline and cocaine.

III. Level of Consciousness and Neuromuscular Status

Alteration of level of consciousness is noted after ingestion of narcotic depressants, sedatives, hypnotics, alcohol, ethylene glycol, carbon monoxide, organophosphates and insecticides.

If patient is restless, delirious and present with psychotic behaviour,suspected agents are plant toxins, like *dhatura* poisoning, alcohol, drugs of abuse like marijuana, cocaine, heroin, methaqualone, sympathomimetics, anticholinergics, steroids and after ingestion of heavy metal.

Depending upon the dose of ingestant, some children may present with hallucinations, myoclonic jerks, agitation and convulsions, particularly in cases of tricyclic antidepressants (amytryptiline, imipramine), camphor, alcohol, organophosphates, plant toxins (water hemlock) and theophylline and carbamezapine).

Gait abnormality, particularly ataxias are noted with alcohol, barbiturates, sedatives, hypnotics (especially benzodiazepines) carbon monoxide and if patient is having hypoglycaemia.

Patient may present with paralysis following ingestion of botulin, heavy metals and plants (poison hemlock).

Antiparkinsonism rigidity, involuntary movement with oculogyric crisis are noted in phenothiazine poisoning.[9]

IV. Examination of the Pupil

Pupillary size gives us clue to the ingestant. *Miosis* may be due to narcotics, organophosphates, plants (muscarinic type of mushroom) ethanol, barbiturates, phenobarbital and clonidine. *Mydriasis* is noted in anticholinergics, amphetamine, cocaine, methanol, LSD (lysergic acid diethylamine), carbamazepine and theophylline.

Further presence of nystagmus guides us to phenytoin, sedatives, hypnotics barbiturates and ethanol ingestion.

It is worthwhile to remember that exposure to poison will not result in poisoning if a poisonous dose does not get into the body. Some may seem well because it is too soon for the effect at the time of examination. Acetaminophen, sustained-release or delayed-release formulations, transdermal patches may have slower onset. Hence, as we are examining, documentation must be made with date and time.

Drug Classification and Symptomatology

Toxicology is the part of the core knowledge necessary for practice of emergency medicine. Classification may be done into drug class, toxidromes[10] or toxic syndromes. Specific symptom complex helps us to identify the drug.

Specific Symptom Complex

SLUDGE – Cholinergics, pilocarpine, OP's
- **S**alivation
- **L**acrimation
- **U**rination
- **D**efecation
- **G**astric **E**mptying

SLUMPED ↑ Anion Gap Metabolic Acidosis
- S – Salicylates
- L – Lactic acidosis
- U – Uremia
- M – Methanol
- P – Paraldehyde
- E – Ethylene glycol
- D – Diabetic ketoacidosis

Laboratory Investigations

Urine, blood and vomitus are sent for toxicology to identify the poison. Drug screening is for medico legal consideration. However, a negative toxicological screen does not rule out a toxic ingestion.

Laboratory studies are dictated by patient's condition.

Blood works should include, besides the routine, estimations of bicarbonates, pH, anion gap, electrolytes, renal function tests, liver function tests, coagulation profile and urine analysis for hemoglobinuria.

ECG is a must in rhythm disorders.

Plain radiograph of chest may be useful in case of ingestion of metals like iron and lead.

Legal Obligations

- Must treat as deemed medically appropriate.
- Contact poison centre for assistance, where available.

- Restrain if necessary; protect the patient from himself.
- Refer all suicide attempts/gestures for psychiatric evaluation.

Principles of Therapy for Drug Poisoning

The ultimate objective for drug poisoning is to prevent the poison from exerting its effects. Principles of therapy include the following:

1. Prevention of drug absorption.
2. Prevention of drug distribution.
3. Alteration of drug metabolism.
4. Enhancement of excretion.
5. Specific pharmacological interventions
   Treatment of shock.
   Treatment of convulsions.

1. Prevention of Drug Absorption

Decontamination of Skin

This is achieved by immediately washing the affected part of the body under cold or lukewarm water for 10 minutes and by removing all contaminated clothes. Speed is important.

Decontamination of Eyes

Wash chemical out of the eyes at once with plenty of cool, clean water before washing the skin. Even a delay of few seconds can make the injury worse. Eyes must be washed for 15-20 minutes, timed with a watch where possible. Do not allow the patient to rub the eyes.

If the pain is severe the patient may need an injection of morphine.

Burns in the eyes will show a yellow stain with drops of fluorescein, in which case infection must be prevented with 1% chloramphenicol eye ointment.

2. Prevention of Drug Distribution

Induction of vomiting to remove poison from stomach by:

a. Mechanical stimulation
b. Ipecac syrup
c. Apomorphine
d. Warm salt water gastric lavage.

Mechanical stimulation is mainly done by tickling the throat.

Ipecac syrup contains emetine that induces emesis by a combined local irritant effect on the gastrointestinal tract and central medullarly stimulation of the chemoreceptor trigger zone. Ipecac syrup should not be given to children under 6 months. Dosage for children 6 months to 12 yrs age is 10 ml, followed by a glass of tepid water or fruit juice. The patient generally vomits 15-20 minutes after the dose, failing which a second dose is administered after 30 minutes; not more than two doses are given.

Vomiting is not induced in a patient when:

- Substance not likely to cause poisoning.
- Four hours has lapsed since the patient has taken the poison.
- If the patient is unconscious or sleepy.
- The ingestant is a chemical that is likely to burn.
- The patient has swallowed a petroleum distillate like kerosene, petrol, gasoline.
- The patient has swallowed a substance that is likely to cause fits. The act of vomiting may start a fit.

Gastric lavage should be considered only in a patient with ingestion of life-threatening agent and the procedure should be undertaken within 60 minutes of ingestion.

Unless a patient is intubated, gastric lavage is contraindicated if airway protective reflexes are lost. It is also contraindicated if a hydrocarbon with high aspiration potential or corrosive substances have been ingested.[11]

Decontamination of the Gastrointestinal Tract (GIT).

This is achieved by binding of the poison by specific chelating agents like EDTA, absorption of poison onto activated charcoal and whole bowel irrigation.

Activated Charcoal

The efficacy of activated charcoal is dependent on the absorption of poison, and is considered if a potentially toxic amount of poison (which is known to be absorbed to charcoal) ingested within the past one hour. Unless a patient has an intact or protected airway, the administration of charcoal is contraindicated.[12]

Activated charcoal is most effective in adsorbing poison with a molecular weight in the range of 100-1000 Daltons. It is a superior alternative to Ipecac and lavage. Single dose of activated charcoal as the sole therapy should suffice as adequate therapy.

The minor risks associated with activated charcoal administration must be weighed against the negligible benefits of therapy when there is a significant time lapse to administration. Furthermore, the physical nature of activated charcoal creates compliance problem in infants.

Initial Dose

Initial dose in Children is 1 g/kg/BW PO, or via nasogastric tube, with a 70% sorbitol solution. The dose should be used in a well mixed slurry ,diluted at least in the proportion of 1 : 4. It is better tolerated if cold.[13]

American Academy of Clinical Toxicology, European Association of Poisons Centres and Clinical Toxicologists (AACT/EAPCCT) has recently challenged GIT decontamination.

Position statement on GI decontamination:

1. This is based on the issues that half-life of gastric emptying is estimated to be 12-20 minutes depending on

Table 65.1: Toxic syndromes

Syndrome	*Manifestations*	*Examples*
Anticholinergic	**Parasympatholytic:** Dry skin/mucous membranes, thirst/dysphagia, blurred vision (near objects), fixed dilated pupils, Tachycardia, hypertension, flushing, scarlatiniform rash, hyperthermia, abdominal distention, urinary urgency and retention. **Central:** Lethargy, confusion, delirium, hallucinations, delusions, ataxia, respiratory failure, cardiovascular collapse, extrapyramidal movements.	Belladonna alkaloids, atropine, scopolamine Synthetic: Glycopyrrolate Other: Antithistamines, tricyclic antidepressants.
Anticholinesterase	**Muscarinic:** Sweating, constricted pupils, lacrimation, wheezing, cramps, vomiting, diarrhea, tenesmus, bradycardia, hypotension, blurred vision, urinary incontinence, excessive salivation. **Nicotinic:** Striated muscle: fasciculations, cramps, weakness, twitching, paralysis, respiratory compromise, cyanosis, cardiac arrest. **Sympathetic ganglia**: Tachycardia, hypertension. **Central:** Anxiety, restlessness, ataxia, convulsions, insomnia, coma, absent reflexes, Cheyne-Stokes breathing, respiratory/circulatory depression.	Organophosphates, carbamate insecticides.
Cholinergic	See anticholinesterases: Nicotinic and Muscarinic.	Acetylcholine, betel nut, bethanecol, muscarine, pilocarpine.
Extrapyramidal	**Parkinsonian:** Dysphonia, dysphagia, oculogyric crisis, rigidity, tremor, torticollis, opisthotonos, shrieking, trismus.	Chlorpromazine, haloperidol, perphenazine, promazine, thioridazine, trifluoperazine.
Hemoglobinopathy	Disorientation, headache, coma, dyspnea, cyanosis, cutaneous bullae, gastroenteritis	Carboxyhemoglobin (carbon monoxide), methemoglobin, sulfhemoglobin.
Metal fume fever	Chills, fever, nausea, vomiting, muscularpain, throat dryness, headache, fatigue, weakness, leukocytosis, respiratory distress.	Fumes of oxides: brass, cadmium, copper, iron, magnesium, mercury, nickel, titanium, tungsten and zinc.
Narcotic	CNS depression, pinpoint pupils, slowed respirations, hypotension. Response to naloxone: pupils may dilate and excitement may predominate.	Codeine diphenoxylate (Lomotil), fentanyl, heroin, morphine, opium, oxycodone.
Sympathomimetic	CNS excitation, convulsions, hypertension, tachycardia.	Aminophylline, amphetamines, caffeine, cocaine, dopamine, ephedrine, epinephrine, fenfluramine, levarterenol, methylphenidate, Pemoline, phencyclidine.
Narcotic withdrawal	Diarrhea, mydriasis, goose bumps, hypertension, tachycardia, insomnia, lacrimation, muscle cramps, restlessness, yawning, hallucinosis.	Cessation of alcohol, barbiturates, benzodiazepines, chloral hydrate, glutethimide, meprobamate, methaqualone, narcotics, opioids, paraldehyde.

From Done AK. Poisoning: A systematic approach for the emergency department physician. In: Tintihalli et al. (ed) *Emergency Medicine* London: McGraw-Hill 1985

the character of the gastric contents. Gastric emptying is clearly complete within 60-100 minutes.

2. Most pediatric poisoning exposures are classified as nontoxic and do not necessitate any intervention.[14]

Cathartics

Osmotic agents like magnesium citrate can be used to induce catharsis in children who are more than 1 year old. The administration of a cathartic alone has no role in the management of the poisoned patient. Its use should be limited to a single dose in order to minimize adverse effects.[15]

Whole Bowel Irrigation (WBI)

WBI should not be used routinely in the management of the poisoned patient. It may be considered for potentially toxic ingestion of sustained release or enteric-coated drugs.

WBI is contraindicated in obstruction, perforations, ileus, unprotected airway and haemodynamic instability.[16]

3. Alteration of Drug Metabolism

This is achieved by:

1. The enhancement of metabolism for drugs inactivated by metabolism e.g. use of thiosulfate in cyanide poisoning.
2. Inhibition of metabolism of drugs that produce toxic metabolites e.g. use of ethanol for methanol poisoning.

4. Enhancement of Elimination/Excretion

A. pH alteration

Urinary alkalinization is helpful in elimination of weak acids such as salicylates, barbiturates and methotrexate. Serum alkalinization is important in preventing tricyclic antidepressant toxicity.

I.V. bolus of 1-2 mEq/kg of $NaHCO_3$ is recommended, followed by continuous infusion of 5% Dextrose in water (D5W) with 132 mEq /kg of $NaHCO_3$ (3 ampoules of $NaHCO_3$ added to D5W to make one liter), and maintenance is done to achieve the goal of a urinary pH of 7 to 8 or blood pH >7.45.

B. Hemodialysis is potentially beneficial for life-threatening ingestion of low molecular weight substances.

5. Specific Pharmacology Intervention

- Receptor competition e.g. nalorphine in morphine overdose.
- By direct chemical antagonism e.g. acid-base.
- Blockade of receptors that cause the toxic effects e.g. atropine in organophosphorus poisoning.
- Restoration of normal function using on agent exerting a direct opposite effect e.g. barbiturate in CNS stimulant poisoning.

Antidotes

Acetylcysteine is given orally in Paracetamol and carbon tetrachloride poisoning in home situation; however, injectable acetylcysteine should be given only in a setting where resuscitation can be given if the patient has an allergic reaction. Dose: Oral, loading dose of 140 mg/kg followed by 70 mg/kg 4 hourly for 17 doses, over a period of 72 hours.

Ascorbic acid is given orally to treat methemoglobinemia from sodium chlorate poisoning.

Atropine intravenously is given in poisoning from carbamate or organophosphorus pesticides. Dose is 0.05 mg/kg every 15 minutes, until full atropinisation is reached. Continuous or intermittent IV infusion of 0.05 mg/kg/hr is maintenance therapy. Respiratory support services should be readily available.

Calcium gluconate solution is injected subcutaneously when hydrofluoric acid has been in contact with skin.

Deferoxamine (desferrioxamine) injection in iron poisoning. Dose: Acute iron poisoning: IM, 1-2 g every 3-12 hours to a maximum of 6 g every 24 hours (500 mg is dissolved in 5 ml water for injection).

Dicobalt edetate, 1.5% solution: for injection in cyanide poisoning is the preferred treatment. Dose: IV injection, 300 mg over 1 minute, followed immediately by 50 mL 50% dextrose, using the same needle.

Dimercaprol (BAL): for arsenic poisoning and lead poisoning. Dose: Deep IM injection, 400-800 mg in divided doses on the first day; 200-400 mg in divided doses on the second and third days; 100-200 mg in divided doses on subsequent days.

4-Dimethylaminophenol (4-DMAP), 5% solution: for injection in cyanide poisoning.

DMPS (dimercaptopropanesulfonate): for arsenic poisoning and lead poisoning.

Ethanol for methanol poisoning, beginning with loading dose of 0.6 g/kg, followed by an ethanol infusion of 66 mg/kg/hr.

Fomepizole is the standard treatment for ethylene glycol. Loading IV dose is 15 mg/kg, maintained on 10 mg/kg every 12 hours for four doses. It is continued till ethylene glycol levels are reduced below 20 mg/dl.

Hydroxocobalamin, 40% solution: for intravenous injection in cyanide poisoning.

Methylthioninium (methylene blue): for cyanosis caused by methaemoglobin in dapsone poisoning.

Naloxone in opioid poisoning, administered IV preferably, with an initial dose of 0.01 mg/kg, followed by a dose of 0.1 mg/kg.

Obidoxime chloride: for poisoning from organophosphorus pesticides. Dose: IV, initially 250 mg (3-5 mg/kg). If a satisfactory response is obtained after the first injection, a further dose should be given once or twice at intervals of 2 hours.

Oxygen, 100%, in carbon monoxide poisoning.

Penicillamine for lead poisoning. Adult dose: Chelation therapy: Oral, usually 0.5-1.5 g daily in 4 divided doses. Paediatric dose: Oral, 20-40 mg/kg daily in 4 divided doses.

Phytomenadione (vitamin K) injection in warfarin poisoning.

Pralidoxime mesilate (P-2-S) or pralidoxime chloride (PAM2): for poisoning from organophosphorus pesticides.

Pyridoxine: for intravenous injection in isoniazid poisoning.

Sodium nitrite, 3% solution, for intravenous injection in cyanide poisoning.

Sodium thiosulfate, 25% solution, for intravenous injection in cyanide poisoning; also given by mouth, with sodium hydrogen carbonate (sodium bicarbonate), to treat methemoglobinemia from sodium chlorate poisoning.

Succimer (DMSA, short for dimercaptosuccinic acid) for arsenic poisoning and lead poisoning.

Supportive Care

It should be determined at the earliest whether the poisoning is life-threatening and already compromising the vital functions.[17]

It is not uncommon for these patients to be in coma, in which case the basic principles of airway maintenance, breathing and circulation are to be upheld. A reliable venous access should be established, and blood samples taken for laboratory estimations. Hypoglycemia must be excluded in any comatose patient and corrected if present. Hypoventilation is avoided by ensuring a clear airway with removal of dentures and secretions. If needed, insertion of an airway or intubation, with mechanical ventilation, are recommended.

Hypotension is most common, due either to volume deletion or venous pooling, frequently necessitating monitoring of central venous pressure and adequate fluid replacement. Renal perfusion has to be maintained, confirmed by an adequate urinary output.

Hypothermia may be associated in comatose patients and a rectal temperature reading should be routinely done.

Cardiac irregularities occur in acute poisoning with various substances; attention has to be given to correction of any aggravating factors such as acidosis, hypoxia and electrolyte and fluid imbalances. Specific treatment has to be instituted.

Convulsions are not uncommon, and should undergo therapy if protracted or recurring frequently. Diazepam (IV) slowly should be administered.

DISCHARGE

Patient must be medically fit prior to discharge. It is important that a formal assessment of suicide and self-harm risk be made. Counseling forms an important aspect on discharge, especially for those with a history of substance abuse. Caregivers must be educated for accidental ingestion. Industries prone to work-related toxic exposures should be made legally responsible to provide adequate safety measures.

REFERENCES

1. Gupta SK, Peshin SS, Srivastava A, Kaleekal T. A study of childhood poisoning at National Poison Information Centre, All India Institute of Medical Science, New Delhi. *J Occup Health* 2003;45;191-196.
2. Lue E. Review of accidental poisoning. *Asian Toxical* 2003;6: 112-120.
3. Ike Izoura, Adebowole Adeoye. *Ann Saudi Med* 2001;21: 13-15.
4. Paritsis N, Pallis D, Deligeorgis D, Doxiadis S, Phylactou C, Vlachonicolis I. An epidemiological study of the factors influencing poisoning in children aged 0-5 years. *Pediatric Perinat Epedemiol* 1994; 8:79-89.
5. Liehelt E.L, De Angelis CD. Evolving trends and treatment advances in pediatric poisoning *JAMA* 1999;282:1113-1115.
6. Bryant S, Singer J. Management of toxic exposure in children. *Emerg Med Clin North Am* 2003;21:101-119.
7. Cardona J, Boussemart T, Berthier M, Oriot D Accidental bleach ingestion in children: results of a survey in 11 anti-poison centres. Proposals for management. *Pediatrics* 1983;48:705-709.
8. Travis SF, Warfield W, Greenbaum BH, Molokisher M, Siegel JE. Spontaneous hemorrhage associated with accidental brodifacoum poisoning in a child. *J Pediatr* 1993;122:982-984.
9. Gupte S, Kaushal RK. Pediatric accidental poisoning. In: Gupte S (ed) *The short textbook of Pediatrics* 10th edn New Delhi: Jaypee Brothers 2004;539-548.
10. Done AK. Poisoning: A systematic approach for the emergency department physician. In: Tintihalli et al (ed) *Emergency Medicine*. London: McGraw-Hill 1985.
11. American Academy of Clinical Toxicology, European Association of Poisons Centers and Clinical Toxicologists. Position statement on gastrointestinal decontamination: Gastric lavage. *J Toxicol Clin. Toxicol* 1997;35:711-719.
12. Bond GR. The role of activated charcoal and gastric emptying in gastrointestinal decontamination: a state-of-the-art review. *Ann Emerg Med.* 2002;39:273-286.
13. Gupte S. Reflections on pediatric accidental poisoning in India. *Asian Toxical:* 2003;6:141-146.
14. American Academy of Clinical Toxicology, European Association of Poisons Centers and Clinical Toxicologists. Position Statement on Gastrointestinal Decontamination: Ipecac. *J Toxicol Clin Toxicol* 1997;35:699-709.
15. American Academy of Clinical Toxicology, European Association of Poisons Centers and Clinical Toxicologists. Position statement on cathartics *J Toxicol Clin Toxicol* 1997;35:743-752.
16. American Academy of Clinical Toxicology, European Association of Poisons Centers and Clinical Toxicologists. Position statement on gastrointestinal decontamination: Whole bowel irrigation. *J Toxicol Clin Toxicol* 1997;35:753-762.
17. Krenzelok EP, Dunmire SM. Acute poisoning review. Resolving the gastric decontamination controversy. *Postgrad Med* 1992;91:179-186.

Anju Kapoor

66 Salicylate Poisoning/Toxicity

INTRODUCTION

Salicylate can be found in hundreds of over-the-counter (OTC) medications. Out of these, Aspirin is the most common salicylate in regular use and so both accidental and suicidal ingestions are common with this drug. The usual pediatric dose of aspirin for fever control and analgesia is 65 mg/kg/day in divided doses every 4-6 hours to a maximum daily dose of 3.6 g.

Toxicity is anticipated when the intake exceeds 150 mg/kg.

Salicylates are also present in oil of wintergreen, salicylate powder and ointment, which when applied on the broken skin may lead to toxicity. Toddlers are most vulnerable to acute salicylate poisoning. The real extent of salicylate poisoning is mostly underestimated due to underreporting or the cases may remain unrecognized.

PHARMACOKINETICS

A salicylate is well absorbed orally. It is a weak acid. So, in acidic environment of the stomach, it precipitates and forms pharmaco-bezoars,[1] a large mass of the drug that further delays the absorption. In toxic ingestion, peak salicylate levels may not be seen until 24 hours after ingestion.

In the serum, salicylate is largely bound to serum albumin and free salicylate is toxicologically active. It is metabolized in the liver mainly by conjugation with glycine and partly by hydroxylation. When large amount is ingested these pathways get saturated prolonging its half-life and elimination. The metabolites are excreted via the kidney. Urine pH influences the renal excretion of salicylate. Being a weak acid it remains in unionized form in the urine that gets reabsorbed in renal tubules. Alkaline urine enhances salicylate excretion by decreasing the reabsorption.

Ingested dose of salicylate and estimated severity[2] are given in Table 66.1.

Table 66.1: Dose ingested and expected severity of poisoning

Dose	Severity
<150 mg/Kg	No toxicity expected
150-300 mg/Kg	Mild–moderate toxicity expected
300-500 mg/Kg	Severe toxicity expected
>500 mg/Kg	Potentially fatal

PATHOPHYSIOLOGY

First response to toxic salicylate ingestion is direct stimulation of respiratory center leading to hyperventilation and respiratory alkalosis, though this phase is less prominent in younger children. To compensate this alkalosis, there is bicarbonate excretion in urine associated with loss of sodium, potassium and water in the urine, which ultimately leads to acidosis, dehydration and hypokalemia.

Later on, due to inhibition of Krebs cycle, uncoupling of oxidative phosphorylation, gluconeogenesis, increase lipid metabolism and inhibition of amino acid metabolism patient develops metabolic acidosis. Thus metabolic acidosis is due to endogenous production of acids rather than salicylate itself. There are three phases of salicylate toxicity (Table 66.2).[3]

Table 66.2: Three phases of salicylate toxicity

Phase 1:	Respiratory alkalosis with alkauria
Phase 2:	Respiratory alkalosis with paradoxical aciduria.
Phase 3:	Metabolic acidosis.

CLINICAL FEATURES

Clinical manifestations depend on the age of the patient, dose ingested and duration of exposure to the drug.[4]

General Appearance

Patient is diaphoretic and hyperventilating. Temperature is increased. Hyperthermia is a sign of severe toxicity.

Central Nervous System

Salicylates are neurotoxic. Patients may develop tinnitus, nausea, ataxia, vomiting, vertigo, headache, mental confusion, convulsion and coma. These changes are known as "salicylate Jag" and are secondary to hyperthermia and altered glucose metabolism.

Cardiovascular System

Tachycardia.

Gastrointestinal System

Direct stimulation of gastric mucosa leads to nausea, vomiting, hematemesis and malena. High doses lead to pylorospasm and decreased gut motility.

Hepatic System

Reye's syndrome is a salicylate induced hepatic disease in children.

Respiratory System

Initially patient will be having tachypnea and hyperpnea followed by kussumaul's breathing secondary to metabolic acidosis. Non-cardiac pulmonary edema may develop.

Fluid and Electrolyte Disturbances

Dehydration, hypokalemia, and hypo/hypernatremia are common. Decreased ionic calcium leading to tetany may develop due to respiratory alkalosis. Hypo/hyperglycemia can also develop. Dehydration upto 5-10% may develop secondary to vomiting and insensible fluid loss (hyperpnea and hyperthermia). Hypokalemia may occur due to primary respiratory alkalosis.

Coagulation System

Patient might develop hemorrhagic tendency due to hypoprothrombinemia, decreased platelet function, production of thromboxane-A2 and inhibition of vitamin K dependent synthesis of clotting factors.

Musculoskeletal System

Rhabdomyolysis can occur due to dissipation of heat.

LABORATORY DIAGNOSIS

Bedside Diagnosis

Qualitative determination of presence of salicylic acid in the urine can be done by ferric chloride test, combining 1 ml of patient's urine to few drops of ferric chloride solution. If salicylate is present, solution will turn to brown-purple color. This test will be positive even after ingestion of one tablet of aspirin. So if this qualitative is positive, quantitative assessment in the serum should be done to confirm the toxicity.

Blood Salicylate Level

This is the best indicator of the severity of intoxication. It should be done 6 hours after ingestion and then repeated every 4-6 hourly for serial estimation and response to therapy (Table 66.3).

Table 66.3: Blood salicylate level and severity of poisoning

Blood salicylate level (at 6 hours)	*Severity of poisoning*
<50 mg/dl	Mild
50-100 mg/dl	Moderate
>100 mg/dl	Severe

After single dose ingestion plasma salicylate levels should be plotted on the done nomogram to monitor the severity of ingestion. Nomogram cannot be used for chronic toxicity.[5]

Other supportive investigations are:

- Complete blood count.
- Prothrombin time- increased.
- Serum electrolyte- hypokalemia, Hyponatremia or hypernatremia.
- Anion gap-high anion gap acidosis is found in salicylate intoxication.
- Blood glucose level-hypoglycemia.
- Arterial blood gas analysis-initially there will be alkalosis followed by acidosis or there can be mixed acid-base abnormality.
- Liver and renal function tests.
- Urine pH- should be monitored closely during treatment.

DIFFERENTIAL DIAGNOSIS

Other conditions with high anion gap are:

- Diabetic ketoacidosis.
- Lactic acidosis.
- Renal failure.
- Methanol toxicity.
- Ethylene glycol toxicity.

TREATMENT OF SALICYLATE POISONING

The basic principles of any poisoning management also apply to the salicylate poisoning. These are the support of airway, breathing, circulation, decontamination and finally the definitive care.

Decontamination

Vomiting is induced with syrup of ipecac if the patient is cooperative, alert and presented within 30 minutes of ingestion.

Thorough gastric lavage is to be done if vomiting is not successful or if patient is obtunded. At the end of the lavage activated charcoal in the dose of 1 gram/kg should be left in the stomach, which will bind the unabsorbed salicylate. Repeat doses of 0.5 gram/kg of activated charcoal can be given every 2-4 hourly to enhance the elimination if toxicity is severe. Intravenous metoclopramide will help the patient in tolerating the activated charcoal. With the initial doses of charcoal cathartic, 4 ml/kg of magnesium citrate can be used in children.

If high serum level is sustained, elimination can be enhanced by whole bowel irrigation with polyethylene glycol/ electrolyte lavage solution at a rate of 500 ml/hour. The end point of irrigation is reached when rectal effluent is clear and serum level of salicylate is decreasing. Formation of drug bezoars poses problem in the elimination.

Fluid and Electrolyte Management

Managing fluid, electrolyte and metabolic disturbances forms the mainstay of treatment because no specific antidote is available. Correction of dehydration is done by crystalloids to replace the fluid loss that can be upto 200 ml/kg.

Acidosis is corrected by giving 1-2 mEq/kg of soda bicarbonate every 1-2 hour. It is also useful in making the urine alkaline (alkaline diuresis).

Though blood sugar level may be normal, a push of dextrose is essential because of presence of neuroglycopenia.

Hypocalcemic tetany is treated with 10% calcium gluconate.

Seizure can be controlled with diazepam (1–.3 mg/kg/ dose) or phenobarbitone (5 mg/kg). Vitamin K should be injected if PT is prolonged.

If patient develops respiratory failure, positive pressure ventilation should be started.

Urinary Alkalization

Alkaline diuresis is very effective in increasing the clearance of salicylate in the urine. By increasing the urine pH to 7.5–8, elimination is increased by 10 folds. Enough fluid should be given to maintain adequate urine output (2-5 ml/kg/hour). Serum electrolyte, ABG and urine pH should be monitored closely during therapy. Blood pH is maintained at 7.45–7.55. Patient should be catheterized. If patient develops hypokalemia, urine cannot be alkalinized effectively because of the compensatory mechanism that leads to increase K^+ absorption in distal tubules associated with H^+ ion excretion, producing aciduria. So adequate potassium should be administered to prevent hypokalemia (maintain serum K^+ >3.5 mEq/L). Acetazolamide should not be used because it will exaggerate the acidosis.

Hemodialysis

It is preferred over hemoperfusion and peritoneal dialysis. It provides the double benefits of removal of salicylate and maintenance of fluid and electrolyte balance.

Indication of hemodialysis are[6]

- Renal failure.
- Persistent CNS manifestations.
- Congestive cardiac failure.
- Non-cardiogenic pulmonary edema.
- Progressive deterioration of the patient's condition.
- Severe acid/base and electrolyte imbalance despite appropriate treatment.
- Hemorrhagic condition.
- Blood salicylate level >100 mg/dl.
- Severe salicylate induced symptoms (e.g. seizure, hyperthermia).

PROGNOSIS

Poor prognostic factors are:

- Prolonged convulsion.
- Severe respiratory acidosis.
- Hypoglycemia.
- Life threatening bleed.

REFERENCES

1. Rodgers GC Jr, Matyunas NJ. Poisonings: Drugs, chemicals and plants. In: Behrman RE, Kliegman RM, Jenson HB (eds) *Nelson Textbook of Pediatrics,* 16th edn. Philadelphia: WB Saunders 2000;2160-2171.
2. Temple AR. Acute and chronic effects of aspirin toxicity and their treatment. *Arch Intern Med* 1981;141:364-369.
3. Waseem M, Gernsheimer JR. Toxicity, salicylate. *Medicine Journal*, July 24 2002, Volume 3, Number 7:http://author.emedicine.com/PED/topic2031.htm.
4. Singh UK, Layland FC, Suman S, Prasad R. Salicylate poisoning. In: *Poisoning in Children.* New Delhi: Jaypee Brothers 2000;106-111.
5. Done AK. Salicylate intoxication: Significance of measurements of salicylates in blood in cases of acute ingestion. *Pediatrics* 1960:26:800.
6. Goldfrank LR, Bresnitz EA, Hartnett L. Salicylates. In: Goldfrank LR (ed) *Goldfrank's Toxicologic Emergencies.* Norwalk: Appleton and Lange 1990: 261-270.

Bhadresh Vyas

67 Paracetamol Poisoning/Toxicity

INTRODUCTION

Paracetamol was first introduced into clinical medicine towards the end of the last century but it attracted little attention and was soon forgotten. There was a resurgence of interest in paracetamol when it was found to be the major metabolite of acetanilide and phenacetin and it was commonly assumed to be responsible for the therapeutic effects of both of these drugs.[1] Paracetamol has since been used increasingly as a substitute for other analgesics such as aspirin and phenacetin.

TOXICITY

Toxicity stems from its saturable metabolism. In therapeutic doses, 60-90% is conjugated to inactive sulphates and glucuronides (e.g. mercaptopuric acid).[2] Saturation of the sulphation path diverts an increased fraction to the reactive/toxic species NABQI (N-acetyl-benzoquinoneimine) whose detoxification rapidly depletes hepatic glutathione stores.

PATHOPHYSIOLOGY

The major target organ in paracetamol poisoning is the liver and the primary lesion is acute centrilobular hepatic necrosis. In children the single acute threshold dose for severe liver damage (which has been arbitrarily defined as elevation of the plasma alanine or aspartate aminotransferase activity above 1000 U/l) is 140 mg/kg and the lethal dose 200 mg/dl[3] but there is marked individual variation in susceptibility. Children under the age of about 6 years appear to be much more resistant than adults, but in any event they rarely ingest enough paracetamol to cause liver damage.[4] Only a small proportion of unselected adult patients who take an overdose of paracetamol are at risk of severe liver damage.

Without specific antidotal therapy, less than 10% would suffer severe liver damage but 1 to 2% will develop fulminant hepatic failure and this is often fatal. One to 2% of patients develop acute renal failure requiring dialysis.[5]

When the patient is first seen, the severity of intoxication with paracetamol cannot usually be determined on clinical grounds alone, as there are no specific symptoms or signs. Consciousness is not depressed unless other drugs have also been taken or there is a very high plasma paracetamol concentration of the order of 6.62 mmol/l (1000 mg/l) with a metabolic acidosis.[6] Nausea and vomiting usually develop within a few hours of ingestion of a hepatotoxic dose of paracetamol and at this stage liver function tests may be normal or only slightly deranged. From about 24 hrs after ingestion (Table 67.1) there may be hepatic tenderness and abdominal pain due to swelling of the liver capsule. Unless hepatic failure develops, there is usually rapid improvement after the third day with eventual complete recovery.

The maximum abnormality of liver function tests is usually delayed until the third day. The characteristic changes include dramatic elevation of the plasma alanine and aspartate transaminase activity from normal values of less than 40 to as much as 10,000 or even 20,000 U/l with mild to moderate increases in the plasma bilirubin concentration and prothrombin time ratio. The sudden dramatic increase in the activity

Table 67.1: Stages (phases) of paracetamol poisoning

Stage	*Time of ingestion (hrs)*	*Clinical feautres*	*Lab investigations*
Stage 1	First 24 hrs	Vomiting, malaise, pallor, diaphoresis	Normal liver enzymes
Stage 2	24-48 hrs	Upper abdominal pain/tenderness	Moderately elevated liver enzymes
Stage 3	48-96 hrs	Symptoms of renal failure Fulminant hepatic failure	Max elevation of liver enzymes (SGPT > 1000), Increased PT, elevated LFT's, centrilobular necrosis
Stage 4	> 96 hrs-2 wks	Stage of resolution	Resolution of LFTs, Normal histopathology of liver

of plasma transaminases is presumably caused by their release from a large mass of necrotic hepatocytes, and the prolongation of the prothrombin time reflects acute impairment of synthesis of the vitamin K-dependent clotting factors. There is little or no increase in the plasma alkaline phosphatase activity unless liver damage is severe or the patient is a chronic alcoholic. Liver biopsies show extensive centrilobular hepatic necrosis with little inflammatory reaction.

In patients who recover, liver function tests become normal within 1 to 3 weeks and follow-up histological examination reveals regeneration, repair and eventually a return to normal appearances. Serial measurements of the prothrombin time probably give the best guide to prognosis.[7] Oliguric renal failure may become apparent within 24 to 48 hr after the overdose of paracetamol, and in this setting it is almost always associated with back pain, microscopic haematuria and proteinuria.

Fulminant hepatic failure may develop in severely poisoned patients from the third to the sixth day. It is characterized by deepening jaundice, encephalopathy, increased intracranial pressure, grossly disordered haemostasis with disseminated intravascular coagulation and hemorrhage,

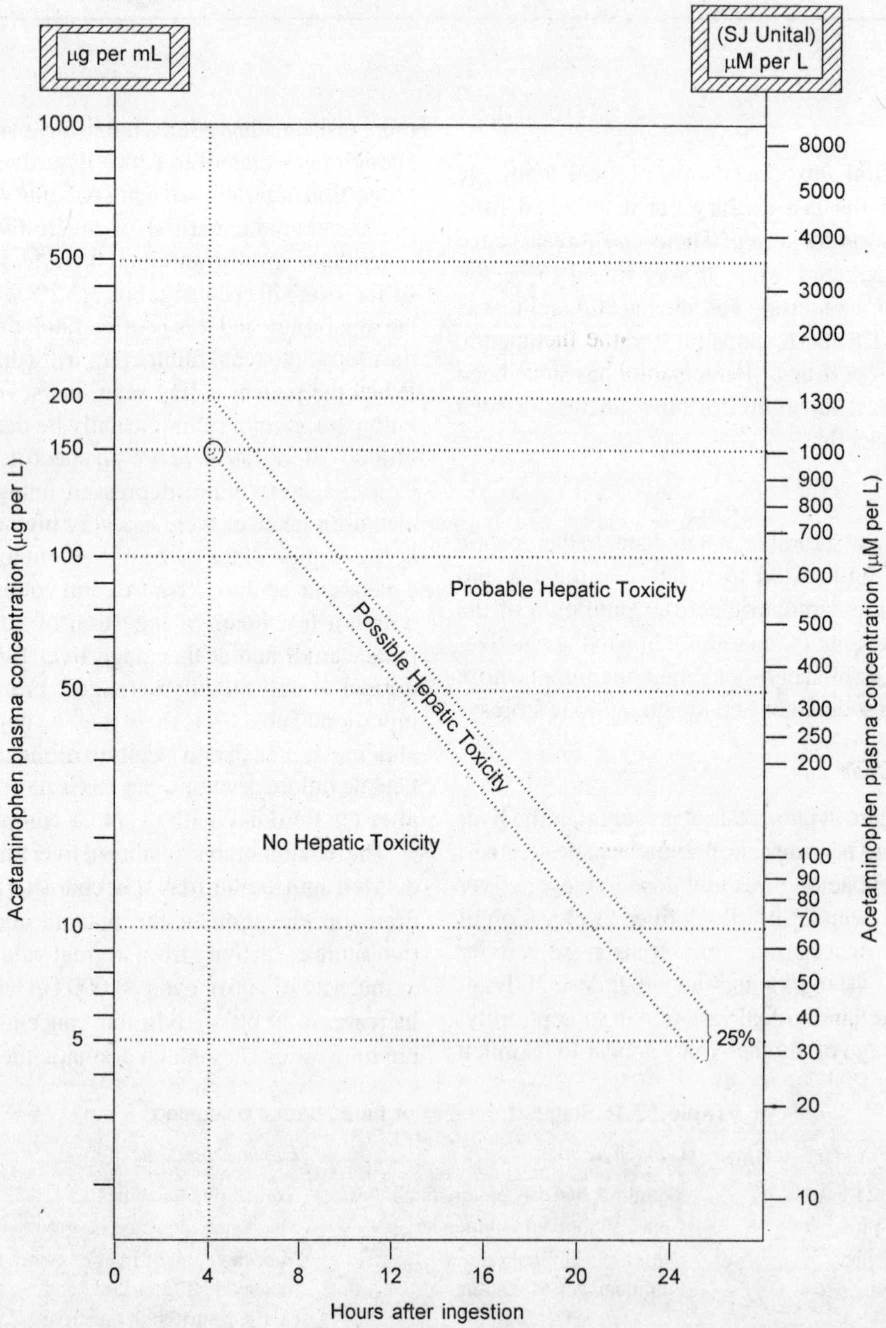

Fig. 67.1: Rumack-Matthew Nomogram for acetaminophen poisoning

hyperventilation, acidosis, hypoglycaemia and renal failure. The prognosis is very poor.

Patients should be considered high risk if they are taking enzyme-inducing drugs (e.g. carbamazepine, phenobarbital, phenytoin, rifampicin, and alcohol) or they are malnourished (e.g. in anorexia, in alcoholism, or those who are HIV-positive).

MANAGEMENT

Gastric aspiration with lavage, or induction of emesis with syrup of ipecac (ipecacuanha), is usually carried out in patients who are thought to have taken at least 100 mg paracetamol/kg within the previous 1-2 hours. Activated charcoal has also been recommended (avoid if planning to give N-acetyl cysteine). Unfortunately, paracetamol is normally absorbed very rapidly, and it is uncommon to obtain a good return of tablet material. Provided that more than 4 hours have elapsed since the time of ingestion, a blood sample should be taken for the emergency estimation of the plasma paracetamol concentration and for baseline measurements of liver function tests, prothrombin time ratio, and plasma urea, creatinine and electrolytes.

Acute oliguric renal failure during the first 24 to 48 hours may be accompanied by severe back and loin pain. Fluid and electrolyte balance must be monitored carefully and dialysis is often necessary. The plasma urea and creatinine concentrations may rise slowly but progressively over a period of many days before renal function recovers.

The onset of acute, possibly fatal, hepatic failure is indicated by a rapid rise of the prothrombin time to a ratio of more than 5.0, gross elevation of the plasma alanine aminotransferase (ALAT) and appearance of mild jaundice within 36 to 48 hours. In such circumstances vitamin K_1 is usually given parenterally and, depending on the results of serial clotting screens, the intravenous administration of clotting factor concentrate or fresh frozen plasma may be necessary to keep the prothrombin time ratio within a safe range. Careful attention must be given to fluid, electrolyte and acid-base balance, and it is important to avoid fluid overload as this will aggravate cerebral edema. Neomycin (1 g every 4 to 6 hours) and lactulose administration by nasogastric tube should be considered, as in the case of acute liver failure from other causes. Hypoglycaemia may occur at any time and should be prevented by intravenous administration of fluids containing glucose. Established acute liver failure should be treated by conventional methods.

N-Acetyl Cysteine Therapy

The maintenance of hepatic glutathione (GSH) concentrations by administration of N-acetylcysteine and promotion of elimination of paracetamol metabolites was first suggested as a treatment for paracetamol poisoning by Prescott and Matthew. Treatment with intravenous N-acetylcysteine is indicated in patients who present within 24 hours of taking paracetamol in overdose and who have plasma paracetamol concentrations above the treatment line. Dosing regimen for oral NAC is in the form of a 5% solution in a soft drink or juice starting with a loading dose of 140 mg/kg followed by a maintenance dose of 70 mg/kg every 4 hours for a total of 17 doses. The intravenous regimen consists of administration of 150 mg/kg made up in 200 ml of 5% dextrose over 15 min, followed by 50 mg/kg in 500 ml of 5% dextrose over 4 hours and 100 mg/kg in 1 liter of 5% dextrose over 16 hours. This regimen effectively prevents liver damage, renal failure and death if started within 8 hr of paracetamol ingestion but efficacy falls off rapidly after this time. If an allergic-like reaction occurs, stop the infusion, give I.V. chlorpheniramine and hydrocortisone, then continue N-acetylcysteine at a lower rate. In substantial overdose (> 125 mg/kg), start acetylcysteine without waiting for plasma levels–the antidote may be discontinued if the levels are found to be in the non-toxic range.

The Rumack-Matthew Nomogram

This estimates the potential for hepatotoxicity from paracetamol poisoning. Patients with concentrations above a line joining plots on a semi-logarithmic graph of 1.32 mmol/l (200 mg/l) at 4 hr and 0.20 mmol/l (30 mg/l) at 15 hr after ingestion (called the "treatment line") have about a 60% chance of developing severe liver damage as defined by elevation of the plasma transaminase activity above 1000 U/l. In patients with concentrations above a parallel line joining 2 mmol/l (300 mg/l) at 4 hours and 0.33 mmol/l (50 mg/l) at 15 hours the probability rises to 90%. In addition, it is also used to indicate the need for N-acetylcysteine (NAC) therapy. It is based on a semi-logarithmic plot of plasma paracetamol levels *vs* time. A plasma level that falls above the treatment line indicates a potential for toxicity and requires NAC treatment. Anyone who uses this nomogram, however, has to understand that the nomogram is applicable only when the poisoning involves a single acute ingestion and that the blood level is drawn between 4 and 16 hours. Blood levels drawn before 4 hours may not represent peak levels since absorption is not complete and those drawn after 16 hours may not be predictive of potential hepatotoxicity or the need for NAC therapy.

Role of Methionine

Treatment with oral methionine is indicated in patients who present within 15 hours of taking paracetamol in overdose and who have plasma paracetamol concentrations above the treatment line. Oral methionine is very safe. Yet, the plasma paracetamol concentration should always be measured. As far as possible, treatment should never be delayed while awaiting the laboratory result. The dose of methionine is 2.5 g (10 × 250 mg tablets) orally repeated 4 hourly to a total dose of 10 g over 12 hours.

Oral Versus Intravenous Route of Antidotes

The obvious advantage of the oral route is that most of the absorbed dose passes directly to the sites of action in the liver. Oral therapy is also simpler and can be given by nonmedical healthcare workers in developing countries. On the other hand, the efficacy of oral treatment may be compromised if absorption is delayed or incomplete as a result of nausea and vomiting. A substantial proportion of severely poisoned patients develop nausea and vomiting within a few hours and it is in these circumstances that effective reliable treatment is most needed. Oral therapy must be given by nasogastric tube in unconscious patients. This route is inappropriate in patients who have been given emetics or oral activated charcoal.

Role of Liver Transplantation

Liver transplantation may have an important role in patients presenting with adverse prognostic factors such as:

- Hepatic failure.
- Prothrombin time > 100 sec.
- Serum creatinine > 3.3 mg/dl.
- ph < 7.3.

REFERENCES

1. Smilkstein MJ, Knapp GL, Kulig KW. Efficacy of oral N-acetylcysteine in the treatment of acetaminophen overdose. Analysis of the national multicenter study (1976 to 1985). *N Engl J Med* 1988;319:1557-1562.
2. Anker AL, Smilkstein MJ. Acetaminophen: Concepts and controversies. *Emerg Med Clin North Am* 1994; 12:335-349.
3. Rpdgers GC Jr, Matyunas NJ. Poisonings: Drugs, chemicals and plants. In: Behrman RE, Kliegman RM, Jenson HB (eds) *Nelson Textbook of Pediatrics*, 16th edn. Philadelphia: WB Saunders 2000;2160-2171.
4. Bond GR, Hite LK. Population-based incidence and outcome of acetaminophen poisoning by type of ingestion. *Acad Emerg Med* 1999;6:1115-1120.
5. Mitchel, Dawson AH, Henry DA, McEwen J. Adverse reactions to N-acetylcysteine during treatment for paracetamol poisoning. *Med J Aust* 1989;50:329-331.
6. Gee P, Ardagh M. Pediatric exploratory ingestions of paracetamol. *N Z Med J* 1998;22;111(1066):186-188.
7. Gray Jones AL. Mechanism of action and value of N-acetylcysteine in the treatment of early and late acetaminophen poisoning: A critical review. *J Toxicol Clin Toxicol* 1998; 36: 277-285.
8. GrayJones AL. Mechanism of action and value of N-acetylcysteine in the treatment of early and late acetaminophen poisoning: A critical review. *J Toxicol Clin Toxicol* 1998;36: 277-285.
9. Harrison PM, Keays R, Bray GP. Improved outcome of paracetamol-induced fulminant hepatic failure by late administration of acetylcysteine. *Lancet* 1990; 335(8705):1572-1573.

Suraj Gupte and Utpal Kant Singh

68 Kerosene Oil Poisoning

Kerosene oil poisoning is by and large the most frequently encountered accidental poisoning amongs toddlers, especially in the lower strata of society that depends on kerosene as a household fuel. In north India, it accounts for about 50% of infants and children brought to hospital for accidental poisoning.[1]

Kerosene certainly is the most common amongs the hydrocarbons (that include a large number of chemical substances found in commercial products) causing accidental poisoning in children.[2]

ETIOPATHOGENESIS

Kerosene oil is a hydrocarbon. Its main danger is aspiration that causes pneumonia (aspiration pneumonuia) with all its complications such as collapse, pneumothorax and pleural effusion.[2-6] As small an aspiration as 1 ml is good enough to cause significant injury. Respiratory problem(s) may be compounded by absorption from the gastrointestinal tract subsequent to a heavy ingestion accompanied by aspiration.

Respiratory involvement has its complications elsewhere as well. Hypoxia may involve the CNS, leading to hypoxic encephalopathy.

Kerosene oil has a fatal dose of 30 ml. With ingestion of this dose or more, fatality occurs within 24 hours.

CLINICAL MANIFESTATIONS

Local manifestations include irritation of oral mucosa. In addition, there may be manifestations secondary to irritation of gastric and esophageal mucosa, say nausea, vomiting and abdominal discomfort.

Clinical features of kerosene poisoning depend on the amount of ingestion. With moderate ingestion, manifestations include choking, cough, respiratory distress and pyrexia. If left unattended, symptoms are likely to show worsening over the next 24 hours. Improvement begins over next 3–8 days. Respiratory symptoms may progress to respiratory failure.

Fever is common. It may persist over the next 7–10 days.

Addition manifestations are headache, euphoria, lethargy/drowsiness, restlessness, muscle twitching, seizures, coma, abdominal pain, cardiac arrhythmias, hemolytic anemia and even acute renal failure. Hepatotoxicity and bone marrow suppression has also been on record.

Physical examination of chest reveals predominantly crepitations with some rhonchi.

INVESTIGATIONS

Chest Radiograph

The only specific investigation required is a chest X-ray. The changes are bilateral, involving multiple lobes. However, the tendency is to involve the lower lobes relatively more widely. Three stages are seen:

Early: Within 6 hours of kerosene ingestion, perihilar midlung field region shows fine punctate mottled densities.

Later: The above-mentioned densities coalesce to form ill-defined densities.

Late: The ill-defined densities further coalesce to form large areas of consolidation within intervening areas of atelectasis.

Finally, such complications as pneumatoceles progressing to pneumothorax, pneumomediastinum, subcutaneous emphysema and pleural effusion may develop in a small proportion of cases.

Interestingly, radiologic changes may be present even without clinical evidence of pneumonia. On the other hand, radiologic findings may be missing during the first 8–12 hours after aspiration.[2] Notably, a chest radiograph may continue to remain abnormal long after clinical recovery. It cannot, therefore, be depended upon as a guide for continuing treatment.

Leukocytosis

It is a common finding but does not always mean presence of a bacterial infection.

MANAGEMENT

Supportive measures are the lifeline of treatment of kerosene oil poisoning.[1-3, 8] The child needs to be observed for at least 24 hours in the hospital for any signs of kerosene toxicity. It is quite unlikely that such a toxicity shall manifest after this period.

Emptying of Stomach

Induction of vomiting (emesis) and/or gastric lavage is contraindicated, except:

- When ingestion of kerosene is massive (> one ml/kg).
- When the child is in coma.
- When kerosene is mixed with pesticides, heavy metals and other toxic substances.

In no case should it ever be done without intubation. Else, there is a risk of aspiration.

Monitoring

The child should be monitored for heart rate, respiratory rate, sensorium and chest signs.

In case of tachypnea, oxygen should be administered.

Antibiotics

Bacterial pneumonia is uncommon. Therefore, prophylactic antibiotic therapy is not recommended.[2] Table 68.1 lists important features of kerosene pneumonia.

Table 68.1: Salient features of kerosene pneumonia

- Causes of aspiration, leading to aspiration pneumonia, in kerosene oil ingestion are:
  - Coughing and gagging at the time of ingestion.
  - Vomiting following ingestion.
  - Absorption of kerosene from the GI tract or skin and its inhalation usually does not cause pneumonia unless it is a very heavy ingestion.
- Chest X-ray usually fails to reveal evidence of pneumonia initially.
- During the course of treatment, chest X-ray cannot be depended upon for guiding therapy as radiologic findings persists for a much longer time.

Nevertheless, risk-benefit should be assessed. Antibiotic shield may well be in order in a child with very little respiratory reserve. Antibiotics are, therefore, indicated in a limited situations (Table 68.2).

Table 68.2: Indications of antibiotic therapy in kerosene ingestion

Definitive

- A proved or highly suspected bacterial pneumonia or some other superimposed or pre-existing infection

Prophylactic

- A very restricted respiratory reserve
- Gross malnutrition
- Immunocompromised state

Steroids

Steroid therapy may be useful only when administered concurrently with the time of aspiration.[7] Else, steroids may prove rather harmful, often enhancing the risk of superadded secondary infection.

Bronchodilators

Bronchodilarors may be of some help in the presence of significant bronchospasm.

Oxygen Therapy

Oxygen therapy is necessary in a subject who develops hypoxemia.

Standard ventilation and extracorporeal membrane oxygenation (ECMO) may need to be resorted to in critical respiratory failure.[6]

REFERENCES

1. Gupte S, Kaushal RK. Pediatric poisoning. In: Gupte S (ed): *The Short Textbook of Pediatrics*, 10th edn. New Delhi: Jaypee Brothers 2004;520-530.
2. Rodgers GC, Jr, Matyunas NJ. Poisonings: Drugs, chemicals and plants. In: Brahman RE, Kliegman RM, Jenson HB (eds): *Nelson Textbook of Pediatrics,* 17th edn, Philadelphia: Saunders 2004;2362-2375.
3. Anas N, Nanasonthi V, Ginsburg CM. Criteria for hospitalizing children who have ingested products containing hydrocarbons. *JAMA* 1981;246:840-843.
4. Mickiewicz M, Gomez HF. Hydrocarbon toxicity: General review and management guidelines. *Air Med* 2001;20:8-11.
5. Meredith TJ, Ruprah M, Liddle A, et al. Diagnosis and treatment of acute poisoning with volatile substances. *Hum Toxicol* 1989;8:277-286.
6. Chyka PA. Benefits of extracorporeal membrane oxygenation for hydrocarbon pneumonitis. *J Toicol Clin Toxicol* 1996;34: 357-363.
7. Colombo JL. Aspiration syndromes. In: Behrman RE, Kliegfman RM, Jenson HB (eds) *Nelson Textbook of Pediatrics,* 17th edn. Philadelphia: Saunders 2004;1427-1428.
8. Singh UK, Leyland FC, Suman S, Prasad R. *Poisoning in Children,* 2nd edn. New Delhi: Jaypee Brothers 2001.

Suraj Gupte and Abdul Quazi

69 DDT Poisoning

INTRODUCTION

Dichloro-diphenyl-trichloroethane (DDT), now called "chlorophenothane", a white powder with slight odor, continues to be extensively employed as a spray against malaria and other diseases.[1,2] Though an environmental pollutant, in view of its benefits in the health program, it continues to be used.

DDT poisoning is frequent in children. It can occur through inhalation, ingestion and skin absorption. Like other hydrocarbons, it can readily cross the placenta and excrete in breastmilk, thereby causing injury to the growing baby in intrauterine life and the breastfed infant.[3] It may even cause reproductive impairment.

CLINICAL MANIFESTATIONS

DDT, when accidentally ingested, may cause serious neurologic manifestations, including confusion, tremors, incoordination, seizures and paresthesia involving lips, tongue and face.[1]

GI manifestations include salivation, vomiting, diarrhoea and abdominal pain.

Inhalation poisoning causes irritation of throat, nose and eyes, cough, blurred vision and pulmonary edema.

MANAGEMENT

Since so far there is no specific antidote for DDT poisoning, treatment is purely supportive and symptomatic, including control of seizures. For controlling convulsions, diazepam, 0.1-0.3 mg/kg (IV) is good enough.

Decontamination of skin and gastrointestinal tract is needed. Skin should be washed with soap and water and contaminated clothes removed.

While doing GI contamination, such substances as castor oil, fats and oils and milk should never be left in the stomach. They are likely to further enhance the absorption of DDT, a chlorinated hydrocarbon, rather than reduce it.[2]

REFERENCES

1. Gupte S, Kaushal RK. Pediatric accidental poisoning. In: Gupte S (ed) *The Short Textbook of Pediatrics*, 10th edn. New Delhi: Jaypee Brothers 2004;539-548.
2. Rumack BH, Dart RC. In: Hay WW, Hayward AR, Levin MJ, Sondheimer JM. *Current Pediatric Therapy*, 6th edn. New York: McGraw-Hill 2003;336-361.
3. Landrigan PJ, Forman JA. Chemical pollutants. In: Behrman RE, Kliegman RM, Jenson HB (eds) *Nelson Textbook of Pediatrics*, 17th edn. Philadelphia: Saunders 2004;2353-2355.

Suraj Gupte and Mohinder Pal

70 Corrosive Poisoning

INTRODUCTION

Corrosives are strong acids and strong alkalis which are highly active irritant that damage the skin and the mucous membrane. They produce not only local inflammation but also actual ulceration of the tissues. They are often responsible for accidental poisoning in children.[1] Occasionally, corrosives have been employed for disfiguring children as well (just as in adults) with malacious intent ("vitriolage").[2,3]

The group includes detergents, washing soda, unslaked lime, toilet and drain cleaners. Both acid (mineral acids: sulphuric acid, organic acids: carbolic acid, oxalic acid, vegetable acid: hydrocyanic acid, salicylic acid) and alkali (caustic potash and soda, ammonium hydroxide).[1] Corrosives are available.

PATHOPHYSIOLOGY

Acidic corrosives produce coagulation necrosis that cause superficial damage. They are capable of causing gastric perforation and peritonitis.

Alkalis cause a deep and penetrating liquefaction necrosis, frequently ending up with severe consequences. They tend to cause grave damage to the esophagus which may be accompanied by mediastinitis and pneumonia.

CLINICAL MANIFESTATIONS

Onset of manifestations is immediate, the breath often smelling strongly in case of carbolic acid ingestion.

These include burning sensation in mouth, throat, esophagus, stomach and abdomen followed by intense thirst, vomiting (often blood stained), drooling and dysphasia. The child specifically refuses taking liquids. Oral burns involving lips, mouth or both may be present.

In severe ingestion, there may be respiratory distress with stridor secondary to glottic edema, esophageal perforation with mediastinitis, gastric perforation with peritonitis.[2,3]

Remote manifestations include respiratory distress, shock and nephrotoxicity presenting as oliguria and anuria. Contracted pupils (miosis) together with cold and clammy skin may be confused with opioid poisoning.

INVESTIGATIONS

In case of carbolic acid, its presence in urine can be demonstrated by Benedit's test or ferric chloride test.

It is useful to do upper GIT endoscopy with fiberoptic endoscope within 24-48 hours and a repeat after 2-3 weeks to ascertain extent of injury caused by the corrosive.

X-rays of chest and soft tissues of neck are indicated in case of respiratory distress.

Baseline barium swallow and upper GI contrast series following treatment and before discharge are needed for documenting esophageal stricture/pyloric stenosis in the long run.

MANAGEMENT[1,2]

A detailed history helps to know about the magnitude of the poison consumed. Neither emesis nor gastric lavage should be done (except in case of carbolic acid i.e. phenol ingestion in which case a soft stomach tube can be passed with care). Likewise, neutralization of offending agent too is best avoided.

- If skin or eyes are exposed to the corrosive, these should be thoroughly irrigated with water followed by local application of castor oil in case of acid ingestion.
- For eye injury, an ophthalmologist should be immediately involved.
- A small amount of water or milk may be given to the child to wash away any residual corrosive from oral mucosa. Then, acid should be diluted by 500 ml of water or milk followed by a demulscent drink (melted butter, white of egg, milk olive oil, barley water).

- H_2 blockers or antacids should be given for 6-8 weeks to prevent secondary injury from reflux of gastric acid into esophagus.
- Steroid therapy to prevent development of esophageal stricture doesn't seem to be well founded.
- Self-dilatation of esophagus is achieved by allowing the child to take liquids as soon as he is in a position to swallow. It cuts down chances of stricture formation. Alternative or additional methods aimed at this are being evaluated.
- Antibiotic shield is recommended in presence of an infection or for prevention of secondary infection.

PROGNOSIS

Acid ingestion causes high mortality. Incidence of late complications from tissue necrosis too is high. If repeated barium studies show stricture, dilatation is initiated with bougies. In case of poor response, esophageal replacement is indicated.[4]

REFERENCES

1. Parikh CK. *Parikh's Textbook of Medical Jurisprudence, Forensic Medicine and Toxicology,* 6th edn. New Delhi: CBS 1999.
2. Dart RC, Rumack BH. Poisoning. In: Hay WW Jr, Hayward AR, Levin MJ, Sondheimer JM (eds) *Current Pediatric Diagnosis and Treatment 16th* edn. New York: Lange/McGraw-Hill 2003; 336-361.
3. Mullick DN, Gupte S. Vitriolage in two adolescents. *Asian J Med Surg* 1974;5:14-15.
4. Rothstein FC. Caustic injuries to the esophagus in children. *Pediatr Clin North Am* 1986;33:665-673.

Praveen C Sobti and Gautam Biswas

71 Organophosphate and Carbamate (OPC)Poisoning

INTRODUCTION

Organophosphate compounds (OPCs) were first synthesized in early 1800s when Lassaigne reacted alcohol with phosphoric acid. Shortly thereafter in 1854, Philip de Clermount described the synthesis of tetraethyl pyrophosphate at a meeting of the French Academy of Sciences. Eighty years later, Lange in Berlin and Schrader, a chemist at Bayer AG, Germany, investigated the use of OPCs as insecticides. However, the German military prevented the use of OPCs as insecticides and instead developed an arsenal of chemical warfare agents (i.e. tabun, sarin, soman). During World War II, in 1941, OPCs were reintroduced worldwide for pesticide use, as originally intended.

COMMON ORGANOPHOSPHATE COMPOUNDS

- Chlorpyriphos (Chlorofos 20, Agrofos 20, Gilphos)
- Diazinon (Agrozion, Zionosul 50)
- Fenitrothion (Folithion, Tik 20)
- Malathion (Maladan, Finit, Cythion)
- Trichlorphon (Diptrenex)
- Glyphosate (Weed off)

Common Carbamates[1]

- Aldicarb (Temik)
- Carbaryl (Sevin 50, Agroyl)
- Propoxur (Baygon)
- Carbofuran (Carbocil 3, Furadan 3G)
- Carbaryl + Gamma BHC (Sevidol)

OPCs and carbamates are extensively used as pesticides for soft-bodied insects in agriculture. They have been imported by India since 1951, but little was known about the nature of these compounds as virulent poison till the Kerala food poisoning tragedy in 1958.[2] Pesticide poisoning is found to be more prevalent in Punjab and West Bengal than in any other states. Accidental poisoning is common, involving 50–90% of children below 5 years of age.[3] Males outnumber females in a ratio of 2.65 : 1.[3] Pesticide poisoning is the most common mode of suicide in some developing countries like India and Sri Lanka. The American Association of Poison Control Centers' National incidence report indicates that pesticide injuries number 70,000-80,000 annually, out of which 3.9% are due to insecticides.

PHYSICAL APPEARANCE

These compounds are available as dusts, granules, or liquids. Some products need to be diluted with water before use and some are burnt to make smoke that kills insects.

TOXICOKINETICS

OPCs and carbamates are absorbed by many routes including transdermal, transconjunctival, inhalational, across the GIT (from residues on floors and carpets, children toys, food and dust) and through direct injection.

The primary mechanism of action of OPCs and carbamates is inhibition of carboxylic ester hydrolases including acetylcholinesterase (AChE) and plasma or butayrl cholinesterase (pseudocholinesterase). Hence, these compounds are called **cholinesterase inhibitors**. AChE is a neuro-transmitter found in CNS, the peripheral nervous system and the skeletal muscles. It is also genetically expressed on the membrane of erythrocytes. Its normal physiologic action is to break down acetylcholine (ACh). OPCs and carbamates inactivate AChE by phosphorylating the serine hydroxyl group located at the active site of AChE. Phosphorylated enzymes degrade very slowly over days to weeks, making the AChE essentially inactive. Once AChE has been inactivated, acetylcholine accumulates in the autonomic nervous system, the somatic nervous system and the brain, resulting in over stimulation of muscarinic and nicotinic receptors as shown in Figure 71.1.

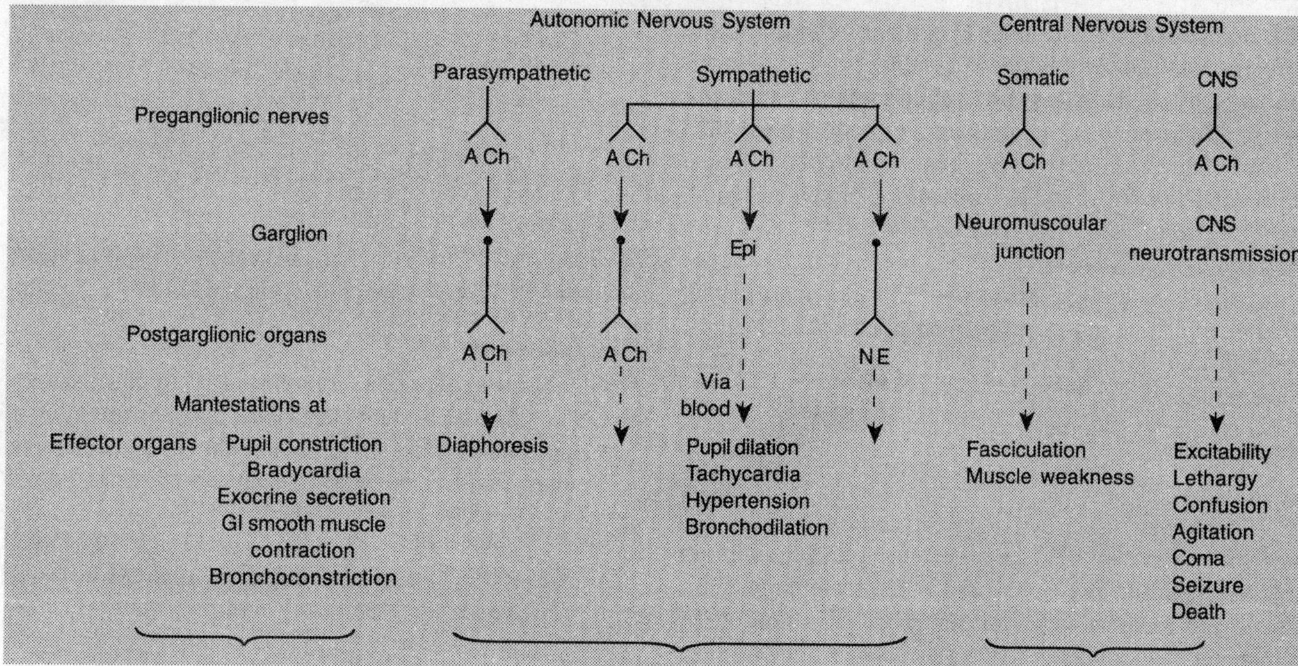

Fig. 71.1: Schematic representation of the autonomic nervous system and effector organ manifestations of OPCs and carbamates toxicity (Adapted from Goldfrank's Toxicologic Emergencies)

Fortunately, both morbidity and mortality associated with carbamates is limited as a result of the transient nature of cholinesterase inhibition and the rapid enzyme reactivation (they hydrolyze spontaneously from the cholinesterase enzymatic site within 48 hours). An important distinction between OPCs and carbamates is that carbamates do not penetrate the CNS to the same extent; resulting in limited CNS toxicity. With respect to all other clinical manifestations, there is little difference between OPCs and carbamates.[4,5]

MORTALITY/MORBIDITY

Worldwide, mortality due to OPCs poisoning varies from 3–25%. The compounds involved most frequently are malathion, dichlorovos and trichlorphon. Mortality rates depend on the type of compound used, the amount ingested, the general health of the patient, and the delay in discovery and transport. Outcome also depends on adequacy of respiratory management, time taken for intubation and for weaning off from ventilatory support.

Age

Study by Dong et al found that 62% of cases were due to accidental ingestion of OPCs by children under the age of 10 years in Zimbabwe.[6] Study by Kara *et al.* found 54.2% of the cases of OPC poisoning were under the age of 20 years in Turkey.[7] In a study of 37 infants and children, Zwiener *et al.*[8] found that ingestion of an improperly stored liquid pesticide was the most common route of intoxication (76% of patients). Study by Weissmann-Brenner *et al.*[9] found that more than one-third of patients (n = 97) were less than 10 years old. Accidental exposure was the cause of intoxication in 51.5% of the patients. Intoxication occurred at home in most patients (67%) and route of intoxication was oral in 65% of them.[9] Emerson *et al*[10] and Agarwal *et al.*[11] found that accidental poisoning with OPCs and carbamates were more likely in children than adults.[11] Emerson et al[10] found men aged 30–50 years were more likely to attempt suicide with OPCs. Agarwal[11] found that most poisonings occur in patients aged 21–30 years. Male, female ratio in the study was 2.1 : 1.

Clinical Features

Zwiener *et al.* found that miosis, excessive salivation, muscle weakness and lethargy were the most common abnormal signs. Tachycardia and seizures occurred in 49 and 22% of patients respectively, and 38% of the children had respiratory insufficiency that required endotracheal intubation and mechanical ventilation.[8] In another study by Sofer *et al.*[12] the main presenting signs and symptoms were severe CNS depression, coma, stupor, dyspnea and flaccidity. Other clinical signs such as miosis, excessive salivation, lacrymation, sweating and G.I. symptoms were less frequent, while fasiculations and bradycardia were uncommon at admission. Signs of carbamate poisonings were indistinguishable from those of OPC poisoning and include signs of myoneural and CNS cholenergic receptor involvement in addition to parasympathetic muscarinic dysfunction. They suggested that clinical presentation of

OPC and carbamate poisoning in early childhood is quite different from those of adults.[12] Lifshitz *et al.*[13] reported similar results in their study of 52 children intoxicated with OPCs and carbamates. Predominant symptoms were related to CNS depression and severe hypotonia. Other clinical signs such miosis, diarrhea, salivation, bradycardia and fasciculations were less frequent while tearing and diaphoresis were not observed. Pulmonary edema developed in 6 patients with OPC poisoning. They concluded that absence of classic muscarinic effects does not exclude the possibility of cholinesterase inhibitor agents poisoning in young children with CNS depression.[13,14]

Most patients become symptomatic between 30 minutes to 2 hours after exposure.[15] In fatal cases the symptoms begin within few minutes and death results in 1-3 hours; in non-fatal cases, the effects last for about 30 hours and fade off in the next 48-72 hours.[2] Onset and duration of action depend on the nature and type of compound, the degree and route of exposure, the mode of action of the compound, lipid solubility and rate of metabolic degradation.

Signs and symptoms of OPC poisoning can be divided into 3 broad categories.[2,4,15,16]

I. *Muscarinic or hollow organ parasympathetic manifestations:*
   - *Gastrointestinal*—Increased salivation, nausea, vomiting, retrosternal pain, abdominal cramps, diarrhea and fecal incontinence.
   - *Cardiovascular*—Bradycardia, hypertension.
   - *Respiratory*—Rhinorhea, bronchospasm, bronchorrhea, cough, wheezing, dyspnea.
   - *Ocular*—Blurred vision, miosis.
   - *Glands*—Increased lacrimation, rhinorrhoea, chromolacryorrhea (shedding of red tears due to accumulation of porphyrin in lacrymal glands), sweating.

     Kerosene or garlic like smell may be observed in the breath and body secretions.

   Mnemonics used to remember the signs and symptoms are:

   i. SLUDGE: Salivation, lacrimation, urination, diarrhea, gastrointestinal distress and emesis

   ii. DUMBELS: Diaphoresis, diarrhea, urination, miosis, bradycardia, bronchospasm, bronchorrhea, emesis, lacrimation and salivation

II. *Nicotinic or autonomic ganglionic and somatic motor (NMJ) effects*

   Nicotinic manifestations include muscle fasciculations, cramping and weakness, twitching, and diaphragmatic failure and can progress to paralysis, areflexia and respiratory failure. Autonomic effects include hypertension, tachycardia, mydriasis and pallor.

III. *CNS effects*

   CNS manifestations include restlessness, emotional liability, headache, tremor, drowsiness, confusion, slurred speech, ataxia, generalized weakness, Cheyne-Stokes respiration, delirium, and coma, absent reflexes, seizures, psychosis and death.

In children less than 3 years, predominant symptoms are vomiting, miosis, salivation and muscle weakness. Seizures are more common (25% of cases) than in adults (3% cases).

Signs and symptoms may be categorized into mild, moderate or severe depending upon the kind of exposure.

Mild Exposure

- GIT-Nausea, anorexia, cramping without diarrhea.
- CNS—Malaise, fatigue, headache, dizziness, tremors of tongue and eyelids, anxiety, minimal muscle weakness.
- Ocular—Miosis, decreased visual acuity.

Moderate Exposure

SLUDGE and/or tremors, muscle fasciculations followed by flaccid paralysis, respiratory muscle weakness, incoordination, confusion, lethargy and anxiety.

Severe Exposure

- SLUDGE.
- CNS—Convulsions, coma, loss of sphincter tone, paralysis, autonomic dysfunction.
- Respiratory—Respiratory insufficiency, pulmonary edema.
- Cardiovascular—Bradycardia, heart block.

MANAGEMENT[2,4,15-19]

Patient should be stripped of his clothing and the clothing discarded, preferably before the patient is transported from the scene, to prevent contamination of the treating personnel and the ambulance. Clothing is considered toxic waste and should be double bagged or washed clean with large amounts of water. Gentle cleaning of skin is recommended; abrading the skin with rigorous rubbing will enhance absorption. The airway should be maintained and adequate oxygenation provided. The treating personnel should be protected with water-impermeable gowns, masks with eyeshields, shoe covers and should use double gloves.

History and Physical Examination

Inquire about possible exposure from recent insecticide spraying in the home, mislabeled or poorly stored insecticides. Look for parasympathetic and CNS signs, muscle weakness or paralysis.

Laboratory Diagnosis

The essential finding in laboratory diagnosis is depression of cholinesterase activity. In acute poisonings, signs and symptoms generally occur after more than 50% of cholinesterase is inhibited, and the severity of symptoms parallels the degree of cholinesterase depression. In mild poisoning, depression in cholinesterase activity occurs up to 20-50% of normal; in moderate poisoning 10-20% and in severe poisoning the activity of enzyme is less than 10%. However, do not wait for cholinesterase results before administering treatment of the patient. Diagnosis of OPC poisoning is usually confirmed retrospectively (4-7 weeks) as the majority of laboratories cannot perform these tests on an urgent basis. Moreover, a single oxime therapy should no longer be considered dogma.

Interpretation of Cholinesterase Levels RBC (True) Cholinesterase

Found in CNS grey mater, RBC and motor end plate. RBC cholinesterase levels are a good reflection of the degree of synaptic inhibition. Used to evaluate unsuspected prior exposure with elevated plasma cholinesterase. Falsely depressed levels of RBC cholinesterase can be found in cases of pernicious anemia, hemoglobinopathies (e.g. sickle cell anemia, thalassemia), use of antimalarial drugs and use of oxalate blood tubes.

Plasma (Pseudo) Cholinesterase

Found in CNS white matter, plasma, liver, pancreas and heart. It is easier to assay, and declines rapidly. Falsely depressed levels of plasma cholinesterase are observed in cases of liver dysfunction (cirrhosis); low protein condition (e.g. malnutrition), genetic deficiency, neoplasia and hypersensitivity reactions. In addition, the use of drugs such as succinylcholine, codeine, and morphine gives falsely depressed values.

RBC cholinesterase is considered the more accurate of the two. However, plasma cholinesterase activity is easier to assay and generally more readily available.

Ancillary Laboratory Testing

- A complete blood count may show leukocytosis with a normal differential count. There may be an increase in the hematocrit, from hemoconcentration due to loss of fluid. There is anion gap acidosis due to poor tissue perfusion.
- Serum glucose may be elevated with hypokalemia and hypomagnesaemia due to catecholamine excess. Blood urea nitrogen (BUN), creatinine and urine specific gravity—determine the patient's hydration status, ABG's—help in monitoring oxygenation status.

Imaging/Special Tests

- *Chest X-ray:* if respiratory difficulty is present.
- *ECG:* prolonged QTc interval (most common; up to 67%), elevated ST segments, inverted T-waves, dysrhythmias, bradycardia, tachycardia, and heart block.
- *CT scan of head:* for altered mental status when diagnosis is uncertain.

Yilmazlar *et al.*[20] investigated 16 patients with OPC poisoning and suggested the use of brain single photo emission computerization tomography (SPECT), together with clinical symptoms and plasma cholinesterase activity to monitor the clinical prognosis of OPC poisoning.

Other Laboratory Tests[1]

P-nitro phenol test: P-nitro phenol is a metabolite of some OPCs (e.g. parathion, ethion) and is excreted in the urine. Its presence in the urine can be used as a confirmation test of OPC poisoning.

Procedure

Steam distill 10 ml of urine and collect the distillate. Add sodium hydroxide (2 pellets) and heat in a water bath for 10 minutes. Production of a yellow color indicates the presence of p-nitro phenol.

This test can also be done on vomitus or gastric lavage contents.

DIFFERENTIAL DIAGNOSIS[4,16]

Mild to moderate exposure:

- Gastroenteritis
- Asthma
- Heat prostration
- Influenza
- Exhaustion
- Hypoglycemia
- Pneumonia
- Venomous arthropods bite (black widow spider, scorpion)
- Non-specific viral syndrome
- Progressive peripheral neuropathy (Guíllain–Barré syndrome)
- Carbon monoxide.

Severe exposure:

- Narcotic overdose
- Coma and miosis
  - Meprobamate, phenothiazine, clonidine, nicotine, carbacol
  - Muscarinic containing mushrooms—cholinergic crisis without nicotinic symptoms
- Metabolic disorders and infections
  - Ketoacidosis, sepsis, meningitis, encephalitis
  - Hypoglycemia
  - Reye's syndrome
- Neurologic disorders
  - Subdural or epidural hematoma
  - Postictal state
  - CVA.

TREATMENT

The patient is treated according to the severity of the symptoms as shown in Figure 71.2.

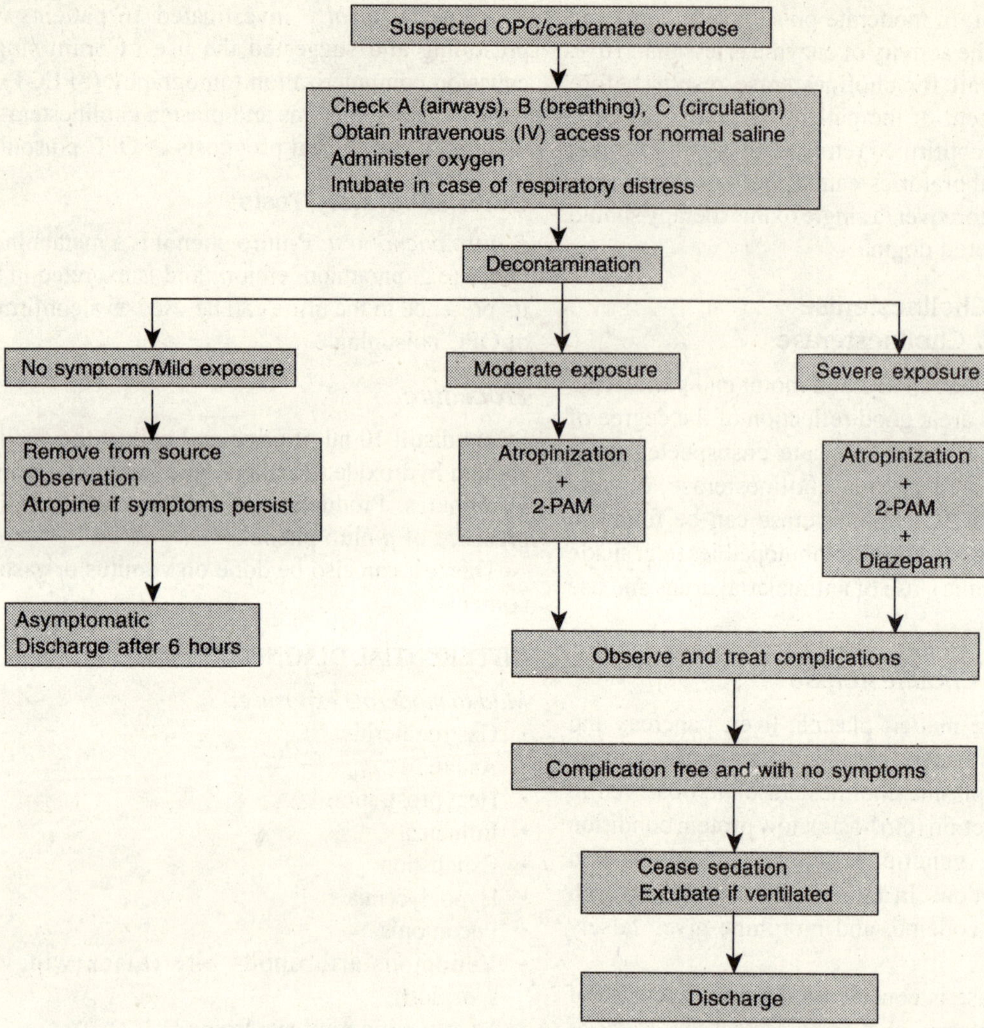

Fig. 71.2: Flow diagram showing treatment of the patient depending upon the severity of exposure

Initial Stabilization

I. *ABCs*

- Maintain airway and oxygenate
- Intubate in case of respiratory distress from laryngospasm, bronchospasm, or severe bronchorrhea.

II. *Decontamination*

- If decontamination was not done earlier, remove the clothes and flush the skin with water.
- Gastric lavage—Gastric emptying should be done with continuous suction via a nasogastric tube. Activated charcoal should be administrated in doses of 1 g/kg.
- Cathartics are unnecessary as intestinal motility is markedly enhanced; any oral treatment will move rapidly throughout the GI tract.
- Patient's with ocular exposures should have copious eye irrigation with normal saline or lactated Ringer's solution. If these are not available tap water can be used.
- Inhalational exposures should be treated with removal from the offending vapor and by administration of oxygen.

Diagnostic Trial

For a few suspected toxins, administration of an antidote or a chelator not only initiates therapy but also assists in the diagnosis of the agent involved. For a suspected case of OPC poisoning, atropine in a dose of 0.1 mg/kg IV can be given in an appropriate PICU setting. Pupillary dilation and decrease in secretions should be looked for.[21]

III. *Atropinization:* Atropine, a postsynaptic muscarinic receptor antagonist, blocks the muscarinic manifestations. It has no effect on nicotinic receptors (on muscle weakness or paralysis) and does not affect the rate of regeneration of inhibited AChE.

Dose: 0.05–0.2 mg/kg IV repeated after every 5–15 minutes.

Once signs of adequate atropinization occur, the dose should be adjusted to maintain this effect for at least 24 hours (maintenance dose 0.02–0.05 mg/kg).

The endpoint to atropinization is clearing up of the secretions from the tracheobronchial tree and drying of most secretions. **Mydriasis is an early response to atropine and is not a therapeutic endpoint.** A common failure of therapy is not maintaining adequate atropinization. Tachycardia is not a contraindication to atropine treatment, as it may be due to hypoxia or autonomic stimulation.

Precautions: Atropine is avoided in patients with Down's syndrome and/or children with brain damage to prevent a hyperactive response. It is also avoided in cardiac arrhythmias, hypertension, peritonitis, hepatic disease, hiatal hernia with reflex esophagitis.

Some authors have recommended the need to maximize oxygenation prior to atropine administration to prevent ventricular dysrhythimias associated with hypoxia. Along with this a cardiac monitor and a defibrillator should be nearby.

Another drug, *glycopyrrolate* may be substituted if there is no evidence of central toxicity. Glycopyrrolate does not penetrate the CNS, and substituting it for atropine eliminates the potential risks of developing central anticholinergic syndrome in a patient with clear sensorium.

Dose: 4-10 mg/kg IV repeated after 3-4 hours, not to exceed 0.2 mg/dose or 0.8 mg in 24 hours.

Precautions: It is recommended for children < 12 years, patients with Down's syndrome, hiatal hernia or hyperthyroidism. It may produce increased intraocular tension, blurred vision, cycloplegia, urinary hesitancy and retention.

IV. *Pralidoxime (2-PAM)*

Pralidoxime, a nucleophilic oxime, regenerates AChE by phosphorylating it at the muscarinic, nicotinic and CNS sites. It may also prevent continued toxicity by scavenging the remaining OPC molecules. Treatment with 2-PAM is most effective, when started early and if used in acute (within 48 hours) rather than chronic OPC poisoning. Once the phosphorylated enzyme has 'aged' then the phosphate group becomes irreversibly bound to the enzyme and oxime therapy is no longer effective.

Dose: 20-40 mg/kg IV dissolved in 0.9% normal saline solution and infused over 15-30 minutes; may be repeated at 1-2 hours if muscle weakness is not relieved, and again after 8-10 hours. IM/SC can be used if IV is not feasible.

Precautions: Rapid IV bolus administration should be avoided as it may cause tachycardia, laryngospasm, muscle rigidity, diastolic hypertension, dizziness and blurred vision. Occasionally respiratory and cardiac arrest may occur.

Atropine and 2-PAM given together are synergistic against the signs and symptoms of cholinesterase inhibition, thus decreasing atropine requirements. Signs of atropinization might occur earlier with addition of 2-PAM to the treatment regimen.

The use of pralidoxime in carbamate poisoning is controversial. It is usually unnecessary but its use is safe, particularly if administered in conjunction with atropine in case of unknown pesticide or in mixed poisoning.[4,15,22-24]

V. *Diazepam*: Addition of diazepam for treatment of seizures and neuropathy improves survival. It decreases the cardiac and brain morphologic damage resulting from OPC seizures.

Dose: 0.05–0.3 mg/kg/dose IV/IM over 2–3 minutes may be repeated after 15–30 min; not to exceed 10 mg.

Precautions—Diazepam must not be used with other CNS depressants, low albumin levels or in the presence of hepatic disease.

VI. Supportive Care
- Suction as required to remove respiratory secretions.
- Treat bronchospasm with atropine and not bronchodilators.
- Intubate and ventilate if necessary.
- The use of other medication, including opiods for sedation, may worsen CNS manifestations and the degree of respiratory depression.
- *Dextrose:* 2-4 ml/kg D 25 of 50% dextrose IV.
- Antibiotics to prevent pulmonary infection.
- Vitamin K may also be given.

ADMISSION CRITERIA

Hospitalization of all symptomatic patients for at least 4-6 days following amelioration of symptoms is recommended because of risk of development of respiratory depression or intermediate syndrome after resolution of an acute cholinergic crisis.

DISCHARGE CRITERIA

Some authors suggest discharge of asymptomatic patients from emergency departments after 6 hours of observation. Follow-up of the case must be certain.

DELAYED AND LONG-TERM NEUROLOGIC SEQUELAE

Intermediate syndrome was described in 1974 with an incidence from 8-49%. It develops in 24-96 hours after resolution of acute cholinergic poisoning symptoms and manifests commonly as paralysis and respiratory distress. Neuromuscular transmission defect and toxin-induced muscular instability play a role in the intermediate syndrome. It may also be due to inadequate treatment of the acute episode especially involving sub-therapeutic administration of oximes or inadequate ventilation. This syndrome involves proximal groups of muscle with relative sparing of distal groups and is characterized by cranial nerve palsies, weakness of neck flexors and proximal limb muscles. It is managed by supportive measures, since it does not respond to oximes or atropine.[1]

Organophosphate-induced delayed neurotoxicity (OPIDN) or polyneuropathy (OPIDP) occurs 1 to 3 weeks after exposure to large doses of certain OPCs. The patient initially complains of symmetric lower extremity weakness and glove and stocking paresthesias, leg cramping and calf pain. Atrophy and paralysis of the peroneal muscles lead to foot drop and eventually ataxia. Steppage gait develops with a positive Romberg sign. The Achilles and ankle jerk reflexes are lost. This ultimately progresses to the upper extremities. In some cases, a bilateral symmetric flaccid paralysis occurs. Sensory symptoms resolve over the ensuing 1–2 months but paralysis remains. Mild cases may recover in over 15 months but severe cases have persistent symptoms including spasticity. This syndrome also does not respond to either oximes or atropine.[4,25,26]

MEDICOLEGAL ASPECTS

- Hospitalizing all symptomatic patients for at least 4-6 days following resolution of symptoms is recommended because of the risk of development of respiratory depression or intermediate syndrome after resolution of an acute crisis.
- Follow-up of cases must be certain and failure to follow up will amount to an act of negligence.
- The symptoms of OPC poisoning can mimic other toxidromes and diseases. The clinician must keep in mind that misdiagnosis is a potential medicolegal pitfall.

REFERENCES

1. Pillay VV. Pesticides. In: Pillay VV (ed) *Handbook of Forensic Medicine and Toxicology*, 12th edn. Hyderabad: Paras Publishing 2001;386-400.
2. Subrahmanyam BV. Inorganic irritant poisons. *Modi's Medical Jurisprudence and Toxicology*, 22nd edn. New Delhi: Butterworths 1999;77–101.
3. Dutta AK, Seth A, Goyal PK, et al. Poisoning in children: Indian scenario. *Indian J Pediatr* 1998;65: 365-370.
4. Aaron CK, Howland MA. Insecticides: organophosphates and carbamates. In Goldfrank LR, Flomenbaum NE, Lewin NA, Weisman RS, Howland RS (eds) *Goldfrank's Toxicologic Emergencies*. 6th edn. Standford: Appleton and Lange 1998;1429-1444.
5. Wagner SL. Diagnosis and treatment of organophosphate and carbamate poisoning. *Occup Med* 1997;12:239-249.
6. Dong X, Simon MA. The epidemiology of organophosphate poisoning in urban Zimbabwe from 1995 to 2000. *Intian J Occup Environ Health* 2001;7:333-338.
7. Kara IH, Guloglu C, Karabulut A, Orak M. Sociodemographic, clinical and laboratory features of cases of organic phosphorus intoxication who attended the Emergency Department in the Southern Anatolian region of Turkey. *Environ Res* 2002;88: 82-88.
8. Zwiener RJ, Ginsburg CM. Organophosphate and carbamate poisoning in infants and children. *Pediatrics* 1998;81:121-126.
9. Weissmann-Brenner A, David A, Vidan A, Hourvitz A. Organophosphate poisoning: a multi-hospital survey. *Isr Med Assoc J* 2002;4:573-576.
10. Emerson GM., Gray NM, Jelinek GA. Organophosphate poisoning in Perth, Western Australia, 1987-1996. *J Emerg Med* 1999;17:273-277.
11. Agarwal SB. A clinical, biochemical, neuro behavioral and socio psychological study of 190 patients admitted to hospital as a result of acute organophosphorous poisoning. *Environ Res.* 1993;62:63-70.
12. Sofer S, Tal A, Shahak E. Carbamate and organophosphate poisoning in early childhood. *Pediatr Emerg Care* 1989;5:222-225.
13. Lifshitz M, Shahak E, Sofer S. Carbamate are organophosphate poisoning in young children. *Pediatr Emerg Care* 1999;15:102-103.
14. Lifshitz M, Shahak E, Bolotin A, Sofer S. Carbamate poisoning in early childhood and in adults. *J Toxicol Clin Toxicol* 1997; 37:25-27.
15. Linden CH, Burns MJ. Poisoning and drug overdose. In: Braunwald E, Fauci AS, Kasper DL, Hauser SL, Longo DL, Jameson JL (eds) *Harrison's Principles of Internal Medicine*, 15th edn. New York: McGraw Hill, 2001;2595-2615.
16. Cole K. Organophosphate poisoning. In: Rosen P, Baskin RM, Hayden SR, Schaider J. Wolfe R (eds). *The 5-minute Emergency Medicine Consult.* Philadelphia: Lippincort Williams and Wilkins 1999;868-869.
17. Olson KR. Poisoning. In: Tierney Jr LM, McPhee SJ, Papadakis MA (eds) *Current Medical Diagnosis and Treatment*, 42nd edn. New York: Lange/McGraw-Hill, 2003;1555-1588.
18. Proudfoot AT, Vale JA, Meredith TJ. Pesticides. In: Weatherall DJ, Ledingham JGG, Warrell DA *Oxford Textbook of Medicine)*, 3rd edn. New York: Oxford University Press 1996;1120-1124.
19. Dart RC, Rumack BH. Poisoning. In: Hay WW, Yayward AR, Levin MJ, Sondheimer JM (eds) *Current Pediatric Diagnosis and Treatment*, 16th eds. New York: Lange/McGraw-Hill 2003;336-361.
20. Yilmazlar A, Ozyurt G. Brain involvement in organophosphate poisoning. *Environ Res* 1997;74:104-109.
21. Wolf AD, Lovejoy FH. Principle of toxin assessment and screening. In: Fuhrman BP, Zimmerman JJ (eds) *Pediatric Critical Care*, 2nd edn. New York: Mosby 1998;1142-1149.
22. Lifshitz M, Rotenberg, M, Sofer S, Tamiri T, Shahak E. Carbamate poisoning and oxime treatment in children; a clinical and laboratory study. *Pediatrics* 1994;93:652-655.
23. Garber M. Carbamate poisoning: The 'other' insecticide. *Pediatrics* 1987;79:734–738.
24. Peduto VA, D'Uva R, Piga M. Carbamate and organophosphate poisoning. *Minerva Anestesiol* 1996;62:33-54.
25. Genel F, Arslanoglu S, Uran N, Dogan N, Altihan F. Late-onset distal polyneuropathy due to acute organophosphate intoxication: Case report. *Turk J Pediatr* 2003;45:67-70.
26. Moretto A, Lotti M. Poisoning by organophosphorus insecticides and sensory neuropathy. *J Neurol Neurosurg Psychiatry* 1998;64:463-468.

Suraj Gupte and HE Peterson

72 Dhatura Poisoning

INTRODUCTION

It is a leading plant poisoning with deliriant effect. The plant grows in waste places all over, especially in the Indian subcontinent.[1]

Accidental dhatura poisoning usually occurs by eating its raw fruit (mistakenly thought to be edible fruit) or seeds (mistakenly thought to be capsicum seeds). In teenagers, dhatura poisoning can occur when employed as an aphrodisiac or when added to country liquor for enhancing its "kick" effect.

Dhatura, in small dose, is often fed in candies or sweets or administered as inhalant to children with the motive of kidnapping.

PATHOPHYSIOLOGY

The active principles in dhatura are toxins, namely hyosclamine, scopolamine and traces of atropine.[2, 3]

The alkaloids are anticholinergic in nature and stimulate the higher centers of brain and motor centers and inhibit secretion of sweat and saliva, dilate cutaneous blood vessels, dilate pupils and stimulate heat regulatory center in the floor of the 3rd ventricle. Initial stimulation soon gives way to depression and paralysis of the vital centers in the medulla.

CLINICAL MANIFESTATIONS

Manifestations of dhatura poisoning, occurring secondary to its anticholinergic nature, are aptly described as "dry as a bone, red as a beet , blind as a bat, hot as a hare and mad as a wet hen". These are secondary to peripheral and central antimuscarineic effects.

Manifestations include dryness of mouth and throat ("dry as a bone") , bitter taste in mouth, flushing of face due to dilatation of cutaneous blood vessels ("red as a beet") dry and hot skin secondary to inhibition of sweat secretions and stimulation of heat regulatory center ("hot as a hare"), dilated pupils i.e. mydriasis with paralysis of power of accommodation ("blind as a bat"), difficulty in speech and swallowing and vomiting. These, in due course, progress to giddiness, delirium ("mad as a wet hen") and ataxia. This is followed by drowsiness, stupor and coma Respiratory center paralysis may prove fatal.

Table 72.1 summarizes the manifestations of dhatura poisoning under **9 Ds.**

Table 72.1: 9Ds of dhatura poisoning manifestations

1. Dryness of mouth and throat ("dry as a bone")
2. Dry hot skin ("hot as a hare")
3. Difficulty in talking
4. Dysphagia
5. Dilatation of pupils ("blind as a bat")
6. Dilatation of cutaneous blood vessels causing flushing ("red as a beet")
7. Drunken (ataxic) gait
8. Delirium ("mad as a wet hen")
9. Drowsiness

DIAGNOSIS

Immediate attention should be on assessment of airway and breathing, and cardiac rhythm and blood pressure ("ABC").

Core body temperature and acid-base and respiratory status (measurement of arterial blood gas tidal volume) should be ascertained.

Chest X-ray should be done when aspiration pneumonia is suspected.

Presence of alkaloids may be tested in the gastric contents.

Mydriatic test consists in instilling a drop of the material suspected of consumption by the child into a cat's eye. It causes pupillary dilatation in about an hour.[2]

MANAGEMENT

Decontamination

It is important to evacuate the unabsorbed poison from stomach by gastric lavage with a weak solution of potassium permanganate ($KMnO_4$) or 4-5% tannic acid.

Within 48 hours of ingestion, even normal saline and large doses of activated charcoal are good enough for gastric decontamination.[3]

Specific Antidote

Physostigmine, 0.02 mg/kg/dose IV slowly over 5-10 minutes period. It is repeated every 1-2 hour but not too often. Alternatively, neostigmine may be given. It is a physiologic antidote.

Supportive Measures

Supportive therapy includes care of airway, breathing, cardiac rhythm and blood pressure, core temperature and fluid, electrolyte and acid-base status.

Seizure control may be achieved with IV diazepam.

Monitoring of urinary output is best achieved by inserting a urinary catheter under aseptic conditions.

Response to treatment is in the form of moistening of tongue and return of pupils to normal size which is the last to occur.[2] Recovery takes a day or two.

REFERENCES

1. Parikh CK. *Parikh's Textbook of Medical Jurisprudence, Forensic Medicine and Toxicology* 6th edn. New Delhi: CBS 1999.
2. Chacko B, Singh T. Poisoning and toxicity. In: Gupte S (ed) *Recent Advances in Pediatrics,* Vol 13. New Delhi: Jaypee Brothers 2004: 252-270.
3. Seldon BS, Curry SC. *Pediatric Emergency Medicine.* Philadelphia: W B Saunders 1995.
4. Dart RC, Rumack BH. Poisoning. In: Hay WW Jr, Hayward AR, Levin MJ, ondheimer JM (eds) *Current Pediatric Diagnosis and Treatment.* 16th edn. New York: Lange/McGraw-Hill 2003: 336-361.

Suraj Gupte, Farooq Ansari and EW Nelson

73 Mushroom Poisoning

INTRODUCTION

Mushroom (derived from French word *musculi*) is an umbrella-shaped wild fungus which grows on decaying vegetable matter, usually in damp places. It is low in carbohydrates and fats and high in proteins.

Since it is not always possible to differentiate edible mushroom from wild inedible (poisonous) mushroom, mushroom poisoning occurs quite often.[1,2]

The various toxins produced by poisonous mushroom are:[2]

- Cyclopeptides (by amanita species)
- Monomethylhydrazine
- Muscarine
- Coprine
- Ibotenic acid
- Psilocybin

Over and above these, some unidentified toxins are also believed to be present.

FACTORS CONTRIBUTING TO MUSHROOM TOXICITY

A number of factors influence the development of toxicity and clinical signs and symptoms following ingestion of toxic mushrooms:[3-6]

- Species ingested
- Stage of maturity
- Time of the year
- Amount ingested
- *Interval since ingestion:* Onset of manifestations rapidly (within 2 hours) points to muscarine toxin whereas delayed onset of symptoms (after 6-48 hours) suggests Amanita poisoning.
- *Individual variation:* Interestingly, a mushroom that is toxic to one person may not be toxic to another.
- *Simultaneous Ingestions:* Drinking alcohol along with certain mushrooms may cause disulfiram-like reaction.
- *Cooking:* It destroys some toxins. However, deadly toxins by Amanita phalloides (responsible for 90% mortality from mushroom poisoning) are not affected by cooking.

AMANITA POISONING (LATE MUSHROOM POISONING)

This is the most common mushroom poisoning, especially the fatal mushroom poisoning.

Pathophysiology

Amanita poisoning causes cellular necrosis in the GIT, acute yellow atrophy of liver and proximal renal tubular necrosis.

Clinical Manifestations

Amanita poisoning causes delayed (6-24 or even 48 hours after ingestion) gastrointestinal symptoms in the form of nausea, vomiting, severe abdominal pain and profuse watery diarrhea followed by icterus, renal failure and coma.

Treatment

Supportive

It comprises aggressive correction of fluid and electrolyte losses and, in advanced stage, attention to liver and renal failure.

Specific

Decontamination is required to remove the toxin rapidly. Oral activated charcoal and lactulose are ideal.

IV penicillin infusion together with silibinin are employed for their synergestic effect to inhibit binding of both toxins and interrupt enterohepatic recirculation of toxins.[2]

Orthotopic liver transplant in advanced liver failure.

MUSCARINE POISONING (EARLY MUSHROOM POISONING)

Pathophysiology

Certain mushrooms (genera *Inacybe* and *Clitocybe*) contain muscarine or related compounds which bind to the post-synaptic receptors. As a result, hyperchilinergic response is produced, causing various clinical signs and symptoms.

Clinical Manifestations

The exaggerated cholinergic manifestations appear within an hour of ingestion and are in the form of excessive sweating, lacrimation and salivation, vomiting, constricted pupils (miosis), urinary and fecal incontinence, broncho-spasm and excessive bronchopulmonary secretions causing respiratory distress.

Management

Specific antidote is atropine sulfate. It is given intravenously, 0.01–0.02 mg/kg/dose,[2] repeated usually every 30 minutes until complete atropnization (mydriasis, dryness of mouth, tachycardia) occurs or symptoms resolve.

Even without therapy, symptoms in most modest poisonings resolve spontaneously.

ANTICHOLINERGIC/HALLUCINOGENIC POISONING (IBOTENIC ACID AND MUSCIMOL POISONING)

Pathophysiology

Ibotenic acid is a hallucinogen. Muscimol is an insecticide having anticholinergic action.

Clinical Manifestations

CNS symptoms appear within 30 min–3 hours following ingestion of the mushroom and include lethargy alternating with agitation, seizures and, infrequently nausea and vomiting. Cholinergic crisis may occur in severe poisoning.

Management

In case of an exaggerated cholinergic response, atropinization is needed.

In case of anticholinergic manifestations, physiostigmine (which is an acetylcholinesterase inhibitor) should be administered for reversing delirium and coma. For seizure control, diazepam may be employed.

INDOLE (MAGIC MUSHROOM) POISONING

Pathophysiology

Certain mushroom contain psychotropic compounds, *psilocybin* and *psilocin*, which are responsible for psychosomatic manifestations.[2]

Clinical Manifestations

These develop within 30 minutes after ingestion and include euphoria, hallucinations, tachycardia and mydriasis. Severe agitation develops in heavy ingestion.

Management

Manifestations, as a rule, are short-lived and subside after 6 hours or so. Diazepam may be administered in case of severe agitation.

REFERENCES

1. Editorial. Mushroom poisoning. *Lancet* 1980;2:351.
2. Salerno DA, Aronoff SC. Nonbacterial food poisoning. In: Behrman RE, Kliegman RM, Jenson HB (eds) *Nelson Textbook of Pediatrics*, 17th edn. Philadelphia: Saunders 2004;2375-2378.
3. Spoerke DG, Rumack BH. *Mushroom Poisoning: Diagnosis and Treatment*, 2nd edn. CRC Press 1994.
4. Lampe KF, McCann MA. Differential diagnosis of poisoning by north American mushrooms with particular emphasis on Amanita phalloides-like intoxication. *Ann Emerg Med* 1987;16:956.
5. Dart RC, Rumack BH. Poisoning. In: Hay WW, Hayward AR, Levin MJ, Sondheimer JM (eds) Current Pediatric Diagnosis and Treatment, 16th edn. New York: Lange/McGraw-Hill 2003;336-361.
6. Nelson EW, Chou E. Accidental poisoning revisited. *S-E Asian J Med Surg* 2003;12:456-463.

Suraj Gupte and Sanjay Wazir

74 Opioid Poisoning

INTRODUCTION

Opioids are opium group of agents and include:

- *Natural alkaloids*: Morphine, codeine
- *Semisynthetic derivatives*: Heroin (brown sugar), hydromorphine, oxycodon
- *Synthetic derivatives*: Butorphanol, fentanyl, levorphanol, pethidine (meperidine), methadone, propoxyphen, pentazocin.[1]

There are three ways in which opioid poisoning can occur:

1. Accidental ingestion
2. Therapeutic mishap
3. Substance abuse.

PATHOPHYSIOLOGY

Also called "somniferous" or "narcotic" agents, their primary pharmacological action is to relieve pain through opioid receptors. Secondary effects include sedation, anxiolysis, vomiting, urinary retention, ileus, respiratory depression and hypotension. It is believed that a combination of mechanisms such as vasodilatation, sympatholysis, vagal-mediated bradycardia and histamine release are responsible for their action.[1,2]

DIAGNOSIS

It is mainly from history and clinical profile. Raw-flesh smell in breath, pin-point immobile pupils, moist perspiring skin with subnormal temperature, weak slow pulse, Cheyne-Stokes respiration, cyanosis, froth from nose and mouth are noteworthy features.

Laboratory support may be in the form of:

- Arterial blood gas hypoxia and hypercapnia
- Hyperamylasemia/hyperlipasemia
- Positive toxicological analysis of blood and urine for opioids.

DIFFERENTIAL DIAGNOSIS

Opioid poisoning needs to be differentiated from:

- Intracranial hemorrhage.
- *Poisonings:* Alcohol, barbiturate, organophosphate, phosphorus, carbolic acid.
- *Metabolic conditions:* Uremic coma, diabetic coma.
- *CNS infections:* Encephalitis, meningitis, encephalopathy, cerebral malaria.
- *CNS conditions:* Epileptic coma, hysterical coma.

CLINICAL MANIFESTATIONS

Clinical manifestations are best considered in three stages: excitement, stupor and narcosis.

The "triad" of respiratory depression, pinpoint pupil and impairment of sensorium is characteristic of opioid poisoning.

Cardiovascular manifestations include arrhythmias in the form of bradycardia, intraventricular conduction defects, heart block, bigemini and nonspecific ST-T wave changes.

In addition, there may be noncardiogenic pulmonary edema. In such a situation, manifestations include respiratory distress, cyanosis, hypoxemia, tachypnea, basal crepitations and acidosis (both respiratory and metabolic).

Hypoxia may cause seizures.

In severe opioid poisoning, there is deep cyanosis, froth escaping from mouth, breath smelling of opium, Cheyne-Stokes breathing (sighing and irregular respiration), weak pulses, nonreacting dilated pupils, coma and respiratory paralysis. Death may occur within 9-12 hours.

MANAGEMENT

The cornerstone of treatment revolves around

- Gut decontamination
- Initial stabilization together with supportive treatment
- Antidote administration

Decontamination

Gut decontamination is of value only following ingestion of an opioid. Measures include.

Induction of vomiting and/or gastric lavage to remove any leftover toxin, ensuring protection of the airway (say by using a cuffed endotracheal tube).

- Administering activated charcoal with a cathartic, and
- Leaving 1-2 g/kg of it in the stomach to safeguard against further absorption of the toxin after lavage is over.

Supportive Measures

Immediate attention to airway, breathing, and cardiorespiratory stabilization are essential; so are the maintenance of fluid, electrolyte and acid-base status.

Endotracheal intubation with oxygen inhalation and, if required, positive pressure ventilation may become necessary.

Seizures may need anticonvulsant therapy.

For cardiac arrhythmia, antiarrhythmiac treatment is needed.

In case of an infection, a suitable antibiotic cover is provided.

Antidote

The specific antidote is naloxone, a specific antagonist, which is very efficacious in reversing the toxicity of opioids immediately. It is administered in a dose of 0.1 mg/kg for weight < 20 kg and 2 mg for weight > 20 kg, repeated every 2-3 minutes until toxicity is reversed or a total cumulative dose of 10 mg has been administered. Since it has a short duration of action, it has got to be administered repeatedly for sustained effect.

While treating opioid poisoning with naloxone in a narcotic-dependent subject, one must remember that the treatment may cause opioid withdrawl syndrome (Table 74.1). The withdrawl syndrome should be managed as shown in Table 74.2.

Alternative antidotes are nalarphine, naltroxone and levallorphan.[3]

Table 74.1: Manifestations of opioid withdrawl syndrome

Initial	Dilatation of pupils	
	Piloerection	
	Profuse sweating	
	Rhinorrhea	
	Myalgia/cramps	
	Lacrimation	
	Anorexia	
Late	*Milder Form:*	Restlessness
		Insomnia
		Hyperthermia
		Tachycardia
		Tachypnea
	Sever Form:	Vomiting
		Diarrhea
		Hyperactive bowel sounds
		Hypertension
		Muscle twitching
		Seizures

Table 74.2: Treatment of opioid withdrawal syndrome

Mild Manifestations

Reassurance.

Moderate-Severe Manifestations

- Readministration of opioid (methadone) on first day followed by gradual withdrawal in increments over 5-10 dats period.
- An alpha$_2$ blocker (usually clonidine 5 mcg/kg with a maximum of 0.3 mg in 2-4 divided doses) for relieving discomfort and pain by inhibiting sympathetic overactivity.
- Appropriate treatment of any superimposed infection.

REFERENCES

1. Parikh CK. *Parikh's Textbook of Medical Jurisprudence, Forensic Medicine and Toxicology*, 6th edn. New Delhi: CBS 1999.
2. Chacko B, Singh T. Poisoning and toxicity. In: Gupte S (ed) *Recent Advances in Pediatrics*, Vol 13. New Delhi: Jaypee Brothers 2004;252-270.
3. Dart RC, Rumack BH. Poisoning. In: Hay WW Jr, Hayward AR, Levin MJ, Sondheimer JM (eds) *Current Pediatric Diagnosis and Treatment 16th edn.* New York: Lange/McGraw-Hill 2003;336- 361.

Suraj Gupte

75 Carbon Monoxide Poisoning

INTRODUCTION

Poisoning with cabon monoxide (CO), a colorless, odorless, nonirritating gas, usually occurs from accidental fire and use of kerosene stove or coal in a closed room.[1] It is a common gas poisoning in Kashmir valley and Shimla Hills where people use bukhari (a sort of heating appliance using coal) in winter.

CO predominantly exerts its adverse effects by binding with hemoglobin and producing carboxyhemoglobin (COHB) which is notorious for producing hypoxia.[1]

PATHOPHYSIOLOGY

CO produces tissue hypoxia by acting through three mechanisms:

- It displaces oxygen and binds to hemoglobin with which it has a 250 times higher affinity. This results in formation of carboxyhemoglobin (COHB).
- It impairs the affinity of hemoglobin to release oxygen to tissues.
- It binds to enzyme, cytochromoe oxidase in tissues, impairing utilization of oxygen.

There may well be additions mechanisms contributing to development of hypoxia by CO.

LABORATORY DIAGNOSIS

It is by measuring levels of carboxyhemoglobin in subject's blood.

CLINICAL MANIFESTATIONS

Manifestations, understandably, depend on the proportion of COHB in blood. Early symptoms are nonspecific (headache, malaise and nausea) which may be confused with the flu.

When COHB is $< 20\%$, manifestations include shortness of breath and dilatation of cutaneous blood vessels.

When COHB is about 20%, manifestations include headache and tightness of frontal region.

When COHB varies between 20 to 50%, manifestations include nausea, vomiting, generalized weakness, visual disturbances, dizziness, confusion and fainting.

When COHB is over 50%, unconsciousness and convulsions and respiratory instability develop.

When COHB is 60 to 80%,CO poisoning ends up fatally.

MANAGEMENT

Decontamination

It is mandatory that the subject is immediately removed from the adverse environments.

Specific Treatment[2-6]

- 100% oxygen inhalation, preferably hyperbaric oxygen, helps to remove hypoxia.
- Ventilatory support in case of hypercarbia and respiratory failure.
- Hyperventilation, diuretics (fursemide, IV) and fluid restriction for cerebral edema.

Note that mild acidos need not be treated. In fact, it is of value in reducing hypoxia by shifting the oxygen dissociation curve to right.

Supportive Treatment

It should be in the form of general supportive therapy, taking care of fluid and electrolyte and acid-base balance, nutrition, etc.

PROGNOSIS

Delayed-onset neurotoxicity may develop in some children with significant exposure, especially when aggressive early treatment could not be offered.[5,6]

REFERENCES

1. Gole AW. *Accidental Poisoning* 2000s. London: Smith and Smith 2001.
2. Liebelt EL. Hyperbaric oxygen therapy in childhood carbon monoxide poisoning. Curr *Opinion Pediatr* 1999;11:259-264.
3. Waisman D, Shupak A, Weis ZG, Melamaid Y. Hyperbaric oxygen therapy in pediatric patients: The experience of the Israel Naval Medical Institute. *Pediatrics* 1998;102:653-658.
4. Meyers RA, Linberg SE, Cowley RA. Carbon monoxide poisoning: The injury and its treatment. *J Am Coll Emerg Physicians* 1979;8:479-488.
5. White SR. Pediatric carbon monoxide poisoning. In: Penney DG (ed) *Carbon Monoxide Toxicity.* New York: CRC Press 2000;463-491.
6. Weaver LK, Hopkins RO, Chan KJ. Carbon monoxide poisoning. *N Engl J Med* 2002;347:1057-1067.

Suraj Gupte

76 Aluminium Phosphide Poisoning

INTRODUCTION

Aluminium phosphide, a powerful rodenticide and pesticide, employed as grain preservative, causes its toxicity by releasing phosphine and carbon monoxide gases on coming in contact with the gastric juice.[1,2] The gases produce disturbances in activities of various body enzymes.

It is available as tablets (brand names Quickphos, Phosphotek, Phostoxin, Alphos, Celphos, Fumigran). Its easy availability contributes to its accidental ingestion by young children. The aforesaid trade preparations contain 56% of active ingredient. Ingestion of a part of the tablet is good enough to cause serious toxicity.

Its symptomatology closely resembles that of zinc phosphide.[3]

CLINICAL MANIFESTATIONS

Aluminium phosphide involves by and large all systems. Foul (decaying fish-like) smell is characteristic.

GIT manifestations include nausea, vomiting, diarrhea, epigastric pain and polydispsia.

Liver may be enlarged but overt icterus is infrequent.

Respiratory manifestations include cough and dyspnoea and ARDS.

Cardiovascular manifestations include hypotension, arrhythmias, myocardial ischemia, myocarditis, pericarditis and CCF.

Renal manifestations include oliguric and nonoliguric renal failure.

Neurologic manifestations include restlessness, anxiety, seizures and coma.

DIAGNOSIS

It is based on:

- History of ingestion
- Characteristic foul smell
- Metabolic acidosis
- *Confirmatory test:* Analysis of blood or gastric fluid for phosphine gas.

MANAGEMENT

Treatment is more or less supportive and symptomatic. No specific antidote is available.

Decontamination

- Gastric lavage with potassium permanganate ($KMnO_4$).
- Activated charcoal administration.
- Cathartics for evacuation of gut.
- IV magnesium sulfate, 200 mg/kg every 4-6 hours reduces organ toxicity.

Supportive

- Oxygen for treating hypoxia.
- Judicious use of IV fluids and vasopressors for combating shock.
- Magnesium sulfate for arrhythmias.
- Sodium bicarbonate for metabolic acidosis.
- Appropriate measures for ARDS.

PROGNOSIS

Mortality depends on:

- Dose of aluminium phosphide consumed by the child, and
- Lag period between ingestion and institution of treatment.

Since after one hour of ingestion, considerable toxicity is already developed, mortality in this poisoning is usually very high.

Cardiac toxicity leading to peripheral circulatory failure is the dominant cause of death.

REFERENCES

1. Parikh CK. *Parikh's Textbook of Medical Jurisprudence, Forensic Medicine and Toxicology,* 6th edn. New Delhi: CBS 1999.
2. Roy E. Less-known pediatric poisonings. *Curr Trends Med* 2002;6:234-239.
3. Roy E, Boyd AS. Aluminium phosphide and aluminium phosphide poisoning in children. *Curr Trends Med* 2004;8:453-454.

B Vishnu Bhat and Prajnya Shenoy

77 Iron Poisoning

INTRODUCTION

Iron is one of the essential nutrients required for the normal growth and development of the human body, being an important component or cofactor of many critical proteins and enzymes.[1] However, when taken in excess, it can lead to a number of harmful effects and lethal complications. Most cases of iron poisoning occur due to an overdose of preparations which are used for supplemental therapy in cases of iron deficiency. The more commonly available preparations include ferrous sulphate, ferrous gluconate and ferrous fumarate, each containing different amounts of elemental iron–ranging from 12–33%.[2] Rarely, the source of the toxic iron may be tanning, inks, dyes and pigments. Poisoning is more often accidental, especially so in children who are attracted to the iron preparations which are available in bright colored and pleasant flavored forms. Poisoning may sometimes be suicidal in older children and adults.

Iron poisoning occurs when the serum iron exceeds the total iron binding capacity (TIBC) resulting in free circulating iron in the blood stream. Elemental iron less than 20 mg/kg is unlikely to be toxic to the body, 20-60 mg/kg leads to mild toxicity, > 60 mg/kg causes moderate to severe toxicity and > 200 mg/kg leads to lethal complications.[3]

CLINICAL MANIFESTATIONS

Clinical manifestations of iron poisoning can be divided into the following four stages:[4]

a. *Stage I:* It occurs 30 minutes to 6 hours postingestion. Features are mostly due to the direct effect of iron on the gastric and small intestine mucosa. These include vomiting, diarrhea, abdominal pain, gastrointestinal hemorrhage, hypotension, pallor and lethargy.
b. *Stage II:* It occurs 6 to 24 hours postingestion. Patient may have mild acidosis, hypotension, oliguria and hyperventilation, but on the whole seems to show an apparent improvement.
c. *Stage III:* It occurs 24-48 hours up to few days after ingestion. Patient develops multi-organ dysfunction involving gastrointestinal, hepatorenal, neurological and cardiovascular systems with coagulopathy, hypoglycemia, convulsions, disorientation, coma and death from hepatic failure.
d. *Stage IV:* It occurs 2-6 weeks after ingestion. It includes complications such as gastric scarring and pyloric obstruction following corrosion of the gastric mucosa.

INVESTIGATIONS

I. *Tests for Estimation of Iron*
   a. *Abdominal Radiograph*: If the history or physical examination suggests the possibility of significant exposure, an X-ray of the abdomen is useful. Presence of a large number of pills on X-ray confirms the exposure and suggests the need for GI decontamination and treatment. Absence of radiological evidence may be reassuring in the setting of minimum clinical features, but does not eliminate the possibility of exposure.[5]
   b. *Serum Iron Level Estimation*: This should ideally be measured between 2 and 6 hours after ingestion.[6] Levels of iron beyond 8 hours after ingestion are misleading because some of the iron becomes intracellular by then. Serum levels of 350-500 mg/dL indicate mild toxicity and > 500 mg/dL indicate severe toxicity.
   c. *Desferrioxamine Challenge Test*: Desferrioxamine is given as an intramuscular injection in a dose of 25 mg/kg. The excess iron chelates to this and the complex is excreted in the urine imparting a reddish 'vin rose' colour to the urine. A negative result does not rule out iron poisoning.[7]
   d. *Qualitative Desferrioxamine Color Test:* Two ml of gastric aspirate is mixed with 2 drops of 30 % hydrogen peroxide in two tubes. Desferrioxamine solution (0.5 ml) is added to one of the tubes and

the colour change is compared with the other control tube. Appearance of an orange to red colour in the test tube indicates a positive test. This test must be performed within 2 hours of the ingestion.[7]

II. *Other Tests in Severe Poisoning*

The following laboratory parameters should be measured at admission and also monitored subsequently:

- Complete Blood count,
- Hemoglobin and hematocrit,
- Blood glucose,
- Serum electrolytes,
- Blood urea nitrogen,
- Liver function tests, and
- Arterial blood gas analysis.

In addition blood grouping and cross matching should be done, in case the need for transfusion of blood products should arise.

MANAGEMENT

Initial Stabilization of the Patient

Airway, breathing and circulatory compromise should be looked for and appropriate airway management and ventilatory support, when required, should be instituted.

Fluid Resuscitation

Most patients with significant intoxication will have some GI fluid losses and will be in at least early stages of shock. Intravenous access should be established immediately at admission. If in shock, a bolus of normal saline (0.9%) should be given followed by continuous infusion of maintenance fluids. If the shock does not get corrected with fluid replacement inotropic support with dopamine may be required. If the blood loss has been significant and patient has marked pallor, whole blood transfusion in a dose of 20 ml/kg is ideal.

Supportive Therapy

Correction of hypoglycemia with dextrose and acidosis with sodium bicarbonate infusion should be done.

Gastric Decontamination

Any patient with significant exposure should have lavage/whole bowel irrigation with normal saline or polyethylene glycol–electrolyte solution at a rate of 0.5 L/hr.[8] After the lavage, 1% solution of sodium bicarbonate or magnesium hydroxide should be added to precipitate the residual iron as insoluble ferrous carbonate or ferrous hydroxide and thereby decrease absorption. Though advocated previously, the use of oral desferrioxamine and addition of desferrioxamine in the lavage fluid has now been abandoned

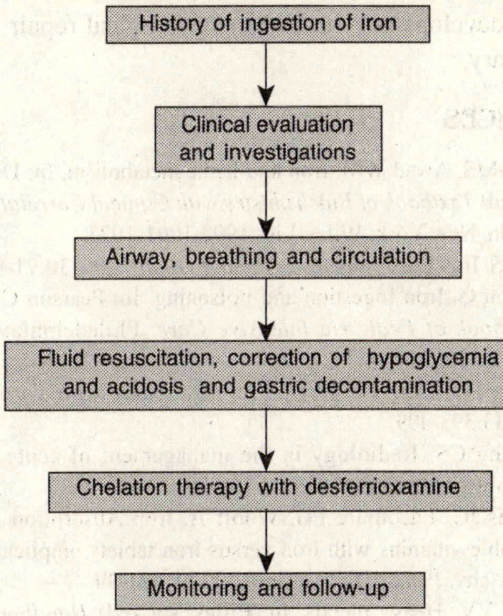

Fig. 77.1: Algorithm for management

because experimental studies have shown that it does not significantly decrease the absorption of iron from the gut.[9] There is no role for activated charcoal in the decontamination because it cannot adsorb metals.

An abdominal radiograph should be taken to assess the efficacy of the decontamination procedures. Sometimes, following a large dose, if a conglomerate of pills forms in the stomach and does not get dislodged with the irrigation measures, removal by gastroscopy or even gastrostomy may become necessary, to prevent hemorrhagic infarction and perforation of the gut.[10]

Chelation Therapy

Desferrioxamine therapy should be initiated in the presence of shock, lethargy, altered mental status, persistent vomiting or diarrhea, hematemesis, metabolic acidosis and when serum iron level is > 350 mg/dL.

The recommended dose for desferrioxamine is 15 mg/kg per hour as continuous infusion to a maximum of 6 g. The most important side effect of desferrioxamine is hypotension and, therefore, careful blood pressure monitoring has to be done. Chelation therapy should be continued till there is a significant resolution of systemic toxicity, especially acidosis and shock. Some centers prefer to continue the infusion for 12–24 hours after the resolution of the vin rose color of urine.[2,3]

Other Modalities

Fulminant hepatic failure not responding to medical management may require emergency liver transplant. In infants, exchange transfusion has been tried to reduce the free iron levels in the blood.

After discharge, the patient has to be followed up for at least upto 2 months to monitor for gastrointestinal scarring.

If patient develops any such scarring, surgical repair may be necessary.

REFERENCES

1. Wells MS, Awad WM. Iron and heme metabolism. In: Devlin TM (ed) *Textbook of Biochemistry with Clinical Correlations*, 3rd edn. New York: Wiley-Liss 1992;1001-1023.
2. Fine JS. Iron Poisoning. *Curr Probl Pediatr* 2000; 30:71-90.
3. Pearson G. Iron Ingestion and poisoning. In: Pearson G (ed) *Handbook of Pediatric Intensive Care.* Philadelphia: WB Saunders 2002;310-311.
4. Banner JW, Tong TG. Iron poisoning. *Pediatr Clin North Am* 1986;33:393-409.
5. Hosking CS. Radiology in the management of acute iron poisoning. *Med J Aust* 1969;1:576-579.
6. Linakis JG, Lacouture PG, Woolf A. Iron Absorption from chewable vitamins with iron versus iron tablets: implications for toxicity. *Pediatr Emerg Care* 1992;8:321-34.
7. Pillay VV. Heavy metals. In: Pillay VV (ed) *Handbook of Forensic Medicine and Toxicology,* 13th edn. Hyderabad: Paras 2003;359-361.
8. Tenenbein M. Whole bowel irrigation in iron poisoning. *J Pediatr* 1987;111:142-145.
9. Henretig FM, Karl SR, Weintraub WH. Severe iron poisoning treated with enteral and intravenous deferoxamine. *Ann Emerg Med* 1983;12:306-309.
10. Venturelli J, Kwee Y, Morris N, Cameron G. Gastrostomy in the management of acute iron poisoning. *J Pediatr* 1982;100:768-769.
11. Devlin TM. *Textbook of Biochemistry with Clinical Correlations,* 3rd edn. New York: Wiley-Liss 1992.
12. Fine JS. Iron poisoning. *Curr Probl Pediatr* 2000;30:71-90.
13. Pearson G. Iron ingestion and poisoning. In: *Handbook of Pediatric Intensive Care*. Philadelphia: WB Saunders 2002; 310-311.
14. Banner JW, Tong TG. Iron poisoning. *Pediatr Clin North Am* 1986;33:393-409.
15. Hosking CS. Radiology in the management of acute iron poisoning. *Med J Aust* 1969;1:576-579.
16. Linakis JG, Lacouture PG, Woolf A. Iron absorption from chewable vitamins with iron versus iron tablets: Implications for toxicity. *Pediatr Emerg Care* 1992;8:321-324.
17. Pillay VV. Heavy metals. In: Pillay VV (ed) *Handbook of Forensic Medicine and Toxicology,* 13th edn. Hyderabad: Paras 2003;359-361.
18. Tenenbein M. Whole bowel irrigation in iron poisoning. *J Pediatr* 1987;111:142-145.
19. Henretig FM, Karl SR, Weintraub WH. Severe iron poisoning treated with enteral and intravenous deferoxamine. *Ann Emerg Med* 1983;12:306-309.
20. Venturelli J, Kwee Y, Morris N, Cameron G. Gastrostomy in the management of acute iron poisoning. *J Pediatr* 1982; 100:768-759.

Accidental Poisoning

Suraj Gupte and O Lee

78 Lead Poisoning

INTRODUCTION

Though the metal, lead, has no beneficial role for the human body, its widespread dissemination in environments poses a constant risk of lead poisoning for the man.

In infants and children known for non-nutritive hand-to-mouth activity, lead poisoning usually occurs when they suffer from pica involving ingestion of lead paint flakes, artist's paints, etc, from inhalation of fumes from batteries and from practice of employing kajal or surma containing black oxide of lead in eyes.[1]

Lead poisoning in children may be acute, chronic or subclinical.

PATHOPHYSIOLOGY

Lead causes toxicity by disturbing the oxidative phosphorylation of the mitochondria. Erythroid precursors, renal tubular cells and cells of central and peripheral nervous system are principally involved.

Three mechanisms are supposed to operate in lead toxicity:

1. *By binding to RBCs (97%) and the plasma fraction (3%) entering cells and inducing toxicity.* Accumulation of protoporphyrin results. A level > 35 mcg/dL is consistent with lead poisoning provided that iron-deficiency anemia (IDD) and recent inflammatory disease are excluded. This effect may be reversible.
2. *By competition with calcium.* Many calcium-binding proteins are known to have greater affinity for lead. Once lead gets bound to these proteins, altered function may cause intracellular and intercellular communication breakdown. Adverse effect on neuromuscular release by lead toxicity is an important example in this behalf. This effect too may be reversible.
3. *By preventing development of normal tertiary structure in brain.* This causes a permanent abnormality when lead toxicity occurs during first few years of life.

CLINICAL MANIFESTATIONS

Manifestations are mainly in relation to three systems, namely *erythrocytes*, kidneys and central and peripheral nervous system.

These include transient abdominal pain, resistant anemia, loss of weight, irritability, vomiting, constipation, headache, personality changes, peripheral neuropathy and ataxia. A blue-black lead-line over the gums (not teeth) is characteristic. Physical development is poor.

Reversible renal tubular disorder (Fanconi-like) may occur.

Cognitive and behavioral problems may also occur depending on blood lead level (BLL). Hyperactivity and aggressiveness may be precursors of juvenile delinquency later in life.[5]

Seizures and raised intracranial pressure (RICP) with papilledema and even coma ("acute encephalopathy") are rather late manifestations.

Subclinical lead poisoning occurs in relatively low-dose exposure to lead. Harmful effects in the form of poor biosynthesis of heme, slow nerve conduction and poor excretion of uric acid occur but are usually not evident clinically.

DIAGNOSIS

The probability of lead poisoning should be actively entertained in the situations enumerated in Table 78.1.

In addition to the clues given by the clinical picture, the following investigations should be done:

- Urine lead level of > 80 mcg/dL/24 hrs is diagnostic.
- Blood lead level (BLL) in symptomatic cases usually exceeds 80 mcg/dL. However, it is now known that as low a level as 10 mcg/dl may be harmful. Ideally, normal BLL should be zero.
- Urinary coproporphyrin or red cell aminolevulinic acid dehydrase levels are also good screening tests.
- Peripheral blood film shows normocytic-hypochromic anemia with reticulocytosis and basophilic stippling of RBCs.

Table 78.1: Situations in which lead poisoning should be suspected

• Hypochromic-microcytic anemia resistant to iron therapy
• Pica
• Recurrent abdominal pain
• Recurrent seizures not responding to appropriate anticonvulsant therapy
• Blue-black lead-line over gums
• Wrist and foot drop
• Regression of milestones after 12-18 months age
• Abnormal behavior of recent origin
• Unexplained altered sensorium with raised intracranial pressure

- X-rays may reveal opaque flakes in the GIT and areas of excessive mineralization or calcification (called "lead lines" although these are not because of deposition of lead) at the metaphyseal areas of bony skeleton.
- Measurement of skeletal lead by X-ray fluorescence.
- Nerve conduction velocity test (NCVT) assists in documenting lead-related peripheral neuropathy.
- Calcium sodium EDTA ($CaNa_2$ EDTA) challenge test. After administration of $CANa_2$ EDTA (IV), urinary excretion of lead in measured in an 8-hour urine sample. Lead excreted/CaNaEDTA ratio of over 0.6 is considered a positive test.
- CSF pressure, proteins and cell count are moderately high.

MANAGEMENT

Decontamination

Total removal of the source of lead exposure is very important and, very often, the only action warranted.

Chelation Therapy

Recommendations in this behalf are listed in Table 78.2.[3,4]

Table 78.2: Recommendations regarding chelation therapy in lead poisoning

Symptomatic Children and Children with Blood Level > 70 mcg/dl
BAL 75 mg/m² every 4 hourly IM
Followed 3-4 hours later by
$CaNa_2$EDTA 1500 mg/m²/day slow IV infusion
Asymptomatic Children with Blood Level 45-69 mcg/dl
$CaNa_2$ EDTA (as above) or by IM route
or
DMSA 350 mg/m² every 8 hourly followed by 2 weeks of therapy every 12 hourly for 19 days in toto.
Symptomatic Children with Blood Level 20-45 mcg/dl
Ca Na $_2$ EDTA or DMSA (as above) after $CaNa_2$EDTA challenge test has turned out to be positive.
Note: In case of unacceptable reactions to DMSA and $CaNa_2$ EDTA and necessity of continued therapy, D-penicillamine may be used (20-30 mg/kg/day for 4-12 weeks) provided that the subject is not allergic to penicillin.

In case of lead encephalopathy, chelation therapy should be supplemented by anticonvulsant agent(s), IV mannitol and dexamethasone for raised ICP and other supportive measures.

REFERENCES

1. Gupte S, Kaushal RK. Pediatric accidental poisoning. In: Gupte S (ed) *The Short Textbook of Pediatrics*, 10th edn. New Delhi: Jaypee Brothers 2004;538-552.
2. Markowitz M. Lead poisoning. In: Behrman RE, Kliegman RM, Jenson HB (eds) *Nelson Textbook of Pediatrics*, 17th edn. Philadelphia: Saunders 2004; 2358-2362.
3. Anonymous. *Preventing Lead Poisoning in Young Children.* Atlanta: Center for Disease Control 1991.
4. Dart RC, Rumack BH. Poisoning. In: Hay WW Jr, Hayward AR, Levin MJ, Sondheimer JM (eds) *Current Pediatric Diagnosis and Treatment 16th edn.* New York: Lange/McGraw-Hill +2003;336- 361.
5. Lanphear BP, Dietrich K, Auinger P. Cognitive deficits associated with blood lead concentrations < 10 mcg/dL in US children and adolescents. *Public Health Rep* 2000;115:521-529.

RK Kaushal

79 Mercury Poisoning

INTRODUCTION

Mercury poisoning still occurs in children because of its widespread use in industry and agriculture.[1-3] It is also a professional hazard for goldsmiths and those dealing with gold and silver ornaments. Mercury vapor poisoning has been reported in family members including children of goldsmiths extracting gold by heating amalgam of gold–mercury.

Mercury exists in three states: elemental mercury (HgO), inorganic mercury salts ($Hg1^+$, $Hg2^+$) and organic mercury (methyl mercury (CH_3 Hg^-). Elemental mercury is present in thermometers, sphygmomanometers, and barometers as liquid metal. It is nontoxic if ingested (absorption < 0.01%) but in vapor form it is completely absorbed from distal airways.

Inorganic mercury salts are found in fungicides, pesticides, disinfectants, antiseptics, pigments and dry batteries, is absorbed from gut to the extent of 10% and excreted mainly in the urine. Inorganic mercurials are corrosive to the GI tract.

Organic mercury in the diet especially fish containing methyl mercury, is a major source of chronic mercury exposure to the general population.

Mercury compounds in the environment derived from industrial waste/effluents are methylated by the soil and water micro–organism. Methyl mercury in the water rapidly acummulates in fish. Methyl mercury is absorbed from the gut to the extent of 90% and exerted mainly in the bile.

Mercury after absorption is distributed in all the tissues. Mercury ion has high affinity for sulfhydryl groups present in enzymes and other tissue proteins, disrupting cellular functions and resulting in multiorgan toxicity.

CLINICAL FEATURES

Acute Mercury Poisoning

It can result from inhalation of high concentration of elemental mercury vapors or acute ingestion of inorganic mercury salts. The inhaled mercury vapors cause an exudative alveolar and interstitial edema, erosion and desquamation of epithelium. The ensuing obstruction is proportionately greater in infants and young children. There is rapid onset of cough, dyspnea, chest pain, fever, chills, nausea and vomiting, diarrhea, acute renal failure, hepatocellular dysfunction, irritability, delirium, seizures, ataxia and visual disturbances. Acute ingestion produces corrosive gastroenteritis presenting within a few hours with nausea, oropharyngeal burns, severe abdominal pain, hematemesis, bloody diarrhea, cardiovascular collapse and acute tubular necrosis.

Chronic Poisoning

It is characterized predominantly by CNS and skin manifestations. Chronic inorganic mercury intoxication produces the classic triad of tremor, neuropsychiatric abnormalities and gingivostomatitis. Renal involvement may be in the form of asymptomatic proteinuria to nephrotic syndrome.

Acrodynia (Pink disease) occurs mostly in children due to idiosyncratic hypersensitivity reaction to repeated ingestions or contact with mercury.[3] Extreme hypotonia, phtophobia, acral rash which is pinkish, papular, pruritic and painful, marked dejection and melancholia are its outstanding features.

Minamata disease is another form of chronic mercury intoxication (methyl mercury) caused by eating contaminated fish and shellfish. Manifestations include disturbances in hand co–ordination, gait and speech, chewing and swallowing difficulties, visual blurring, tremors, rigidity, seizures and clouding of consciousness.

Infants exposed *in utero* are the most severely affected with low birth weight, microcephaly, profound mental retardation, abnormal movements, deafness, blindness and seizures.

LABORATORY FINDINGS

The diagnosis is based on characteristic clinical features, history suggestive of exposure and elevated blood or urine levels of mercury. Levels < 2 mg/L in the blood and < 10 mg/L in 24 hour urine are considered normal.

X-ray chest in inhalation injury is helpful in knowing the extent and follow up of the pulmonary lesions.

X-ray abdomen may reveal ingested mercury.

Proteinuria of varying grades suggest renal dysfunction.

MANAGEMENT

Principles of management include prompt removal from source of poisoning, aggressive stabilization of vitals and supportive care, decontamination and chelation therapy.

In acute inhalation intoxication, careful monitoring of respiratory status administration of IV fluids, oxygen and prophylactic antibiotics are the mainstay of treatment.

After acute oral exposure treatment consists of removal of mercury from stomach by gastric lavage with normal saline. Correction of fluid and electrolyte imbalance, peritoneal or haemodialysis for acute renal failure, hydroxyzine and chlorpromazine may be useful for restlessness. Whole bowel irrigation may be used to remove any radiopaque material remaining in the GT tract.

British antilewisite (BAL) or dimercaprol is the chelator of choice.[4] It is an oily preparation administered intramuscularly, given in a dose of 5 mg/kg for first injection and 3 mg/kg every four hourly for 2 days, then tapered to every six hourly for one day and then every 12 hourly for seven days. It protects kidneys if given within 3 hours of ingestion.

If BAL is not available, D–penicillamine, an oral chelator, can be used in a dose of 100 mg/kg in 4 divided doses to a maximum of 1000 mg daily for upto 1–2 weeks.

Succimer (DMSA) is another orally administered water–soluble derivative of BAL, which can be used for chelation in the dose of 30 mg/kg divided in 3 daily doses for first 5 days followed by 20 mg/kg in two divided doses for next 2 weeks. A gap of 1-2 weeks between courses of chelation is recommended.

Besides this, symptomatic treatment in the form of anticonvulsants and good nourishing diet should be used. The CNS damage being irreversible, survivors need rehabilitation and long–term care.

REFERENCES

1. Gote CS. Heavy metal poisoning. In; Behrman RE, Kliegman RM, Jenson HB (eds) *Nelson Textbook of Pediatics*, 16th edn. Philadelphia: WB Saunders 2000;2154-2156.
2. Soni JP, Singhania RV, Bansal A, Rathi G. Acute mercury vapor poisoning. *Indian Pediatr* 1992;29: 365-369.
3. Gupte S, Kaushal RK. Pediatric accidental posisoning. In: Gupte S (ed) *The Short Textbook of Pediatrics*, 10th edn. New Delhi: Jaypee Brothers 2004;539-548.
4. Boyer M, Lasek RW. Heavy metals. In: Reisdroff EJ, Roberts MR, Wiegenstein JG (eds) *Pediatric Emergency Medicine*, 9th edn. Philadelphia: WB Saunders 1993;757-758.

Accidental Poisoning

Bhadresh Vyas

80 Barbiturate Poisoning/Toxicity

INTRODUCTION

Barbiturates are a class of organic compounds that were developed in the late 19th century for the treatment of anxiety and insomnia. Barbiturates are used mainly as intravenous (IV) anesthetics, as anticonvulsants, and in the resuscitation of patients with cerebral injuries. Barbiturates also are used commonly in combination with other substances for the treatment of gastrointestinal illness and migraine.

CLASSIFICATION (ON BASIS OF DURATION) AND LETHAL DOSE[1]

Ultra short-acting barbiturates (e.g., thiopental, thiamylal, methohexital) are highly lipid soluble and penetrate the CNS within minutes of an IV injection. Their effects generally last less than 30 minutes; these agents are used mainly for the induction of anesthesia. *Fatal doses* are around 1 g.[2]

Short-acting barbiturates (e.g., secobarbital, pentobarbital) cross the blood-brain barrier and affect the CNS within 10-15 minutes of ingestion. Their effects generally last 3 hours. Traditionally, they have been prescribed as sedative-hypnotics, but their abuse potential precludes their use as first-line agents. **Fatal doses** range from 1-2 g.[2]

Intermediate-acting barbiturates (e.g., amobarbital, butalbital, butabarbital, aprobarbital) cross the blood-brain barrier and affect the CNS within 30-60 minutes of ingestion. Their effects generally last as long as 6 hours. These barbiturates traditionally were prescribed as sedative-hypnotics, but their abuse potential precludes their use as first-line agents. *Fatal doses* range from 2-3 g.[2]

Long-acting barbiturates (e.g., phenobarbital, mephobarbital) are much less lipid soluble, have virtually no acute mood-altering effects, and have the least potential for abuse. They are used mainly as anticonvulsants, and their effects last as long as 12 hours. *Fatal doses* range from 3-4 g.

PATHOPHYSIOLOGY

Barbiturates suppress the activity of all excitable tissue, including the CNS, the peripheral nervous system, and the cardiovascular system. They also depress gastrointestinal function and have a number of effects on hepatic function. Their effects on the respiratory system are due mainly to CNS inhibition. Their effects on GABA result in prolongation of the duration of opening of GABA-gated chloride channels,[3] leading to hyperpolarization of the membrane and suppression of neurotransmission.

HISTORY

In massive overdoses, patients present with coma accompanied by cardiorespiratory collapse and are unable to provide their history. Other substances often are used concomitantly. Every effort should be made to identify the ingested substance and the circumstances of ingestion. Search for corroborating evidence (e.g., empty bottles, pill count), patient's immediate history of present illness (e.g., the timing of presumed overdose, congestions, history of recent trauma.[4] Try to identify signs and symptoms immediately preceding the comatose state (e.g., fever, headache, slurred speech, ataxia, syncope, seizures, chest pain, palpitations, dyspnea, abdominal pain, vomiting, diarrhea, bleeding).

EXAMINATION

- Vital signs
  - *Temperature:* Hypothermia as low as 31°C often occurs and is due to depression of the thermoregulation center and reduced muscle activity.[5] Exposure to a cold environment may worsen the extent of the hypothermia.
  - *Pulse:* Bradycardia is due to depression of the sympathetic ganglia. Early in the course of barbiturate poisoning, the presence of coingestants or hypoxia may result in tachycardia.
  - *Respiration:* Bradypnea is due to depression of the neurogenic respiratory drive. At high doses, the hypoxic drive is eliminated, resulting in apnea. In the presence of hypoxia and acidosis, the patient may exhibit rapid, shallow breathing and Cheyne-Stokes respirations.
  - *Blood pressure:* Hypotension is due to vasodilation and direct myocardial depression, indicating a significant ingestion. Central nervous system: In the absence of coingestions and structural brain disease, barbiturates depress the CNS in a predictable manner.

Mild toxicity presents with disorders of mentation, slurred speech, loss of coordination, and ataxia.

Severe intoxication presents with stupor and additional neurologic dysfunction.

In massive overdoses, the patient becomes deeply comatose, hypotonic, and areflexic. The brainstem reflexes, including the corneal and oculovestibular reflexes, may be obliterated, and the electroencephalogram (EEG) may exhibit periods of electrical silence.

- Eyes
  - The ocular examination reveals nystagmus and a dysconjugate gaze.The pupils usually appear normal but may be small and reactive to light.
- Gastrointestinal system
  - Barbiturates reduce gastrointestinal muscle tone and peristaltic function, resulting in gastric dilatation with delayed gastric emptying and ileus with bowel distention. Bowel distention may become so severe as to cause bowel necrosis.
  - Physical examination findings include a succussion splash, decreased bowel sounds, and abdominal distention.
- Renal system
  - Barbiturate overdose may result in urinary retention. Poisoning with short-acting barbiturates may result in high output of dilute urine, much like diabetes insipidus.
  - Hemodynamic instability and shock may lead to acute tubular necrosis, which is manifested by azotemia, volume overload, hyperkalemia, and acidosis.
- Skin
  - Approximately 6% of patients with barbiturate poisoning and 50% of patients with lethal poisoning develop tense, clear, bullous skin lesions of unclear etiology.[6] These lesions commonly occur on the hands, knees, and buttocks within 24 hours of ingestion and heal very slowly.
  - The lesions are not specific to barbiturates and occur with other CNS depressant overdoses and with carbon monoxide poisoning.

INVESTIGATIONS

Barbiturate Levels

Blood levels may be obtained to confirm the diagnosis, but they are not reliable in predicting the severity of the overdose because they do not reflect brain concentrations accurately. This is due to a number of different factors, including protein binding, plasma pH, and liver function. Analysis of arterial blood gases determines the presence of acidosis, hypoxia, hypercarbia, and carboxyhemoglobin. The analysis of electrolytes and glucose determines the presence of disorders of glucose, sodium, and calcium, which may cause coma. Blood urea nitrogen and creatinine may be used in the differential diagnosis of coma and in monitoring renal complications of barbiturate poisoning. Urinalysis and urine pH may be useful in determining the presence of myoglobin, renal failure, and the monitoring of forced alkaline diuresis. Elevated plasma ammonia levels may suggest the presence of hepatic encephalopathy. Liver enzymes, prothrombin, and activated partial thromboplastin time aid in the diagnosis of liver disease, which may have significant impact on the metabolism of barbiturates. CBC may suggest an infectious etiology for coma or an infectious complication of barbiturate overdose.[7]

Chest X-ray

Radiographic evaluation of the chest in comatose patients may be invaluable in the diagnosis of bronchopneumonia, aspiration pneumonia, atelectasis, and ARDS.

CT Scan

A CT scan of the brain is indicated in all comatose patients with suspected trauma, stroke, hemorrhage, or mass lesion in the brain.

Electroencephalogram

- In massive barbiturate poisoning, the EEG may be isoelectric and unresponsive to all stimuli, simulating brain death. These abnormalities may last as long as 24-28 hours, and, in the absence of hypoxia, cortical necrosis and head injury are completely reversible.
- Because barbiturates and other sedative-hypnotics have predictable effects on the EEG, the pattern of EEG waves may be used to evaluate the depth of coma and the progress of patients in the intensive care unit. Seven EEG grades have been identified in barbiturate toxicity.
- The grading of barbiturate poisoning may be based on Matthew EEG findings (Table 80.1).

Table 80.1: Matthew EEG grades

Grade	Findings
Grade I	Alpha rhythm with beta waves and a few theta waves
Grade II	Predominant theta waves with some alpha, beta, and delta waves
Grade III	Predominant delta waves mixed with some theta waves
Grade IV	Delta waves with occasional isoelectric intervals
Grade V	Suppression alternating with burst activity of several seconds
Grade VI	Suppression with occasional burst activity of one half second
Grade VII	Isoelectric

MEDICAL CARE

The management of barbiturate poisoning cases is supportive. Airway protection, cardiovascular support, and the immediate identification and treatment of correctable metabolic and structural abnormalities have a great impact on patient survival. Once the patient is stabilized, gut decontamination and elimination enhancement are performed.

Airway Support

- Patients with barbiturate poisoning exhibit severe CNS depression with loss of airway protective reflexes and a 40% risk of aspiration pneumonia. Assessment and stabilization of the airway must be performed early in the course of poisoning, and mechanical ventilation with oxygenation must be provided immediately.
- Positive pressure ventilation should be used with caution and only when necessary to maintain adequate oxygenation because barbiturates impair reflex cardiovascular adjustments to inflation of the lungs.

Cardiovascular Support

- Hypotension, which is due to vasodilation and direct myocardial depressant effects, responds to crystalloid bolus infusions and rarely requires vasopressors.
- When adequate crystalloid solution have been infused and the patient remains hypotensive, vasopressors (e.g., dopamine, norepinephrine) may be initiated, and a search for other causes of shock must be conducted.

Decontamination and Elimination

- Once the patient is stabilized, drug removal is performed. Orogastric intubation and lavage are indicated for life-threatening overdoses that present soon after ingestion and those that are symptomatic.
- Activated charcoal, which is emerging as the most effective decontamination procedure for most substances, is indicated for barbiturates, and the use of multiple doses of activated charcoal has been advocated for life-threatening phenobarbital overdoses.
- Elimination of the weakly acidic barbiturates that have poor lipid solubility (e.g., phenobarbital [pKa 7.2]) may be enhanced through alkalinization of the urine. The alkaline medium increases the ionization of the drug and decreases its permeability, thereby enhancing its urinary excretion.
- Multidose activated charcoal may be better than forced alkaline diuresis. For example, the elimination half-life of phenobarbital may be reduced from 148 to 19 hours with multidose activated charcoal, whereas alkaline diuresis only reduces it to 47 hours.
- Gut decontamination: The value of gastric lavage in the setting of overdose has recently been questioned, especially in cases of delayed presentations. However, lavage may be indicated for acute, life-threatening, massive overdoses and for drugs that reduce gastrointestinal motility. Orogastric lavage should be performed only in patients with protected airways.

Elimination Enhancement

- *Activated charcoal:* In general, barbiturates adsorb well to activated charcoal. Their enterohepatic recirculation may be reduced substantially when multiple doses of activated charcoal are administered 2-4 hours apart.
- *Forced alkaline diuresis*
  - Phenobarbital is a long-acting barbiturate with a pKa of 7.2 and a half-life of 96 ±12 hours. This agent is absorbed slowly from the gastrointestinal tract and is eliminated slowly from the blood. While most of an ingested dose undergoes hepatic metabolism, as much as 30% may be excreted unchanged in the urine. In severe poisoning, coma may persist for 72 hours. Because of its pKa, alkalinization of the pH ionizes most of the phenobarbital and enhances its urinary excretion.
  - Forced alkaline diuresis may be achieved by adding 2-3 ampules of sodium bicarbonate (44.6 mEq per ampule) to 1 L of dextrose 5% in water solution (D5W). The rate of infusion, started at 30 ml/kg/h, is guided by urinary pH, which should be maintained between 7.5 and 8. Potassium replacement becomes of utmost importance in this setting because hypokalemia promotes bicarbonate ion retention and prevents bicarbonate excretion, thereby interfering with alkalinization of the urine.
- *Extracorporeal drug removal:* Hemodialysis or hemoperfusion is indicated for phenobarbital poisoning in the presence of renal failure with anuria (precluding the use of forced diuresis) and shock with ileus (precluding the use of multidose activated charcoal). This method of elimination enhancement has no role in poisonings with short-acting barbiturates.

Other Measures

- Hypothermia may be treated with passive rewarming and continuous monitoring of the temperature. Patients rarely may require active rewarming maneuvers.
- Complications of barbiturate poisoning and complications of therapy must be monitored continuously.

REFERENCES

1. Coupey SM. Barbiturates. *Pediatr Rev* 1997;18:260-264.
2. Singh UK, Layland FC, Suman S, Prasad R. *Poisoning in Children* New Delhi: Jaypee Brothers 1998.
3. Amitai Y, Degani Y. Treatment of phenobarbital poisoning with multiple dose activated charcoal in an infant. *J Emerg Med* 1990;8:449-450.
4. de Boer WB, Kendall PA, Breheny FX. Alpha coma and barbiturate poisoning. *Anaesth Intensive Care* 1989;17:503-504.
5. Pond SM, Olson KR, Osterloh JD, Tong TG. Randomized study of the treatment of phenobarbital overdose with repeated doses of activated charcoal. *JAMA* 1984;251:3104-3108.
6. Ellenhorn MJ. Sedative-hypnotic drugs. In: *Ellenhorn's Medical Toxicology.* Philadelphia: Lippincott, Williams and Wilkins 1997;684-687.
7. Bertino JS, Reed MD. Barbiturate and nonbarbiturate sedative hypnotic intoxication in children. *Pediatr Clin North Am* 1986;33:703-22.

Praveen C Sobti and Gautam Biswas

81 Phenothiazine Poisoning/Toxicity

INTRODUCTION

Drugs are the most frequent cause of acute poisoning in children and mostly involve children less than 6 years of age.[1-6] In a data collected from eight hospitals in India, Dutta *et al.*[7] found a very high incidence of toxicity due to drugs/medicine intake: New Delhi 66.8% of all poisoning cases admitted, Punjab 41.6% and Shimla 35%. The commonest group of drugs involved was phenothiazines followed by antipyretics, anti-epileptics and iron preparations.

Phenothiazines have been widely used for their antiemetic, antipsychotic sedative properties for many years. In pediatric practice, phenothiazines are used for anxiety, tension, difficulty in concentration, sleep disturbance, and behavioral disorders such as agitation, hyperactivity or aggressiveness.

Phenothiazines arc classified into three groups (Table 81.1).

Table 81.1: Classification of phenothiazines

Group	*Example*
	Aliphatic Chlorpromazine
	Trifliupromazine
Piperazine	Trifluoperazine
	Prochlorperazine
	Perphenazine
	Fluphenazine
Piperidine	Thioridazine
	Mesoridazine

TOXICOKINETICS

Phenothiazines are completely absorbed from the GI tract. The average systemic bioavailability is approximately 60%. The relative distribution volume is about 10l/kg and protein binding is high i.e. more than 95%. Excretion is mainly *via* feces (50%) but also *via* the kidneys (30%) as metabolites; less than 4% is excreted in the unchanged form. Plasma elimination half-life is approximately 10 hours. Toxic and potentially fatal dose is between 15-150 mg/kg depending on the agent ingested. Peak plasma levels are attained within 2-4 hours of oral ingestion. Cardiovascular toxicity peaks in 10-15 hours and dystonic reactions occur from 5-18 hours to 72 hours after ingestion.

MECHANISM OF ACTION

The phenothiazines have inhibitory effects on a variety of receptors, including dopaminergic, cholinergic, alpha$_1$ and alpha$_2$-adrenergic, histaminic and serotonergic receptors ($5HT_2$). The dopamine-receptor blocking activity in the limbic system is thought to account for their neuroleptic activity, and the anti-psychotic activity is probably mediated through serotonergic receptors. There are six distinct dopamine receptor subtypes: D_1, D_{2A}, D_{2B}, D_4, and D_5. Most clinically effective neuroleptic agents have a high affinity for D_2 and D_3 receptors. Phenothiazines bind with high affinity to D_1 and D_2 receptors and D_3 and D_4 receptor subtypes. They also depress the release of hypothalamic and hypophyseal hormones. The thioxanthenes are derivatives of the phenothiazine. The thioxanthenes and the butyrophenones (such as haloperidol) are similar pharmacologically to the phenothiazines. Most neuroleptics are considered safe even when taken in significantly high doses. Deaths are rare and most frequently associated with thioridazine and mesoridazine overdosage.

SIGNS AND SYMPTOMS

Depressed levels of consciousness and dystonia were the most common presenting signs (90.7% and 51.2%, respectively) found by James *et al.*[4] Mild poisoning was characterized by somnolence, tremor, ataxia and dysarthria. Severe intoxication presented with coma and ventricular arrhythmias in a study done by Schurch *et al.*[8] The most frequent features seen by Le Blaye *et al.*[9] in a review of 227 cases of thioridazine poisoning were impairment of consciousness and arrhythmia.

Toxic manifestations can be divided into CNS and non-CNS effects.[10-15]

Non-CNS Effects

- *Cardiovascular*—orthostatic hypotension, ventricular tachycardia, torsades de pointes (ventricular tachycardia in which QRS morphology twists around the baseline), ventricular fibrillation, atrioventricular block
- *Gastrointestinal*—dry mouth, decreased colonic motility resulting in constipation, pseudo-obstruction
- *Ocular*—mydriasis, visual acuity, visual fields and color vision perception may be altered
- *Genitourinary*—urinary retention, priapism
- *Hematologic*—agranulocytosis, aplastic anemia, leukopenia, eosinophilia, thrombocytopenia, anemia, pancytopenia
- *Hepatic*—cholestatic jaundice.

CNS Effects

- Depression, agitation, seizures, somnolence and coma.
- Behavioral reactions—oversedation, impaired psychomotor function, paradoxical effects such as agitation, excitement, insomnia, bizarre dreams, toxic confusional states.
- Extrapyramidal signs manifest with a wide variety of presentation and with a 00000000 duration of onset lasting from one day to several weeks (Table 81.2).

Table 81.2: Extrapyramidal signs and symptoms of phenothiazine toxicity

Presentation	*Time of onset*	*Signs and symptoms*
Dystonia (acute)	1-5 days	Oculogyric crisis Torticollis Retrocollis Opisthotonuos Tortipelvis Laryngeal dystonia Jaw, tongue, lip and throat spasms Buccolingual grimacing Hyperthermia (rarely)
Akathisia	5-60 days	Muscular discomfort Restlessness Inability to sit still
Parkinsonism (akinesia)	5-30 days	Bradykinesia Shuffling gait Resting tremor Rigidity Mask-like expression Pill rolling Perioral tremor "Rabbit syndrome"
Neuroleptic malignant syndrome (NMS)	Several weeks	Rigidity Autonomic dysfunction Hyperthermia Altered mental status Catatonia
Tardive dyskinesia	Several months	Involuntary buccolinguo-masticatory movements Choreoathetoid movements

DIAGNOSIS[10-15]

History and Physical Examination

- Inquire about possible ingestion of drug and poorly stored medications.
- Monitor vital signs with significant exposure.

Laboratory Investigations

Plasma levels of phenothiazine do not correlate well with clinical signs and symptoms.[10]

Qualitative Calorimetric Tests[10,16]

Positive urine phenothiazine colorimetric testing suggests the presence of phenothiazine. For *ferric chloride test*, a 10% solution of fresh ferric chloride [5 to 10 drops] is added to 10 ml of acidified urine. On boiling, it turns purple green in the presence of phenothiazines.

The Forrest test or Phenistix reagent strip test may also be used.

Ancillary Laboratory Testing

- Electrolytes, BUN, creatinine, glucose.
- Liver function tests for significant overdose.
- Urine analysis: Dip for myoglobin if neuroleptic malignant syndrome (NMS) is suspected.
- CPK level if NMS is suspected.

Imaging/Special Tests

- *ECG:* Increased QT, QRS and PR intervals (QRS > 100 msec, QT > 450 msec), non- specific ST and T wave changes, right-axis deviation
- *Abdominal radiograph:* An abdominal radiograph may help confirm a deliberate overdose, as some unabsorbed phenothiazines are radiopaque. Absence of visible tablets does not rule out the possibility of ingestion.

DIFFERENTIAL DIAGNOSIS

It includes overdose with the following class of drugs:

- Tricyclic antidepressants
- Antihistaminics
- Cocaine
- Amphetamine.

TREATMENT[10-15]

There is no specific antidote for acute phenothiazine poisoning. Therefore, treatment is directed at minimizing the amount of drug absorbed, eliminating the absorbed drug from the body and combating the toxic effects of the over dose. Symptoms rapidly resolve with parenteral antihistaminics, anticholinergics or benzodiazepines.

Initial Stabilization

ABCs

Administer supplemental oxygen. Intubation may be necessary in case of respiratory depression. In severe poisoning, management in an intensive care unit (ICU) with cardiac monitoring is essential.

Diagnostic Trial

For a suspected case of phenothiazine poisoning, administration of diphenhydramine (dose: 1-2 mg/kg, maximum 25 mg) results in not only resolution of dystonia or oculogyria but also assists in the diagnosis.

Emesis—Do not induce emesis due to the risk of development of seizures and sedation.[11,13]

Gastric Lavage—If the pharyngeal and laryngeal reflexes are present and if less than 4 hours have elapsed since ingestion, a lavage must be done followed by administration of activated charcoal (dose: 1 g/kg). It may be beneficial even upto 6 hours. Gastric lavage in an unconscious patient must not be attempted unless cuffed endotracheal intubation has been performed to prevent aspiration and pulmonary complications.

For children greater than 1 year old: Sorbitol in a dose of 0.5-l g/kg or a 35% solution mixed in the activated charcoal slurry may be used.

Catharsis: Following gastric lavage, a saline cathartic (sodium or magnesium sulfate) may be introduced and left in the stomach.

Diuresis: Encourage diuresis with the administration of IV fluids assisted, if necessary, by mannitol solution given slowly IV in a dose of 5 ml/kg initially, followed by 2 ml/kg every 6 hourly for 2 days.

Exchange transfusion: Exchange transfusion may be indicated to remove most of the circulating drug which is strongly bound to plasma proteins. Peritoneal dialysis and hemodialysis have been found to be ineffective because of protein binding and large volume of distribution.

Correction of hypotension Elevate the foot end of the bed. Give adequate IV fluids (0.9% NS). If a vasopressor is needed to manage refractory hypotension, a mixed α and β adrenergic receptor agonist such as epinephrine or dopamine should not be used. Since phenothiazines are potent α-adrenergic antagonists, β-adrenergic stimulation will cause peripheral vasodilatation, further worsen the blockade-induced vasodilatation and hypotension. Treatment of resistant hypotension is done with norepinephrine.

Dose: 1-2 mg/kg/minute (titrated to blood pressure).

Management of Ventricular Dysrhythmia

Administration of sodium bicarbonate is an appropriate intervention to treat the toxicity from this drug. Plasma alkalinization is said to be the mainstay of treatment. Supraventricular dysrhythmias are usually managed supportively. Ventricular dysrhythmias are treated with lidocaine or phenytoin (often ineffective).

Dose: Lidocaine: Loading dose—1 mg/kg IV repeated after 5-10 minutes. (3 mg/kg max); maintenance dose: 2–4 mg/min IV.

Phenytoin: 15-20 mg/kg IV (loading dose).

Avoid Class I antidysrhythmics as they may cause exacerbation of phenothiazine's quinidine-like effect. Treatment with physostigmine salicylate reverses central as well as peripheral anticholinergic abnormalities caused by phenothiazine, but should not be used in patients with conduction abnormalities. Temporary pacing (atrial stimulation) is often required.

Dystonic Reactions Administer diphenhydramine or benztropine mesylate.

Dose: Diphenhydramine—1 mg/kg IV
Benztropine—1–2 mg IV (1 mg/min)

Malignant hyperthermia Administer dentrolene or bromocriptine.

Dose: Dantrolene—2.5 mg/kg IV
Bromocriptine—5 mg

Seizures Treat seizures initially with diazepam. Phenobarbital or phenytoin can be used for persistent seizures.

Dose: Diazepam—0.2–0.5 mg/kg IV, repeat after 10–15 minutes
Phenobarbital—15–20 mg/kg IV (loading dose)
Phenytoin—15–20 mg/kg IV (loading dose).

General Supportive Measures

- Good nursing care is of prime importance, particularly in the comatose patient, and should include regular observation and accurate recording of the vital signs and depth of coma, maintenance of a free airway, frequent turning and other routine measures usually adopted with unconscious patients.
- Careful supervision and recording of fluid intake and output is essential.
- Hypothermia may occur in phenothiazine intoxication, maintain normal body temperature and avoid overheating.
- Attention should be paid to the fact that phenothiazines are capable of potentiating CNS depressants (e.g., anesthetics, analgesics, hypnotics, antihistamines, opiates etc.).

Admission Criteria

- Overdose with CNS excitation, sedation, vital sign abnormalities or extrapyramidal effects.

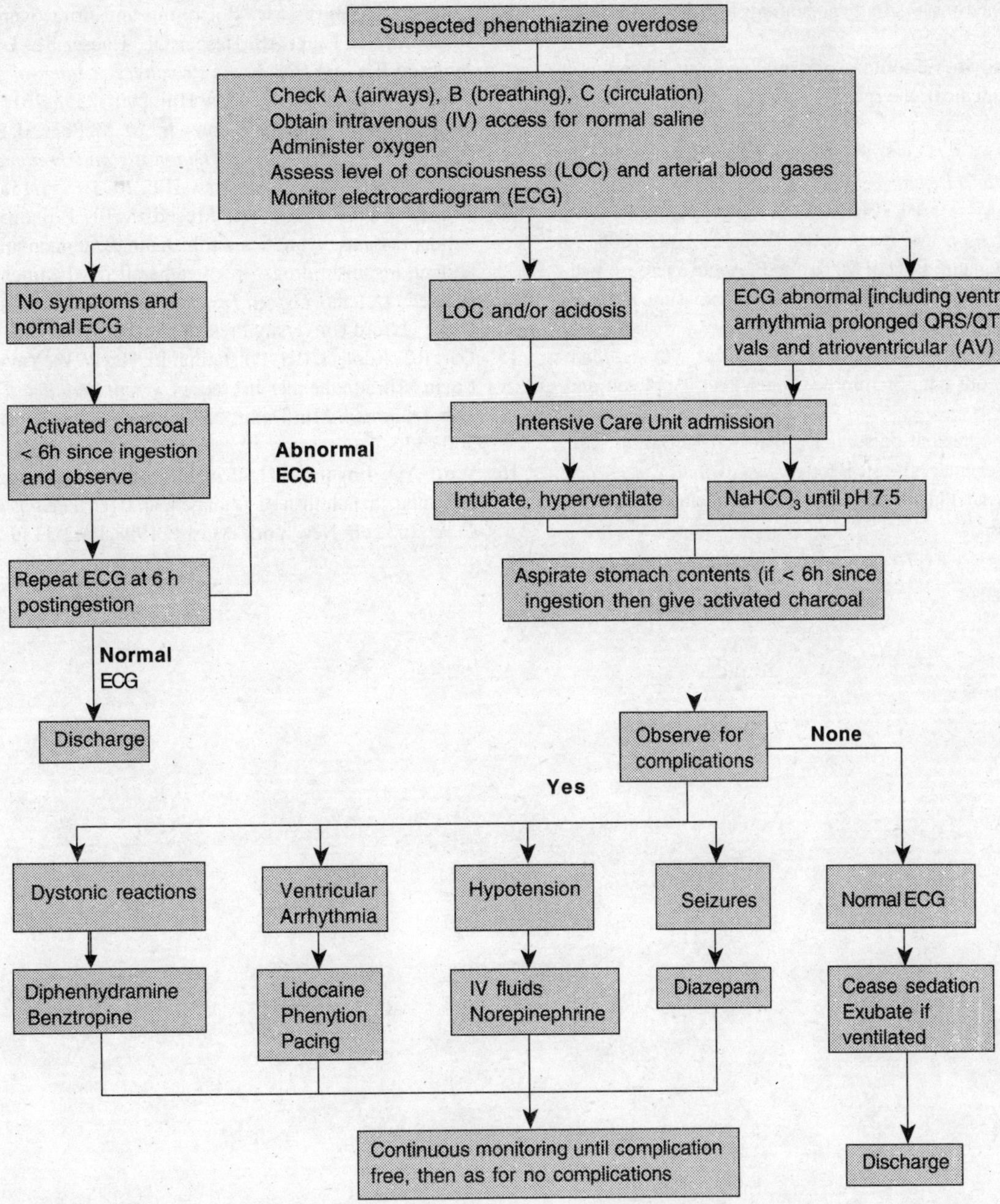

Fig. 81.1: Flow diagram showing treatment in a case of acute phenothiazine poisoning

- Any patient presenting with ECG abnormalities, such as conduction delays and dysrhythmias or hemodynamic instability must be admitted.
- All other patients should be placed on a cardiac monitor and observed for a minimum of 6 hours.

Discharge Criteria

If the patient is alert, has had adequate gastric detoxification and has remained asymptomatic for 6 hours and a repeat ECG is normal he is fit for discharge.

Figure 81.1 provides an algorithm on steps involved in treatment of acute phenothiazine poisoning.

REFERENCES

1. Jaraczewska W, Kotwica M. Acute poisoning with drugs. A review of the data collected at The National Poison Information Center during the period 1991-1995. *Przegl Lek* 1997;54: 737-740.
2. Buch NA, Ahmed K, Sethi AS. Poisoning in children. *Indian Pediatr* 1991;28:521-524.
3. Greenblatt DJ, Allen MD, Koch-Weser J, Shader RI. Accident poisoning with psychotropic drugs in children. *Am J Dis Child* 1976;130:507-511.
4. James LP, Abel K, Wilkinson J, Simpson PM, Nichols MH. Phenothiazine, butryrophenone and other psychotropic medication poisonings in children and adolescents. *J Toxicol Clin Toxicol* 2000;38:615-623.

5. Lifshitz M, Gavrilov V. Acute poisonings in children. *Isr Med Assoc J* 2000;2:504-506.
6. Surpure J, Lall Sb. Editorial: Accidental pediatric poisoning-a preventable medical emergency. *Indian J Pediatr* 1998;65: 363-364.
7. Dutta AK, Seth A, Goyal PK. Poisoning in children: Indian scenario. *Indian J Pediatr* 1998;65:365-370.
8. Schurch F, Merier PJ, Wyss PA. Acute poisoning with thioridazine. *Dtsch Med Wochenschr* 1996;121:1003-1008.
9. Le Blaye I, Donatini B, Hall M, Krupp P. Acute overdose with thioridazine: a review of the available clinical exposure. *Vet Hum Toxicol* 1993;35:147-150.
10. Lewin NA. Neuroleptic agents. In: *Goldfrank's Toxicologic Emergencies*, 6th edn. Stamford, Connecticut: Appleton and Lange, 1998;943-952.
11. June R. Phenothiazine poisoning. In: Rosen P, Baskin RM, Hayden SR, Schaider J. Wolfe R (eds) *The 5- Minute Emergency Medicine Consult.* Philadelphia: Lippincort Williams and Wilkins 1999;868-869.
12. Linden CH, Burns MJ. Poisoning and drug overdose. In: Braunwald E, Fauci AS, Kasper DL, Hauser SL, Longo DL, Jameson JL (eds) *Harrison's Principles of Internal Medicine,* 15th edn. New York: McGraw Hill, 2001;2595-2615.
13. Olson KR. Poisoning. In: Tierney Jr LM, McPhee SJ, Papadakis MA (eds). *Current Medical Diagnosis and Treatment,* 42nd edn. New York: Lange/McGraw-Hill, 2003;1555-1588.
14. Proudfoot AT, Vale JA, Meredith TJ. Poisoning from antidepressants, hypnotics, antihistamines, anticonvulsants and antiparkinsonism drugs. In: Weatherall DJ, Ledingham JGG, Warrell DA (eds). *Oxford Textbook of Medicine*, 3rd edn. New York: Oxford University Press 1996;1058-1062.
15. Dart RC, Rumack BH. Poisoning. In: Hay WW, Yayward AR, Levin MJ, Sondheimer JM (eds) *Current Pediatric Diagnosis and Treatment*, 16th edn. New York: Lange/McGraw-Hill 2003;336-361.
16. Wolf AD, Lovejoy FH. Principle of toxin assessment and screening. In: Fuhrman BP, Zimmerman JJ (eds) *Pediatric Critical Care,* 2nd edn. New York: Mosby, 1998;1142-1149.

Accidental Poisoning

B Vishnu Bhat and B Adhisivam

82 Naphthalene Poisoning

INTRODUCTION

Naphthalene poisoning or mothball toxicity is not an uncommon poisoning among children. Naphthalene was introduced by Rossback as an internal antiseptic for typhoid fever in 1841 and as an antihelminthic in 1842 and the early cases were the result of intoxication secondary to this.[1,2] Nowadays, Naphthalene and paradichloro benzene (PDB), commonly found in moth repellent products such as mothballs, flakes, lavatory bowl cleaners and diaper pail deodorizers, causes accidental poisoning among children following oral, dermal or inhalation exposure. Life-threatening hemolysis due to naphthalene poisoning has been documented. An early diagnosis, emergency decontamination and adequate supportive care are important aspects of the management.

BACKGROUND

Both naphthalene and PDB are white crystalline solids at room temperature. Mothballs with naphthalene appear dry whereas those containing PDB look wet and oily. PDB is more soluble in turpentine than naphthalene and this has been suggested as a useful test to help differentiate between these two compounds. As PDB is less toxic and does not induce hemolysis, it is more commonly used than naphthalene.

Naphthalene is well absorbed following oral exposure. It can also be absorbed through the skin or following inhalation. Naphthalene is metabolised in the liver to alpha–naphthol, beta naphthol and their quinones. Although the parent compound is devoid of hemolytic properties, alpha naphthol produces hemolysis.[3,4]

Naphthalene toxicity cases reported in literature are usually accidental and occasionally suicidal or homicidal. Schafer[4] described a fatal case involving a 6 day old female exposed for 3 days to diapers and blankets that had been stored in naphthalene. Vales et al reported hemolysis following inhalation in 21 greek newborns and young infants exposed to clothing stored in naphthalene mothballs.[5] Newborns are unable to conjugate naphthalene metabolites effectively and are more susceptible to hemolysis. They also have thinner skin and subject to application of baby oil, which promotes dermal absorption. As naphthalene is lipophilic, the presence of a fatty meal in the stomach could increase its absorption. Moreover, patients with G-6-PD deficiency are more susceptible to hemolysis.[4,5] Chronic toxicity from oral naphthalene has occurred in children mistaking mothballs for candy. Chronic naphthalene pica during the third trimester of pregnancy has resulted in toxicity in the mother and the fetus.[6]

CLINICAL MANIFESTATIONS

After ingestion, vomiting, diarrhea, and fever appear in 1 to 2 days followed on the third to fifth day by an acute hemolytic crisis as evidenced by pallor, mild jaundice and pigmented urine. Five to six days after ingestion, the hemolytic process ends and if the patient survives this stage, the recovery is rapid.[7]

Hematological changes occurring in severe cases lead to a Heinz-body hemolytic anemia and a sharp fall in hemoglobin level. There is often a concurrent leukocytosis. Reticulocytosis follows with subsequent gradual restoration of the normal blood values. A blood smear may show red cell fragmentation and anisopoikilocytosis. Hemoglobinuria and methhemoglobinaemia may also occur.[7,8]

MANAGEMENT

A small mothball ingestion needs ipecac syrup induced emesis preferably within 2 hours of ingestion.

If larger quantities have been ingested, ipecac induced emesis should be followed by activated charcoal and cathartics. Milk or fatty meals, which will facilitate naphthalene absorption, should be avoided 2-3 hours after ingestion.

Screening for hemolysis should include hematocrit and blood smears for at least 1 week after exposure. If fulminant toxicity occurs, blood transfusion may be needed.

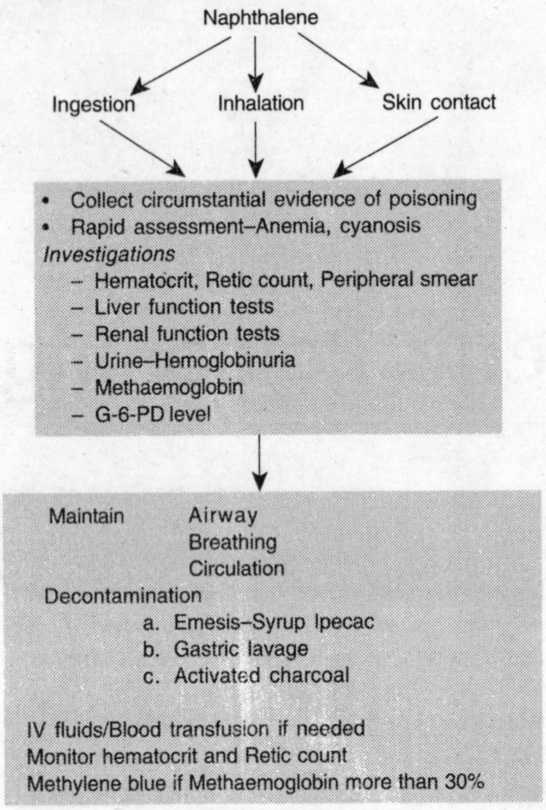

Fig. 82.1: Algorithm for management of naphthalene toxicity

Judicious use of intravenous fluids with alkalinisation may prevent acute renal failure and precipitation of hemoglobin in renal tubules. If a patient presents with cyanosis, methemoglobinemia should be suspected.

Treatment with methylene blue may be indicated if symptoms of hypoxia are severe or if methemoglobin levels exceed 30%.[9]

PREVENTION

PDB moth repellents are a safer alternative in that it has a low order of acute and chronic toxicity. However, it is carcinogenic in rodents. Proper dry-cleaning and storage of clothes in sealed containers can keep out moths and the use of chemicals like naphthalene can be avoided. Given their toxic potential and the large number of ingestions children with every year, they should be banned.[10]

REFERENCES

1. Gidron E, Leuren J. Naphthalene poisoning. *Lancet* 1956;1:228-230.
2. Smillie WG. Betanaphthol poisoning in the treatment of hookworms. *J Am Med* Assoc 1920;74:1503-1506.
3. Zinkham WH, Childs B. A defect of glutathione metabolism in erythrocytes from patients with a naphthalene-induced hemolytic anemia. *Pediatrics* 1958; 22:461-471.
4. Schafer WB. Acute hemolytic anemia related to naphthalene. Report of a case in a newborn infant. *Pediatrics* 1951;7: 172-174.
5. Valaes T, Psyros AD, Phaedron F. Acute hemolysis due to naphthalene inhalation. *J Pediatr* 1963;63:904-915.
6. Anziulewicz JA, Herman JD, Chiarulli EE. Trasplacental naphthalene poisoning. *Am J Obst Gynecol* 1959;78:519-521.
7. Ostlere L, Amos R, Wass JA. Hemolytic anemia associated with ingestion of naphthalene containing anointing oil. *Postgrad Med J* 1988;64:444-446.
8. Santhanakrishnan BR, Ranganathan G, Raju BV. Naphthalene-induced hemolytic anemia with hemoglobinuria. *Indian J Pediatr* 1973;40:195-197.
9. Siegel E, Wason S. Mothball toxicity. *Pediatr Clin North Am* 1986;33:369-374.
10. Todisco V, Lamour J, Finberg L. Hemolysis from exposure to naphthalene moth balls. *N Eng J Med* 1991;325:1660-1661.

Section XIV

Surgical Emergencies

Anup Mohta

83 Acute Abdomen

INTRODUCTION

Acute abdomen in children can occur due to wide variety of causes. Evaluation of abdominal pain in children poses a major challenge for the clinician. The diagnosis in infants and small children can be really difficult due to lack of clarity in history and physical signs that are nonspecific and difficult to elicit. It is important to reach the diagnosis at the earliest so that need of surgery can be decided in order to avoid morbidity and mortality due to delay.

PATHOPHYSIOLOGY

Acute abdominal pain arises from three nervous pathways.[1]

a. Parietal pain
b. Visceral pain and
c. Referred pain

Parietal pain arises from noxious stimulation of the parietal peritoneum and is transmitted by somatic nerves. This may occur due to ischemia, inflammation and stretching of parietal peritoneum. It is usually sharp, discrete, localized and increased by coughing or movement. The retroperitoneal lesions do not generate parietal pain.

Visceral pain occurs due to stimulation of a viscus by tension, stimulation or stretching. Since visceral nerves are bilateral, unmyelinated and enter the spinal cord at multiple levels, pain is dull, poorly localized and felt in the midline.

Referred pain is felt in remote areas supplied by the same dermatome as the diseased organ. It occurs due to sharing of central pathways for afferent neurons from different sites. For example, a patient of pneumonia may present with abdominal pain because T9 dermatome is shared by lungs and abdomen.

CAUSES

Common causes of abdominal pain include medical problems while surgical causes are present in small a percentage of cases.[2] In infants and young children, complications of various congenital abnormalities are more common causes of abdominal pain where as acquired disorders are more common in older children and adolescents.[3] Various causes of acute pain in abdomen are summarized in Table 83.1.

DIAGNOSIS

The three main considerations for a clinician should be:

a. Age and sex of the patient
b. Duration of symptom
c. The presence of other symptoms/signs related to specific organ systems.

History

An accurate history and detailed examination will provide more information than a multitude of investigations. The chronological order of appearance and progress of each symptom must be obtained.[4]

Age

Newborns to 2 years of age: Common causes of abdominal pain include medical conditions like acute viral gastroenteritis, pneumonia, colic, and constipation while major surgical causes are midgut volvulus associated with malrotation and intussusception.

Neonates, more so than older children, with unrecognized intestinal obstruction deteriorate rapidly, show an increase of associated morbidity and mortality and appropriate surgical treatment becomes more hazardous.[5] Early diagnosis depends largely on the prompt detection of obstructive manifestations by the clinician and the subsequent accurate interpretation of radiographic findings and other investigations, leading to definitive treatment, which should always be preceded by appropriate resuscitation of the child.

Children (2-12 years of age): Acute appendicitis is the most important cause of acute abdomen in this age group. Medical causes include urinary tract infections, gastroenteritis, constipation, recurrent abdominal pain syndrome, pneumonia etc.

Table 83.1: Causes of abdominal pain according to age

	Inflammatory/Infection	*Mechanical*	*Functional*	*Others*
Neonate	Gastroenteritis Omphalitis UTI*	Midgut volvulus	Colic	Milk intolerance
Infant	Gastroenteritis UTI	Midgut volvulus Intussusception Incarcerated hernia Trauma/abuse	Colic Constipation	Milk intolerance
Preschool	Gastroenteritis UTI Pneumonia Appendicitis	Midgut volvulus Intussusception Urinary calculi Incarcerated hernia	Constipation	Trauma/abuse H-S Purpura** Diabetic ketoacidosis Pepic ulcer
School age/Adolescents	Appendicitis Mesenteric adenitis Gastroenteritis Pancreatitis PID$/testicular pathology	Midgut volvulus Urinary calculi Trauma/abuse	Constipation RAP#	H-S Purpura Diabetic ketoacidosis Peptic ulcer

* Urinary tract infection
** Henoch-Schönlein purpura
\# Recurrent abdominal pain
$ Pelvic inflammatory disease

Adolescents: Appendicitis still remains major diagnosis in this age group. In an adolescent female, mittelschmerz, pelvic inflammatory disease and ectopic pregnancy should be considered.

Pain: The nature of the pain and its onset should be elicited carefully. Children who cannot verbalize usually present late and associated symptoms may not be noticed. Many times, infants react to pain as a change in behavior, persistent crying, irritability, sleeplessness and poor feeding.[6] Localization of pain in small children is not exact.

Colicky pain signifies obstruction of a gastrointestinal tract, urinary tract or hepatobiliary tract. Patients with severe pain lasting over 4-6 hours are more likely to have a surgical cause. Sudden pain that is aggravated by jerks or bumps while riding is suggestive of peritoneal irritation.

Associated symptoms: Pain usually precedes vomiting in surgical conditions. Any child with bilious vomiting should be considered to have acute intestinal obstruction unless proved otherwise. Urinary symptoms like dysuria, frequency and urgency suggest urinary tract infection.

Gynecologic history: In pubertal girls, complete gynecological history is important. History regarding menstrual cycle, sexual activity and contraception should be ascertained.

Drugs: Some drugs like erythromycin, salicylates and lead can cause abdominal pain and thus a history of past drug intake becomes important.

Physical Examination

Physical examination should be complete and should begin as the child walks in to the room. Change in gait is suggestive of pain in the hip joint and psoas abscess. It is helpful to sit by the patient and talk to him for few minutes before starting examination to gain confidence. General physical examination should be completed first while procedures like pharyngeal examination and rectal examination should be done last. Attitude of the child is an important guide to pathology. An active child rarely has peritonitis. Hydration status and vital signs of the patient should be assessed. One should look for tongue furring, jaundice and characteristic spots of Henoch-Schönlein purpura.

Abdominal examination: The breathing pattern of the patient is noted and chest examination is done. On abdominal examination, note should be made of distention, any previous scars and visible bowel loops and peristalsis. The child is requested to point to site of maximum tenderness. The abdominal palpation is begun from the normal area while gaining confidence of the child. It is useful to distract the child by talking during examination to differentiate between voluntary guarding and rigidity. Abdominal examination is not complete without examination of hernial sites.

Rectal and pelvic examination: These should be performed only when these are likely to provide some information that is not elicited on abdominal examination.[7,8] Only experienced clinician should do these so as to gain maximum information from these and if a decision has been made to refer the child to a specialist, it should not be done by primary care physician. Rectal examination may provide information on tenderness, presence of mass, fecal matter, melena and sphincter tone. Intussusceptum may be felt on rectal examination. In an adolescent girl, purulent cervical discharge, tenderness and adnexal mass suggest pelvic inflammatory disease.

It is a formidable challenge for a clinician to identify the cause in a neurologically or immunologically impaired child suspected to have acute abdomen.[9] They require constant vigil and repeated examination to reach a diagnosis. Sound surgical judgment helps to avoid unnecessary therapeutic delay due to inattention or indecision.

INVESTIGATIONS

Investigations help to confirm the diagnosis that is made on basis of detailed history and examination but cannot replace them. These should be done according to the history and clinical findings.

Laboratory Investigations

1. *Complete blood count:* Leukocytosis and toxic granulations suggest presence of infection in the body.
2. *Urinalysis:* It helps to diagnose urinary tract infection and stone.
3. Pregnancy test is advocated in postmenarchal girls.

Radiological Investigations

Different radiological investigations can be used to ascertain the cause of acute abdomen.[10-12]

Plain film radiograph of abdomen and chest is important in a case of acute abdomen. Distribution of gas in the bowel, free gas under dome of diaphragm, air fluid levels, mass lesions, calcification and outline of psoas muscle are noted. A chest X-ray should be done to rule out pneumonia.

Ultrasonography has become the mainstay of diagnosis in emergency settings. It is readily available, is less expensive, does not cause radiation exposure and can be done at bedside in severely sick patient. But, it is highly operator dependent and findings may be obscured by gaseous distention. Questions to be addressed are status of the organs, lymphadenopathy, free fluid, mass lesion, bowel wall thickness and intestinal peristalsis.

Computed tomography is more accurate but involves radiation and may require contrast. It should be done in selected settings. Mostly an intravenous contrast enhanced CT examination without oral contrast is carried out in case of acute abdomen.

Laparoscopy: Diagnostic laparoscopy plays a significant role in the evaluation of acute abdominal pain. In addition to confirming or ruling out a diagnosis, it has the advantage of performing definitive therapeutic intervention at the same time.[13] There are a wide variety of acquired or congenital conditions for which minimal access techniques provide advantage of cost-effective diagnosis and therapy with minimal discomfort for the patient.[14] Laparoscopy may be used as the primary invasive intervention in patients with abdominal pain where facility and expertise exists.

MANAGEMENT

The general measures that are taken in a patient with acute abdominal pain are:

1. Intravenous fluids are necessary when the pain is severe and associated with vomiting. Any child who is likely to be suffering from surgical cause is kept nil orally.
2. Nasogastric intubation is done where intestinal obstruction is suspected. Sometimes it may be indicated in acute pancreatitis.
3. Antibiotics may be administered as and when indicated. Routine use is not justified.
4. *Pain relief:* The practice of providing analgesia for children with acute abdominal pain is divergent between primary emergency physician and pediatric surgeons.[15] Some surgeons are less likely to provide analgesia for children with acute abdominal pain. The perceived disapproval of providing analgesia to children with acute abdominal pain by pediatric surgeon is considered a barrier influencing primary emergency medicine practice. Intravenous morphine provides significant pain relief to children with acute abdominal pain without adversely affecting the examination and it does not affect the ability to identify patients with surgical conditions.[16]
5. Definitive treatment depends on the final diagnosis and may require surgical intervention.

Different Conditions Causing Acute Abdomen

Infantile Colic

It is a common cause of abdominal pain in first month of life. Infants suffering from colic scream and draw up their legs up against their abdomen. Relief may occur after some time.

Malrotation and Volvulus

This condition is one of the most important emergencies in children, especially neonates, that requires a very high index of suspicion for early diagnosis in order to prevent bowel ischemia.

Rapid elongation of midgut is associated with herniation outside with subsequent return and fixation by the 12th week of gestational life. Failure of fixation results in mobile or subhepatic cecum. The bowel may undergo volvulus due to short mesentery. It is most commonly seen in the neonate but may occur at any age.

The generally healthy child presents with sudden onset of bilious vomiting.[17] As the level of obstruction in midgut volvulus is high, abdominal distention may occur only in about 30 percent cases. Untreated child rapidly goes into shock and peritonitis.

In absence of peritonitis, contrast studies may be done to confirm diagnosis. In case of a suspected volvulus, no time should be spent on diagnostic investigations. The child should be taken up for urgent laparotomy after aggressive resuscitation. The rotated bowel is untwisted and base of mesentery is widened. There is no need to fix the cecum in right iliac fossa.

In case of frankly gangrenous bowel, resection and anastomosis is done.

Appendicitis

Acute appendicitis is the most common and important cause of acute abdomen in children. There is history of pain arising in the umbilical region which that shifts to right iliac fossa to be finally localized at McBurney's point. This indicates irritation of parietal peritoneum. The pain is associated with vomiting and fever, in that order. Vomiting preceding pain is more suggestive of gastroenteritis. Anorexia may be present. If there is delay in diagnosis, perforation rate may be higher and professional delay has been found to be a cause of increase in incidence of perforated appendices.[18]

On examination, there is pain in the right iliac fossa and percussion may reveal rebound tenderness. In case of perforation of appendix, there will be diffuse tenderness suggestive of peritonitis. In late presentation, there may be formation of an appendicular mass. It may be required to re-examine the patient at intervals in doubtful cases. Complete blood counts and urinalysis are helpful at times but normal counts in presence of classical history and signs do not rule out appendicitis. The clinician has to weigh the significance of the signs and symptoms to differentiate between acute appendicitis and nonspecific abdominal pain.[19]

Ultrasonography is useful diagnosis. It may demonstrate distended appendix, localized ileus and peri-appendiceal fluid.[12] An appendicolith may be identified. An appendicular abscess or mass can be diagnosed. Pre-operative focused appendiceal CT with colon contrast has not been found to increase the accuracy in diagnosis of appendicitis when compared with patients diagnosed by history and clinical examination and laboratory investigations. But it may be useful in presence of atypical history and examination.[20] Treatment of acute appendicitis is emergency appendicectomy. This can be performed by open surgery or by laparoscopic method. A standard protocol for management of acute appendicitis helps to reduce hospital stay and complications.[21] An appendicular mass is managed conservatively followed by interval appendicectomy 3-6 months later.

Intussusception

Intussusception is invagination of bowel (intussusceptum) in to lumen of adjacent bowel loop (intussuscepiens). This leads to intestinal obstruction and subsequent interference with mesenteric blood supply and necrosis if not treated.

Various types include ileo-colic (commonest), ileo-ileal and colo-colic. Peak age for intussusception is 6 to 12 months and it is uncommon in neonatal age. Most cases are idiopathic but history of preceding viral illness, gastroenteritis or respiratory illness may be available. Intussusception in older children is more likely to be associated with a lead point like Meckel's diverticulum, invaginated appendix or polyp.

The hitherto healthy child presents with sudden onset colicky abdominal pain that may be associated with facial pallor and bilious vomiting. In between attacks, the child is calm and healthy. Later, the child may pass blood mixed mucus (red currant jelly stools).

Abdominal examination may reveal a palpable mass in the abdomen in about 85 percent cases. In late stages, mass may be palpable on rectal examination or it may prolapse out of the anus. Bowel ischemia and necrosis leads to peritonitis and abdominal examination will reveal guarding and rigidity with rebound tenderness. Delayed presentation is associated with features of septicemia and shock.

Plain X-ray abdomen may show coiled spring sign due to air trapped between intussusceptum and intussuscipiens. Later, features of intestinal obstruction may be apparent. Ultrasonography is now considered a very good modality and when properly performed, it obviates the need of contrast studies.[22] It can also be used to assess the completeness of reduction of intussusception by air or contrast. Contrast enema is still considered confirmatory investigation in many centers.

After correction of fluid and electrolyte imbalance, treatment aims at reduction of the intussusception. This may be done by non-operative means like air or barium reduction under radiological control. It should not be attempted when signs of peritonism are present. In case of failure or lack of facility, surgical exploration and reduction is done. Gangrene requires resection of the affected bowel.

Mesenteric Adenitis

It is an important cause of acute abdomen in older children and is due to enlargement of mesenteric lymph nodes. A history of gastrointestinal or upper respiratory tract infection with high fever is usually available. Examination reveals tenderness in the right lower abdomen due to inflation of non-suppurating inflammation of lymph nodes in the mesentery. In contrast to appendicitis, it produces tenderness that may shift with change in posture. Treatment is usually conservative with symptomatic relief and antibiotics.

Complicated Inguinal Hernia

Complicated inguinal hernia is the commonest cause of mechanical intestinal obstruction in children. Obstruction and strangulation of the bowel presents with abdominal pain and bilious vomiting. Delay in diagnosis can occur due to failure to look at the hernial sites and difficulty in making a diagnosis. Early diagnosis and emergency surgical reduction of hernia followed by herniotomy is necessary.

Meckel's Diverticulum

Meckel's diverticulum is the remnant of the vitello-intestinal duct on the antimesenteric border of the small intestine. It is usually present within 2 feet of the ileocecal junction. It may be present as acute abdomen at any age due to complications like acute inflammation; perforation and peritonitis; lead point for intussusception and acute intestinal obstruction due to volvulus around a band between Meckel's diverticulum and umbilicus. It is difficult to diagnosis this entity pre-operatively and confirmation is usually made on exploratory laparotomy for intestinal obstruction. Complicated Meckel's diverticulum should be removed at surgery.

Gastroenteritis

It is the most common cause of pain in children. Gastrointestinal symptoms, including vomiting, are caused by a variety of infective organisms in children and include viruses like rotavirus, adenovirus and enterovirus and bacteria like E. coli, Yersinia and Shigella.[23] The pain may be severe and is associated with severe diarrhea and vomiting. Many of these infections are self-limiting and resolve within a week, but others are potentially much more serious in their consequences. Investigation is dictated by the likely causative organism, given the age and presentation of the child. Yersinia, Campylobacter and Salmonella may produce symptoms difficult to distinguish clinically from appendicitis.

Acute Pancreatitis

Acute pancreatitis is inflammation of pancreas associated with variable local and systemic inflammatory response. Its incidence in childhood is unknown. Diagnosis is difficult in small children because of non-specific clinical features.[24]

Idiopathic pancreatitis is the commonest group seen although trauma is the most common recognized cause of pancreatitis in childhood. Other causes include infections, biliary tract disease, drugs, metabolic and hereditary diseases. Acute autodigestion of pancreas leads to local and systemic inflammatory response.

Usual presenting feature is sudden onset severe abdominal pain in the epigastrium and upper lateral quadrants. The pain may radiate to and back. Nausea and vomiting usually follow. Hypovolemia and shock can occur along with multiorgan failure in late cases.

Diagnosis is confirmed by hyperglycemia, hypocalcemia, elevated LDH and other liver function test. Serum amylase and lipase are markedly raised. Serum trypsinogen and alpha-1-antitrypsin have good sensitivity. Abdominal X-ray can be used to rule out other causes of acute abdomen. Ultrasound is useful but CT scan is the best investigation to assess and identify edema, necrosis, abscess and pseudocyst formation. Treatment is generally supportive with nasogastric drainage and intravenous fluids initially. Use of antibiotics is advocated in high risk groups. Enteral feeding should be started early and parenteral nutrition reserved for those who do not tolerate the former. Mortality is about 10-15 percent. Surgical intervention is needed for management of complications like pancreatic necrosis, abscess and pseudocyst.

Peptic Ulcer Disease

Peptic ulcer disease in childhood presents most commonly as abdominal pain is a responsible for about 15-20 percent cases of abdominal pain.[25] It may be primary or secondary peptic ulcer disease. It is the secondary peptic ulcers, usually due to underlying disease or drugs that are more acute in onset. Peptic ulcers can present as complications including perforation.[26]

Urinary Tract Infection

Urinary tract infection (UTI) is a common infection in children and causes acute morbidity. Its incidence is higher in girls than the boys. Majority of cases are caused by gram negative bacteria. Some of the cases present as acute abdominal pain that can be associated with fever, vomiting, lethargy and symptoms of systemic sepsis.[27] Urinary symptoms include burning, urgency, frequency and flank pain. Urine may be turbid or foul smelling. Untreated UTI can be associated with vesicoureteric reflux and results in renal scarring.

Urinalysis and urine culture examination are necessary for diagnosis. Antibiotic therapy is given according to culture sensitivity reports. Therapy may be oral in uncomplicated UTI while complicated UTI necessitates use of parenteral administration.

Patients should be evaluated by ultrasonography, micturating cystogram and Dimercaptosuccinic acid scan (DMSA) for assessment of renal damage after treatment of initial infection.

Miscellaneous Surgical Causes

Abdominal tuberculosis is a common cause of intestinal

obstruction in India and may present as acute abdomen in case of acute intestinal obstruction or perforation of bowel.[28]

Round worms are a common cause of acute abdomen in children. These can cause acute intestinal obstruction due to impaction of worms in the lumen.[29] Untreated, there may be peritonitis due to pressure necrosis and perforation.

Primary pyogenic psoas abscess is an important cause of abdominal pain in India.[30] It is associated with fever, inability to use the affected limb and fixed flexion deformity at the hip. Diagnosis is made by ultrasound examination. Treatment includes surgical drainage and appropriate antibiotics.

Hirschsprung's disease may present with enterocolitis and acute intestinal obstruction in neonatal age.[31] If not treated, it may lead to perforation and peritonitis.

Acute cholecystitis and cholelithiasis can cause acute abdominal pain in some children.[32]

Psychosomatic Disorders

The cause of acute and recurrent abdominal pain may not be identified in many children even after repeated examination and investigation. A careful psychosocial history and assessment by a psychologist is helpful in such cases.[34] Caution should be exercised before labeling a child to be suffering from psychosomatic disorder. The acceptance by parents of a biopsychosocial model of illness is important for the resolution of recurrent abdominal pain in children.[35]

Surgical Referral

Surgical consultation in patients with acute abdominal pain is indicated in following situations:

1. Severe increasing pain with progression
2. Deterioration in general condition
3. Bile stained or feculent vomiting
4. Involuntary abdominal guarding and rigidity
5. Rebound abdominal tenderness
6. Masking of liver dullness suggesting free gas
7. Signs of acute blood loss into abdomen
8. Significant abdominal trauma
9. Suspected surgical cause
10. Abdominal pain without obvious etiology.

When to operate immediately and when to observe and when not to operate at all represents the major challenge for the pediatric surgeon.[35] The acute abdomen is a clinical diagnosis and other diagnostic modalities have only a supportive role. The decision to operate is based on the results and thorough and, if required, repeated clinical examination.

REFERENCES

1. Leung AKC, Sigalet DL Acute abdominal pain in children. *Am Fam Physician* 2003;67:2321-2326.
2. Reynolds S, Jaffe D, Lavigne J. Abdominal pain in pediatric emergency department. *Pediatr Emerg Care* 1988;4:297.
3. Neblett WW 3rd, Pietsch JB, Holcomb GW Jr. Acute abdominal conditions in children and adolescents. *Surg Clin North Am* 1988;68:415-430.
4. Spitz L, Kimber C. Acute abdomen. The history. *Semin Pediatr Surg* 1997;6:58-61.
5. Hajivassiliou Ca C. Intestinal obstruction in neonatal/pediatric surgery. *Semin Pediatr Surg* 2003;12:241-253.
6. D'Agostino J. Common abdominal emergencies in children. *Emerg Med Clin North Am.* 2002;20:139-153.
7. Scholer SJ, Pituch K, Orr DP, Dittus RS. Use of rectal examination on children with acute abdominal pain. *Clin Pediatr* (Phila) 1998;37:311-316.
8. Jesudason EC, Walker J. Rectal examination in pediatric surgical practice. *Br J Surg* 1999;86:376-378.
9. Bansard DD, Haase GM. Acute abdomen. Special considerations for the neurologically and immunologically impaired child. *Semin Pediatr Surg* 1997;6:92-99.
10. John SD. Imaging of acute abdominal emergencies in infants and children. *Curr Probl Pediatr Adolesc Health Care* 2001;31:319-353.
11. Mishra DS, Magu S, Sharma N, Rattan KN, Tewari AD, Rohilla S. Imaging in acute abdomen. *Indian J Pediatr* 2003;70:15-19.
12. Carty HML. Pediatric emergencies: non-traumatic abdominal emergencies. *Eur Radiol* 2002;12:2835-2848.
13. Salky BA, Edye MB. The role of laparoscopy in the diagnosis and treatment of abdominal pain syndromes. *Surg Endosc* 1998;12:911-914.
14. Lobe TE. Acute abdomen. The role of laparoscopy. *Semin Pediatr Surg* 1997;6:81-87.
15. Kim MK, Galustyan S, Sato TT, Bergholte J, Hennes HM. Analgesia for children with acute abdominal pain: a survey of pediatric emergency physicians and pediatric surgeons. *Pediatrics* 2003;112:1122-1126.
16. Kim MK, Strait RT, Sato TT, Hennes HM. A randomized clinical trial of analgesia in children with acute abdominal pain. *Acad Emerg Med* 2002;9:281-287.
17. Torres AM, Ziegler MM. Malrotation of the intestine. *World J Surg* 1993;17:326-331.
18. Hatch EI Jr. The acute abdomen in children. *Pediatr Clin North Am* 1985;32:1151-1164.
19. Williams NMA, Johnstone JM, Everson NW. The diagnostic value of symptoms and signs in childhood abdominal pain. *J R Coll Surg Edinb* 1998;43:390-392.
20. Stephan AE, Segev DL, Ryan DP et al. The diagnosis of acure appendicitis in pediatric population: To CT or not to CT. *J Pediatr Surg* 2003;38:367-371.
21. Emil S, Laberge JM, Mikhail P et al. Appendicitis in children: A ten year update of therapeutic recommendations. *J Pediatr Surg* 2003;38:236-242.
22. Daneman A, Navarro O. Intussusception. Part 1: A review of diagnostic approaches. *Pediatr Radiol* 2003;33:79-85.
23. Blakelock RT, Beasley SW. Infection and the gut. *Semin Pediatr Surg* 2003;12:265-274.
24. Mehta DI. Acute and chronic pancreatitis in children. *Indian J Pediatr* 1999;66:S81-S86.
25. Hassal E. Peptic ulcer disease and current approaches to Helicobacter pylori. *J Pediatr* 2001;138:462-428.

26. Mohta A, Shrivastava UK, Gupta BP, Gupta A. Perforated duodenal ulcer in a child. *Indian Pediatr* 2002;39:578-79.
27. Hari P, Mantam M, Bagga A. Management of urinary tract infection. *Indian J Peditatr* 2003;70:235-239.
28. Talwar S, Talwar R, Chowdhary B, Prasad P. Abdominal tuberculosis in children: An Indian experience. *J Trop Pediatr* 2000;46:368-370.
29. Mohta A, Bagga D, Malhotra CJ, Chadha R, Kumar A, Arora MP. Intestinal obstruction due to round worms. *Pediatr Surg Int* 1993;8:226-228.
30. Kadambari D, Jagdish S. Primary pyogenic psoas abscess in children. *Pediatr Surg Int* 2000;16:408-410.
31. Klein MD, Coran AG, Wesley JR, Drongowski RA. Hisrchsprung's disease in the newborn. *J Pediatr Surg* 1984;19: 370-374.
32. Lobe TE. Cholelithiasis and cholecystitis in children. *Semin Pediatr Surg* 2000;9:170-176.
33. Alfvén G. One hundred cases of recurrent abdominal pain in children: diagnostic procedures and criteria for a psychosomatic diagnosis. *Acta Pœdtr* 2003; 92:43-49.
34. Crushell E, Rowland M, Doherty M, et al. Importance of parental conceptual model of illness in severe recurrent abdominal pain. *Pediatrics* 2003;112:1368-1372.
35. Gauderer MWL. Acute abdomen. When to operate immediately and when to observe. *Semin Pediatr Surg* 1997;6:74-80.

Anup Mohta and Medha Mohta

84 Burns

INTRODUCTION

Burns, wounds that are characterized by coagulative necrosis of the tissues, are a major preventable cause of morbidity and mortality in children. These also impose an enormous financial burden on the medical care system. These are the second most common cause of accidental death and most common cause of accidental death at home.

ETIOLOGY AND EPIDEMIOLOGY

Various causes of burn injuries can be classified as follows:

1. Thermal burns
   - Flame
   - Scalds
   - Contact
2. Inhalation injuries
   - Airway injuries
   - Lung injuries
   - Systemic intoxication
3. Electrical burns
4. Chemical burns
   - Acid
   - Alkali
   - Organic hydrocarbons
5. Cold injury
   - Freezing cold injury
   - Non-freezing cold injury
6. Radiation burns

Pediatric burns constitute about 13-17 % of the total admissions in burn wards in India.[1,2] Scalding is the commonest cause of burns in children.[3] Infants can receive scald injury due to hot water in the bath. Toddlers are usually affected due to spillage of hot water, milk, oil or food over them. Flame injuries are more common in preschool children. Kitchen is the most common place where such injury is inflicted in Indian homes.

Electrical cord injuries are also very common in toddlers as they tend to play with them due to their inquisitive nature. Adolescents are often involved in fire injuries and high voltage electrical injuries.

Child abuse is another aspect of burns injury. Evidence of previous abuse, symmetrical injuries, multiplicity of injuries, burns to back of hands, single parent and poor socio-economic status point towards child abuse.

Higher incidence of burns has been noticed in winters because of:

- Increased indoor activities
- Increased consumption of hot drinks
- Use of hot water for bath
- Use of fire to keep warm
- Festivities and marriages with use of lighting and fire crackers in winter season.[2]

TYPES OF BURNS

Superficial/first degree burns: The epidermis is involved with trauma to deeper layers and nerves. It is characterized by redness, edema and pain.

Partial thickness/second degree burns: The epidermis and dermis both are injured. Blistering occurs and the site is painful.

Full thickness/third degree burns: The epidermis, dermis and nerve endings are all destroyed. The wound is painless.

CLASSIFICATION OF BURNS

Minor

- First degree burns, or
- Second degree burns less than 10% of body surface, or
- Third degree burns less than 2% of body surface. No area of face, feet, hands or genitalia is involved.

Moderate

- Second degree burns 10-20%, or
- Burns on face, hands, feet or genitalia, or
- Third degree burns less than 10% body surface area, or
- Smoke inhalation.

Severe

Second degree burns more than 20%, or third degree burns more than 10% body surface area.

PATHOPHYSIOLOGY

Skin is the largest organ in the body and constitutes about 15% of the total body weight.

Pathology of the Burn Wound

At the point of heat contact from where heat cannot be conducted away, the tissues die. This central area is called 'zone of coagulative necrosis'. Surrounding this, there is a zone of tissue where there is damage to the microcirculation but the injury is not severe enough to cause immediate cell death. This is called 'zone of stasis'. In unfavorable conditions and with inadequate resuscitation, it may transform into zone of necrosis. Beyond this, there is 'zone of hyperemia' which is due to tissue response to injury by inflammation, cytokine release and increased blood flow. This returns to normal as the healing occurs.[4]

The extent of injury, in depth or size is determined by the intensity of heat source, the duration of exposure and thickness of exposed skin.

Burn injuries cause various pathophysiological changes in the body.[5]

Intravascular Volume

The intravascular volume is depleted in all burns, its extent being greatest in burns involving the dermis. The loss of plasma takes place from the site of burns and rest of the circulatory system.

Burn Edema

Endothelial destruction in the region of burns permits exudation of plasma from the intravascular space. The microcirculation is likely to be affected by release of locally released mediators like histamine, prostaglandin, thromboxane A_2 and oxygen radicals.

Non-burn Edema

Hypoproteinemia has been implicated as the main cause of edema distant from the site of burn.

The combination of burn and nonburn edema can be dangerous around head and neck where it can cause swelling of face, tongue and supraglottic structures. The edema reaches its peak at 24-36 hours and early intervention is required to secure airway while it is still possible.

Metabolism

There is massive and sustained release of catecholamines, glucagons and corticosteroids. Insulin production may be overwhelmed and result in hyperglycemia. Children with burns of 10% or more show a period of normothermia followed by rapid rise in temperature 5-8 hours after the accident which reaches its peak by 10-12 hours and remains so for up to 24 hours. This could be cytokine-mediated in response to gut derived organisms, bacterial fragments or toxins.

Respiratory Function

In the child the narrowest part of airway is at cricoid ring. Any edema of the glottic or supraglottic structures secondary to edema of neck or direct thermal injury from swallowed fluids is poorly tolerated in the child. In the presence of increased metabolic rate, the airway may prove inadequate. The child demonstrates hypoxia with reduced pulmonary perfusion. As temperature rises and metabolic rate increases, the child responds to increasing carbon dioxide load by increase in respiratory rate.

Cardiovascular Function

The large losses from the intravascular compartment are compensated by progressive peripheral and splanchnic vasoconstriction and the cardiac output is maintained. Without rapid resuscitation, a fall in cardiac output with development of anaerobic respiration occurs in the patient. Fluid administration opens up peripheral vascular bed, peripheral resistance decreases and cardiac output increases.

Renal Function

Kidneys are damaged by sustained hypovolemia along with systemic hypoxia. After an electric burn or a burn with massive muscular damage, resultant myoglobinuria or hemoglobinuria blocks the tubules and reduces renal function.

The quantity and quality of urine should be monitored at all stages of treatment as kidney not only provides homeostasis but also is a valuable indicator of adequate resuscitation. Renal blood flow must be maintained with low dose dopamine and urine flow stimulated by appropriate colloid and crystalloid solutions with administration of diuretics if necessary.

Hepatic Function

Hepatic functions are remarkably well preserved till late after burn injury.

Gastrointestinal Function

Hypovolemia results in gastric atony and some degree of paralytic ileus. A nasogastric tube must be inserted in all patients with burns of more than 10% to reduce pooling of gastric secretions. Severe gastric ulcerations are said to be more common in children than adults. Occult blood loss may be reduced by administration of antacids and enteral feeding as soon as possible following restoration of intravascular fluid volume.

Hemopoiesis

Hemoglobin falls from the time of injury and is proportionate to the area of burn surface. Loss occurs because of:

- Heat destruction
- Loss by consumption and clotting in a full thickness burn
- Increased fragility, and
- Increased removal by reticuloendothelial system. This loss is compounded by suppression of hemopoiesis until the burn is healing.

MANAGEMENT

The burn care aims to preserve life and function with physical, psychological and social rehabilitation. Care of burn patient consists of adequate initial resuscitation followed by early surgery aimed at rapid and definitive wound closure. Nutritional support, early rehabilitation and continuous psychosocial care are very important.

Immediate Care

At the site of injury, the burning agent should be removed as soon as possible or patient should be moved away and burning process stopped. Hot clothes should be removed. For immediate cooling, cold tap water is used. Universal precautions should be observed when contact with blood or body fluids is expected.[6]

Attention should be given to airway, breathing and circulation. Particular attention is given to airway especially in cases of closed space burns. 100% oxygen should be given and resuscitation fluids started as soon as possible after securing intravenous access. In case of problem in finding suitable peripheral vein, femoral or intraosseous transfusion can be given. In patients associated with falls or blast injuries, cervical spine immobilization is done till injury to cervical spine is ruled out.[7] All the rings and jewellary should be removed to avoid tourniquet effect. The wound should be covered and hypothermia avoided. A nasogastric tube is passed and indwelling urinary catheter is introduced to empty urinary bladder and record hourly urine output.

In case of chemical injury, the wound should be thoroughly cleansed with copious amount of running water. It is important to keep the lavage site drained to remove the earlier washings so that effluent does not come in contact with uninjured area. Room temperature should be 31-33°C and lavage fluid should be at or near body temperature. All garments with chemical should be cut away and not taken off over the extremity/head to avoid further damage.

Indications for Ventilation

Prolonged nasotracheal intubation and ventilation are known to increase morbidity in burn patients. But there are certain specific indications for ventilatory support in these children.[5]

1. Suspected inhalation injury.
2. Scalds and burns of head and neck in which rapid development of edema indicates securing of airway.
3. Electric burns with an entry or exit wound on the head or neck.
4. Incipient septicemia with pulmonary shunting.
5. Following massive infusions associated with excision and grafting to stabilize ventilation while child organizes fluid shifts between compartments.
6. Hypoxemia.
7. Inability to clear secretions.
8. Increased intracranial pressure from hypoxic brain injury.
9. Tracheostomy has been shown to be associated with a very high incidence of infection resulting in morbidity and mortality and is not recommended routinely. Recently it has been found to be useful in severely burnt children by some authors as it secures airway and is better for ventilator management of these children.[8]

Estimation of Extent of Burns

Measurement of area of the burned body surface is important as it has a bearing on patient management in terms of fluid resuscitation, decision for admission, chances for developing infection and prognosis. Wallace's Rule of Nine is not applicable in pediatric age group because of different relative surface area of body parts. Most commonly, Lund - Browder Charts are used for calculation of affected body surface (Table 84.1).

In emergency situations patient's palm with finger represents roughly 1% of the body area.

Admission Criteria

Pediatric patients with following should be admitted for management:[9]

- Any burns to hands, feet, face or perineum
- Partial thickness burns more than 10% or full thickness burns more than 2%
- All electrical injuries and
- Suspected cases of child abuse.

Monitoring During Acute Phase

During acute phase patients are monitored continuously for:

- Sensorium
- Respiration
- Blood pressure
- Body temperature
- Urine output
- Other fluid loss
- Body weight.

Laboratory Investigations

Investigations that need to be performed at admission and during stay in the hospital are:

- Complete blood count (CBC)
- Biochemical profile

- Urinalysis
- Chest radiograph
- Wound swabs and blood culture
- Arterial blood gases
- Carboxyhemoglobin levels
- Electrocardiography

Last three are required if electrical or inhalation injury is suspected.

Fluid Management

In view of the extensive fluid loss from the wound and sequestration as burn and non-burn edema, fluid administration is the mainstay of resuscitation of a burn patient. Intravenous fluid administration is indicated in all patients with burns more than 10% total body surface area (TBSA). Various formulae are used to calculate the requirements.[9]

Parkland formula: Lactated Ringer's solution 4 ml per kilogram body weight per TBSA burned should be given over 24 hours. Half of the calculated volume is administered over first 8 hours after injury and the rest is given during the next 16 hours. Towards the end of 24 hours fresh frozen plasma 0.5 ml per kilogram per TBSA burned should be infused.

Brooke's formula: It recommends 2 ml of lactated Ringer's solution per kilogram per percentage of TBSA burned over first 24 hours.

Shriners Burn Institute (Galveston) regimen: Fluid requirements for the first 24 hours can be met with a solution of lactated Ringer's solution at 5000ml/m^2 TBSA burned plus 2000 ml/m^2 TBSA for maintenance. Half of the calculated volume is given over first 8 hours after injury and the rest given over next 16 hours. Albumin is added after 12 hours in order to keep levels above 2 gm/dl.

Mount Vernon regimen:[5] From the time of injury, the resuscitation period is divided into six periods. Equal volumes of plasma are given in each of the successive periods of 4, 4, 4, 6, 6 and 12 hours. The volume of plasma per period is estimated by formula:

$$\frac{\text{Total \% of burns (excluding erythema)} \times \text{weight (kg)}}{2} = \text{volume of plasma (ml)}$$

Metabolic water requirements are met with 5% dextrose. One-half to two-thirds of normal requirements may be given as sodium chloride solution 0.45% + dextrose 5%. Potassium can be added to this fluid if required.

Hypertonic Saline solution: Hypertonic saline solution is given to the patients with second and third degree burns larger than 10% of TBSA. During the first day post burn, 5 ml/percent TBSA burned/kg body weight are administered decreasing it to 3 ml and 1 ml on the second and third post burn days. It is administered at a constant rate over time. Hypertonic saline resuscitation decreases net fluid intake, increases lymph flow and peripheral perfusion and causes less edema. But it can lead to hypernatremia, hyperosmolar coma, alkalosis and renal failure. Care should be taken that serum sodium should not exceed 160 mEq/dl.[7]

Resuscitation formulae are guidelines only and each given situation may require modification depending upon clinical and biochemical parameters. Deep burns and inhalation injury require higher amounts of fluids. Adequacy of fluid resuscitation is assessed by monitoring urine output which should be maintained at 1-2 ml/kg/hour. Other helpful parameters are vital signs like pulse, blood pressure and mental status.

Pain Management

Pain control in pediatric burn patients is one of the most neglected areas. There is difference in perception of pain by the child and the clinician, as well as from patient to patient.[10, 11] Attempts at assessing pain are limited by patient's vocabulary and previous experiences with pain and discomfort. Pain affects not only the afflicted but also the care givers including the family.

Pediatric patients with burn injury experience two types of pain.

a. *Background pain:* This refers to unpleasant sensations during rest or during activities when no procedure is being conducted.
b. *Procedural pain:* This is the pain associated with wound care, dressing change, skin grafts or other interventions.

Aggressive pain management should start immediately. Pain can be controlled by pharmacologic and non-pharmacologic methods.[12] Comprehensive pain management takes care of child's changing responses over the time. An anesthesiologist should be involved at first dressing change who then, based on the response, can help the burn team plan adequate pain relief protocol for the particular patient.

Intravenous morphine in dose of 0.1-0.2 mg/kg is the most commonly used drug for control of wound care pain, breakthrough pain and background pain. It can be administered as intermittent bolus injections, continuous infusion or with patient controlled analgesia. Other commonly used intravenous analgesics are tramadol, fentanyl, ketamine and pentazocine. Acetaminophen with codeine is also very commonly used.[13] Trimeprazine is useful for providing background sedation and reduction of itching.

Treatment protocol should allow for as much patient participation as possible during procedures. Parental presence during treatment is also beneficial. Distraction, music/art therapy and relaxation therapy are other useful non-pharmacologic measures used for management of pain in burn patients. Psychological intervention techniques are an important adjunct to pharmacologic methods and their integration into standard burn care can improve pain control for pediatric patients with burn injuries.

The control of pain continues to be a challenge that demands staff expertise and awareness, family education and cooperation and continued research.

Wound Management

After admission, the wounds are gently cleaned and thoroughly washed with soap and water. All devitalized tissue and foreign bodies are removed. All the blisters should be opened as the blister fluid acts as an excellent growth media for bacteria. Escharotomy is carried out immediately in circumferential burns of extremities and chest.

Infection of the burn wound can usually be controlled with topical antibiotics. Ideal topical agent should be painless and non-allergenic, prevent desication, penetrate eschar, and achieve bacteriologic control. It should not inhibit re-epithelialization and damage viable tissue. Silver sulphadiazine meets most of these criteria. Combination of cerium nitrate with silver sulphadiazine has been shown to improve results.[9] Other topical antibiotics that have been used are mefenamide, silver nitrate, povidone-iodine, nitrofurazone and neosporin/bacitracin preparations.

Dressings aim to minimize pain, absorb exudates and debris, shield the burns from secondary infection and provide protection during transport.

Application of bilaminar temporary skin substitute has been found to decrease pain, analgesic requirement, wound healing time and hospital stay.[17] Use of collagenase for debridement results in shorter hospital stay, reduced overall need of surgery and blood transfusion.[18]

Morbidity and mortality have decreased with aggressive treatment protocols. Early burn wound excision is a safe therapeutic approach and is better than treatment with silver sulphadiazine and delayed excision. Excision of full thickness and deep partial burns has been shown to shorten hospital stay, limit number of painful debridements and dressings and reduce total hospital cost.[19-21]

There are three techniques of wound excision. Sequential excision involves daily sessions of debridement with guarded knife to remove firmly adherent eschar. This results in a granulating scar that can be grafted. The second method entails primary excision of the burn wound down to fascia. Blood loss is less with this technique but it is inferior in its cosmetic results. Tangential excision, the third method, involves the removal of sequential thin layers of burn eschar till a viable tissue bed is reached. This requires more clinical judgment for identifying the correct level. It also causes more blood loss.[9]

Positioning is a very important aspect of wound care. While edema, inflammation and immobility hamper the function; exercise, elevation, proper splinting and early closure of the wound limits disability. The extremity should be splinted in position of function.

Most freshly excised wounds can be grafted immediately with skin grafts. Meshed grafts can be used if donor area is small. Culture epithelial autografts and human cultured keratinocytes have been used with success for post-excision wound cover. Other techniques used for postburn reconstruction are Z-plasty, local and free flaps and skin expansion.[20, 22, 23]

Head, face and neck burns are problematic for the pediatric population not only because of potential deformities but also because of effect on growth and development of these areas.[24]

Recombinant human growth hormone has been used to promote wound healing and decrease protein loss.[25] Insulin given in pharmacologic doses improves net protein balance and accelerates wound healing.

Corneal burns require attention by ophthalmologist. These are managed by debridement, topical antibiotics, cycloplegia and pressure patching.

Infection

Total burned surface area, catheter use and ventilation are the variables that determine development of infections in burn patients.[14]

Most efficacious infection control method in burn care is considered to be early wound excision followed by grafting.[15] Delay in wound excision allows the wound to be colonized by bacteria and fungi.

Pseudomonas, Staphylococcus aureus and Klebsiella are the most common species associated with burns wounds. Multidrug resistant Acinetobacter has also been found to be an important cause of nosocomial infection.[16]

Topical antibiotics are used to prevent proliferation of microorganisms. Indications for systemic antibiotics include:[7]

a. Sepsis
b. Massive wound infection
c. Chondritis
d. Inhalation injury with documented infection
e. Keratinocytes
f. Non-burn related infection
g. Impaired immune system.

Transfer of the Patient

Smaller burns may be treated on outpatient basis. Its advantages include less cost, less chances of exposure to nosocomial infections and a more normal environment for the child. Pre-requisites for home treatment include pain controlled with oral analgesics, no wound infection and no apparent complications.

The patients with large burns area or critical illness need to be transferred to nearest specialized burns treatment unit.

Before transfer, following should be ensured:

a. Information regarding transfer should be given to the concerned burns unit where patient is being sent.
b. Complete examination of the patient should be done.
c. Oxygen is provided during transfer.
d. Airway is secured in consultation with an anesthesiologist in case of suspected inhalation injury,
e. Adequate intravenous access should be secured and fluid resuscitation is started.
f. Burn wound should be covered and steps are taken to prevent hypothermia.
g. Adequate analgesia is given.
h. Nasogastric tube and urinary catheter are inserted.
i. All findings and interventions are documented and sent with the patient.
j. Patient should be sent with a trained escort.

Nutrition in Burns Patients

The burn wound causes severe catabolism which can only be modulated and not reversed. The therapeutic aims of nutritional support should be to prevent body weight losses of more than 10%. There is overwhelming evidence that enteral route is the preferred method of providing nutritional support to burn patient.[26] Total parenteral nutrition increases stress response, endotoxin translocation and causes impaired mucosal immunity. Enteral route, on the other hand, provides better regulation of inflammatory cytokines, decreases intestinal permeability, preserves intestinal mucosal barrier and reduces chances of enterogenic infections. Enteral feeds through a nasogastric tube should be started as soon as possible after fluid resuscitation is achieved.

Inhalation Injury

It is a potential life-threatening situation and is responsible for 30-80% deaths in burn cases. Presence of following features suggests inhalation injuries:

- History of closed space exposure to burns/fumes
- Exposure to blast
- Collapse, restlessness, irritability
- Hoarseness or change in voice/harsh cough
- Stridor
- Burns to face, head and neck area
- Singing of nasal hairs
- Soot in sputum/saliva
- Inflamed oropharynx
- Raised carboxyhemoglobin levels
- Deteriorating pulmonary function.

Inhalation injury due to burns consists of three components:

- *Airway injury:* This occurs due to hot gases, steam or flames. This leads to upper airway swelling with subsequent airway obstruction.
- *Lung injury:* It occurs because of inhalation of products of combustion causing chemical injury to lung parenchyma.
- *Systemic intoxication:* Absorption of products of combustion at the alveolar level leads to systemic toxicity. It is mainly due to carbon monoxide and cyanide which cause inhibition of cellular metabolism.

The diagnosis of inhalation injury is confirmed by bronchoscopic examination and Xenon-133 pulmonary ventilation scan. Carboxyhemoglobin levels more than 10% suggest presence of inhalation injury.

All patients should be given 100% oxygen that increases carbon monoxide elimination. Humidification of inspired air, oxygen supplementation and good pulmonary toilet are important components of treatment. Pressure controlled ventilation in combination with permissive hypercapnia is useful in these patients.[15]

Electrical Injuries

Electrical injury is infrequent but potentially devastating form of multisystem injury with high morbidity and mortality. Electric burns account for about 2-3% of all burns in children.[27] Children are mainly exposed to injuries at home which are usually associated with electrical and extension cords for appliances. Second common source is the unprotected wall outlets. Damage due to lightening is uncommon in children. Sports like kite-flying [28] have also been described as unusual means of electrical injury.

The type and extent of an electric injury depends on the intensity of current, duration of contact with the source of current and resistance of tissues to the current. Pathway of current through the body determines the organ systems involved in the damage and thus the severity of injury. A vertical pathway of current through the axis of body involves virtually all the systems and is the most dangerous.[27]

Access to the victim poses threat to the rescuer who should take care to avoid contact with source of current. During triage, special attention is required to assess the subjects of lightening who may become transiently apneic due to transient paralysis of respiratory centre and may be given up for dead.

A patient of electric injury may require cardio-respiratory resuscitation alongwith management of acute multiple trauma. Fluid requirements are higher in these patients due to extensive injuries. All the body systems should be assessed for any evidence of injury. CT scan of the head is indicated in lightening injuries. Preventive steps for stress ulcers should be undertaken. In case of high voltage injury, evaluation for rhabdomyolysis and myoglobinuria is required.

COMPLICATIONS OF BURNS

Various complications of burns are given in Table 84.1.

Table 84.1: Important complications of burns

Early	*Late*
1. Hypovolemia	1. Hypertrophic scar
2. Shock	2. Contracture
3. Infection	3. Psychological trauma
4. Hemorrhage	4. Secondary hemorrhage
5. Hematemesis (Curling ulcer)	
6. Sloughing of mucus membranes	

Toxic shock syndrome is a relatively rare but important condition as it is a cause of mortality in superficial burns.[5] The diagnosis depends upon 5 out of the following 6 criteria being fulfilled.

- Temperature of 38.9°C or more.
- Erythematous macular rash.
- Systolic blood pressure less than 90 mmHg or less than 5th percentile for age in children.
- Involvement of three or more organ systems.
- Reasonable evidence of absence of systemic infection.
- The evidence of desquamation of palms and soles during recovery phase.

The illness is because of colonization of the burn area by *Staphylococcus aureus* in patients who have no natural immunity. Blood culture for organism is negative as clinical syndrome is caused by absorbed toxins.

Successful treatment depends upon recognition before cardiovascular deterioration is established. Beta-lactamase resistant anti-staphylococcal antibiotics are started.

PROGNOSIS

Conventional thinking has been that children, especially less than 48 months in age have higher mortality but now with improved care for burn patients, most children should survive with minimal morbidity.[29,30]

Degree of physical disability depends on various factors which are:

Intrinsic: Anatomic location of burns, depth of injury, quality of healing, genetic predisposition for scar formation, physiological contractile forces, maturation and age of the patient

Extrinsic: Treatment intervention such as wound excision and grafting; patient and parental compliance with positioning, exercises and efforts to reduce edema.

Constant pressure is the most effective way of decreasing the incidence of hypertrophic scar formation.

PREVENTION

Burns are unfortunate accidents that occur due to momentary inattention but result in consequences that last a lifetime. The patient is scarred physically and emotionally while the parents and caregivers are affected by feeling of guilt and concern.[31]

Most effective treatment of burns is their prevention. Prevention programs should be targeted at high risk areas. Public education and effective legislation are important components of burn management.

Some measures suggested for prevention of burns are:[2]

1. Unsupervised use of firecrackers by children should be prohibited.
2. Keep the matches, lighters and electrical appliances out of reach of children. Low level switches and sockets should be kept covered.
3. Kitchens should be made safe and small children should not be allowed in them.
4. Mothers and care takers should avoid handling hot liquids while with small children.

Table 84.2: The Lund and Browder chart for estimation of burns area [32]

	Age (years)					
	0-1	1-4	5-9	10-14	15	Adult
Head	19	17	13	11	9	7
Neck	2	2	2	2	2	2
Anterior trunk	13	13	13	13	13	13
Posterior trunk	13	13	13	13	13	13
Buttock	2.5	2.5	2.5	2.5	2.5	2.5
Genitalia	1	1	1	1	1	1
Upper arm	4	4	4	4	4	4
Lower arm	3	3	3	3	3	3
Hand	2.5	2.5	2.5	2.5	2.5	2.5
Thigh	5.5	6.5	8	8.5	9	9.5
Leg	5	5	5.5	6	6.5	7
Foot	3.5	3.5	3.5	3.5	3.5	3.5

5. Children should not be left in the bathrooms unattended.
6. Food should be kept in center of table and not at the edge.

REFERENCES

1. Ahuja RB, Bhattacharya S. An analysis of 11,196 burn admissions and evaluation of conservative management techniques. *Burns*. 2002;28:555-561.
2. Mukerji G, Chamania S, Patidar GP, Gupta S. Epidemiology of pediatric burns in Indore, India. *Burns* 2001;27:33-38.
3. Kumar P, Chirayil PT, Chittoria R. Ten years epidemiological study of pediatric burns in Manipal, India. *Burns* 2000;26: 261-264.
4. Kay A, Rickard R. Burn injury. In Gwinnutt CL, Driscoll PA (eds) *Trauma Resuscitation: The Team Approach*, 2nd edn. Oxford: BIOS Scientific Publishers 2003;253-272.
5. Lord WD. The severely burned child. In: Healy TEJ, Cohen PJ (eds) *Wylie and Churchill-Davidson's A Practice of Anesthesia*, 6th edn. London: Edward Arnold 1995;1061-1078.
6. Mlcak R, Cortiella J, Desai MH, Herndon DN. Emergency management of pediatric burn victims. *Pediatr Emerg Care* 1998;14:51-54.
7. Meuli M, Lochbühler H. Current concepts in pediatric burn care: general management of severe burns. *Eur J Pediatr Surg* 1992;2:195-200.
8. Palmieri TL, Jackson W, Greenhalgh DG. Benefits of early tracheostomy in severely burned children. *Crit Care Med* 2002; 30:922-924.
9. Sharp RJ. Burns. In Aschcraft KW, Murphy JP, Sharp RJ et al (eds) *Pediatric Surgery*, 3rd edn. Philadelphia: WB Saunders 2000;159-175.
10. Beushausen T, Mücke K. Anesthesia and pain management in pediatric burn management. *Pediatr Surg Int* 1997;12:327-333.
11. Henry DB, Foster RL Burn pain management in children. *Pediatr Clin North Am* 2000;47:681-698.
12. Martin-Herz SP, Thurber CA, Patterson DR. Psychological principles of burns wound pain in children. II: Treatment application. *J Burn Care Rehabil* 2000;21:458-472.
13. Martin-Herz SP, Patterson DR, Honari S, Gibbons J, Gibran N, Heimbach DM. Pediatric pain control practices in North American Burn Centers. *J Burn Care Rehabil* 2003;24:26-36.
14. Gastimeier P, Weigt O, Sohr D, Rüden H. Comparison of hospital-acquired infection rates in pediatric burn patients. *J Hosp Infect* 2002;52:161-65
15. Wolf SE, Debroy M, Herndon DN. The cornerstones and directions of pediatric burn care. *Pediatr Surg Int* 1997;12: 312-320.
16. Singh NP, Goyal R, Manchanda V, Das S, Kaur I, Talwar V. Changing trends in bacteriology of burns in the burns unit, Delhi, India. *Burns* 2003;29:129-132.
17. Barret JP, Dziewulski P, Ramzy PI, Wolf SE, Desai MH, Herndon HN. Biobrane versus 1% silver sulphadiazine in second degree pediatric burns. *Plast Reconstr Surg* 2000;152:62-65.
18. Özcan C, Orkan E, Çelik A, Çördük N. Enzymatic debridement of burn wound with collagenase in children with partial thickness burns. *Burns* 2002;28:791-794.
19. Herndon DN, Spies M. Modern burn care. *Semin Pediatr Surg* 2001;10:28-31.
20. Meuli M, Lochbühler H. Current concepts in pediatric burn care: Surgery of severe burns. *Eur J Pediatr Surg* 1992;2: 201-204.
21. Barrett JP, Herndon DN, Modulation of inflammatory and catabolic responses in severely burned children by early burn wound excision in the first 24 hours. *Arch Surg* 2003;138: 127-132.
22. Tamisani AM, Ferreti S, Sangiorgio. Critical reflections on the use of human cultured keratinocytes in the children with burns. *Eur J Pediatr Surg* 1992;2:223-226.
23. Germann G, Cedidi C, Hartmann B. Post-burn reconstruction during growth and development. *Pediatr Surg Int* 1997;12: 321-326.
24. Staley M, Richard R, Billmire D, Warden G. Head/Face/Neck Burns: Therapist considerations for the pediatric patients. *J Burn Care Rehabil* 1997;18:164-171.
25. Ramirez RJ, Wolf SE, Barrow RE, Herndon DN. Growth hormone treatment in burn patients- a safe therapeutic approach. *Ann Surg* 1998;228:439-448.
26. Andel H, Kamolz L, Hörauf K, Zimpfer M. Nutrition and anabolic agents in burned patients. *Burns* 2003;29:592-595.
27. Koumbourlis AC. Electrical injuries. *Crit Care Med* 2002;30 S424-S430.
28. Tiwari VK, Sharma D. Kite-flying: A unique but dangerous mode of electrical injury in children. *Burns* 1999;25:537-539.
29. Sheridan RL, Remensnyder JP, Schnitzer JJ, Schulz JT, Ryan CM, Tompkins RG. Current expectations for survival in pediatric burns. *Arch Pediatr Adolesc Med* 2000;154:245-249.
30. Sheridan RL, Schnitzer JJ. Management of high risk burns pediatric burn patient. *J Pediatr Surg* 2001; 36:1308-1312.
31. Burd A. Paediatric burn prevention. *Burns* 2003; 29:596-598.
32. Warden GD. Outpatient care of thermal injuries. *Surg Clin North Am* 1987;67:147-57.

Anup Mohta

85 Head Injury

INTRODUCTION

Traumatic brain injury is a leading cause of death and acquired disability in pediatric age group. It is a significant socioeconomic problem in India.

EPIDEMIOLOGY

Common causes of head injury in pediatric age group include fall from height, motor vehicle accidents, falling objects and assault. While falls are the most common cause of head injury in India, motor vehicle accidents (MVA) is the leading cause in western countries.

Falls have been classified as high level or low level, high level falls being those occurring from heights greater than 15 to 20 feet. Common sites of fall are from roof, window, balcony or stairs. In India, a common cause of falls is playing on the unsafe roofs and falling accidentally as while flying kites. There is higher incidence of intracranial injuries in patients with low level falls due to lack of time for protection by stretching hands by the falling person. Approximately 50% deaths occurring after high level falls are due to head injury.[1,2]

Motor vehicle accident is the commonest cause of head injury in children older than 14 years of age because of age-related risk-taking behavior. Effective child restraint devices are not used or are inappropriately used to a large extent. Also teenagers are least likely to wear seat belt.[3]

Gunshot injuries are getting more common nowadays and occur due to getting caught in cross fire, accidental gunshots and suicidal injuries. Trans-hemispheric injuries are more common and most of the deaths occur in pre-hospital period.[4]

Risk factors for pediatric head injuries are age, sex and socioeconomic status.[2] Boys are more likely to suffer from head injury as compared to girls.[5,6] Nearly half the patients are in 0-4 years age group. Children under two years of age are more likely to suffer from head injury due to abuse or neglect.

PATHOPHYSIOLOGY

Brain injury is the most common cause of acquired disability and mortality during childhood. Anatomically, children have a different brain water content, myelination pattern, cerebral blood volume, larger relative head mass, and weaker cervical structure as compared to adults. The biomechanical milieu of the child's brain lends to injuries of deep white matter, punctuate hemorrhages, brain swelling and linear non-depressed fractures rather than mass lesions. Physiologic differences in cerebral blood flow and metabolism due to differences in oxygen content, oxygen delivery, auto-regulatory mechanisms and neurotransmitter receptor expression affect brain injury in children in a unique manner.[7]

There are two phases of traumatic head injury. Primary injury is because of the damage sustained at the time of impact and is proportional to magnitude, duration and nature of the mechanical force. This occurs due to compression of brain over bony skull or disruption of axons by acceleration-deceleration and shearing forces at the time of impact. Expanding mass lesions within brain parenchyma can lead to increased intracranial pressure (ICP), transtentorial herniation and brain stem distortion.

Secondary injury includes intracranial or systemic events such as hypotension or hypoxia. These occur in response to primary injury resulting in complex intracellular biochemical cascades due to release of oxygen radicals, neurotransmitter excitotoxicity, lipid peroxidation and cellular calcium entry. Excitotoxicity is defined as the action of excitatory neurotransmitters like glutamate and aspartate in the propagation of injury within the central nervous system. There is a strong correlation of excitatory amino acids with young age, poorer outcome and child abuse.[8]

Cerebral perfusion pressure (CPP), defined as difference between mean arterial pressure (MAP) and ICP, is an important determinant of cerebral injury. Decrease in CPP due to hypotension caused by shock or primary cardiac injury, or increase in ICP due to hemorrhage or cerebral edema leads to cerebral ischemia and neuronal death.

CLINICAL EVALUATION

Mechanism of trauma and signs and symptoms following injury are assessed.

These include nature of injury, circumstances of accident, any drug intake and neurological findings such as loss of consciousness, lucid interval or neurological deficits. Associated historical features of importance are amnesia, disorientation, vomiting, and seizures.

Cervical spine should be stabilized in an injured child till cervical spine injury is ruled out. Primary trauma survey aims to establish adequate airway (A-airway), ensure adequate ventilation (B- breathing) and gain venous access to start volume resuscitation (C-circulation). Level of consciousness should be determined (D-disability).

Secondary trauma survey includes complete neurologic evaluation and should be completed once the patient is stable.

INITIAL MANAGEMENT

Airway may be occluded by blood, mucus, foreign body or injuries and should be cleared. Ventilation should be assessed and assisted ventilation may be required. Ventilation and airway management is adjusted to maintain arterial blood gas values so that pCO_2 is in the 35 ± 5 mmHg range, pO_2 is greater than 100 mmHg and oxygen saturation is greater than 100 percent.[7] Indications of endotracheal intubation include airway obstruction, absence of airway protective reflexes, abnormalities in respiratory rate or rhythm, co-existing thoracic or pulmonary pathology, clinical evidence of raised ICP and prior to inter-hospital transfer. Intubation should be performed by an experienced physician.[9]

Hypotension at presentation in head injured patients is more likely to be due to associated injuries and search should be made for any thoracic or abdominal trauma. Hemodynamic balance is maintained with isotonic intravenous solution and packed red blood cells to maintain normal serum electrolyte values, hemoglobin of more than 9 g/dl and hematocrit more than 28 percent. This reduces brain edema and optimizes oxygen delivery.

Neurologic examination is usually done by Glasgow Coma Scale (GCS). Adult GCS system has been modified to suit the pediatric population (Table 85.1) and is widely used for initial assessment and monitoring.[10] Posturing of the extremities, pupillary size and reaction to light is assessed. Examination of the head may demonstrate signs of raised intracranial pressure (ICP) or signs of skull fracture like palpable depression or crepitus, discoloration over mastoid, black eyes, or CSF rhinorrhea.

Child Under 2 Years

Children under two years form a special group of patients. Younger patients have higher incidence of intracranial injuries and are difficult to assess. Guidelines have been designed for management of these children.[11]

Table 85.1: Glasgow coma scale (modified for children)

Sign	*Score*
Eye opening	
Spontaneous	4
To verbal command	3
To pain	2
No response	1
Best motor response	
Obeys verbal commands	6
Localizes to pain	5
Withdraws to pain	4
Flexion response to pain	3
Extension response to pain	2
No response	1
Best verbal response	
Oriented	5
Confused	4
Inappropriate words	3
Non specific sounds	2
No response	1

Classification of head injury according to modified Glasgow coma scale CS:

Mild head injury	:	GCS 13-15
Moderate head injury	:	GCS 9-12
Severe head injury	:	GCS 3-8

a. In younger children threshold for obtaining imaging studies should be low. Clinical predictors of intracranial injury include skull fracture, altered mental status, focal neurological findings, scalp swelling, younger age, inflicted injury, and head injury with no clear history of trauma. Incidence of skull fracture in younger children with intracranial injuries ranges from 60-100%.

b. The greater the severity and number of historical symptoms and physical signs, the stronger the consideration for obtaining a radiological investigation. Greater force of collision, fall from greater heights or on hard surface, more pronounced physical findings suggest higher risk of intracranial injuries.

c. Patients should be considered high risk if they have depressed mental status, focal neurological signs, acute skull fracture by clinical or radiological examination, irritability or bulging fontanel. A child with a seizure, progressively worsening vomiting or loss of consciousness for longer than 1 minute should undergo CT examination.

d. A neurosurgeon should be consulted for any child with intracranial injury noted on CT and for any child with depressed basilar or widely diastatic fracture. Child with isolated simple fracture (a single fracture that has margins not separated by more than 3 mm, is restricted to single bone, and has no associated intracranial injury on CT) may be discharged if they meet the discharge criteria.

e. Younger children with large scalp swellings and fractures resulting from a high energy mechanism are more likely to develop delayed complications.

Seizures

Post-traumatic seizures (PTS) occur due to epileptogenic focus resulting due to hemorrhage, contusion or other lesion secondary to head injury. PTS is defined as 'early' onset (occurring within a week of injury) or 'late' onset (occurring after one week of injury). Post-traumatic seizure can be a serious complication of head injury because this can cause secondary brain damage through increased metabolic requirements, raised intracranial pressure, cerebral hypoxia and/or excessive release of neurotransmitters.

This makes the monitoring of the patient more difficult due to postictal neurological deterioration and may lead to delay in treatment of intracranial lesions.

Incidence of PTS has been reported to be 7-21%. Infants under 2 years of age, low GCS scores (less than 8) and long duration of unconsciousness are more prone to develop PTS.

The incidence of early PTS among patients with GCS less than 8 is much higher than patients with GCS 13-15.[12,13] Suitable management of children with severe head injury must include adequate prophylaxis with antiepileptic drugs for immediate and early PTS.

Child Abuse

Infants having head injury and persistent neurologic deficit without any history of significant trauma are more likely to be victims of abuse. Cases in which history changes or the injury is blamed on home resuscitation efforts are also likely to represent child abuse.[14] Child abuse must be considered in all children under two years of age, especially belonging to lower socioeconomic status, who present with acute subdural hematoma in the absence of a history of motor vehicle accident.[15] Head injury is a major cause of morbidity and mortality in the abused children and is associated with higher incidence of severe intracranial injuries. Retinal hemorrhages occur in 20-60 percent cases. Child abuse leads to heavy economic burden on the society as they have more severe injuries and longer period of hospital stay, require more intensive care time and undergo more diagnostic work-up.

Imaging Techniques

The risk of sustaining injury that is visible on imaging studies in the acute period is approximately 20- 45 percent. Around 43 percent victims have skull fracture, 58% intracranial hemorrhage (ICH) and over 50 percent have cerebral edema.[16]

Computed tomography (CT) is the modality of choice for the evaluation of acute neurologic presentations or hemorrhage in pediatric trauma. It is widely available and less expensive as compared to magnetic resonance imaging (MRI), can accommodate life-support equipment, traction and monitoring devices and is easy to obtain. It is useful for detection of acute or subacute hemorrhage, scalp injury and pneumocephalus as well as other neurologically significant conditions like hydrocephalus, midline shift, masses and mass effect, ischemia and hernia-that require rapid detection for treatment.[17] Disadvantages of CT include exposure to ionizing radiation, transport of the child away from the direct supervision of emergency physicians, frequent requirement of sedation hampering neurologic evaluation, additional health care cost and increased time for emergency room evaluation.

Role of MRI in head injury is complimentary to CT scan. It provides better delineation of abnormal brain anatomy and function in injured pediatric brain. It has improved sensitivity for detection of intracranial injury like edema, hematoma, contusion, diffuse axonal injury and brain edema. Sequelae of head trauma are better assessed with MRI.

Cerebral blood flow and volume in trauma patients can be assessed with CT perfusion, MR perfusion or transcranial Doppler imaging.

Contrary to convention, neither loss of consciousness nor mildly altered sensorium is a sensitive indicator with which to select patients for CT scanning. Therefore, a liberal policy of CT scanning is warranted for pediatric patients with high-risk injury mechanism. It may be the most cost-effective method of managing minor pediatric head trauma.[18]

Cross table lateral X-ray of cervical spine should be done in all patients over 3 years of age with altered mental status, neurologic deficit or neck or back pain to rule out associated cervical spine injury.

Admission Criteria

Hospitalization of all mild head injury patients is not recommended. Children with mild to moderate head injury are admitted if they have persistent malaise, abnormal neurologic physical findings or abnormal radiologic findings on X-ray or CT scan.[7] Patients with a normal CT scan and a normal neurological examination at the time of discharge can be managed as outpatients.[19] There is a growing propensity for admitting children for 24 hours for admission even when there is a negative workup.[5] As it is stressful for the child and family and increases the cost, unnecessary admissions should be avoided.

In a metropolitan area, pediatric patients with severe traumatic brain injury should be transported directly to a pediatric trauma center if available.[20]

Resuscitation

Primary brain injury is not amenable to treatment therefore fundamental goals of resuscitation in a head injured child are directed towards preventing secondary brain damage due to hypoxia, hypotension and raised intracranial pressure.

Child should be nursed in neutral position or with the head end of the bed raised to up to 30° if there is no shock. This may help to reduce intracranial pressure.

Intracranial hypertension, though difficult to diagnose in infants, is associated with decreased survival. Presence of open fontanel and/or sutures does not preclude intracranial hypertension or negate utility of monitoring of ICP. Physician may choose to monitor ICP in patients with traumatic mass lesions or in whom serial neurologic examination is precluded by sedation, neuromuscular blockade or anesthesia. Intracranial pressure is monitored and treated with a combination ventricular catheter, fiberoptic or strain gauge transducer which allows simultaneous recording of ICP and therapeutic CSF removal.[7, 20] Treatment of ICP is initiated if it rises above 20 mm Hg.

Three accepted forms of therapies to reduce intracranial pressure are available:[20]

a. Ventricular drainage if a ventricular drain is available,
b. Mild hyperventilation with pCO_2 maintained above 30mmHg,and
c. Use of boluses of Mannitol (0.25-1 gm/kg). Alternatively hypertonic saline (3%) in a dose of 0.1-1.0 ml/kg/hr may be used to reduce ICP.

Second tier therapies include large decompressive craniectomy, barbiturate therapy, perfusion pressure management (artificial elevation of systemic arterial blood pressure), hypocarbia to decrease pCO_2 below 30 mmHg, limited periods of induced hypothermia (temperature more than 30°C) and controlled lumbar drainage. Unilateral decompressive craniectomies improve outcome and decrease mortality when these are performed within 6 hours of injury.[20,22] High dose barbiturates may be considered in hemodynamically stable patients with salvageable severe head injury and refractory intracranial hypertension. The use of steroids is not recommended for improving outcome in patients with severe brain injury.

Traditional teaching has been that patient should be kept euthermic but it has been shown that use of moderate hypothermia in the treatment of acute traumatic brain injury helps to prevent long-term cognitive and motor impairment.[23] Moderate hypothermia (rectal temperature maintained between 32-34°C) administered within 6 hours of acute traumatic brain injury in children in conjunction with conventional intracranial hypertension management and maintained for 48 hours results in decreased severity of intracranial pressure. One single therapeutic measure may not provide the degree of neuroprotection that will provide significant functional improvement in clinical outcome.

In the absence of intracranial injuries on neuroimaging, antiepileptic prophylaxis is not recommended.[19]

There is no role of antibiotics unless a ventricular catheter has been inserted for ICP monitoring or there is history of CSF rhinorrhea.

Management of Specific Injuries[24]

a. *Scalp injuries:* Scalp injuries are commonly seen in pediatric head injury. As scalp has a rich vascular supply, any laceration can lead to profuse bleeding. Simple lacerations are primarily sutured after cleaning and debridement. Healing is usually good.
b. *Concussion:* It is defined as transient loss of consciousness. Some children may suffer from irritability, post-traumatic amnesia and occasionally behavioral problems.
c. *Contusion*: Contusions are areas of brain injury due to primary impact and are commonly seen in temporal, frontal and occipital lobes. These may enlarge over time. Functional outcome is usually good.
d. *Hemorrhage:* Common types of intracerebral hemorrhage are intracerebral hematoma, epidural hematoma (EDH), subdural hematoma (SDH) and subarachnoid hemorrhage. While treatment of most intracerebral hematomas is conservative, symptomatic epidural hematomas are treated by emergency clot evacuation. Subdural hematomas (SDH) with mass effect require management of intracranial hypertension by surgical drainage. Outcome of patients with SDH is worse than EDH due to underlying brain damage and resultant raised intracranial pressure. Treatment of subarachnoid hemorrhage is conservative.
e. *Fractures:* Most of the skull fractures are linear and do not require any active management. Leptomeningeal cyst or growing fracture occurs in association with a dural tear when torn meninges become interposed between the fracture segments. With pulsation of CSF, the meninges herniate through the fracture site, widening it over time. Leptomeningeal cyst tends to occur with thin, mobile membranous bones and is, therefore, common in the parietal and frontal bones of children under three years of age. Surgical intervention is required for management of growing fractures or leptomeningeal cysts.
f. Diffuse axonal injuries occur due to disruption of axonal pathways in corpus callosum, deep nuclei, basal ganglia and thalamus due to acceleration/deceleration and shearing forces. Functional outcome of these injuries is poor.

Discharge Criteria

Child may be considered for discharge after appropriate evaluation, with imaging, observation and neurosurgical consultation if indicated.

a. The child has no significant extracranial injures or other indications for admission.

b. The child easily alerts and has normal neurologic examination.
c. There is no suspicion of abuse or neglect.
d. The child lives in a relatively close proximity to health care and has reliable caretakers who are able to return if necessary.

Caregivers of any child who is sent home should be advised to bring the child back to medical facility if there is drowsiness, loss of unconsciousness, persistent vomiting or convulsions, severe headache, unusual weakness or change in behavior.

PROGNOSIS

The outcome of children with brain injury depends on the nature of the primary damage and on how well secondary brain damage can be limited. Appropriate critical care management at the scene and in hospital can prevent secondary brain damage that would otherwise result from cerebral reactions.[25] Outcome of a head injury patient also depends on the type of injury, its severity, age of the patient, systemic illness and extracranial injuries. Acute brain stem lesions, focal disruption of white fibers at pontomedullary junction or from avulsion of midbrain perforating vessel due to acute congestion or edema of supratentorial hemisphere leads to instant death while late deaths occur due to acute inflammatory processes.[26]

Patients who have a GCS of less than 8 have a poor outcome. Prognostic value of GCS may be increased by presence of hypoxia on admission, and CT scan features of subarachnoid hemorrhage, diffuse axonal injury and brain swelling.[27] Decerebration and flaccidity have the worst prognosis.

The teaching that children always have a better outcome than adults after a severe head injury, regardless of mechanism of injury, is a myth. Children involved in motor vehicle accidents are as likely to die from severe head injury as adults. Improved results in some studies may be due to referral patterns, GCS scoring errors, time to treatment and reporting errors.[28]

Some avoidable factors that lead to increased mortality and morbidity in pediatric head injury are aspiration, missed intracranial pathology or delay before diagnosis, associated injuries, severe cerebral edema and hazards of inter-hospital transfers.[29]

Strict guidelines should be followed to decide about brain death in patients. At the same time, severity and irreversible nature of brain injury in neurotrauma patients are more easily definable by history, physical examination and neuroimaging than in neurological disorders such as hypoxic injury. Unnecessary long observation periods have disadvantages for family, the hospital and the society.[30]

REHABILITATION

Rehabilitation of the child with a head injury is an important component of management as traumatic brain injury may have lasting effects on development and maturation.[31] It allows the child the necessary experiences to stimulate neuronal reorganization following traumatic brain injury and maximize recovery. Although injury-related and treatment-related factors are critical during the early stages of recovery, patient-related factors such as age-at-injury, developmental achievement at time of injury, maturation, and family involvement and resources impact the later stages of recovery.

Early rehabilitation prepares the family for the child's long-term recovery and developmental needs. Involvement and training of family members early in the recovery process is critical for successful long-term outcome as they can ensure treatment compliance, follow-through with treatment recommendations, maintain treatment gains and in generalizing treatment effects beyond the medical settings.

PREVENTION

As traumatic brain injury is a serious socioeconomic problem, it is important to take necessary preventive steps.

The children should not be allowed to play without supervision especially on roofs and balconies. Proper play grounds need to be provided so that they do not play on the roads. Educational programs are important aspects for avoiding accidents. Use of helmets has been shown to reduce the risk of brain injury substantially among bike riders of all ages. Reasons for nonuse include fashion issues, discomfort and lack of knowledge regarding the protective effect of helmets. There are almost no guidelines for child passenger safety. Legislations need to be passed to ensure safety criteria in vehicles for children. Legislation is more cost-effective than education programs.[3]

REFERENCES

1. Wang MY, Kim KA, Griffith PM, Summers S, McComb JG, Levy ML, Mahour GH. Injuries from falls in the pediatric population: An analysis of 729 cases. *J Pediatr Surg* 2001;36:1528-1534.
2. Sharma M, Sharma AK. Mode, presentation, CT findings and outcome of pediatric head injury. *Indian Pediatr* 1994;31:733-739.
3. Dowd MD, Keenan HT, Bratton SL. Epidemiology and prevention of childhood injuries. *Crit Care Med* 2002; 30(Suppl):S385-S392.
4. Coughlan MD, Fleggan AG, Semple PL, Pet er JC. Craniocerebral gunshot injuries in children. *Child's Nerv Syst* 2003;19:348-352.
5. Murgio A, Andrade FA, Sanchez Muñoz MA, Boetto S, Leung KM. International multicenter study on head injury in children. *Child's Nerv Syst* 1999;15:318-321.

6. Ghooi AM, Khanna T, Gupta MM. An analysis of 500 cases of head injury in children. *Indian J Pediatr* 1976;43:191-197.
7. Faillace WJ. Management of childhood neurotrauma. *Surg Clin North Am* 2002;82:349-363.
8. Glass TF. Treatment of pediatric traumatic brain injury: A broad path to a narrow gate. *J Pediatr* 2001; 138:1-3.
9. Noah ZL, Hahn YS, Rubenstein JS, Aronyk K. Management of the child with severe brain injury. *Crit Care Clin* 1992;8: 59-77.
10. Teasdale G, Jennet B. Assessment of coma and impaired consciousness. *Lancet* 1974;11:81.
11. Schutzman SA, Barnes P, Duhaime AC, Greenes D, Homer C, Jaffe D et al. Evaluation and management of children younger than two years old with apparently minor head trauma: Proposed guidelines. *Pediatrics* 2001;107:983-993.
12. Chiaretti A, Benedictis RD, Polidori G, Piastra M, Iannelli A, Rocco CD. Early post-traumatic seizures in children with head injury. *Child's Nerv Syst* 2000;16:862-866.
13. Ratan SK, Kulshreshtha R, Pandey RM. Predictors of posttraumatic convulsions in head injured children. *Pediatr Neurosurg* 1999;30:127-131.
14. Hettler J, Greenes DS. Can the initial history predict whether a child with head injury has been abused? *Pediatrics* 2003; 111: 602-607.
15. Dashti SR, Decker DD, Razzaq A, Cohen AR. Current patterns of inflicted head injury in children. *Pediatr Neurosurg* 1999;31:302-306.
16. Woodcock RJ, Davis PC, Hopkins KL. Imaging of head trauma in infancy and childhood. *Semin Ultrasound CT MR* 2001;22:162-182.
17. Poussaint TY, Moeller KK. Imaging of pediatric head trauma. *Neuroimag Clin North Am* 2002;12:271-294.
18. Simon B, Letourneau P, Vitorino E, McCall J. Pediatric minor head trauma: Indications for computed tomography revisited. *J Trauma* 2001;51:231-238.
19. Savitsky EA, Votey SR. Current controversies in the management of minor pediatric head injuries. *Am J Emerg Med* 2000;18:96-101.
20. Society of Critical Care Medicine. Guidelines for the acute medical management of severe traumatic brain injury in infants, children, and adolescents. *Crit Care Med* 2003;31(6 Suppl): S407-491.
21. Rekate HL. Head injuries: management of primary injuries and prevention of secondary damage. *Child's Nerv Syst* 2001;17: 632-634.
22. Hejazi N, Witzmann A, Fae P. Unilateral decompressive craniectomy for children with severe brain injury. Report of seven cases and review of the relevant literature. *Eur J Pediatr* 2002;161:99-104.
23. Biswas AK, Bruce DA, Sklar FH, Bokovoy JL, Sommerauer JF. Treatment of acute traumatic brain injury in children with moderate hypothermia improves intracranial hypertension. *Crit Care Med* 2003;30:2742-2751.
24. Gruber DP, Brockmeyer DL, Walker ML. Head injuries in children. In: Ashcraft KW, Murphy JP, Sharp RJ, Sigalet DL, Snyder CL (eds) *Pediatric Surgery,* 3rd edn. Philadelphia: Saunders 2000;217-229.
25. Chiaretti A, De Benedictis R, Della Corte F, Piastra M, Viola L, Polidori G, Di Rocco C. The impact of initial management on the outcome of children with severe head injury. *Childs Nerv Syst.* 2002;18:54-60.
26. Ratan SK, Pandey RM, Kulshreshtha R, Ratan J. Risk factors for mortality within first 24 hours of head injury. *Indian J Pediatr* 2002;69:573-577.
27. Ong L, Selladurai BM, Dhillon MK, Atan M, Lye MS. The prognostic value of the Glagow coma scale, hypoxia and computerized tomography in outcome prediction of pediatric head injury. *Pediatr Neurosurg* 1996;24:285-291.
28. Johnson DL, Krishnamurthy S. Severe pediatric head injury: Myth, magic, and actual fact. *Pediatr Neurosurg* 1998;28: 167-172.
29. Sharples PM, Storey A, Aynsley-Green A, Eyre JA. Avoidable factors contributing to death of children with head injury. *BMJ* 1990;300:87-91.
30. Chang MY, McBride LA, Ferguson MA. Variability in brain death declaration practices in pediatric head trauma patients. *Pediatr Neurosurg* 2003;39:7-9.
31. Beaulieu CL. Rehabilitation and outcome following pediatric traumatic brain injury. *Surg Clin North Am* 2002;82:393-408.

Section XV

Ophthalmic Emergencies

Vijaya Wali and RK Sharma

86 Pediatric Ocular Emergencies

INTRODUCTION

In terms of loss to society of productive human beings due to visual impairment, childhood blindness contributes significantly. The total number of blind years suffered by a blind child is more than those suffered by a person who becomes blind in adulthood or in the old age. Though accurate data on the prevalence of childhood blind ness are not available but according to one of the studies,[1] the causes of childhood blindness are congenital globe anomalies (microphthalmos/ anophthalmos) in 25%, retinal diseases (mostly retinitis pigmentosa) in 22.2%, optic atrophy in 16.7%, cataract/ lens related in 15.3%, corneal opacities in 11.1% (including vitamin A deficiency in 5.5%), glaucoma in 4.2%, amblyopia due to high refractive error in 2.8%, and abnormality of higher visual pathway in 2.8%. The proportion of these causes of childhood blindness may be different in other studies and different in different states. These causes can be grouped under different heads like congenital, intrauterine, perinatal and natal causes. Out of these the blindness due to corneal opacities, vitamin A deficiency, glaucoma, refractive error, and trauma etc. are preventable to some extent if not treatable.

Pediatric ocular emergencies include number of disorders, which may provide detrimental to vision or fatal to life if not managed in time. Hence, a thorough clinical examination of a child by an ophthalmologist consequent to any ocular complaint is essential. Delay in reporting to a qualified person and then a further delay in referral to an ophthalmologist may lead to irreversible loss of the word vision. Emergency, may not be interpreted as an accident. Considering a problem requiring an urgent attention as an emergency is a step in the right direction.

Depending upon these factors, there are numerous conditions, which are to be treated urgently. So to say, for an ophthalmologist a baby of one day, reporting with complaints of watering is an emergency because it may be one of the earliest presentation of congenital glaucoma, which may cause permanent blindness subsequently. But congenital and neonatal problems are not considered here.

MELTING CORNEA (XEROPHTHALMIA, KERATOMALACIA)

Keratomalacia is a rapid destructive liquefactive necrosis of the corneal with perforation and extrusion of the contents of the eye. This may result in adherent leukoma, anterior staphyloma or phthisis bulbi. All this can be prevented by diagnosing vitamin A deficiency by seeing conjunctival xerosis, Bitot's spot and marked dryness or roughening of the area in the eye. A child presenting to a pediatrician with protein-energy malnutrition may seek his attention for poor general health only. Keratomalacia may go unnoticed because nutritional ulcers are not associated with classical reaction of corneal ulcer. Early diagnosis and referral to an ophthalmologist can prevent the child from having life long darkness.

A survey of blind school students in 9 Indian states revealed that 18.6% of the blindness was due to vitamin A deficiency and another 3.2% due to measles which precipitates vitamin A deficiency.[2] On the other hand, vitamin A deficiency contributed to only 5.5% of the childhood blindness in a population-based survey in West Godavari district of Andhra Pradesh.[3] The magnitude of childhood blindness due to vitamin A deficiency probably varies considerably in different parts of India. This may be related to variations in socioeconomic status. Vitamin A deficiency also contributes to child mortality,[4] which can be reduced with vitamin A supplementation.[5]

There are global initiatives to eliminate this public health problem in the affected areas.

In India, programs include:

i. Vitamin A supplementation for preschool children with the first dose being given at 9 months of age with measles immunization.
ii. Food-based strategy including nutritional education. There are no recent population-based data regarding the extent of vitamin A deficiency as a public health problem in India, or on the effectiveness of vitamin A supplementation and nutrition education programmes.

In India, nearly 6 percent of children under 6 years have ocular signs of Vitamin A deficiency, and 30-40 thousands get blinded every year. Awareness has to be increased amongst pediatrician and ophthalmologists that the preferred way to treat vitamin A deficiency is with oral supplementation rather than intramuscular injection, except in cases of severe vomiting and diarrhea. All children suffering from vitamin A deficiency must be administered a single oral dose of 200,0000 IU of vitamin A on diagnosis followed by another dose of 200,0000 IU, one to four weeks later.

OCULAR TRAUMA

Ocular trauma most commonly causes loss of vision in one eye. Though good data on the prevalence of childhood blindness due to trauma in India are not currently available, it is a fact that monocular vision loss due to trauma may not be negligible in children. Andhra Pradesh Eye Disease Study's[6] statistics indicates that in an urban population 3.97% people showed some clinical evidence or gave a history of ocular trauma. Blindness due to trauma was noted in 0.60% population. In 55% the trauma causing blindness was sustained before 15 years of age and in 92.1% before 40 years. Another study[7] by the same centre indicated that the reason for enucleation was trauma in 13% subjects. Another 25% had staphylomas, 34% of which were related to childhood trauma.

Most ocular trauma in children occurs as a part of everyday activities. A child may sustain injury playing game outdoors or with toys and at times by negligence on the part of kith and kins. Ignorance, lack of awareness, typical childhood behavior makes children more susceptible to injuries in general. Trauma to eye can be blunt, penetrating, perforating or a trauma with retained intraocular foreign body. Chemical injuries represent a true form of ocular emergency and need extraordinary and immediate attention; treatment should be initiated even before undertaking a detailed history. Ocular injury with callously disposed hypodermic needles as part of hospital waste, has recently been noticed with increasing frequency in children.

Blunt Ocular Trauma

Being hit by a ball, stone, a marble ball of fist, tennis ball or a small rubber (cosco ball) causes more severe injury to eye ball as compared to a bigger sized ball which damages the bony orbital boundaries more often. Though quite often it is the black eye or ecchymosis, which is common but thorough examination of the eye is needed to know the true extent. Other features may be severe subconjunctival hemorrhage, conjunctival and corneal lacerations, iris tears, subluxated or dislocated lens, hyphaema, traumatic cataract, retinal detachment or even fracture of orbital floor.

Suspition, early diagnosis and treatment are essential to preserve the anatomical and functional status of eye. Inappropriate and unwanted handling of the eyeball after sustaining injury can cause more harm than benefit. Once the eyeball is ruptured a slight increase in intraocular pressure by forced blinking even, can be sufficient to complete the unfinished task of expulsion of eyeball contents. The best approach by any one first attending to a child with any type of ocular trauma (except chemical trauma) is to just apply a pad and bandage and refer to an ophthalmologist. Putting any kind of ointment into the eye is contraindicated. There is a common practice to apply hot fermentation to any painful site. In blunt trauma causing black eye care is taken to apply cod compresses. In any case, diminution/ loss of vision following a trivial trauma invites urgent attention from ophthalmologist.

Penetrating Ocular Trauma

In children full evaluation of trauma should be done by an ophthalmologist preferably under sedation and detailed history of mode of injury from the parents should be sought. An innocuous looking hole might actually be an extensive laceration with poor visual prognosis. A grossly chemosed conjunctiva or a subconjunctival hemorrhage not only is indicative of scleral rupture but occasionally also masks it. All traumatized eyes, even those with little evidence of penetrating injury, should be deemed to contain an IOFB unless proved otherwise. Common causes of perforating injuries are pencil/pen knife, pair of scissors, sewing needle, knitting needles, kroshia, iron nails, thorn/pointed twigs, glass pieces or any other thing which has a pointed tip or edge, fire cracker injuries and road traffic accidents. A trauma with a vegetative source is more likely to be fungal infected. Injuries with bow and arrow are special to mention in Indian subcontinent. Its incident increases in festival season of Dusshera and Diwali.

First aid treatment of such cases is to do patching of the eye by a sterilized eye pad available in the market and urgently referring to ophthalmologist for earliest management. The timing of injury and the time elapsed between injury and seeking expert advice—in hours—is of utmost importance, not only from the point of view of final visual outcome but it also holds immense medicolegal value. Unwanted handling of the eye to assess the wound and using dry sun sterilised cotton, ointments should be avoided. No oral medicines should be administered and patient should be asked to remain fasting further on. Using of home remedies like honey, surmaa, kajal, alyan, and boric wash need to be condemned.

Management of penetrating wound may require, at times, multiple surgeries to restore anatomical and functional status of the eye.

Attempts can be made to minimize visual loss in children due to trauma by:

- Increasing public awareness about risk of vision loss due to trauma.
- Legislation to restrict dangerous toys and fireworks.
- Legislation to impose strict hospital waste disposal regulations to prevent injury with hypodermic needles.

- Encouraging the public to seek early treatment for eye injuries, promote closer liaison between pediatricians, obstetricians and ophthalmologists to facilitate easier cross referral regarding childhood disorders.
- Training of ophthalmologists in the skills necessary to effectively manage ocular trauma.

Small foreign bodies, in the form of dust/carbon particle can cause corneal abrasion. Persistent irritation, watering, red eye and photophobia need consultation with ophthalmologist. Foreign body may be too small to be visible to naked eye but sufficient to cause permanent damage to corneal.

Chemical Injuries

Chemical injuries to eye form the real emergency in ophthalmology. Acids and alkalis form major chunk of ocular chemical burns.

Alkali injuries are more commonly encountered. They are extensively used in industries and in various household as cleansing agents, like fertilizers, refrigerants (ammonia); drain cleaner (sodium hydroxide), causative potash (potassium hydroxide), sparklers and fireworks (magnesium hydroxide), white wash, cement, plaster (lime). Alkali injuries tend to be more severe than acid injuries because of the quick penetration into the eyes.

Acid burns are often confined to the ocular surface and tend to produce superficial damage. Most acid injuries are minor and heal with little are no ocular damage. Trauma mostly occurs from contact with weak acids or dilute strong acid. Common source are industrial cleaners, battery acid (sulphuric acid), fruit and vegetable preservatives, bleach refrigerants (sulfurous acid), and vinergar (acetic acid).

Chemical injuries represent a true form of ocular emergency and need extraordinary and immediate attention. The most important component of occur chemical burns is the initiation of irrigation the sooner the better. Any available bland solutions can be used. Sterile solutions like normal saline, ringer lactate or buffer solutions are preferred as water may cause minor cellular damage owing to its hypotonicity. Irrigation should be carried out for about half an hour or more.

Thermal Injuries

Basic management of the burnt skin of lids and adnexal structure is as usual. Minimum structural deformity is the aim to prevent consequential scarring and lifelong epiphora. Trauma to the cornea is of utmost importance. So, a child sustaining burn injuries of face must be referred at the earliest to an ophthalmologist for specialized care after first aid management of reducing the immediate temperature. Thermal trauma can be because of ghee and oil/spilling in kitchen, blast injuries secondary to IED and battery explosions, cracker injury, simple fire of any origin, etc.

DEFECTIVE VISION AND EYE STRAIN

It is better to consider it as a relative emergency. There are few data available on the prevalence and types of refractive errors in children in developing countries but, in the USA, the prevalence of vision problems is estimated to be 5-10%, while the prevalence of amblyopia is 1-5% in children.[8] In a study in India, 5.1% of children in schools head a visual acuity of < 6/12 in the better eye.[9] Uncorrected refractive error are thought to be a common cause of visual impairment during childhood in India. 2.8% of the childhood blindness in the population based assessment in Andhra Pradesh was caused by amblyopia associated with uncorrected high refractive error.[1] The frequency of vision testing needs to be linked to the availability of resources. If conditions are favorable, children should be screened once during the primary school years (6-11 years) and once during early adolescence (12-14 years). This is the ideal for developing countries.

Teachers and parents should be taught to look for symptoms and signs, which indicate refractive errors. They can observe if children hold books unusually close to their eyes, sit close to the TV, rub their eyes frequently or twist or tilt their heads to favor one eye. Any child having headache or having eyestrain should be screened for vision testing. Children scoring low in the exams, not taking interest in outdoor activities or frequent blinking too point towards refractive errors. Refractive errors have best prognosis if treated in time, roughly speaking under twelve years of age.

Deviation of eye to one or other direction or misalignment should be considered seriously and not merely a weakness of muscles in younger age. Sometimes diarrhea or associated debilitating disease may be a precipitating cause for underlying strabismus. Any squinting eye can go blind or any blind eye can be squinting. After assessing the cause of squint (strabismus), excluding the organic causes (like intracranial space occupying lesion), the management revolves around refraction, surgery and orthoptic exercises. The result are best if strabismus management is done below the age of 11-12 years. Common practice of wait and watch policy and leaving the child to grow or the child is too young to undergo surgery has to be discouraged.

WHITE REFLEX IN PUPILLARY AREA

Normally pupillary area in children and very old is slightly grey in colour because of internal reflection but if there is a white reflex in pupillary area the child should not be immediately referred to an ophthalmologist for detailed evaluation. White reflex may be because of cataract or it may be amaurotic cat's eye reflex which is a golden yellow reflection behind the pupillary area in a blind eye.

Cataract and lens related causes contributed to 15.3%[3] of childhood blindness in the population based assessment and 12.3% in the blind school study.[2] Cataract may be congenital due to chromosomal abnormalities, metabolic disorders e.g. galactosemia, intrauterine infections because of rubella or other maternal diseases during pregnancy. It can be acquired also because of trauma and infections. It may present as nuclear, cortical or dense opacity seen as a white reflex from the papillary area. Removal has to be done earliest, so as to permit development of appropriate retinal fixation and cortical visual responses. Intraocular lens implantation is essential to prevent amblyopia of the operated eye.

Glioma (retinoblastoma) and non malignant but sight-threatening pseudoglioma (metastatic endophthalmitis, persistent hyperplastic primary vitreous, toxocariasis, Coat's disease, retinal astro-cytoma, Norrie's disease) also present as white reflex.

Retinoblastoma is the most common primary intraocular malignancy in children appearing between 2nd–4th year of life. Ninety percent cases are diagnosed within three years of life the incidence of which has increased to approximately one in 15,000-20,000 live births.

Retinoblastoma is sporadic in 60% of cases and hereditary in 40% of cases. It usually presents as unilateral but may be bilateral (hereditary). Most common presenting sign is a white reflex from pupillary area detected by parents or the pediatrician. Strabismus is the second common presentation. Apparent intraocular inflammation and secondary glaucoma may be present in some cases. Other modes or presentation are unilateral proptosis, pupillary dilatation and diminution of vision. Various ways of treating to either save the eye or life are:

- If the eye can be saved with useful vision, choice is radiotherapy.
- Enucleation is the treatment of choice to prevent spread of tumour and save life.
- Chemotherapy as an adjunct for long-term surgery.
- Chemotherapy or photocoagulation for smaller lesion.

The factors that are helpful in the management of childhood cataract, glaucoma, and retinoblastoma are:

- Early identification and referral.
- Surgical management by trained specialists.
- Long-term follow-up by specialists to manage complications.
- Effective refractive error correction to prevent amblyopia.

To deal effectively with these causes of childhood blindness, the following issues need to be addressed:

i. Increase public awareness that a white reflex from the eye or a hazy/enlarged appearance of the front of the eye in a child requires immediate attention by an ophthalmologist.
ii. Have adequate number of trained ophthalmologists to deal with these causes based on needs assessment in India.
iii. Have reasonable pediatric support services, including anesthesia and effective refractive correction, in selected centres for managing childhood cataract, glaucoma, and retinoblastoma.
iv. Address to known etiology for some cases of cataract, e.g., rubella.

INFLAMMATION

Acute infections of conjunctiva and adnexa which can involve any age group needs attention in general but orbital cellulitis at times may present as an ocular emergency in children. Orbital cellulitis may be preseptal of may involve tissues behind the orbital septum. Strepto and staphylococcal infections are common but H. influenza may also precipitate it, especially children with sinusitis. There may be proptosis, chemosis, and conjunctiva, with limitation of movements and loss of vision. It is a life threatening condition and needs emergency treatment. Besides parenteral antibiotics surgical drainage of contiguous abscess or sinus infection is needed.

Certain childhood diseases like juvenile rheumatoid arthritis or ankylosing spondylitis or psuedotumors of the orbit primarily lead to iridocyclitis or intermediate uveitis. This condition is to be treated with topical periocular or systemic steroids and mydriatic, cycloplegics to prevent various sequelae or iridocyclitis and loss of vision. So, any child, in consultation with the pediatrician for such systemic diseases if has red eyes, pain, diminution of vision watering etc., should not be taken as granted to have conjunctivitis like problem and treated but referred to ophthalmologist for the expert opinion. On the other hand, every red eye should not be put on steroid-antibiotic combinations which can cause more harm than benefit to a child by causing glaucoma or cataract as a side-effect.

REFERENCES

1. Deshmukh A. Childhood blindness in the Third world. *J Pediatr Adolesc* 2002;7:118-127.
2. Rahi JS, Sripathi S, Gilbert CE, Foster A. Childhood blindness in India: causes in 1318 blind school children in nine states. *Eye* 1995;9:6545-6550.
3. Dandona L, Williams JD, Williams BC, Rao Gn. Population-based assessment of childhood blindness in southern India. *Arch Ophthalmol* 1998;116:545-546.
4. Sommer A, Tarwotio I, Hussaini G, Susanto D. Increased mortality in children with mild Vitamin A deficiency. *Lancet* 1983;ii:5855-5888.
5. Sommer A, Tarwotjo I, Djunaedi E, West Jr KP, Loeden AA, TIlden R, et al. Impact of Vitamin A supplementation on childhood mortality: A randomised controlled community trial. *Lancet* 1986;i:1169-1173.
6. Dandona L, Dandona R, Srinivas M, et al. Ocular Trauma in an Urban Population in Southern India. The Andhra Pradesh Eye Disease Study. *Clini Experim Ophthalm* 2000;28(5):350-356.
7. Vemuganti GK, Jalali S, Honavar SG, Shekhar GC. Enucleation in a Tertiary Eye Care Centre in India. *Eye* 2001;15:760-765.
8. Community Pediatric Committee. Vision screening in infants and children. *Pediatr Child Health* 1998;3:261-262.
9. Kalikivayi V, Naduvilath T, Bansal Ak, Dnadona L. Visual impairment in school children in Southern India. *Indian J Ophthalmol* 1997;45:129-134.

Section XVI

ENT Emergencies

Aniece Chowdhary

87 Foreign Bodies

INTRODUCTION

The vulnerability of the child to accidentally or intentionally lodge objects in the numerous orifices and cavities of the head and the critical physiologic importance of the upper airway, makes foreign bodies a subject of major importance when discussing the otolaryngologic emergencies.[1-3] Clinical features due to foreign body lodgement in ENT area not only depend upon the anatomic site involved but also on the age of the patient and the degree of obstruction and inflammatory response produced by the foreign body, symptoms ranging from asymptomatic to acute life threatening condition. Also, the point to be stressed is the possibility of multiple foreign bodies in same or different orifices, especially in mentally abnormal and psychotic patients.

FOREIGN BODIES IN THE NOSE

Common vegetable foreign bodies are peas, beans, dried pulses, nuts, cotton wool, pencil pieces etc. Mineral matter may be parts from metal and plastic toys, pebbles, beeds etc. Button batteries may also be inserted in the nose. Animate foreign bodies are the screw worms and their larvae, maggots and roundworm.

The inert foreign bodies may remain in the nose for years, without any symptomatology. Others, however lead to inflammation and infection of the mucosa, leading to purulent, foul–smelling discharge often tinged with the dark blood. These features are usually unilateral except in animate infestations. Ultimately, granulation tissue is formed and there may be ulceration of mucosa and occasionally necrosis of bone or cartilage. Vegetative foreign bodies are known to cause brisk inflammatory reaction. If a foreign body is buried in granulation tissue or firmly impacted, it may act as a nucleus for concretion and becomes a 'rhinolith' which is usually seen near the floor of nose and is radio-opaque Maggots and leach usually give rise to a severe inflammatory reaction and, if untreated, may also involve the sinuses, orbits, adjoining skin, meninges and brain.

With inanimate foreign bodies the suspicion usually arises because of unilateral, foul smelling, purulent nasal discharge and in children these symptoms must be regarded as due to a foreign body until proved otherwise. Frequently, the foreign body is seen on anterior rhinoscopy after suction and application of vasoconstrictor nasal drops. X-rays are of limited use, because most foreign bodies are radiolucent. Management includes removal of the foreign body under controlled, atraumatic conditions in cooperative or anesthetized patients. Soft foreign bodies or those with a thin free edge, can be easily grasped and removed with crocodile or Tilley's forceps. Solid and round foreign bodies are removed using a Jobson Horne's probe, bent slightly at the tip, by passing the probe beyond the foreign body and drawing slowly forward towards oneself. Presence of second concomitant foreign body in some nostril or other nostril is always ruled out. Otoscope or nasal endoscope can be utilized for this examination. Systemic antibiotics are advised to cover secondary rhinosinusitis. General anaesthesia with cuffed tube is indicated in children, uncooperative patients and posteriorly placed foreign bodies because of risk of pushing it back into the nasopharynx or chances of brisk hemorrhage.

Infestation with maggots and screw worms are treated by instilling 25% chloroform solution or turpentine oil nasal drops which suffocate the larvae followed by manual removal under local anesthesia or general anaesthesia.

FOREIGN BODY IN EAR

Ear is the most common site for foreign bodies in young children, who not only insert objects in their ears but also into the ears of their sibs. Foreign body usually lodges just lateral to the bony–cartilaginous junction of external auditory canal, but can also get lodged in the isthmus of the canal, or may penetrate through the drum into the middle ear cavity. On examination, small smooth object especially pebble, beed, popcorn kernel is seen which is difficult to grasp and may be more than one. Usually foreign bodies are asymptomatic but some cause secondary otitis externa, bloody–purulent discharge and insects are the most troublesome. Obstructed foreign bodies cause decreased hearing.

Radiology has no role except in case of penetrating foreign bodies to assess the depth of penetration especially in the presence of inner ear damage. Diagnosis is usually straight forward with either the child complaining of otalgia or the parents being aware of foreign body insertion, bringing the patient to the ENT surgeon. Soft foreign bodies e.g., cotton wool, paper etc. can be removed with crocodile or Tilley's forceps while solid foreign body e.g. a beed can be taken care of with a hook or Jobson Horne probe, which is passed beyond the foreign body and gently pulled forward. Otherwise, removal is usually achieved with syringing with water at body temperature in cooperative children. In other removal is done under general anesthesia using micro–aural crocodile forceps or other micro hooks. In presence of tissue reaction induced by the foreign body, subsequent treatment of otitis externa is required.

Insects may be drowned with olive oil and then syringed out.

FOREIGN BODY IN OROPHARYNX/HYPOPHARYNX

Sharp objects like fish bones and pins are prone to become ledged in palatine or lingual tonsils. Dental prosthesis or teeth may get dislodged accidently and get impacted, especially after a road traffic accident. Patient gives a history of initial gagging episode which may be absent in children. Other features are odynophagia, with correct side localisation but level is poorly localised. Patient may complain of ipsilateral otalgia. Dysphagia and drooling are less common presenting features. A large foreign body impacted in hypopharynx will in addition cause obstruction of the airway leading to dyspnea (air hunger) and stridor (noisy breathing) on inspiration along with intercostal, suprasternal and substernal retractions. Mostly foreign bodies are easily seen in oropharynx and tongue base. X-rays are helpful in metallic foreign bodies. Thin bones, nonferrous metal objects and fish bones (cartilaginous) are usually not seen in X-ray film.

Removal can be achieved under local or topical anesthesia in cooperative patients.[2] Otherwise, general anesthesia is preferred and direct laryngoscopic examination is done and removal achieved with forceps.

Foreign body in Esophagus

Over 90% of ingested foreign bodies pass uneventfully through the gastrointestinal tract. If a foreign body fails to pass through, holding most commonly occurs in the esophagus. There are four anatomic sites of narrowing in the oesophagus, namely the postcricoid region, level of the aortic arch, the level of the left main bronchus and the level of the diaphragmatic hiatus, with maximum impaction at cricopharyngeal level (80%). Impaction may also occur at the sites of pathologic narrowing e.g. strictures, stenosis, tumours and malignancies.

Clinical features range from asymptomatic patient to obscure, unusual clinical symptomatology. There may be history of ingestion of foreign body with acute symptoms of coughing, choking, excessive salivation, dysphagia or vomiting. With chronic esophageal foreign bodies, there is edema of tracheoesophageal wall, leading to tracheal airway symptoms like biphasic stridor. In some, wheeze, recurrent pneumonia, anorexia, haematemesis or pyrexia of unknown origin (PUO) are the presenting feature.

Diagnosis is confirmed on PA and lateral X-ray of the chest in radio–opaque foreign bodies. In doubtful cases barium esophagogram or CT scan may be required. Radiograph of neck and chest after swallowing small cotton ball soaked with barium, which may stick to the foreign body can help to localize the radiolucent foreign bodies.

Removal is done using direct esophagoscopy under general anesthesia. Sometimes, rounded objects can be dislodged by means of a Foley balloon catheter. Button batteries deserve immediate attention because of risk of erosion of esophageal wall.

AIRWAY FOREIGN BODIES

Choking on foods has been the cause of 2500–3900 deaths per year in USA. It is the sixth most common cause of accidental deaths. Approximately 55% of aspirated foreign bodies involve the respiratory tract in children of 6 months to 4 years of age, boys more likely to aspirate than girls by almost 2:1 ratio. The peak incidence of inhaled foreign bodies in early childhood is because of two reasons:

i. The exploring nature of the young child who is often partially edentulous and has a tendency to place any object in the mouth, the solid object entering the pharynx elicits a startle response permitting the foreign body to enter the open larynx during forced inspiration.
ii. High incidence of upper respiratory tract infection makes the young children mouth breathers. Also due to the presence of coughing, the inhalation of food particles may easily occur with the sharp intake of breath following a bout of cough.

Majority of inhaled foreign bodies in adults lodge in right bronchial tree because of its width which is more than the left bronchus and the interbronchial septum which projects to the left. But in the young children, there is equal distribution of foreign bodies between right and left bronchi because the above-mentioned anatomical differences are less pronounced. A minority of foreign bodies (< 4%) impact in the larynx, if they are too large to pass through or if they have an irregular shape or have sharp edges which can catch on the laryngeal mucosa, the common offenders being egg shells, glass fragments or plastics.

Stridor is the most common feature seen which may be inspiratory (laryngeal) or biphasic (indicating subglottic or upper tracheal impaction). Voice may be hoarse especially in glottic foreign bodies. Patient may also present with aphonia indicating complete impaction. Cough may be the presenting feature especially in subglottic foreign bodies.

In case of foreign bodies in one bronchi, obstruction ranges from none to partial or complete. Partial obstruction produces hyperinflation of lung distal to obstruction (obstructive emphysema) while complete obstruction produces atelectasis of distal lung.

Majority of patients with inhaled foreign bodies give a definite history of choking, followed by paroxysmal coughing. After the initial paroxysm of cough, the tracheobronchial mucosa becomes tolerant to foreign body and the cough ceases, delaying the diagnosis. Approximately in 1/3rd of children, the accident of aspiration is neither observed nor suspected, leading to increased morbidity. Other common features are wheeze, predominantly unilateral, unexplained persistent fever, persistent or recurrent lobar pneumonia. Acute respiratory distress is uncommon but most alarming presentation, seen mainly in laryngeal foreign body which may also manifest as pain in root of neck or over the larynx. But the most common difficulty encountered in laryngeal foreign body is the delay in diagnosis.

Prolonged impacted foreign bodies may complicate into bronchial suppuration, bronchial ulceration and granulation tissue formation, bronchial stenosis, peribronchial and peritracheal lymphadenopathy with compression of the bronchi, pneumonitis, atelectasis, obstructive emphysema, pneumomediastinum, pneumothorax, hemoptysis and variable degree of airway obstruction.

Diagnosis is confirmed by radiography of soft tissue neck and PA view of chest. Radio-opaque foreign body is obvious on X-rays, while radiolucent foreign bodies are always suspected in patients with atelectasis or recurrent, prolonged or migratory pneumonia. Inspiratory and expiratory chest X-rays are important in diagnosing obstructive emphysema. Also the mediastinal shift is seen which is towards site of lesion with atelectasis, away from site of lesion in obstructive emphysema. In cases of uncooperative patients, right and left lateral decubitus X-rays are done where absence of volume loss on dependant side is seen with partially obstructive foreign body. Videofluroscopy of lateral view of neck can be done in suspected cases.

For the removal of foreign bodies, there is no substitute for open rigid endoscopes. Other techniques like pounding the throat and Heimlich's procedures are dangerous, because they may cause further impaction and possible total obstruction not present prior to these attempts.

Laryngeal or large tracheal foreign bodies are dealt as dire emergencies with facilities for emergency tracheostomy. Sometimes these may have to be delivered through the tracheostome. Laryngeal foreign bodies are usually removed by direct laryngoscopy in majority of cases but in few cases during the induction of anesthesia, foreign body may cause total respiratory obstruction and may warrant emergency tracheostomy or cricothyrotomy. Small tracheal and bronchial foreign bodies are removed using the rigid bronchoscopes under general anesthesia. These may be taken as elective procedures, in the absence of any respiratory distress. Rarely a bronchial foreign body may require thoracotomy and bronchotomy.[3]

REFERENCES

1. Huxlay EW. *Pediatric ENT Review* 2nd edn. London: Smith and Smith 2003.
2. Anthony A, Barter AE. Foreign body management in ENT practice. *Br Bull Otolaryngol* 1999;11:212-216.
3. Ronald, AM. Foreign body in ENT passages in children. *J Medical Sci* 2002;14:112-119.

Aniece Chowdhary

88 Airway Obstruction

INTRODUCTION

Airway obstruction is a frequent emergency in infants and children.[1,2]

A clinical history prior to the initiation of management of acute airway obstruction may be helpful. In the previously normal and asymptomatic patient the possibility of foreign body aspiration is real and must be exluded by questioning the patient, family or friends and by performing a quick physical examination. In stable patients, indirect laryngoscopy or flexible fibreoptic examination of the upper airway can be useful to assess the laryngeal function. X-ray lateral view of neck, chest, radiography and blood gas analysis are indicated only if time permits.

OPTIONS FOR INTERVENTION

1. Medical management.
2. Heimlich manoeuvre and positioning manoeuvres.
3. Nasopharyngeal/oral airway and intubation.
4. Surgical intervention.

Medical Management

It is indicated when respiratory distress is because of oedema secondary to injury, infective process or in neoplastic conditions. It includes oxygen inhalation, steroids or antibiotics. Oxygen is given via a face mask using a humidifier; providing 50% inspired oxygen. The humidification provides liquification of secretions. Steroids help to reduce edema, by using hydrocortisone in dose of 100 mg stat and 50 mg every 8 hourly for 24-48 hours. A short course of antibiotics is given in the dose of 1 million units of penicillin every 6 hourly I/V for 3-5 days.

Heimlich Manoeuver and Positioning Maneuvers

a. *Heimlich maneuver:* Acute airway obstruction by a food bolus or any foreign body is dislodged by Heimlich maneuver. The approach is from behind a standing patient. Sudden pressure is applied by rapid squeezing motion in the epigastrium, against the xiphoid region of sternum, with the clenched fists, thereby making the residual air in the lungs to expel the foreign body.

   Alternatively, in a supine patient, kneel beside the patient and apply the epigastric pressure with the palms of the hand. If the manoeuvre fails, proceed to cricothyrotomy in adolescent adult or tracheostomy in the young child. Forced ventilation in the form of mouth-to-mouth or Ambu bag often provides some ventilation to the lungs, while surgical intervention of the airway is being performed.

b. *Positioning maneuvers:* These are useful in the unconscious patients who present with upper airway obstruction due to flaccidity of the tongue and pharyngeal muscles.

   i. *Lateral–prone position:* In the absence of cervical spine injury, turn the patient on his side and place the head sideways and down without a pillow, allowing the tongue to fall away from posterior pharyngeal wall and secretions to drain by gravity from the mouth.

   ii. *Head maneuver:* Is performed by lifting up the back of the neck while gently pressing the top of the head back and toward the shoulder. This is not advisable in possible cervical spine injury. This position is for mouth to mouth respiration.

   iii. *Jaw thrust maneuver:* Is performed by placing the fingertips of each hand behind and beneath the angles of the mandible and lifting the mandible forward. This position is used for mask to mouth ventilation.

In case of conscious patients, who present with severe upper airway obstruction from the base of tongue or larynx the following maneuver is performed to provide some temporary relief till such time that a more secure airway is established.

Patient is asked to sit up which improves the pulmonary function and decreases upper airway edema. Patient is also advised to lean forward from the hips and then extend the head from the upper neck so that chin comes up and forward which open the airway to its maximum extent, providing good pulmonary ventilation.

Airways and Intubation

a. *Airways (oral/nasopharyngeal):* These overcome the problems related to the prolapse or relaxation of the palate and the base of the tongue and may provide a well tolerated, fully adequate airway.
   i. *Nasal airway:* Is better tolerated in the conscious or semiconscious patient, or who has sustained a mild to moderate head injury with obtundation but with normal respiratory drive. Insertion of nasal airway is made easy by instillation of topical nasal decongestant drops (otrivin/nasivion nasal drugs) and lubrication of the airway device.
   ii. *Oral airway:* Is curved and semirigid, and can be used to bypass obstruction in the nose or mouth. It is used primarily in the unconscious patient to help hold the tongue forward and can also be used in semiconscious intubated patient to prevent him from occluding the tube by bitting it. It also facilitates sectioning of secretions.
   iii. *Esophageal airway:* This is inserted 'blind' into the esophagus and balloon is distended. Air is insufflated through the device into the hypopharynx with presumptive ventilation. Nowadays, this is not recommended because it can lacerate the esophageal mucosa and increase the supraglottic edema, thereby increasing the problem.

b. *Intubation:* In the patients, in whom respiration has ceased but upper airway obstruction is not suspected e.g. cardiopulmonary arrest, perform the mouth-to-mouth or mask-to-mouth respiration, maintain effective cardiac output and intubate the patient after he has been well oxygenated for several minutes.
   i. *Endotrachael intubation:* Mask-to-mouth or mouth-to-mouth ventilation is performed till equipment required for intubation (laryngoscope, endotracheal tubes with stylet, suction) are available. Patient is positioned in 'sniffing position' i.e. lower chin and head are slightly extended. Laryngoscope is inserted with the left hand into the right side of the mouth so that the tongue is pushed to the left of the laryngoscope blade. The curved blade of laryngoscope is slided around the base of tongue into the vallecula which is lifted up and away from the operator. This manoeuver lifts the epiglottis up and out and the glottic chink is visible. With the right hand, endotracheal tube with sylet is inserted into the mouth and through the vocal cords. As the tube passes through the cords, stylet is removed. Suction is used to clear the secretions. If the obstruction is considered to be lower down, then a rigid bronchoscope is passed to inspect the subglottic area and trachea.

      In case of difficult intubation, do not struggle but ventilate the patient with a mask until oxygenation improves before attempting intubation again. In case of failed intubation, a laryngeal mask airway can be inserted.
   ii. *Blind nasal intubation:* Is indicated in presence of trismus, cervical spine injuries, severe mandibular injuries, distortion or masses in the oral cavity. The patient should have good spontaneous respiration because the tube is guided by breath sounds. Being a blind procedure, it requires lot of expertise on the part of the performer. It can cause epistaxis, retropharyngeal mucosal laceration and sinusitis.
   iii. *Combitube:* Can be used where skilled persons are not available. It can be inserted blindly.

Surgical Intervention

a. *Transtracheal ventilation:* It requires oxygen under pressure (50 lbs per sq. inch), connecting hose with luer–lok connectors, and a 16 guage plastic sheeted needle. The needle is directed through the circothyroid membrane and is attached to the oxygen line. Patient can be fully ventilated with this technique for 30 minutes, providing rapid control in the emerging setup, till more definitive procedures can be introduced.
b. *Tracheostomy (Tracheotomy):* Indication–(5 R's)
   - Respiratory obstruction because of any cause
   - Respiratory failure due to any aetiology
   - Respiratory paralysis
   - Removal of retained secretions from respiratory system
   - Reduction of dead space

   Elective tracheostomy is performed when the upper airway is potentially at risk. Any major operation in the mouth, pharynx and the larynx warrants elective tracheostomy till swallowing function improve. Mechanical respiratory insufficiency occurs in drug intoxication, head and chest injuries, neurological diseases, chronic obstructive airway diseases. The patients require intermittent or continuous positive pressure ventilation.

   The care of tracheostomy tube includes:
   - Fixation of the tracheostomy tube.
   - Periodic change of tube, removal of secretions, humidification.

- Care of the inflatable cuff, periodic deflation to avoid ischaemic necrosis induced by pressure of the cuff.
- Breathing exercises, dressing and nursing.

Complications of tracheostomy include:

- Accidental decannulation.
- Pneumothorax, more common in infants because of high pleural apices into the neck.
- Bleeding: Immediate bleeding is usually from the anterior jugular veins. Delayed bleeding is usually from erosion of innominate artery especially in a low placed tracheostomy.
- Tracheitis sicca, which can cause bleeding and crusting.
- Mucus plug retention can cause acute respiratory obstruction.
- Aerophagia in young children can cause gastric distention and vomiting and requires nasogastric tube decompression.
- Apnea and cardiac arrest due to sudden loss of CO_2 drive.

REFERENCES

1. Henry C. Airway obstruction in infants and children. *Asian Chron Pediatr* 2002;6;61-68.
2. Huxlay EW. Pediatric ENT Review. London: Smith and Smith 2003.

Aniece Chowdhary

89 Earache

INTRODUCTION

Earache (otalgia) is a common pediatric symptom, usually on account of inflammation of the middle ear or the external ear.[1,2] At times, it may be a referred pain due to involvement of teeth, temperomandibular joint or pharynx. Ear rubbing or pulling accompanied by crankiness, irritability, poor sleep and fever may be the only manifestation of earache in young children.[2]

Etiology

Pain in the ear can be due to problems occurring locally in the ear or referred to it from remote areas.

A. Local Causes

1. *External ear:* Furuncle, impacted wax, otitis externa, otomycosis, myringitis bullosa, herpes zoster, and malignant neoplasms.
2. *Middle ear:* Acute otitis media, eustachian tube obstruction, mastoiditis, extradural abscess, aero-otitis media, and carcinoma middle ear.

B. Referred Causes

As ear receives nerve supply from Vth (auriculotemporal br.), IXth (tympanic br.) and Xth (auricular br.) cranial nerves; and from C_2 (lesser occipital) and C_2 and C_3 (greater auricular), pain may be referred from these remote areas.

1. Via Vth cranial nerve:
   a. *Dental:* Caries tooth, apical abscess impacted molar, malocclusion.
   b. *Oral cavity:* Benign or malignant ulcerative lesions of oral cavity or tongue.
   c. *Temporomandibular joint disorders:* Bruxism, osteoarthritis, recurrent dislocation, ill-fitting denture.
   d. *Sphenopalatine neuralgia.*
2. Via IXth cranial nerve:
   a. *Oropharynx:* Acute tonsillitis, peritonsillar abscess, tonsillectomy. Benign or malignant ulcers of soft palate, tonsil and its pillars.
   b. *Base of tongue:* Tuberculosis or malignancy.
   c. *Elongated styloid process.*
3. Via Xth cranial nerve. Malignancy or ulcerative lesion of: vallecula, epiglottis, larynx or laryngopharynx, oesophagus.
4. Via C_2 and C_3 spinal nerves. Cervical spondylosis, injuries of cervical spine, carries spine.

C. Psychogenic

When no cause has been discovered, pain may be functional in origin but the patient should be kept under observation with periodic re-evaluation.

Otalgia is a *symptom.* It is essential to find its cause before specific treatment can be instituted.

MANAGEMENT

In case of earache secondary to ASOM which has failed to respond to treatment with antibiotics and decongestants (both systemic and topical), it is advisable to do myringotomy to drain collected pus and promote early healing of the ear drum.

For earache due to otitis externa or furunculosis, treatment is in the form of antibiotics, analgesics and local packing with icthymol glycerine. The latter has hydroscopic and antiseptic action.

When earache is because of otomycosis (say *Aspergillus niger*), local debris should be cleaned followed by instillation of 1% clotrimazole and systemic antihistaminics.[1]

In case of wax, first ceruminolytics should be instilled to soften it and then it is removed by suction, syringing or ear probe.[2]

REFERENCES

1. Hayward AR, Levin MJ, Sondheimer JM (eds) *Current Pediatric Therapy*, 16th edn. New York: Lange/McGraw-Hill Johnson CE, Kelley P, Friedman N, Chan K, Berman S. Ear, nose and throat. In: Hay WW Jr. 2003;17-491.
2. Chowdhary A, Gupte S. Pediatric ear, nose and throat (ENT) problems. In: Gupte S (ed) *The Short Textbook of Pediatrics*, 10th edn. New Delhi: Jaypee Brothers 2004;670-678.

Aniece Chowdhary

90 Epistaxis

INTRODUCTION

Bleeding from nose is one of the most common complaints in all age groups, with a prevalence rate of 10-12%. Anterior epistaxis is more common in children and young adults while posterior nasal bleed is mostly seen in older patients with arteriosclerosis or hypertension. Epistaxis is more common during hot dry climates with low humidity.

Etiology

In clinical practice, only few cases of epistaxis are due to well defined primary cause as lister in Table 89.1. Otherwise in maximum patients, epistaxis is without any obvious causative factor and thereby known as idiopathic epistaxis. Nose–blowing, sneezing, coughing, straining, upper respiratory tract infection, all can increase the vascular pressure suddenly or mucosa can get inflammed, more vascular and friable and thus contribute to bleeding in an epistaxis prone patient.

Trauma is the most common cause of epistaxis which may be blunt trauma to the nose or digital trauma (nose picking), the later is most common cause in children.[1-3] Fear and anxiety due to bleeding and the pain associated with epistaxis management may further elevate the BP causing a vicious cycle. Bleeding disorders may present clinically as epistaxis in children with leukemias, idiopathic thrombocytopenia purpura (ITP), Von–Willebrand's disease or chemotherapy induced thrombocytopenia. In the end of the list, it is worthwhile to mention the tumours of nasopharynx, sinuses, nasal septum, lateral nasal wall and nasal vestibule which may not be visualized until the bleeding has stopped and edema has subsided.

VARIOUS BLEEDING SITES

Various sites of bleeding from the nose are described as below:

i. *Nasal septum:* Kisselback's plexus (Little's area); at the antero–inferior part of septum; 90% of anterior epistaxis arise from this site; bleeding polypus of septum arises from here (also bleeding can occur behind a spur).

ii. *Inferior turbinate and nasal floor.*

iii. *Woodruff's plexus:* In the lateral wall of inferior meatus posteriorly. These vessels originate from posterior pharyngeal wall and are venous in origin.

Table 90.1: Cause of epistaxis

A. Local :	– Inflammatory	Rhinosinusitis, nasal polyposis, chronic infections like T.B., syphilis, rhinoscleroma.
	– Trauma	Iatrogenic, facial trauma, foreign body, surgery.
	– Idiopathic	Little's area, Woodruff's plexus.
	– Eoplastic	Benign e.g. angiofibroma, inverted papilloma, malignant e.g. squamous cell C/A, olfactory neurobalstoma, melanoma.
	– Drug/Inhalants	Cocaine, tobacco, heroin, wood–dust, cannabis etc.
	– Miscellaneous	Wegner's granulomatosis, midline granuloma.
B. Systemic :	– Coagulation disorders	Hemophilia, specific factor deficiency.
	– Thrombocytopenia	Bone–marrow aplasia, hypersplenism, DIC.
	– Platelet dysfunction	Von–Willebrand's disease, leukemia, uraemia, bypass surgery.
	– Drugs	Aspirin, anti-coagulants, immunosuppression, alcohol, chloramphenicol chemotherapy.
	– Miscellaneous	Liver failure, hypothyroidism, Vitamin K deficiency.

iv. *Above middle turbinate:* From anterior ethmoidal artery especially in hypertensive patients.

v. *Middle meatus:* Spontaneous bleeding from polypoidal swelling, may be neoplasia.

vi. *Diffuse:* Both from septum and lateral nasal wall, it is seen in bleeding diathesis or general systemic dysfunction.

vii. *Nasopharynx:* Seen in angiofibroma, carcinoma of nasopharynx.

viii. *Sinuses:* Rarely spontaneous bleeding from the vessels of antrum or ethmoidal sinuses.

MANAGEMENT

It includes a history taking regarding bleeding tendencies. History of trauma, site of bleed, recurrent attacks of sinus infection, sino–nasal surgery or any drug intake (aspirin, anticoagulants) is obtained. The examination of patient includes monitoring of vital signs, and I/V line. Blood is also arranged. The laboratory tests include a complete blood count, bleeding and clotting time and platelet count. Deficiencies in clotting factors are less common and are screened with a prothrombin time (PT) and partial thromboplastin time (PTT). PT measures the extrinsic clotting system and PTT measures the intrinsic clotting factors, specially the factor VIII, IX, XI and XII. Specific factor assays of all the known clotting factors can be performed when indicated. Liver and renal function test are also undertaken if indicated. After a posterior nasal pack is placed, arterial blood gas (ABG) analysis is advisable.

The management of epistaxis at any age group is done by resuscitating the patient, establishing the site of bleed, stopping the bleeding and treatment of the cause. In the young, resuscitation is uncommon and therefore pinching of nostrils bilaterally with firm pressure by the thumb and forefingers for 5–10 minutes, is the time–honoured method of stopping the venous bleed from the caudal end of the septum. Unilateral pressure may be applied with the thumb on the ala–nasai of the affected side and the middle finger behind the angle of the jaw on the opposite side. This allows the patient's one side of the nose and the mouth for respiration. Patient is asked to sit down with head and neck leaned slightly forward because lying supine will cause the blood to drain into the pharynx and results in spitting of the blood or swallowing and subsequent vomiting, creating more anxiety, increasing the BP and thereby causing more bleeding. Ice–packs or damp clothes on the forehead or back of the neck has no role to play. After these initial measures, nasal examination is performed, which includes anterior and posterior rhinoscopic examination, flexible and rigid endoscopy.

In the absence of any obvious local disease, attention is turned to the septum which will often reveal an engorged vein, a micro-aneurysm or only prominent vessels in the Little's area itself. Cotton pledget soaked in topical anaesthetic agent with vasoconstrictor (2 or 4% xylocaine with adrenaline) is placed against the bleeding site for approximately 4–5 minutes which stops or slows the bleeding site is done with silver–nitrate soaked cotton–tipped applicator or by fused beed of chromic acid. Occasionally, trichloroacetic acid (TCA) can also be used. Chromic acid beed is made by picking up a crystal of chromic acid on the end of a metal probe and heating the metal in a spirit lamp close to the crystal which melts and fuses into a smooth beed. The applicator is placed firmly against the area to allow the chemical to work without the blood washing away the chemical cautery and sometimes suction can be used alongwith to keep the area clean. Care must be taken not to touch the skin, which causes a smarting, but if happens, thick paste of sodium bicarbonate should be applied. In case of failure of chemical cautery, electro cautery is used, in which repeated applications are made to adjacent areas because of the presence of submucosal excursions of small arterioles with anastomotic connection in Little's area, which are taken care of. Whichever method is adopted, patient is instructed to keep the area moist with antibiotic ointment or vaseline, blowing one nostril at a time and avoiding nose picking.

In cases of major anterior epistaxis, oxycel pledgets, tampons or anterior nasal packing is indicated. Oxycel pledgets are packed when bleeding site is identified under the inferior or middle turbinate and oxycel is packed from the floor of nose, tightly under the turbinate, thereby obviating the need of total anterior nasal pack. Nasal tampons are simplest way to pack the nose which consist of a desiccated, compressed sponge which when inflated with any water–based fluid, expands dramatically. Insertion is very simple. Lift the tip of nose and slide the lubricated tampon into the nasal cavity along the floor of nose and inflate with water or saliva. Tampon is secured with a stitch passed through the tampon which is then taped to the face. If specific bleeding site cannot be identified, the nose is packed firmly on the side of bleed with petroleum–soaked gauze, or vaseline gauze or BIPP (bismuth iodoform paraffin paste) pack, packing is done in horizontal layers beginning along the floor of nose as shown in Figure 90.1. The pack should be 25 mm wide for adults and 12 mm wide for children, and 1 metre should be prepared for each side, if both sides require packing. Topical anesthesia with 4% xylocaine is essential.

A thudicums speculum is inserted and the gauze is placed in a layered fashion into the nasal cavity using Tilley's dressing forceps. The first 10 cm should be folded double and inserted along the floor of the nose and the nasal cavity

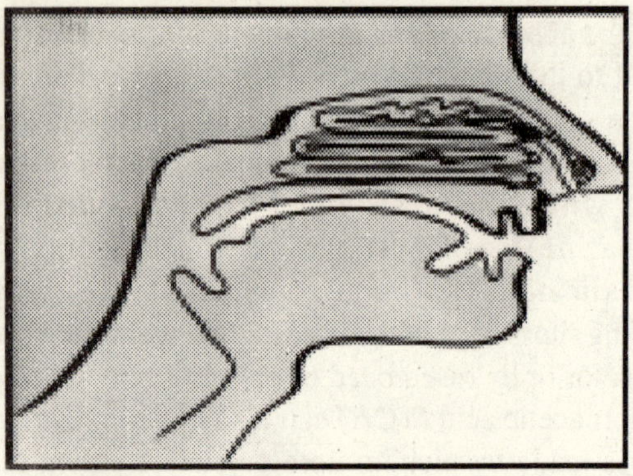

Fig. 90.1: Anterior nasal packing

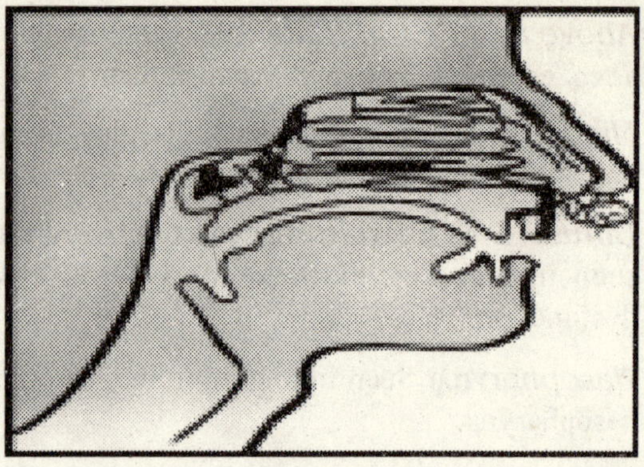

Fig. 90.2: Anterior and posterior nasal packing

packed, as tightly as possible and as far backwards and upwards as possible. This, being a painful procedure, should always be done in a good light and as rapidly as feasible. Prophylactic antibiotics are adviced to prevent sinusitis. Pack is removed after 48 to 72 hours. On removal of the pack, sometimes there is a slight ooze mild oozing due to irritation and the inflammatory response of the nasal mucosa which stops without any further treatment. If not, gentle application of a thin layer of oxycel pledgets controls it. If significant bleeding occurs during pack removal, immediate reinsertion of fresh pack is done.

Humidification and the avoidance of further trauma from nose blowing, picking, or scratching are mandatory for a week, heavy work and sports are avoided for 2 weeks after pack removal.

Posterior epistaxis: When the bleeding is posterior (or both anterior and posterior) an additional post nasal pack is advisable which may be a balloon catheter (e.g. Foley's) (Fig. 90.2). Foley's catheter is inserted along the floor of nasal cavity on the bleeding side until the catheter tip is just visible below the soft palate. The balloon is inflated with 15 ml of sterile water or air and then withdrawn to impact on the choana.[2] Figures 90.1 and 90.2 demonstrate "anterior" and "anterior and posterior" packings.

Concurrent Management

- Assess bloodloss and monitor BP and pulse.
- IV line maintained.
- Bed rest with head elevation is advised.
- Humidification of the room along with low flow oxygen by face mask for patients with posterior packing.
- Broad spectrum antibiotics with adequate hydration.
- Blood cross–matched for transfusion, if required.
- Hematologist, physician consultation sought as and when the situation warrants.
- Vitamin C, vitamin K and calcium supplementation.

REFERENCES

1. Wurman LH. Epitaxis. In: Gates GA (ed) *Current Therapy in Otolaryngology, Head and Neck Surgery*, 5th edn. St Lois: CV Mosby 1994;354-359.
2. Hayward AR, Levin MJ, Sondheimer JM (eds) *Current Pediatric Therapy*, 16th edn. New York: Lange/McGraw-Hill Johnson CE, Kelley P, Friedman N, Chan K, Berman S. Ear, nose and throat. In: Hay WW Jr, 2003;17-491.
3. Chowdhary A, Gupte S. Pediatric ear, nose and throat (ENT) problems. In; Gupte S (ed) *The Short Textbook of Pediatrics*, 10th edn. New Delhi: Jaypee Brothers 2004;670-678.

Aniece Chowdhary

91 Caustic Ingestion

INTRODUCTION

Caustic ingestion accidentally or intentionally results in significant morbidity and mortality and continues to be a common and controversial problem faced by otolaryngologists. Caustic ingestion has a bimodal presentation, peak occurring in children (accidental) and in adulthood (suicidal). Caustic agents burn the muscosa of aerodigestive tract, alkaline agents being more common than acids. Alkalies cause damage by way of liquefactive necrosis resulting in rapid and deep burns. The damage continues as long as the alkali is in contact with soft tissue. The acidic product ingestion causes gastric and esophageal injury.

ALKALINE BURNS

Common alkaline agents include Lyes (Sodium hydroxide, potassium hydroxide), miniature or disc batteries, hair relaxers, ammonia and clinitest tablets. Solids (crystalling form) are usually spit out by a child before large amounts are ingested. Therefore, liquid alkalies carry much greater risk of severe esophageal and gastric burns. Also solids usually do not reach the stomach owning to gastroesophageal sphincter spasm while liquids can cause transmural necrosis of the stomach and small intestine. Bleaches cause mild to moderate gastrointestinal irritation with symptoms such as nausea, vomiting and diarrhoea. Mucosal ulceration usually does not occur with bleaches except with concentrated ammonia solutions. Esophageal injury and stricture formation after ingestion of household bleech is very rarely seen.

Symptoms and signs include:

- Burning sensation in the mouth and chest (esophagus).
- Dysphagia and increased salivation leading to drooling and vomiting which may be blood stained.
- Stridor due to laryngeal swelling secondary to aspiration.
- Mouth or pharynx may have white patches or inflammed ulcerated mucosa–in the presence of two or more symptoms (vomiting drooling or stridor) there is a 50% chance of an associated esophageal burn.
- Esophageal perforation, mediastinitis and/or shock.
- Clinically, 25–70% of oropharyngeal burns do not have associated esophageal burns. The reverse is also true and 15% of esophageal burns have a normal oral cavity and oropharyngeal findings.

Management

Initial management of the caustic ingestion patient follows a standard emergency protocol as under:

- Securing an airway.
- Cardiovascular support.
- I/V line to be commenced and blood samples sent for complete blood count and electrolytes (including ABG, if indicated).
- Urine analysis is also done.
- Keeping the patient on "nil orally".
- Determine the type and amount of caustic agent ingested and whether the patient has aspiration, emesis or respiratory distress by asking relevant questions from patient or attendants.
- Note vital signs and perform complete physical examination and look for any skin burns due to agent spilled onto the clothing.
- Any obvious skin or oral cavity burns should be washed with a copious amount of water.
- Flexible fiberoptic nasopharyngolaryngoscopy is most helpful in determining the presence of upper airway injury.
- X-ray chest routinely and abdominal radiography, if indicated.

Water or milk can be administered to dilute or neutralize the agents unless immediate surgery is planned.

Induction of vomiting, gastric lavage, emetics are contraindicated as they may cause further damage. Also contraindicated is acid ingestion to neutralize an ingested base because of risk of exothermic chemical reaction which can increase the internal trauma.

- Role of nasogastric tube is controversial and usually not recommended.

- Hoarseness and stridor indicate possible damage to pharynx, larynx or trachea. Such patients may require tracheostomy.
- Acute chest or abdominal pain indicates a possible viscus perforation usually seen in an adult who has ingested large amount of a strong acid or base in a suicidal bid and may require emergency laparotomy with possible esophagogastrostomy.
- Ingestion of miniature or disc batteries require emergency management because leakage from them can cause perforation within hours. If the battery is lodged in esophagus as seen on a radiograph the patient is directly taken to the OT for emergency esophagoscopy. If the battery is in the stomach it can be allowed to pass and patient is kept under a general surgeon's observation. If not detected in stools within 4 days, a repeat X-ray is done. As long as the battery continues to progress through the GIT. no intervention is required but constant checkup from a general surgeon is mandatory.
- Bleach ingestion rarely causes significant esophageal injury and many of these patients can be sent home directly from the emergency room depending on the clinical status.
- Attempted suicide patients require urgent psychiatric consultation and preventive precautions.
- After taking care of the emergency, subsequent evaluation and management of injury of upper aerodigestive tract especially oesophagus is initiated. Definitive evaluation of esophagus should be performed 12–48 hours after the injury. Some surgeons prefer to wait for at least 24 hours before esophagoscopy but is unlikely that a significant burn will be missed if the oesophagoscopy is performed only 12 hours after ingestion.

Role of Endoscopy: Ideally, every known or suspected case of ingested strong acid or base (except bleach) should undergo esophagoscopy under general anaesthesia by an experienced endoscopist unless there are contraindications for esophagoscopy like impending airway obstruction, evidence of esophageal perforation such as mediastinitis or shock.

Much is written in literature regarding 'pros and cons' of rigid versus flexible endoscopy. Rigid esophagoscopy has always been preferred by ENT surgeons and carries no extra risk of perforations in experienced hands. Esophagoscopy is performed cautiously and not distal to a visualized full thickness burn. If it is encountered, a nasogastric tube or esophageal stent is passed. Flexible gastroduodenoscopy should always follow rigid esophagoscopy in case of any suspicion of gastric injury.

If esophagoscopy is not possible, contrast, barium–radiography is helpful in diagnosing esophageal injury. Mild injury patients show delayed passage of contrast or edematous esophageal mucosal folds and linear ulcerations while severe injury reveals either a rigid, narrowed esophagus, a dilated atonic oesophagus or an esophagus showing increased irritability and uncoordinated peristaltic activity. Also an esophagogram is helpful in evaluation of esophagus distal to the level of most proximal circumferential burn which was the most distant point of direct visualization at esophagoscopy, in case flexible gastroduodenoscopy after rigid esophagoscopy has not been carried out.

Further management depends upon degree of burns. If esophagoscopy reveals no burn or only minor first degree burn (erythema and/or oedema of the mucosa), patient is adviced only topical antibiotic ointment) and local oral hygiene for oral burns. When oral ulcer heals satisfactorily and allows eating, patient can be discharged and kept on follow–up in OPD. Patients with second degree burns (2° burns : full thickness injury to the mucosa, including bleb information, sloughing or ulceration) are given steroids (prednisone 1 mg/kg, BW, twice daily for two weeks and then tapered over another 4 weeks) in order to decrease collagen deposition with subsequent fibrosis during healing. Antibiotics (ampicillin, cephalosporins or clindamycin) for a period of 10–14 days alongwith antacids and H_2 blockers are given for 2–4 weeks. I/V fluids with correction of electrolyte–imbalance are advised, followed by oral clear liquid diet and subsequently soft diet when swallowing is possible. Repeat barium oesophagogram is performed at 3 weeks of caustic ingestion. On detection of esophageal stricture, esophageal dilatation procedure is commenced. For circumferential 2nd degree and all 3rd degree burns (3° burns: full thickness esophageal injury, with perforation into or through the muscular layer), a nasogastric tube or esophageal stent (Ryle's tube) is left in place for 6 weeks. Antibiotics alongwith antacids and H2 blockers and pro–kinetic agents (cisapaide) are used. Severely burnt patients are kept in hospitals for long time due to risk of massive hemorrhage as a result of esophagogastic necrosis.

If stricture becomes evident, serial dilators are commenced which may be carried out either in anterograde method (e.g., mercury filled Maloney Bougies) or by Tucker retrograde method via gastrostomy.

Role of thoracic and/or gastric surgeon: Their opinion is sought in cases of:

- Severe esophageal necrosis with risk of esophageal perforation and major blood vessel rupture;
- Progressive and/or complete esophageal stricture.

The surgeon can opt for total esophagectomy with replacement with either gastric pull up, colon–interposition or jejunal free flap.

- Also surgical intervention is required for correction of hiatus hernia due to shortening of esophagus secondary to stricture formation.

Important point to be kept in mind during follow–up in higher risk of developing squamous cell carcinoma of oesophagus due to caustic ingestion induced esophageal injury and that the late onset dysphagia may be due to stricture, tumour or both.

ACID BURNS

Hydrochloric, sulphuric and nitric acids are most common agents ingested. Acids cause a coagulation necrosis upon exposure to mucosa, whereby a coagulum forms at the interface between agent and mucosa reducing further penetration of the agent into the muscle layers. Acids are less likely to cause severe esophageal burns but more commonly involve the gastroduodenal region which on healing produce gastric outlet obstruction. Clinically, patient presents with burning sensation in the mouth, chest and abdomen with dysphagia and hematemesis. Oral examination may reveal inflammed mucosa with whitishslough covered ulcerated areas. On palpation of abdomen, acute abdominal signs may be elicited.

Initial management includes checking vials, IV fluids and supportive care. Neutralization of acid with sodium bicarbonate, lavage and emetics are contraindicated. Prophylatic antibiotics and steroids are not indicated. Cutaneous burns are treated in the conventional way. Patient is closely monitored for signs of gastric perforation when laprotomy is required.

During follow-up, upper gastrointestinal contrast (barium) radiography is performed 3–6 weeks post ingestion of acid to look for gastric outlet obstruction where general Surgeon's consultation and intervention is warranted.[2]

REFERENCES

1. Huxley EW. *Pediatric ENT Review*, 2nd edn. Londn: Smith and Smith 2003.
2. Sondheimer JM. Gastrointestinal tract. In: Hayward AR, Levin MJ, Sondheimer JM (eds) *Current Pediatric Therapy*, 16th edn. New York: Lange/McGraw-Hill Johnson CE, Kelley P, Friedman N, Chan K, Berman S. Ear, nose and throat. In: Hay WW Jr, 2003:614-646.

Aniece Chowdhary

92 Facio-maxillary Trauma

INTRODUCTION

Facio-maxillary trauma is most commonly the result of road traffic accidents and physical combat.[1,2] The foremost intervention in any facio-maxillary trauma will include "ABCDE" as explained below:

1. Maintenance of an adequate "airway" and assess and establish "breathing" so that ventilation is effective.
2. Control sources of "blood loss" and maintain the circulation.
3. Maintain the alignment of neck in case there is unstable "cervical spine" injury.
4. Assess the level of consciousness and neurological "dysfunction".
5. "Expose" the patient to identify all other injuries.

Definitive treatment of facial injury is always the second priority. In initial examination, always look for posterior displacement of tongue due to mandibular fracture, posterior-inferior displacement of the maxilla, paradoxical chest movements due to flail chest segment, laryngotracheal framework trauma. These all warrant establishment of a safe airway and effective ventilation by means of endo-tracheal ventilation or tracheotomy.

Bleeding from nose or mouth in semiconscious/comatosed patient will justify timely intervention by means of nasal pack, balloons, catheters, sutures or arterial ligation.

SCALP AND FACIAL INJURIES

In scalp, skull fracture and presence of any foreign body is looked for. In face, facial nerve injury and underlying bony injuries are checked.

Direct pressure application to the bleeding site controls most of scalp hemorrhage temporarily. Large vessels are caught with hemostat and ligated. Scalp laceration with multiple point ooze is best controlled by using a 2-0 nylon running silk taking large, deep bites.

The wound is explored under local anaesthesia or general anaesthesia and copious irrigation with saline is done to remove the dirt and foreign matter. Non-viable tissue is debrided and wound is closed in layers. Antibiotics are given emperically and tetanus prophylaxis is advised as per the immune status which includes tetanus toxoid 0.5 ml in one arm and human tetanus immune-globulin 250 units in the other arm, if immune status is unknown.

In cases of avulsions, small wounds are closed primarily while local flaps are used for other cases.

NASAL FRACTURES

Trauma to nose will cause the damage depending upon the direction. In the frontal plane, the force of impact will determine the extent of injury. In mild frontal trauma, there is injury to the cartilagineous vault causing its separation and avulsion injury along with posterior dislocation of the septum. In moderate frontal trauma, deviation of a nasal septum is encountered. In severe frontal trauma, there is in addition the adjacent structural involvement like frontal process of maxilla, ethmoid labyrinth, lacrimal bones, cribriform plate and orbital plate of frontal bones. Also seen is collapse and telescoping of septal fragments.

Lateral impact injuries are more common, causing depression of ipsilateral nasal bone, may also involve nasal process of maxilla and pyriform margin. Also seen is lateral displacement of contralateral nasal bone with fractured or dislocated septum.

Isolated nasal trauma presents with pain, tenderness and swelling along with epistaxis and external nasal deformity. The radiology of nasal bones is unnecessary because of its limited role in management planning which depends on degree of external and internal deformity on anterior rhinoscopy. Reduction of fracture is done within 3-7 days for children and within 5 to 10 days for adults. Closed reduction is the standard treatment for most fractures, performed under L.A. or G.A., where direction of force is applied in reverse of causative trauma force, bony nasal pyramid is reduced first followed by reduction and stabilization of septum. "Walsham forceps" are used to grasp and manipulate the nasal into correct position. "Asch forceps" are used to elevate the dorsum and disimpact the septum simultaneously. This is followed with nasal packing for 2-3 days with 0.5 inch vaseline soaked packs which provides internal splinting. Dorsum is splinted with plaster cast or prefabricated splint which is removed after 7 days.

In case of nasoethmoid fractures, in addition, external fixation devices (like lead or silastic splints) are used which prevents with nasal collapse and telescoping of fractured segments. Open reduction of fractured nasal bone is done in selected cases.

Some times, mild nasal trauma leads to septal hematoma only especially in children because of bleeding in the subperichondrial planes, on both sides of the septum. It is immediately evacuated or drained by means of hemi or full transfixation incision, followed by bilateral anterior nasal packing to prevent recurrence. If septal hematoma persists for 3-4 days, it can lead to irreversible damage to the septal cartilage because of ischaemic necrosis leading to saddle nose deformity and retraction of columella.

EAR TRAUMA

Ear examination is usually missed as a part of multiple trauma patients but its morbidity is high if neglected.

1. External Ear Trauma

i. *Hematoma:* of auricle is managed by aspiration or by incision and drainage. For I & D, incision is made in the helicasulcus and hematoma is milked out. Some surgeons prefer not to close the wound, while some keep a drain routinely. Contours of pinna are packed with cotton wool soaked in betadine or saline, or use a through and through mattress suture tied over a bolster in order to encourage the skin to adhere to the underlying cartilage. Mastoid bandage along with broad spectrum antibiotics against staphylococcus are advised.

ii. *Laceration:* of the auricle is closed primarily after adequate cleansing and foreign body debris removal. Associated cartilage damage is repaired as per the clinical situation. Small pieces can be sacrificed, but a large piece of avulsed cartilage with intact perichondrium is placed in the wound and given soft tissue cover over it.

iii. *Avulsion:* If a piece of auricle is nearly avulsed but attached by a skin remnant, it is reapproximated primarily if the blood flow is adequate. If the blood supply is poor, the avulsed piece is sacrificed. Delayed repair is indicated if major portion of auricle has been avulsed or when there is significant exposed cartilage without any viable skin. In these patients, cartilage is buried into the postauricular pocket or abdominal pocket for 7-10 days and grafted at a later date. Broad spectrum antibiotics are adviced.

2. Middle Ear Trauma

It includes tympanic membrane perforation with or without ossicular disruption and occasionally associated with dizziness.

Most of the traumatic tympanic membrane perforations are seen in anterior–inferior quadrant of the pars tensa. If clean there are managed conservatively and 95% of them heal spontaneously. Antibiotics and topical ear drops are avoided. The contaminated injuries are cleaned of any foreign debris and adviced oral as well as topical antibiotic drugs. No surgical intervention is required immediately and patient is advised to keep the ear dry. If perforation does not heal on its own, planned myringoplasty is done as a cold surgery.

Posterior-superior quadrant tympanic membrane perforations are usually associated with ossicular disruptions (incudostapedial joint separation). Management is similar as described above and the hearing mechanism is repaired at a later stage as a planned surgery (ossiculoplasty or tympanoplasty).

Occasionally there is subluxation of incus on the stapes superstructure or displacement of the stapes into the vestibule, causing vertigo, nausea and vomiting and nystagmus beating away from the injured side. Management includes the labyrinthine sedatives and antiemetics and bed rest. Surgery is indicated if there is suspicion of fistula between inner and middle ear.

3. Inner Ear Injury

Is because of temporal bone fractures which may be longitudinal (due to direct trauma to parietal or temporal bone) or transverse (trauma directed at the occiput).

In longitudinal fracture, the fracture line extends from external ear canal anteromedially along the anterior edge of the petrux apex to the foramen lacerum and foramen ovale. Conductive hearing loss is most common presentation because of tympanic membrane perforation, hemotympanum, CSF in the middle ear and/or ossicular disruption. Facial nerve injury occurs in 20% of cases, usually at the geniculate ganglion and horizontal portion of the nerve. In transverse fracture, the fracture line extends from the jugular foramen through the internal auditory canal to the foramen lacerum leading to nerve deafness and associated facial nerve injury (50% cases). Management of facial nerve injury includes CT scan of the temporal bone (high resolution, both coronal and axial cuts) to locate the site of fracture, topognostic tests to determine the site of injury and electrical nerve test to determine the physiologic status of facial nerve. Clinically, progression from partial to complete paralysis, loss of tearing, submandibular salivary flow rate less then 25% of normal, indicate unfavourable signs and warrant surgical exploration and nerve decompression and/or nerve repair at the earliest.

If facial nerve function does not recover after 1 year, facial hypoglossal anastomosis or facial slings, is indicated.

Management of 'acute vertigo' includes:

- Strict bed rest in a quiet room and administration of vestibular suppressants like:
  - i/v diazepam (5-20 mg) in 3–5 min. provides most rapid relief of symptoms (in a large vein in order to minimize the possibility of vein sclerosis). More drug can be added to the i/v bottle and infused slowly if severe symptoms recur and dose can be titrated by observing its effect on the nystagmus, turning both the nystagmus and vertigo sensation on or off by slowing or quickening the i/v rate Promethazine hydrochloride (Phenargen, Avomine) 25-50 mg i/m, or prochlorperazine (Stemetil) 12.5-25 mg i/m can also be used as vestibular suppressants as well as for the control of accompanying nausea and vomiting. Ondansetron (Emeset) may also be used to control nausea and vomiting.
  - i/v fluid and electrolyte replacement is another important aspect to be considered for the management of acute vertigo.

Maintenance therapy is given once the acute phase is over. Diazepam is generally given on a short-term basis (2, 5 or 10 mg, 6-8 hourly), depending on the severity of the patient's symptoms and level of anxiety. Meclizine (Diligan) in dose of 12.5 to 25 mg, 6-8 hourly or Dimenhydrinate (Gravol) in dose of 50-100 mg, 6-8 hourly can be used.

Promethazine (Avomine, Phenargen) 25 mg, 6-8 hourly and Prochlorperazine (Stemetil) orally or by rectal suppository at 25 mg b.d. dosage, are also useful for the control of nausea and vomiting on an OPD basis.

Management of posttraumatic nerve deafness is unfortunately, not possible because of permanent damage. Although there is some spontaneous recovery of the high frequency loss that often accompanies longitudinal fracture there is little possibility of recovery of any useful hearing following transverse fractures. Only point to be stressed is to document the hearing loss (conductive, sensorineural or mixed) on the case file, as per the tuning-fork tests and pure tone audiometry (bed side if possible) from the medico-legal point of view.

CSF OTORRHOEA

CSF leak may manifest through ear as CSF otorrhoea when ear drum is perforated or may press the myheustachian tube to the nasopharynx in presence of intact ear drum. On examination, if drum is intact, there may be air fluid level as a meniscus or air bubbles but seigalization is contraindicated to prevent pneumocephalus. Patient is made to lean forward to look for rhinorrhoea, which on white cloth reveals a ring sign with the CSF having a further diffusion point than blood.

In cases of perforated drum, careful suction and cleaning of external ear canal with sterile instruments under microscope is performed. Management includes keeping the ear dry and keep in gasterile cotton plug in the external ear canal, elevation of patient head to 30 degree angle and bed rest. No topical ear drops are adviced. Oral antibiotic prophylaxis is adviced. CSF otorrhoea usually resolves spontaneously within 72 hours. If there is no improvement after 7-10 days surgical intervention is indicated.

CSF RHINORRHOEA

Approximately 25% of fractures of sinuses are associated with CSF rhinorrhoea and therefore should always be suspected even in presence of minor facial trauma. Mostly it is due to anterior cranial fractures, through ethmoid root or cribriform plate or CSF may pass through fractured posterior table of frontal sinus. Patient may present with intermittent or continuous watery or blood stained rhinorrhoea, provoked or increased by straining or change in posture. Mostly patient complain of continuous headache secondary to low pressure.

Management includes avoidance of straining and nose blowing, advising head elevation and bed rest with antibiotic prophylaxis. Surgical intervention for repair of dura is indicated after 7-10 days if CSF rhinorrhoea does not resolve spontaneously following the said measures.[3]

REFERENCES

1. Huxley EW. *Pediatric ENT Review*, 2nd edn. Londn: Smith and Smith 2003.
2. Goodyear A, Morris E. Accidental injuries in pediatrics. *J Matern Child Hlth* 2001;5:124-132.
3. Rudy AS. CSF rhinorrhea in children. Asian Med Bull 2003;7:21-25.

Aniece Chowdhary

93 Neck Trauma

INTRODUCTION

Neck trauma may be penetrating wounds or blunt injuries. The later may be of low or high velocity. Penetrating wounds are usually caused by knives, bullets, agricultural tools etc. High velocity blunt trauma is due to injuries caused by road traffic accidents (steering wheel or dashboard), low velocity trauma is due to blow injury (fist or foot) or as a result of sports injury (karate, basketball, racing, golf and cricket balls, hockey sticks etc.).[1,2]

The presentation is usually life–threatening and may end with permanent airway or voice changes. Clinical presentation also depend upon the associated neck injuries like cervical spine fractures or vascular injuries, compound fractures of laryngotracheal framework, respiratory distress and shock.

ACUTE LARYNGOTRACHEAL TRAUMA

Clinical manifestations of trauma are: In case of simple contusions, pain and hoarseness along with tenderness of thyroid cartilage is seen. Edema and possible hematoma of endolarynx can be visualized on laryngoscopic examination of larynx if patient has no airway distress. If a patient has cricoarytenoid dislocation alongwith, there is usually dyspnoea, dysphagia and slight aspiration. Laryngeal examination shows edema of arytenoid area and aryepiglottic fold, abnormal arytenoid position, bowing and decreased mobility of vocal cord.

The hyoid bone fracture presents with pain and odynophagia. Bleeding into the paraglottic space causing swelling of base of tongue with supraglottic edema and respiratory distress. On palpation, hyoid area is tender and swollen with bony crepitus.

Extent of trauma to thyroid and cricoid cartilage is determined by the degree of their calcification and thus, on the age of patient. If the thyroid cartilage is pushed backwards over the cervical spine, then it splays apart and there is no fracture with an elastic thyroid cartilage. If force is more, the cartilage will usually split down the front or in down the prominence and with inherent elasticity of cartilage, it will spring back into place with little damage or disruption of anterior commissure. There may be bleeding in the paraglottic space and posterior displacement of the epiglottis. The calcified thyroid cartilage on compression injury, shatters like an egg with the loss of thyroid eminence. Arytenoids get sandwiched between thyroid cartilage and cervical spine and may get dislocated. Cricoid being the only complete ring in the respiratory tract behaves differently with tendency to resorption and ultimately stenosis, thereby reducing the airway lumen. Cricoid defects are most difficult to repair. Patient's symptomatology includes pain, mild to severe dyspnoea, stridor, hoarseness or aphonia, odynophagia and hemoptysis. External neck examination may reveal subcutaneous emphysema, tenderness, palpable fracture of thyroid cartilage, ecchymosis of skin and loss of landmarks of external larynx. Endoscopic examination of larynx reveal edema or hematoma, distortion of normal anatomy, mucosal tears of larynx or posterior pharynx, bleeding, exposed cartilages and vocal cord weakness or displacement.

Laryngotracheal separation may be the most disastrous injury leading to death at the roadside. Sometimes, enough lumen may remain for the patient to breathe long enough to reach the hospital. Several tracheal rings may be damaged along with shearing of cricotracheal membrane. Symptoms are usually severe dyspnoea, pain aphonia or hoarseness, hemoptysis. On examination there is severe airway distress, subcutaneous emphysema, tenderness, ecchymosis and head posturing forwards to breathe.

Assessment

One should always suspect airway injuries in every patient of road traffic accidents who present with dyspnoea and dysphonia. Surgical emphysema limited to neck is almost pathognomic of airway breach. Plain radiographs of neck are helpful in confirming the presence or absence of air in soft tissues, fractures of laryngeal framework and cervical spine injuries. X-ray chest is done to look for mediastinal, emphysema and/or pneumothorax. Laryngograms in absence of airway distress, demonstrates mucosal tears. A CT scan axial plane helps to localize the fracture sites. Larygoscopic examination is mandatory in all patients, usually indirect, direct under GA or by flexible laryngoscopy.

Management

Immediate airway management is the first line of treatment. Intubation can be attempted in semiconscious or unconscious patients but because of distorted larynx, tracheostomy is always preferred which may have to be performed in sitting or semi-sitting position in some patients. In inexperienced, cricothyroidectomy may be a safer and quicker option in casualty ward. Depending upon extent of injuries, definite treatment is initiated which is as follows:

i. *Contusions:* If there is no respiratory distress or fracture or any evidence of intraluminal bleed or tracheal damage, patient can be kept on bed rest with or without steroids or steam inhalation and head elevation.
ii. *Fracture of hyoid bone:* may need only symptomatic treatment, rarely open reduction and interosseous wiring of major fracture is done.
iii. *Thyroid and cricoid cartilage fractures:* Require open reduction, repair of laceration and stent placement, along with tracheostomy. Bleeding in the laryngeal space may be dealt with opening of these spaces and then obliterating them with quilting sutures. In presence of a significant bleeding in the larynx, it is opened by way of midline laryngofissure and drainage of clot is achieved. Drains are not kept in these spaces. Principle of minimal debridement is followed. Any exposed cartilage is covered with mucosa which may get resorbed later on, forming a scaffold for firm fibrous tissue. Dislocated arytenoids are relocated usually within 48 hours.
iv. Laryngotracheal separation is dealt with tracheostomy, open reduction, suturing of cartilage and stenting of airway. Recurrent laryngeal nerves are explored and if found severed, reanastomosis can be done but with doubtful outcome. Damaged tracheal rings can be excised followed by laryngeal drop to end anastomosis.

Broad spectrum antibiotics are always administered to prevent infection from mucosal tears and subcutaneous emphysema and to help avoid stenosis. Steroids are used for laryngeal edema. Feeding is achieved via nasogastric tube to prevent aspiration and to bypass the dysphagia.

CERVICAL SPINE INJURY

Any trauma to the neck may be associated with cervical spine injury resulting in fracture or dislocation. The condition may become life-threatening from neurogenic shock or it may cause quadriplegia. Patient complains of neck pain and neck swelling. On examination, there is tenderness over cervical vertebrae, paraplegia or quadriplegia and dyspnoea.

X-ray AP or lateral view of cervical spine with arms and shoulders pulled caudally will reveal dislocated vertebrae and/or increased thickness of retropharyngeal space. Management includes immobilization of head and neck airway establishment usually tracheostomy by experienced ENT surgeon and neurosurgical intervention in form of tongs and traction.

INJURY OF MAJOR VESSELS IN NECK

Blunt trauma is an unusual cause for major vessel rupture. Penetrating injuries especially bullet are mostly associated with injuries to the vessels, without being clinically evident and this aspect of acute trauma to the neck needs to be suspected in every patient, which deserves immediate exploration or if no emergency exists, and arteriogram.

Clinically, patient presents with pain, swelling tenderness and ecchymosis of skin or pharynx and airway distress. Swelling is usually static in hematomas but progressive in arterial or jugular vein injury. Imaging includes X-ray film of neck (AP or lateral) to determine in trajectory crosses near the path of any of the major vessel and arteriogram. Soft tissue injury with hematoma which in static and patient in without dyspnoea or shock, can be managed conservatively. Arterial injury or jugular vein injury needs urgent exploration of neck with repair or ligation offending vessels.

INJURY TO PHARYNX AND ESOPHAGUS

The upper GIT injuries in the form of contusion, laceration or rupture in the wall may be because of blunt trauma or penetrating injuries which may not be obvious initially. Since the complications can be fatal it is important to recognize and treat them properly. Clinical features are pain, mild to moderate dysphagia, hemoptysis, edema or hematoma of the pharynx, subcutaneous emphysema. Patient may be initially asymptomatic but later on manifests fever, odynophagia, neck abscess formation, mediastinitis and purulent discharge from the injury site. Diagnosis is confirmed by soft tissue X-ray films (AP or lateral views) in which free air and/or retropharyngeal thickening is seen. CT scan helps in accurate localization of injury site. Direct laryngoscopy and oesophagoscopy by skilled endoscopist is done to confirm the finding.

Management includes nothing peroral, intravenous antibiotics, neck exploration followed by repair and minimal debridement if required.

INJURY TO SUBMANDIBULAR GLAND AND THYROID GLAND

In the submandibular gland, most important structure is the facial artery because it can lead to significant bleeding and hematoma formation, while trauma to thyroid is unlikely to produce any significant thyroid dysfunction. Major concern in thyroid gland injury is bleeding because of high vascularity. Management requires exploration and debridement of the wound. Also trachea and oesphagus are looked for any injury. In case of thyroid tissue loss, attempt is made to save some of thyroid gland and one or more of parathyroid glands.

REFERENCES

1. Huxley EW. *Pediatric ENT Review*, 2nd edn. London: Smith and Smith 2003.
2. Goodyear A, Morris E. Accidental injuries in pediatrics. *J Matern Child Hlth* 2001;5:124-132.

ENT Emergencies

Aniece Chowdhary

94 Deep Neck Infections

INTRODUCTION

The morbidity and mortality in any head and neck infection depends upon many parameters, including virulence, pathogenicity and antibiotic sensitivity of the invading organism and the host factors (age, general health and immunologic capability of the host).[1,2] The deep neck infections, although uncommon, may have life-threatening sequelae despite antibiotic therapy.

ANATOMIC CONSIDERATIONS

An understanding of the anatomic relationships of the fascial planes and potential spaces of the neck is essential for the surgical management required for most deep neck (Fig. 94.1) infections. The cervical fascia consists of fibrous connective tissue that ensheaths the organs, muscles, nerves and vessels of the neck, binding them into functional units and thereby forming planes and potential compartments. The "tube within tube" concept helps one to visualise the three layers of the deep cervical fascia namely the superficial, middle and deep layer.

Superficial layer of deep cervical fascia is a clear continuous sheet of fibrous tissue, surrounding the neck and enclosing two glands, two muscles and two spaces (the rule of two). Two glands are a submandibular on each side, two muscle on each side are the trapezius and sternocleidomastoid and the two spaces are the suprasternal space of Burns and posterior triangle. The middle or visceral layer of deep cervical fascia surround the esophagus, trachea, larynx and thyroid. The deep layer surround the paraspinous muscles of the neck. Each of the three layers contribute to the carotid sheath as it courses through the neck.

The deep layer consists of two divisions, the alar and the prevertebral layer. The alar layer lies anterior to the prevertebral and posterior to the visceral (middle) layer, forming the posterior wall of retropharyngeal space and anterior wall of prevertebral or danger space. The retropharyngeal space extends from skull base till T_1 and

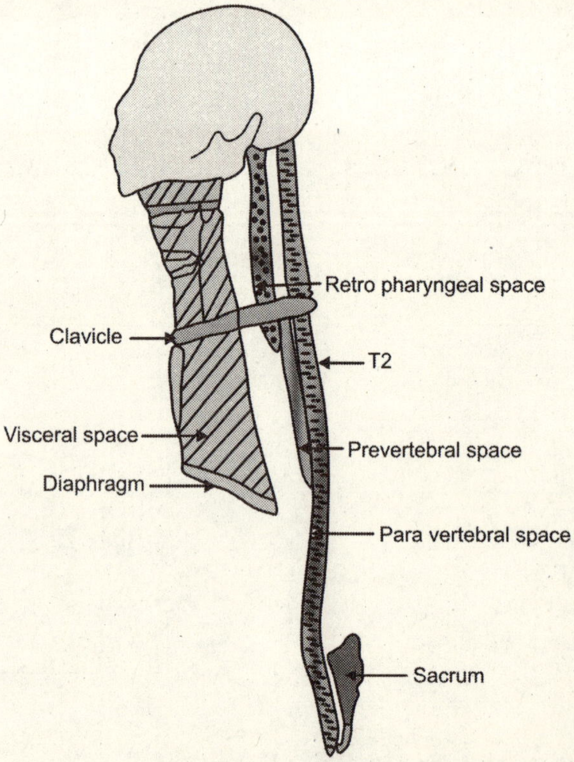

Fig. 94.1: Deep neck spaces

T_2 level. The prevertebral layer form the posterior wall of prevertebral space and anterior wall of paravertbral space, extending from skull base to coccyx. The surgical importance is when an abscess forms in a space, spread to other spaces occurs along planes of least resistance because of the interrelationship and continuity of all the layers of deep cervical facia and the potential spaces.

INFECTION OF SPACES INVOLVING THE ENTIRE LENGTH OF NECK

i. Retropharyngeal abscess: Retropharyngeal space lies behind the hypopharynx and the esophagus, extends superiorly from the base of skull and inferiorly upto the superior mediastinum to the level of T_1–T_2 where middle and deep layers of cervical fascia fuse. Retropharyngeal abscess occurs most frequently in infants and young children. Infection springs from nasal chambers, posterior nasal sinuses, adenoids and nasopharynx to involve the retropharyngeal lymph nodes. Other causes include foreign bodies piercing the posterior esophageal wall, esophageal rupture, vertebral fractures, syphilis, upper respiratory tract infection and dental infections. Infection in ear, nose and throat spreads via lymphatics to retropharyngeal lymph nodes, which are found in greatest numbers in children under the age of four and account for relatively greater incidence of retropharyngeal abscesses in this age group. Symptoms of this abscess in children differ from those in adults. Most common organisms are Group A streptococcus, staphylococcus aureus, aerobic and anaerobic pharyngeal microorganisms. In children, most common features are drooling, fever, dysphagia, interference with breathing and torticollis. Usually no trismus is present and laryngeal oedema may occur. X-ray soft tissue neck reveals air in the retropharyngeal soft tissues or widening of prevertebral area. Normally the retropharyngeal tissue on lateral plain X-ray is equal to width of the body of C_2 in small children. The classical appearance of retropharyngeal abscess is a unilateral (postero-lateral) swelling of the posterior pharyngeal wall, which may push the palate forward, because of midline fascia dividing the retropharyngeal space and restricting the abscess to one side.

Surgical management is done mainly by external approach, while the peroral approach is indicated in selected patients.

Peroral approach: indicated in early retropharyngeal abscesses with no respiratory obstruction. Head is kept in extreme 'Rose' position and mouth gag is utilized and incision and drainage is done. Tracheostomy is indicated in presence of airway obstruction.

External approach: is indicated in larger retropharyngeal abscess, paravertebral and prevertebral, carotid sheath abscess where anterior external approach is employed. A transverse incision is made along the anterior border of sternomastoid muscle at the desired level between the hyoid bone and the sternum. The sternocleidomastoid muscle and carotid sheath are retracted laterally, and the thyroid gland and superior thyroid pedicle is retracted medially, exposing the abscess at the level of hypopharynx and abscess is opened. If abscess extends down, finger dissection can be carried into mediastinum along the oesophagus and a drain is left in place. Another external approach is posterior approach, incision is made behind the sternomastoid muscle avoiding the carotid sheath and abscess is entered from the fascia behind the sternomastoid muscle.

INFECTION OF SPACES ABOVE THE HYOID BONE

i. *Submandibular space:* Involvement of this space occur mainly in dental or periodonal infections submandibular gland or súppuration of submandibular lymph nodes, leading to Ludwig's angina. Streptococci and staphylococci are the commonest organisms but Vincent's organism and common spirochetal commensals of the mouth may be primary or secondary invaders. Ludwig's angin (original described by ludwig in 1836) usually presents a patient in acute distress with characteristic finding–the tissues of the floor of mouth are greatly swollen and extremely inflammed, displacement of the tongue upward and backward towards the palatal vault, wooden like induration at first confined to the submandibular compartment, trimus, hoarseness and dyspnea. this highly virulent infection is a cellulitis and not a true abscess and can cause rapid death from upper airway obstruction or mediastinitis if it descends past the hyoid. Wide surgical drainage is indicated and airway is managed with tracheostomy. Trismus and hypopharyngeal mucosal oedema contraindicate preliminary intubation. Transverse incision is made in submental space and carried down to the deep fascia of the mylohyoid muscle. Mylohyoid muscle is divided perpendicular to the course of its fibres and drain is kept. If the infection localizes to the floor of mouth above the mylohyoid line, intra oral drainage is sometimes possible.

ii. *Parapharyngeal space:* This space is most commonly involved in children because of portals of infection here are most often from the pharynx, tonsils and adenoids, teeth, parotid glands, and the lymph nodes that drain the nose and pharynx. Also uncommon cause is Bezold's abscess (mastoiditis leading to abscess in inner aspect of mastoid tip). It presents as a rapidly growing unilateral tender neck mass obliterating the angle of the mandible with high grade fever. Staphylococcus aureus, streptococcus sp. and anaerobic bacteria are most common causative organisms. Other clinical features are trimus due to medial pterygoid muscle irritation, medial displacement of tonsil and lateral pharyngeal wall, toxicity and altered sensorium. Plum color of the swollen oral mucosa indicates submucosal hemorrhage suggesting arterial erosion. Externally, there is swelling in the neck with ill defined margins, absence of fluctuation but with pitting oedema of neck, mostly seen in patients with diabetes, nephritis, tuberculosis or AIDS. Ear hemorrhage is a grave prognostic sign of vascular involvement. Hemorrhage due to the erosion of internal carotid artery may occur and may require immediate surgical intervention. The proper time for surgical drainage depends on the stage of infection which can be monitored effectively by CECT scan. Rarely the abscess ruptures spontaneously and drains externally. It should be drained surgically, even when no complication has occurred. However, no drainage attempt should be made during the stage of phlegmon formation (cellulitis), when antibiotics alone are sufficient (clindamycin, chloramphenicol, metronidazole, cefoxitin, or imipenem, and combination of a penicillin plus a beta–lactamas inhibitor are more appropriate antibiotics). Surgical drainage by submaxillary approach can be accomplished by a modification of the Mosher–T shaped incision.

iii. *Masticator space or masseteric space abscess:* is a subperiosteal abscess and cellulitis of the mandible and soft tissue and may involve the fascial sling containing the muscles of mastication (i.e. masseter, pterygoid and the temporalis muscle). There is a brawny induration over the area of angle and body of the mandible externally, which may resemble the swelling of parapharyngeal abscess. Trismus is marked, oral cavity and oropharynx are swollen with tonsil displacement. Incision and drainage is achieved via intraoral approach or by external incision made below the horizontal ramus of mandible posterior to facial artery, carrying it down till the periosteum and blunt dissection is carried on each side of the mandible.

iv. *Parotid space:* The parotid space formed by the superficial layer of deep cervical fascia, is not a true anatomic space, many fascial septa run vertically through it. A parotid space abscess is actually an infection of the gland with loculated micro–abscesses, most common pathogen being staphylococcus. The patient presents with erythematous skin and a swollen parotid gland with high grade fever and tenderness but with absence of trismus or swelling of lateral pharyngeal wall. Stenson's duct usually reveals a purulen flow on massage. Surgical drainage is necessary when antibiotics are unsuccessful and achieved via "Furstenberg incision, where multiple incision are made through the fascia parallel to the branches of fascial nerve and opening of space with a blunt clamp.

v. *Peritonsillar space:* This space is between superior constrictor muscle and tonsil capsule. Peritonsillar or paratonsillar abscess (quinsy) is rare in young and is commonly seen after puberty. Clinically patients present with severe pain, fever, dysphagia or odynophagia, trismus and 'hotpotato' voice. On oral examination there is erythema and enlargement of the offending tonsil with medial deviation of tonsil and edema of soft palate. Most common cause for hospitalization is dehydration. Abscess is drained intraorally.

REFERENCES

1. Roy E. Infections of head and neck. *Austr Clin Med Surg* 1999;3:453-487.
2. Roy E, Brown CA. Infections (deep) in neck. *Carrib J Surg* 2002;11:432-438.

Section XVII

Dermatological Emergencies

Praveen C Sobti, Alka Dogra and Aman Dua

95 Dermatological Emergencies

INTRODUCTION

Cutaneous lesions may be the major or sole complaint in a significant proportion of children seeking emergency care. It is the pediatrician or the family physician who sees these patients first. The diagnosis and treatment may be confused by more sensitive reaction patterns, or tendency towards vesicle and bulla formation and therapeutic dosages and regimens that frequently differ from those of adults. This chapter attempts to provide a practical approach to the assessment and initial management of the common dermatological emergencies.

APPROACH TO THE CHILD WITH A DERMATOLOGIC EMERGENCY

Accurate diagnosis of cutaneous disease in infants and children, as in adults, is a systematic process that requires careful inspection, evaluation and some knowledge of dermatologic terminology, morphology and differential diagnosis.

Quick assessment of the child's condition can be made by noting the following:

a. Nature of lesions—blisters, erosions or petechiae.
b. Percentage of skin involvement—skin surface area.
c. General condition of the child.

One must note the nature of the lesions. The most serious emergencies are usually associated with raw areas and blisters involving large areas of the skin. These children require immediate hospitalisation and intensive care.

Another clue to the seriousness of a child's disease is how ill the child appears. It can be a useful clue in situations where the skin lesions are limited in extent but cause morbidity because of associated abnormalities. Conversely a child with an extensive eruption may be quite cheerful as in viral exanthems.

On the basis of initial assessment, pediatric dermatological emergencies can be classified as per Table 95.1.

Table 95.1: Classification of pediatric dermatological emergencies

a. *Hypersensitivity Reactions*
   i. Urticaria, angioedema, anaphylaxis.
   ii. Toxic epidermal necrolysis.
   iii Erythema multiforme, Stevens Johnson syndrome.
   iv. Exanthematous drug eruptions.
   v. Acute irritant and allergic contact dermatitis.

b. *Bullous disorders*
   i. Chronic bullous dermatosis of childhood.
   ii. Epidermolysis bullosa.
   iii. Pemphigus.

c. *Infections*
   i. *Viral Exanthems*
      – Varicella (Chickenpox).
      – Rubeola (Measles).
      – Rubella (German measles).
   ii. *Bacterial Infections*
      – Bullous impetigo.
      – Staphylococcal scalded skin syndrome.
      – Cellulitis/necrotizing fascitis.

d. *Vasculitis*
   i. Henoch-Schönlein (anaphylactoid) purpura.
   ii. Purpura (petechiae, Ecchymosis).

e. ***Hereditary Causes***
   i. Harlequin fetus, collodion Baby and other congenital icthyosis

HYPERSENSITIVITY REACTIONS

Urticaria, Angiodema, Anaphylaxis[6]

These are manifestations of the Type-I hypersensitivity reactions. Acute urticaria is perhaps the most common dermatological emergency and is characterized by itchy, erythematous, edematous wheals which may develop over large areas of the skin (Fig. 95.1). Individual skin lesions usually subside within a few minutes to a few hours (maximum 24 hours). However, new lesions may continue to erupt. Mucous membranes may be involved and there may be swelling of the lips, tongue and larynx (angiodema);

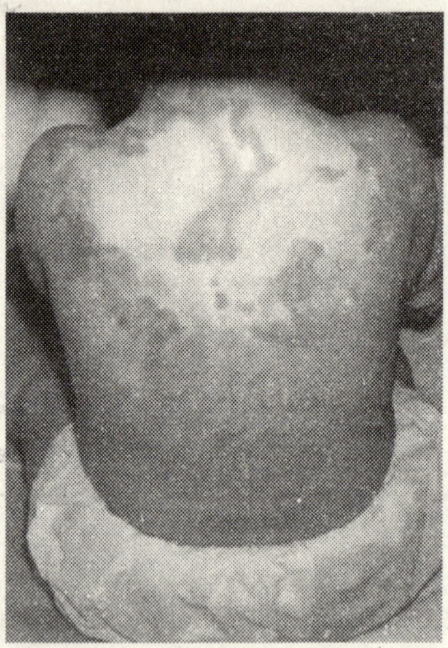

Fig 95.1: Acute urticaria
(See for colour figure plate 1)

which can cause respiratory distress. The wheals may be accompanied by fever, abdominal pain and syncope depending on the severity of attack. When the process develops very rapidly, it constitutes anaphylactic shock which is characterised by hypotension, bronchoconstriction, urticaria and syncope. The condition may be fatal unless managed properly. Anaphylactic shock usually develops following an injection or an insect bite.

Management

The most common cause of urticaria in children under 6 months of age is cow's milk allergy. In childhood, it is the worm infestation taking the lead. One must fully investigate the patient and get complete hemogram routine urine and stool examination. For acute urticaria, patient should be given an adequate dose of antihistamines. This usually consists of 2 different drugs e.g. Pheniramine and cetrizine given 3-4 times and 1-2 daily doses, respectively. It is expected that acute urticaria will be substantially controlled within 24 hours. In anaphylactic shock, as soon as possible, patient must be given oxygen inhalation and injection adrenaline (1 in 1000), 0.01 ml/kg IM. An intravenous line should be set up. Patient should be observed over the next 15 minutes and an injection of adrenaline repeated if no improvement is there. Injection pheniramine maleate 1.5 mg/kg IV or IM should be given along with injection hydrocortisone 2 mg/kg IM or IV.

Toxic Epidermal Necrolysis (TEN)[2,13,16,17]

It is a severe acute blistering disease that has a high mortality rate without treatment. It is generally considered to be a hypersensitivity reaction to drugs such as thiacetazone, sulphonamides, phenytoin, barbiturates, penicillin, non-steroidal anti-inflammatory agents (NSAIDs) among the others. The reaction generally develops within 2-3 weeks of starting the drug in a non-sensitized person but may develop within hours if the patient is already sensitized to the drug. TEN can occur at all ages though most patients are young adults.

The eruption begins abruptly as tender, erythematous maculas accompanied by vesiculation and bullae. Large areas of the erythematous skin develop a characteristic brown black discoloration. This necrotic skin peels off easily to leave large raw areas. Mucous membrane involvement is nearly constant and is generally severe. Mucosae of mouth, eyes, genitialia, esophagus and brachial tree may be involved. Ocular lesions carry a high risk of sequelae such as corneal scarring and blindness. There is marked toxemia and high grade fever. Complications include super-added bacterial infections and septicemia, hypovolemic shock, acute tubular necrosis, glomerulonephritis, broncho-pneumonia, pulmonary edema and gastrointestinal bleeding.

Management

The immediate stoppage of all the drugs that the patient has been taking is the most important part of the management of TEN. It is emphasized that suspecting and stopping only one of the drugs being taken is extremely dangerous because a mistake in identifying the drug can lead to worsening of the condition. If a drug is essential, a chemically unrelated substitute should be used. Nursing and supportive care is provided. Prednisolone is administered in an initial dose of 1.5-2 mg/kg daily. The condition of the patient is closely monitored over a period of 24-48 hours for the appearance of new lesions and persistence or appearance of erythema at the periphery of lesions. Erythema on the palms and soles persists much longer than elsewhere and should not be used to titrate therapy. If these signs are present, an increase in the daily dose by 0.5-1 mg/kg of prednisolone equivalent is made and the same dose is controlled. The dose is then abruptly halved every 2-3 days and withdrawn completely over a period of 10-14 days.

Some workers advocate that corticosteroids should be avoided in the treatment of TEN. However, we have had good results with corticosteroid therapy and would advocate a high dose, short duration regimen to rapidly control the disease.

Stevens-Johnson Syndrome[2,17]

Stevens-Johnson syndrome is an uncommon reaction pattern that is usually triggered by drugs like thiacetazone, sulphonamides, phenytoin, barbiturates, pencillin, non-steroidal anti-inflammatory agents among the others or certain infections (pharyngitis, pneumonitis, herpes labialis, hepatitis). Target lesions i.e. erythematous lesions with a blue-black center are a distinctive features. Other organs may be affected like mouth, eyes, male genitalia and mucous membrane. New crops of lesions continue to appear upto

10 days or even 3-4 weeks. In the absence of target lesions, the difference between SJ syndrome and TEN is largely subjective. In addition, a thorough search must be made to look for a focus of infection which may be cause of the reaction and must be treated appropriately. In patients who have herpes simplex infection, acyclovir 5 mg/kg 8 hourly, intravenously or 200 mg five times a day orally should be administered.

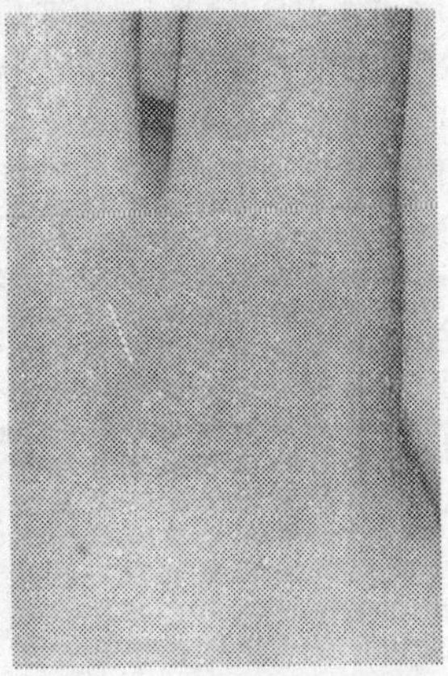

Fig. 95.2: Erythema multiforme—typical target lesions over knuckles *(See for colour figure plate 1)*

Exanthematous Drug Eruption[15,18]

This is the most common pattern of drug eruption and can be caused by a number of drugs including sulfonamides, penicillins, anticonvulsant and antitubercular agents. Characteristically, a symmetrical itchy macular and papular eruption rapidly spreads to involve the entire cutaneous surface including the plasmas and soles. Initially the lesions are discrete but soon coalesce into large patches. The mucosal surfaces may be involved. Fever may sometimes accompany the rash. The rash usually continues to spread if the drug is not stopped. Conversely, it becomes statis or begins to regress within 24 hours of stopping the drug. If left untreated, the rash can proceed to exfoliative dermatitis. The development of a generalised, symmetrical, rapidly progressive, erythematous eruption should prompt a detailed interrogation for drug intake and the timing of the intake in relation to the rash. A system-by-system questioning for symptoms and the treatment taken is often rewarding as most patients omit to mention over-the counter preparations and self-prescribed medications unless specifically questioned. The major differential diagnosis is a viral exanthem. Drug history can usually be elicited and the characteristic patterns of viral exanthem is lacking.

Management

All drugs being taken when the rash developed must be stopped. It is risky to try to guess and stop only one drug because an error may lead to worsening of disease. If a particular drug is essential, a chemically unrelated substitute may be used. Most patients will require systemic corticosteroid therapy in a dose of 0.5 to 1 mg/kg prednisolone daily. The rash can be controlled in 24-48 hours as evidenced by fading of erythema and lack of new lesions. At this stage, the dose of prednisolone can be halved every 2-3 days and withdrawn over 7-10 days. Antihistamines are not effective in treating exanthematous drug eruptions. They only provide symptomatic relief of itching.

BULLOUS DISORDERS

Chronic Bullous Dermatosis of Childhood[3,10]

This auto-immune bullous disorder is characterized by tense, clear vesicles and bullae that may develop anywhere on the skin but have a predilection for the peri-oral and genital skin. The blisters often develop in a ring arranged around a central active or healed blister; this is known as the "string of pearls" appearance (Fig. 95.3). In our experience, the blisters are often impetiginized and may be mistaken for impetigo contagious or infective dermatitis at presentation till a fresh crop of tense vesicles gives lead to the diagnosis. A biopsy reveals a subepidermal blister and direct immunofluorescence demonstrates a linear band of IgA along the basement membrane zone.

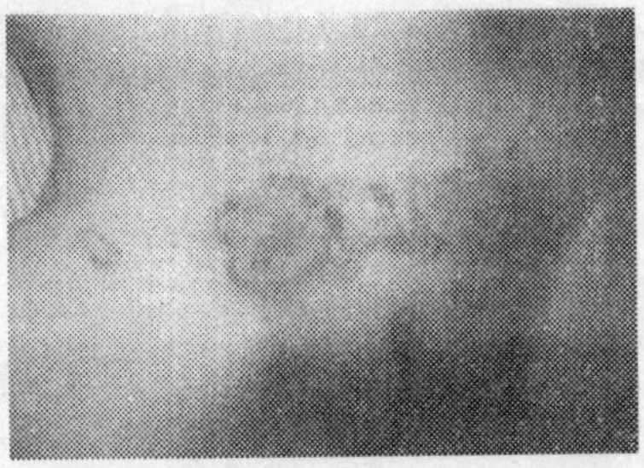

Fig. 95.3: Chronic bullous dermatoses of childhood—Cluster of jewels with new bullae forming over older lesions *(See for colour figure plate 1)*

Management

Treatment with dapsone 25-50 mg daily and a low dose of corticosteroids (0.5-1 mg/kg) controls the blisters. The corticosteroids may be tapered over 2-4 weeks. Dapsone should be continued for 3-6 months. Recurrences may develop and should be treated similarly. The disease remits spontaneously by puberty in most children.

Epidermolysis Bullosa[21]

Multiple clear and/or hemorrhagic blisters on the hands and feet and the knees and elbows are suggestive of epidermolysis bullosa. (Fig. 95.4a and b). Blisters are present at or soon after birth in severe varieties of the disease and are often accompanied by erosions. Extensive erosions of the skin may lead to overwhelming infections. In some neonates, epidermolysis bullosa is accompanied by other anomalies such as pyloric atresia.

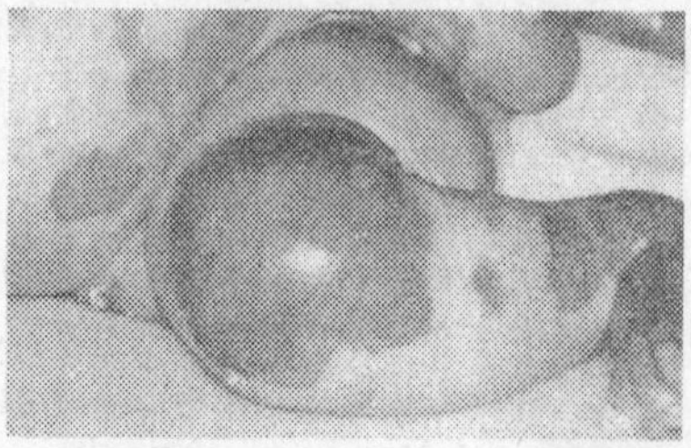

Fig. 95.4a: Extensive erosion in a neonate with Epidermolysis bullosa simplex (Dowling—Meare) *(See for colour figure plate 1)*

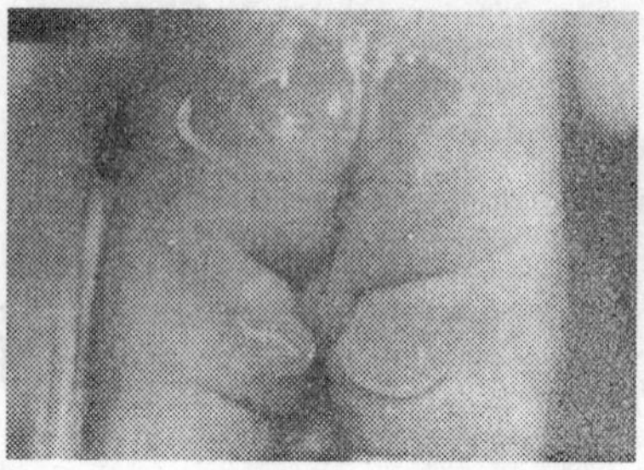

Fig. 95.4b: Junctional epidermolysis bullosa (Herlitz) *(See for colour figure plate 1)*

Management

Supportive care is necessary. Trauma is to be avoided. The role of high dose oral steroids is controversial but some workers feel it may be life saving. Associated anomalies should be managed appropriately.

Pemphigus[3,12]

Pemphigus is an auto immune blistering disorder that manifests as flaccid bullae which usually occur on apparently normal skin. The bullae rupture easily leaving large, raw areas which have a tendency to extend peripherally. Spontaneous healing is very slow. The normal skin can be peeled off easily with gentle pressure (Niklosky's sign). In over half of the patients, ulcers in the mouth precede the appearance of cutaneous lesions and eventually almost all patients develop oral mucosal lesions. Giemsa staining (Tzanck Smear) of the scraped material obtained from the base of the freshly ruptured bullae when examined under the microscope reveals the presence of characteristic acantholytic cells i.e. large round epidermal cells with prominent nucleus and loss of contact with surrounding cells. The diagnosis is confirmed by skin biopsy.

Management

The general principles of treatment of diseases with extensive erosions apply to patients with pemphigus. Corticosteroids are the mainstay of therapy—dexamethasone pulse therapy, dexamethasone 50 mg infused in 5% dextrose on 3 consecutive days, every 4 weeks. In the initial few weeks, most patients also require a daily dose of oral corticosteroids such as prednisolone 0.5-1 mg/kg. As the disease becomes inactive, the daily dose can be reduced and stopped but the pulses of dexamethasone are continued for a period of 9 months after complete clinical remission. In our experience, this regime gives long-lasting remissions.

An alternative schedule consists of using 1-2 mg/kg day or a higher dose of prednisolone or equivalent steroid. The daily dose can be increased by 1 mg/kg daily if there is no clinical response as indicated by continued appearance of new lesions, and extension of the old lesions. The dose of steroids should be maintained till all lesions have completely healed. The dose is then gradually tapered and the patient maintained on the minimal required dose. The side effects of daily corticosteroid therapy are more severe as compared to pulse therapy. In addition, patients are usually unable to completely stop therapy and require a small daily dose of corticosteroids indefinitely.

INFECTIONS

Viral Exanthems[4,15] (Varicella, Rubella, Rubeola etc.)

Several viral infections are associated with a rash. Macular and papular erythematous lesions develop over one part of the skin surface and gradually spread to involve other parts of the body over 2-3 days. Initial lesions may fade while new lesions continue to develop. In varicella characteristic vesicular lesions on an erythematous base in a centripetal fashion is characteristic (Fig. 95.5). Mucosal lesions may be seen and occasionally precede the skin eruption. Constitutional symptoms such as fever, myalgia and malaise usually accompany the eruption, but may sometimes precede the rash.

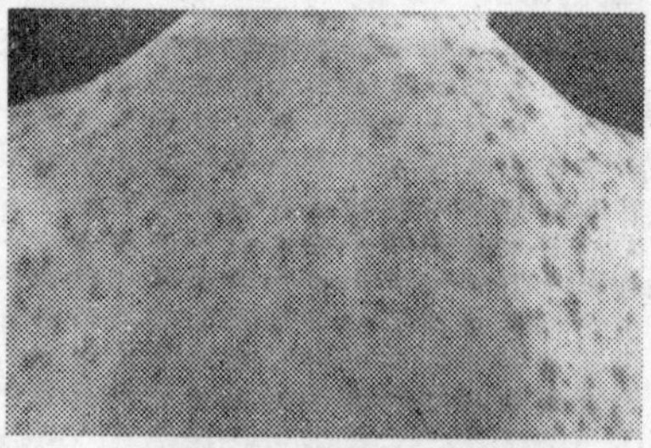

Fig. 94.5: Varicella *(See for colour figure plate 2)*

Occasionally, it may be very difficult to differentiate a viral exanthem from an exanthematous drug eruption, especially if the patient was taking drug(s) before the onset of the rash. However, spread of the rash in a sequential manner and the development of similar eruptions in other family members or in the community may provide a clue to the diagnosis. Usually, most viral exanthems subside in about 2 weeks with fine scaling and some post-inflammatory pigmentation.

Management

Antipyretics and analgesics like paracetamol may be prescribed for the relief of fever and myalgias. If a drug eruption cannot be reliably excluded, and the patient has already been taking these drugs, chemically unrelated substitutes should be advised.

Bacterial Infections

Bullous Impetigo[20]

Bullous impetigo is a contagious, superficial bacterial infection of skin caused by staphllococcus aureus, Streptococcus pyogenes or a mixture of both. The disease commonly affects infants and children. Lesions begin as clear vesicles and flaccid bullae which soon turn into pustules and rupture to form yellow brown crusts (Fig. 95.6). Face, especially the area around the nose and month and extremities are commonly affected sites. Extensive areas of the skin may be involved. The lesions remain discrete and even when numerous, generally cause little systemic disturbance. Mucosal lesions do not occur. A Gram stained smear from the blister fluid shows the presence of staphylococci and/or streptococci.

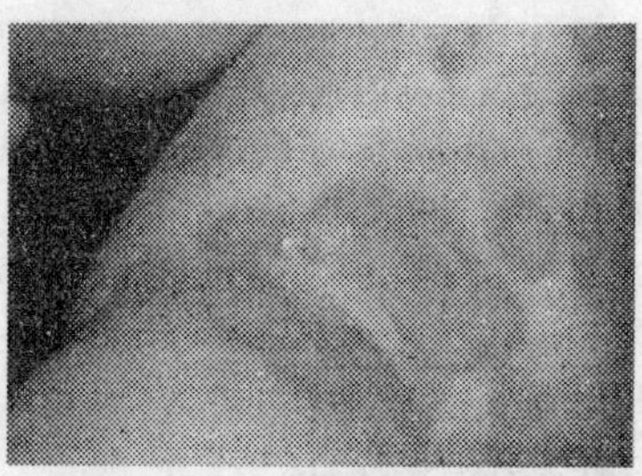

Fig. 95.6: Bullous impetigo after disruption of bullae *(See for colour figure plate 2)*

Management

Systemic antibiotics should be administered for a period of 5-7 days. Cloxacillin, amoxycillin-clavulanic acid, cephalexin and erythromycin are effective choices. The crusts should be removed thoroughly with the help of soap and water. A proper maintenance of hygienes and cleanliness must be emphasized.

Staphylococcal Scalded Skin Syndrome (SSSS)[9]

It is an uncommon but serious condition caused by "epidermolytic toxin" liberated by some strains of *Staphylococcus aureus*. It is characterized by tenderness, erythema and peeling of skin (Fig. 95.7). The condition occurs almost exclusively in infants and young children. It usually begins from perioral areas and flexures and may spread to involve the entire skin. Toxemia may sometimes be associated. Mucosae are not usually affected. The underlying staphylococcal infection is usually occult (conjunctivitis, pharyngitis, otitis media) or sometimes obvious as boils or umbilical sepsis.

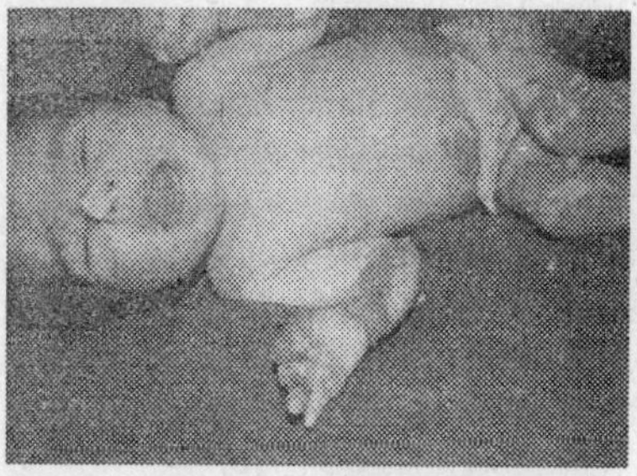

Fig. 95.7: Staphylococcal scaled skin syndrome *(See for colour figure plate 2)*

Management

The condition is treated by appropriate antibiotics effective against staphylococci, including the penicillinase producing strains. Cloxacillin 100 mg/kg/day, intravenously is generally the preferred choice. Amoxycilline with clavulanic acid and vancomycin are useful alternatives. The use of corticosteroids is contraindicated.

Cellulitis/Necrotizing Fascitis

Infection of the deep dermis and subcutaneous tissue by Staphylococcus aureus and Streptococcus pyogenes leads to cellulitis. This may develop *de novo* or around a preexisting lesion. Redness, warmth, tenderness and swelling of a localised area usually over the lower limb develops rather rapidly. The area is usually considerably swollen and hot. The overlying skin is red and may show blisters (Fig. 95.8a to d). The draining lymph nodes are tender and enlarged. Some patients develop more severe damage with necrosis of skin surrounded by inflammatory zone of erythema and blistering. Lesions progress with extension of the necrosis. Constitutional symptoms may be severe in these patients.

Management

If seen early, cellulitis can be managed by rest and elevation of the part and systemic antibiotic therapy. Bed rest is advised. The affected limb should be elevated on a pillow and kept immobile as far as possible. Systemic antibiotic therapy should be aggressive; amoxycililn with clavulanic acid 30-45 mg/kg/day (amoxycillin base), cloxacillin 100 mg/kg/day or cefaxolin 50-100 mg/kg/day are effective choices for parenteral therapy. Treatment should be continued for 10-14 days as the lesions resolve slowly. Oral therapy is substituted once toxemia is controlled. Surgical debridement is mandatory when necrosis develops. Early and complete debridement facilitates healing which may require a split skin graft if the excised area is large. Aggressive parenteral antibiotic therapy should be instituted

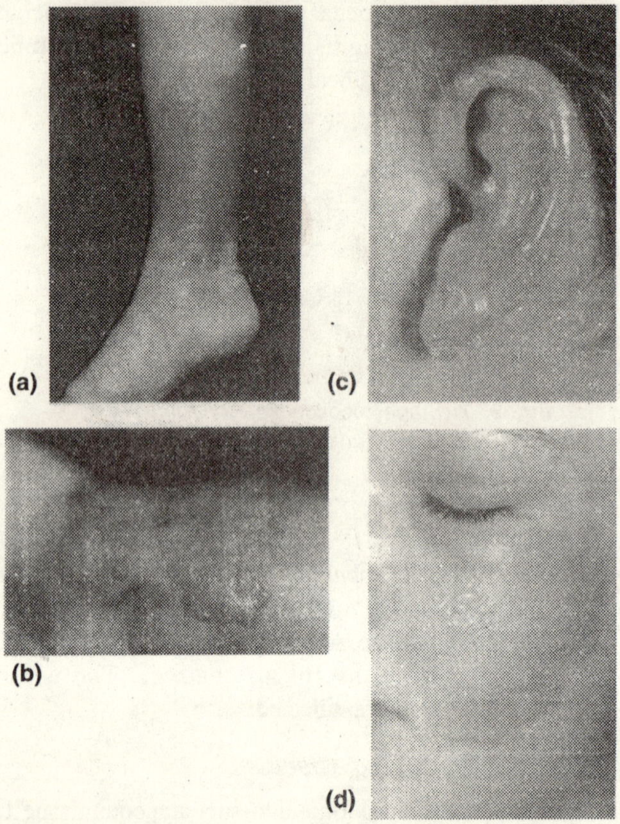

Figs 95.8a to d: Cellulitis (a) Lower leg (b) Extensor aspect of elbow (c) Pinna (d) Face
(See for colour figure plate 2)

as soon as possible. A suggested combination is intravenous therapy with crystalline penicillin 200,000 units/kg/day, cloxacillin 100 mg/kg/day and metronidazole 30-45 mg/kg/day to provide effective coverage against anaerobes.

VASCULITIS

Purpura (Petechiae, Ecchymosis)[19]

Purpuras represent small bleeds into the skin. Clinically, the lesions are non-blanchable, pink to red spots that fade over 5-7 days with light hyperpigmentation. They may be caused by a bleeding diathesis or a vasculitis. Purpura due to a bleeding disorder is recognized by the random distribution of lesions determined by the site of skin injury. Purpura itself is bland and unaccompanied by erythema or edema. Mucosal bleeds may also be seen. Large purpuras may be noticed at the sites of injection or venipunctures. The presence of a hematoma at the site of injury or a hemarthrosis provides additional clues. The child may have bled from other sites such as the nose or the gut. Purpura due to a hypersensitivity vasculitis is characterized by the development of lesions mainly on the legs. Lesions also develop on the buttocks and forearms. The trunk, head and face are usually spared. Purpura is bright red, has a blanchable component, and is accompanied by edema and infiltration, which leads to the lesions being raised i.e. "palpable purpura".

Henoch-Schönlein (Anaphylactoid) Purpura

In Henoch-Schönlein syndrome, purpuric lesions are raised above the surface giving a typical flea-bitten appearance over the extensor surfaces of legs and buttocks. In addition, the child may have pain and swelling of the joints, abdominal pain, hematemesis, melena and hematuria. A history of an upper respiratory tract infection or drug intake should be sought. When purpura is accompanied by fever, the possibility of a septic vasculitis or a hemorrhagic fever must be considered.

Management

If purpura is due to a bleeding disorder, urgent evaluation and appropriate therapy are recommended. Purpura fulminans should be treated with fresh frozen plasma (10 ml/kg), repeated as required. Platelet transfusions may be necessary. The underlying condition should be treated. In patients with septicemia, ceftriaxone or cefotaxime (100-200 mg/kg/day) should be started while awaiting blood culture reports. The antibiotic regimen can be modified, if necessary, when the culture reports become available. Purpura due to hypersensitivity vasculitis requires treatment if the skin lesions are severe, if there is renal involvement or severe articular symptoms. Prednisolone in a dose of 0.5-1 mg/kg/day is administered for 2-4 weeks. In dengue and other hemorrhagic fevers, intravenous fluids and other supportive measures form the mainstay of therapy.

HEREDITARY CONDITIONS

Harlequin Fetus, Collodion Baby and Other Congenital Icthyosis[1,22]

Thick scales over the entire skin are a characteristic feature of some genodermatoses. The degree of scaling and the deformity varies from condition to condition. The most severe cases are exemplified by harlequin fetus in which the neonate is encased in a tough sheath of scales (Figs 95.9a and b). Prominent fissures develop between the scales. The stretch produced by the scales leads to ectropion, eclabion and crumpling of the ear. Collodion baby, non-bullous and bullous ichthyosiform erythroderma and lamellar ichthyosis show a similar clinical picture with minor clincal variations in the degree of erythema, stretching of the skin and the presence or absence of blisters (Figs 95.10a and b).

Management

Severely affected neonates are usually very ill and may be dehydrated and hypothermic. In spite of intensive nursing care, many of these babies die in the first few days of life.

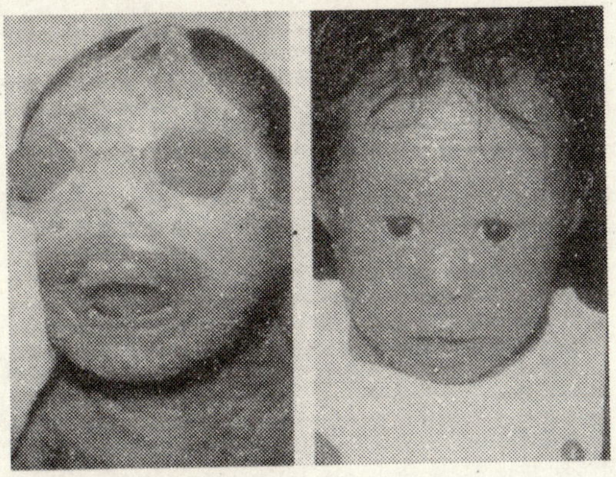

Figs 95.9a and b : (a) Harlequin ichthyosis; neonatal period (b) Same patient; aged 18 months
(See for colour figure plate 3)

In those who survive, emollients such as coconut oil or petroleum jelly may be used to relieve the stretching of the skin. In recent eyars, oral retinoids such as acitretin, 0.5 mg/kg have been used in these conditions with a significant reduction in scaling and hyperkeratosis. Since relapse may occur once retinoids are stopped, the drug needs to be continued indefinitely or administered intermittently whenever hyperkeratosis recurs. Unfortunately, acitretin is expensive and not freely available in our country.

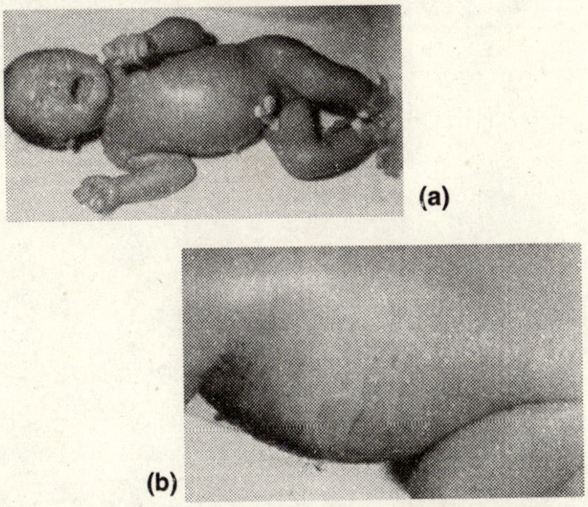

(a)

(b)

Figs 95.10a and b: (a) Collodion (lacquered) baby, aged 2 days. The membrane shed within 5 days, non-bullous ichthyosiform erythroderma was evident age 2 weeks (b) Same patient as in (a) Peeling of collodion membrane aged 2 days.
(See for colour figure plate 3)

REFERENCES

1. Akiyama M. Severe Congenital ichthyosis of the neonate. *Int J Dermatol* 1998;37:722-728.
2. Bastuji-Garin S, Rzany B, Stern RS, Shear NH, Naldi L, Roiyeaiu JC. Clinical classification of cases of toxic epidermal necrolysis, Steven Johnson syndrome, and erythema multiforme. *Arch Dermatol* 1993;129:92-96.
3. Cotell S, Robinson ND, Chan LS, Autominunne blistering skin diseases. *Am J Emerg Med* 2000;18: 288-299.
4. Frienden IJ, Resnick SD Childhoold exanthems old and new. *Pediatr Clin North Am* 1991;38:859-887.
5. Goldberg GN, Hansen RC, Lynch PJ Necrotizing fascitis in infancy; report of three cases and review of the literature. *Pediatr Dermatol* 1984;2:55-63.
6. Greaves MW, sabroe RA, ABC of Allergies. Allergy and the skin 1 Urticava. *Brit Med J* 1998;316:1147-1150.
7. Lacour M, Mehta–Nikhar B, Athuton DJ, Harper JI. An appraisal of acitretin therapy in children with inherited disorders of keratinization. *Br J Dermatol* 1996;134:1023-1029.
8. Leung DYM, Rodes AR, Geha RS, Schneider L, Ring. Atopic dermatitis (Atopic Eczema). In Fitzpatrick TB, Eisen AZ, Wolff K, Freeberg IM, Austen KF (eds) *Dermatology in General Medicine*, 4th edn. New York: McGraw-Hill 1993;1543-1564.
9. Lyell A The staphy lococcal scalded skin syndrome in historical perspective emergency of dermopathic strains of staphylococcus aureus and discovery of epidermolytic toxin. A review of events up to 1970. *J Am Acad Dermatol* 1983;9:285-294.
10. Marsden RA, Me Kee PH, Bhogal B, Black MM, Kennedy LA. A study of benign chromic bullous dermatosis of childhood and comparison with dermatitis herpetiformis and bullous pemphigoid occurring in childhood. *Clin Exp Dermatol* 1980;5;159-176.
11. Mortz CG, Anderson KE Allergic Contact dermatitis in children and adolescents. *Contact Dermatitis* 1999; 41:121-136.
12. Pasricha JS, Khaitan BK, Raman RS, Chandra M Dexamethasone–Cyclophosphamide pulse therapy for pemphrgus. *Int J Dermatol* 1995;34:875-882.
13. Pasricha JS, Khaitan BK, Shantharaman R, Mital A, Girdhar M. Toxic epidermal necrolysis. *Int J Dermatol* 1996;35:523-527.
14. Pruszkowski A, Bodermer C, Fraitag S, Teillac–Hamel D, Amorie JC, de Prost Y. Neonatal and infantile erythroderma A reterospective study of 51 patients. *Arch Dermatol* 2000;136: 875-880.
15. Raman M, Verma KK, Khaitan BK Exanthematous eruptions. *Natl Med J Indra* 1998;11:226-230.
16. Rohrer TE, Ahmed AR. Toxic epidermal necrolysis. *Int J Dermatol* 1991;30:457-466.
17. Schopf E, Stuhimer A, Rzany B, et al. Toxic epidermal necrolysis and Steven Johnson syndrome. *Arch Dermatol* 1991;127:839-842.
18. Sharma VK, Dhai S. Clinical pattern of cutaneous drug eruption among children and adolescents in north India. *Pediatr Dermatol* 1995;12:178–183.
19. Shetty AK, Pesselle BC, Ey JL, Cornea H, Galen WK, Gedalia A Infantile Henoch-Schönlein purpura. *Arch Fam Med* 2000;9:553-556.
20. Tunnessen WW Jr. Practical aspects of bacterial skin infections in children. *Pediatr Dermatol* 1985;2:255-265.
21. Uitto J, Eady R, Fine JD, Feder M, Dart J. The DEBRA International Visioning/Consensus Meeting on Epidermolysis Bullosa: Summary and recommendations. *J Invest Dermatol* 2000;114:734-737.
22. Williams MLK, Lynich PJ Geveralized disorders of cornifications: The ichthyoses. In: Same WM, Lynch PJ (eds) *Principles and Practices of Dermatology*. New York: Churchill Livingstone 1996;379:396.

Section XVIII

Psychosocial Emergencies

Nitin Gupta and Parthasarathy Biswas

96 Psychiatric Emergencies

INTRODUCTION

Psychiatric emergencies in children are those conditions where there is a direct or immediate threat to themselves or others or where children exhibit distressing or disruptive psychiatric or behavioral symptoms that need immediate attention.[1] Emergencies in children occur in a variety of settings. Hence, clinicians must be familiar with not only the most common emergencies but also the approaches to assessment and disposition of such cases as all such emergencies warrant a unique set of considerations as they span a variety of scientific disciplines.[2] For example, some psychiatric conditions such as severe depression can result in fatalities if not properly recognized or treated. Literature has shown that almost 50% of completed suicides in children had a contact with a physician within 1 week to 6 months preceding the event.[3-5] A child may develop acute symptoms of psychiatric disorders such as acute psychosis, anorexia nervosa, conduct disorder etc, which could be so distressing that immediate contact is necessary. There are a number of rare yet serious medical conditions with early stage manifestations that can mimic behavioural or psychiatric disorders. Conversely, some psychiatric conditions manifest with somatic symptoms that the pediatrician in an emergency setting may be asked to evaluate.[6] Also children with psychiatric conditions, particularly those on psychotropics, warrant special attention when they are brought to pediatric emergency settings as they have a wide range of adverse side-effects and drug interactions that can cause significant mortality and morbidity if not appropriately recognized or managed.[6] All these are broadly considered as emergencies. Apart from parents, sometimes teachers, and pediatricians and on rare occasions the police or other social agencies may refer children for emergency help.[1] Cases of psychiatric and behavioural emergencies are taken to hospitals in the general medical emergency rooms or to pediatric or psychiatric services.

Nevertheless, a large number of these clinical problems remain unrecognized and unattended by people and professionals in the community which results in increase in of distress, disease and eventually leading to death.

CONCEPTUAL ISSUES

The patients who attend pediatric emergency settings may present with 4 different types of psychiatric emergencies. *These are:*

1. True psychiatric emergencies.
2. Neurological disorders that present with psychiatric manifestations.
3. Side effects of psychotropic medications that have direct implications for emergency assessment and management.
4. Psychiatric disorders that present with somatic symptoms.

1. The pure psychiatric emergencies *are those that are arising entirely out of an underlying psychiatric disorder or are a manifestation of a psychiatric disorder.*

   For example, children may present with the following:

   i. Severe depressive episode with suicidal tendencies
   ii. Dissociative disorders
   iii. Anxiety and panic disorders
   iv. Child abuse–physical and/or sexual
   v. Post traumatic stress disorder
   vi. Conduct disorder
   vii. Drug abuse
   viii. Anorexia Nervosa
   ix. Psychotic disorders

   Clinical manifestations of these disorders is varied and may take various forms irrespective of the diagnosis, for example:

   i. Fits or impaired consciousness
   ii. Abnormal behaviour
   iii. Suicidal behaviour such as bodily harm, poisoning, drug over dosage
   iv. Aggression and violence
   v. Paralysis (or paresis), loss of bodily sensations
   vi. Refusal to eat and severe weight loss

vii. Hyperventilation
viii. Acute anxiety and panic.
ix. Acute pain
x. Non-accidental injuries and neglect

2. Neurological disorders that present with psychiatric manifestations.
There are several neurological and medical disorders that mimic psychiatric disorders or have psychiatric symptoms as their prodromal or initial presentation. Amongst them most common is delirium and it has to be differentiated from psychosis. Also, a number of rare neurological disorders herald their onset with psychiatric manifestations. Some diseases that may present with behavioural changes include: Tourette's syndrome, subacute sclerosing panencephalitis, Vitamin deficiencies (including Niacin, thiamine and vitamin B_{12}), Juvenile Huntington's disease, AIP (acute intermittent prophyria), Guillian Barré syndrome, CNS lupus (lupus cerebritis), Encephalitis, intra-cerebral space occupying lesion etc.
3. Side effects of psychotropic drugs (iatrogenic)
Children with psychiatric disorders particularly those who are on psychotropic medications, may several adverse effects and drug interactions that can cause significant morbidity and mortality if not recognized or appropriately managed in the emergency department. For example, tricyclic anti-depressants (e.g. imipramine) have a side-effect profile that includes sedation, orthostatic hypotension and anticholinergic side-effects, but most significant is their potential for mortality in over dose. Selective serotonin reuptake inhibitors (e.g. fluoxetine) have fewer side effects and are relatively safe. Amongst anti-psychotics, conventional typical anti-psychotics can cause numerous side-effects i.e. sedation, orthostatic hypotension, extrapyramidal symptoms etc; most fatal being the neuroleptic malignant syndrome. Mood stabilizing agents like lithium, carbamazepine and valproic acid also have neurological, nephrotoxic and hepatotoxic side effects.
4. Psychiatric disorders that may present as a medical or neurological disease.

Somatoform disorders include several disorders, which are characterized by an overwhelming concern for physical appearance, physical symptoms or disease within the context of normal morphology and good health. They can be differentiated from the factitious disorders or malingering by the fact that these patients have little or no awareness or understanding into the basis of their complaints and tend not to achieve any observable/tangible gain. Somatoform disorders include somatization disorder, conversion disorder, persistent somatoform pain disorder, hypochondriasis, and body dysmorphic disorder (APA 1994).[7] Patients with somatization disorders focus intensely on their symptoms, with little concern for the underlying disease processes. Hypochondriasis includes patients with intense fear of having an underlying fatal illness but persevere less with their symptoms. Conversion disorder patients present with variety of acute neurological pathologies like fits, paralysis, aphonia etc that is inconsistent with the actual central and peripheral nervous system functioning. Patients with pain disorders experience pain that is severe and persistent enough to disrupt their daily functioning. Body dysmorphic disorder is characterized by an excessive concern for a defect in their appearance, which is more imaginary than real.

DESCRIPTION OF TYPES

True Psychiatric Emergencies

Suicidal Behavior

Children can present to the emergency department after threatening or attempting to commit suicide. In fact, threatened suicide or unsuccessful suicidal attempts are the most common emergencies seen in child psychiatry.[8] These patients require admission into the hospital for close observation. Suicide occurs rarely in patients younger than 10 years but the incidence increases progressively with age; finally reaching adult rates by late adolescence.[9,10] Suicidal behaviour in children may present itself in form of bodily harm (wrist slashing, poisoning, drug over dosage) while violent means like hanging and shooting are rare.[11] In many instances, suicidal behavior is seen as an attempt to achieve some goal or the patient's last effort to get some relief from intolerable stressors.

It is important to remember that some children are successful in their attempt. Community surveys estimate that approximately 9% of adolescents and 1% of preadolescents report attempts at suicide.[8] The incidence in male and female subjects is equal in childhood and early adolescence. In 1991 (the most recent year for complete records of US vital statistics) age specific suicide rates for children aged 5-14 yrs was 0.7/100,000 as compared to 13.1/100,00 in the age group 15-24 yrs. The rates were greatest for white males followed by white females and non-white females. Males tend to have higher rates of completed/successful suicide than females; the most common method being use of firearms.[12] Females attempt suicide 3 times more than males, most commonly by ingestion.[12]

Relevant risk factors for a successful suicide attempt include—the presence of psychiatric disorder, a past history of one or more suicide attempts, lack of mental health treatment and the presence of a firearm at home.[9,10] Suicidal behaviour in children is indicative of the presence of severe psychopathology and is a pervasive maladaptive step so as to attract attention of the dysfunctional family.[1] In one postmortem study, 90% of children who committed suicide-met criteria for either depression, conduct disorder,

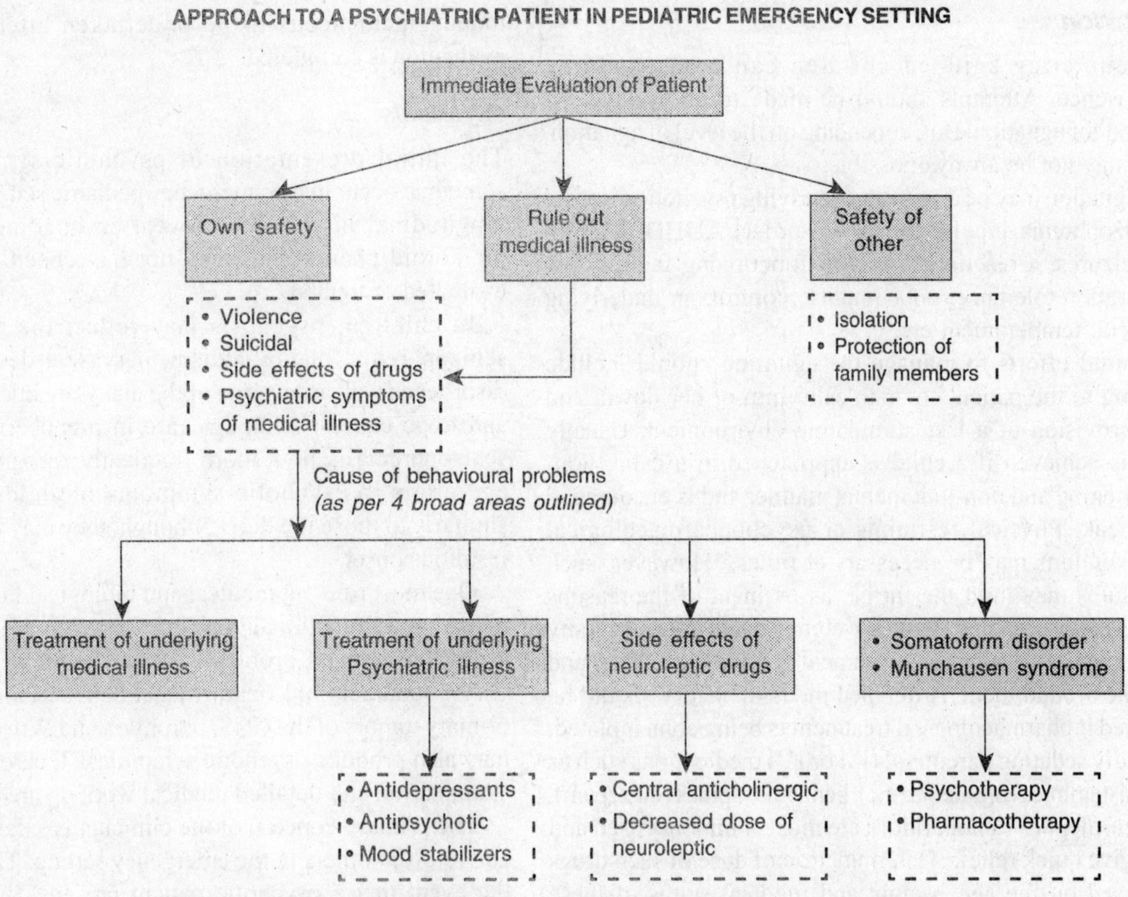

Fig. 96.1: Algrithmic approach to a pediatric-cum-psychiatric emergency

or substance abuse.[10] Other studies have yielded similar high figures, with high presence of comorbid diagnoses.[13] Children under age of 14 years are not as likely to have been previously diagnosed with a psychiatric disorder, and often attempt suicide secondary to a specific life event but fear its consequences.[5] Approximately 50% of children who committed suicide have had contact with health care systems within 1 to 6 months prior to the event.[3-5]

As with adults, numerous factors must be evaluated so as to assess the risk for suicide. However, it should be kept in mind that these factors may vary from individual to individual. The most essential component is-assessment of intent. Even in the absence of a high degree of lethality, true intent must be considered as a major risk factor. Intent must be explored keeping the developmental perspective in mind, as most children below the age of 10 years do not understand the finality of death. However this does not, by definition, render young children at low risk.[14] Another important factor to consider is the nature of the current attempt (i.e. degree of planning, lethality of the method and possibility of rescue). Other important risk factors are-history of attempts by family members or friends, exposure to stories about suicide through media, symptoms of major depression (especially depressed mood and ideas of hopelessness/helplessness), symptoms of psychosis, bipolar disorder and conduct disorder; violent or aggressive behaviour, self injurious behaviour and presence of a recent stressor or significant psychological loss.

Evaluation of the family is an important aspect in determining risk of suicide in children; of utmost importance being the relationship of primary care givers with such children. Additional risk factors could be—parental psychopathology like depression, substance abuse, and antisocial personality disorder as well as neglect or physical/sexual abuse.[15]

As with any emergency, the primary concern is to maintain safety of the child and others. Therefore, treatment of a child's self-injury or medical consequences of poisoning requires emergency hospitalization. Once the medical conditions are taken care of, psychiatric management is warranted. Inpatient treatment is required for highly suicidal patients. Before discharge, care should be taken that the principal caregivers are supportive and responsible so that recurrences does not occur. In this aspect, high surveillance is of utmost importance. Further specialized treatment should be carried out with help of psychiatrist where the malfunctioning family should be integrated with the child's treatment that is focused on the underlying psychiatric morbidity.

Agitation

Encountering agitated children can be a troubling experience. Attempts should be made to understand the reason for agitation. But, depending on the level of agitation, this may not be always possible.

Agitation may be due-to an underlying psychotic disorder (schizophrenia, bipolar affective disorder), ADHD, delirium or seizures; a reaction to the malfunctioning family; low frustration tolerance, poor impulse control, an underlying difficult temperament etc.

Initial efforts to manage the agitation should include talking to the patient so as to calm him or her down, and the provision of a less stimulating environment. Usually this is achieved if a child is approached in a calm, non-threatening and non-judgmental manner and is encouraged to speak. Physical restraints or psychopharmacological interventions may be necessary at times.[1] However, such measures may limit the further assessment of the reasons for agitation, but this must be weighed against the necessity of maintaining a safe environment for these children and people around them. A detailed medical history should be elicited if pharmacological treatment is being contemplated. Rapidly sedating parenteral (IM or IV) medications such as antihistaminics (promethazine), benzodiazepines (diazepam), or neuroleptics (haloperidol), are most commonly used and this give quick relief.[2] Determination of dose of such drugs is based on the age, weight and medical status of these children. Drugs may also be chosen on basis of past history of good response to that particular drug. Assessment should be made of the degree to which children are really in control of their emotions and behaviour. The therapist should make active efforts in order to understand and resolve their problems during the sessions. The emergency management must be followed by a long term psychiatric treatment.

Aggression

Aggression or dangerous behaviour is a common presenting problem accounting for nearly 25% of child and adolescent emergency psychiatric evaluations.[8] Unlike agitated (or violent) patients, the described behaviours may not be observed directly by the evaluator. Hence, a great deal of assessment comes from history and information from parents though these children are unlikely to give an accurate report of their own behaviour, but their thought content is most crucial. Attempts should be made to understand whether violence is in response to psychotic symptoms (i.e. auditory hallucinations or delusions) or due to homicidal ideation. In addition, one needs to ascertain the accurate diagnosis, severity of attempt, use of weapons, history of injury to self or others, physical fights, arrests, indications suggestive of intent, response to limit setting, lethality, destruction of property and the presence of precipitants v/s impulsive acts. Appropriate immediate and long-term management needs to be undertaken after the above evaluation is completed.

Psychosis

The initial presentation of psychotic symptoms can sometime occur in the emergency pediatric setting. A proper longitudinal history may reveal an ongoing insidious, premorbid change that may not have been recognized, evaluated or treated.[8]

In children, psychosis may reflect the presence of schizophrenia, mania, autism, pervasive developmental disorder as well as any one of the many organic, neurologic and toxic causes. Although rare in prepubertal children, schizophrenia is now more frequently recognized in this age group.[16] Psychotic symptoms in children present similarly to those in adults although, they may have a more insidious onset.

One must rule out medical and biological factors before assuming a "functional" origin of psychosis.[8,16,17] Neurologic and medical problems e.g meningitis, encephalitis, CVA, subarachnoid hemorrhage, seizures, metastatic or primary tumors of the CNS, porphyria and Wilson's disease may also produce psychotic symptoms. A careful physical examination and detailed medical work up are essential.

The primary concern of the clinician is safety of patient and relevant others in the emergency setting. Thereafter, in the event that a psychotic patient presents in an acutely agitated state, psychopharmacological intervention or physical restraint may be necessary. Agents that can be employed are neuroleptics (haloperidol, olanzapine etc) or, in some cases, benzodiazepines. One must take into account the individual's medical status, age, weight, and prior history of response to medications.

Eating Disorders

Eating disorders like anorexia nervosa (AN) and bulimia nervosa (BN), are relatively common in adolescent girls (sex ratio = 10:1). Yet, they can also occur in boys and in prepubertal children.[18,19] It is a rare, life threatening emergency condition encountered in prepubertal patients. Diagnosis may be difficult to establish if the child denies the symptoms, especially of purging or laxative abuse. As secondary amenorrhoea is a common presenting symptom in AN, establishing a diagnosis in the premenarchal child may also be difficult. However, body weight of less than 85% of the expected body weight should raise the suspicion.[18] A high index of suspicion should be present for AN when a patient presents with a history of food avoidance coupled with poor weight gain and expressed concerns about appearance.

The long-term mortality rate for AN is 15-20%[16,20] and those for BN patients are not available. A child with clinical diagnosis of AN or BN presents in the pediatric emergency with significant medical or physical complications and thus may indicate a severe form of illness.

Common complications commonly include dehydration, electrolyte abnormalities, impaired cardiovascular function, neuro-endocrine abnormalities with oral, esophageal and gastric damage caused by vomiting.[16] Impaired cardiovascular function and ECG changes are seen and most deaths occur due to cardiac complications leading onto ventricular arrhythmias.

A comorbid psychiatric diagnosis (most commonly depression) is present in upto 73% of patients with AN and 60% with BN.[16] Indications for hospitalization in such cases are-severe depression, suicidality, medical complications and weight loss of ³ 20% or more of ideal body weight.

Laboratory evaluation includes measurement of complete blood count, BUN, electrolytes, calcium, magnesium, albumin-protein and creatinine. Treatment should be initiated only after the patient's cardiac and electrolyte status have been assessed. Treatment of these patients is difficult. First and foremost one needs to treat the medical complications. The psychological management of the disorder is lengthy and multifaceted. The gravity of the condition needs to be explained to the family members. The need for continuous treatment in form of psychotherapy, behavior therapy, family therapy and pharmacotherapy (SSRI, TCA etc) should be explained.

Substance Abuse

Recent statistics confirm that children of increasing younger age are using alcohol and illegal substances.[16] Substance abuse is associated with significant morbidity, mortality and often coexists with psychiatric disorders. When a patient presents to the paediatric emergency department with acute intoxication, maintaining patient and staff safety with medical stability are the primary concerns.[8] For example, patients with respiratory depression, cardiac or neurological abnormalities, or acute agitation must be rapidly assessed and managed.

After the acute intoxication has cleared, one should then treat the psychiatric condition after a thorough psychiatric assessment.

Physical Abuse or Neglect

Abused or neglected children often present first to pediatric emergencies because of physical and medical sequalae of abuse and neglect. The sequele include-multiple injuries like burns, bruises, ruptured viscera, spinal fractures, head and eye injury etc.[15] Neglect is observed in the following areas viz. medical care, safety and or lack of supervision, physical neglect (lack of food and shelter), educational neglect and emotional neglect.

Risk factors include multiple family stressors like violence between parents; social isolation, parental drug abuse, inappropriate expectations from children, child poverty, unemployment and overcrowding.[15]

Psychiatric or psychological sequalae vary widely and can have acute or delayed presentation. These include depression, suicide attempts, posttraumatic stress disorder [a condition characterized by reliving of past traumatic experiences], adjustment disorder, aggressive and self-destructive behaviour, academic failure and difficulty in trusting others.

The primary concern remains of the child's safety. Often pediatricians have to work in close unison with the social worker and outside agencies. Follow-up psychiatric services are determined on a case-to-case basis.

Sexual Abuse or and Rape

The true incidence and prevalence of sexual abuse and rape cannot be estimated due to under-reporting. Sibling incest is the most common form. However, father-daughter or stepfather-daughter incest is also commonly reported.[21] Girls are 4-5 times more commonly abused than boys.[22] Sexual abuse in families is often kept a secret in contrast to rape, which is committed by a stranger where emergency evaluation is often sought immediately.

Risk factors for incest in a family include-social isolation, a dominating father or mother, marital problems amongst parents, substance abuse amongst parents and blurring of interpersonal boundaries. Significant psychiatric sequalae can be seen in such children. They may present with conduct disorder, anxiety disorders (including PTSD), depressive disorders, conversion disorders, substance abuse, aggressive behaviour, sexual promiscuity, academic failure, sexual orientation problems and sleep disturbances.[22] These children usually come to pediatricians or pediatric gynecologist for advice.

The American Academy of Child and Adolescent Psychiatry (AACAP) has set up certain practice parameters for assessment and evaluation of such patients.[23] The main focus of treatment is protection of such patients. The place of treatment may be hospitalization or out of home placement depending on the severe medical or psychiatric risk and ability of parents to take care of the child.

Acute Anxiety and Panic

Acute anxiety can occur as a symptom presentation in many psychiatric disorders. It is usually characterized by acute palpitations sweating, trembling, choking, dizziness, numbness, tingling sensation, hyperventilation, fainting or acute chest pain. During a panic (or acute anxiety) attack, the patient experiences a discrete period of intense fear or discomfort that peaks in about 10 mins. It is accompanied by a fear of impending death or doom. Such episodes may occur in patients with panic disorder, other anxiety disorders, phobias, school phobia, separation anxiety disorder etc.

Children who have experienced severe catastrophic events may develop extreme fear of similar situations. They mentally relive such situations and have dreams and flashbacks regarding the catastrophic events.[1]

Separation anxiety disorder is commonly seen in young children who have just joined school or have been separated from their attachment figures.

Patients presenting with panic attacks need to be thoroughly investigated for any underlying medical disorder e.g. mitral valve prolapse, epilepsy, pheochromocytoma, etc. Children with such disorders should be placed in a calm, comfortable and non-threatening environment to reduce their distress. Oral or parentral anxiolytics (e.g. lorazepam) may be useful. A very vital component in the treatment of such cases is the reassurance of the family and the child. Psychotherapy play therapy are useful modalities along with pharmacotherapy (e.g. fluoxetine, imipramine etc.).

Medical/Neurological Diseases that May Present with Psychiatric Manifestations

Whenever a child presents in the pediatric emergency with atypical features, one must ascertain whether the symptoms are psychiatric or organic in origin. One of the most common conditions with which children present is delirium. The most common differential diagnosis of delirium is psychosis. Awareness of subtle differences between the two conditions can help the pediatrician to differentiate between them. Delirium is characterized by disorientation, altered sensorium and deficits in attention and concentration. It tends to have a fluctuating course. This is in contrast to patients with psychosis who would be oriented with a largely preserved concentration, attention and memory. Delirious patients have disorganized and fleeting perceptual disturbances, often in the form of visual hallucinations with an evening worsening of symptoms (sun-downing effect). In psychosis, hallucinations are often fixed, persistent and well organized.

Delirium is often under diagnosed in children, especially the mild types where it is misdiagnosed as behavioural abnormalities.[24] The criteria for diagnosing delirium will be different in children, because a very young child may not be oriented to time or location, or have the verbal skills necessary for describing their subjective state.[25] Instead the child may be very irritated or agitated. Slow wave EEG pattern is indicative of delirium in adults. However, a similar pattern may be seen in normal children. Therefore such findings need to be interpreted with caution in children.[26,27]

Once the diagnosis of delirium is established its cause needs to be determined. There are a host of medical and neurological causes of delirium. Illicit drugs, anticholinergics, barbiturates, anticonvulsants and benzodiazepines have been implicated in the etiology of delirium.

Apart from delirium, a number of rare neurological diseases can have their onset with psychiatric manifestations. These include-Wilson's disease, Tourette's syndrome, subacute sclerosing panencephalitis, Vitamin deficiency states, Juvenile huntingson's disease, Acute intermittent porphyria, Guillian Barré syndrome and CNS lupus.

Drug (Psychotropic) Induced or Iatrogenic

Antidepressants

a. *Tricyclic antidepressants (TCA)*: these drugs have common side effects of sedation, orthostatic hypotension, and anticholinergic effects and they can be fatal in cases of overdose. The most common causes of fatality include-cardiac arrhythmias, hypotension or decreased seizure threshold leading onto seizure activity. It has been seen that levels of > 1000 mg/ml are indicative of toxicity though lower levels have also led onto toxicity.[28] Cardiac monitoring should be done in such cases as QT^c interval >0.10 secs can cause ventricular arrhythmias. Recent advances in management of TCA overdose include the use of drug specific antibodies.[29]

Selective Serotonin Reuptake Inhibitors (SSRI): SSRIs like fluoxetine, sertraline, paroxetine, fluvoxamine etc have few side effects. They are relatively safe in patients with cardiac problem. Fatalities occur only when there are interaction between MAO inhibitors and SSRIs called the "serotonin syndrome".[30] Also, SSRIs are known to inhibit the Cytochrome P_{450} system leading onto possible toxic levels of the co-administered drug most commonly with terfenadine, astemizole, TCAs, antipsychotics, theophylline, carbamazepine, and phenytoin.[31]

MAO inhibitors: These include phenelzine and tranylcypromine. They act by blocking the breakdown of biogenic amines. So patients on these medications must restrict their dietary intake of tyramine and dopamine containing foods in order to avoid accumulation of amines that can result in a hypertensive crisis (with secondary intracranial bleeding), hyperpyrexia, tachycardia, diaphoresis, tremulousness or cardiac arrhythmias. Foods that need to be avoided include aged cheese, cured meat and fish extracts, wine, beer, chocolates and coffee. Treatment of hypertensive crisis involves blockade of the a-adrenergic receptors with phentolamine or sodium nitroprusside.

Deaths usually occur when children on MAO inhibitors are given meperidine for pain management due to autonomic catastrophic reactions. Symptoms of this idiopathic autonomic catastrophic reaction include hyperthymia, muscle rigidity, myoclonus, mental status changes, convulsions, unstable vitals, coma and death. SSRI's, clomipramine, bupoprion, dextromethorphan and propoxyphene can also cause similar reactions. The safe period after which SSRI's or meperidine can be given is 14 days after stopping MAO inhibitors.

Antipsychotics: Conventional antipsychotic medications are thought to work by blocking the centrally acting dopamine transmission in the mesolimbic system. However by blockage of the nigrostriatal system and effects on the pituitary gland leads onto the various side effects. Newer "atypical" antipsychotics act by having complex actions on both dopaminergic and serotonergic systems. These antipsychotics have been used not only in schizophrenia and mania but also in other conditions like Tourette's syndrome, Sydenham's chorea. Nowadays, they are used for other conditions like- conduct disorders, borderline personality disorder, mental retardation and autism in order to control aggression in these conditions.

Side-effects: Neurological adverse effects of antipsychotic medications occur as a consequence of the blocking of basal ganglia and typically present as movement disorders and extrapyramidal symptoms. The incidence of these side effects is different for adults and children. However, much of the data about the children is anecdotal and the exact epidemiology is not known. The general dictum is that the "high potency" drugs like haloperidol have high propensity to cause extrapyramidal side-effects whereas the "low potency" ones like thioridazine have more of anticholinergic side effects.

Amongst the acute extrapyramydal side-effects seen in children, the most common are acute dystonic reactions where patient experiences spasms of a particular group of muscles like those of head and neck. Oculogyric crisis (upward deviation of the eyes) is diagnostic of dystonic reactions. Childhood dystonic reactions can be generalized and severe and can involve the arching of the back, which can be confused with meningismus in the pediatric emergencies. The neck and eye muscles are not as frequently affected as other muscles.[32,33] Children can present in emergencies with dysphonia and airway compromise due to laryngeal spasms.[34,35] Treatment of acute dystonic reactions consist of intramuscular or intravenous diphenhydramine followed by prophylaxis with anticholinergic agents like trihexiphenidyl and benztropine.[32,33] This is of prime importance in laryngeal dystonias. Persistent or tardive dystonic reactions have also been seen in children.

Acute akathisia and drug induced parkinsonism are two common side effects though such patients usually do not land up in the pediatric ICU. The former is characterized by inner restlessness, which is extremely distressing, and the later is characterized by symptoms similar to the Parkinson's disease (bradykinesia, tremors, rigidity and postural instability). Treatment includes decreasing the dose of neuroleptic medication with addition of propranolol.

Tardive dyskinesias are usually seen after long term antipsychotic use. However, this condition is not an emergency.

Neuroleptic malignant syndrome is a rare but potentially fatal condition. It presents with muscle rigidity, fever, autonomic instability, increase in CPK-MM enzyme levels and leucocytosis. The lethality of this condition is due to the profound muscle breakdown, myoglobinuria, consequent renal failure, disseminated intravascular coagulation, aspiration pneumonia and cardiorespiratory arrest. This condition occurs most commonly within 2 weeks of the start of intravenous high potency neuroleptic or after a sudden hike in parenteral preparations of neuroleptic medications. Other medications that have been implicated are- lithium, metoclopromide, and tricyclic antidepressants. Treatment includes immediate discontinuation of the offending agent and care in an intensive care unit for continuous monitoring of hydration and renal functions. Intravenous fluids will decrease the concentration of myoglobin in the urine. Cooling blankets should be used to take care of the hyperthermia. Medications like bromocriptine, amantadine and levodopa have been used to tackle the CNS effects.[36] Dantrolene, a direct stimulating muscle relaxant helps by decreasing the calcium influx across the sarcoplasmic reticulum.

Blood dyscrasias due to "atypical" antipsychotics like clozapine has been seen in 1.5-3% of patients. Data for children is however not available. Due to this particular side effect, weekly estimation of leucocytes needs to be done. An absolute neutrophil count of less than 1000/cumm warrants immediate stoppage of clozapine.

Mood stabilizers: Lithium is used as a mood stabilizer for treatment of bipolar affective disorder. The common side-effects are nausea, vomiting, diarrhoea, anorexia. The neurological side-effects seen are-tremors and pseudotumor cerebri. The nephrological side-effects include polyuria, nephrotic syndrome and elevated serum creatinine. Hypothyroidism, cardiac toxicity, acne, psoriasis, hypercalcemia are other side effects.[37] Carbamazepine has diplopia, drowsiness and ataxia as side effects. Blood dyscrasias occur rarely; aplastic anaemia and agranulocytosis are rare side-effects. Hepatotoxicity and exfoliative dermatitis may also occur; so periodic LFT and blood counts need to be done. Valproate can cause tremors, gastrointestinal side effects, alopecia, ataxia and weight gain. Rarely it can also cause hepatotoxicity.

Stimulants: The CNS stimulants like methylphenidate, dextroamphetamine and pemoline used in treating ADHD can cause anorexia, weight loss, exacerbation of tics. Pemoline can also cause transient increase of liver enzymes and rarely fulminant liver failure.

Psychiatric Diseases that may Present as Medical or Neurological Diseases

i. *Somatoform disorders:* Epidemiological studies of children are sparse. However, upto 50% of children do go to the physicians with recurrent pain that does not have any "organic" cause.[38-40] Some of these children come from overprotective families and have experienced a significant illness or traumatic event in the recent past. The pediatrician can reach a reliable diagnosis if he looks for lack of physical findings, recent stressors, symptom fluctuations, variation in pain with distraction, multiple visits to the pediatric emergencies with vague, poorly defined complaints in the patient.[38,39] In children, somatoform disorders have an equal sex ratio but females are more likely to have persistent complaints and visit the pediatricians more frequently.[38] Conversion disorder, though rare in children, occurs more frequently in females. A host of symptoms like syncope, pseudocyses, globus hystericus, involuntary movements, blepharospasm, torticollis, astasia-abasia, weakness, blindness, anesthesia and deafness can be seen in patients with conversion disorder. When such patients are brought to the pediatric emergency the parents are usually extremely anxious and tense. The first step involves the reassurance of the patient and parents. A properly conducted interview where the examiner assumes a non-threatening and friendly attitude towards the patient may help in revealing the details about the concerns and fears of the child. An attempt should be made to explore for physical causes, yet avoid unnecessary investigations, and it is mandatory to involve the psychiatrists and psychologists in the treatment of such patients.

ii. *Factitious disorder and malingering:* Classificatory systems like the DSM-IV[7] and ICD-10[41] defines factitious disorder to be characterized by physical or psychological symptoms that are intentionally produced or feigned in order to assume the sick role. In malingering the person has specific secondary gains (like drug seeking, avoiding police custody) in his mind. The incidence of these two conditions in children is unknown. One study was done to determine whether simulated deficits faked by children be detected using neuropsychiatric testing, and it was found that the testing could not determine whether symptoms were faked or not.[42] The conditions that are most commonly feigned are mental retardation, organic impairment, psychosis, dementia, amnesia etc. Primary goal in treatment of factitious disorders are to reduce the patient's disease dissimulation and the over utilization of medical services. Multidisciplinary approach is usually taken. Rather than angrily rejecting the patient as a fraud psychiatrist should extend an offer help. Pharmacotherapy of factitious disorders is largely limited to treatment of comorbid Axis 1 disorder. SSRIs have been used to reducing impulsivity. Psychotherapy of such patients are aimed at treating underlying personality disorder (e.g. Cluster B personality disorders). Supportive psychotherapy may be effective in containment of symptoms.[11]

iii. *Munchausen's by proxy:* Munchausen's by proxy is a term given when the caregiver simulates or induces illness in the child with the purpose of increasing the contact with pediatricians. It is a form of child abuse and has high morbidity, the mortality rate being 9%. Video-recording of the patient and disappearance of the symptom can ascertain the diagnosis with separation from the caregiver. Such a diagnosis is difficult to make in the pediatric emergencies as it may take more than 6 months to be sure of the diagnosis.[43] In many situations child's safety can be assured by his removal from home, at least temporarily. Criminal prosecution of the mother may be indicated as well. Medical care of physical problems of the child and treatment of psychological problems (e.g. separation anxiety in spite of abuse) needs to be done. However, no author as yet has described a consistently effective or specific treatment program for factitious disorder by proxy.

CONCLUSION

Emergencies in child psychiatry are not uncommon. These psychiatric and behavioral emergencies present themselves in a variety of ways which could be life threatening. In all types of emergencies there occurs the breakdown of family functioning that requires restoration. In order to achieve this a comprehensive assessment of the patient's biological, physical, psychological and family factors are necessary. In emergency situations the therapist should be non-judgmental, empathic and sensitive. The environment should be non-threatening and less stimulating. Ventilation catharsis and reassurances can be extremely beneficial. Drugs have a limited role unless there are medical complications and severe mental illnesses. Psychiatric consultation in an emergency setting, and psychiatric hospitalization, is often necessary.

Future research should generate epidemiological data for childhood psychiatric emergencies. Psychopharmacological research into the management of patients with acute agitation.

Aggression and violence needs to be undertaken. Finally, the development of successful strategies to prevent psychiatric emergencies in children and adolescents are equally important.

REFERENCES

1. Malhotra S. Psychiatric and behavioral emergencies. In: *Child Psychiatry in India*, 1st edn. New Delhi: Macmillan India 2002;170-186.

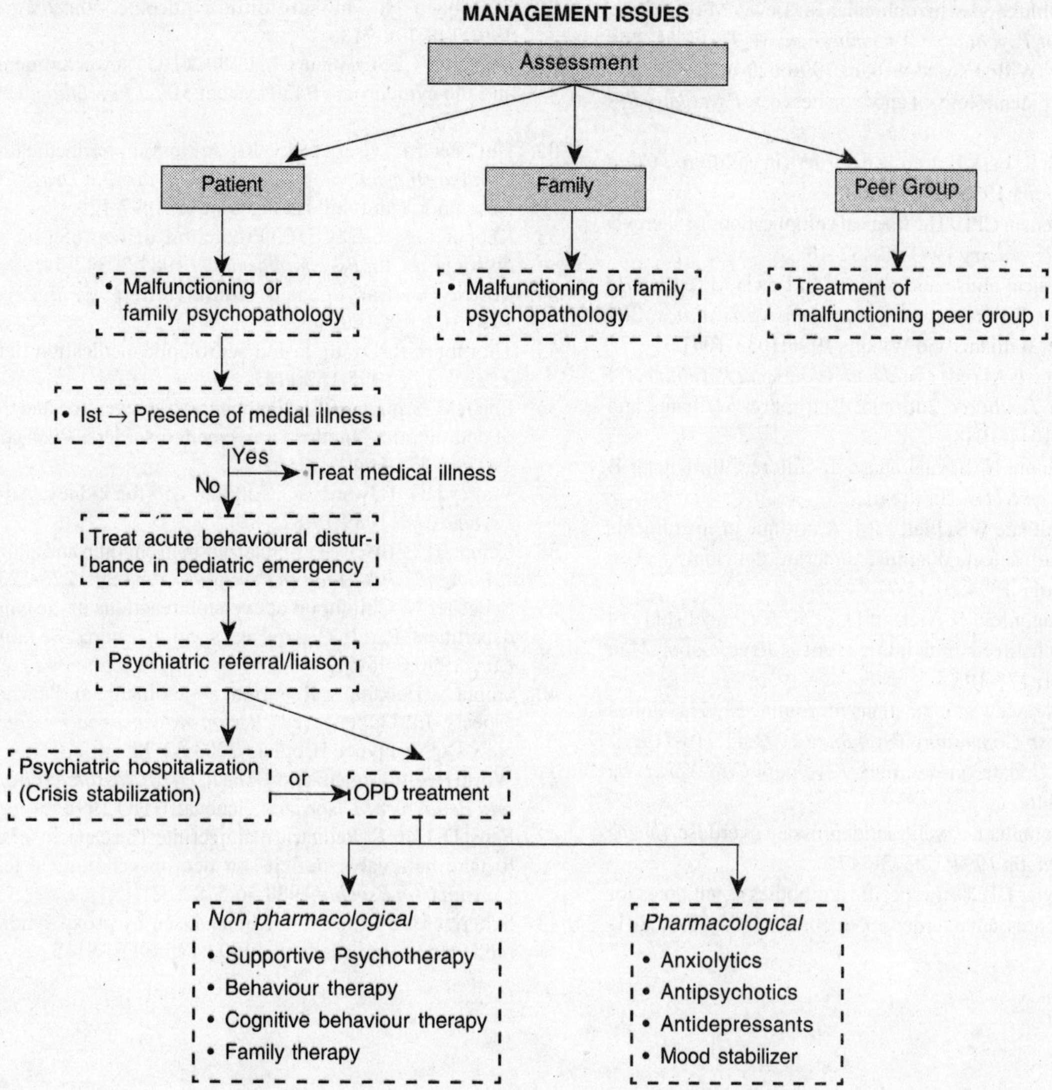

Fig. 96.2: Management issues in a pediatric-cum-psychiatric emergency

2. Halamandaris PV, Anderson TR. Children and adolescents in the psychiatric emergency setting. *Psychiatr Clin North Am* 1999;22:865-874.
3. Murphy GE. The physician's responsibility for suicide II. Errors of omission. *Ann Intern Med* 1975;82:305-309.
4. Barraclough B, Brunch J, Nelson B, et al. A hundred cases of suicide: Clinical aspects. *Br J Psychiatry* 1974;125:355-373.
5. Scaffer D, Gould MS, Fisher P, et al. Psychiatric diagnosis in child and adolescent suicide. *Arch Gen Psychiatry* 1996;53:339-348.
6. Slater N, Constantino JN. Pediatric emergencies in children with psychiatric conditions. *Pediatr Emg Care* 1998;14:42-50.
7. American Psychiatric Association. *Diagnostic and Statistical Manual of Mental Disorders*, 4th edn. Washington: American Psychiatric Association 1994.
8. Tomb D. Child psychiatric emergencies. In Lewis M (ed) *Child and Adolescent Psychiatry: A Comprehensive Textbook*, 2nd edn. Baltimore: Williams and Wilkins 1996;629-635.
9. Brent DA, Parker JA, Goldstein CE, et al. Risk factor for adolescent suicide. *Arch Gen Psychiatry* 1988;45: 581-588.
10. Kellerman Al, Rivara FP, Somes G, et al. Suicide in the home in relation to gun ownership. *N Engl J Med* 1992;327:467-472.
11. Kaplan HI and Sadocks BJ. Psychiatric emergencies in children. In: *Pocket Handbook of Emergency Psychiatry Medicine*. New Delhi: BI Publications 1993;50-63.
12. Pfeffer C: Suicidal behaviour in children and adolescents: Causes and management. In: Lewis M (ed) *Child and Adolescent Psychiatry: A Comprehensive Textbook,* 2nd edn. Baltimore: Williams & Wilkins 1996;666-673.
13. Henriksson MM, Aro HM, Marttunen MJ, et al. Mental disorders and comorbidity in suicide. *Am J Psychiatry* 1993;150:935-940.
14. Zwillich T: Child Suicide risk: Assess parents. *Clin Psychiat News* 1998;6:18.
15. Dulcan M, Martin D. *Concise Guide to Child and Adolescent Psychiatry*. Washington: American Psychiatric Press 1999.
16. Sadka S. Psychiatric emergencies in children and adolescents. In: Allen M (ed) *Growth and Specialization of Emergency Psychiatry*. San Francisco: Jossey-Bass Publishers 1995;65-77.

17. Volkmar F: Childhood schizophrenia. In: Lewis M (ed) *Child and Adolescent Psychiatry: A Comprehensive Textbook*, 2nd edn. Baltimore: Williams and Wilkins 1996;629-635.
18. Wakeling A. Epidemiology of anorexia nervosa. *Psychiatry Res* 1996;62:3-9.
19. Bryant–Waugh R, Lask B. Eating disorders in children. *J Child Psychol Psychiatry* 1995;36:191-202.
20. Sharp CW, Freeman CPL. The medical complications of anorexia nervosa. *Br J Psychiatry* 1993;62:452-462.
21. Kaplan S. Physical abuse and neglect. In Lewis M (ed) *Child and Adolescent Psychiatry: A Comprehensive Textbook*, 2nd edn. Baltimore: Williams and Wilkins 1996;1033-1041.
22. Green A. In: Lewis M (ed) *Child and Adolescent Psychiatry: A Cmprehensive Textbook*, 2nd edn. Baltimore: Williams and Wilkins 1996;1041-1048.
23. Malhotra S, Gupta N. Sexual abuse in children. In: Kumar B (ed) *Textbook on STDs*. (In press).
24. Smith MJ, Breitbart WS, Platt MM. A critique of instruments and methods to detect, diagnose and rate delirium. *J Pain Symptom Manage* 1994;10:35-77.
25. Prugh DG, Wagonfeld S, Metcalf D, et al. A clinical study of delirium in children and adolescents. *Psychosom Med* 1980;42(Suppl):177-195.
26. Boutros NN. A review of indications for routine EEG in clinical psychiatry. *Hosp Community Psychiatry* 1992;43:716-719.
27. Lipowski ZJ. Update on delirium. *Psychiatr Clin North Am* 1992;15:335-346.
28. Pimental L, Trommer L. Cyclic antidepressant overdose. *Emerg Med Clin North Am* 1994;12:533-547.
29. Pentel PR. Keyler DE. Drug specific antibodies as antidotes for tricyclic antidepressant overdose. *Toxical Let* 1995;82-83:801-806.
30. Sternbach H. The serotonin syndrome. *Am J Psychiatry* 1991;148:705-713.
31. Nemeroff CB, DeVane CL, Pollock BG. Newer antidepressants and the cytochrome P450 system. *Am J Psychiatry* 1996;153: 311-320.
32. Hollister LE, Csernansky JG. Antipsychotic medications, In: *Clinical Pharmacology of Psychotherapeutic Drugs*, 3rd edn. New York: Churchill Livingstone 1990;97-125.
33. Keeper GA, Casey DE. Prediction of neuroleptic-induced dystonia. *J Clin Psychopharmacol* 1987;7: 342-345.
34. Murray V. Laryngeal dystonia [letter]. *Br J Psychiatry* 1995;167:168-169.
35. Thornburn R. Dystonia and neuroleptic medication [letter]. *Br J Psychiatry* 1995;167:114.
36. Ebadi M, Srinivasan SK. Pathogenesis, prevention and treatment of neuroleptic—induced movement disorders. *Pharmacol Rev* 1995;45:575-604.
37. Waller DG, Edwards JG. Lithium and the kidney. An update. *Psychol Med* 1989;19:825-831.
38. Campo JV, Fritsch SL. Somatization in children and adolescents. *J Am Acad Child Adolesc Psychiatry* 1994;33:1223-1235.
39. Schecker N. Childhood conversion reactions in the emergency department. Part II. General and specific features. *Pediatr Emerg Care* 1990;6:46-51.
40. Gupta N, Lobana A. Recurrent abdominal pain: Psychological aspects. In: Gupte S (ed) *Recent Advances in Pediatrics–13*. New Delhi: Jaypee Brothers 2003;62-75.
41. World Health Organization. *The ICD-10 Classification of Mental and Behavioral Disorders*. Geneva: WHO 1992.
42. Faust D, Hart K, Pediatric malingering: The capacity of children to take believable deficits on neuropsychological testing. *J Consult Clin Psychol* 1988;56:578-582.
43. Scherier HA, Libow JA. Munchausen by proxy syndrome: A modern pediatric challenge; 1994;125: S110-S115.

Praveen C Sobti, Gautam Biswas and Ashima Taneja

97 Child Abuse and Neglect

INTRODUCTION

Children are the world's most valuable resources or assets, our "future", but children's rights are largely ignored throughout the world often with a tragic outcome. The vulnerability of children, from infancy and throughout their childhood, dependency on adults for safety and ongoing nurturing, puts them at risk of neglect and maltreatment. Extreme forms of maltreatment, including child soldiers, children of war, child prostitution, child physical abuse, child sexual abuse, child labor etc. are generally abhorred and attempts are made to prevent such abuse in most countries. One of the major problems in estimating the scope of the issue is that only a very small number of respondents are able to provide substantiated data about the number of children reported for abuse.

Child maltreatment, regardless of the severity, can pose a serious risk to the immediate and long-term physical, psychological and spiritual health of children. In some instances, it can be life threatening and can even cause death.[1,2] The visible and invisible scars of child abuse in the past prevents many people from achieving their full potential, thereby draining our global society of much good —while fomenting a spirit of mistrust, anger and hatred, which impacts each of our lives. Child Abuse and Neglect Prevention is still a new field—and many approaches and methods of treatment remain controversial.

DEFINITION[3-5]

Child abuse can be defined as causing or permitting of any harmful or offensive contact to a child's body; and/or any communication or transaction which humiliates, shames, or frightens a child.

Legal Definition

The Child Abuse Prevention and Treatment Act,1974 of United States, defines child abuse and neglect as "at a minimum, any recent act or failure to act on the part of a parent or caretaker, which results in death, serious physical or emotional harm, sexual abuse or exploitation, or an act or failure to act which presents an imminent risk of serious harm." The Act defines sexual abuse as "the use, persuasion, or coercion of any child to engage in any sexually explicit conduct (or any simulation of such conduct) for the purpose of producing any visual depiction of such conduct, or rape, molestation, prostitution, or incest with children..." As a result of the Child Abuse Amendments of 1984, the Act also includes as child abuse, the withholding of medically indicated treatment for an infant's life-threatening conditions.

MAJOR TYPES OF ABUSE[3-5]

- Physical abuse
- Sexual abuse
- Emotional abuse
- Neglect (physical, educational and emotional).

Physical abuse of children includes any non-accidental physical injury caused by the child's caretaker. The abuse might take place in single or repeated episodes. It refers to the beating or battering of a child and includes poisoning, burning, hitting, kicking, biting, punching, shaking, throwing, stabbing, choking or any other harmful force or restraint. The most common cause of child abuse-related deaths is head injuries. Physically abusive behavior is often justified in the name of discipline.

Sexual abuse: Sexual abuse is inappropriate sexual behavior with a child. It includes fondling a child's genitals, making the child fondle the adult's genitals, intercourse, incest, rape, sodomy, exhibitionism indecent exposure, and commercial exploitation through prostitution or the production of pornographic materials. To be considered child abuse these acts have to be committed by a person responsible for the care of a child (for example a babysitter, a parent, or a daycare provider) or related to the child. If a stranger commits these acts, it would be considered sexual assault and handled solely by the police and criminal courts.

Sexual abuse may take place within the child's immediate family (referred to as incest) or at the hands of adult caretakers outside the family, e.g. a relative (aunt, cousin, or grandfather), family friend, or a teenage neighbor.

Commercial or other exploitation of a child refers to use of the child in work or other activities for the benefit of others. This includes, but is not limited to, child labor and child prostitution.

Emotional abuse (also known as: verbal abuse, mental abuse, and psychological maltreatment) is commonly defined as acts of commission and omission which are judged on the basis of community standards and professional expertise, to be potentially damaging psychologically. This can include parents/caretakers using extreme and/or bizarre forms of punishment, such as confinement in a closet or dark room or being tied to a chair for long periods of time or threatening or terrorizing a child. This type of abuse is the most difficult form of child maltreatment to identify because the signs are rarely physical.

Neglect is the failure to provide for the child's basic needs. Neglect can be physical, educational, or emotional. In general, neglect is an act of omission.

- *Physical neglect* can include not providing adequate food or clothing, appropriate medical care, supervision, or proper weather protection (heat or cold). It may include abandonment.
- *Educational neglect* includes failure to provide appropriate schooling or special educational needs, allowing excessive truancies.
- *Emotional neglect* includes the lack of any emotional support and love, never attending to the child, drug and alcohol abuse including allowing the child to participate in drug and alcohol use.

PREVALENCE OF CHILD ABUSE AND NEGLECT

Child abuse is found in all societies and is almost always a highly guarded secret, wherever it takes place. In countries with reliable mortality reporting, WHO estimates that as many as one in 5,000 to one in 10,000 children under the age of five dies each year from physical violence, although much lower rates are also noted.[6] In the same countries, from one in 1,000 to one in 180 children are either brought to a health care facility or are reported to child welfare services as a consequence of abuse every year.[6] According to interviews of children or young adults in Finland, the Republic of Korea and the USA, from 5 to 10% of all children experience physical violence during childhood.[6] In America, the most accurate scientific studies, based on lengthy interviews, report that 30% of men and 40% of women remember having been sexually molested during childhood—defining "molestation" as actual genital contact, not just exposure. About half of these are incestuous, and the other half with others, but with the complicity of caretakers in at least 80% of the cases. The seduction occurred at a much earlier age than had been previously assumed, with 81% occurring before puberty and an astonishing 42% before the age of 7.[7] A recent Canadian study by Gallup comprising of 2,000 adults has reported incidence rates almost exactly the same as those found in the United States.[7] In England, a recent BBC "Child Watch" program asked its female listeners—a large though admittedly biased sample—if they remembered sexual molestation, and, of the 2,530 replies analyzed, 83% remembered someone touching their genitals, 62% recalling actual intercourse.[7] In Germany, the Institut für Kindheit has recently concluded a survey asking West Berlin school children about their sexual experiences, and 80% reported having been molested.[7]

FATALITIES[4,8,9]

In US, approximately 1,300 children died of abuse or neglect during the year 2001, a rate of 1.81 children per 100,000 children in the population. Youngest children were the most vulnerable. Children younger than 1 year accounted for 41% of child fatalities, and 85% of child fatalities were younger than 6 years of age (Fig. 97.1).

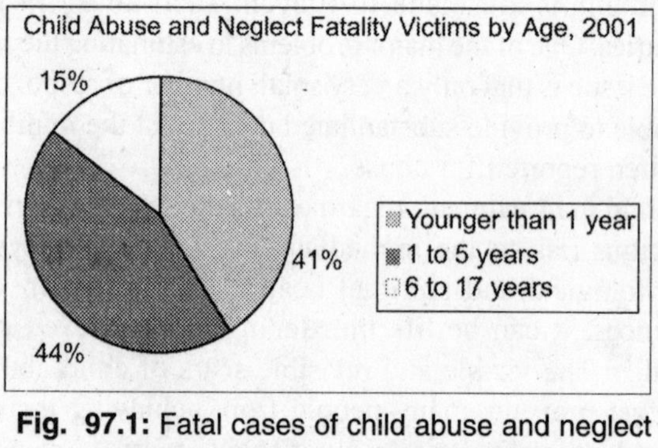

Fig. 97.1: Fatal cases of child abuse and neglect according to the age of the victims

Indian Scenario[10]

According to a study released in 1997 by the Sakshi Violence Intervention Centre, based on a survey done with 350 school girls in New Delhi, India:

- 63% of the girls had experienced child sexual abuse at the hands of family members.
- 25% of the girls had either been raped, forced to masturbate the perpetrator, or forced to perform oral sex.
- nearly one-third of the girls said the perpetrator had been a father, grandfather or male friend of the family.

In a 1999 report by the Tata Institute of Social Sciences, a study done in 1994 and 1995 with 150 minor-age girls in

Mumbai showed 58 of the girls surveyed had been sexually abused before the age of 10. Of this number, 50 had been abused by a family member or friend of the family.

Another study was done in 1997 by RAHI, a Delhi-based organization. This study focused on 1,000 English-speaking middle and upper class women living in Delhi, Mumbai, Chenai, Kolkata and Goa. Majority were graduate and undergraduate students. Findings from this study showed 76% of respondents had been sexually abused as children; 31% of these by someone they knew and 40% by a family member. While 48% had been abused by a single abuser, 52% had been abused by two or more abusers - meaning the majority of women had multiple perpetrators. Abuse for 11% of the survivors occurred once in their lives while 42% were subjected to the abuse many times at different times of their lives either by the same abuser or different abusers at different times. Fifty percent of the abuse took place when the survivors were under 12 years of age, 35% had been abused between 12-16 years of age. Victims were almost always in the care or company of some family member, caretaker or known person. Sixty-eight percent of those who had been abused were living in nuclear families, 16% in families that included grandparents, and 15% in extended families that comprised other relatives. Fifty-four percent of the survivors had told someone about the abuse compared to 36% who did not. Most of those who disclosed did so voluntarily. Thirty percent told a friend, 26% told their mothers, 12% told a sister, 9% told both parents. The main reasons given for not telling anyone about the abuse were: wanting to forget it happened (23%), fear of what people would think of them (14%), self-blame for the abuse (11%), and not having anyone to trust (11%). Only 3% did not tell because the abuser had threatened them. The overwhelming responses to disclosure of abuse by the victims were anger at the perpetrator, disbelief in the victim, and denial. The actions that followed most often did not involve confrontation of perpetrator. Only 2% sought professional help from a therapist or a counselor.

According to this study the most often cited long-lasting effects of the sexual abuse were lack of self-confidence, inability to express feelings, inability to trust people and feeling angry at the world most of the time. Other effects included: avoiding sex or compulsively seeking it out, experiencing chronic aches and pains, use of drugs and alcohol.

A 1996 study done in Bangalore by Samvada with high school students showed 47% of respondents had been sexually abused; 62% of whom had been raped once and 38% of whom had suffered repeated violation. Where vaginal and/or oral penetration were involved, 32% of the girls had been under age. Where abuse did not involve penetration, 13% had been under age 10. Sixty-four percent of those, whose abuse involved penetration made total disclosure, 20% made partial disclosure. Self-blame went up as the "seriousness" of the abuse increased; 37% of those who were molested blamed themselves compared to 50% of those whose abuse involved penetration. Where families placed great emphasis on virginity and equated it with purity, virtue and family honor, the victims felt greater sense of shame, self contempt, anger, and felt compelled to keep quiet about the abuse.

Many of the respondents who feared the person abusing them continued to feel it at the present time. Those who felt anger wished they could retaliate. Those whose desire for revenge (or justice) did not materialize began feeling helpless. Asked what they expected as a result of the abuse, 31% called for prevention; 17% said society needed to talk about sex; 13% said women should fight back compared to 3% who said girl children should learn martial arts; 8% said victim assistance should be available; 14% said abusers should be punished; 1% said abusers should be helped.

FACTORS ASSOCIATED WITH ABUSE AND NEGLECT[11-18]

Major factors which increase the probability of maltreatment occurring in a child's life, are shown in Table 97.1.

SIGNS AND SYMPTOMS[3,4,19,20]

Physical signs of abuse or neglect are those that can actually be seen. Whether mild or severe, they involve the child's physical condition. Frequently the child presents in the emergency with physical signs like bruises, bone injuries, or evidence of lack of care and attention manifested in conditions such as malnutrition.

Behavioral clues may exist alone or may accompany physical indicators. They might be subtle clues, such as a "sixth sense" that something is wrong, or sexual behaviors in young children indicating sexual knowledge not ordinarily possessed by young children, for example, sexual aggression toward younger children.

Common signs that may help the pediatrician to detect that an incidence of child maltreatment has occurred:

- Delay in bringing the child for medical attention
- Injuries that are clearly older than claimed lack of explanation for an injury
- Inconsistency between the severity of the injury and the explanation offered
- Injuries in uncommon areas of the body for children
- Explanations for injuries that do not match the developmental capabilities of the child
- Extreme diaper rash and/or scars from old sores
- A parent or caregiver attributing an injury or accident to a child's sibling.

Table 97.1: Factors associated with child maltreatment

Parent/Caregiver	*Child*	*Situation*	*Level of support*
• History of childhood maltreatment • Alcohol and/or drug addiction • Mental illness • Illiteracy • Lack of parenting skills • Tradition and superstition • Rural-urban migration	• Living with a disability • Serious behavioral problems • Born prematurely • Conceived at a time of parental stress • Health problems like allergies, mood swings, or hyperactivity with learning disabilities	• Low socio-economic status • Unemployment • High-risk communities • Single-parent • Population growth • Political instability • Weak implementation of legal provisions	• Lack of community support • Social isolation

RECOGNIZING CHILD ABUSE[3,4]

The child has learning problems (or difficulty in concentrating) that cannot be attributed to specific physical or psychological causes, is overly compliant, passive, or withdrawn, is always watchful, as though preparing for something bad to happen, has not received help for physical or medical problems brought to the parents' attention, lacks adult supervision and does not want to go home.

The parent shows little concern for the child and perceives the child as entirely bad, worthless, or burdensome. The parent and child rarely touch or look at each other, consider their relationship entirely negative and state that they do not like each other.

Signs and symptoms according to type of abuse
The following are some signs often associated with particular types of child abuse and neglect These types of abuse are more typically found in combination than alone. *A physically abused child, for example, is often emotionally abused as well, and a sexually abused child also may be neglected.*

Signs of Physical Abuse[20,21]

- Has unexplained burns, bites, bruises, broken bones, or black eyes
- Has fading bruises or other marks noticeable after an absence from school
- Seems frightened of the parents and protests or cries when it is time to go home
- Shrinks at the approach of adults
- Reports injury by a parent or another adult caregiver

Possibility of physical abuse when the parent or adult caregiver:

- Offers conflicting, unconvincing, or no explanation for the child's injury
- Describes the child as "evil," or in some other very negative way
- Uses harsh physical discipline with the child
- Has a history of abuse as a child

Signs of Sexual Abuse[22-24]

- Has difficulty walking or sitting
- Reports nightmares or bedwetting
- Experiences a sudden change in appetite
- Demonstrates bizarre, sophisticated, or unusual sexual knowledge or behavior
- Becomes pregnant or contracts a venereal disease, particularly if under age 14
- Reports sexual abuse by a parent or another adult caregiver

Possibility of sexual abuse when the parent or adult caregiver:

- Is unduly protective of the child
- Is secretive and isolated
- Is jealous or controlling with family members

Signs of Neglect[25]

- Lacks needed medical or dental care, immunizations, or glasses
- Is consistently dirty and has severe body odor
- Lacks sufficient clothing for the weather
- Abuses alcohol or other drugs
- States that there is no one at home to provide care

Possibility of neglect when the parent or adult caregiver:

- Appears to be indifferent to the child
- Seems apathetic or depressed
- Behaves irrationally or in a bizarre manner
- Is abusing alcohol or other drugs

Signs of Emotional Maltreatment[25]

- Show extremes in behavior, such as overly compliant or demanding behavior, extreme passivity, or aggression
- Is either inappropriately adult (parenting other children, for example) or inappropriately infantile (frequently rocking or head-banging, for example)
- Is delayed in physical or emotional development
- Has attempted suicide
- Reports a lack of attachment to the parent

Possibility of emotional maltreatment when the parent or adult caregiver:

- Constantly blames, belittles, or berates the child
- Is unconcerned about the child and refuses to consider offers of help for the child's problems
- Overtly rejects the child.

ASSESSMENT OF ABUSE AND NEGLECT

Typically, the complexity of cases involving child maltreatment requires multidisciplinary input. Many communities have established teams to assist in the assessment of child abuse and neglect cases. These teams may include a pediatrician, a gynecologist, a psychiatrist, a forensic expert, a child protective services (CPS) caseworker, a law enforcement officer, an educational psychologist, a child development specialist, a substance abuse specialist, and other social service professionals. In conducting an assessment, the therapist needs to tap the resources of the team. Adopting a multidisciplinary method when evaluating this problem will also lessen the anxiety facing the examining physician and provide a better outcome for the child, parents, and community. If a team does not exist, consultation with professionals representing the key disciplines is strongly recommended.

The pediatrician needs to be able to talk explicitly about sexuality with the child, the family, and with other professionals. Children who have been sexually abused need to feel comfortable talking about the maltreatment, feelings of shame, injuries, secondary gains, sexuality, and sexual feelings. It is important for the therapist to be able to explain these processes to the child and the parents in a language they can relate to and understand. A therapist who is comfortable clarifying adolescent slang terms or a young child's descriptive phrases for his/her body parts or behavior will help the child feel comfortable when talking about a difficult subject.

Trust is a difficult issue for many abused and neglected children. A child who has been physically or sexually abused by a known or trusted person may be cautious in developing relationships. An abused child needs to form a trusting relationship with the doctor; that relationship must be secure enough to allow the child to begin to explore the actual abuse.

When staff is changing diapers or helping children go to the toilet, they might see bruises or burns that were covered by clothing. Often, abusive parents are consciously or unconsciously aware that the signs of their abuse need to be concealed so they dress their children in long sleeves or long pants. Injuries to the abdomen or the head, which are two particularly vulnerable spots, often go undetected until there are internal injuries. Injuries to the abdomen can cause swelling, tenderness, and vomiting. Injuries to the head may cause swelling, dizziness, blackouts, retinal detachment, and even death. In particular, bilateral black eyes could be an indication of bleeding in the brain. Another sign to look for is bruises at various stages of healing, as if they are the result of more than one incident. The ages of bruises[26] can be detected by the following consecutive colors:

- Red–within 24hours
- Blue (deoxy-hemoglobin)–24 hours to 3 days
- Black-purple to brown (hemosiderin)–4th day
- Green tint, dark (hematoidin)–5 to 6 days
- Pale green to yellow (bilirubin)–7 to12 days

However, it is more difficult to detect the color of bruises in children of dark brown color.

The physical signs of sexual abuse include child's torn, stained, or bloody underclothing or bruises or bleeding in the child's external genitalia, vaginal, or anal area. If a child says that it hurts to walk or sit or if he/she complains of pain or itching in the genital area, a doctor should take note and watch to see if it is a recurring condition. A child who has been sexually abused is often concerned that any invasive sexual contact, especially vaginal or anal penetration, may have caused internal damage. The child may also fear having contracted sexually transmitted disease.[27]

Medical examination of sexually abused children or adolescents aims at:[28,29]

i. Identifying clinical evidence of genital or extragenital lesions,
ii. Diagnosing sexually-transmitted infections or pregnancy,
iii. Addressing the child's fear and anxiety regarding test results,
iv. Using information and services for the child if the tests results are positive,
v. Evaluating the need for medical care, psychological support, and social investigation.

Laboratory investigations usually include tests for sperm, bacteriological cultures from all sites, testing for HIV, HCV and HBV antibodies, and the detection of pregnancy (for detail examination and findings refer to Suraj Gupte's *Recent Advances in Pediatrics, Vol 13*). The issues of body integrity, sexual or physical adequacy, injury or scarring, and concerns about any changes in the body that might have resulted from abuse and neglect need to be explored with the child. Symptomatic behavior such as encopresis, enuresis, or psychosomatic aches and pains are also important to identify and explore during therapy.

PHYSICAL HEALTH CONCERNS

Children often have a number of health or health related concerns that are generated by abuse or neglect. A child who has been physically abused may complain of difficulties opening and closing his/her mouth[30], noting that he/she was slapped or hit on the side of the head. The child may also complain of earaches or stomachaches, fearing that these areas of the body were damaged when the child was beaten. The child may have lost teeth or hair. He/she may have broken bones or internal injuries that require a hospital stay.

Sexually Transmitted Diseases and Fear of Acquired Immunodeficiency Syndrome (AIDS)[27]

Sexually transmitted diseases are not an uncommon

occurrence in child sexual abuse. Generally, diseases are determined at the time of the medical exam and treated with appropriate medication. Currently, few cases have been documented of human immunodeficiency virus (HIV) infection through sexual abuse. However, the increasing incidence of both HIV infection and sexual abuse suggests the need to follow guidelines for HIV-antibody testing of pediatric victims of sexual abuse. A child who is known not to have experienced rectal, vaginal, or oral exposure to semen or HIV-positive body fluids can be assumed to be safe.

Sexual and Physical Adequacy

Some children worry that their bodies have been damaged by the sexual or physical abuse and that they are somehow inadequate compared to nonabused children. Issues of strength, body and muscle development, and size are especially important to children who have been physically abused. A sexually abused girl often worries about "virginity" and that partners in future relationships will be able to tell that she has been sexually assaulted. Some girls fear they will not be able to have children.

Pregnancy

Although pregnancy is a very rare occurrence among sexually abused children, the fear of pregnancy, the desire for an abortion, or the reality of carrying a fetus to term and undergoing delivery of the baby all provide a concrete focus for victims' fear of the body being affected or damaged by the experience.

Scarring and Permanent Damage

Some children have scars or disfigurement from the abuse or neglect. Damage may serve as a continual stimulus, reminding the child of the maltreatment. These reminders need to be acknowledged and discussed in therapy.

Encopresis and Enuresis

Encopresis and enuresis may be behavioral indicators of abuse. Some victims have never managed to control elimination or their bladders, but other children, who were toilet-trained, become enuretic or encopretic with the onset of abuse. The former situations often are ones of chronic family dysfunction and chronic sexual abuse. In the latter, the incontinence is regression to an earlier developmental stage. The encopretic or enuretic behavior may be related to regression, anxiety, and misperceptions about the abuse and how the body functions. This behavior may also be an attempt to make the victim unappealing to protect against future assault.

Psychosomatic Complaints

In the absence of any medical evidence, persistent fears and concerns that the child or the child's body is somehow "damaged" or less desirable than before the abuse require interventions suitable to psychosomatic complaints or stigmatization. Psychosomatic complaints can include headaches, stomachaches, feelings of tiredness or exhaustion, and vague aches and pains, hypochondriasis and excessive blinking. A child who has difficulty articulating his/her anger, fear, relief, loss, or sadness may develop aches and pains that express his/her discomfort. Psychosomatic complaints can often be identified as the child recounts the details of the assault(s).

Intervention with regard to these health concerns requires that the pediatrician should address concerns about the body by having the child undergo a thorough medical exam; explore the child's embarrassment about injuries, possible envy of children who are not disfigured, and fear of rejection because of appearance; help the child who is disfigured by the abuse express his/her anger and sense of loss of a healthy and normal body; help the child develop responses to questions about their injuries that do not elicit fear, rejection, or pity; and help the child develop an identity that is based on behavior and accomplishments, rather than on body image.

He should clarify anatomy, purpose, and function of the genitalia and sex organs; explain theories of sexuality and sexual orientation to the children his/her parents; clarify age-appropriate interactions and intervene to protect the child if he/she is being exploited or abused; integrate the experience of sexual abuse and pregnancy; give appropriate perinatal anticipatory guidance for women who have a history of sexual abuse; address issues of guilt, blame, and responsibility; and address decisions made regarding care of the baby; offer support and encouragement to support the child's decision to refrain from engaging in sexual activity until he/she is physically and emotionally ready for the experience and provide information on safe sex, sexual health care, and birth control to sexually active teenagers.[31,32]

The counselor should help the child recognize the connection between his/her experience of abuse and his/her body sensations and facilitate the expression of emotions about abusive or neglectful experiences, including loss and depression; and support the child's need for nurturance and attention. There should be a change of attitude from punitive to therapeutic (with long term goals of rehabilitation) and increase quality child abuse and neglect prevention training for all professionals working with children and families.[33,34]

CONSEQUENCES[35-50]

It has been suggested that the severity of the consequences a child experiences as a result of maltreatment are related to the length and severity of the abuse and the relationship of the abuser to the victim.

Therefore, long-term severe abuse perpetrated by a parent

tends to produce more detrimental effects than shorter-term, less severe abuse by a stranger. The primary consequence of child maltreatment is the development of "dysfunction" within the developing child-that is, the "functioning" of abused children is set apart or becomes difficult as a result of having experienced abuse and/or neglect. Dysfunction may result in immediate impairment, problems in adjusting to the abusive experience, or it may occur as problems later in development. Therefore, the goal of therapeutic intervention is to address the problems or conflicts within the child's current functioning and/or conflicts that are likely to impair functioning in the future.

Child maltreatment can affect all aspects of a child's life, physical, sexual, psychological, behavioral, academic, interpersonal and subsequent violence (Table 97.2).

Behavioral Consequences[51,52]

Maltreated children are known to display the following behavioral problems like developmental delays, clinging behavior, extreme shyness and fear of strangers, troubled socialization with peers-constant fighting or socially undesirable behaviors, such as bullying, teasing or not sharing and poor school adjustment and disruptive classroom behavior

There is a growing understanding among researchers that child maltreatment is associated with a host of behavioral problems that manifest themselves in adolescence in form self-destructive behavior such as self-mutilation or burning, truancy and running away behavior, delinquency and prostitution, eating disorders, such as anorexia, bulimia or obesity—primarily among female victims, suicide and suicide attempts.

Academic Consequences[53,54]

One of the most destructive consequences of child maltreatment may be the detrimental effect on a child's school performance. Maltreated children demonstrate reduced intellectual functioning, perform very poorly in school; display lower overall school performance test scores and lower language, reading and math scores, grade repetitions, disciplinary referrals and a high number of suspensions, working and learning at below average levels and weaker orientation to future vocational and educational goals compared to non-maltreated children.

Interpersonal Consequences

Child maltreatment can interfere with a person's ability to develop meaningful and appropriate relationships from childhood through to adulthood. Victimization reduces social competence and limits empathic ability, both of which are necessary to establish satisfying relationships with others. Maltreated children have been known to display insecure attachments to parents and caregivers, loss of close friends, difficulty in trusting others, relationship problems, such as overly sexualized or overly conflicted relationships and chronic dissatisfaction with adult relationships and fear of intimacy.

Subsequent Violence

Victims of child maltreatment often become further victimized as adolescents and adults and/or become violent themselves toward their own children and in intimate relationships. Adults and adolescents who report a history of child maltreatment may demonstrate maltreatment of their own children, a history of being a victim of a violent assault by a non-family member during adolescence, perpetrating dating violence in adolescence and/or spousal violence in adulthood, becoming a victim of an assaultive partner (most often a male abuser) and/or the victim of additional sexual assaults.

Generalized Consequences

While the consequences of maltreatment were discussed collectively, one can generalize a link between certain consequences and specific forms of maltreatment. Females tend to display more inward consequences, such as suicidal ideation, eating disorders, low self-esteem and psychological

Table 97.2: Long-term consequences of child maltreatment

Physical consequences	*Sexual consequences*	*Psychological consequences*
• Permanent neurological damage • Sensory, and/or psycho-motor • Delay in motor skills, even gross	• Dissociation, nervousness commonly associated with post-traumatic stress disorder (PTSD) • Engaging in open or excessive masturbation, excessive sexual curiosity and frequent exposure of the genitals problems • Simulated sexual acts with siblings and friends, inappropriate sexual behavior such as breast or genital grabbing motor skill deficits • Premature sexual knowledge, sexualized kissing in friendships • Risk for teenage pregnancy or sexually transmitted diseases • Increased risk of revictimization	• Extreme and repetitive nightmares • Anxiety, perception of low selfesteem • Unusually high levels of anger and aggression • Feelings of guilt and shame • Sudden phobias, such as a fear of darkness or water • General fearfulness and a specific fear of others of the same gender as the abuser • Depressive symptoms, long bouts of sadness, social withdrawal • Feelings of stigmatization • Dissociation, intrusive thoughts, suicidal ideation • Distorted cognition, such as chronic perceptions of danger and confusion, illogical thinking

disorders, while males tend to display more out-ward consequences, such as increased aggression, delinquency and spousal abuse.

Consequences of Neglect

A form of neglect that affects infants and young children is nonorganic failure to thrive (NFTT). Failure to thrive may occur when a child does not grow or develop during the first 3 years of life. Failure to thrive is the diagnosis if the child's height, weight, or head circumference is less than the third percentile. The diagnosis of nonorganic failure to thrive caused by emotional deprivation or physical neglect is supported if the infant gains 1.5 ounces a day for 1 week in a "safe" environment (for example, the hospital).[55]

Infants and young children may also exhibit behavioral signs of this type of neglect. Infants may be unresponsive and withdrawn. They do not respond to their caregivers' smiles and coos. They rarely cry or express any kind of frustration. When caregivers try to interact with these infants, they look away, actively cover their faces with a hand, or turn away to face the wall or some other inanimate object. The infants tend to scan their environment, not focusing on any single person or object.

Physical problems associated with a significantly reduced caloric intake indicate that neglected children tend to make significant gains in both weight and nutritional status after identification and implementation of a medically related treatment regimen. However, throughout their childhood (and probably adulthood) their stature remains short and their physical health is identified as somewhat fragile.

PREVENTION

Remember the "Five Rs" (courtesy Prevent Child Abuse America):[56]

1. Remember risk factors.
2. Recognize warning signs.
3. Report suspected abuses or neglect (Fig. 97.2).
4. Raise the issue.
5. Reach out to kids and parents.

CONCLUSION

While research does link maltreatment with a myriad of detrimental outcomes for children, longitudinal research is still needed to truly improve our understanding. There is a clear absence of data that outlines development from infancy to adulthood in maltreated children. While maltreatment needs to be understood as an extremely serious social problem simply for the immediate impact it has on children, findings of longitudinal research will be important in improving the identification and management of maltreatment victims. Children who have been maltreated tend to fare much worse in life than those who have not.

In order that children achieve proper developmental milestones, they need to have countless skills and aptitudes, the capacity for trust and empathy with others, impulse control; the ability to focus attention, control aggression, accept reasonable adult authority, develop an internalized sense of values; a sense of membership in society, an identification with its value system and finally a sense of hope and confidence about the future.

Child maltreatment makes the attainment of these attributes extremely difficult, if not impossible. Early identification, treatment and reporting of cases of maltreatment will offer an abused or neglected child the chance to overcome many of the otherwise likely consequences of maltreatment.[57]

REFERENCES

1. Baker AM, Craig BR, Lonergan GJ. Homicidal commotio cordis: the final blow in a battered infant. *Child Abuse Negl* 2003;27:125-130.
2. Ransom GH, Mann FA, Vavilala MS, Haruff R, Rivara FP. Cerebral infarct in head injury: Relationship to child abuse. *Child Abuse Negl* 2003; 27(4):381-392.

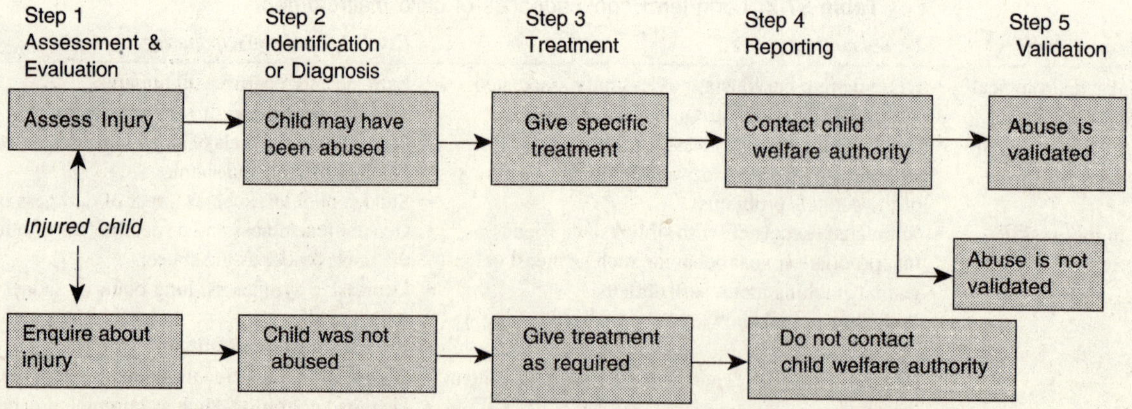

Fig. 97.2: Multi-step process of identification and reporting of child maltreatment

3. National Clearinghouse on Child Abuse and Neglect Information. Child Abuse and Neglect State Statutes Elements: Reporting Laws Number 1. Washington, DC: US Department of Health and Human Services, December 31, 2000.
4. National Clearinghouse on Child Abuse and Neglect Information. Child fatalities resource listing. Available online at URL: http://www.calib.com/nccanch (Accessed May 2003).
5. World Health Organization. Child Abuse and Neglect. Fact Sheet. Available online at URL: http://www.who. int/inf-fs/en/fact.
6. Child abuse: Statistics, research, and resources. Available online at URL:http://www.jimhopper.com/abstats.
7. DeMause L. The history of child abuse "The Evolution of Childhood." *J Psychohistory* 1998;25:216-236.
8. Sedlack, AJ, Broadhurst DD (1996). The third national incidence study of child abuse and neglect (NIS-3). Washington, DC: US Department of Health and Human Services.
9. U.S. Department of Health and Human Services, Children's Bureau (2003). Child maltreatment 2001. Washington, DC: US Government Printing Office.
10. Virani P: Child sexual abuse in India. *Bitter Chocolate* New Delhi Penguin Books 2000;5-34.
11. Svedin CG, Back C, Soderback SB. Family relations, family climate and sexual abuse. *Nord J Psychiatry* 2002;56:355-362.
12. Sidebotham P, Heron J. Child maltreatment in the "children of the nineties:" the role of the child. *Child Abuse Negl* 2003;27: 337-352.
13. Weissman AM, Jogerst GJ, Dawson JD. Community characteristics associated with child abuse in Iowa. *Child Abuse Negl* 2003;27:1145-1159.
14. Brown J, Cohen P, Johnson JG, Salzinger S.A longitudinal analysis of risk factors for child maltreatment: Findings of a 17-year prospective study of officially recorded and self-reported child abuse and neglect. *Child Abuse Negl.* 1998;22;1065-1078.
15. Harrington D, Dubowitz H, Black M, Binder A. Maternal substance use and neglectful parenting: Relations with children's development. *J Clin Psychol* 1995;24:258-263.
16. Magura S, Laudet AB. Parental substance abuse and child maltreatment: Review and implications for intervention. *Children and Youth Services Review*. 1996;18:a193-220.
17. Dunn MG, Tarter RE, Mezzich AC, Vanyukov M, Kirisci L, Kirillova G. Origins and consequences of child neglect in substance abuse families. *Clin Psychol Rev.* 2002;22:1063-1090.
18. Johnson CF. Child maltreatment 2002: recognition, reporting and risk. *Pediatr Int.* 2002;44:554-560.
19. Paavilainen E, Merikanto J, Astedt-Kurki P, Laippala P, Tammentie T, Paunonen-Ilmonen M. Identification of child maltreatment while caring for them in a university hospital. *Int J Nurs Stud* 2002;39:287-294.
20. Giardino AP, Hudson KM, Marsh J. Providing medical evaluations for possible child maltreatment to children with special health care needs. *Child Abuse Negl* 2003;27(10):1179-1186.
21. Warner JE, Hansen DJ. The identification and reporting of physical abuse by physicians: A review and implications for research. *Child Abuse Negl* 1994;18:11-25.
22. Kini N, Brady WJ, Lazoritz S. Evaluating child sexual abuse in the emergency department: clinical and behavioral indicators. *Acad Emerg Med.* 1996;3:966-976.
23. Laourinz JHC, Powel GJ: Physical abuse, sexual abuse, neglect of child. In Kaplan MI, Sadock BJ (eds): Comprehensive Textbook of Psychiatry, 6th edn. Baltimore: William and Wilkins, 1994;2455-2469.
24. Farley M, Patsalides BM. Physical symptoms, posttraumatic stress disorder, and healthcare utilization of women with and without childhood physical and sexual abuse. *Psychol Rep* 2001;89:595-606.
25. Glaser D. Emotional abuse and neglect (psychological maltreatment): A conceptual framework. *Child Abuse Negl* 2002;26:697-714.
26. Subrahmanyam BV. Injuries by mechanical violence. In. *Modi's Medical Jurisprudence & Toxicology.* 22nd edn. New Delhi: Butterworths, 1999;333-359.
27. Conard LA, Blythe MJ. Sexual function, sexual abuse and sexually transmitted diseases in adolescence. *Best Pract Res Clin Obstet Gynaecol* 2003;17:103-116.
28. Rey C, Chariot P, Alvin P, Werson P. Medical examination of sexually abused children and adolescents. *Arch Pediatr* 1998;5:1378-1382.
29. Dammeyer MD. The assessment of child sexual abuse allegations: using research to guide clinical decision making. *Behav Sci Law* 1998;16:21-34.
30. Serrano Garcia MI, Tolosa Benedicto E, Forner Navarro L. Oral lesions due to child abuse. Identification of the problem and role of the professional. *Med Oral* 2001;6:276-289.
31. Sarywitz KJ, Mannarino AP, Berliner L, Cohen JA: Treatment for sexually abused children and adolescents. *Am Psychol* 2000;55:1040-1049.
32. Roussillon JA. Adult survivors of childhood sexual abuse: suggestions for perinatal caregivers. *Clin Excell Nurse Pract* 1998;2:329-337.
33. Briere J, Elliott DM. Prevalence and psychological sequelae of self-reported childhood physical and sexual abuse in a general population sample of men and women. *Child Abuse Negl* 2003;27:1205-1222.
34. Feehan M, Nada-Raja S, Martin JA, Langley JD. The prevalence and correlates of psychological distress following physical and sexual assault in a young adult cohort. *Violence Vict* 2001;16:49-63.
35. Romito P, Crisma M, Saurel-Cubizolles MJ. Adult outcomes in women who experienced parental violence during childhood. *Child Abuse Negl* 2003;27: 1127-1144.
36. Collin-Vezina D, Cyr M. Current understanding about intergenerational transmission of child sexual abuse. *Child Abuse Negl* 2003;27:489-507.
37. McGee R, Wolfe D, Olson J. Multiple maltreatment, attribution of blame, and adjustment among adolescents. *Dev Psychopathol* 2001;13:827-846.
38. Romans S, Belaise C, Martin J, Morris E, Raffi A. Childhood abuse and later medical disorders in women. An epidemiological study. *Psychother Psychosom.* 2002;71:141-150.
39. Fergusson DM, Lynskey MT. Physical punishment/ maltreatment during childhood and adjustment in young adulthood. *Child Abuse Negl* 1997;21:617-630.
40. Silverman AB, Reinherz HZ, Giaconia RM. The long-term sequelae of child and adolescent abuse: A longitudinal community study. *Child Abuse Negl* 1996; 20:709-723.
41. Malinosky-Rummell R, Hansen DJ. Long-term consequences of childhood physical abuse. *Psychological Bulletin* 1993;114:68-79.
42. Reissing ED, Binik YM, Khalife S, Cohen D, Amsel R. Etiological correlates of vaginismus: sexual and physical abuse, sexual

knowledge, sexual self-schema, and relationship adjustment. *J Sex Marital Ther* 2003; 29:47-59.

43. Quas JA, Goodman GS, Jones D. Predictors of attributions of self-blame and internalizing behavior problems in sexually abused children. *J Child Psychol Psychiatry* 2003;44:723-736.
44. Gajowy M, Simon W. Child abuse, neglect and pregnancy losses—combination and its psychological sequel. *Psychiatr Pol* 2002;36(6):911-927.
45. Siegel JA: Aggressive behavior among women sexually abused as children. *Violence Vict* 2000;15: 235-255.
46. Swanston HY, Parkinson PN, Oates RK, O Toole BI, Plumkett AM, Shrimpton S: Further abuse of sexually abuse children. *Child Abuse Negl* 2002;26(2):115-127.
47. Mian M, Marton P, LeBaron D. The effects of sexual abuse on 3 to 5-year-old girls. *Child Abuse Negl* 1996; 20:731-745.
48. Smith C. The link between childhood maltreatment and teenage pregnancy. *Social Work Research* 1996;20:131-141.
49. Moody CW. Male child sexual abuse. *Pediatr Health Care* 1999;13:112-119.
50. Teicher MH, Andersen SL, Polcari A, Anderson CM, Navalta CP, Kim DM. The neurobiological consequences of early stress and childhood maltreatment. *Neurosci Biobehav Rev* 2003;27:33-44.
51. de Paúl J, Arruabarrena MI. Behavior problems in school-aged physically abused and neglected children in Spain. *Child Abuse Negl* 1995;19:409-418.
52. Gushurst CA. Child abuse: behavioral aspects and other associated problems. *Pediatr Clin North Am* 2003;50:919-938.
53. Kendall-Tacket KA, Eckenrode J. The effects of neglect on academic achievement and disciplinary problems: A developmental perspective. *Child Abuse Negl* 1996;20:161-169.
54. Kurtz PD, Gaudin Jr JM, Wodarski JS, Howing PT. Maltreatment and the school-aged child: School performance consequences. *Child Abuse Negl* 1993; 17:581-589.
55. Munkel WI. Neglect and abandonment. In: Monteleone JA (ed.) *Recognition of child abuse for the mandated reporter.* St. Louis, MO: GW Medical Publishing, Inc: 1996;115.
56. Peddle H, Wang CT, Diaz J, Reid R. Current trends in child abuse prevention and fatalities: The 2000 fifty State survey. Chicago: *Prevent Child Abuse America.* 2002.
57. Hendry E. Engaging general practitioners in child protection training. *Child Abuse Review* 1997;6:60-64.

Section XIX

Procedures in Pediatric Emergency Complex

MNG Nair and SK Jatana

98 Sedation Analgesia

INTRODUCTION

In order to provide optimum comfort control to a critically ill child, in the strange and unpredictable environs of Pediatric Intensive Care Unit (PICU), a great degree of skill and planning due to the inherent disadvantages of excessive exposure to visual, auditory and tactile stimuli, absence of simple effective methods of comfort assessment and extreme variability in the response of children to methods adopted is mandatory.

Currently, sedation/analgesia is considered an integral part of PICU protocols for quite a few reasons.

Firstly, it is well documented that perception of pain in children is as much as in adults. Though more difficult to manage compared to adults, it is mandatory to provide adequate comfort control measures to critically ill children.

Secondly, the child also needs protection against the tremendous stress response and excessive motor activity resulting from the physiological stress of the illness , which may interfere with intensive care.

Thirdly, failure to provide adequate sedation and analgesia to control the stress response has been seen to be associated with increased complications and mortality.[1]

This chapter reviews various aspects of optimum comfort control in PICU with special emphasis on sedation plan, organization and provision of services, various steps in the conduct of sedation, different pharmacological agents in use and non pharmacological methods like hypnosis.

SEDATION AND ANALGESIA : DEFINITIONS

The term, *Sedation*, means administration of agents to depress the level of consciousness. Sedation is a continuum, varying from a state of conscious sedation where the patient is awake, responds to commands meaningfully and has intact airway protective reflexes, to a state of general anesthesia.[2] Same dose of the drug may produce different degrees of sedation in different children. The child may pass from one state to the other with unexpected rapidity and ease with progressive deterioration of airway reflexes. Conscious sedation, in conjunction with analgesia, provides cooperation and anxiolysis and may not be the desired goal in PICUs. Deep sedation is a state in which the child is not able to respond meaningfully to stimuli with probable suppression of airway protective reflexes.

Ideally the child should remain sedated, should be arousable by vigorous stimulation, and should have a stable natural airway during the procedure. However, it is easier said than achieved without crossing the line to general anesthesia. Deep sedation is also associated with features of disinhibition at times when one should keep in mind the possibilities of hypoxia band hypercarbia.

The term, *analgesia*, means ablation or blunting of pain sensation.

TYPES OF SEDATION ANALGESIA

Types of sedation/analgesia in pediatric intensive care may be broadly grouped as follows:

- Short-term procedural sedation/analgesia.
- Long-term sedation/analgesia as an adjunct to pediatric intensive care.
- Off-site procedural sedation/analgesia e.g. for MRI, CT scan etc.

CONDUCT OF SEDATION ANALGESIA

In this behalf, the first and foremost essential task is to identify the requirement of an individual child for sedation, analgesia or both. Children who are deeply sedated or unconscious may perceive painful stimuli. In general, therefore, all painful procedures require analgesia. Sedation alone does not block pain. In many invasive procedures like suturing of a small wound, addition of a sedative also allays fear and anxiety.

Evaluation of the Patient

Any child who is to undergo sedation must have a thorough medical evaluation to determine what underlying conditions if any will affect the choice of the agent, the prescription, and the plan.[3,4]

Airway and Respiratory System

The ease or difficulty of securing a patent airway and endotracheal intubation should be ascertained. Presence of hyperreactive airway disease and recent respiratory illness add to the risk of laryngospasm. In case of any doubt, the airway should be secured before sedating the child.

Cardiovascular Status (Including State of Hydration and Intravascular Filling)

Sedation results in diminution of sympathetic outflow leading to decrease in heart rate and peripheral vascular resistance which further compromises tissue perfusion which will be more pronounced in an already compromised cardiovascular system. Adequate volume repletion to achieve haemodynamic equilibrium is mandatory in case of hypovolumia before any sedation is administered.

Drug Metabolism

Factors affecting drug metabolism like liver cell function, renal function, and the serum proteins should be evaluated as they influence the distribution, and elimination and thereby the choice of the sedative/analgesic.

Safeguard Against Aspiration

Risk of aspiration (full stomach, gastroesophageal reflux, loose teeth etc) should be assessed.

Personnel: Close monitoring for early detection of adverse events and prompt institution of corrective measures, are the only means to avoid any catastrophe. It is not possible for the intensivist to perform the procedure and also observe the child for early warning signs at the same time. Therefore, it is essential to have a trained physician or nurse to monitor the child, attend to the airway, administer the drugs and record all clinical data and other important events.[2,4] However, as the intensivist is responsible for the safe conduct of the procedure, including sedation/analgesia, the monitoring person should be in constant touch with the intensivist throughout the procedure. In off-site procedures, the treating pediatrician will remain responsible for the conduct of sedation and should be available throughout.

Monitoring

All children receiving sedatives should have basic monitoring to assess the adequacy of respiration and cardiovascular status.[2, 4]

Bedside Monitoring

Basic monitoring with heart rate (HR), blood pressure (BP) (frequently and with bolus doses of medication), pulse oximetry, respiratory rate (RR), electrocardiogram (ECG) (especially in the presence of cardiac disease).

Remote Monitoring in Offsite Procedures

As movements of the chest wall continue even in the presence of respiratory obstruction, impedance respiratory monitors based on movement of the chest are not effective. In situations where close observation of the patient is difficult observation of a moving breathing bag is essential to monitor adequate air flow in and out of the lungs. However, it is preferable to do the procedure under general anaesthesia using MRI compatible equipment because of difficult access and adverse effect of even the slightest movements on the result of the investigation. Measurement of End tidal carbon dioxide ($EtCO_2$) and pulse oximetry are other means of assessing the adequacy of gas exchange and oxygenation.

Supplementary Oxygen

Supplementary oxygen, suction, equipment for Intermittent positive pressure ventilation (IPPV), laryngoscopes, endotracheal tubes of appropriate sizes should be available at hand.

PHARMACOLOGICAL INTERVENTIONS

The goals of sedation/analgesia-anxiolysis, cooperation, amnesia, immobility and lack of awareness are behavioral or emotional parameters. Nevertheless, pharmacological intervention is often required. The ideal approach should be a sedative/hypnotic for sedation, an anxiolytic for anxiety, and an analgesic for pain. The role of pharmacological therapy should be to deliver an effective concentration of the drug (therapeutic window) to its desired site where it produces the desired clinical effects. A large variability exists in the response of any child to various drug dosages. It is, therefore, essential to provide the right drug to the right problem at the right time in the right dosage.

The common pharmacological agents used in sedation/analgesia act by binding to the target organs, mainly the nervous system. They can be broadly grouped by their action Table 98.1.

Table 98.1: Available pharmacologic agents for sedation analgesia in children

Sedation alone	Benzodiazepines
	Chloral hydrate
	Barbiturates
Analgesia with mild sedation	Opioids
	Ketamine
Analgesia alone	Local anesthetics

Table 98.2: Benzodiazepines[6]

Preparation	Short term action: Dose (mg/kg) Sedation	Hypnosis	Effect: Onset	Peak	Duration	Sustained action
Diazepam	0.1-0.15; 2-3 min	0.15-0.3	<60 sec	1-2 min	15-30 min	0.1-0.15 mg/kg 4-6 hr
Midazolam	0.05-0.1; 2-3 min	0.1-0.2	<60 sec	3-5 min	15-30 min	0.5-4 μg/kg/min
Lorazepam	0.05	0.1	2-3 min	20-30min	1-2 hrs	0.4-1μg/kg/min

Benzodiazepines

Benzodiazepines (which have sedative, anxiolytic, muscle relaxant and anticonvulsant minus analgesic actions) are the most frequently used sedatives in PICU. The three most commonly used agents are diazepam, midazolam, and lorazepam (used for managing benzodiazepine dependence).

Benzodiazepines have a sedative-hypnotic, muscle-relaxant, anxiolytic and anticonvulsant effects due to distinct mechanism of action. Except for two effects, almost all effects of benzodiazepines result from their action on the CNS. The action on peripheral tissues of these drugs, when administered intravenously in therapeutic dosage, can lead to coronary dilatation and in high dosages to neuromuscular blockade. Recent evidence suggests that the specific pharmacological properties of benzodiazepines are due to their action on specific subunits of $GABA_A$ receptors.[5] However, they are unreliable hypnotics and have no analgesic effect. They are particularly useful in managing agitation and mild to moderate procedural discomfort.

Children's response to benzodiazepines is highly variable. Side-effects include lassitude, increased reaction time, motor incoordination, confusion, impairment of mental and motor functions and anterograde amnesia. Headache, blurred vision, nausea and vomiting may occur in some patients. At higher doses such as used for endoscopy procedures, benzodiazepines can cause respiratory depression and respiratory acidosis. The effect may be profound and apnea may occur when combined with anesthetic drugs or other sedatives like opioid agonists and barbiturates.[5] The potential hypotensive action of benzodiazepines especially midazolam after bolus administration, warrants cautious use in children with unstable hemodynamics.

A majority of effects of these drugs can be reversed or prevented by flumazenil, an imidazobenzodiazepine, which competes with benzodiazepine for attachment to the receptor.[5] Flumazenil can be given only intravenously and the primary indications for its use are management of overdosage of and reversal of sedative effects produced by benzodiazepines.

The dosages of benzodiazepines are given in Table 98.2.[6]

Chloral Hydrate

It is the oldest synthetic hypnotic and a commonly used drug in the past in pediatric practice for sedation in children undergoing diagnostic, dental and other painful and uncomfortable procedures. It is irritating to the skin and mucous membrane. Hence, if given undiluted and on empty stomach, can result in unpleasant taste, epigastric distress and vomiting. This agent is relatively free from side-effects, though it may produce malaise, light-headedness, nightmares, ataxia. Idiosyncratic reaction may rarely occur in some patients and they may become disoriented and incoherent. Acute poisoning can result in hepatoxicity[5] Table 98.2 gives the dosages.[6]

Triclophoss

It is the monosodium salt of phosphate ester of trichloroethanol. It is stable and less irritating. However, it can cause hepatotoxicity. For sedation it can be given in the dosage of 20 mg/kg/dose. It can be combined with paracetamol for obtaining an additional mild analgesic effect.

Barbiturates

Barbiturates are very potent hypnotics and anticonvulsants and large doses result in a state of general anesthesia. However, barbiturates have been more or less replaced by benzodiazepines in PICUs, because of their cardiorespiratory depressant effect, development of dependence and hepatic enzyme induction. Dosages are shown in Table 98.3.[6]

Table 98.3: Sedatives other than benzodiazepines[6]

Preparation	Short term action: Dose (mg/kg) Sedation	Hypnosis	Effect: Onset	Duration	Sustained action
Chloral hydrate	20-25	60-75	20-25min	1-2 hrs	Not recommended
Pentobarbital	2-4	2-4	1-2 min	1-2 hrs	1-4 mg/kg/hr
Thiopental	0.5-2	0.5-2	<30 sec	10-15 min	Not recommended
Propofol	0.5-2	25-100 μg/kg/min	<30 sec	5-10 min	Not recommended yet

Opioid Agonists

Opioid agonists continue to be the most frequently used agents for pain control in PICU. Morphine and most other opioid agonists used clinically act by binding to m opioid receptors in central and peripheral nervous systems. Opioids are capable of blocking transmission of pain impulses at multiple levels by virtue of the wide distribution of opioid receptors in the brain, spinal cord and the periphery. They produce analgesia and affect mood and rewarding behavior. Analgesia occurs at low doses and sedation and hypnosis at higher doses. Analgesia occurs without affecting consciousness of the patient and is a very useful feature. Pain relief by opioid agonist is relatively selective and does not affect other sensations. They are more effective in relieving continuous dull pain than intermittent sharp pain.[7] There is a wide variation in the analgesic response from individual to individual. Undesirable effects of opioids include:

- Dysphoria and agitation especially in pain free children
- Nausea and vomiting
- Miosis
- Dose-dependant respiratory depression (especially when combined with benzodiazepines)
- Hypotension
- Anti-peristaltic activity
- Generalized muscle rigidity
- Tolerance, dependence and withdrawal syndrome.

Common uses of opioids are:

- Brief sedation analgesia for short painful procedures
- Acute distress behavior during mechanical ventilation
- Maintenance sedation/analgesia. Morphine infusion remains the mainstay in maintenance/sedation analgesia. Patient controlled analgesia may be a most useful method of opioid administration in older children.[8]

Opioids are not effective in neuropathic pain and pain due to infiltration. Because of the long elimination phase, the synthetic opioid derivative methadone is ideally suited for management of opioid withdrawal. Dosages are shown in Table 98.4.[6]

Propofol

Propofol, a substituted phenol has shown great promise for use in adults because of dose dependant pharmacological effects, minimal accumulation, and rapid clearance from the system and absence of active metabolites.[9] However, more evidence is required before propofol is accepted in PICUs because of potent cardiovascular and respiratory depressant effects.

Ketamine

Ketamine, initially introduced as an intravenous anesthetic agent, has unique properties that make it useful for certain pediatric procedures and for anesthetizing patients at risk for hypotension and bronchospasm. After administration, it rapidly produces a hypnotic state that is different from other anesthetic agents. It produces analgesia and amnesia and though the patient can move his limbs, eyes are open and may have spontaneous respirations but he does not respond to commands. This state is called dissociative anesthesia. Therefore, ketamine is a dissociative sedative/analgesic which produces sedation, analgesia and amnesia. Minimal doses produce anxiolysis. Profound analgesia is achieved with 1/5th to 1/10th of anaesthetic dose.

Rapid onset and short duration of action make it the ideal sedative/analgesic for short painful procedures, intravenous route being the most preferable one. No other drug offers as many desirable pharmacodynamic effects (amnesia, analgesia, sedation, cardiovascular stability) as ketamine. It has the added advantage of being effective when administered enterally (orally/rectally).[10] Ketamine infusion may be preferable for sustained analgesia and sedation, when traditional opioid-benzodiazepine combination shows adverse effects.

However, the following pharmacological effects should be considered before the decision to use ketamine is taken. It can cause dose dependant respiratory depression, cardiovascular stimulation, effect on pulmonary vascular resistance, rise in intra-cranial and intra-ocular tension. It can cause emergence delirium, which is characterized by hallucinations, vivid dream and illusions.[11] Table 98.5 shows the dosages used.[6]

USE OF LOCAL ANESTHETICS

In case the child is sedated adequately, as is in most of the cases, it is always better to avoid the use of an additional systemic agent for analgesia and use a local anesthetic agent. Contraindications for the use of local anesthetics are rare

Table 98.4: Opioid agonists[6]

Preparation	*Short Term Administration*		*Long-Term Administration*				
	Dose		*Clinical effect (min)*			*Dose (mcg/kg/min)*	
	Analgesia	*Sedation*	*Onset*	*Peak*	*Duration*	*Analgesia*	*Sedation*
Morphine	0.05-0.1 mg/kg 5-10 min	0.1-0.15 mg/kg 5-10 min	5-10	20-30	3-4 hrs	0.2-0.4	> 0.4
Fentanyl	0.5-1 μg/kg 2-4 min	1-4 μg/min 2-4 min	2-3	4-5	30-60	0.5- 2	> 2
Alfentanil	3-5 μg/kg 2-3 min	5-7.5 μg/kg 2-3 min	< 1	1-2	10-15	0.5- 1	1-3
Methadone	0.1-0.2 mg/kg		10-20	60-120	6-12 hrs	0.05-0.1 mg/kg	4-12 hrs

Table 98.5: Ketamine[6]

Route	Dose (mg/kg)s	Short-term administration: Clinical effects: Onset	Peak	Duration	Sustained administration
IV	0.5-1(analgesia) 1-2 (sedation)	<60 sec	1-2 min	10-15 min	0.5-2 mg/kg/hr
IM	2-4	1-2 min	2-4 min	30-60 min	
Oral	6-10	10-15 min	20-45 min	2-3 hrs	
Rectal	6-8	5-10 min	10-20 min	2-3 hrs	

and judicious use of a local anesthetic may significantly reduce the dose of the sedative and side effects. Local anesthetics can be administered parenterally, transdermally, or by iontophoresis.[12] Large doses cannot be used because of the toxicity and on absorption, these agents can have important effects on central nervous system, autonomic ganglia, neuromuscular junctions and the muscle itself. Hence, to avoid over dosage, it is necessary to calculate the maximum permissible dose and load the drug before its administration. Dosages are shown in Table 98.6.[13]

Table 98.6: Local anesthetics

Preparation	Dose (< 6 months)	Dose (>6 months)
Lidocaine with epinephrine 1:200,000	5 mg/kg	7 mg/kg
Bupivacaine with epinephrine 1:200,000	1.6 mg/kg	2.5 mg/kg

Regional blockade (penile block, digital nerve block, regional nerve block) is a very useful method of analgesia, where repeated painful procedures like dressings and wound debridement are required. It is also very useful in conditions like chest injuries with rib fractures where sedation may be hazardous. It is essential to consult an experienced pediatric anesthesiologist when regional blockade is contemplated and placement of a catheter when repeated/continuous blockade is planned. Risk of infection, catheter migration, neurologic injury and numb limb should be kept in mind.

ORAL SUCROSE/GLUCOSE

Oral sucrose/glucose when administered to neonates and small infants orally in the concentration of 25-50%, has shown to produce analgesia adequate for very short procedures like heel pricking.[14] Administration of oral sucrose/glucose (a disaccharide), raises the pain threshold, presumably mediated by endogenous opiods and could be used for that purpose.

HYPNOSIS

The goals of sedation-anxiolysis, amnesia, immobility and lack of awareness all being emotional parameters, behavioural techniques like hypnosis have been attracting attention in recent times. Children are excellent subjects for hypnosis and hypnosis may become a powerful adjunct to pharmacological agents in sedation/ analgesia in PICUs.[15]

OFFSITE PROCEDURES

Sedation/analgesia for offsite procedures like MRI, CT scan, etc, pose special problems because of the strange environment, limited access and visibility of the patient making monitoring difficult. Where general anesthesia is not feasible, remote monitoring based on a moving breathing bag or measurement of end tidal carbon dioxide if intubated may be necessary. Proper planning of a strategy with availability of skilled staff and a sedation cart (MRI compatible in case of MRI imaging) is mandatory.

CONCLUSION

Since painful procedures often become mandatory in critically ill children, sedation and analgesia are 'critical' components of critical care and for performing practical and diagnostic procedures in children. No single agent, which satisfies all criteria is available at present. A careful system approach, with active cooperation amongst the pediatrician, intensivist and anesthesiologist can minimize the complications and provide maximum comfort to the child in PICU. The protocol should have flexibility to suit the needs of individual child patient.

REFERENCES

1. Little LA, Koenig JC, Newth CJL. Factors affecting accidental extubations in neonatal and pediatric intensive care patients. *Crit Care Med* 1990;18:163-165.
2. American Academy of Pediatrics, Committee on Drugs. Guidelines for monitoring and management of pediatric patients during and after sedation for diagnostic and therapeutic procedures. *Pediatrics* 1992;89:1110-1115.
3. Maxwel LG, Deshpande JK, Wetzel RC. Pre-operative evaluation of children. *Pedatr Clin North Am* 1994;41:39-110.
4. American Academy of Pediatrics, Section on Anesthesiology. Evaluation and preparation of pediatric patients undergoing anesthesia. *Pediatrics* 1996;98: 502-508.
5. Charney SD, Mihic SJ, Harris RA. Hypnotics and sedatives. In: Hardman JG, Limbird LE, Gilman AG (eds) *Goodman and Gilman's The Pharmacologic Basis of Therapeutics*, 10th edn. New York: McGraw Hill 2001;400-421.

6. Holman GA. Analgesia and Sedation in Pediatric critical care. In: Fuhrman PB, Zimmerman JJ (eds) *Pediatric Critical Care*, 2nd edn. 1998;1363-1379.

7. Gutstein HB, Huda A. Opioid analgesics. In: Hardman JG, Limbird LE, Gilman AG, (eds) *Goodman and Gilman's, The Pharmacologic Basis of Therapeutics,* 10th edn. New York: McGraw Hill 2001;579-591.

8. Berde CB, Lehn BM, Yee JD, Sethna NF, Russo D. Patient controlled analgesia in children and adolescents: a randomized prospective comparison with intramuscular administration of morphine for postoperative analgesia. *J Pediatr* 1991;118: 460-466.

9. Mirenda J, Broyles G. Propofol as used for sedation in ICU. *Chest* 1995;108:539-548.

10. Gutstein HBJohnson KL, Heard MB, Gregory GA. Oral ketamine pre-anesthetic medication in children. *Anesthesiology* 1992;76:28-33.

11. Evers SA, Crowder CM. General Anesthetics. In: Hardman JG, Limbird LE, Gilman AG (eds) *Goodman and Gilman's The Pharmacologic Basis of Therapeutics*, 10th edn. New York: McGraw Hill 2001;346-347.

12. Arrowsmith J, Campbell C. A comparison of local anesthetics for venepuncture. *Arch Dis Child* 2000; 82:309-310.

13. Polaner DM. Sedation analgesia in the pediatric intensive care unit. *Pediatr Clin North Am* 2001;48: 695-714.

14. Skogsdal Y, Eriksson M, Schoclin J. Analgesia in newborns given oral glucose. Acta *Pediatr* 1997;86; 217-220.

15. Chen E, Joseph MH, Zeltzer LK: Behavioral and cognitive interventions in the treatment of pain in children. *Pediatr Clin North Am* 2000; 47:513-525.

Sanjay Wazir and Akash Deep Arora

99 Pulse Oximetry and Capnography

INTRODUCTION

According to the American Academy of Pediatrics (Committee on Hospital Care, 1991-92 Guidelines), CO_2 and O_2 monitoring must be performed on all patients receiving care in level I and II Pediatric Critical Care centers.[1]

In the past, the only method to quantify the adequacy of ventilation and oxygenation was by assessment of arterial blood gas (ABG). While ABGs remain the gold standard, limitations also exist. ABGs require either a painful, time consuming procedure or an invasive arterial line to obtain a specimen for evaluation. Further, ABGs have other drawbacks such as the amount of time before analysis and hyperventilation due to pain during percutaneous sampling. ABG's provide intermittent data which limits its use in documenting transient events.

Noninvasive monitors such as pulse oximetry to determine oxygenation, and transcutaneous CO_2 ($PctCO_2$) monitoring and end-tidal CO_2 monitoring (capnography) to monitor the CO_2 status of critically ill infants and children are, therefore, becoming increasingly popular.

Reliance on cyanosis in the recognition of arterial hypoxemia is subjective. An eleven percent of a group of experienced clinicians could not detect cyanosis in healthy individuals when the arterial oxygen saturation had been reduced to 75%.[2] Pulse oximetry has recently been suggested to be a fifth vital sign in pediatrics.[3] Besides the use in anesthesia and Pediatric Intensive Care, oximetry has also been used as a screening device for detecting cyanotic heart disease in asymptomatic newborns.[4]

PULSE OXIMETRY

History

Oximetry measurements can be traced to the early 1930s when German investigators reported the use of an "ear oxygen meter" that used red and infrared light to compensate for changes in tissue thickness, blood content, light intensities and other variables.[5] In 1964, a San Francisco surgeon developed a self-calibrating, 8-wavelength oximeter that was marketed by Hewlett Packard in the 1970s.[6] This system was very large, expensive but allowed for continuous noninvasive monitoring of arterial oxygenation. In the late 1970s, the Biox Corporation in Colorado made significant advances in pulse oximetry, 2-wavelength measurements. They first introduced the use of Light Emitting Diodes (LED's) for the red and infrared light sources.

Today, there are many manufacturers of pulse oximeters. All offer a variety of different oximeter boxes with SpO_2 (oxyhemoglobin) and pulse rate readings, waveform displays, alarms, etc. While the boxes and the displays may differ, all use a similar principle of measuring oxyhemoglobin saturation by two wavelengths of light in the red and infrared range.

Principles

The relationship between the absorption of light and the amount of absorbent (Beer-Lambert law) was published in 1851 which states that the concentration of an unknown solute dissolved in a solvent can be determined by the amount of light absorption. The relationship can be expressed as:

$$L_{(trans)} = L_{(in)} e^{-a}$$
$$a = DC\mathring{a}$$

$L_{(in)}$ is the amount of incident light, D is the distance through which the light travels, C is the concentration of a substance (i.e., hemoglobin) , a is the absorption coefficient and $L_{(trans)}$ is the intensity of the transmitted light through a substance. The absorption coefficient is the constant.

The principle of pulse oximetry is based on the red (600-750 nm wavelength) and infrared light (850-1000 nm) absorption characteristics of oxygenated and deoxygenated hemoglobin. Oxygenated hemoglobin absorbs more infrared light and allows more red light to pass through. Deoxygenated (or reduced) hemoglobin absorbs more red light and allows more infrared light to pass through (Fig. 99.1).

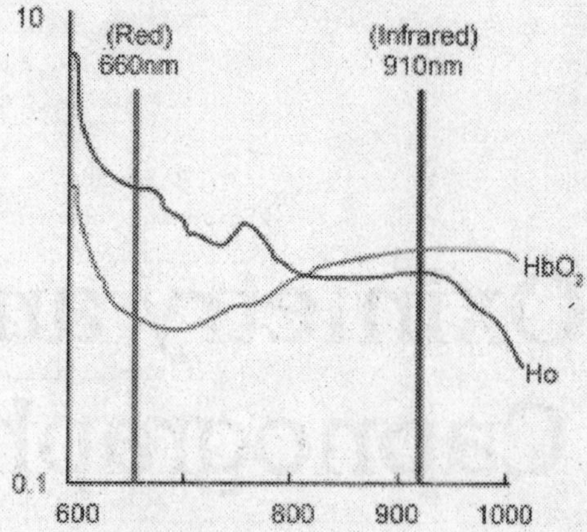

Fig. 99.1: Principle of pulse oximetry
(See for colour figure plate 3)

Pulse oximetry uses a light emitter with red and infrared LEDs that shines through a reasonably translucent site with good blood flow.

Typical sites of application are (i) finger (ii) toe (iii) pinna (top) and (iv) lobe of the ear. Infant sites are the foot or palm of the hand and the big toe or thumb. Opposite the emitter is a photodetector that receives the light that passes through the measuring site (Fig. 99.2).

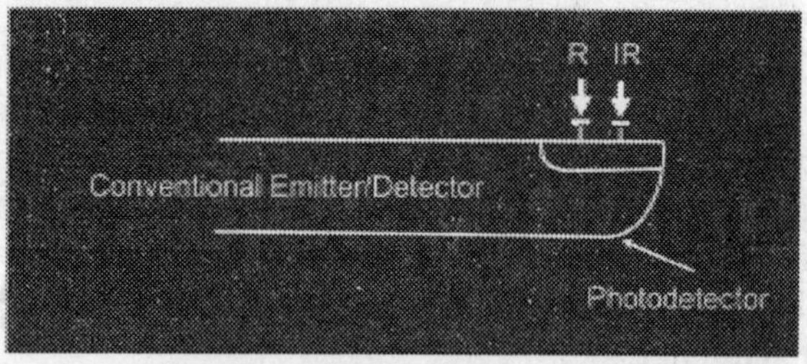

Fig. 99.2: In pulse oximetry, opposite the emitter is a photodetector
(See for colour figure plate 3)

There are two methods of sending light through the measuring site: transmission and reflectance. In the transmission method, as shown in the Figure 99.2, the emitter and photodetector are opposite to each other with the measuring site in-between. The light can then pass through the site. In the reflectance method, the emitter and photodetector are next to each other on top of the measuring site. The light bounces from the emitter to the detector across the site. The transmission method is the most common type used.

At the measuring site, there are constant light absorbers that are always present. They are skin, tissue, venous blood, and the arterial blood. However, with each heart beat the heart contracts and there is a surge of arterial blood, which momentarily increases arterial blood volume across the measuring site. This results in more light absorption during the surge. If light signals received at the photodetector are looked at 'as a waveform', there should be peaks with each heartbeat and troughs between heartbeats. If the light absorption at the trough (which should include all the constant absorbers) is subtracted from the light absorption at the peak then, in theory, the resultants are the absorption characteristics due to added volume of blood only; which is arterial. Since peaks occur with each heartbeat or pulse, the term "pulse oximetry" was coined (Fig. 99.3).

After the transmitted red (R) and infrared (IR) signals pass through the measuring site and are received at the photodetector, the R/IR ratio is calculated. The R/IR is compared to a "look-up" table that convert the ratio to an SpO_2 value. Most manufacturers have their own look-up tables based on calibration curves derived from healthy subjects at various SpO_2 levels. Typically a R/IR ratio of 0.5 equates to approximately 100% SpO_2, a ratio of 1.0 to approximately 82% SpO_2, while a ratio of 2.0 equates to 0% SpO_2.

$$\text{R/IR Ratio} = \frac{\text{Pulsatile absorption (red)/baseline absorbance (red)}}{\text{Pulsatile absorption (infrared)/ baseline absorbance (infrared)}}$$

CLINICAL APPLICATIONS

Pulse Oximetry can be used to monitor oxygenation status (e.g. mechanical ventilation, intubation, surgery, etc), to titrate F_iO_2 (Increase F_iO_2 in hypoxemia or decrease F_iO_2 in weaning) and to verify ABG accuracy (Compare O_2 saturation readings to rule out venous sample).

FALLACIES AND LIMITATIONS

SpO_2 has good correlation with arterial oxygen saturation (SaO_2) when the SaO_2 is 95% or greater. SpO_2 become less accurate as SaO_2 decreases and overestimation of a patient's oxygenation status may result. The accuracy of pulse oximetry can be affected by the following factors:

Dyshemoglobins

The presence of abnormal hemoglobins affects the accuracy of oximeter.

Methemoglobinemia

Methemoglobin is a form of hemoglobin in which iron has been oxidized and is no longer capable of transporting oxygen. This can occur with exposure to nitrates, nitrites, phenacetin, pyridium, sulfonamides, or benzocaine. In a study in dogs it was seen that with increasing MetHb, the oxygen saturation decreased till it reached a plateau of 85%, then becoming independent of MetHb levels.[7] This phenomenon occurs because MetHb absorbs light at both 660 nm and 940 nm and when MetHb increases, the red and infrared light absorption increases and drives the ratio towards unity, which according to the calibration scale corresponds to a saturation of 85%.

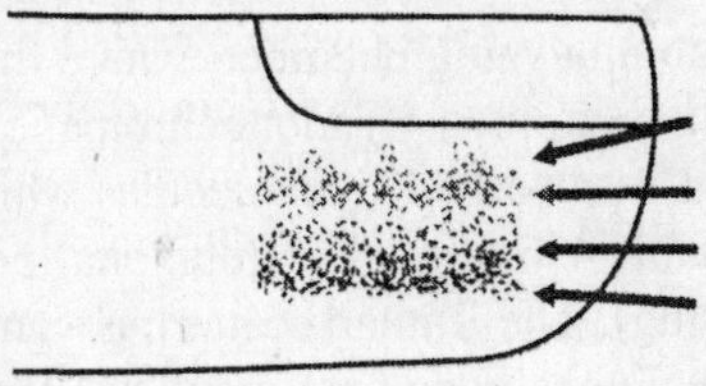

Fig. 99.3: Various light absorbers
(See for colour figure plate 4)

Carboxyhemoglobin

Study of effect of CO inhalation on pulse oximeter in dogs showed that oximetry overestimated O_2 saturation in presence of carboxyhemoglobin.[8] This occurs because COHb absorbs light similar to oxyHb at 660 nm whereas has minimal absorption at 940 nm and hence oximeter interprets COHb as oxyHb and gives falsely high values. This is in clinical correlation that in CO poisoning the blood is cherry red.

Fetal Hemoglobin

HbF has similar absorption characteristics as adult Hb. Hence, its presence does not alter the accuracy of oximeter[9] and this enables the device to be used in even the tiniest of newborns where HbF concentrations are very high.

Dyes

Scheller *et al.*[10] evaluated the effects of bolus doses of methylene blue, indigocarmine and indocyanine green on pulse oximeter. They found that these intravenous dyes cause low values to be recorded by the oximeter. This occurs because any substance present in pulsatile blood that absorbs light at 660 nm or 940 nm were not present at the time of generating calibration curves in the volunteers.

Anemia

Because the pulse oximeter depends on the absorption characteristics of Hb, anemia can be expected to affect the oximeter values but in practice, it does not become a problem unless Hb < 5 g%. What is more clinically relevant is that despite the adequate saturation the oxygen carrying capacity of the blood is reduced.

Low Perfusion States

In shock, for instance, there is small pulsatile signal, the pulse oximeter will amplify that signal in the process the background noise will also get amplified. The oximeter will analyze this noise and generate SpO_2 from it. Tremper *et al.*[11] showed that hypotension was associated with loss of signal or decreased accuracy.

Venous Pulsations

These are seen in situations like tricuspid regurgitation and complete heart block. Oximeter interprets this as arterial pulsations and, hence, displays lower saturation values.[12,13]

Motion Artifacts

One of the ways in which these artifacts can be taken care of is by increasing the averaging time so that if the averaging time is more, the effects of small changes can be lessened and vice versa.[14] Most of the pulse oximeters allow users to set the averaging time. Newer oximeter now use sophisticated algorithms to assess the signal ratio and check the validity of saturation change by assessing its rate of change. If the rate of change is very fast which is usually seen due to a motion artifact, this is given a lower weightage.[15]

Interference from Lights

Excessive light from number of sources can interfere with the accuracy.[16] This problem has been addressed in some oximeters by use of alternating red and infrared LED. When red LED is turned on first, the detector produces a current resulting from red LED and the light. When the infrared LED is switched on current represents infrared signal plus ambient light. Finally, both the LEDs are switched off and the detector analyzes signal from ambient light only. This sequence is repeated hundreds of time per second. However, flickering lights could still be a problem. In practice, covering the sensor with opaque shield can minimize the artifact.[17]

Hyperoxia

As the oxyHb curve flattens out at higher paO_2, the oximeter cannot detect hyperoxia[18] which could be detrimental in some situations like newborns.

Other Factors

Other factors that have been shown to affect the accuracy are–nail polish/thickened or artificial nails,[19] radiofrequencies e.g. from mobile phones and edema of the skin.

Whenever a discrepancy exists between the pulse oximeter reading and the ABG, or the reading does not match the patient's clinical presentation, the pulse oximeter should not be used as an evaluation tool.

CAPNOGRAPHY

Capnography is a graphic record of CO_2 concentration in respiratory gases as a function of time. Capnometry means the measurement of concentration without the waveform record. The concentration of CO_2 in the expired air towards the end of tidal volume i.e. $ETCO_2$ most closely represents the alveolar CO_2 which in turn is supposed to reflect the arterial CO_2. The devices measure $ETCO_2$ in torr (normal 38 mm Hg) or volume concentration (5%) by dividing the $ETCO_2$ in torr by atmospheric pressure.

METHODS OF DETERMINATION OF ALVEOLAR CO_2

A capnographic device incorporates one of two types of analyzers: mainstream or sidestream. Mainstream analyzers insert a sampling window into the ventilator circuit for measurement of CO_2 whereas a sidestream analyzer aspirates gas from the ventilator circuit, and the analysis occurs away from the ventilator circuit. The major advantage of mainstream analysis is the fast response time between actual CO_2 sampling and the display update. The disadvantage of the mainstream adapter is its excessive weight on the endotracheal tube as well as the additional deadspace in the ventilator/ patient circuit. With mainstream sampling, water condensation does not affect analysis; however, secretion buildup on the cell windows can affect the accuracy. A mainstream analyzer also tends to be more frequently handled than the sidestream sensor as the clinician must disconnect it manually to suction the patient. A sidestream analyzer (aspirating analyzer) places the analyzing mechanism safely within the monitor and draws a sample via a tubing connected at the patient's airway (e.g., endotracheal tube). The major advantage with sidestream analysis is the ease of handling and it can be attached to other patient devices (e.g., cannulua, mask). The major disadvantage is that with periodic aspiration of air samples, secretions and water can be drawn into the sampling tube and cause an occlusion. Analyzers utilize infrared, mass or Raman spectra, or a photoacoustic spectra technology.

Infrared Spectrography

Infrared spectrographs are more compact and less expensive than the other methods of measurement. This has been the most popular technique for monitoring CO_2. The wavelength of IR rays exceeds 1.0 milli micron while the visible spectrum is between 0.4 and 0.8 milli microns. The IR rays are absorbed by polyatomic gases (non-elementary gases such as nitrous oxide (N_2O), CO_2, and water vapour. Carbon dioxide selectively absorbs specific wavelengths (4.3 milli microns) of IR light. Since the amount of light absorbed is proportional to the concentration of the absorbing molecules, the concentration of a gas can be determined by comparing the measured absorbance with the absorbance of a known standard.

Raman Spectrography

Raman spectrography uses the principle of "Raman Scattering" for CO_2 measurement. The gas sample is aspirated into an analyzing chamber, where the sample is illuminated by a high intensity monochromatic argon laser beam. The light is absorbed by molecules which are then excited to unstable vibrational or rotational energy states (Raman scattering). The Raman scattering signals (Raman light) are of low intensity and are measured at right angles to the laser beam. The spectrum of Raman scattering lines can be used to identify all types of molecules in the gas phase.

Mass Spectrography

The mass spectrograph separates molecules on the basis of mass to charge ratios. A gas sample is aspirated into a high vacuum chamber (10^{-5} mmHg) where an electron beam ionizes and fragments the components of the sample. The ions are accelerated by an electric field into a final chamber, which has a magnetic field, perpendicular to the path of the ionized gas stream. In the magnetic field the particles follow a path wherein the radius of curvature is proportional to the charge:mass ratio. A detector plate allows for determination of the components of the gas and for the concentration of each component.

Photoacoustic Spectrography

Photoacoustic gas measurement is based on the same principles as conventional IR-based gas analyzers: the ability of CO_2 and N_2O and anaesthetic agents to absorb IR light. However, they differ in measurement techniques. While Infra-red spectrography uses optical methods, PAS uses an acoustic technique.

The changes in the $ETCO_2$ are reflection of changes in CO_2 production, pulmonary blood flow, alveolar ventilation (Tables 99.1 and 99.2).

Capnography is superior to capnometry because

- Waveform can detect if the alteration in PCO_2 is because of sampling errors.
- Underlying disease process can be differentiated e.g. CO_2 rise can occur both in asthma and central hypoventilation but these can be differentiated based on shape of the curve.

NORMAL CAPNOGRAPH (Fig. 99.4)

The capnographic recording is done at 2 speeds i.e. 7 mm/ sec and 0.7 mm/sec. For routine clinical practice high speed capnograph is used. However, more accurate information is obtained by the other method where PCO_2 changes are recorded against the volume of expired gases rather than time, so called single breath test SBT-CO_2.

Phase 1

Flat portion of the curve at the ground level represents the inhalation. Hence, no CO_2 is detected.

Table 99.1: PETCO$_2$ increased

CO_2 output	*Pulmonary perfusion*	*Alveolar ventilation*	*Technical errors*
Fever	Increased cardiac output	Hypoventilation	Exhausted CO_2 absorber
Malignant hyperpyrexia	Increased blood pressure	Bronchial intubation	Inadequate fresh gas flows
Sodium bicarbonate		Partial airway obstruction	Leaks in breathing system
Tourniquet release		Rebreathing	

Table 99.2: PETCO$_2$ decreased

CO_2 output	*Pulmonary perfusion*	*Alveolar ventilation*	*Technical errors*
Hypothermia	Reduced cardiac output	Hyperventilation	Circuit disconnection
	Hypotension	Apnea	Sampling tube leak
Pulmonary embolism	Partial airway obstruction	Malfunction of ventilator	
	Cardiac arrest	Accidental tracheal extubation	

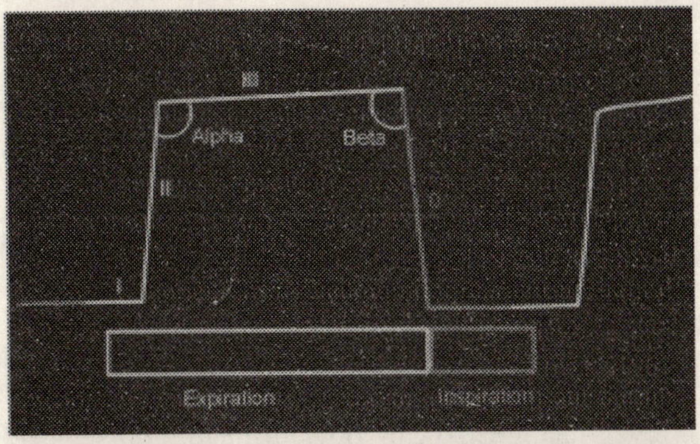

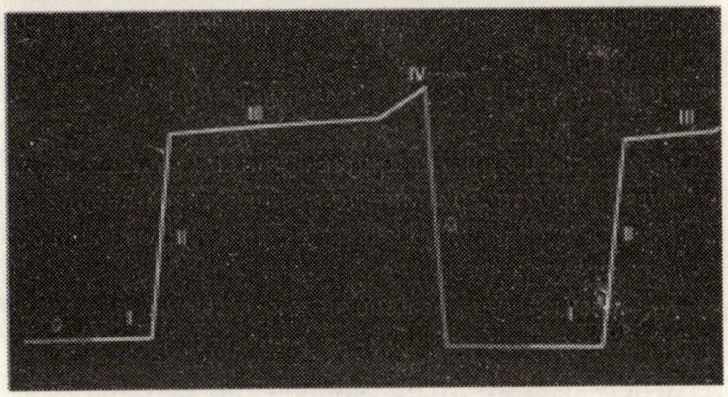

Fig. 99.4: Normal capnograph
(See for colour figure plate 4)

Phase 2

Rapid upswing with increase in CO_2 levels represents early expiration where there is gradual replacement of the dead space with alveolar air.

Phase 3

It represents the alveolar air and hence the slope is a plateau. The plateau is not a horizontal line but is rising continuously and sometimes there is a sudden rise towards the end representing the phase 4. This occurs because:

- There is a cyclical variation in alveolar PCO$_2$ because CO_2 is continuously being excreted into alveolar gas during respiration.
- Delayed emptying of alveoli with low V/Q (high PCO$_2$).

The angle between the phase II and the phase III, which has been referred to as α angle is thus an indirect indicator of the V/Q status of lung. The angle between the phase III and phase 0 is called the β angle and represents the ET CO_2 point.

Phase 0

Phase 0 occurs with the start of inspiration and CO_2 rapidly declines to zero.

ABNORMALITIES IN THE CAPNOGRAPHY

We need to evaluate the following in a capnogram:

Phase I

Is the CO_2 zero (normal baseline) or elevated? Elevated baseline suggests rebreathing. Other causes of abnormal baseline during mechanical ventilation include spontaneous breathing or inadvertent chest compressions.

Phase II Upstroke

Is there evidence of slow prolonged exhalation? It can occur with asthma.

Phase III

Is there evidence of uneven emptying of the lungs? The slope of the plateau i.e. angle, reflects the V/Q status of the lung.

Phase IV

Is the plateau top smooth? The irregularities of the surface top can be caused by inadequate paralysis (curare effects), cardiac oscillations or water in the ventilator circuit.

Phase 0

Is the downstroke steep (β angle) or is there evidence of slow inspiration as may occur with depression of the central respiratory drive?

CLINICAL USES OF CAPNOGRAPHY AND CAPNOMETRY IN PEDIATRIC PRACTICE

1. *Noninvasive Predictor of $PaCO_2$:* By far the most important use of capnography is its noninvasive ability to provide an instantaneous clue to the level of CO_2 in the arterial blood. In infants and children breathing spontaneously, the $PETCO_2$ values range from 36-40 mmHg.[20] In infants and children the (a-ET)PCO_2 gradient can vary from -0.65 mmHg to 2.4 mmHg. In preterm infants the gradient may be 3.5 mmHg.[21] Alveolar hypoventilation increases $PaCO_2$ as well as $PETCO_2$.
2. *Apnea Monitor:* During apnea of either type, the CO_2 concentration at the sampling site falls rapidly and can be instantaneously detected by capnography. Therefore, CO_2 monitoring serves as a reliable apnea monitor in neonates, infants and children.[22]
3. *Airway Obstruction*: In severe airway obstruction such as bronchial asthma and laryngotracheobronchitis, the shape of the capnogram can be altered, with a prolongation or slanting of phase II and increased slope of phase III, the expiratory plateau. With adequate treatment, the capnogram reverts to normal.
   Therefore the effectiveness of bronchodilator treatments in a child with asthma, and racemic epinephrine treatments in the child with stridor can be assessed from the capnography.[23]
4. *P(a-et)CO_2 Gradient as an Indicator of Pulmonary Disease:* The P(a-et)CO_2 gradient (difference) between these two measurements is about 2 mm Hg in normal children. For critical patients, a gradient of 5 mm Hg is considered acceptable. The P(a-et) CO_2 gradient is primarily affected by alveolar deadspace ventilation, presence of pulmonary disease, and changes in mechanical volume and modality. Table 99.3 lists some specific conditions that increase the P(a-et) CO_2 gradient.

Table 99.3: Factors that increase the P(a-et)CO_2 gradient

Clinical condition	*Factors*
Ventilation	Increased deadspace ventilation, positive pressure ventilation.
Perfusion	Decreased cardiac output, Decreased pulmonary perfusion, Cardiac arrest, Pulmonary embolic disease.
Temperature	Hyperthermia, Hypothermia

The (a-et) PCO_2 is an indicator of V/Q mismatching resulting from pulmonary disease. In neonates with respiratory disease, the P (a-ET)CO_2 difference becomes wider, as for example, in infants with bronchopulmonary dysplasia, where the gradient may be as much as 9 mmHg.[21] The angle in the capnogram increases with increasing V/Q mismatch.

5. *Placement and Displacement of Endotracheal Tube:* When used with the standard techniques of chest auscultation, CO_2 monitoring is probably the best way to detect esophageal intubations and displacement of endotracheal tube. $PETCO_2$ would decrease resulting in a flat capnogram. Recently, $PETCO_2$ detectors, which change color on exposure to 4% CO_2 have been used successfully to confirm ETT placement in children.[24]
6. *Mechanical Ventilation*
   a. *Noninvasive Monitoring of Adequacy of Mechanical Ventilation*
   In intubated infants with normal respiratory and cardiovascular physiology, $PETCO_2$ values approximate $PaCO_2$ values. In older children though, $PETCO_2$ values are lower than $PaCO_2$ by 2-5 mmHg.[25] Changes in $PETCO_2$ can often be regarded as indicative of changes in $PaCO_2$. It is prudent to establish the relationship of $PETCO_2$ to $PaCO_2$ initially by blood gas analysis. Thereafter, changes in $PaCO_2$ may be assumed to occur in parallel with those in $PETCO_2$, thus avoiding repeated ABGs.
   b. *Integrity of Ventilation*
   Capnography can identify disconnections in the ventilatory circuit instantaneously before O_2 and CO_2 levels change in the blood. During the course of IPPV in children with no spontaneous breathing, $PETCO_2$ falls to zero instantaneously following the disconnections in the circuit and sounds an alarm. Corrective measures can be instituted immediately before irreversible damage is caused by prolonged hypoxia. However, in children breathing spontaneously, circuit disconnections distal to CO_2 sampling site (towards the child) can be identified instantaneously as CO_2 concentration falls to zero in the sampling adaptor, whereas, circuit disconnection proximal to the sampling site may not be detected instantaneously as $PETCO_2$ values depends on the adequacy of spontaneous breathing. If spontaneous breathing is adequate, the $PETCO_2$ values remain normal, whereas, $PETCO_2$ values may rise gradually if spontaneous breathing is inadequate, and thereby alert the physician. Capnography is also useful in giving an early warning of CO_2 retention caused by faulty ventilators and wrong connections.
   c. *Weaning*: Capnography along with pulse oximetry can be used to monitor alveolar ventilation during weaning from mechanical ventilation. Using ABG's alone may not be an adequate guide to decide on weaning because occasionally pain from blood sampling will cause patients to hyperventilate and, thus, decrease the PCO_2 level in the blood, which may not be a true indicator of patients ventilatory status. Capnography can be used to evaluate the trend of $PaCO_2$, breathing pattern,

and, more importantly, the consistency of breathing before extubation.[26] Ventilator rates can be gradually decreased to the lowest point at which the patient can comfortably breathe and maintain adequate alveolar ventilation. If the child becomes distressed and increases the work of breathing, or $PETCO_2$ rises, ventilatory rates can be returned to the previously acceptable settings. Evaluation of CO_2 waveforms produced by spontaneous ventilation during weaning gives information about the depth and consistency of spontaneous ventilation. The stability of $PETCO_2$ and increasing similarity of capnograms `between the patient and the ventilator breaths indicate the patient's readiness to wean from the mechanical ventilation.[23]

7. *$PETCO_2$ as a noninvasive monitor of pulmonary blood flow:* A reduction in the cardiac output (pulmonary blood flow) produces high V/Q ratio (increased alveolar dead space) resulting in lower $PETCO_2$ and an increased $P(a-E_T)CO_2$ gradients. As pulmonary blood flow increases, thereby improving V/Q ratio, the $PETCO_2$ increases and $(a-E_T)PCO_2$ gradient becomes small. Thus, $PETCO_2$ is a function of cardiac output for a given ventilation.[27] Hence, $PETCO_2$ is a noninvasive monitor of pulmonary blood flow. Utilizing this principle, $PETCO_2$ monitoring can be used to monitor the effectiveness of cardiopulmonary resuscitation. During cardiac arrest, circulation ceases and $PETCO_2$ gradually disappears, reappearing only when circulation is restored either by effective cardiopulmonary resuscitation or cardiac function. $PETCO_2$ monitoring enables the physician to change the technique of Pediatric Advanced Cardiac Life Support to produce effective pulmonary circulation.[28]
8. *CO_2 Production:* If a child is unable to alter minute ventilation sufficiently, increased CO_2 production will be manifested by an increase in $PETCO_2$ whereas decrease CO_2 production will be manifested by decreased $PETCO_2$. Malignant hyperpyrexia, sepsis, thyrotoxicosis, seizures, shivering, bicarbonate injection and parenteral nutrition increases CO_2 production and increase $PETCO_2$ whereas hypothermia leads to a decrease in $PETCO_2$. Hence, increasing $PETCO_2$ may be an early warning sign of an impending hypermetabolic crisis.[29]

COMPLICATIONS

Capnography with a clinically approved device is a safe, noninvasive test, associated with few hazards. With mainstream analyzers, the use of too large a sampling window may introduce an excessive amount of dead space into the ventilator circuit.[30] Care must be taken to minimize the amount of additional weight placed on the artificial airway by the addition of the sampling window or, in the case of a sidestream analyzer, the sampling line.

LIMITATIONS OF THE DEVICE

It is important to note that although the capnograph provides valuable information about the efficiency of ventilation (as well as pulmonary and coronary perfusion), it is not a replacement or substitute for assessing the $PaCO_2$. The difference between $PetCO_2$ and $PaCO_2$ increases as dead-space volume increases. In fact, the difference between the $PaCO_2$ and $PETCO_2$ has been shown to vary within the same patient over time.[31]

FACTORS AFFECTING RELIABILITY

1. The infrared spectrum of CO_2 has some similarities to the spectra for both oxygen and nitrous oxide.[32] High concentrations of either or both oxygen or nitrous oxide may affect the capnogram.
2. The breathing frequency may affect the capnograph. High breathing frequencies may exceed the response capabilities of the capnograph. In addition, the breathing frequency, above 10 breaths/min, has been shown to affect devices differently.
3. The presence of Freon (earlier used as a propellant in metered dose inhalers) in the respiratory gas has been shown to artificially increase the CO_2 reading of mass spectrometers.[33] A similar effect has not yet been demonstrated with Raman or infrared spectrometers. Contamination of the monitor or sampling system by secretions or condensate, a sample tube of excessive length, a sampling rate that is too high, or obstruction of the sampling chamber can lead to unreliable results.

CONCULSION

In conclusion, the pulse oximetry and capnography have become important in pediatric critical care and can avert many a life-threatening situations. They provide continuous and noninvasive means of monitoring oxygenation and ventilation obviating the need for repeated invasive monitoring. Although these instruments are fairly reliable, the gold standard still remains the ABG which should be resorted to whenever there is doubt.

REFERENCES

1. American Academy of Pediatrics. Guidelines and levels of care for pediatric intensive care units (American academy of pediatrics: Committee on Hospital Care). *Crit Care Med* 1993; 7:1077-1086.
2. Comroe J, Botelho S. The Unreliability of cyanosis in the recognition of arterial anoxemia. *Am J Med Sci* 1947;214:1-6.
3. William R, Carolyn S, Emily L, Larry J. Pulse oximeter as a fifth pediatric vital sign. *Pediatrics* 1997;99:681-686.
4. Koppel R, Druschel C, Carter T, Goldberg B, Mehta P, Talwar R et al. Effectiveness of pulse oximetry screening for congenital heart disease in asymptomatic newborns. *Pediatrics* 2003;111:670-671.

5. Hillikan GA. The oximeter, an instrument for measuring continuously the oxygen saturation of arterial blood in man. *Rev Sceint Instruments* 1942;13:434-444.
6. Flick M, Block A. In vivo continuous arterial oxygen saturation measurements by oximetry. *Am Rev Respir Dis* 1976;113:126.
7. Barker S, Tremper K, Hyatt J. Effect of methemoglobinemia on pulse oximetry and mixed venous oximetry. *Anesthesiology* 1989;70:112-117.
8. Barker S, Tremper K. The effect of carbon monoxide inhalation on pulse oximetry and transcutaneous PO_2. *Anesthesiology* 1987;66:677-679.
9. Rajdurai V, Walker A, Yu V, Oates A. Effect of Fetal hemoglobin on the accuracy of pulse oximetry in preterm infants. *J Pediatr Child Health* 1992;28:43-46.
10. Scheller M, Unger R, Kelner H. Effects of intravenously administered dyes on pulse oximetry readings. *Anesthesiology* 1986;65:435-436.
11. Tremper K, Hufstedler S, Barker S, Adams A. Accuracy of a pulse oximeter in critically ill adult: effect of temperature and hemodynamics. *Anesthesiology* 1985;63;A175.
12. Marks J. Systolic Venous Waves Cause spurious signs of arterial hemoglobin desaturation. *Anesthesiology* 1989;71:158-160.
13. Sterwart K, Rowbottom S. Inaccuracy of pulse oximetry in patients with severe tricuspid regurgitation. *Anesthesia* 1991;46:668-670.
14. Ohmeda B III. Pulse Oximeter. *Operating/Service Manual.* Ohmeda: Boulder 1987;24.
15. Wukitsch H, Tobler D, Pologe J, Patterson M. Pulse oximetry. An analysis of theory, technology and practice. *J Clin Monit* 1988;4:299-301.
16. Monowell L. Ambient light affects pulse oximeters. *Anesthesiology* 1987;67:864-865.
17. Siegel M, Gravenstein N. Preventing ambient light from affecting pulse oximetry. *Anesthesiology* 1987;67:864-865.
18. Tremper K, Barker S. Pulse oximetry. *Anesthesiology* 1989;70:98-108.
19. Welch J, DeCesare M, Hess D. Pulse oximetry. Instrumentation and clinical applications. *Respir Care* 1990;35:584-601.
20. Curley M, Thompson J. End tidal CO_2 monitoring in critically ill infants and children. *Pediatr Nurs* 1990;16:397-403.
21. Dumpit F, Brady J. A simple technique for measuring alveolar CO_2 in infants. *J Appl Physiol* 1978;45:648-650.
22. Magnan A, Philip-Joet F, Rey M, Reynaud M, Poori F, Arnand A. End tidal CO_2 analysis in sleep apnea syndromes. Conditions for use. *Chest* 1993;103:129-131.
23. Nuzzo P, Anton W. Practical applications of capnography. *Respir Ther* 1986;12-17.
24. Kelly J, Wilhoit R, Brown R, James R. Efficacy of the FEF colorimetric end-tidal carbon dioxide detector in children. *Anesth Analg* 1992;75:45-50.
25. Sivan Y, Eldadah M, Cheah T, Newth C. Estimation of arterial carbon dioxide by end-tidal and transcutaneous PCO_2 measurements in ventilated children. *Pediatr Pulmonol* 1992;12:153-157.
26. Henry AE, Kinsley A. Capnography today. *Pediatr Aids* 1978;11:130-137.
27. Leigh MD, Jones JC, Mottley HL. The expired carbon dioxide as continuous guide of the pulmonary and circulatory systems during anesthesia and surgery. *J Thoracic and Cardiovasc Surg* 1961;41:597-610.
28. Falk J, Rackow E, Weil M. End-tidal carbon dioxide concentration during cardiopulmonary resuscitation. *N Engl J Med* 1988;318:607-611.
29. Baudendistel L, Goudsouzian N, Cote C, Strafford M. End-tidal CO_2 monitoring: its use in the diagnosis and management of malignant hyperpyrexia. *Anaesthesia* 1984;39:100-103.
30. Block F, McDonald J. Sidestream versus mainstream carbon dioxide analyzers. *J Clin Monitor* 1992;8:139-141.
31. Russel G, Graybeal J. End tidal carbon dioxide as an indicator of arterial carbon dioxide in neurointensive care patients. *J Neurosurg Anesth* 192;36:245-249.
32. Ammann E, Galvin R. Problems associated with the determination of carbon dioxide by infrared absorbtion. *J Appl Physio* 1968;25;333-335.
33. Elliot W, Reamer D, Goldman D, Philip J. The effects of bronchodilator inhaler aerosol propellents on respiratory gas monitors. *J Clin Monitor* 1991;7:175-180.

Ravinder K Gupta and Ritu Gupta

100 Practical Procedures

INTRODUCTION

Several procedures are unique to the pediatric patient in the emergency settings.

Consent should be obtained when appropriate but one should not delay life-saving procedures. Preparing a child for a procedure may facilitate the process and must be related to the child's age, developmental status, and ability to understand the procedure in terms of what the child will feel, taste, see, or smell, while making the child as comfortable as possible.

BACKGROUND

Medical and traumatic illnesses progress rapidly in the pediatric patient. The vast majority are treatable with appropriate and timely intervention and may be expected to leave the child without sequelae and with a full life ahead.

Emergency care of the pediatric patient continues to evolve; the unique knowledge, skills, experience, equipment, and facilities are increasingly available to the clinician and patient in the prehospital and hospital setting. The pediatric patient is seen in a variety of emergency settings. Approximately 25 to 35% of patients in general emergency department are pediatric, presenting problems ranging from benign, self-limited conditions to those that are life threatening. The major pediatric triage categories are mentioned in Table 100.1.

ARTERIAL PUNCTURE

Arterial punctures are used routinely to obtain heparinized blood for arterial blood gas (ABG) determinations.

The radial artery is the preferred site because of its stability and lack of an accompanying vein. It is entered tangentially, with the artery being localized by placing fingers proximal and distal to the point of entry (Fig. 100.1). The brachial artery may be entered at its most superficial point at the median side of the antecubital fossa. The superficial temporal artery is useful in the infant. The artery located and immobilized by one finger while the puncture is made often with a scalp vein needle instead of a straight needle.

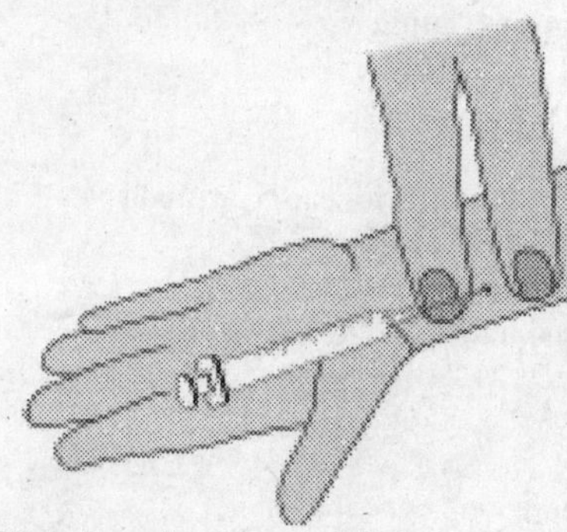

Fig. 100.1: Localization of radial artery for puncture

The dorsalis pedis, posterior tibial and the femoral arteries are other options.

VENOUS INFUSION

Obtaining venous access in the pediatric patient requires familiarity with potential sites and techniques, as well as expertise and patience. The choice of technique may require modification because of the nature of the injury or illness and the patient's condition, size, and fluid requirements.

PERIPHERAL VEIN PERCUTANEOUS PUNCTURE

The preferred sites are the antecubital vein, veins on the dorsa of the hand and foot, and, in the child less than 2 years of age, the scalp. The external jugular or femoral vein also may be used.

The patient is immobilized to the extent necessary. Extremities require careful immobilization with tape (Fig. 100.2). Hands may be better positioned if a small amount of cotton or gauze is placed under the wrist when using veins on the dorsum of the hand.

Procedure

Cleanse the area to be entered. Shave the area if necessary (e.g., the head). Apply a tourniquet proximal to the point of venous access. On the head a rubber band may serve as

Table 100.1: Major pediatric triage categories

*Emergent**				*Urgent+*
Abnormal vital signs				
Age	Systolic BP (mmHg)	Pulse (beats/min)	Respiration (breaths/min)	Abuse, child
0-2 yr	< 60	< 80	< 15 or > 40	Abuse, sexual
2-5 yr	< 70	< 60	< 10 or > 30	Acute symptoms in child < 2-3 mo
> 5 yr	< 90	< 50	< 5 or > 25	Behavioral alteration
Respirations				Bite, poisonous snake
Irregular				Bleeding, moderate
Apneic				Dehydration
Labored				Drowning (near)
Pulse				Eye : alkali, acid, or chemical burn
Irregular				Fever ≥ 40°C
Dyshythmic				GI hemorrhage
Coma				Headache : acute and severe
Cyanosis				Hypertension
Status epilepticus				Hyperthermia
Multiple or major trauma				Neck pain or stiffness
Head				Pain : acute and severe
Loss of consciousness				Poisoning
Altered mental status				Rash (isolate patient)
Changing or asymmetric neurologic findings				**SIDS (near)**
Cerebrospinal fluid leak				
Depressed fracture				
Neck or spinal injury				
Chest				
Abdomen				
Orthopedic				
Two or more long bone fractures				
Pelvic fracture				
Potential neurovascular compromise				
Amputation				
Major burn				
Bleeding : acute and significant				

* If none of these emergent or urgent conditions is present, the patient should be appropriately screened and treated according to normal facility flow patterns unless there is a complicating condition.

+ May be emergent, depending on patient's condition. Repeat visits or very anxious parents may require that the visit be categorized as urgent.

the tourniquet. Place a small amount of tape at one point on the rubber band to facilitate removal of the tourniquet (Fig. 100.3).

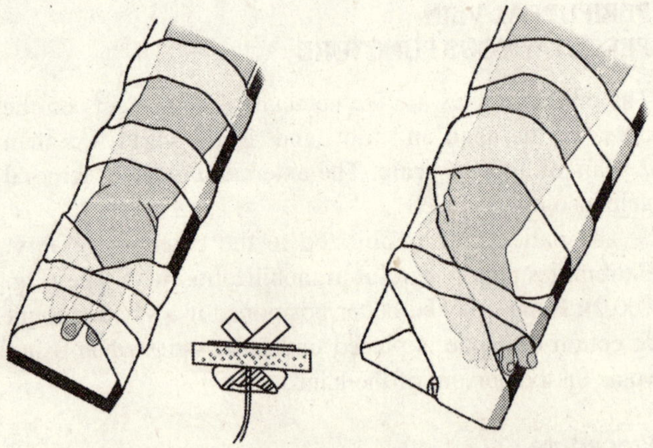

Fig. 100.2: Immobilization of extremity for ercutaneous venous puncture. Scalp vein needle taping

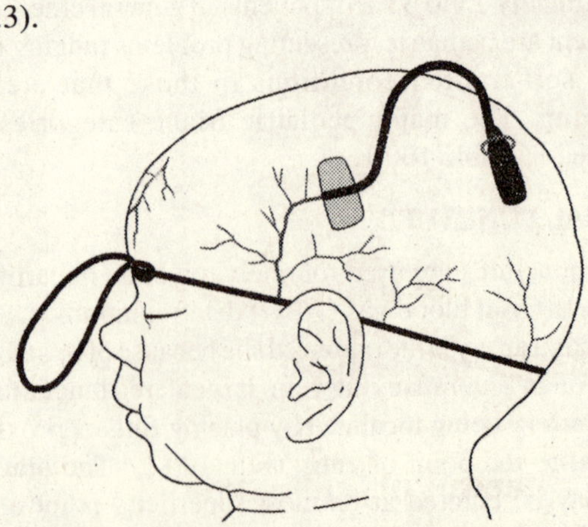

Fig. 100.3: Rubber band tourniquet applied to the scalp

The choice of needles and cannulas is based on personal preference. Scalp vein needle may be used in all areas except for veins overlying joints. The inherent problem is the lack of true stability of the needle after it is inserted. Before inserting the needle, flush with saline solution leaving the syringe attached until the skin is punctured. Once the skin is entered, remove the syringe to permit a flashback on entering the vein. Insert the needle tangentially through the skin approximately. Grasp the needle by the winged tags. Advance the needle gently until the vein is entered and a flashback is visible. Unless the vein is large, do not thread the needle further. Place a 1cm wide tape over the needle at the point of entry to provide initial stabilization, and loop a second piece around the winged tags. The needle should be flushed intermittently to ensure patency and position. Tape the needle carefully to minimize movement.

An IV infusion set should be attached after the patient is stabilized. In children less than 5 years of age, there should always be a volume-limiting device in line to prevent excessive fluid administration.

VENOUS CUTDOWN

The greater saphenous vein located anterior to the medial malleolus and medial to the anterior tibial tendon is the ideal site.

The foot is immobilized with careful visualization of the malleolus.

After cleansing, draping and infiltrating locally with 1% lidocaine, apply a tourniquet. Make a 1 cm transverse incision perpendicular to the vein, usually one finger breadth above and one finger breadth anterior to the medial malleolus. Bluntly dissect down to the tibia in the direction parallel to the vein and identify the vein. Free the vein, and place two 3-0 Vicryl or silk sutures loosely around it. The distal suture is ligated to control venous return. The proximal suture is tied after the venous catheter has been place. At this time it is left loose (Fig. 100.4).

Some clinicians have recommended a more rapid approach. An incision from the posterior border of the malleolus is extended anteriorly to the 'shin' or the anterior border of the tibia. A curved closed hemostat pointing downward is scraped along the tibia from the anterior to the posterior aspect of the incision. All tissue is picked up and the hemostat is turned upward and opened. The saphenous vein is identified. Another approach includes identification and isolation of the vein and subsequent cannulation using a guide wire technique.

Select the appropriate size catheter. Using the proximal suture for traction, make a small flap incision in the anterior third of the vein with a no. 11 scalpel blade. The vein also can be cannulated by direct puncture, which does not require ligation. Insert the catheter with traction from the proximal tie while elevating the vein flap. Remove the tourniquet and ensure that there is free flow. Secure the catheter by tightening the proximal tie. Begin the IV infusion.

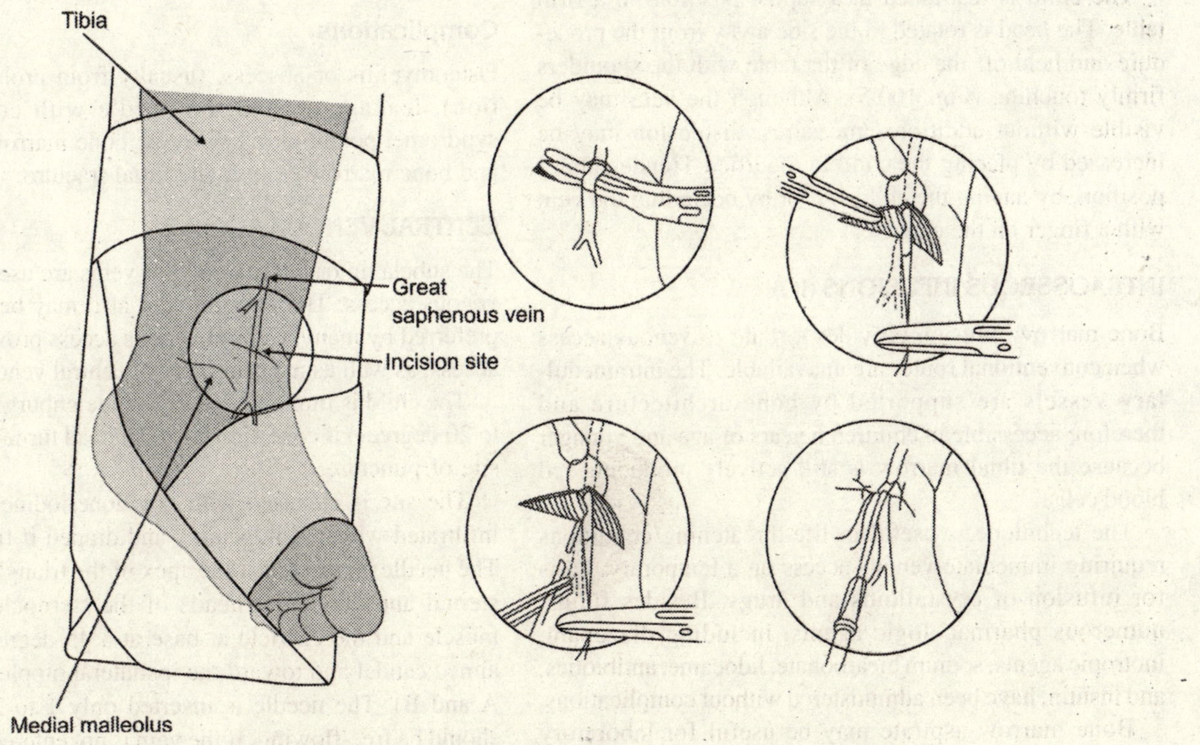

Fig. 100.4: Method for great saphenous vein cutdown at the ankle

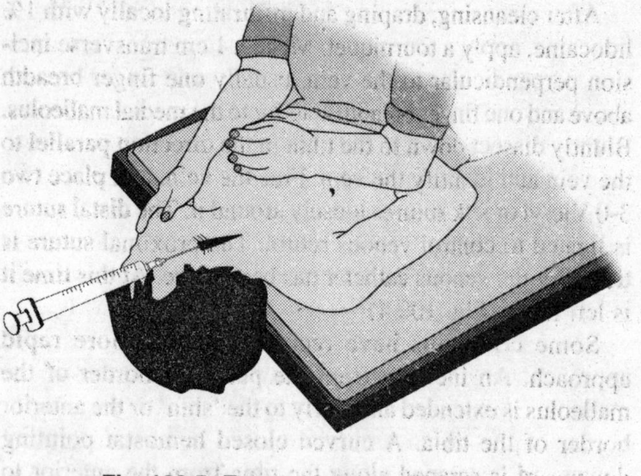

Fig. 100.5: External jugular vein puncture

Close the wound with 4-0 Vicryl or Dexon sutures (some prefer silk or nylon), and further secure the catheter by extensive taping. Cover with sterile dressing.

EXTERNAL JUGULAR VEIN PUNCTURE

The external jugular vein is easily accessible in children whose necks are not unduly short or obese. The vein courses from the angle of the mandible to the middle of the clavicle over the sternocleidomastoid muscle. The vein may be used for venipuncture, as well as for establishing peripheral or central venous access.

The child is restrained in a supine position on a firm table. The head is rotated to the side away from the procedure and held off the edge of the table with the shoulders firmly touching (Fig. 100.5). Although the vein may be visible without additional measures, distension may be increased by placing the child in modified Trendelenburg position, by having the child cry, or by occluding the vein with a finger on the clavicle.

INTRAOSSEOUS INFUSIONS (IO)

Bone marrow infusion provides a route to venous access when conventional routes are unavailable. The intramedullary vessels are supported by bone architecture and therefore accessible in children 6 years of age and younger because the tibial marrow is still actively producing red blood cells.

The technique is useful in life-threatening conditions requiring immediate venous access on a temporary, basis for infusion of crystalloids and drugs. Besides fluids, numerous pharmacologic agents, including diazepam, inotropic agents, sodium bicarbonate, lidocaine, antibiotics, and insulin, have been administered without complications.

Bone marrow aspirate may be useful for laboratory studies such as blood culture and electrolytes.

The patient is immobilized in the supine position. It is often useful to position a small sandbag under the leg, immediately behind the operative site. Restrain the leg. 18 to 20 gauge spinal needles with stylet or a small 15 to 18 gauge bone marrow trephine needle can be used.

Strict aseptic technique must be maintained. Local infiltration with lidocaine is desirable. The needle is inserted perpendicular to the skin or at a 45 to 60 degree angle away from the epiphyseal plate (Fig. 100.6). The proximal tibia or distal femur is preferred. A screwing motion is used to push the needle through the cortex. The needle is in the marrow when there is a lack of resistance after the needle passes through the cortex and stands upright without support. Bone marrow is aspirated by the syringe, and the infusion flows smoothly.

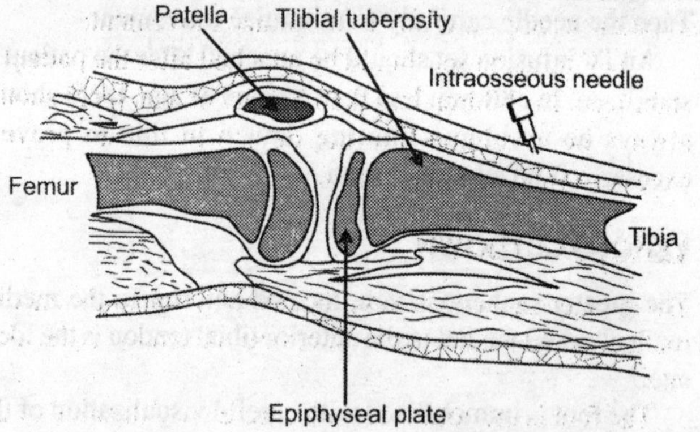

Fig. 100.6: Intraosseus insertion of needle

Complications

Osteomyelitis or abscess, (usually from prolonged insertion), leakage around the needle with compartment syndrome, potential injury to the bone marrow cavity, fat and bone marrow emboli and tibial fracture.

CENTRAL VENOUS ACCESS

The subclavin or internal jugular veins are used for central vegous access. The femoral vein also may be used and is preferred by many. Central venous access provides venous access, as well as measurement of central venous pressure.

The child is immobilized in Trendelenburg position (15 to 20 degrees) if condition permits, head turned away from site of puncture.

The site is cleansed with povidone-iodine (Betadine)-infiltrated with 1% lidocaine, and draped if time permits. The needle is inserted at the apex of the triangle created by sternal and clavicular heads of the sternocleidomastoid muscle and the clavicle at base at a 45-degree angle and aimed caudal and toward the ipsilateral nipple (Figs 100.7 A and B). The needle is inserted only 1 to 2 cm; blood should be free-flowing. If the vein is not entered, the needle is withdrawn and redirected slightly more laterally. Once the vein is entered, the needle is left in place while the attached syringe is removed. The guidewire is then inserted through the needle. The needle is then removed over the guidewire. A small cut is made at the point of skin entry and the catheter is inserted according to the manufacturer's directions.

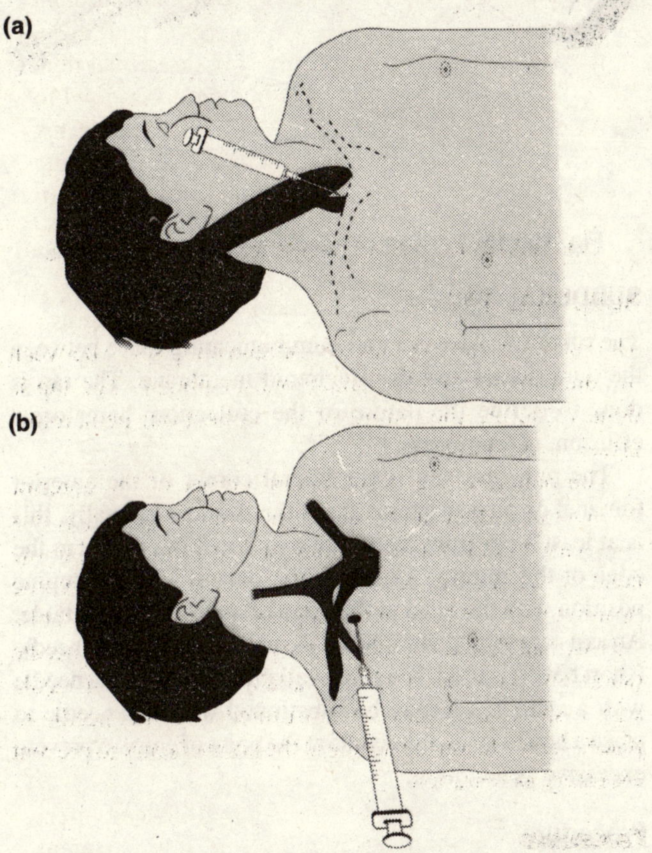

Figs 100.7a and b: (a) Internal jugular vein puncture and (b) Subclavian vein puncture

Femoral Vein

The femoral vein may be cannulated by locating the femoral pulse and inserting a needle 2 cm distal to the inguinal ligament and 0.5 cm medial. The remainder of the approach using a guidewire is similar to other routes.

The IV infusion is attached with an inline manometer to measure central venous pressure (CVP). The catheter is secured with suture through the skin and wrapped around the catheter. A sterile dressing is applied. CVP can be determined.

Cautions

A bright–red blood return indicates that an artery has been punctured. If unable to advance the catheter, remove the needle and catheter together. Never withdraw the cannula through the needle. The right side usually is preferred, because the dome of the lung is lower on the right, it is a more direct path to the right atrium, and there is a smaller thoracic duct on the right.

Complications

These include pneumothorax, hemothorax, hydrothorax, air or catheter embolization, and brachial plexus injury.

LUMBAR PUNCTURE

Lumbar punctures (LP) commonly are performed to exclude central nervous system (CNS) infection. It is important to exclude potential increased intracranial pressure on the basis of history and physical examination before performing the LP.

The patient should be placed at the edge of a firm examination table and maintained in a position with the neck flexed and the knee drawn upward (fetal position) (Fig. 100.8).

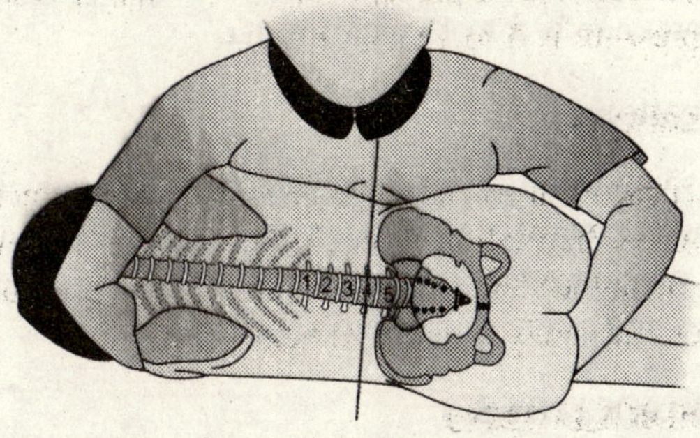

Fig. 100.8: Position for lumbar puncture

The shoulders and back of the patient should be perpendicular to the table. An alternative position for the small infant is to have the patient sitting flexing the thighs up to the abdomen (Fig. 100.9). This is recommended only if the holder and clinician are experienced with this approach. In the preterm infant, the optimal position is either the lateral recumbent one with the hips flexed and partial neck extension or the upright position. Full flexion of the neck may cause hypoventilation.

The patient's back is cleansed with a surgical solution, using povidone-iodine (Betadine), and then draped. Steri-drapes are particularly useful, because they are adherent and do not obscure the landmarks. The puncture is at the intersection of the line joining the superior portion of the iliac crest with the spine. This point is the spinuous process of L4. The needle is optimally inserted at L3-L4 but may be inserted one space above or below. The needle should be inserted perpendicular to the back and aimed toward the umbilicus. In the younger child it is advisable to puncture the skin and allow the child to calm down and then to reassess the position before proceeding. It is advisable to frequently remove as the needle with stylet is advanced.

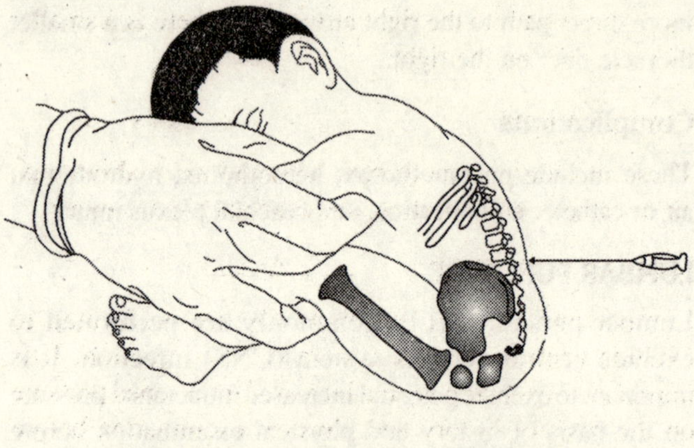

Fig. 100.9: Site for lumbar puncture with infant in a sitting position

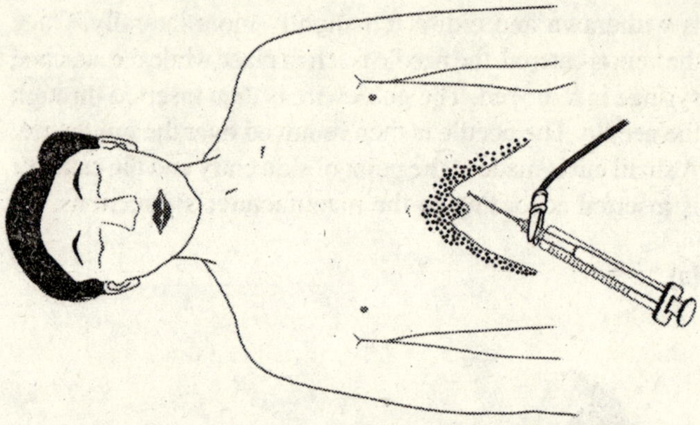

Fig. 100.10: Position of needle for pericardiocentesis

A three-way stopcock and manometer are attached to the spinal needle and the pressure can be determined. Normal relaxed pressure is 5 to 15 cm of water.

Complications

Cardiorespiratory arrest, infection secondary to introduction of pathogens, herniation through the foramen magnum because of antecedent increased intracranial pressure), headaches and rarely spinal cord hematoma.

PERICARDIOCENTESIS

Fluid collection in the pericardial sac, whether it results from effusion, infection, or hemorrhage, may be removed in the acute situation for both diagnostic and therapeutic reasons by pericardiocentesis. An echocardiogram may be an important diagnostic tool in a stable patient to establish the presence of an effusion.

The patient is supine, leaning backward at a 45-degree angle, supported by the bed or pillows. The left subxiphoied is used, with the needle aimed cephalad and backward toward the tip of the left scapula (Fig. 100.10). Some authorities recommend aiming the needle toward the right scapula.

An 18 or 20 gauge metal spinal needle (7.5 cm) is attached to a three-way stopcock and 20 ml syringe.

Procedure

After preparing, cleaning, and draping the patient, the needle is inserted slowly under negative pressure through the puncture site, penetrating the diaphragm. As the pericardium is entered, there is a distinct "pop". As little as 2 ml may be temporarily effective at relieving tamponade and improving cardiac output. Vital signs should be monitored throughout the procedure. Ultrasound may facilitate this procedure.

Complications

Pneumothorax, coronary artery injury or myocardial laceration, dysrhythmias and bleeding.

SUBDURAL TAP

The subdural space is a non-communicating space between the dura matter and the arachnoid membrane. The tap is done to define the nature of the collection: hematoma, effusion, or empyema.

The puncture site is the lateral corner of the anterior fontanel or further lateral along the suture. Optimally, this is at least 5 cm from the midline or 1 to 2 cm lateral to the edge of the anterior fontanel. The patient is in the supine position with the head at the edge of an examination table. An assistant should immobilize the patient. A subdural needle (short bevel) is used. If it is unavailable, a short spinal needle with a short bevel may be substituted with this needle to place a hemostat on the needle at the point of entry to prevent excessive penetration.

Procedure

The anterior two-thirds of the scalp are shaved and surgically scrubbed. Meticulously, the needle is inserted slowly at a right angle to the skin surface with total finger control. It is advanced slowly with the stylet in place until there is a sudden decrease in resistance, usually associated with a "pop", representing penetration of the dura. The stylet is removed, and up to 15 to 20 ml of fluid is allowed to drain by gravity, avoiding aspiration. Normally, there are only a few drops in this space. Sometimes none is obtained. In most cases the procedure is repeated on the other side. If excessive fluid is present or reaccumulates, repeat taps may be necessary over a period of time.

Complications

Infection, bleeding from small vessels and injury to the cerebral cortex.

SUPRAPUBIC ASPIRATION

Suprapubic aspiration is a safe method to obtain urine from the newborn and infants less than 2 years of age, because the distended bladder in this age–group is primarily intra-abdominal.

The infant's bladder must be full. Determining that the diaper has been dry for 45 minutes is good evidence of a full bladder. The patient is restrained in the supine position. The site is 2 cm (a fingerbreadth) above the symphysis.

Procedure

Cleanse the suprapubic area with povidone-iodine (Betadine). Identify the pubic bone without contaminating the area of puncture. Insert a 4 cm, 22-gauge needle attached to a 5 ml syringe at midline, angling the needle 10 to 20 degrees cephalad and advancing it through the skin under negative pressure at all times (Fig. 100.11). Entry into the bladder is indicated by return of urine.

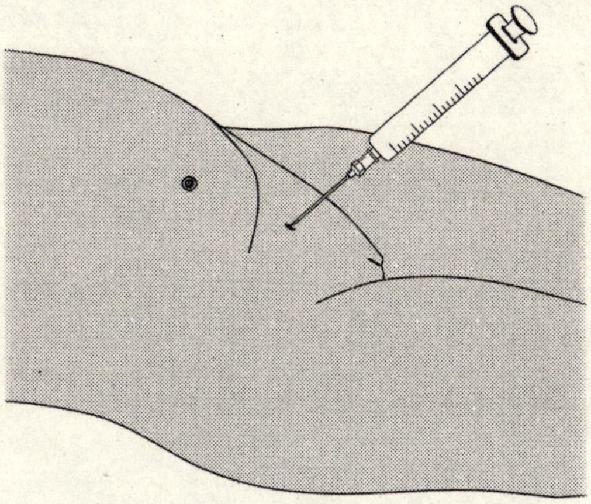

Fig. 100.11: Suprapubic aspiration

Complications

Gross hematuria, anterior abdominal wall abscess; bowel puncture peritonitis is uncommon.

THORACENTESIS

Thoracentesis is indicated to remove pleural fluid for diagnostic or therapeutic reasons or in the emergency treatment of a pneumothorax pending placement of a chest tube.

For posterior or posterior-lateral approaches to fluid removal, the patient sits in a flexed position, leaning forward against a bed stand or chair back. Small infant may be held in the 'burping' position.

If the patient is too ill to sit, the procedure may be performed with the patient lying on the involved side on a firm surface with a portion of the lateral chest wall extending over the edge of the bed. An alternative for gaining access to the lateral chest wall is for the patient to lie across two beds or examination tables with the involved side down.

The site of puncture depends on the location of the pleural fluid. If a pneumothorax is being decompressed before placing chest tube venting is done at the second or third intercostal space at the midclavicular line (Fig. 100.12). An 18 or 19 gauge needle with a short bevel attached to a three-way stopcock and 10 ml syringe is used. If fluid is expected, plastic tubing is attached to the sidearm of the stopcock to facilitate removal of fluids.

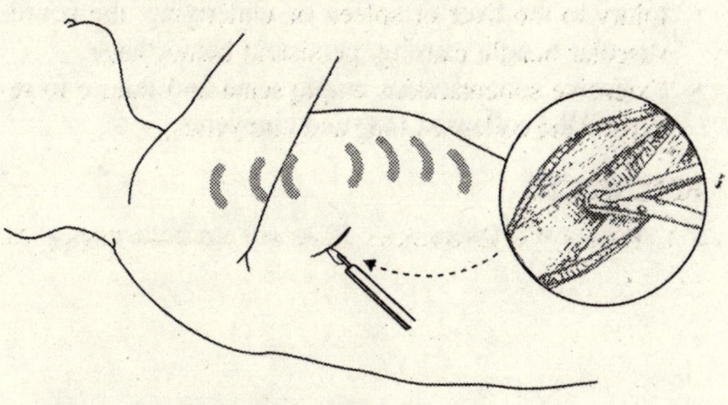

Fig. 100.12: Placement of chest tube

Procedure

The patient is prepared and draped, and 1% lidocaine is infiltrated locally. With sterile technique the needle or catheter over needle is inserted, passing over the superior edge of rib under negative pressure, and advanced slowly. There is a sudden decrease in resistance once the pleural space is reached. A hemostat should be placed on the needle at the skin to prevent further penetration once the pleural space is entered. Fluid is aspirated the volume reflecting cardiopulmonary status and the therapeutic goals of the procedures.

THORACOSTOMY

Chest tubes are used for the treatment of pneumothorax or hemothorax, often before making a definitive radiologic diagnosis.

PROCEDURE

The area is prepared, draped, and locally infiltrated with 1% lidocaine down to the rib and along the subcutaneous tissue to be tunneled. The skin is incised with a scalpel parallel to the long axis of the rib. The incision should be adequate to permit manipulation of the tube (3 to 5 cm). The area is bluntly dissected down to the rib with a clamp or scissors. If tunneling is desired, the dissection is continued across the intercostal space above the incision site and over the next rib. A clamp is then curved over the superior edge of the rib, dividing the intercostal muscles down to the parietal pleura, which is penetrated. The thoracostomy tube is grasped at the tip by a curved clamp and advanced through the tunnel and intercostal space into the chest. It is directed posteriorly and apically. The inter-space is entered superior to the rib to avoid injuring the neurovascular bundle. The tube is attached to an underwater seal. If there is a continuous air leak or an associated hemothorax, additional pleural suction may be needed up to 15 to 25 cm water. The tube is sutured in place and dressed with a sterile covering, often including a petrolatum soaked gauze as an air seal.

Complications

- Injury to the liver or spleen or underlying, the neurovascular bundle causing, persistent hemorrhage.
- Extensive subcutaneous emphysema and failure to re-expand the collapsed lung and empyema.

REFERENCES

1. Hughes WT. Emergencies: Fluid and metabolic therapy. In: Taeusch HW, RO Christiansen, Buescher ES (eds) *Pediatric and Neonatal Tests and Procedures*, Philadelphia: WB Saunders 1996;251-302.
2. Rosen P. Procedures. In: Barkin RM, Rosen P (eds) *Emergency Pediatrics*, 4th edn. St. Louis: Mosby 1993:747-763.
3. Vatwani V, Gupte S. Practical pediatric procedures. In: Gupte S (ed) *The Short Textbook of Pediatrics*, 10th edn. New Delhi: Jaypee Brothers. 2004;733-746.
4. Proter FL, Miller JP, Cole FS. A controlled clinical trial of local anaesthesia for lumbar puncture in newborns. *Pediatrics* 1991;88:663.
5. Ellis RW, Strauss LC, Wiley JM. A simple method of estimating cerebrospinal fluid pressure during lumbar puncture. *Pediatrics*1992;89:895.

Section XX

Drugs in Pediatric Emergencies

Puneet Pooni

101 Drugs and Dosages in Pediatric Emergencies

Unless otherwise indicated, the IV route is preferred. In an emergency, intraosseous administration is an acceptable alternative when IV access cannot be obtained within 90 seconds or after three attempts to establish IV access. Endotracheal route of administration can be used for some drugs, such as epinephrine, atropine, naloxone, and lidocaine (LANE). A recommended method of endotracheal delivery is to administer the *drug* with or dilute in 1 to 5 ml of isotonic saline through a catheter inserted to the tip of the endotracheal tube and then giving positive pressure ventilation. This method may enhance absorption from the lung.

Dosage should be individualized, and the patient's age, weight, underlying illness, concurrently administered drugs, and known hypersensitivity should be taken into consideration.

A practitioner who uses a neuromuscular blocking agent ("muscle relaxant") must be qualified to maintain the patient's airway through bag and mask ventilation and endotracheal intubation. Once the patient has received the muscle relaxant, there is no longer any respiratory effort.

In a patient who is hypovolemic, rapid IV administration of barbiturates (such as thiopental) may be risky because of the cardiac depressant and vasodilator effects of barbiturates. Ketamine is a better choice in this circumstance, as it does not cause hypotension. In case of bronchial asthma patients also ketamine is preferred as it is a bronchodilator also.

Conversely, a patient with a closed head injury would benefit from the use of barbiturates and/or lidocaine and fentanyl because this would reduce cerebral blood flow and cerebral oxygen consumption and therefore intracranial pressure. Following head injury, ketamine therapy increases cerebral blood flow and intracranial pressure and, hence, should be avoided. Combining drugs with different modes of action may be advantageous. For example, adding a benzodiazepine or narcotic to the regimen may prolong the effect and/or enable a reduction in the dose of ketamine or barbiturate required to sedate.

Following is the list of drugs used in along with dosages.

Acetaminophen

Indication: Pain/fever.

Dose: 15 mg/kg/dose repeated 4-6 hours.
Post-operative pain PO 20 mg/kg/dose q6h for 48 hours.

N-Acetylcysteine

Indication: Acetaminophen overdose.

Dose: IV 48 hours loading dose 140 mg/kg over 1 hour diluted in D5W, maintenance 70 mg/kg/dose over 1 hour repeated q4h, dilute in D5W and infuse over 1 hour.

Caution: IV therapy may cause skin rashes and anaphylaxis, these may be treated with diphenhydramine and epinephrine.

Acetazolamide

Indications: Slows progression of hydrocephalus in patients who are not good candidates for surgery. Renal tubular acidosis to alkalinize the urine.

Dose: Hydrocephalus 5 mg/kg/dose given every 6 hours IV slow push or PO, increase as tolerated to 25 mg/kg/dose.

RTA 5 mg/kg/dose every 8-12 hours.

Note: IV is painful; causes hypokalemia at higher doses.

Acyclovir

Indications: Herpes simplex infection, varicella zoster infection with CNS and pulmonary involvement; HS encephalitis.

Dose: 10 mg/kg/dose give every 8 hr, infuse over 1 hour IV, duration 10-21 days.

Albumin

Indications: Hypovolemia, symptomatic hypoalbuminemia.

Dose: For hypovolemia 10-20 cc/kg of 5% albumin given IV push over 30 min–1 hr. For hypoalbuminemia 1 g/kg/ dose of 25% albumin given by slow infusion.

Note: Rapid infusion may cause pulmonary edema or circulatory overload.

Caution: In severe anemia and CHF.

Adenosine

Indication: Paroxysmal supraventricular tachycardia.

Dose: Initial dose: 0.10 mg/kg as rapidly as possible followed by flush of the IV catheter with 2-5 ml saline. *Subsequent doses*: If there is no response within 30 seconds, increase by 0.05 mg/kg until single dose of 0.30 mg/kg is reached. Maximum single dose, 12 mg.

Note: The antidote for profound bradycardia is aminophylline, 5 to 6 mg/kg over 5 minutes. *Atropine is contraindicated.* A defibrillator must be immediately available.

Albuterol

Indication: Status asthmaticus (acute severe asthma), bronchospasm.

Dose: 0.1 to 0.15 mg/kg by nebulization. Repeat as needed.

Note: 0.02 to 0.03 ml/kg of 5 mg/ml solution with normal saline to make 3 ml total in nebulizer; maximum single dose, 2.5 mg. Administration can be repeated and dose adjusted until desired clinical effect or symptomatic tachycardia. Oxygen is the preferred gas source for nebulisation. Supplemental oxygen should be considered when compressed air driven nebulizers are used or when oxygen flow rate dictated by nebulizer is inadequate.

Allopurinol

Indications: Hyperuricemia (secondary to malignancy, inborn errors of purine metabolism, large tissue breakdown or renal failure).

Dose: 10 mg/kg/day divided 1-3 doses/day PO.

Amikacin

Indications: Gram-negative organisms resistant to gentamicin.

Dose: 15-30 mg/kg/day divided bid or tid IV/IM.

Note: Caution in renal compromise.

Amphotericin B

Indications: Disseminated fungal disease.

Dose: test dose 0.1-0.25 mg/kg IV on first day over 6 hours. Subsequently increase gradually to 0.5-1.0 mg/kg/day IV as single infusion over 6-8 hr. Cumulative dose 15-30 mg/ kg given over a month.

Note: Protect against light.

Caution: May cause fever, vomiting, hypokalemia, and renal toxicity.

Aminophylline

*Indication:*Acute asthma.

Dose: Loading dose IV 6 mg/kg slowly over 20-30 min, if patient received previous theophylline then 3 mg/kg IV maintenance dose continuous infusion (mg/kg/hr) 1 month-1 year 0.2-0.7, 1-9 yrs 1, 9-16 yrs 0.8.

Amiodarone

Indication: Atrial and ventricular arrhythmias.

Dose: Loading dose PO 10-20 mg/kg/day for 7-14 days. IV 5mg/kg/dose over 1 hour. Repeat if required or 25 mcg/ kg/min × 4 hrs. maintenance dose PO 5-10mg/kg/day once daily. IV 5-15 mcg/kg/min by continuous infusion.

Note: IV loading dose can cause hypotension and bradycardia.

Amlodipine

Indication: Hypertension in renal disease PO 0.1-0.2 mg/ kg/dose once daily up to 5 mg/day. Maximum 10 mg/day.

Amoxycillin

Indication: Mild to moderate infections PO 25-50 mg/kg/ day divided q8h. Acute otitis media PO 80-90 mg/kg/day divided q8h. Endocarditis Prophylaxis 50 mg/kg PO 1 hr before procedure.

Amoxy/clavunate

Indication: Otitis media, respiratory tract infections.

Dose: 40 mg/kg amoxycillin, 10 mg/kg clavulanate q8h for 10 days.

Ampicillin

Indication: Meningitis IM/IV 200-300 mg/kg/day divided q6h.

Other IM/IV 100-150 mg/kg/day divided q6h.

Azithromycin

Indications: Otitis media/pneumonia.

Dose: PO 10 mg/kg on day one and then 5 mg/kg/day daily for 4 additional days.

Note: Concomitant use with digoxin may elevate serum digoxin levels and result in cardiac arrhythmias.

Atenolol

Indication: Hypertension.

Dose: 1-2 mg/kg/day Caution: CI in bradycardia, heart block, CCF, asthma.

Atracurium

Indications:

1. Neuromuscular blockade to facilitate mechanical ventilation.
2. Emergency intubation.

Dose: IV: A dose of 0.3-0.6 mg/kg will provide relaxation for 20-40 minutes. Supplemental doses should be 5-10 mg.

Note: This drug does not alter the level of consciousness or provide analgesia or amnesia. This agent may be used for emergency intubation when succinylcholine is contra-indicated. It is a short acting relaxant, which is rapidly broken down by the body. This makes atracurium very predictable as it wears off rapidly compared to the longer acting relaxants.

Caution: Ventilatory support is necessary. Personnel with skills in airway management must be present and prepared to respond when this agent is administered. Age-appropriate equipment for suctioning, oxygenation, intubation, and ventilation should be immediately available. Atracurium precipitates (comes out of solution) in an alkaline pH and it should never be mixed with thiopentone. Always flush the vein with saline if using the two drugs at induction.

Atropine Sulfate

Indication:

1. Symptomatic bradycardia

   Dose: Intramuscular (IM): 0.02 to 0.04 mg/kg
   Intratracheal: 0.02 to 0.04 mg/kg
   IV: 0.02 mg/kg.
   Minimum single dose, 0.1 mg
   Maximum single dose, 0.5 mg for child, 1.0 mg for adolescent.
   This dose may be repeated once.

   Note: Oxygenation and ventilation are essential first maneuvers in the treatment of symptomatic bradycardia. Epinephrine is the drug of choice if oxygen and adequate ventilation are not effective in the treatment of hypoxia-induced bradycardia. If administered through an endotracheal tube, follow the dose with or dilute in saline flush (1 to 5 mL) based on patient size.

2. Anticholinesterase poisoning

   Dose: IV: 0.05 mg/kg, repeat as needed for clinical effect

   Note: Anticholinesterase poisonings may require large doses of atropine or the addition of pralidoxime.

Aztrenam

Indications: Third line drug for life-threatening infections with susceptible gram negative aerobic organisms, especially pseudomonas.

Dose IV/IM 90-120 mg/kg/day divided q608h.

Note: can be used in patients who are allergic to cephalosporins.

Bicarbonate, Sodium.

Indication:

1. Metabolic acidosis
2. Tricyclic antidepressant overdose.
3. Hyperkalemia,
4. Hypermagnesemia

Dose: IV: 1 to 2 mEq/kg (1 ml/kg of8.4% solution)

Caution: Administer slowly because bicarbonate solution is hyperosmotic.

Note: Routine initial use of sodium bicarbonate in cardiac arrest is not recommended. However, sodium bicarbonate may be used in cases with documented metabolic acidosis after effective ventilation has been established.

Bretylium

Indication: Acute ventricular fibrillation.

Dose: IV/IO 5 mg/kg/dose undiluted by rapid IV pushover one minute, followed by additional doses of 10 mg/kg/dose at 15-30 min intervals until a maximum dose of 30 mg/kg.

Note: Use only in refractory ventricular arrhythmias, can cause significant hypotension. avoid extravasation.

Budesonide

Indication: Asthma.

Dose: 3 mo-12 yr Neb: Initial dose is 0.25-1 mg bid.

Note: Use gas flow rate of 6-10l/min and nebulisation time 10-15 min, total volume 4 ml, rinse after inhalation.

Calcium Chloride

Indication:

1. Ionized hypocalcemia
2. Hyperkalemia
3. Hypermagnesemia
4. Calcium channel blocker toxicity.

Dose: IV: 20 mg/kg (if using 10% $CaCl_2$, dose is 0.2 mL/kg). Inject slowly. Repeat dose as necessary for desired clinical effect.

Caution: Stop injection if symptomatic bradycardia occurs. Extra vascular administration can result in severe skin injuries.

Calcium Gluconate

Indication: Same as for calcium chloride ionizes as rapidly as calcium chloride and may be substituted using three times the dose of calcium chloride (mg/kg).

Dose: IV: 60 mg/kg (if using 10% gluconate, dose is 0.6 mL/kg). Inject slowly. Repeat dose as necessary for desired clinical effect.

Caution: Same.

Captopril

Indication: Hypertension and CHF.

Dose PO: begin with 0.1 mg/kg first dose, and increase to 0.3-0.5 mg/kg/dose repeated 6-8 hour. Maximum 6 mg/kg/day.

Note: Administer on an empty stomach, tablets can be crushed to make 1 mg/ml. Dose adjusted in renal failure.

Carbamazepine

Indication: Anticonvulsant of choice in partial seizures.

Dose: PO Initial 10 mg/kg/day, maintenance 20-30 mg/kg/day.

Carbenicillin

Indications: Infections by sensitive Pseudomonas aeruginosa and Proteus.

Dose: IV/IM 400 mg/kg/day every 6 hours.

Note: Rapid resistance develops if used alone. Inactivates aminoglycosides when mixed in same IV bottle or tubing.

Cefaclor

PO 20-40 mg/kg/day q8h.

Cefexime

PO 8 mg/kg once daily or divided q12h.

Note: Does not cover staphylococcus aureus adequately.

Cefotaxime

Indication and Dose: Meningitis IM/IV 200-300 mg/kg/day divided q6h.

Other IM/IV 100-200 mg/kg/day divided 6-8 hours.

Note: Good gram negative coverage (except pseudomonas).

Ceftazidime

Indication and Dose: Meningitis IM/IV 150 mg/kg/day divided q8h.

Other IM/IV 100-150 mg/kg/day divided q8h.

Ceftriaxone

Indication and Dose: Meningitis IV 100 mg/kg once or divided q12h (maximum 4 gm/day).

Other 50-100 mg/kg/day q12-24h (maximum 2 gm/day).

Cefuroxime

IV/IM 75-150 mg/kg/day divided q8h

Note: Not recommended for meningitis.

Cephalexin

PO 25-100 mg/kg/day q8h.

Chloral Hydrate

Indication and Dose: Sedative dose PO/PR 5-15 mg/kg/dose, repeat q8h.

Hypnotic for procedures PO/PR 50-75 mg/kg/dose, maximum 100 mg/kg/dose.

Note: Dilute oral dose with water to avoid gastric irritation. Lacks analgesic effects, so causes paradoxical excitement in patients with pain.

Chloramphenicol

Indication and Dose: Meningitis IV 100 mg/kg/day divided q6h.

Other 50-100 mg/kg/day divided q6h (maximum 4 gm/day).

Note: Monitor CBC for dose dependent or idiosyncratic bone marrow depression.

Chloroquine

Dose: 10 mg/kg (base) stat followed by 5 mg/kg after 6 hours, then 5 mg/kg od for 2 days.

Note: Give parenteral in case of persistent vomiting or severe illness, IV preparation to be diluted with 10 ml/kg of isotonic saline and infused over 3-4 hours.

Clindamycin

IM/IV 25-40 mg/kg/day divided q6-8h
PO 10-30 mg/kg/day divided q6h

Caution: Give slowly IV, thrombophlebitis, hypotension and cardiac arrest can occur with rapid IV injection.

Ciprofloxacin

PO 10-205 mg/kg bid, IV 5-105 mg/kg.

Cloxacillin

IM/IV 100-200 mg/kg/day divided q6h
PO 50-100 mg/kg/day divided q6h
Charcoal, Activated

Indication: Acute ingestion of selected toxic substances.

Dose: 1 to 2 g/kg.

Note: Administer as slurry or down a nasogastric tube. Iron, lithium, alcohols, ethylene glycol, alkalies, fluoride, mineral acids, and potassium do not bond to activated charcoal.

Caution: Commercially available preparations of activated charcoal often contain a cathartic, such as sorbitol. Fatal hypernatremic dehydration has been reported after repeated doses of charcoal with sorbitol. Nonsorbitol-containing products should be used if repeated doses are necessary.

Desmopressin

Indication: Diabetes Insipidus.

Dose: PO 0.05 mg tid, maximum of 1.2 mg/day.
Intranasal 3 mo-12 yr 5-30 mcg/24 hour once daily or bid.

Dexamethasone

Indication:

1. Emergency treatment of elevated intracranial pressure due to brain tumor
   Dose: IV: 1 to 2 mg/kg as a loading dose.
   Maintenance dose 1 mg/kg/24 hours.
2. Croup
   Dose: IV, IM, or
   PO: 0.6 mg/kg dexamethasone, 1 dose/d, or 2 mg/kg/ 24 h of prednisone.
   Further dosing and route of administration determined by clinical course.

Diazepam

Indication: Status epilepticus.

Dose: IV: 0.1 mg/kg every 2 minutes.

Maximum dose, 0.3 mg/kg (maximum 10 mg/dose).

Rectal: 0.5 mg/kg up to 20 mg.

Note: Do not give as IM injection.

Caution: There is an increased incidence of apnea when combined with other sedative agents or when given rapidly. One must be prepared to provide respiratory support. Monitor oxygen saturation.

Diazoxide

Indication: Hypertensive crisis.

Dose: IV: 1 to 3 mg/kg rapid IV push.

Note: Alternative regimen: 3 to 5 mg/kg IV over 30 minutes. This is reported to result in fewer problems with hypotension or hyperglycemia.

Digoxin

Indication: CHF, cardiac arrhythmias.

Dosage: Total digitalizing dose given in divided portions as 1/2 initially followed by 1/4 and 1/4 at 8 hrs intervals.

Age	*IV (mcg/kg)*	*Oral (mcg/kg)*
< 2 yr	30-40	40-50
2-10 yr	20-30	30-40
>10 yr	8-12	10-15

Maintenance dose daily divided into q12h (<10 yr) or once daily >10 yr. Start maintenance dose 12 hrs after last portion of digitalizing dose.

Age	*IV (mcg/kg)*	*Oral (mcg/kg)*
< 2 yr	8	10
2-10 yr	6	8
>10 yr	2-3	2.5-5

Caution: Side effects are more in case of renal impairment, hypokalemia, hypomagnesemia, hypercalcemia, and arrhythmia. Monitor serum levels (optimum serum levels 1.3-2.7 nmol/L or 0.8-2.0 g/L.

Diphenhydramine

Indication:

1. Acute hypersensitivity reactions.
2. Dystonic reactions.

Dose: IV or IM: 1 to 2 mg/kg.

Maximum dosage, 50 mg.

Note: May cause sedation, especially if other sedative agents are being used. May cause hypotension.

Dopamine

Indication: Continued shock after volume resuscitation.

Dose: IV infusion: 2 to 20 μg/kg/min. A widely recommended starting dosage is 10 μg/kg/min. Titrate to desired clinical effect.

Note: Preparation of infusion solution: 6 mg × body weight (kg) diluted to 100 mL. Infuse at 10 mL/h = 10 μg/kg/min using a constant infusion pump.

Caution: Extravascular administration can result in severe skin injuries. Tachycardia can occur with higher doses increasing myocardial oxygen demand.

Dobutamine

Indication: Impaired cardiac contractility.

Dose: IV infusion: 5 to 25 μg/kg/min. A widely recommended starting dosage is 10 μg/kg/min. Titrate for desired clinical effect.

Note: Preparation of infusion solution: 6 mg × body weight (kg) diluted to 100 mL. Infuse at 10 mL/h = 10 μg/kg/min using a constant infusion pump.

Caution is the same as with dopamine.

Enalpril

Indication: CHF

Dose: PO 0.1-0.5 mg/kg/day once daily or bid. IV 0.005-0.01 mg/kg/dose q8-24h.

Epinephrine

Indication:

1. Cardiac arrest or profound bradycardia, asystole, ventricular fibrillation, or pulseless electrical activity:

   Initial Dose: IV: 10 µg/kg (0.01 mg/kg)

   Intraosseous: 10 µg/kg (0.01 mg/kg)

   Endotracheal: 100 µg/kg (0.10 mg/kg)

   Note: 10 µg/kg = 0.1 mL/kg of 1:10 000 dilution 100 µg/kg = 0.1 mL/kg of 1:1000 dilution.

   If administered through an endotracheal tube, follow the dose with saline flush or dilute in isotonic saline flush (1 to 5 mL) based on patient size.

   Subsequent doses: given every 3 to 5 minutes

   IV: 100 µg/kg (0.1 mg/kg)

   Intraosseous: 100 µg/kg (0.1 mg/kg)

   Endotracheal: 100 µg/kg (0.1 mg/kg)

   Note: For subsequent doses of epinephrine, a dosage up to 200 µg/kg (0.2 mg/kg) may be given.

2. Anaphylaxis

   Dose: Subcutaneous (SC): 10 µg/kg per dose (maximum 3 doses)
   IV: 10 µg/kg per dose: 10 µg/kg = 0.01 mL/kg of 1:1000 dilution or 0.1 mL/kg of a 1:10 000 dilution

   Note: Repeat the SC dose every 20 minutes while attempting IV access. Indication:

3. Continued shock after volume resuscitation

   Dose: IV infusion: 0.1 to 3.0 µg/kg/min. Start at lowest dose and titrate for desired clinical effect.

   Note: Preparation of infusion solution: 0.6 mg × body weight (kg) diluted to 100 mL. Infuse at 1 mL/h = 0.1 µg/kg/min using a constant infusion pump.
   Caution: Extravasation can result in tissue necrosis injuries.

4. Status asthmaticus, bronchospasm

   Dose: SC: 10 µg/kg per dose 10 µg/kg = 0.01 mL/kg of 1:1000 dilution. Maximum single dose, 300 µg (0.3 mL of 1:1000 dilution).

   Note: Albuterol administered by inhalation is now considered the agent of choice for treatment of acute exacerbations of asthma. Dose can be repeated SC every 20 minutes if needed for clinical effect. Total of 3 doses.

5. Laryngotracheobronchitis:

   Dose: Racemic epinephrine, 2.25% inhalation solution

   0-20 kg: 0.25 mL in 2 mL with normal saline administered by nebulizer 20-40 kg: 0.50 mL in 2 mL with normal saline administered by nebulizer > 40 kg: 0.75 mL in 2 mL with normal saline administered by nebulizer.

   Note: L-Epinephrine: An equal volume of 1% L-epinephrine (1:100) is approximately equivalent in biologic activity to 2.25% racemic epinephrine; one can be substituted for the other in equal volumes for inhalation. Alternatively, 5 mL of 1:1,000 L-epinephrine is equivalent to 0.5 mL of 1:100.

Fentanyl

Indication: Pain.

Dose: IV: 0.5 µg to 2.0 µg/kg. Repeat dose as necessary for clinical effect.

Note: Higher doses may be necessary if the patient is tolerant. Rapid administration of fentanyl has been associated with both glottic and chest wall rigidity even with dosages as low as 1 µg/kg. Therefore, fentanyl should be titrated in slowly over several minutes.

Caution: There is an increased incidence of apnea when combined with other sedative agents, particularly benzodiazepines. Naloxone should be ready. Monitor the patient's vital signs and oxygen saturation.

Flumazenil

Indication: Benzodiazepine intoxication.

Dose: IV: 5 to 10 µg/kg (up to 100 µg/kg has been used). Maximum dose, 1 mg.

Caution: Duration of action is shorter than most clinically important benzodiazepines. Resedation may occur. May precipitate acute withdrawal in dependent patients; use drug with caution as its use may be associated with seizures. Patients who receive flumazenil should be continuously observed for resedation for at least 2 hours after the last dose of flumazenil.

Fosphenytoin

Indication: Status epilepticus (same as phenytoin).

Dose: Always in phenytoin equivalents (pe) 10 to 20 mg PE/kg (same as phenytoin).

IM or IV: 1 to 3 mg PE/kg/min; maximum rate 150 mg PE/min.

Note: Data are currently being collected on children less than 6 years of age. Itching is a common and controllable by reducing flow rate.

Caution: Rate of infusion should not exceed 3 mg PE/kg/min. Heart rate should be monitored and the rate of infusion reduced if the heart rate decreases by 10 beats/minute (same as phenytoin).

Frusemide

Indication:

1. Fluid overload
2. Congestive heart failure

Dose: IV, IM: 1 mg/kg

Gentamicin

IV/IM 5-7.5mg/kg/day q8h or once daily.

Note: Once daily dosing may be appropriate in children who are otherwise stable vs. fluid balance and renal function.

Glucagon

Indication:

1. Hypoglycemia due to insulin excess

   Dose: Adult and adolescent: 0.5 to 1.0 mg SC, IM, IV; repeat every 20 minutes.

   Pediatric: 0.025 mg/kg up to 1.0 mg SC, IM, IV; repeat the dose every 20 minutes if needed for clinical effect. Total of 3 doses.

   Note: An attempt should be made to provide a simultaneous IV glucose infusion.

2. Beta-blocker or calcium channel blocker overdose

   Dose: Adolescent

   IV: 2 to 3 mg followed by a 5 mg/h infusion.

   Pediatric

   IV: 0.025 to 0.05 mg/kg followed by 0.07-mg/kg/h infusion.

Glucose

Indication: Hypoglycemia.

Initial Dose: IV: 250 to 500 mg/kg.

Maintenance Dose: Constant infusion of 10% dextrose in water at a rate of 100 mL/kg/24 hour (7 mg/kg/min). Older children may require a substantially lower dose. The rate should be titrated to appropriate glucose values.

Note: 250 to 500 mg/kg = 2.5 to 5.0 mL/kg of D10% 250 to 500 mg/kg = 1.0 to 2.0 mL/kg of D25% 250 to 500 mg/kg = 0.5 to 1.0 mL/kg of D50%.

Glucose levels should be determined before and during administration. If large volumes of dextrose are administered, include electrolytes to prevent hyponatremia and hypokalemia.

Haloperidol

Indication: Psychosis with agitation.

Dose: IM, IV: 0.1 mg/kg, may repeat hourly as necessary. Maximum single dose, 5 mg.

Note: Hypotension and dystonic reactions may occur.

Heparin

Indication: Anticoagulation.

Loading dose IV 75 units/kg IV bolus over 10 min, maintenance infusion 15-25 units/kg/hours.

Note: Monitor PTT 4 hour after load and adjust dose to keep in range 60-85 sec. Antidote is protamine 1mg/100 units received in the last 4 hours.

Low molecular weight heparin->2 months 1mg/kg/dose q12h.

Hydralazine

Indication: Hypertension.

Dose: IM/IV 0.1-0.2 mg/kg/dose repeated q4-6h, maximum 20 mg/dose.

Ibuprofen

Indication and Dose: Analgesic/antipyretic PO 5-10 mg/kg/dose q6h, maximum daily dose 40 mg/kg/day.

JRA PO 30-50 mg/kg/day in 4 divided doses.

Indomethacin

Children 2-14 yr PO/PR 2-4 mg/kg/day divided tid with meals.

Note: Monitor liver functions.

Insulin, Regular

Indication:

1. Diabetic ketoacidosis

Dose: SC: 0.25 to 0.5 unit/kg per dose

IV infusion dose: 0.05 to 0.1 unit/kg/hour.

Note: Blood glucose levels should be closely monitored. Appropriate fluid and electrolyte therapy are also required in treating diabetic ketoacidosis.

2. *Hyperkalemia*

Dose: IV: 0.1 unit/kg with 400 mg/kg glucose. Ratio of 1 unit of insulin for every 4 g of glucose.

Note: Potassium levels in blood or serum should be monitored.

Imipenem

Indications: Effective against most gram-negative and gram-positive bacteria, both aerobes and anaerobes, including Pseudomonas aeruginosa.

Dose: IV 20 mg/kg/dose every 12 hours.

Note: Should be reserved for use against resistant organisms.

Ipecac Syrup

Indication: Acute ingestion of selected toxic substances.

Dose: Oral (PO): 6-month-old to 1-year-old = 10 mL >1 year old = 15 mL

Adolescent/young adult = 30 mL.

Caution: Not to be used when patient is suffering from central nervous system depression or if having seizures. Contraindicated in caustic and hydrocarbon ingestion. Patients who ingest pesticides or other chemicals that may have a hydrocarbon base may need to have emesis induced.

Note: Administer with 120 to 180 mL of fluid; 90% effective in inducing vomiting within 25 minutes of first dose. May repeat once. Activated charcoal is now considered the first line therapy for most oral ingestions treated in the hospital setting.

Ipratropium Bromide

Indication and Dose: In h 0.5-1 ml diluted in 3 ml normal saline via nebulizer q4-6h. MDI 1-2 puffs tid-qid.

Note: can be mixed with albuterol (salbutamol).

Isoproterenol

Indication: Bradycardia, heart block, bronchodilator .

Dose: IVI 0.025-1mcg/kg/min.

Kayexalate (Sodium Polystyrene Sulfonate)

Indication: Treatment of hyperkalemia.

Dose: Adolescents

PO: 15 g (60 mL) 1 to 4 times/day

Rectal: 30 to 50 g every 6 hours

Children PO: 1.0 g/kg every 6 hours.

Rectal: 1.0 g/kg/dose every 2 to 6 hours (for small children and infants use lower doses by using the practical exchange ratio of 1 mEq K^+/g of resin).

Ketamine

Indication:

1. Sedation/analgesia
   Dose: IM: 1 to 2 mg/kg
   IV: 0.5 to 1 mg/kg
2. Adjunct to intubation
   Dose: IV: 1 to 2 mg/kg

Note: Laryngospasm associated with ketamine is usually reversed with oxygen administration and positive pressure ventilation. Atropine or other antisialogogue should be used to prevent increased salivation.

Caution: Be prepared to provide respiratory support. Monitor oxygen saturation. Avoid use in patients with increased intracranial pressure or increased intraocular pressure.

Labetalol

Indication: Hypertensive crisis.

Dose: IV 0.2-1 mg/kg/dose. Maximum 20 mg/dose IVI 0.25-3 mg/kg/h.

PO 1-2 mg/kg/dose.

Note: Combined alpha and beta-blocker. Use with caution in asthma, cardiogenic shock, CHF, heart block and liver dysfunction.

Lactulose

Indication: Acute hepatic encephalopathy.

Dose: PO/NG Infants 2.5-10 ml/day div tid-qid Children 40-90 ml/24 h div tid-qid. Normally 1 ml/kg/dose (6-8h).

Note: Increase dose until watery diarrhea occurs, then reduce dose to produce 2-3 soft stools per day.

Lidocaine

Indication:

1. Ventricular arrhythmia

   Dose: IV: 1 mg/kg as a single dose slowly, repeat every 5 to 10 minutes to desired IV infusion: 20 to 50 µg/kg/min

   Endotracheal: 1 mg/kg.

   Note: If administered through an endotracheal tube, follow the dose with saline flush or dilute in isotonic saline flush (1 to 5 mL) based on patient size. A reduced infusion rate should be used in patients with a low cardiac output. Excessive dosage may result in myocardial depression, hypotension, central excitation, and seizures.

   Caution: Contraindicated in complete heart block and wide complex tachycardia due to accessory conduction pathways.
2. To attenuate airway reflexes before endotracheal intubation or airway manipulation in patients with elevated intracranial pressure.

   Dose: 1 mg/kg IV as a single dose 30 seconds before airway instrumentation.

Lorazepam

Indication:

1. Status epilepticus
2. Adjunct for intubation.

Dose: IM or IV: 0.05 to 0.1 mg/kg Repeat doses every 10 to 15 minutes for clinical effect.

Caution: There is an increased incidence of apnea when combined with other sedative agents. Be prepared to provide respiratory support. Monitor oxygen saturation.

Magnesium Sulphate

Indication and Dose: Hypomagnesemia or hypocalcemia IM/IV initial dose 25-50 mg/kg/dose (0.1-0.2 mmol/kg/dose) 4-6 h for 3-4 doses may repeat if necessary.

Note: Monitor blood pressure and respiratory rate during IV infusions. 50% magnesium sulphate is hyperosmolar (4000 mOsm/kg). Dilute IV doses to 1% (10 mg/ml)-10% (100 mg/ml) solution and infuse over 1-4 hours at maximum rate 150mg/min. Maintenance dose is 30-60 mg/kg/day Caution; Signs of toxicity include CNS depression, decreased tendon reflexes, respiratory paralysis and heart block.

Mannitol

Indication: Increased intracranial pressure.

Dose: IV: 0.25 g/kg given over a 15-minute infusion.

Note: A larger dose (0.5 g/kg given over 15 min.) may be appropriate in an acute intracranial hypertensive crisis. In conjunction with mannitol, other measures to control intracranial pressure such as hyperventilation, barbiturates, and muscle relaxation (using a neuromuscular blocking agent) should be considered.

Caution: Rapid administration may cause hypotension, hyperosmolality, and elevated intracranial pressure.

Meperidine

Indication: Pain.

Dose: IV or IM: 1 to 2 mg/kg. Repeat dose is necessary for clinical effect.

Note: Higher doses may be necessary if patient is tolerant.

Caution: There is an increased incidence of apnea when combined with other sedative agents, particularly benzodiazepines. Be prepared to administer naloxone. Monitor the patient's vital signs and oxygen saturation. Be prepared to provide respiratory support.

Methylprednisolone

Indication:

1. Asthma/allergic reaction
   Dose: IV: 1 to 2 mg/kg every 6 hours.
2. Spinal cord injury
   Dose: IV: 30 mg/kg over 15 minutes. In 45 minutes begin a continuous infusion of 5 to 6 mg/kg/h for 23 hours.
3. Croup
   Dose: IV: 1 to 2 mg/kg of methylprednisolone, then 0.5 mg/kg every 6 to 8 hours.

Midazolam

Indication:

1. Adjunct for endotracheal intubation or for sedation/ anxiolysis (while on ventilator also).
   Dose: IV: 0.05 to 0.2 mg/kg given over several minutes.
2. In status epilepticus
   Dose: Start with 2 mcg/kg/min, increase to 4,8,16,24 every min till seizures are controlled then continue the infusion for 48 hours after the last seizure before tapering off.

Caution: There is an increased incidence of apnea when combined with other sedative agents. Be prepared to provide respiratory support. Monitor oxygen saturation.

Milrinone

Indication: Inadequate cardiac output with high systemic or pulmonary vascular resistance, cardiogenic shock (particularly post-operative CHF and dilated cardiomyopathy), septic shock.

Dose: Loading-50-75 mcg/kg, Infusion 0.5-0.75 mcg/kg/ min.

Note: Monitor for hypotension during loading dose, consider infusion without loading dose. Causes less tachycardia as compared to other vasopressors.

Caution: May cause thrombocytopenia, so monitor platelets, and long half-life with increases toxicity in renal failure.

Morphine Sulfate

Indication: Pain, infundibular spasm ("Tet Spell" or cyanotic spell in cyanotic congenital heart disease), and sedation in patients on mechanical ventilation.

Dose: Pain IV/IM/SC 0.1-0.2 mg/kg/dose every 2-4 hours. Cyanotic infant 0.05 mg/kg/dose.
Continuous infusion 0.04-0.07 mg/kg/hr IV. Repeat dose as necessary for clinical effect.

Note: Higher doses may be necessary if patient is tolerant.

Caution: There is an increased incidence of apnea when combined with other sedative agents, particularly benzodiazepines. Be prepared to administer naloxone. Monitor the patient's vital signs and oxygen saturation. Be prepared to provide respiratory support.

Naloxone

Indication: Respiratory depression induced by opioid.

Dose: IV, IM: 0.1 mg/kg from birth until age 5 years or 20 kg of weight. Thereafter, the minimum dose is 2.0 mg. Doses may be repeated as needed to maintain opiate reversal. IM absorption may be erratic.

Note: This dosage is indicated for acute opiate intoxication. Titration to effect with lower initial doses (0.01 mg/kg or 10 µg/kg) should be considered for other clinical situations, e.g., respiratory depression during pain management.

Caution: May induce acute withdrawal in opioid dependency. Patients who receive naloxone should be continuously observed for renarcotization for at least 2 hours after the last dose of naloxone.

Naproxen

Indication and Dose: Analgesic > 2 yrs PO/PR 10 mg/kg/ day divided q12h.
Anti-inflammatory, JRA PO 10-20 mg/kg/day bid.

Note: Use cautiously in patients with GI, renal or cardiac disease and those patients taking oral anticoagulants.

Nifedipine

Indication: Hypertension.

Dose: PO/SL 0.25-0.5 mg/kg/dose q1-3h.

Children >20 kg 5-10 mg/dose.

Note: For pediatric doses, puncture capsule and administer a portion by counting drops or withdraw contents of capsule in insulin syringe. Each 5 mg capsule contains 0.1 ml of nifedipine 50 mg/ml.

Nitroprusside

Indication: Hypertensive crisis.

Dose: IV: 0.5 to 10 μg/kg/min. Start at the lowest dosage and titrate for the desired clinical effect. Administer through low dead space system or as close to IV catheter as possible to prevent accidental bolus injection.

Note: Preparation of infusion solution: 6 mg × body weight (kg) diluted to 100 mL D5W. Infuse at 1 mL/h = 1 μg/kg/min using a constant infusion pump. Bottle, burette, or syringe pump but not the IV tubing should be covered with protective foil to avoid breakdown by light.

Caution: Administration may result in profound hypotension. Patients should be closely monitored. Blood pressure should be continuously monitored with an arterial line. Cyanide toxicity can result from large doses and/or prolonged infusions. Patients should be closely monitored for the development of metabolic acidosis. Patients with decreased renal function may be at increased risk.

Omeprazole

Indication: Refractory gastroesophageal reflux disease.

Dose: PO 0.7-3.3 mg/kg/day once daily.
Children < 3 yr PO 10 mg daily in the morning >3 yr PO 20 mg once daily in the morning.

Note: May use a simplified omeprazole solution (SOS) 5 mg/ml in $NaHCO_3$ or crush tablet and mix in water to give down feeding tube, take before meals.

Ondansetron

Indication Chemotherapy induced nausea and vomiting.
Dose: IV 0.15 mg/kg/dose. PO 0.2 mg/kg/dose.

Note: Use only in severe cases of vomiting may cause headache, seizures, bronchospasm, tachycardia, hypokalemia, constipation, and diarrhea.

Oxygen

Indication:

1. Hypoxemia and/or respiratory distress
2. Carbon monoxide poisoning
3. Shock.

Dose: 100% by nonrebreather mask initially or endotracheal tube; wean as tolerated.

Note: The administration of supplemental oxygen should be considered during EVERY pediatric emergency.

Pancuronium

Indication:

1. Neuromuscular blockade to facilitate mechanical ventilation.
2. Emergency intubation

Dose: IV: 0.1 mg/kg.

Note: This drug does not alter the level of consciousness or provide analgesia or amnesia. This agent can be used when succinylcholine is contraindicated. Pancuronium is a long-acting neuromuscular blocker that requires ventilatory assistance for at least 1 hour. Satisfactory conditions for endotracheal intubation will generally occur 2 to 3 minutes after administration.

Caution: Ventilatory support will be necessary. Personnel with skills in advanced airway management must be present and prepared to respond when this agent is administered. Age-appropriate equipment for suctioning, oxygenation, intubation, and ventilation should be immediately available.

Paraldehyde

Indication and dose: Anticonvusant PR 0.3-0.5ml/kg/dose diluted to 50% with mineral oil or vegetable oil. Repeat dose in 20 min if not effective and then q2-4h.

Note: Do not use outdated or discolored solutions. It will dissolve plastic, use within 5 min of preparation or use glass syringe.

Pencillamine Various heavy metal poisonings (not first line drug).

PO 20-40 mg/kg/day qid.

Penicillin G benzathine Group A streptococcal upper respiratory tract infection 25000 units/kg IM once.
Prophylaxis for Rheumatic fever 25000 units/kg IM q3-4 weeks.

Note: Administer undiluted by deep IM injection into anterolateral aspect of thigh. Shake well before use, do not administer IV.

Pencillin G procaine Children <12 yrs IM 25000-50000 units/kg/day once daily or divided q12h. Children >12 yrs IM 60,000 units/day once or q12h.

Note: same as above.

Pencillin G sodium IV/IM 100,000-250,000 units/kg/day divided q4-6h.

Piperacillin

Indications: Broad-spectrum coverage of hospital acquired infections.
Dose: 50-100 mg/kg/dose IV over 30 min 6-8H. Can be given IM.

Phenobarbital

Indication: Status epilepticus.

Dose: IV: 20 mg/kg. Maximum dose, 100 mg. Repeat dose once if necessary for clinical effect after 15 minutes.

Caution: There is an increased incidence of apnea when combined with other sedative agents. Be prepared to provide respiratory support. Monitor oxygen saturation.

Phenylephrine

Indication: Infundibular spasm ("Tet Spell").

Dose: 5 to 20 µg/kg push then followed by infusion at 0.1 to 5.0 µg/kg/min.

Caution: Blood pressure must be carefully followed and dose titrated to effect.

Phenytoin (Diphenyl hydantoin sodium)

Indication: Status epilepticus.

Dose: IV: 10 to 20 mg/kg initial dose.
Maximum initial dose, 100 mg.
Maximum rate of administration, 50 mg/min or 1 mg/kg/min, whichever is less.

Note: Should be diluted in normal saline to avoid precipitation.

Caution: Rate of infusion should not exceed 0.1 mL of undiluted preparation per kg/min. Heart rate should be monitored and the rate of infusion reduced if the heart rate decreases by 10 beats/minute.

Pralidoxime

Indication: Organophosphate insecticide poisoning.

Dose: Loading dose 20-40 mg/kg/dose by slow infusion over 30 min. Maintenance dose is not well established, a continuous infusion of 9-19 mg/kg/hr has been recommended.

Note: If weakness and fasciculations persist repeat loading doses after 1 hr. Treatment is most effective if started within 24-36 hrs of poisoning.

Prednisolone

Indication: Acute asthma, anti-inflammatory.

Dose: 1-2 mg/kg/day in 1 or 2 divided doses.

Note: 5 mg of prednisolone = 20 mg of hydrocortisone. Infrequent (4 times per year) short courses (< 5 days) of high dose glucocorticoids do not need tapering. Give with food to avoid gastric irritation.

Procainamide

Indication: Wide complex tachycardia.

Dose: IV: Start at 3 to 6 mg/kg/dose over 5 minutes not to exceed 100 mg to a titrated maximum of 15 mg/kg/loading dose.

Maintenance dose, 20 to 80 µg/kg/min (0.02 to 0.08 mg/kg/min); maximum, 2 g/24 h.

Caution: If 50% QRS widening or hypotension occurs during loading dose, the remainder of the loading dose is held, and the maintenance dose is delayed until these signs have resolved.

Prochlorperazine

Indication: Antiemetic.

Dose: Children >2 yr and 9 kg IM 0.13 mg/kg/dose by deep IM injection tid-qid.
PO/PR 0.4 mg/kg/day divided tid or qid.

Note: Children are very susceptible to extrapyramidal effects, use lowest possible dose and do not use IV route.

Promethazine

Indication and Dose: Antihistamine PO 0.125 mg/kg/dose q4-6h or 0.5 mg/kg at bedtime.
Antiemetic IM/IV/PO 0.25-1 mg/kg/dose q4-6h.
Preoperative sedation IM 0.5-1 mg/kg/dose.

Propofol

Indication: Resistant Status epilepticus (after trial of phenytoin, phenobarbitone, midazolam infusion).

Dose: 1-2 (3-4) mg/kg, rate of 5-10 mg/min (1-5 mg/kg/hr).

Note: Rapid acting, advantage over barbiturates-causes less hypotension, more rapid onset of action with rapid elimination.

Caution: May cause metabolic acidosis.

Propranolol

Indication:
Tachyarrhythmias Children IV 0.01-o.15 mg/kg/dose
Infundibular spasm ("Tet Spell").

Dose: IV: 0.01 to 0.02 mg/kg per dose infused over 10 min in 5% dextrose in water.
Maximum initial dose, 1.0 mg.
Tetrology maintenance PO 0.5-4 mg/kg/day divided tid or qid.

Note: Oxygen should be administered first. Morphine is also an effective treatment for infundibular spasms. Phenylephrine is another adjunct for reversal of infundibular spasm. Use is contraindicated in congestive heart failure. Avoid in patients with a history of bronchospasm.

Ranitidine

Indication: Gastroesophageal reflux disease/peptic ulcer disease.

Dose: Children PO 2-6 mg/kg/day divided q12h.
IV 3-6 mg/kg/day divided q6-8h.

Quinine

Indication: Chloroquine resistant malaria.

Dose: 25 mg/kg/day PO div 8h for 3-7 days.
IV 10 mg/kg (1 hr infusion in normal saline) followed by continuous infusion of 0.02 mg/kg/min until oral therapy can be given.

Note: Monitor ECG, blood pressure and glucose in patients.

Rocuronium

Indication:

1. Neuromuscular blockade to facilitate mechanical ventilation.
2. Emergency intubation

Dose: IV: 0.8 to 1.2 mg/kg.

Note: This drug does not alter the level of consciousness or provide analgesia or amnesia. Alternative to succinylcholine for rapid intubation when succinylcholine is contraindicated. Duration of block is generally 30 to 45 minutes and is dose-dependent. Satisfactory conditions for endotracheal intubation will generally occur 45 to 60 seconds after administration.

Caution: Ventilatory support is necessary. Personnel with skills in airway management must be present and prepared to respond when this agent is administered. Age-appropriate equipment for suctioning, oxygenation, intubation, and ventilation should be immediately available.

Salbutamol (*See* Albuterol)

Spironolactone

Indications diuresis, used in combination with other diuretics in CHF.

Dose 1.0-3.0 mg/kg/day PO given 24h or bid.
Note: hyponatremia and hyperkalemia may be seen.

Succinylcholine

Indication: Neuromuscular blockade for emergency intubation or treatment of laryngospasm.

Dose: 1 to 2 mg/kg IV 4 to 5 mg/kg IM.

Caution: Contraindicated with previous history of malignant hyperthermia, severe burns, spinal cord injury, neuromuscular disease, or myopathies. When these contraindications exist use a nondepolarizing muscle relaxant such as rocuronium. Ventilatory support is necessary. Personnel with skills in airway management must be present and prepared to respond when this agent is administered. Age-appropriate equipment for suctioning, oxygenation, intubation, and ventilation should be immediately available.

Note: Atropine, 0.02 mg/kg (minimum dose, 0.1 mg), should be combined with or precede succinylcholine to prevent bradycardia or asystole. Satisfactory conditions for endotracheal intubation generally occur 30 to 45 seconds after IV administration and 3 to 5 minutes after IM administration. If cardiac arrest occurs immediately after administration of succinylcholine, hyperkalemia must be suspected and treatment for this condition initiated.

Terbutaline

Indication: Asthma

Dose: PO 0.075 mg/kg/dose tid or alternatively <12 yr : 0. 625-1.25 mg/dose tid >12 yr 2.5-5 mg/dose tid.

Caution: Tremors, palpitations, restlessness, headache, muscle cramps, nervousness.
No advantage over salbutamol.

Ticarcillin: *Indications*: Severe infections with Pseudomonas and Proteus.

Dose: IM/IV 200-300 mg/kg/day divided q4-6h, maximum 24 gm/day.

Note: Extended spectrum penicillin. Each gram contains 5.2 mmol (120 mg) of sodium. Minimum dilution is 100 mg/ml, inject over at least 10 min.

Tobramycin IM/IV 5-7.5 mg/kg/day divided q8h.

Thiopental

Indication:

1. Adjunct to intubation

   Dose: IV: 4 to 6 mg/kg.

   Note: A lower dose may be used if other sedatives/ narcotics have been administered.

   Caution: IM administration leads to tissue necrosis. Be prepared to provide respiratory support. Monitor oxygen saturation. High doses are associated with hypotension and apnea. Use with caution in patients with cardiac compromise or hypovolemia.
2. Control of intracranial hypertension
   Dose: 1 to 2 mg/kg, repeated as necessary.

Valproic Acid

Dose: PO 15 mg/kg/day, increase weekly by 5-10 mg/kg up to 30-60.
Caution: Hepatic dysfunction.

Vancomycin

Indication: Bacterial infections by resistant Staphylococcus aureus.

Dose: IV 40 mg/kg/day divided q6h, maximum 2 gm/day. Meningitis 60 mg/kg/day divided q6h, maximum 4 gm/day.
Antibiotic associated colitis PO50 mg/kg/day divided q6h.

Note: Minimum dilution for IV by peripheral line is 5 mg/ml and by central line 10 mg/ml. Red man syndrome may occur with rapid infusions.

Vecuronium

Indication:

1. Neuromuscular blockade to facilitate mechanical ventilation.
2. Emergency intubation

   Dose: IV: 0.1 mg/kg.

   Note: This drug does not alter the level of consciousness or provide analgesia or amnesia. This agent may be used for emergency intubation when succinylcholine is contraindicated. Satisfactory conditions for endotracheal intubation generally occur 1.5 to 2.0 minutes after administration.

   Caution: Ventilatory support is necessary. Personnel with skills in airway management must be present and prepared to respond when this agent is administered. Age-appropriate equipment for suctioning, oxygenation, intubation, and ventilation should be immediately available.

Verapamil

Indication: Supraventricular tachycardia.

Dose: IV 0.1-0.2 mg/kg/dose, give over 2-3 min, repeat after 30 min.

Note: For children >1 yr with narrow complex tachycardia who fail to convert on adenosine.

Caution: Not recommended for use in children <1 yr because of hypotension and sudden death.

REFERENCES

1. Berlin CM, McCarver CDJ, Notterman DA,Ward RM, Weismann DN, Wilson GS et al. Drugs for Pediatric Emergencies. *Pediatrics* 1998;101:e13.
2. American Academy of Pediatrics and American College of Emergency Physicians, Joint Task Force on Pediatric Life Support. *APLS: The Pediatric Emergency Medicine Course*. Elk Grove Village, IL: American Academy of Pediatrics 1993.
3. KidSTAT Plus (CD-ROM). Elk Grove Village, IL: American Academy of Pediatrics 1996.
4. American Heart Association, Subcommittee on Pediatric Resuscitation. *Pediatric Advanced Life Support*. Dallas, TX: American Heart Association 1994.
5. American Academy of Pediatrics. Guidelines for monitoring and management of pediatric patients during and after sedation for diagnostic and therapeutic procedures. *Pediatrics* 1992;89:1110-1115.
6. Baldwin GA. Drug dosage guidelines in infants and children. In: *Handbook of Pediatric Emergencies*. Philadelphia: Lippincott Williams and Wilkins 2001;592-667.
7. Bradley JS, Nelson JD. *Nelson's Pocket book of Pediatric Antimicrobial Therapy*. Philadelphia: Lippincott Williams and Wilkins 2002.
8. Gupte S, Smith R. Pediatric Drug Directory, 8th edn. New Delhi: Jaypee Brothers 2001.
9. Hazinski MF, Zaritsky AL, Nadkarni VM, Schexnayder SM, Berg RA Fluid therapy and medications for shock and cardiac arrest. In: PALS Provider Manual. Elk Grove Village, IL:American Academy of Pediatrics with American Heart Association. 2002;127-154.

Appendices

Appendices

APPENDIX I

COMMONLY EMPLOYED PREFIXES, SYMBOLS AND DECIMAL FACTORS

Prefix	*Symbol*	*Decimal factor*
Mega/million	M	10^6
Kilo	k	10^3
Hecto	h	10^2
Deka	d_a	10^1
Deci	d	10^{-1}
Centi	c	10^{-2}
Milli	m	10^{-3}
Micro	u	10^{-6}
Nano	n	10^{-9}
Pico	p	10^{-12}
Fento	f	10^{-15}

APPENDIX II

COMMONLY EMPLOYED SYMBOLS

Symbol	*Interpretation*
$>$	Greater than...
$\geq$	Greater than or equal to...
$<$	Less than...
$\leq$	Less than or equal to...
$\pm$	Plus/minus...
$=$	Approximately equal to...

APPENDIX III

NORMOGRAM FOR ESTIMATING SURFACE AREA

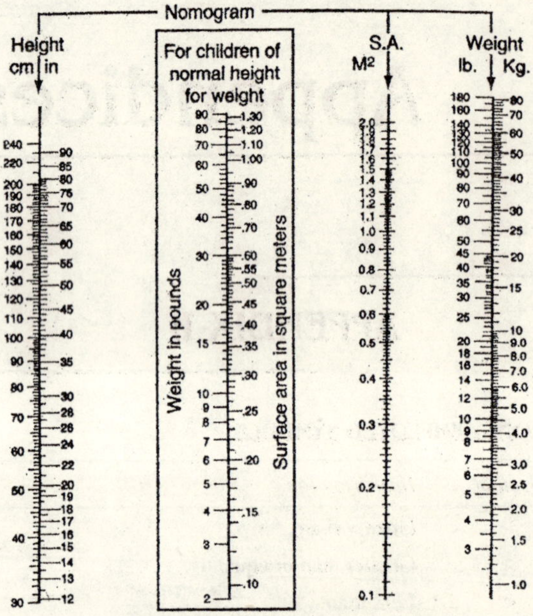

Alternative (Mosteller's formula):

$$\text{Surface area (m}^2) = \sqrt{\frac{\text{Height (cm)} \times \text{Weight (kg)}}{3600}}$$

Fig. A3.1: Note that surface area is indicated where a straight line connecting the height and weight levels interacts the surface area column. In case the subject is of an average size, surface area may be calculated from weight alone (enclosed area). *Courtesy: Nelson Textbook of Pediatrics, 17th edn. Philadelphia: Saunders 2004*

APPENDIX IV

USEFUL EQUATIONS IN INTENSIVE CARE

Serum Osmolarity

$$= 2\,(\text{Na}) + \frac{\text{Blood glucose}}{18} + \frac{\text{BUN}}{2.8}$$

Alveolar Air Equation

$$PAO_2 = FiO_2\,(Pb - 47) - \frac{PaCO_2}{R}$$

Alveolar Arterial Oxygen Gradient

$$A - a\,(O_2) = (FiO_2\%\ 100) \times (Pb - 47\ \text{mmHg}) - (Pa\ CO_2/0.8) - (Pa\ O_2)$$

Where

PAO_2 stands for partial pressure of alveolar oxygen

Pb stands for atmospheric barometric pressure (sea level)

47 stands for water vapor pressure

$PaCO_2$ stands for partial pressure of arterial carbon dioxide

R stands for respiratory quotient which is 0.8

Alveolar Resistance Equation

Pressure = Flow × resistance

$$\text{Resistance} = \frac{8\ \text{nl}}{\text{Pie r4}}$$

In other words, resistance is inversely proportional to 4th power of radius.

Where

Pie denotes 22/7

r radius

l length

n viscosity

Oxygen Content Equation

$CaO_2 = PaO_2 \times 0.003 + Hb\ (g)\ \%\ sat \times 1.36$

Oxygen Delivery Equation

$DO_2 = C1 \times CaO_2 \times 10$ normal 620 (ml/min/meter sq)

Oxygen Consumption

$VO_2 = C1 \times (Ca\ O_2 - C_vO_2) \times 10$ 120–200 (ml/min/meter sq)

Oxygen Extraction

$$OE = \frac{CaO_2 - C_vO_2}{Ca\ O_2} \times 10$$

Shunt Equation

$$\frac{Q_s}{Q_t} = \frac{C_CO_2 - CaO_2}{C_cO_2 - C_v\,O_2}$$

Systemic (Qp) to Pulmonary Shunt (Qs)

$$\frac{Q_p}{Q_s} = \frac{SaO_2 - SmvO_2}{SpvO_2 - SpaO_2}$$

Systemic Vascular Resistance Index (SVRI)

$$SVRI = \frac{MAP - CVP}{CI} \times 80 \quad 800\text{–}1200 \text{ dynes/sec/cm 5}$$

Pulmonary Vascular Resistance Index (PVRI)

$$PVRI = \frac{MPAP - PCVP}{CI} \times 80 \quad 20\text{–}120 \text{ dynes/sec/cm 5}$$

Where

MPAP	stands for	mean pulmonary artery pressure (15 mmHg, systemic 25, diat 10 mmHg)
PCWP	stands for	pulmonary capillary wedge pressure (9 mmHg, range 8-12 mmHg)
MAP	stands for	mean arterial pressure which is calculated by multiplying the systemic pressure plus 2 and 1/3rd of diastolic pressure.
SaO_2	stands for	arterial oxygen saturation
$SmvO_2$	stands for	mixed venous oxygen saturation
$SpvO_2$	stands for	pulmonary venous oxygen saturation
$SpaO_2$	stands for	pulmonary venous oxygen saturation
CI	stands for	cardiac index (cardiac output/surface area 3.2–5.2 L/msq)
CcO_2	stands for	pulmonary capillary oxygen content
CvO_2	stands for	venous oxygen content
SVI	stands for	stroke volume index CI × 1000/hour; 37-47/beat/m_2

APPENDIX V

USEFUL BIOSTATISTICS

Standard Deviation : Interpretation

One plus/minus	68.3%
Two plus/minus	95.4%
Three plus/minus	99.7%

Probability (p value)

< 0.001	Highly significant
< 0.01	Very significant
< 0.05	Significant
> 0.05	Insignificant

Sensitivity

$$\frac{\text{True positive}}{\text{True positive + False positive}}$$

Specificity

$$\frac{\text{True negative}}{\text{True negative + False positive}}$$

Positive Predictive Value

$$\frac{\text{True positive}}{\text{True positive + False positive}}$$

Negative Predictor Value

$$\frac{\text{True negative}}{\text{True negative + False negative}}$$

False Negative Rate

$$\frac{\text{False negative}}{\text{True positive + False negative}}$$

False Positive Rate

$$\frac{\text{False positive}}{\text{False negative + False positive}}$$

APPENDIX VI

USEFUL CONVERSIONS

Conversion to SI Units from Old Units

Component	*Old Units*	*SI Units*
CSF and other body fluid cell count	per mm (cu mm)	$\times 10^6$/L
Urine culture colony count	per ml	$\times 10^6$/L
Antibiotic assay	mcg/ml	mg/L

Conversion of Milliograms (mg) per 100 ml to Milliequivalents (mEq) per Liter of Plasma

$$\text{Sodium (Na)} = \frac{\text{mg/100 ml} \times 10}{\text{23 (atomic weight)}} \times \text{1 (valency)} = \text{mEq/L}$$

$$\text{Potassium (K)} = \frac{\text{mg/100 ml} \times 10}{39} \times \text{1 (valency)} = \text{mEq/L}$$

$$\text{Calcium (Ca)} = \frac{\text{mg/100 ml} \times 10}{40} \times \text{2 (valency)} = \text{mEq/L}$$

$$\text{Chloride (Cl)} = \text{mg/100 ml} \times 10 \times \text{1 (valency)} = \text{mEq/L}$$

Standard Factors for Rapid Conversion of Milligrams per 100 ml to Milliequivalents per Liter

Sodium (Na)	0.435
Potassium (K)	0.257
Calcium (Ca)	0.5
Magnesium (Mg)	0.833
Bicarbonate (HCO_3)	0.455
Chloride (as NaCl)	0.150
Phosphate (HPO_4)	0.58
Sulfate (SO_4)	0.625

Temperature

Conversion of °C to °F = 9/3 × °C = °F

Conversion of °F to °C = 5/9 (°F–32) = °C

Inches to Centimeters

1 inch = 2.54 cm

1 cm = 0.39 inch

Minim to Milliliter

1 minim = 0.06 ml

1 ml = 15 minims

Equivalent Imperial and Meteric Quantities

1	grain	=	65 mg
1	ounce	=	28 g
1	pound	=	453 g
2.2	pounds	=	1 kg

APPENDIX VII

REFERENCE LABORATORY VALUES/RANGES

The information supplied here is a compilation from various sources.[1-3] The values generally refer to the pediatric and adolescent age groups excluding neonates.

Hematology

Component	*Specimen*	*Reference values*
Bleeding time (BT)	Whole blood	1-7 min
Clotting time (CT)	Whole blood	5-8 min ; room temp 5–15 min when glass tubes are employed; in case of silicone tube, it is prolonged 30 min
Activated partial thrombo-plastin time (APTT)	PIC	25–35s; infants < 90s
Factor I (Fibrinogen)	Whole blood (citrated)	Infants and Older children 125–300 mg/dL; Adolescents 200–400 mg/dL
Factor II	Plasma (citrated)	
Factor IV (Iodizedcalcium)	Serum, plasma (heparinized), whole blood (heparinized)	4.8–4.92 mg/dL
Factor V	Plasma (citrated)	0.5–2.0 U/mL (0–150% of normal)
Factor VII	65–135 % of normal	
Factor VIII	Plasma (citrated)	65–145% of normal
Factor VIII antigen	Plasma (citrated)	50–200% of normal

M for Males and F for Females

Contd...

Contd...

Component	*Specimen*	*Reference values*	
Factor IX	Plasma (citrated)	60–140% of normal	
Factor X	Plasma (citrated)	60–130% of normal	
Factor XI	Plasma (citrated)	65–135% of normal	
Factor XII (Fibrin stabilizing factor)	Whole blood	65–150% of normal	
Fibrin degradation products (D-dimer)	Plasma (citrated)	207 (68–494) mcg/L in adolescents	
Fibrinogen	—— See Factor 1 ——	—— See Factor 1 ——	
Prothrombin time (PT)	Whole blood	11–15 seconds	
Thrombin time	Whole blood (citrated)	2 second	
RBC count	Whole blood	1 month	2.7–4.9 million/cu mm (× 10^{12}/L)
		3–6 months	3.1–4.5 million/cu mm (× 10^{12}/L)
		7 months–2 yrs	3.7–5.3 million/cu mm (×10^{12}/L)
		2–6 yrs	3.9–5.3 million/cu mm (× 10^{12}/L)
		6–12 yrs	4.0–5.2 million/cu mm (× 10^{12}/L)
		12–18 yrs	**M**: 4.5–5.3 million/cu mm (× 10^{12}/L)
			F: 4.1–5.1 million/cu mm (× 10^{12}/L)
Hemoglobin	Whole blood	1 month	10–15 g/dL
		2 month	9–14 g/dL
		6–12 yr	11.5–15.5
		12–18 yr	**M**: 13.0–16.0
			F: 12.0–16.0
Packet cell volume (PCV)/ Hematocrit	Whole blood	2 months	28–42 %
		6–12 yrs	35–45 %
		12–18 yrs	**M**: 37–49 %
			F: 36–46 %
Hemoglobin A	Whole blood	> 95%	
Hemoglobin A_2	Whole blood	1.5–3.5% in adolescents but less in infancy	
Hemoglobin F	Whole blood	1 month	55–85 %
		2 months	31–75 %
		3–4 months	2–9 %
		6 months	2–5 %
		Adolescents	< 2 %
Erythrocyte sedimentation/ Rate (ESR)	Whole blood	Infant & children 0–13 mm 1st hour	
		Adolescent	**M**: 0–9 mm 1st hour
			F: 0–20 mm 1st hour
Reticulocyte count	Whole blood	0.5–1.5% of erythocytes	
Total leukocyte Count	Whole blood	1 month	5.0 –19.5 thousand/mm^3
		1–3 months	5.0–17.5 thousand/mm^3
		4–7 yrs	5.5–15.5 thousand/mm^3
		8–13 yrs	4.5–13.5 thousand/mm^3
		Adolescents	4.5–11.0 thousand/mm^3
Platelet count	Whole blood	150–400 thousand/mm^3	
Biochemistry			
Bilirubin (total)	Serum/plasma	0. 0.2–0.8 mg/dL	
Bilirubin (conjugated/direct)	Serum	0–0.3 mg/dL	
Alanine aminotransferase (AAT). Syn: Serum glutamic pyruvic transaminase (SGPT)	Serum	5–45 U/L	

Contd...

Contd...

Component	*Specimen*	*Reference values*	
Asparate aminotransferase (AST). Syn: Serum glutamic oxaloacetic transaminase (SGOT)	Serum	1–9 years	15–55 U/L
		> 10 years	5–45 U/L
Alkaline phosphate	Serum	1–9 years	145–420 U/L
		10–11 years	130–560 U/L
		12–13 years	**M**: 200–495 **F**: 105–420
		14–15 years	**M**: 130–525 **F**: 0–230
		> 16 years	**M**: 65–260 **F**: 50–130
Acid phosphatase	Serum	< 3 ng/ml	
Ammonia	Whole blood	1–12 months	18–74 mc mol/L
		1–14 years	17–68 mc mol/L
		> 14 years	19–71 mc mol/L
Protein (total)	Plasma	1–7 years	6.1–7.9 g/dL
		8–12 years	6.4–8.1 g/dL
		13–19 years	6.6–8.2 g/dL
Albumin	Plasma	< 5 years	3.9–5.0 g/dL
		> 5 years	4.0–5.3 g/dL
Glucose (random)	Serum	60–100 mg/dL	
Glucose (postprandial)	Serum	< 120 mg/dL	
Glucose tolerance test (GTT)	Serum	Fasting	Normal 70–105 mg/dL Diabetic 126 mg/dL
		60 min	Normal 120–170 mg/dL Diabetic 200 mg/dL
		90 min	Normal 100–140 mg/dL Diabetic 200 mg/dL
		120 min	Normal 70–120 mg/dL Diabetic 200 mg/dL
Ketone bodies (qualitative)	Serum	Nil	
Ketone bodies (quantitative)	Whole blood	1–12 months	0.1–1.5 mmol/L
		1–7 years	0.8–1.5 mmol/L
		7–15 years	0.6–0.9 mmol/L
Amylase	Plasma/serum	30–100 U/L	
Antistreptolysin O titer	Serum	2–5 years	120–160 Todd Units
		6–9 years	240 Todd Units
		10–12 years	320 Todd Units
Alpha-1-antitrypsin	Serum	1–9 years	147–245 mg/dL
		> 9 years	152–317 mg/dL
C-reactive protein	Serum	2–12 years	67–1800 ng/ml
Creatine phosphokinase (CRP)		Serum	5–130 U/L
Creatinine kinase isoenzyme	Serum	0–2 %	
Creatinine	Serum/plasma	Infant	0.2–0.4 mg/dL
		Child	0.3–0.7 mg/dL
		Adolescent	0.5–1.0 mg/dL
Creatinine clearance	Serum/plasma/urine		**M**: 97–137 ml/min/1.73 m^2 **F**: 88–128 ml/min/1.73 m^2
Uric acid	Serum	1–5 years	1.7–5.8 mg/dL
		6–11 years	2.2–6.6 mg/dL
		> 12 years	**M**: 3.0–7.7 mg/dL **F**: 2.7–5.7 mg/dL

Contd...

Contd...

Component	*Specimen*	*Reference values*	
Urea nitrogen (BUN)	Serum/plasma	Infant	5–18 mg/dL
		Child	5–18 mg/dL
		Adolescent	7–18 mg/dL
Thyroxine (total)	Serum	1–12 months	6.1–14.9 mcg/dL
		1–3 years	6.8–13.5 mcg/dL
		3–10 years	5.5–12.8 mcg/dL
		> 10 years	4.2–13.0 mcg/dL
Triiodothyroxine (total)	Serum	1–5 years	100–260 ng/dL
		5–10 years	90–240 ng/dL
		10–15 years	80–210 ng/dL
		> 15 years	115–190 ng/dL
Thyroid-stimulating hormone (TSH)	Serum	1–5 months	1.5–9.1 U/L
		> 5 months	0.7–6.4 U/L
Thyrotropin-releasing hormone (hTRH)	Plasma	5–69 pg/mL	
Iron	Serum	22–184 mcg/dL	
Total iron-binding capacity (TIBC)	Serum	Infant	100–400 mcg/dL
		Later	250–400 mcg/dL
Ferritin	Serum	1 month	200–600 ng/mL
		2–5 months	50–200 ng/mL
		> 6 months	7–140 ng/mL
Transferrin	Serum	95–385 mg/dL	
Lead	Whole blood (heparinized)	Child	< 10 mcg/Dl
		Adolescent	< 40 mcg/dL
Magnesium	Plasma (heparinized)	> 2 years	1.5–2.3 mg/dL
Calcium (total)	Serum	Child	8.8–10.8 mg/dL
		Adolescent	8.4–10.2 mg/dL
Calcium (ionized)	Serum, plasma (heparinized), whole blood (heparinized)	4.8–4.92 mg/dL	
Chloride (total)	Serum	5–130 mmol/L	
Sodium	Serum, plasma	Infant	139–146 mmol/L
		Child	138–145 mmol/L
		Adolescent	136–146 mmol/L
Potassium (total)	Serum	1–2 months	3.0–7.0 mmol/L
		2–12 months	3.5–6.0 mmol/L
		> 1 year	3.5–5.0 mmol/L

REFERENCES

1. Nicholson JF, Pesce MA. Reference ranges for laboratory tests and procedures. In: Behram RE, Kliegman RM, Jenson HB (eds): *Nelson Textbook of Pediatrics*, 17th edn. Philadelphia: Saunders 2004;2396-2427.
2. Wordsworth E. *Pediatric and Adolescent Laboratory Procedures*, 3rd edn. London: Smith and Smith 2004.
3. Gupte S. Useful normal laboratory values. In: Gupte S (ed): *The Short Textbook of Pediatrics*, 10th edn. New Delhi: Jaypee Brothers 2004;775.

APPENDIX VIII

SELECT WEBSITES

A. Highly Recommended

1. International Pediatric Criticare

www. Internpedcrit.edu

This is an excellent website for pediatricians involved in emergency care of infants and children, providing most recent recommendations on management of critically sick children. There is incorporation of instructive case studies which assist in formulating effective and state-of-the-art therapeutic strategies. Nevertheless, it is accessible on payment of high charges which becomes its handicap for most of the aspirants interested in free sites.

2. Pediatric Education Network

http:pededunet.org

This paid website provides a unique platform for not only academic information on pediatric emergency care and other aspects of child health but also a most satisfying medium for academic interaction. You can get in touch with senior consultants from around 200 pediatric centers around the globe for state-of-the-art knowledge and guidelines.

3. Nelson Textbook of Pediatrics Online

www.nelsonpediatrics.com

This interactive and state-of-the-art webebsite provides not only the whole contents of the celebrated book but also ongoing weekly updates, pediatric guidelines, case studies (case of the month, radiologic case study, visual diagnosis case) and weekly review question-answers. This enhances the reference power of the treatise. Notably, a CD-Rom and passcode serves as the access key. On top of all that, there are patient instruction handouts for over 200 pediatric entities, pediatric medication tables, laboratory reference values table, updated journal abstracts and links to Pediatric Guidelines, Cochrane Database, MMWR Growth Charts, Vaccination and Immunization Schedules.

4. British Pediatric Surveillance Unit

http:members.rediff.com/meduldu/fle.htm

This Royal College of Pediatrics and Child Health (United Kingdom) sponsored website makes available valuable details about uncommon as well as newly emerging childhood illnesses with special reference to emergency and criticare pediatrics. Also provided by the site is the Newsletter of the Royal College of Pediatrics and Child Health.

5. Indian Pediatrics

www.Indianpediatrics.net

This site is free, providing full text electronic version of the journal of the Indian Academy of Pediatrics, *Indian Pediatrics*. It is a very valuable site especially for pediatric residents and other scholars and practitioners looking for state-of-the-art information on pediatric scenario in India.

6. Indian Journal of Pediatrics

www.ijpediatricsindia.org

Indian Journal of Pediatrics (IJP) is the oldest Indian journal in the field of pediatrics, published monthly from New Delhi. This site provides its electronic version. The material in the site includes original articles, updates, symposia, clinical briefs, abstracts from the leading journals, etc.

7. Synopsis

www.pedsynopsis.com

This website hosts the electronic version of the quarterly journal *Synopsis*, a current survey of world literature in pediatrics from Detroit, USA, and provides in depth reviews and summaries with authoritative commentaries on articles on topical issues and the "Morning Report at Children's Hospital, Michigan" which indeed makes a very interesting and useful reading.

8. Children with Diabetes

www.childrenwithdiabetes.com

This website provides wealth of information which the pediatrician would like to communicate to young children suffering from diabetes mellitus as also to their families for better management. It is, therefore, a favorite site for recommendation to the interested parties.

RECOMMENDED WEBS

1. American Academy of Pediatrics: Position Papers and Practice Guidelines

   www.aap.org/policy/pcyhome.cfm
2. American Diabetes Association

   www.diabetes.org
3. National Institute of Diabetes and Digestive and Kidney Diseases

   www.niddk.bih.gov
4. American Academy of Pediatrics

   www.aap.org/
5. Children's Nutrition Research Center

   www.bcm.tmc.edu/cnrc
6. Pedinfo

   www.uab.edu/pedinfo/
7. American Board of Pediatrics

   www.abp.org
8. Commonwealth Association of Pediatric Gastroenterology and Nutrition

   www.capgan.org/

Index